Intravenous Therapy

Clinical Principles
and
Practice

Intravenous Therapy
Clinical Principles and Practice

General Editor:

Judy Terry, BSN, CRNI
Director, IV Therapy
Moses H. Cone Memorial Hospital
Greensboro, North Carolina

Associate Editors:

Leslie Baranowski, RN, BSN, CRNI
Clinical Manager, IV Therapy Services
Roseville Hospital
Roseville, California

Rose Anne Lonsway, MA, CRNI
President, RDB & Associates
Painesville, Ohio

Carolyn Hedrick, BSN, CRNI
Assistant Director, IV Therapy
Moses H. Cone Memorial Hospital
Greensboro, North Carolina

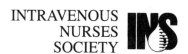

INTRAVENOUS
NURSES
SOCIETY

W.B. SAUNDERS COMPANY
A Division of Harcourt Brace & Company
Philadelphia London Toronto Montreal Sydney Tokyo

W.B. Saunders Company
A Division of
Harcourt Brace & Company

The Curtis Center
Independence Square West
Philadelphia, Pennsylvania 19106

Library of Congress Cataloging-in-Publication Data

Intravenous therapy: clinical principles and practice / Intravenous
Nurses Society; general editor, Judy Terry; associate editors, Leslie
Baranowski, Rose Anne Lonsway, Carolyn Hedrick.

    p.   cm.

Includes index.

ISBN 0–7216–4267–5

1. Intravenous therapy.   2. Nursing.   I. Terry, Judy.
II. Intravenous Nurses Society.

[DNLM: 1. Parenteral Nutrition—methods.   2. Parenteral
Nutrition—nursing.   WY 150 I61 1995]

RM170.I59 1995   615′.6—dc20

DNLM/DLC   95–11495

INTRAVENOUS THERAPY: CLINICAL PRINCIPLES AND PRACTICE   ISBN 0–7216–4267–5

Printed in the United States of America.

Last digit is the print number: 9   8   7   6   5   4   3   2   1

FOREWORD

This textbook, a project of the Intravenous Nurses Society (INS), is an authoritative text on the clinical practices of IV therapy. It is useful to nurses, physicians, pharmacists, students, and other members of the health care community involved in the clinical practices of IV therapy. Principles and practices described in this textbook are applicable to all practice settings, such as acute care and subacute long-term care facilities, home infusion settings, and physicians' offices. This information can be used to develop IV policies, practices, and procedures. The Intravenous Nurses Society's *Standards of Practice* would be helpful in supplementing these principles and practices.

The textbook is also an excellent resource in preparing for the Intravenous Nurses Certification Corporation's (INCC) examination. INCC is a national credential-granting organization mandated for the public benefit and protection to assess, validate, and document the clinical eligibility and continued clinical competency of nurses delivering intravenous therapy in all practice settings. The Corporation supports education and ongoing research and validates the reliability of credential-granting mechanisms and their relationship to the clinical practice. INCC promotes recognition of its credentialed nurses and programs to the public, to other health care organizations, and to the nursing profession.

The INS is a national nursing organization representing over 10,000 IV nurse specialists who practice in both acute care and home infusion settings. The mission of the INS is to promote excellence in intravenous nursing through standards, education, public awareness, and research. Its ultimate goal is to ensure access to the highest quality, cost-effective care for all individuals requiring, and patients receiving, intravenous therapies in all practice settings worldwide.

The Intravenous Nurses Society is located at Two Brighton Street, Belmont, Massachusetts 02178; telephone number (617) 489–5205; FAX number (617) 489–0656.

MARY LARKIN
Chief Executive Officer
Intravenous Nurses Society

PREFACE

The practice of intravenous (IV) therapy is a multifaceted, vitalizing process. Within the scope of medicine, it is a specialty that plays an extensive role in the care of patients. IV therapy incorporates the clinical needs of the patient and the physician's treatment plan with valuable input from many other health care providers.

As the practice of intravenous therapy expands, there is an increasing need for additional information, from the basic to the more sophisticated. This is evidenced by the questions that are continuously posed about the many facets of IV therapy. *Intravenous Nursing: Clinical Principles and Practice* was developed with this need for information in mind—the past, the present, and the future of intravenous therapy.

Beginning with the history of intravenous therapy, a journey into the past is followed by a discussion of the practice of IV therapy today and the professionals providing this care. The legal and ethical aspects of IV practice in addition to maintenance of quality care are reviewed.

No discussion of IV therapy would be complete without laying the foundation on which the specialty exists. This includes anatomy, physiology, and control of infection. Once an illness exists, various treatments are used to achieve the desired patient care outcomes. Intravenous-related treatment involves a host of different modalities, such as parenteral fluids, blood and blood components, pharmacologic agents, nutritional fluids, antineoplastic agents, and pain medications.

The technology and procedures used to provide IV therapy are described. Technology involves the selection and preparation of various types of equipment. The discussion of procedures begins with assessment of the patient and follows through to documentation. Important considerations for patient assessment, treatment, monitoring, complications, and patient education are addressed.

Because certain patients require different IV therapy approaches, information on providing care for children and older adults is included. Also, with IV-related treatment no longer being administered solely in the hospital setting, the provision of care in other surroundings is discussed.

Intravenous therapy is similar to other areas of medical care. Once an order is written, there is always a question about the degree of excellence of care being provided. This concern leads to a discussion of research. Finally, after considering the past and present of IV therapy, predictions for the future of the specialty are given.

Our intent has been to provide answers to the many questions and concerns related to the practice of IV therapy. This text can help ensure that quality care is delivered, and that those in the IV nursing profession are positioned for the many profound changes that are occurring and will continue to occur. The valuable assistance and expertise of all those who contributed to this text are greatly appreciated.

JUDY TERRY
LESLIE BARANOWSKI
ROSE ANNE LONSWAY
CAROLYN HEDRICK

ACKNOWLEDGMENTS

The specialty of intravenous therapy encompasses a variety of areas, including physiologic aspects, IV agents, equipment, nursing care, special considerations, and professional issues. Incorporating this vast array of information into a textbook is an enormous undertaking that has been accomplished only through the efforts of many dedicated individuals.

First, I would like to acknowledge Rose Anne Lonsway for initiating the project. Leslie Baranowski and Carolyn Hedrick, Associate Editors, and Donna Baldwin were instrumental in guiding and completing this endeavor.

Throughout the process, there have been many professionals who were willing to review the various chapters. Special thanks go to the five nurses who helped with the final review:

Maxine Acevedo, RN, MPA, CRNI
Administrative Coordinator
IV Therapy/Nutrition Support
University of California, Davis Medical Center

Lynn C. Hadaway, BS, RNC, CRNI
Clinical Nurse Educator
Menlo Care, Inc.

Gloria Pelletier, CRNI
Coordinator, Pharmacy/I.V. Programs
Southern New Hampshire
Regional Medical Center

Lynn Phillips, RN, MSN, CRNI
Instructor of Nursing
Butte Community College

Ofelia Santiago, RN, BSN, CRNI
Nurse Manager
Caremark

Without the contributing authors, there would be no textbook. Their willingness to give of their time and expertise is greatly appreciated.

I would like to thank the Chief Executive Officer and Board of Directors of the Intravenous Nurses Society for giving me the opportunity to work on this project. Special appreciation goes to Daniel Ruth, Editor, Nursing Books at W.B. Saunders Company, for his guidance throughout the development of the book.

Finally, I would like to thank my department head, Judy Crouch, R.Ph., secretaries, Linda Ravel and Gerri Carpenter, the IV therapy staff, and my family, for their patience and support in bringing this project to fruition.

JUDY TERRY, BSN, CRNI

CONTRIBUTORS

Maxine Acevedo, MPA, CRNI
I.V. Therapy Administrative Coordinator, I.V. Therapy/Nutrition Support, University of California, Davis Medical Center, Sacramento, California
Patient Assessment

Mary C. Alexander, CRNI
Intravenous Staff Nurse, Massachusetts General Hospital, Boston, Massachusetts
Product Selection and Evaluation

Diane L. Baker, CRNI
President, Baker & Associates Health Care Consultants, Seattle, Washington
Documentation

Donna R. Baldwin, MSN, CRNI
Assistant Executive Director, Trinity Health Care Services, Memphis, Tennessee
Quality Management
Legal Aspects of Intravenous Nursing
Pharmacology
Intravenous Therapy in Alternative Settings
Research

Leslie Baranowski, RN, BSN, CRNI
Clinical Manager, Intravenous Therapy Services, Roseville Hospital, Roseville, California
The Intravenous Therapy Department
Future of Intravenous Therapy

Deborah B. Benvenuto, RN, CRNI
Intravenous Therapy Department, Massachusetts General Hospital, Boston, Massachusetts
Intravenous Therapy in Alternative Settings

Rebecca L. Kochheiser Berry, RN, MS
Healthcare Communications Consultant, Buffalo Grove, Illinois
Patient Education

Carol Bolinger, MSN, CRNI, OCN
Pediatric Oncology Nurse Practitioner, Primary Children's Hospital, Salt Lake City, Utah
Research

Ann M. Corrigan, BSN, MS, CRNI
Department Manager, Oncology Services, Cobb Hospital and Medical Center, Austell, Georgia
History of Intravenous Therapy

Mary Ann Doyle, CRNI, MS, OCN
Oncology Clinical Nurse Specialist, Holy Family Medical Center, Des Plaines, Illinois
Oncologic Therapy

Beth Fabian, BA, CRNI
Intravenous Therapy Coordinator, V.A. Medical Center, Ann Arbor, Michigan
Intravenous Therapy in the Older Adult

Carolyn D. Ford, MSN, CRNI
Clinical Nurse Manager, Visiting Nurse Association, Louisville, Kentucky
Parenteral Nutrition

Dawn G. Frederick, BSN, CRNI
Oncology Nurse Clinician, Ellis Fischel Cancer Center, Columbia, Missouri
Intravenous Therapy Equipment: Preparation, Maintenance, and Problem Solvin

Anne Marie Frey, BSN, CRNI
Clinical Nurse III, Intravenous Team, Children's Hospital of Philadelphia, Philadelphia, Pennsylvania
Intravenous Therapy in Children

Linda A. Grace, RN, BS, CRNI
President, Partners Consulting Group, Newport Beach, California
Intravenous Therapy in the Home

Lynn C. Hadaway, BS, RNC, CRNI
Clinical Nurse Educator, Menlo Care, Inc., Menlo Park, California
Anatomy and Physiology Related to Intravenous Therapy

Carolyn Hedrick, BSN, CRNI
Assistant Director, Intravenous Therapy, Moses H. Cone Memorial Hospital, Greensboro, North Carolina
Infection Control
Parenteral Fluids

Brenda L. Jensen, BSN, CRNI
Assistant Manager, Pharmacy/IV Services, University of Missouri Hospital and Clinics, Columbia, Missouri
Types of Intravenous Therapy Equipment
Intravenous Therapy Equipment: Preparation, Maintenance, and Problem Solving

Jim Johnson, Pharm D, BCPS
Infectious Disease Pharmacist, Moses H. Cone Memorial Hospital, Greensboro, North Carolina
Infection Control

Edie Jonas, RN, BSN, PHN, CRNI
Employee Health Coordinator, Roseville Hospital, Roseville, California
The Intravenous Therapy Department

Rose Anne Lonsway, MA, CRNI
Director, Research and Development, Meridia Home Health, Mayfield Village, Ohio
Fluids and Electrolytes
Patient Assessment

Donna Lee Mantel, Esq., RN, BSN, JD
Certified Civil Trial Attorney; Adjunct Professor, Seton Hall University, South Orange, New Jersey
Legal Aspects of Intravenous Nursing

Terri A. Miller, CRNI
Staff Nurse, Intravenous Therapy, University of Kansas Medical Center, Kansas City, Kansas
Hemodynamic Monitoring

Lorys F. Oddi, EdD, RN
Professor, School of Nursing, Northern Illinois University, DeKalb, Illinois
Ethics

Gloria Pelletier, CRNI
Coordinator, Pharmacy Intravenous Programs, Southern New Hampshire Regional Medical Center, Nashua, New Hampshire
Intravenous Therapy Calculations

Maxine Perdue, BSN, CRNI
Director of Intravenous Therapy Services, High Point Regional Hospital, High Point, North Carolina
Intravenous Complications

Roxanne Perucca, BSN, CRNI
Intravenous Therapy Clinician, University of Kansas Medical Center, Kansas City, Kansas
Infection Control
Obtaining Vascular Access
Intravenous Monitoring and Catheter Care
Changing and Discontinuing Intravenous Therapy

Christine A. Pierce, RNC, BSN, CRNI, CNSN
Clinical Manager, HCM Health Care, Meridia Health System, Cleveland, Ohio
Intravenous Nursing as a Specialty

David Schuetz, Pharm D, MS
Outpatient Home Infusion Pharmacist, Roseville Hospital Home Infusion Services, Roseville, California
Intravenous Therapy in Alternative Settings

Barbara St. Marie, MA, CRNI
Pain Management Coordinator, Anesthesiology, P.A. at North Memorial Medical Center, Minneapolis, Minnesota
Pain Management

Judy Terry, BSN, CRNI
Director, Intravenous Therapy, Moses H. Cone Memorial Hospital, Greensboro, North Carolina
Fluids and Electrolytes
Infection Control
Parenteral Fluids
Future of Intravenous Therapy

Becky J. Tomaselli, CRNI, CNSN
Infusion Program Manager, Olsten Kimberly Quality Care, Orlando, Florida
Intravenous Therapy in the Home

Cora Vizcarra, RN, BSN, CRNI
Regional Clinical Manager, Homedco Infusion, Indianapolis, Indiana
Parenteral Nutrition

Jane A. Weir, BA, BSN, CRNI
Charge Nurse, Intravenous Therapy Department, Massachusetts General Hospital, Boston, Massachusetts
Blood Component Therapy

Corinne Wheeler, CRNI, CPNP
Practice Development, St. Vincent Hospital and Health Care Center, Indianapolis, Indiana
Intravenous Therapy in Children

REVIEWER LIST

Maxine Acevedo, RN, MPA, CRNI
  I.V. Therapy Administrative Coordinator
  I.V. Therapy/Nutrition Support
  University of California, Davis Medical Center
  Sacramento, CA

Cynthia C. Chernecky, RN, PhD
  Vice President of Research and Development
  H.E.L.L.O., Inc.
  Alpharetta, GA

Mary Crandall, RN, BSN
  Nursing Department
  Mount Sinai Medical Center
  Miami Beach, FL

Lynn M. Czaplewski, RN, CRNI
  IV Training Consultant
  Caremark, Inc.
  New Berlin, WI

Judi R. Davis, MS, RD, LD, CNSD
  American Dietetic Association
  ASPEN
  Arlington, TX

Lynn C. Hadaway, BS, RNC, CRNI
  Menlo Care, Inc.
  Menlo Park, CA
  Southern Regional Medical Center
  Riverdale, GA

Sue Masoorli, RN
  President
  Perivascular Nurse Consultants, Inc.
  Rockledge, PA

Donna Murphy, CRNI
  Deaconess Home Health Care
  Boston, MA

Madonna Jean Owen, RN, CRNI
Nursing Department
Holy Family Hospital
Spokane, WA

Gloria Pelletier, CRNI
Coordinator, Pharmacy I.V. Programs
Southern New Hampshire Regional Medical Center
Nashua, New Hampshire

Lynn Dianne Phillips, RN, MSN, CRNI
Nursing Department
Butte Community College
Croville, CA

Darnell Roth, RN, AA, CRNI
D/R Intravenous Therapy Consulting, Inc.
St. Louis, MO

Fe San Angel, BSN, CRNI, OCN
The Cedars-Sinai Comprehensive Cancer Center
Los Angeles, CA

Ofelia L. Santiago, RN, BSN, CRNI
Nurse Manager
Caremark, Inc.
Wichita, KS

Armand S. Serrecchia, RN, MS, BSN
Department of Nursing
VA Medical Center
Brockton, MA

Golden T. Soileau, RN, MSN, MA
College of Nursing
McNeese State University
Lake Charles, LA

Becky J. Tomaselli, RN, CRNI, CNSN
Infusion Program Manager
Olsten Kimberly Quality Care
Orlando, FL

CONTENTS

SECTION IV

SECTION V

Intravenous Therapy

Clinical Principles
and
Practice

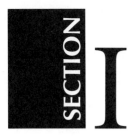

SECTION I

. . . .

INTRODUCTION

CHAPTER 1 Ann M. Corrigan, BSN, MS, CRNI

History of Intravenous Therapy

• •

▬▬ **Early Experiments**
Nineteenth Century
Twentieth Century
Advances in Agents
Advances in Equipment
Nurse's Role in Intravenous Therapy

• •

Intravenous therapy as we know it today is a technical, highly specialized form of treatment. It has evolved from an extreme measure used only on the most critically ill to a therapy used for almost 90% of all hospitalized patients. No longer confined to the hospital, intravenous therapies are now delivered in alternative care settings such as the home, skilled nursing facilities, and physician offices. Intravenous (IV) therapy refers to the parenteral administration of fluids and medications, nutritional support, and transfusion therapy. Although the major advancements in IV therapy occurred in the past 150 years, the practice of using veins to inject substances essentially began in the seventeenth century.

EARLY EXPERIMENTS

The first documented use of blood as a treatment was in 1492, when blood from three young boys was administered to Pope Innocent III.[1] It was not until 1615, however, that the concept of infusing blood from one person to another was considered again, by Libavious,[1] but at that time it was still impossible in practice. This concept constituted the beginning of intravenous therapy. It was several centuries before person-to-person transfusion became possible, and even longer before it became a safe practice.

In 1628, William Harvey's experimental work with blood expanded on the findings of earlier physicians.[2] As a result, the theory of circulation was developed, which led to an understanding of blood flow and of the presence and importance of valves. This new information about the circulatory system led others to experiment with injecting substances into the vascular system to observe the effect on the recipi-

ent. One of the earliest to document this type of experiment was Sir Christopher Wren, of England. In 1656, he experimented with injecting opium and wine into the veins of dogs using a quill and an animal bladder.[2, 3] The first successful injection into humans was accomplished in 1662, by J. D. Major.[2]

About this time, Richard Lower presented a paper before the Royal Society in England on intravenous feeding and blood transfusion in dogs. He was able to demonstrate his transfusion theory with a successful animal-to-animal transfusion,[3] and, in 1666, Lower attempted the first known animal-to-human transfusion.[3]

The first documented transfusion is credited to Jean Baptiste Denis. In 1667 Denis, a physician to the French royalty, successfully transfused 9 ounces of lamb's blood into a 15-year-old boy suffering from madness.[2, 4, 5] Subsequent transfusions to the boy were not successful, and resulted in the first transfusion reaction. The initial success of Denis, however, led to the promiscuous use of transfusions, with fatal results. As a result of the many fatalities, the church and the French parliament banned the transfusion of blood from animals to humans in 1687.[2]

During these early trials with transfusion therapy, scientists and physicians used feather quills (sometimes with metal tips), animal veins, and animal bladders. This equipment has been described in a 1670 Amsterdam publication, *Clysmatic Nova.*[3]

Following the 1687 edict banning blood transfusions, little growth in the field of intravenous therapy was noted for the next 150 years. The one significant event in the eighteenth century occurred in 1795 when Philip Syng Physick, from the University of Edinburgh, noted that the use of blood transfusions in obstetric hemorrhage had some success in decreasing mortality from this complication.[5] It must be remembered, however, that the success or failure of these transfusions was totally without scientific understanding, and can only be considered luck.

NINETEENTH CENTURY

Intravenous therapy, as practiced today, had its beginnings in the nineteenth century, which was a time of rapid advancement in medicine. A first major accomplishment occurred in 1818, when James Blundell performed the first man-to-man transfusion in London.[3, 5] In 1834, Blundell again used human blood to transfuse women during childbirth who were threatened by hemorrhage.[2] Blundell is further credited with the correlation between blood loss and hypoxemia during hemorrhage.

One complication of early transfusions was blood clotting during the transfusion. In 1821, Jean Louis Prevost, a French physician, experimented with preventing this coagulation. Prevost and Jean B. Dumas were the first to use defibrinated blood in animal transfusion.[2] By 1875, Landois had discovered lysing between the serums of different animals, which later resulted in an understanding of antigen-antibody reactions.[6]

The cholera epidemic of 1831 in Leith, Scotland, was an important event in the advancement of intravenous therapy. During this epidemic, Thomas Latta experimented with infusing a saline solution into a patient who ''apparently had reached the last moments of her earthly existence and now nothing could injure her. Indeed, so entirely was she reduced that I feared that I shall be unable to get my apparatus ready, ere she expire.''[2, 7] Latta successfully treated the patient, who eventually recovered and survived. The success of the saline injection led to extensive use of this therapy during the epidemic, but these efforts met with only limited success.

Further work continued and, in 1843, Claude Bernard, a French physiologist, experimented with injecting sugar solutions into dogs. For the next two decades he continued to experiment and infused not only sugar solutions but also egg whites and milk into animals, with some success.[3, 7] During this time, Bernard also discovered that cane sugar, injected intravenously, soon appeared in the urine, whereas ingested sugar, which was acted on by gastric juices, disappeared.

In 1852, the importance of protein in relation to nitrogen balance, weight gain, and general well-being was first observed by Bidder and Schmidt and confirmed by Voit in 1866.[7] This correlation between protein and health led to the concept of nutritional support, although the effect of this relationship would not be fully known for another 75 to 100 years.

During the 1860s, major advances were made that would have an impact on intravenous nursing and on all of medicine. In 1860, Louis Pasteur developed the germ theory of disease, and demonstrated that fermentation and putrefaction result from the growth of germs.[8] Building on this theory, Joseph Lister, professor of Surgery at the University of Glasgow, hypothesized that microbes might be responsible for wound suppuration. He further postulated that infection could be prevented by destroying organisms and preventing contaminated air from coming into contact with the wound.[2, 4, 8] In 1867, Lister published the results of his studies using carbolic acid spray as an antiseptic.[2, 8] He initially used the spray as a dressing material and eventually advanced to using carbolic acid as a soak for the hands and ligatures and for cleaning the site prior to surgery.[8] Lister's work led to the use of cleaner instruments in surgery and provided the framework for the theory of antisepsis and asepsis.

Many physicians, including Lawson Tait of London, observed strict rules of cleanliness without understanding the implications. In France, surgeons continued to focus on the use of antisepsis during procedures instead of asepsis.[4] It wasn't until the early 1900s that the principle of asepsis was fully understood. By then, it was common practice for everything coming into patient contact to be sterile.

The use of gloves for procedures was introduced in 1889, when William Halsted of Johns Hopkins Hospital had the Goodyear Rubber Company make a pair of rubber gloves for his operating room nurse.[4, 9] This nurse, who Halsted later married, was allergic to the hand rinse being used prior to procedures (a corrosive sublimate), and Halsted's only intention was to protect her hands.[9] The use of gloves became popular, and by 1899 rubber gloves were being used on all clean cases. Today, gloves are used not only to protect the patient but also to protect the practitioner. The gloves used in health care today are no longer made of rubber but are composed of various synthetic materials.

The last half of the nineteenth century also saw advances in the field of nutritional support. In 1869, Menzel and Perco of Vienna wrote a paper on the use of fat, milk, and camphor injected subcutaneously.[3, 7] By 1878, the use of oil and a protein extract to treat a patient suffering from anorexia nervosa was reported by Krug, and cow's milk was being injected for volume expansion and nutritional support.[3, 7] Hodder, of Canada, used cow's milk to correct fluid and nutritional losses caused by cholera.[3] Although the results were generally considered good, Hodder was subsequently barred from the practice of medicine by his colleagues. The successful administration of a glucose solution is credited to Biedl and Krause, in 1896.[7]

TWENTIETH CENTURY

For almost 250 years, experiments with injecting different substances into the body had yielded limited results. As with most of medicine, the major advances that would bring intravenous therapy to its current level of sophistication occurred in the twentieth century. By this time, the use of saline and glucose solutions was a more widely accepted practice, although they were still used only on the critically ill patient. Equipment was cleaned and sterilized between uses as a routine measure with the advent of heat sterilization in 1910, and with the medical profession's acceptance that everything coming into contact with the patient needed to be sterile. The discovery of pyrogens in 1923 led to measures that helped eliminate them from fluids and drugs. Dr. Florence Seibert of the Phipps Institute in Philadelphia solved the serious problem of pyrogenic reactions to intravenous infusions in 1925, thus paving the way for safer practice.[3, 4]

Advances in Agents

Early in the twentieth century, Landsteiner discovered naturally occurring antibodies in the blood that led to a reaction when mixed with blood from another subject. This discovery eventually led to the identification of the ABO blood groups in 1901.[6, 10] By 1907, Reuben Ottenberg began using blood type differences as a basis for donor selection. By 1908, Epstein had set forth the hypothesis that ABO blood groups are inherited.[5, 10] Even with this information, transfusion therapy was still potentially fatal. Matching donor and recipient blood types helped reduce the incidence of transfusion reactions, but coagulation during the procedure continued to be a problem. During World War I, Oswald Robertson introduced the use of preserved anticoagulant blood and, by 1915, sodium citrate was being used successfully as an anticoagulant in blood transfusions.[5]

Levine and Stetson discovered the anti-Rh antigen in 1939 and, in 1941, Levine and Burnham recognized that the anti-Rh antigen is responsible for alloimmunization during pregnancy and causes hemolytic disease of the newborn.[6] These developments were important steps in the safe transfusion of blood. An understanding of the effects of the anti-Rh antigen led to the decreased risk of hemolytic disease for children.

World War II is important in the history of transfusion therapy because the practice was used more widely during this time than ever before. Out of necessity, blood was being administered to the wounded troops in an effort to save more lives. Plasma was the first component to be used, and new techniques for the separation of plasma were developed in 1941.[5] It was soon recognized, however, that plasma transfusions could not meet all the needs of the wounded. By 1943, red blood cells were being salvaged and transfused. A filter was subsequently developed to help screen out fibrin clots.[5]

Today, transfusion therapy is a common medical practice. Blood can be separated into many different components and each component is administered to correct a specific deficiency. Improved techniques make it possible to obtain, test, store, and administer these components. The risk of transfusion therapy has diminished as a result of the discovery and understanding of antigen-antibody reactions and of the development of improved methods for detecting bloodborne diseases. Administration sets, filters, infusion and warming devices, and other types of equipment are constantly being modified and improved. Pharmaceutical agents, such as erythropoietin, are being developed to stimulate the body's own production of blood, thereby reducing the need for transfusions and further reducing risks.

During the twentieth century, advances were also being made in the area of nutritional support. Between 1904 and 1906, research on maintaining nitrogen balance for general well-being was conducted, and the rectal administration of protein for nutrition was documented. By 1918, Murlin and Riche were experimenting with the administration of fats to animals as a source of nutrition.[4] The 1930s were a period of intense experimentation in nutritional support. In 1935, Emmett Holt of Baltimore administered an infusion of cottonseed oil, and is credited with the first infusion of a fat emulsion.[3, 4] The administration of a hydrolyzed casein solution was first attempted by Henriques and Anderson in 1913.[4] In 1936, Dr. Robert Elman attempted further administrations of this solution. By 1939 Elman, along with Weiner, infused a solution of 2% casein hydrolysate and 8% dextrose without adverse effects.[7] Following this success, various protein hydrolysates were studied and, in 1940, Schohl and Blackfan infused synthetic crystalline amino acids into infants.[2] By 1944, Helfich and Abelson provided nutritional support to a 5-day-old infant with a solution of 50% glucose and 10% casein hydrolysate, alternated with a 10% olive oil–lecithin emulsion.[7]

Stanley Dudrick's name is synonymous with parenteral nutrition. With the assistance of Dr. Harry Vars, Dudrick conducted a series of experiments on beagle puppies in an attempt to support them totally by the parenteral route.[3] By the early 1970s, Dudrick had proven the effectiveness of protein and dextrose solutions for nutritional support. Today, primarily because of Dudrick's work, patients can receive total nutrition through the intravenous route and survive diseases and conditions that had formerly resulted in death.

The use of fat emulsions as a caloric source was also investigated, but the severe adverse reactions encountered with the intravenous administration of these substances led the Food and Drug Administration (FDA) to ban their use in the United States in 1964. However, fats were still being administered in Europe, and an emulsion derived from soybean oil was developed.[7] This refined product, which produced no significant side effects, led the FDA to reverse its ban on the intravenous administration of fat emulsions in 1980, and soybean and safflower oil emulsions were approved for intravenous administration.

Advances in Equipment

The advances in fluids and medications used for intravenous administration continue today. Medical science has provided the information necessary for us to replace and maintain the body's fluid and electrolyte balance, to maintain or improve nutritional status, and to treat many disease states intravenously. The technology for administering IV fluids and medications has also advanced since Sir Christopher Wren used the quill, vein, and bladder of an animal for his treatments.[8]

The crude apparatus of Wren was later replaced by metal needles, rubber tubing, and glass containers. Originally, the equipment was designed to be reused, and required cleaning and eventually sterilization between uses. The technology for refining plastics has done much for the improvement of intravenous therapy equipment. Administration sets were the first pieces of intravenous equipment to use the plastic, polyvinyl chloride. Solution manufacturers soon developed plastic containers for fluids. Today, most solutions come in plastic containers.

Devices for accessing the vein have also progressed rapidly in the last 50 years. Metal cannulas, crude metal needles that required cleaning and resharpening between uses, were first used in the nineteenth century. Problems with infiltration, however, led to the development of the plastic cannula in 1945.[2] These first catheters were made of flexible plastic tubing that required either a cutdown or needle for introduction into the vessel. In 1950, the Rochester needle was introduced by Gautier and Maasa, and revolutionized the intravenous catheter.[2] Today, this over-the-needle type of catheter is used to deliver almost all peripheral infusions.

The metal needle is still available, but it is now a disposable device modified for short-term use. It has plastic attachments at the hub to assist in handling, and a short piece of plastic tubing is attached. Another piece of equipment available for infusion therapy is the through-the-needle device, which allows the plastic catheter to be threaded into the vein through the needle after venipuncture has been completed. This device was first introduced in 1958 and its successors are used today, especially for peripherally inserted central lines.[2]

Today intravenous cannulas, both metal and plastic, are

available in varying sizes (gauges) to deliver different therapies. Gauges range from a large lumen (12 gauge) to a neonatal size (27 gauge). Cannulas are also available in varying lengths, from 0.75 to 30 inches or more. The length is generally determined by the route of administration, peripheral or central, and the size and age of the patient. The Intravenous Nurses Society recommends that the shortest length, smallest gauge cannula be used to accommodate the therapy prescribed.[11]

Prior to 1949, intravenous therapy could be administered only through a peripheral vein. At that time Meng and colleagues documented the use of a catheter placed in the central venous system of a dog for administering a hypertonic dextrose and protein solution.[7] The subclavian puncture for accessing the central veins was more frequently used after its description by Aubaniac from Vietnam in 1952.[3] In 1967, Dudrick adapted the subclavian approach for the administration of high concentrations of dextrose and proteins, which produced minimal side effects caused by the tonicity of the solution.[3]

Further expansion on this concept led to the development of a catheter that is placed in the subclavian vein and then tunneled under the subcutaneous tissue to exit on the chest wall. Originally designed for use with children, this catheter became known as the Broviac catheter. A size appropriate for adults, the Hickman catheter, was developed soon after. The evolution of the Hickman-Broviac catheter has allowed for the administration of therapies over long periods of time, with minimal technical complications. It has also revolutionized intravenous therapy by allowing safer administration of solutions in the home setting.

The 1980s saw further evolution of the use of central venous access with the introduction of the totally implanted system. This system consists of the central catheter, which is still placed by percutaneous puncture into the subclavian vein and then tunneled under the subcutaneous tissue, but the catheter end is attached to a device referred to as a port that is placed under the subcutaneous tissue on the chest wall. Access to this port is by puncture through the skin with a specially designed needle to the portal septum.

Peripheral catheters primarily consist of a single lumen, although experiments have been carried out with dual-lumen peripheral catheters. Central catheters—percutaneous, tunneled, and ports—are available in both single-lumen and multilumen design. The multilumen design makes it possible for multiple therapies to be delivered through one device, thus sparing the patient from numerous venipunctures.

To make the delivery of intravenous therapy safer, various infusion devices have been developed. Filters were first used in 1943 to screen out fibrin clots during blood transfusions.[5] Filters are now of two types, screen and depth, and are available in a number of micron sizes. Filters remove particulate matter from the infusion and, depending on the micron size, can also eliminate air and remove endotoxins.

In addition to filters, infusion devices that allow for the closer regulation of flow rate have been developed. Prior to the use of this technology, infusions were administered by gravity pressure and the flow rate was regulated primarily by a screw or roller clamp on the administration set. The development of electronic infusion devices has improved the accuracy of administration. Factors that affect flow rate, such as head height and internal pressure, can be overcome by the use of these devices.

The first infusion device developed was the syringe pump, and the quantity of solution it delivered depended on the syringe size used. It was used primarily to administer fluids at a slow rate, especially to infants and children. This type of device is still available and is frequently used to control medication administration. The concept of the syringe pump was modified further to allow large volumes of fluid to be administered. The controller, first developed by IVAC in 1972, allows for gravity infusion but controls it through a drop-counting system that sets off an alarm when the number of drops deviates from the preset number.[2] Subsequently, infusion pumps were designed to deliver a solution at a prescribed rate under positive pressure. Infusion device technology now allows the user to adjust the pressure setting to administer the therapy under varying conditions. Infusion devices can also deliver simultaneous or multiple infusions at prescribed intervals.

Ambulatory infusion devices currently available allow for continuous or intermittent infusions outside the hospital setting. These devices allow patients to receive necessary therapy while maintaining a normal life style as much as possible. The quality of life for many patients has been dramatically improved by the use of these ambulatory devices.

Another technologic advance that has improved the quality of patient care is the patient-controlled analgesia (PCA) pump. This enables patients to control their pain by allowing them to administer their pain medication as they need it. This method of control has proven especially effective in postoperative pain management.

During the 1970s, the administration of pain medication was expanded by alternative routes. As early as 1976, Yaks and Rudy had demonstrated the successful administration of morphine directly into the subarachnoid space of animals.[12] In 1977, Wang proved that an intrathecal injection of morphine provides profound relief in humans.[12] Today, the intrathecal and epidural routes have proven effective for the administration of specific therapies, especially the control of postoperative and cancer pain. The intrathecal route has also been used for administering some antineoplastic agents.

A method of fluid administration that regained some popularity in the 1980s, especially for emergency fluid resuscitation in pediatrics, is intraosseous administration. The bone marrow as a route for transfusion was first advocated by Drinker in 1922.[13] In the 1940s, Tocantins established the basis for the widespread use of this technique for fluid administration,[13] but it was used only briefly. By the late 1950s, intraosseous infusion had fallen into obscurity. The resurgence of this method of administration occurred as a result of advances in pediatric resuscitation and its use is generally limited to young children in the emergency setting. The successful use of this type of administration has proven it to be an important advancement in intravenous therapy.

Nurse's Role in Intravenous Therapy

By the 1980s, administering intravenous fluids and medications had become a specialized practice involving not only the introduction of fluids and medications into the circulatory system, but also into the bone marrow and epidural and intrathecal spaces. Nursing involvement in the practice of intravenous therapy is relatively new; it is only since the 1940s that nurses have been allowed to perform intravenous procedures. Prior to this, nursing's only role in intravenous therapy was in assisting physicians with venipuncture and the administration of fluids.[14] Massachusetts General Hospital of Boston was the first to allow a nurse, Ada Plumer, to be responsible for the administration of intravenous therapies.[14] Plumer became the first IV nurse, and she eventually developed the first IV team.

Intravenous nursing is now a technical, highly specialized field that requires advanced clinical knowledge and technical expertise. Nurses involved in the practice of intravenous therapy need to be knowledgable in the areas of technical and clinical applications, fluid and electrolytes, pharmacology, infection control, pediatrics, antineoplastic therapy, transfusion therapy, parenteral nutrition, and quality assurance to perform their duties competently. The professional practice of intravenous nursing was formally recognized in 1980, when the United States House of Representatives declared January twenty-fifth as IV Nurse Day.

Several professional organizations for intravenous therapy have been established over the last 25 years. The Intravenous Nurses Society, founded in 1973, promotes the specialty practice of intravenous nursing. It seeks to educate the practitioner and protect the public through the development of the *Intravenous Nurses Standards of Practice.*[11] The Intravenous Nurses Certification Corporation also seeks to protect the public by developing and administering a certification-recertification program that meets judicial, regulatory, and professional testing standards.

The administration of fluids and medications has improved considerably since 1492. Advances continue to be made in this practice—in the equipment used, in the fluids and medications administered, and in the techniques used to deliver them. Those involved in the delivery of intravenous therapies must remain current in the field to provide their clients with high-quality care.

References

1. Tasel HF, Pineda AH. Autologous Transfusion and Hemotherapy. London: Blackwell Scientific, 1991.
2. Weinstein SM. Plumer's Principles and Practice of Intravenous Therapy, 5th ed. Boston: Little, Brown and Co., 1993.
3. Rombeau JL, Caldwell MD. Parenteral Nutrition, Vol 2. Philadelphia: W.B. Saunders, 1986.
4. Lyons AS, Petrucelli RJ. Medicine: An Illustrated History. New York: Harry N. Abrams, 1987.
5. Rutman RC, Miller WV. Transfusion Therapy Principles and Policies, 2nd ed. Rockville, MD: Aspen, 1985.
6. Mollison PL. Blood Transfusion in Clinical Medicine, 5th ed. London: Blackwell Scientific, 1972.
7. Grant JP. Handbook of Total Parenteral Nutrition, 3rd ed. Philadelphia: W.B. Saunders, 1992.
8. Wenzel R, ed. Prevention and Control of Nosocomial Infections. Baltimore: Williams & Wilkins, 1987.
9. Bennett JV, Brachman PS. Hospital Infections, 3rd ed. Boston: Little, Brown and Co., 1992.
10. Rice RR, Sanger R. Blood Groups in Man, 6th ed. London: Blackwell Scientific, 1975.
11. Intravenous Nurses Society. Intravenous Nursing Standards of Practice. Belmont, MA: Intravenous Nurses Society, 1990.
12. Zenz M. Epidural opiates for the treatment of cancer pain. Recent Results Cancer Res 1984; 89:107–114.
13. Rosetti VA, Thompson BM, Miller J, et al. Intraosseous infusions: An alternative route of pediatric intravascular access. Ann Emerg Med 1985; 14:885–889.
14. Sager DP, Bomar SK. Intravenous Medications. Philadelphia: J.B. Lippincott, 1980.

CHAPTER 2

Intravenous Nursing as a Specialty

Christine A. Pierce, RNC, BSN, CRNI, CNSN

It has been nearly 500 years since Sir William Harvey, an English physician generally considered to be the father of modern medicine, described completely and accurately the circulatory system.[1] His widespread lecturing in Europe caught the attention of his fellow physicians but also reached those in other professions. Through his discovery and the work of individuals such as Sir Christopher Wren, an architect who together with a chemist produced the first hypodermic needle,[2] the bloodstream became readily accessible. Experimentation with the intravenous injection of many substances resulted.

Success was slow to arrive. In 1687, a fatal attempt at animal-to-human blood transfusions led to an edict from church and parliament prohibiting further such experimentation.[3] Nearly 150 years passed before James Blundell, an English obstetrician, resurrected the idea of transfusion therapy. In 1834, recognizing that hemorrhage often claimed the lives of young women during childbirth, he identified a successful treatment by transfusing human rather than animal blood.[3] Refinements occupied another century until, in 1940, Drs. Karl Landsteiner and Alexander Wiener discovered the Rhesus blood group system. Today, blood and blood products are routinely administered in various practice settings, with few reported complications.

While the details of safe transfusions evolved, advances were simultaneously occurring in other areas. Robert Koch, along with such predecessors and contemporaries as Ignaz Semmelweiss, Louis Pasteur, and Lord Joseph Lister, forged ahead in the field of bacteriology, developing the process of pasteurization, principles of asepsis, and the drying and staining method of examining bacteria. In 1895, Wilhelm Röntgen discovered x-rays and established the foundations of radiology.[1] Saline was identified as a reasonable treatment for dehydration, and the caloric value of dextrose was recognized, but it was not until 1923 that the discovery and elimination of solution pyrogens made intravenous fluid administration safer and more frequent. Preceding 1940, the administration of IV solutions remained the domain of the physician and, because it was considered to be a major procedure, was reserved for use only in the most critically ill.[3] From the mid- to the late twentieth century, progress would explode.

The rapid technologic advances of World War II and the resultant health care needs of the soldiers stimulated medical innovation. This war, as well as those subsequently fought in Korea and Vietnam, necessitated large-scale fluid resuscitation, multiple medication infusions, improved methods of venous access, and disposable and more creative forms of medical supplies to treat those surviving atrocities that previously had led inevitably to death. The steel needle gave way to the flexible catheter, reducing infiltration. Glass bottles were replaced by nonvented plastic containers, reducing both the risk of air embolism and airborne contamination. By 1952, the percutaneous approach to subclavian vein catheterization was described in France,[3] permitting both central venous access for infusion and the monitoring of central venous pressure.

Advances in understanding fluid and electrolyte balance and human nutritional needs were also occurring. In the mid-1870s, Hodder and Thomas discovered that the intravenous infusion of cow's milk into humans could expand intravascular volume and provide nutritional support. Because the freshness of the milk was believed to be a critical factor, cows were often brought to the steps of the hospital and milked on site,[4] an interesting forerunner to today's total parenteral nutrition and lipid solutions delivered to the patient's refrigerator.

From the dawn of the twentieth century, experimentation with amino acids, sugar, and fat continued. In 1968, in the Department of Surgical Research at the University of Pennsylvania, Dr. Stanley Dudrick successfully achieved normal growth and development in children and maintenance in adults using intravenous dextrose and amino acids as their sole nutritional source.[4] This classic work marked the beginning of the clinical applications of IV nutritional support.

And where was nursing in these continuing attempts to use the human bloodstream as a route to calm and cure? It is fitting that Boston, home of "America's first trained nurse" in 1863,[1] should also attain notoriety for the development of the infusion nursing specialty. In 1940, the Massachusetts General Hospital in Boston developed a new nursing position, which included the following general responsibilities:

Administering intravenous solutions and transfusions
Cleaning and sharpening needles
Cleaning infusion sets
Maintaining patent needles and unobstructed infusion flow[1]

Although the emphasis was on technical performance and the prerequisite of being able to perform a venipuncture successfully, this new nursing role established initial autonomy from the physician and the specialty title of "Intravenous Therapist."

Over the ensuing 50 years, the role of the nurse in infusion therapy has evolved to the IV practitioner of the 1990s, no longer the technician but a multifaceted specialist capable of integrating holistic principles of medicine, nursing, management, marketing, education, and quality improvement into the patient's plan of care. The past 10 years have seen particularly rapid growth of the intravenous nursing specialty, as evidenced by

- Publication of the National Intravenous Therapy Association's (NITA) recommendations of practice (1980)
- Recognition and establishment of IV Nurse Day by the United States House of Representatives (October 1, 1980), declaring that January twenty-fifth of each year be nationally celebrated in honor of IV nurses
- Offering of the first national Certification Examination for Intravenous Nurses (March, 1985)
- Development by the Centers for Disease Control and Prevention (CDC) of "universal precautions" to reduce the risk of transmitting the human immunodeficiency virus (HIV) and hepatitis B virus (HBV) to health care workers
- Evolution of the multibillion dollar home infusion business, delivery of which is predicated on infusion specialty nursing practice

Today, over 80% of hospitalized patients receive some form of intravenous therapy during their stay, and many continue that therapy after discharge. Pharmacologic and technologic advances provide the patient with improved quality of care but concurrently demand a more specialized and detailed nursing knowledge base to offset risks and maximize value. Factors such as the growing elderly population, the economic need to service patients outside the hospital, and the proposed changes of health care reform, provide expanding possibilities for the prepared and flexible infusion nurse. The pursuit of continuing education, attainment of specialty certification, and involvement with the professional organizations affiliated with infusion care all bode well for the successful infusion practitioner of the next century.

PROFESSIONAL ORGANIZATIONS

One November day in 1972, two Boston IV nurses, Ada Plumer and Marguerite Knight, wrote an organizational letter requesting interested individuals to join in forming the American Association of IV Nurses (AAIVN). By the time 16 charter members assembled in Baltimore on January 25, 1973, there was already some concern that the use of "nurse" in the organization's name would restrict membership to nurses exclusively, when the proposed bylaws were more expansive.[5] They subsequently decided to name the organization the National Intravenous Therapy Association (NITA). Its stated purpose was to standardize the specialty practice of IV nursing and to ensure the provision of quality, cost-efficient patient care.

Over the next 6 years, NITA expanded rapidly. The addition of new members facilitated local chapter formation and affiliation with other national organizations. In 1979, the demands of rapidly increasing membership heralded the need for a professional full-time staff to work collaboratively with elected and appointed officials. A national office was established in Cambridge, Massachusetts, only a few miles from where it is now located.

By 1987, many milestones had been achieved within NITA. The "Standards of Practice," unifying the specialty approach to infusion nursing practice, were developed in 1980 and revised in 1983. In response to rapid changes in health care and emerging technology, the standards served to increase the recognition of the intravenous specialty nationwide. In October 1980, the United States House of Representatives acknowledged the practice of IV therapy as an independent specialty, and declared January twenty-fifth of each year to be National IV Nurse Day. The first specialty certification examination was offered in 1985, and successful candidates were awarded the designation of CRNI (Certified Registered Nurse, Intravenous).

Although nurses composed 99% of NITA's membership in the mid-1980s, there remained some confusion among fellow professionals, consumers, and legislators about what group this organization represented. In 1987, a letter from one of NITA's own CRNIs highlighted her experience in the "Nurse in Washington Internship Program" and stated that NITA would be recognized by other professional nursing organizations only if the word "nurse" were reflected in the name.[5] In 1987, by a majority vote of the members, NITA officially became the Intravenous Nurses Society (INS). This name was chosen to reflect the organization's nature and focus more accurately.

The INS is now composed of over 8000 members in 54 local chapters. Of these, 93.5% are registered nurses and 6.5% are other professionals, including physicians, pharmacists, and licensed practical nurses. Of the registered nurse members, 30% hold the CRNI credential.[6] Fewer than 1% are international members, but the growing interest in global initiatives is evidenced by the establishment of a Professional Intravenous Nurses Society in Australia (1992) and the 1993 visit to Japan by the INS president. A crucial purpose for international activities, beyond the INS mission of excellence and quality worldwide, is to ensure that products and devices manufactured for United States markets meet acceptable standards of IV therapy.[6]

The *Intravenous Standards of Practice* were revised for the second time in 1990, and a third version is to be published in 1995 to keep pace with the escalating changes in this specialty. INS publishes a peer-reviewed journal bimonthly, highlighting clinical, management, ethical, and technologic issues. To ready its members for the opportunities and challenges of the twenty-first century, INS has recently revised its Mission Statement and developed a Values Statement. The Intravenous Nurses Society's strategic plan is comprised of seven key areas: professional development, membership, public awareness, research, global initiatives, administration, and finance, positioning the organization well within the changing environment of health care reform and offering its members a wide range of professional support services in their daily practice.[7]

Intravenous Nurses Society Mission Statement

The Intravenous Nurses Society exists to promote excellence in intravenous nursing through standards, education, public awareness, and research. INS's ultimate goal is to ensure access to the highest quality, cost-effective care for all individuals requiring and patients receiving intravenous therapies in all practice settings worldwide.

Twenty years of INS success have "contributed significantly to the growth and recognition of the specialty of IV nursing and its ongoing goal of quality health care in this country," according to Mary Larkin, Chief Executive Officer, INS.[5] Now, on the eve of the next century, the organization is prepared not only to develop the IV specialty, but to fashion it into a collaborative practice with other nursing specialties for the holistic welfare of its consumers worldwide. "Nursing is an independent profession that is held accountable for serving the public. The authority for nursing is based upon a contract with society that is derived from a complex social base. Within the context of this contract, society grants the profession considerable autonomy to manage its own affairs."[8]

SCOPE OF PRACTICE

Basic nursing education is designed to prepare the nursing generalist, someone with a global approach to nursing practice. Although there currently exist three primary education entries to registered nursing practice—associate degree, diploma, and baccalaureate degree—all are designed to provide entry level nurses with a foundation on which to build more specialized practices in their areas of competence and interest. The advance of nursing practice is heralded by specialization, requiring knowledge and skills within a circumscribed area, in a more detailed format than the generalist. Although specialization can be achieved by continuing formal education at the graduate level and beyond, it is also a product of concentrated study, continuing education, and skill development in a specific area of clinical interest. The practice of intravenous nursing is specialization. Let us now examine the scope of this role more closely.

The intravenous nurse is a registered nurse who has acquired knowledge and skill in intravenous nursing and is committed to the provision of safe, high-quality intravenous nursing care to the patient. The intravenous nurse's practice is based on the following seven major assumptions:

The nursing process is pervasive in the practice of intravenous nursing. Its cyclical format of assessment, problem identification, intervention, and evaluation underscores the ongoing expansion of knowledge and practice in this, as in all, specialties. Continuously using outcomes to refine data collection and problem identification results in improved and innovative plans of care. It causes a paradigm shift from the role of technician to the expansive role of colleague and collaborator. This enables the intravenous nurse to interact with other members of the health care team, particularly those who regulate or influence nursing practice.

Education and research should have a place within the practice of all intravenous nurses. Research is the foundation for nursing's own body of knowledge, a general prerequisite to its recognition as a profession. It is this distinct knowledge base that sets nursing apart from medicine and the social and biologic sciences, and it is the nurse's responsibility to contribute to this base on an ongoing basis. Sharing information through presentation and publication ensures the dissemination of practice-based specialty learning, and encourages an influx of new practitioners into that specialty. Only then can collaborative nursing truly exist.

COMPETENCIES

The practice setting for intravenous therapy delivery is as disparate as the patient populations served by this specialty. From the hospitalized neonate to the geriatric client in an extended care facility, there are many locations and clinical diagnoses served by intravenous nurses. A critical care setting may find the nurse transfusing blood products and interpreting hemodynamic data gained from transvenous monitoring. Another nurse may be in a suburban home, training a mother to administer total parenteral nutrition to her toddler.

A colleague is fighting downtown traffic to reach a working executive in time to perform a cassette change on an ambulatory antibiotic pump, while yet another is recommending vascular access device alternatives to the new oncology patient being seen in the physician's office. At first glance, the scenes appear uniquely different. What is consistent, however, is the basic competencies of the nurse: that combination of knowledge, skills, and abilities necessary to fulfill the role of a nurse administering intravenous therapy.

In defining those competencies for intravenous nursing, the authors of the revised *Intravenous Nursing Standards of Practice* considered 14 major areas: (1) clinical; (2) communication; (3) patient education; (4) technology; (5) continuing education; (6) legal; (7) quality assurance; (8) research; (9) consultation; (10) supervision; (11) clinical management; (12) certification; (13) budgetary process; and (14) intravenous nursing teams.[8]

Basic competencies are intended to serve as guidelines for the practicing nurse and to assist in the design of orientation and continuing education programs. They provide a valid basis for professional intravenous nursing practice.

Clinical. The registered nurse shall be proficient in all clinical aspects of intravenous nursing, with validated competency in clinical judgment and practice.

Intravenous nursing is defined as the utilization of the nursing process as it relates to fluids and electrolytes, infection control, oncology, pediatrics, pharmacology, quality assurance, technology and clinical application, parenteral nutrition, and transfusion therapy. The practice of intravenous nursing encompasses the nursing management and coordination of care to the intravenous patient in accordance with state statutes, the INS *Standards of Practice,* and established institutional policy. This practice also includes, but is not limited to, the following:

1. Validation of the physician's order for parenteral therapy
2. Initiation, monitoring, and termination of parenteral therapies
3. Preparation of parenteral solutions with the addition of medications in the absence of an admixture service
4. Recognition of medication and solution incompatibilities
5. Administration and monitoring of antineoplastic agents
6. Administration and monitoring of investigational drugs
7. Administration and monitoring of parenteral nutrition
8. Administration and monitoring of blood/blood components
9. Performance of venous and arterial punctures
10. Performance of phlebotomies
11. Maintenance of intravascular site, tubing, and dressing
12. Maintenance of established infection control and aseptic practices
13. Initiation of intravenous therapy in emergency situations
14. Thorough knowledge and proficient technical ability in the use of parenteral equipment
15. Evaluation, care, and maintenance of parenteral equipment
16. Observation and assessment of all adverse reactions and complications related to parenteral therapy and the initiation of appropriate nursing intervention
17. Documentation associated with the preparation, administration, and termination of all forms of parenteral therapies

Communication. The registered nurse shall have verbal and written communication skills to facilitate the translation of ideas and facts to persons within and beyond the scope of the specialty.

Patient Education. In keeping with the holistic approach to patient care, it is the registered nurse's responsibility to educate the patient and significant others about the prescribed therapy. The education of the patient and assessment of the patient's comprehension are documented, communicated to the appropriate person(s), and stored in a system that is accessible for the retrieval of information.

Education and the teaching of intravenous therapy occur within the health care facility and/or the home. The effectiveness of teaching methods is evaluated periodically and continually assessed by the registered nurse.

Technology. Technology in intravenous nursing is continually advancing. The registered intravenous nurse shall continually evaluate and control regimens and products for clinical application used in this nursing specialty. The nurse shall be cognizant of all new technologic advances and shall participate in the evaluation, selection, and implementation of these products in the clinical setting.

Continuing Education. Continuing education is essential to sustain and advance intravenous nursing. Active participation in continuing education programs is vital for the continued growth of this specialty and the nursing profession. Information obtained from continuing education programs should be shared with colleagues in collaborative disciplines to improve care. Continuing education is required for all nurses.

Legal. Nursing standards for the delivery of intravenous therapy

1. Establish a framework for monitoring the care given and the products used in the delivery of intravenous therapies.
2. Provide a frame of reference that allows distinctions to be made regarding malpractice, product failure, or an unfortunate medical result.
3. Assist in resolving ethical conflicts between the intravenous nurse's duty to the patient and the nurse's position as an employee of a health care facility.

Adherence to nursing standards for the delivery of intravenous therapy

1. Reduces the risk to the patient of unnecessary trauma or complications.
2. Assists the medical profession by reducing the risk of malpractice claims against the physician, nurse, hospital, or other medical facility.
3. Assists manufacturers by reducing the risk of product liability claims against their company.

Quality Assurance. The patient receiving intravenous nursing care is assured quality care through the nurse's compliance with outcome criteria. All registered nurses are responsible for quality assurance as it relates to this specialty. Observation of the patient's condition and re-evaluation of the nursing care plan shall be done on a continual basis. Documentation of pertinent statistics relative to intravenous therapy shall be maintained. Deviation from optimal care in intravenous nursing practice requires corrective action. All intravenous policies and procedures shall be reviewed and/or revised annually and approved by a member of the medical staff.

Research. Research is an inherent component of intravenous nursing that allows the continual investigation, validation, and development of this nursing practice. Through the dissemination of research results, the art and science of the intravenous nursing specialty are advanced.

Consultation. The registered nurse is an essential consultant to the health care profession, the family, the community, and related industries. The principal concerns of this consultation are patient advocacy and the delivery of safe and optimal intravenous nursing care.

Supervision. Registered nurses shall be aware of basic management skills, capable of supervising others, and held accountable for all work performed under their supervision.

Clinical Management. Clinical management encompasses all aspects of the nursing process. The goal of clinical management is to meet the needs of the patient and to achieve the established therapeutic outcome.

Certification. Although certification of registered nurses who practice in the specialty of intravenous nursing is voluntary, registered nurses practicing in this specialty should consider obtaining certification and maintaining the CRNI credential, because this certification validates competency and a continuum thereof.

Budgetary Process. Responsibility is required for the financial aspects of intravenous patient care to manage costs while rendering quality care. The registered nurse should be actively involved in and accountable for establishing and maintaining the budgetary process. This process shall include but is not limited to the allocation of monies encompassing staffing, education, and products used in intravenous nursing.

Intravenous Nursing Teams. Clinical data have demonstrated that intravenous nursing teams are cost effective because of their efficient and effective use of equipment, and because intravenous nurses practice at high productivity levels. Intravenous nursing teams provide high-quality patient care through more frequent monitoring of intravenous treatment modalities, thereby significantly decreasing the risk of complications related to intravenous therapy. The types of invasive procedures performed by intravenous nurses require theoretic and clinical knowledge and technical skill. These teams must be managed by a registered nurse who meets the criteria established for a clinical intravenous nurse specialist. The team should have a physician advisor who is a nursing advocate. This physician should provide consultation and approve procedures. The intravenous nursing team should be established as an independent department under administration and should have a close relationship with other departments, including but not limited to the departments of nursing, infection control, and pharmacy.

Educational Requirements

Currently, the Intravenous Nurses Certification Corporation (INCC) does not require the Bachelor of Science in Nursing (BSN) degree, but at both the entry and specialist levels recommends it for intravenous nursing practice. As defined in the revised *Intravenous Standards of Practice,* the complete entrance requirements for intravenous specialty practice at the entry level are as follows:

1. Licensure: registered nurse.
2. Level of academic achievement: the Intravenous Nurses Society recommends the BSN degree.
3. Suggested experience: entry into the practice requires 2 years' medical-surgical nursing experience.
4. The nurse must demonstrate behavioral characteristics such as accountability, reliability, initiative, and sound judgment.
5. The nurse must demonstrate effective communication and technical skills.

The entrance requirements at the specialist level are as follows:

1. Licensure: registered nurse.
2. Level of academic achievement: the Intravenous Nurses Society recommends the BSN degree.
3. Suggested experience: the nurse must have 1 year's experience in the specialty practice of intravenous nursing. One year is defined as 1600 hours in the care and delivery of intravenous therapies to patients within the last 2 consecutive years.
4. The nurse must demonstrate behavioral characteristics such as accountability, reliability, initiative, and sound judgment.
5. The nurse must demonstrate effective communication and technical skills.[8]

Additionally, the standards describe the detailed curriculum and implementation of that curriculum that is thought to best prepare the intravenous nurse specialist.[8] The following discussion highlights those recommendations.

Establish Objectives

The registered nurse wishing to practice in this specialty should undertake a course of study that is based on outcome criteria established by behavioral objectives from the cognitive, affective, and psychomotor domains.

The educational program objectives are accomplished through planned instructional methodology, which should include the following:

1. Assignment of appropriate instructional materials
2. Presentations, discussions, demonstrations, practice sessions, and audiovisual aids
3. Clinical experience under direct and indirect supervision
4. Validation of competency in both theory and practice
5. Evaluation of academic and clinical experience with feedback sessions
6. Planned continuing education programs

Evaluation

To ensure that the nurse can function safely as an intravenous nursing specialist in an ongoing capacity, an evaluation process should be established and include the following:

1. A measure of the registered nurse's knowledge through the use of tests, both oral and written, and satisfactory completion of a comprehensive examination at the end of the orientation program
2. A measure of the registered nurse's behavior and attitudes according to measurable criteria incorporated in a personal evaluation form
3. A measure of the registered nurse's ability to perform the technical tasks of the specialty through direct and indirect observation of performance in the clinical areas.

Theoretic and Clinical Components

It is necessary for the nurse to establish proficiency in both the clinical and theoretic knowledge of intravenous nursing to function successfully as a specialty practitioner. The clinical aspects (see earlier, Competencies) must be supervised until proficiency is determined to be acceptable by observation, return demonstration, and competent clinical judgment. The time frame for clinical internship-preceptorship should be adequate to allow the nurse to function independently and to exhibit an acceptable level of judgment and skill. This time should be stated clearly in institutional or agency policy.

The theoretic aspects should provide a formalized instruction program to enhance both written and verbal communication skills and to expand knowledge in key content areas. It includes the nurse's knowledge and understanding of institutional as well as intravenous departmental policies, and an awareness of the nurse's responsibilities to the patient, employer, nursing profession, other health care professionals, community, and intravenous department.

Curriculum Content Areas

There are nine major areas proposed for a comprehensive theoretic curriculum in intravenous nursing (Table 2–1).[8] It is logical that these same topics should serve as the basis for the professional certification examination offered through the INCC as an assessment of specialty knowledge. Before embarking on a discussion of certification, it is necessary to take a more detailed look at each content area and to understand the specific objectives needed to determine competency within that subject. The following descriptions are taken from the revised *Intravenous Standards of Practice.*[8]

Fluid and Electrolyte Balance. This curriculum should provide the registered nurse with an understanding of the nature, pathophysiology, clinical manifestations, and principles of maintenance, replacement, and/or corrective therapy. This curriculum should be approached on the basis of separate body systems and their related diseases to acquaint the registered nurse with the major objectives of therapy.

Infection Control. The curriculum of infection control should include but not be limited to a general overview of microbiology, specific instructions on microorganisms pertaining to intravenous therapy, transmission of disease-causing organisms, preventive measures, precautions, and aseptic technique.

Oncology. This curriculum should include but not be limited to a knowledge and understanding of the cell cycle, types of cancer, purpose of therapy, such as curative or palliative, assessment of laboratory values, antineoplastic agents and their indications for use in both single and combined therapy, and all related aspects of antineoplastic agent use, such as dosing, anticipated side effects, potential complications, administration and safe handling of these agents, patient education, nursing interventions, and the dying process.

Pediatrics. This curriculum should provide the registered nurse with information regarding the safe administration of parenteral therapy to the pediatric patient and should include but not be limited to growth and development, fluid and electrolytes related to the pediatric population, appropriate intravenous solutions, special considerations in delivery systems, treatment modalities, such as dosing and site selection, and psychologic implications.

Pharmacology. This curriculum should address classifications of medications, including investigational drugs administered by the parenteral route. The knowledge and understanding of intravenous drugs should include but not be limited to indications for use, pharmacologic properties, contraindications, dosing, clinical mathematics, anticipated side effects, potential complications and antidotal therapy, compatibilities, stabilities, and any other special considerations.

Quality Assurance–Risk Management. This curriculum should include structural components, legal aspects, criteria to measure outcome based on policy and procedure, participation in the process, such as planning, implementation, evaluation, and monitoring for desired outcomes, and standards of practice.

Technology and Clinical Application. This curriculum should prepare the registered nurse as a competent specialist in the skills, techniques, and clinical aspects of delivering parenteral therapies. Educational aids and actual equipment shall be used in this instruction. Hands-on practice sessions should be offered. The instruction of skills and techniques should be interactive.

This education should present the proper function, usage, care, and maintenance of supplies and equipment used in the delivery of parenteral therapies. Knowledge and understanding of potential hazards and possible complications related to the use of supplies and equipment should be included.

This instruction should provide in-depth focus on the vascular system and its interrelatedness to all other body systems. Additionally, a thorough knowledge and understanding of the neurologic system should be included, with emphasis on the layers and compartments of the spinal cord and brain and the diffusion of medication across this system. The nurse

Table 2–1

Content Areas: Intravenous Nursing Curriculum

Area	Curriculum
1	Fluid and electrolyte balance
2	Infection control
3	Oncology
4	Pediatrics
5	Pharmacology
6	Quality assurance–risk management
7	Technology and clinical applications
8	Parenteral nutrition
9	Transfusion therapy

must have a complete awareness, knowledge, and understanding of all the encompassing applications of parenteral therapies and must be able to recognize complications and initiate interventions to achieve desired patient outcomes.

Parenteral Nutrition. This curriculum should provide the registered nurse with knowledge of indications for use, types, and composition of solutions available, patient assessment, and administration and termination techniques. This instruction should emphasize patient education, metabolic processes, potential complications, and measures to ensure desired outcomes.

Transfusion Therapy. This curriculum should provide the registered nurse with knowledge of immunohematology, blood grouping, blood and blood components, equipment, and reactions. The registered nurse shall be knowledgeable about the selection and protection of blood donors, the fractionation of blood into its components, and the laboratory testing required for the determination of compatibility. Emphasis shall be placed on the administration of blood, its cellular components and plasma derivatives, and the recognition and management of any adverse reactions.

CERTIFICATION

The history of certification actually spans the greatest portion of the twentieth century, although most are familiar with it as a buzz word of the last 5 years. Believed to have first been used as a credentialing measure for public health nurses as early as 1912,[9] certification was created out of concern for the inadequacy of hospital-based training for diversified roles. The nurse was required to complete a particular program of postgraduate education to be awarded a certificate. By the late 1950s, the American Nurses Association (ANA) began to examine a certification mechanism that would acknowledge achievement in various areas of clinical practice.[9] They identified certification as a method for regulating and protecting specialized practice, but also claimed it to be an effective method for ensuring expert quality to the public. It was not until 1974 that the ANA began certifying registered nurses officially, and then it was only for three practice areas.[10] By 1987, that number had grown to 17, and today the ANA offers certification in 23 specialties.

Soon, other organizations began examining the idea of certification for their area of specialty practice. One of the earliest was the American Association of Critical Care Nurses (AACN). Begun in 1976, this certification program awards the CCRN credential and currently has the greatest number of certified nurses in any specialty.[10] In 1984, there were only 85,000 certified nurses nationwide.[10] Between 1985 and 1990, 20 new certifications were developed, resulting in 60 choices and bringing the total of certified nurses to nearly 250,000.[11] Just what does certification mean today, and why are nearly 15% of all employed nurses following their ''RN'' with some credential?

The primary goal of certification has been and still remains consumer protection. Historically used to declare someone qualified to perform, this credential now identifies those who practice on a higher, more sophisticated level than that determined by license.[12] By design, licensure ensures only a minimal degree of competency. It is the oldest mechanism by which occupations are regulated in the United States and was

defined by the Department of Health, Education and Welfare as ''. . . the process by which an agency of government grants permission to an individual to engage in a given occupation, upon finding that the applicant has obtained the minimal degree of competency necessary to ensure that public health, safety and welfare will be reasonably protected.''[12] Professional nurses are licensed to practice under the Nurse Practice Act within each state. Licensure is mandatory, but certification is voluntary.

Certification is the process by which a nongovernmental agency or association grants recognition to an individual who has met certain predetermined qualifications specified by that agency or association. Such qualifications may include the following: (1) graduation from an accredited or approved program; (2) acceptable performance on a qualifying examination or series of examinations; and/or (3) completion of a given amount of work experience.[1] Licensure then addresses competence for the general practice of nursing, whereas certification signifies competence in specialized professional practice based on the acquisition of additional knowledge and skills. Certification by professional nursing organizations is available to those licensed nurses who have met the predetermined standards or criteria specified by that association or agency for specialty practice.[9] Although each specialty group has its own objectives, goals of these certification programs generally include the following:

- Assessment of advanced knowledge and skill
- Demonstration of excellence in practice
- Insurance of the public's welfare
- Standardization of the qualifications necessary for specialty practice
- Advancement of the knowledge and standards of the specialty[13]

It is clear that certification programs instill a system of accountability that directly affects the quality of care consumers can expect to receive. Certification not only protects the public but the nurse as well by providing control over a specific sphere of practice and limiting the inward migration of those who are unqualified. It provides control to the professional association granting the credential by forcing it to establish a clear identity, define the area of practice, and set performance standards.[12]

The last 5 years have witnessed a virtual explosion in the number of certification programs and nurses participating in the credentialing process. There are a number of reasons for this trend. It has been shown that over time, voluntary processes have the tendency to become institutionalized and legalized, and that voluntary agencies with no legal power may gain access to power through rules and regulations that are subsequently developed.[12] An example of power without law is the need to have successfully passed the survey from the Joint Commission on Accreditation of Healthcare Organizations (JCAHO), a voluntary accreditation process, to qualify for Medicare reimbursement—a necessary fiscal survival mechanism. Already, Pennsylvania requires 50% of emergency department and intensive care nurses to have been or actively be preparing for certification before their institution can become a trauma center.[10] In the psychiatric–mental health specialty, certification creates nurse eligibility for third-party reimbursement,[14] and the advanced roles of nurse anesthetist, nurse midwife, and nurse practitioner require certification to practice. As trends continue toward increased professionalism and accountability to quality care for health care consumers, certification is certain to gain even more popularity. There is a growing effort by nursing organizations and associations to tie direct reimbursement by third-party payers to care delivered by certified nurses, and health care organizations are beginning to recognize their need to support nurses seeking certification, if only for long-term institutional survival.[13]

Beyond the predicted employment and financial implications of certification, and the obvious consumer benefits, there are many additional motivations for a nurse to seek credentialing. The literature is filled with reports of increased job satisfaction, improved self-esteem, employment opportunities, clinical advancement, and the pride of peer recognition and respect, all attributable to certification.[12–14] Although informal surveys and spot checks suggest that most hospitals do not directly increase nursing salaries as a result of certification, some provide a one-time bonus or use the credential as a component of advancement on the clinical ladder, ultimately leading to higher compensation.[10] Others encourage and reward their nurses by providing on-site review courses and paid workshop days during test preparation, refunding test fees for successful passing, and recognizing achievement with certificates, publication of names of successfully certified nurses in the organization's newsletter, and provision of new name pins with the certification designation clearly printed.[13]

The INS, then known as the NITA, offered the first national certification examination for intravenous nurses on March 23, 1985. At 17 sites around the country, 540 registered nurses sat for this examination. Successful completion led to the CRNI designation. This examination has been offered annually ever since, extending the CRNI credential to thousands of intravenous nurses in a variety of practice settings.

Today, the responsibility of preparing and administering the certification examination rests with the Intravenous Nurses Certification Corporation (INCC), a separate corporation from the INS. Although working collaboratively within the intravenous specialty, these organizations have different missions: the INS focuses on its membership (see earlier) and the INCC is concerned with the public and its protection. The national board of examiners for the INCC consists of registered nurses who have passed the certification examination, received the designation CRNI, and are widely recognized as experts in the content areas of the examination. This board works in conjunction with a psychometrician in the areas of test development, administration, and evaluation.[15] To become certified, a registered nurse involved in the specialty practice of intravenous therapy must achieve a passing score on the written INCC certification examination. The following eligibility criteria must be fulfilled prior to submitting application for testing:

1. An active current license as a registered nurse in the United States or Canada
2. A minimum of 1600 hours of experience as a registered nurse in intravenous nursing within the last 2 consecutive years prior to the date of testing

---

Intravenous Nurses Certification Corporation Mission Statement

The Intravenous Nurses Certification Corporation (INCC) exists for the public benefit and protection by assessment, validation, and documentation of the clinical eligibility and the continued clinical competency of nurses delivering intravenous therapy modalities in all practice settings worldwide. INCC supports education and ongoing research, and validates the reliability of credentialing mechanisms and their relationship to clinical practice. INCC promotes the recognition of its credentialed nurses and programs to the public, to other health care organizations, and to the nursing profession.

INCC was created to develop and administer a credentialing program that meets judicial, regulatory, and professional testing standards.

Currently, specialty certification is considered voluntary. However, programs must exist for public protection and not violate antitrust legislation by restraining trade or restricting competition. Eligibility criteria for participating in credentialing programs cannot be overly restrictive. Valid certification examinations must be flexible and open to innovation, as evidenced by empiric data that show a correlation with clinical experience, and they must reflect the skills and knowledge of the content areas being assessed. Challenges to the validity of certification can be reviewed by the courts to ensure that they are fair and nondiscriminatory.

"Intravenous nursing" is defined as the technology and clinical application of intravenous therapies in the areas of fluid and electrolyte therapy, pharmacology, infection control, pediatrics, transfusion therapy, antineoplastic therapy, parenteral nutrition, and quality assurance (see earlier). Registered nurses functioning as educators, administrators, or researchers in the intravenous nursing specialty meet the experience criterion if they have spent the equivalent of 1600 hours in their position within the last 2 consecutive years prior to the date of application.[15]

The Examination

Preparation for the examination is best undertaken with a well-defined plan, implemented months in advance of the actual testing date. Because of the variables in individual practice settings and clinical situations encountered, the nurse should not rely exclusively on work experience to prepare for this broad-based examination. It is helpful to assemble reference material that includes a comprehensive, basic nursing text as well as publications specific to the intravenous specialty practice and test content areas. A number of helpful publications and a recommended bibliography are available through the INS and INCC.

Once the study materials have been gathered, the nurse should plan to devote a specific amount of time each day for reading and review. Some nurses find it helpful to form a study group with colleagues who are also preparing for the test. This can be particularly helpful if the group members represent different areas of expertise and can share information. Certification review courses are offered in conjunction with national INS educational programs and may occasionally be presented by a local INS chapter. Some nurses find this classroom instruction structure to be most familiar and comfortable. Other certified nurses should be sought out in the work place and asked to act as mentors. A successful CRNI can offer much advice and guidance for test preparation, and enjoys the opportunity to serve as a recognized expert in the intravenous specialty.

There are nine major content areas covered on the certification examination (see earlier). The content tested is identical to that recommended for the basic curriculum of intravenous nursing,[8] and should serve as the foundation for any intravenous nursing practice. Candidates who successfully pass this examination are awarded the CRNI designation.

Recertification

Recertification is required every 3 years. To become recertified, one must be an active CRNI, possess a current RN license, and be able to document 1000 hours of experience as a clinical registered nurse in the specialty practice of IV therapy within the 3-year certification period. The nurse must document either 40 recertification units during this 3-year certification period, or successfully complete the certification examination in the third year of certification.[16] Recertification units are awarded through attendance at INS-sponsored continuing education programs that address this specialty practice. General nursing education credits do not currently apply toward recertification credit.

ROLE DELINEATION: BENEFITS OF THE INFUSION NURSE SPECIALIST

The CRNI credential identifies the intravenous nurse as a highly knowledgeable and skilled practitioner in the delivery of intravenous therapies, indicates that the practitioner is prepared to be accountable for his or her professional development, and serves as objective and measurable evidence of clinical expertise in a specialty practice.[17] From the public point of view, the designation of certified infusion specialist ensures that the nurse has been educated to provide IV services and should be selectively sought, much as board-certified physicians comprise medical subspecialties.[17] Physician colleagues evaluate the CRNI from a perspective of minimal risk and high patient satisfaction, convinced that certain com-

plex infusion therapies should only be handled by the infusion specialist,[18] and are selectively requesting these nurses in hospital and alternate site settings. The CRNI has shown positive outcomes in facility and agency quality management, and has decreased liability and risk in areas of high-volume, high-technology procedures. IV specialty nurses have extended that benefit to manufacturers by using products as intended, in a safe and appropriate manner.[17]

Not surprisingly, use of the certified infusion specialist has also proven cost-effective. A CRNI requires less orientation and in-service time, and can also have a positive impact on equipment and supply costs by proper and effective utilization. In an ever-expanding philosophy of total quality management (TQM) and continuous quality improvement (CQI), the process of specialty credentialing becomes more important daily. Within that environment, the certified infusion nurse is prepared to serve as a benchmark against which all those in infusion nursing practice can be evaluated.

References

1. Kelly LY. Dimensions of Professional Nursing, 4th ed. New York: Macmillan, 1981: 21, 23, 41, 412.
2. Phillips LD. Manual of I.V. Therapeutics. Philadelphia: F.A. Davis, 1993:3.
3. Plumer AL, Consentino F. Principles and Practice of Intravenous Therapy, 4th ed. Boston: Little, Brown and Co., 1987:3–5.
4. Grant JP. Handbook of Total Parenteral Nutrition, 2nd ed. Philadelphia: W.B. Saunders, 1992:1, 3.
5. Larkin M. From the editor. NITA 1987; 10(5):319.
6. Larkin M. Chief Executive Officer's report. JIN 1993; 16:210.
7. Intravenous Nurses Society. Strategic Plan. Boston: Intravenous Nurses Society, 1993.
8. Intravenous Nurses Society. Revised Intravenous Nursing Standards of Practice. JIN (suppl) 1990; 511–514, 551.
9. Beecroft PC, Papenhausen JL. Certification for specialty practice? Clin Nurse Specialist 1984; 3:161.
10. Collins ML. Certification: Is the payoff worth the price? RN 1987; 50(7):36, 38, 39.
11. Fickeissen J. 56 ways to get certified. Am J Nurs 1990; 90(3):50.
12. Crudi C. Credentialing for I.V. nurses. NITA 1984; 7(3):234–236.
13. Simpson KR. A specialty certification incentive program: Cost versus benefits. J Nurs Staff Dev 1990; 6(4):180–182.
14. Winter EJS, et al. Is certification for you? Nursing '92, 1992; 22(1):88, 93.
15. Intravenous Nurses Certification Corporation. Professional Certification for Intravenous Nurses: Information on Examination. Boston: Intravenous Nurses Certification Corporation, 1993:1, 2.
16. Wolfram C. The benefits of professional credentialing. JIN 1991; 14:362.
17. Interview: A conversation with Paul Creager. JIN 1992; 15:34.
18. Interview: The value physicians place on nursing certification: The Journal speaks with George Ritter, M.D. JIN 1992; 15:237.

CHAPTER 3

The Intravenous Therapy Department

Leslie Baranowski, RN, BSN, CRNI
Edie Jonas, RN, BSN, CRNI

. . . .

. . . .

The challenge in the health care industry in the United States is to deliver the highest quality of care to the greatest number of people, using all available resources in the most cost-effective manner. With each related advance in technology and with each breakthrough in health care intervention, the challenge becomes greater and the solution more complex. The evolution of management in health has seen this large and ever-growing industry move into a new realm. In the past, the budget management of a facility was often a matter of determining where and how to use the available funds. Payment was based on charges, so attention to volume and operational costs was primary. The components of higher operational costs and decreased payment have changed the focus of management. As in the past, it is mandatory to the success of an institution for managers to be astute in all aspects of health industry standards. The emphasis for nurse managers has changed from managing the delivery of care to managing the fiscal aspects as well.

The delivery of nursing care has been affected dramatically. There are approximately 35 million hospital admissions each year in this country.[1] One aspect of nursing care that has felt the greatest impact is the delivery of intravenous therapy. The percentage of hospitalized patients receiving intravenous therapy has increased greatly, from the 50% average reported in 1981,[2] to 80 to 90% in most acute care facilities in 1994. Maintaining quality and cost effectiveness in delivering this aspect of care alone is of great concern. Criteria for the justification of hospital admission often include the clinical necessity for an IV line or intravenous medications. Although it is not a criterion for remaining in the hospital after the acute phase of illness, as it once was, it is rare to find a patient who has not had intravenous therapy by the end of a hospitalization.

The impact of the shortages in registered nurses, who manage most aspects of IV therapy administration and IV access, has led to changes in the ways nursing care is delivered. There are more demands on the time of the RN at the bedside for complicated patient care needs. Also, there are time demands for assessing present needs and planning for safe and appropriate care outside the acute care hospital environment as soon as feasible. Clearly, in the acute care environment, a benefit of the specialized skills of an IV team is enhancement of the process for managing patient care.

Increasingly, high costs of hospital care and decreasing reimbursements make earlier discharge to alternative settings a necessity. There remains the need to provide the necessary intravenous therapies for recovery after the acute phase of illness in alternative settings. The demand for providing complicated intravenous therapies outside the zones of acute care has expanded the role of the nurse in the area of infusion therapy. Quality of care requires expertise in the specialty practice of intravenous therapy.

Advances in health care delivery and related technologies, along with the adoption of healthier life styles, have led to an increase in life expectancy, raising the average age of the hospitalized patient. This population has frequent and more acute illnesses, requiring complicated therapies, and these all affect the increasing need for complex care and nursing interventions. Models of care that offer relief for some routine, high-volume tasks a nurse must perform are being used. Such models often incorporate the use of unlicensed personnel to provide routine care, such as bathing and feeding patients, under the direction of the RN. Clerical staff and computerization are commonly used to assist the RN in the documentation and communication aspects of unit management and patient care coordination. Advances in technology, such as automated vital signs monitoring and infusion monitoring devices, are commonplace necessities. The complex treatment modalities prescribed almost always include intravenous therapies. Specialized nursing management of IV therapy has often been delegated to teams of intravenous nurse specialists. IV specialists offer the means for maintaining consistency and quality in IV nursing care throughout the acute care facility. Their early assessments and interventions have an impact on the discharge planning of IV therapy needs. Even the most complicated IV therapy needs can be met in the outpatient and home setting by these specialists in IV therapy.

Formerly, in acute care facilities, there was reimbursement for the ancillary (versus routine) services provided by an IV team. The financial incentive, in addition to the cost savings realized with decreased clinical complications and decreased time and materials used when IV care was managed by specialists, increased the incentive for implementing hospital IV teams. When the government's prospective payment system (PPS) for hospitals was implemented in 1983,[4] reimbursement could no longer be assumed, IV teams were at risk, and the justification for these specialty nurses and their services came under the close scrutiny of a cost-benefit analysis. The maintenance of existing and the establishment of new IV teams remain a financial challenge for institutions, although there is ample evidence of the potential benefits to the patients and facility. The commitment to quality in any setting requires careful analysis of how close adherence to standards in practice has an impact on patient outcomes.

ORGANIZATION OF THE INTRAVENOUS THERAPY DEPARTMENT

Determining where to place an IV team within the organizational structure of an acute care institution is a strategic decision because of the impact it can have on the functions and success of the team. Each organization is unique and requires individualized assessment of needs to make the best decision for placing the IV team so that it has the most positive effect on operations and outcomes. Because of the wide range of differences in institutional environments, the role of the IV team within that environment varies greatly from one organization to the next.

Placement of the IV Team

An IV team may logically report to any one of various departments. For example, the team may report directly to administration or to a particular physician within the institution. It may be placed under the direction of the blood bank, the pharmacy, or the nursing service. Each organizational method is associated with distinct advantages and disadvantages that must be carefully weighed. The major consideration is to strive for an organizational structure that enhances the ability of the IV team to meet its own established objectives, goals, and standards of care in this specialty nursing practice while remaining cost effective. The ability to have a positive impact on the maximum volume of patient outcomes must be preserved. The positive impact of an IV team within an organization directly relates to the scope of services offered. It is also important for the team to strive to be in a position that allows for autonomy and independence.[5]

Nursing Division

At first glance, because IV teams are made up of nurses, it would seem logical that the team should report to the nursing department or division. However, it has been found that an IV team's ability for maximum function is enhanced when it can perform as an autonomous unit, distinct from general nursing services and responsibilities, and not related to the specialty of IV nursing. Specialization in nursing is the advancement in an area of practice requiring specific and advanced knowledge and skills. IV nurses are nurses, and need

to retain that professional identity, but it can be more effective to have the IV team, with its specialized practice and levels of competency, report to a department other than nursing. An appropriate choice would be a department that offers the advanced expertise and knowledge required in IV specialty practice.[5] Another concern with having the IV team reporting to nursing is that a typical function and daily need of nursing services is to move or float nurses to other nursing departments or functions within the hospital to resolve staffing problems or shortages. However, in order for the IV team to perform at an optimal level, and for maximum benefit of the IV nurse's specialty skills to the patient and the organization, the IV nurse should be assigned exclusively to IV-therapy related functions, with no crossover into other general nursing activities.

It is important to note that there are successfully operating, high-quality IV teams presently reporting to nursing departments. Advantages may be seen in retaining the intravenous nurse specialist's sense of participation with peers in activities and programs for nurses.

Administration

The concerns regarding the limitations encountered with the placement of IV teams within the nursing division are significant. In many environments it may be most advantageous for the intravenous therapy team to be established as an independent department that reports directly to the administration or to a medical director. This allows for the autonomy and independence critical for the team to achieve its objectives and goals, and to maintain its standards of practice. When the intravenous therapy team is established as an independent department under administration, it is important that a close relationship be maintained with other departments, such as nursing, infection control, and pharmacy.

The optimum placement of the IV team in the organizational structure, as recommended by the Intravenous Nurses Society (INS), is as an independent department, reporting to the administration, to allow the team the autonomy to function independently.[5] The structure of the IV therapy department is determined, to a great extent, by the services offered and the practice setting.

This positioning has many advantages in terms of autonomy and maximum utilization of the IV team expertise. One disadvantage that must be considered is how this positioning isolates the IV nurse from the nursing care team. It is essential that the IV nurse be an active participant in the nursing care team to meet the patient care objectives of providing timely and effective intravenous therapy in the most appropriate setting, without complications. The attention given to how and where the IV team should integrate with the nursing care team is ongoing. The models of care used in nursing departments change with, for example, the service demand and resources. It is important for the IV team to function within these models to have the most positive impact on patient care outcomes and prevent repetition of services. This is setting- and service-dependent, but contributes to the success of the IV team and the organization.

Physician

It may also be appropriate for an IV team to report directly to a physician with a specific interest in IV therapy. This physician should provide consultation to the team and to the patients receiving IV therapy. The physician should review and approve the IV therapy department policies and procedures, because most IV procedures are medical procedures requiring the guidance only a physician can provide. Any staff physician with an interest in IV therapy and who is a nursing advocate can direct the team.[3] Some potential candidates for this role would be the Chief of Staff, the Chief of Medicine, the Director of the Blood Bank, the Director of Anesthesia, and the Director of Infection Control. If a team does not report directly to a physician, it remains important that they have a physician who is designated as a medical advisor.

Blood Bank

Other appropriate alternatives for placement of an IV team include departments that provide a service, or multiple services, related to intravenous therapy practice. For example, the blood bank director may be a good alternative because of the way in which transfusion services relate to IV therapy. The complexity of present transfusion therapy options and issues, along with advances in the technology available for administration, make this an area with an increasing need for nursing expertise. Quality monitoring, utilization monitoring, and new approaches to transfusion therapy have greatly increased the necessity for the involvement of IV nurses in this aspect of care. If a team is not actively involved with the delivery and administration of blood components, reporting to the blood bank may not be a realistic or appropriate choice.

Pharmacy

Many IV teams are placed under the pharmacy department because of the interrelatedness of IV therapy and the administration aspects of IV admixtures, solutions, and medications. Working with the delivery of IV medications and solutions is an integral function of all IV teams. An association with the pharmacy affects the organizational structure and the workload responsibilities of the IV team in various ways. Some teams play an active role in the preparation of large-volume parenteral admixtures and piggyback medications. This can provide the pharmacy with more effective management of IV medications from the time they are ordered until they are administered. In contrast, many teams that report to the pharmacy are not involved with the actual preparation of medications, because this duty is now frequently delegated to pharmacy technicians. There are other benefits afforded to the team reporting to pharmacy; for example, IV team nurses can gain expertise with regard to drugs.

There are many instances in IV drug and fluid administration in which drug compatibilities, drug interactions, and filtration needs require specific administration supplies or intravascular access. Other areas to be considered in drug administration are side effects, expiration dates, and admixture procedures.[6] The pharmacy staff has the benefit of the IV nurse's expertise with IV access devices and their use and maintenance requirements. Advanced intravenous drug administration knowledge can be equated with the prevention of IV drug-related complications. An association with the pharmacy is valuable and necessary for the IV team manag-

ing outpatient or home infusion therapies. Interaction with the IV nurse specialist gives the pharmacy staff the opportunity to participate more directly in IV-related patient care. The pharmacy director's membership on the Pharmacy and Therapeutics Committee is an asset to the IV therapy team. IV teams often use the Pharmacy and Therapeutics Committee as the hospital's body for approval of policies and procedures, because the committee is chaired by a physician.[5] The director of the pharmacy and the chairperson of the Pharmacy and Therapeutics Committee can be IV team advocates on the medical staff. Potential conflicts and problems that may be associated with reporting to the pharmacy include the fact that the pharmacy director, like the nursing department executive, cannot approve the medical policies and procedures that guide the IV team practice. If there is not a strong commitment to the goals and objectives of the IV team, the department director's priorities, in time of conflict and resource allocation, might lean more heavily on the needs of the pharmacists and pharmacy operation issues. There are successful IV teams that are part of the pharmacy department, and many home infusion agencies have a pharmacist as the general manager.

Impact of Shared Governance

Regardless of the department to which an IV team reports, a close relationship with other hospital divisions is essential. In many hospital environments, establishing the communication necessary to ensure this close relationship may not be accomplished easily. In recent years, the development of shared or collaborative governance professional practice models has provided an alternative to the typical hierarchic management structures that exist in most institutions. These practice models provide staff nurses with the opportunity to share the responsibility and accountability for the nursing organization and involve the establishment of committees in which nurses from the various areas of the hospital are responsible for activities such as setting standards for their practice, developing policies and procedures, and evaluating the quality of practice and its outcomes. This offers obvious advantages to IV teams that report to the nursing division but has real and potential advantages to teams that are not within the nursing division.

The IV team that actively participates in shared governance models provides itself with all the associated opportunities and advantages and allows for a strong communication system that would otherwise not be available to an ancillary department. Involvement offers decision making at the unit level and for hospital-wide concerns. Participation in shared governance activities strengthens the IV nurse's ties to the nursing structure and allows for increased visibility and enhanced value of the team to the nursing division. It provides IV nurses with the opportunity to have a voice in the nursing organization, not just about IV issues, but about all facets of nursing. The viability of an IV team rests on the value the institution places on the department's contribution to hospital goals, and on meeting department-specific goals. Shared governance also allows for the development of strong, unit-based groups for quality assurance, education, and policy and procedure formulation and review.[7] When a shared governance model is not practiced in an institution, it remains important that the IV team members interact with other members of the health care team to provide safe, high-quality intravenous therapy.

The INS scope of practice advocates the collaboration and/or participation of the IV nurse in committees that regulate the practice of intravenous nursing.[3] The IV team must become actively involved on committees or task forces relevant to the specialty practice of intravenous nursing. For example, it is important for a representative from the IV therapy department to participate in groups such as pharmacy and therapeutics, infection control, nutritional support, transfusion therapy, safety, quality assurance, and risk management.

Organization in the Alternative Setting

Historically, the provision of IV therapy was managed in the hospital, but it has become more common to continue this care outside the traditional hospital-based practice area. The diagnostic related group (DRG) system initially, and the rapidly increasing costs associated with hospitalization, have influenced the decrease in lengths of stay and created the need for quality care in many settings. Intravenous therapy treatment modalities are now carried out in various other settings, including but not limited to homes, extended care facilities, clinics, hospital outpatient facilities, outpatient surgical centers, ambulatory care centers, and physicians' offices. The delivery of IV therapies in these various settings has opened new doors and presented new challenges for providing the safe, expert care that these patients require.

In particular, the delivery of infusion therapies in the home environment has expanded tremendously over the past few years, and gives no indication of slowing. Increasingly complex therapies, such as total parenteral nutrition (TPN), pain control, chemotherapy, and prenatal and cardiac regimens[8] are now being delivered safely in the home setting as patients are being discharged after shorter hospitalizations. As a result, IV nurses now practice regularly in alternative care settings, and this rapidly growing industry has recognized the need for adherence to established standards and the role of IV nurse specialists in the initiation and management of infusion care. The IV nurse specialist is crucial in these environments, in which independent thinking and excellent technical skills are of paramount importance. Playing an integral role in managing IV care in these settings allows the IV practitioner to control the quality of care and adhere to established standards for all intravenous therapy patients. The INS supports alternative site approaches to meet patient care needs, and believes that all intravenous therapy patients are entitled to receive the standard of care outlined in the *Intravenous Nursing Standards of Practice,* without regard to setting.[3]

The development of outpatient infusion centers has become a critical link between the hospital and home care settings, providing for the infusion needs of ambulatory patients. Some infusion centers are incorporated within physicians' offices, community home infusion agencies, or the hospital itself. In the hospital setting, to provide appropriate staffing for the provision of services, an outpatient infusion service should be established as an extension of the IV therapy department.

An additional alternative care setting is the skilled nursing facility (SNF), which is now faced with the challenges of caring for residents requiring complex treatments, such as IV therapy.[9] Ideally, it is preferable for SNFs to consider the implementation of IV teams. If a team is not practical, an IV nursing specialist should be considered to manage the program. This may not be a realistic alternative for all SNFs, but an IV specialist resource can contribute by developing educational programs and acting as a consultant for the nursing home staff. SNFs are now more actively contracting with institutions and organizations with IV therapy specialists to provide their infusion needs or to act as a resource for the development of their infusion care practices.

Depending on the alternative site practice environment, the organizational structure varies. Surgical and ambulatory care centers and physicians' offices are typically structured so that the intravenous therapy clinician reports directly to a physician or the director of nursing.

The organizational structure of home infusion companies varies depending on the size; for example, the administrator or operational manager may be a pharmacist or nurse who works closely with an IV nursing director. The presence of the IV nurse specialist in management in home infusion organizations is essential to ensure the quality of IV nursing care delivered. Hospital-based outpatient infusion centers can be most efficiently managed by the in-hospital IV team manager. Hospital-based home infusion departments may also be managed by the in-hospital IV team director or placed under the direction of the home health department, depending on how services can best be coordinated.

ORGANIZATION WITHIN THE DEPARTMENT

The organizational structure and roles of the various management and staff members who comprise the IV team vary depending on the size of the department and hospital, functions and services provided by the team, hours of service, and budgetary constraints. It is critical to ensure that an IV team has precisely the right staff and is the right size to perform its services. Typically, IV teams are comprised of a management or supervisory position, nursing staff, and an educational coordinator. However the team is organized, concise position descriptions for all members of the team are essential, and should be reviewed annually and revised when necessary.

IV Nurse

Entry level requirements for the registered nurse entering the intravenous nursing specialty include current licensure and a minimum clinical experience of 2 years of recent medical-surgical nursing experience that included the opportunity to apply principles and practices of intravenous therapy.[3] In addition, the INS recommends the Bachelor of Science degree in nursing. For entry at the specialist level, it is suggested that the nurse have 1 year of experience in the specialty practice of intravenous nursing. According to the 1994 eligibility criteria for Intravenous Nurse Certification, 1 year is defined as 1600 hours in the care and delivery of intravenous therapies to patients within the last 2 consecutive years. It is also important for all IV team members to obtain national certification in the specialty of intravenous nursing (CRNI) through the Intravenous Nurses Certification Corporation. Although professional nursing certification is a voluntary credential, having team members who are certified validates the competency and advanced skill level of the staff. Certification enhances the professional credibility of the nurses and demonstrates the high level of commitment they have to their specialty practice. Credentialed nurses also demonstrate the health care provider's commitment to seek and retain the most qualified nurse clinicians.[10]

IV teams are usually staffed with registered nurses for optimal utilization and functioning because of the types of invasive procedures performed by intravenous nurses. These require the level of theoretic and clinical knowledge of that licensure level, along with expert technical skill. The use of RNs on IV teams has been an especially important result of the patient care delivery models that have been implemented in many institutions in response to changes in the health care reimbursement structure. To enhance efficiency, the new care delivery models are structured with increased numbers of nonlicensed technical staff who are cross-trained to deliver services and care as directed by the professional nurse. As a result, the role of the RN is less in hands-on care and more in managing the overall care plan. The extra support of an IV RN can therefore be very valuable to the RN now managing many more patients and with much of direct patient bedside care often being delivered by nonlicensed personnel. The educational background and skill levels of the IV nurse specialist who is an RN are needed more than ever to ensure quality of care in the delivery of intravenous therapies. Even though the use of RNs may be optimal many IV teams have also found it beneficial as well as necessary to use licensed vocational (LVNs) and/or licensed practical nurses (LPNs) from a cost-effective standpoint. Consideration must be given to the associated limitations in job functions of the LVN-LPN when thinking of using them in the role of the IV nurse. IV therapy–related practice guidelines for the LVN-LPN vary according to state-specific licensure, and may be further restricted by institutional policy. When an LVN-LPN is a member of the IV team, all functions must, as defined in their licensure, be under the supervision of the RN on the IV team or on the individual patient care unit where the LVN-LPN is performing IV care. LVNs-LPNs are limited in their role regarding IV therapy and may not perform advanced technical procedures, such as peripherally inserted central catheter (PICC) insertions. After completion of specific education and training requirements, the LVN-LPN may be permitted to perform venipuncture, monitor IVs and sites, and administer specific solutions and blood products.

Because of the specialized nature of IV therapy, the success of the department depends on the selection of nurses. IV nurses must be conscientious regarding all aspects of their duties and show evidence of good communication and teaching skills, integrity, reliability, accountability, initiative, and creativity. Mental and emotional stability are important characteristics as a result of the often stressful situations that may arise and the frequent need for setting priorities.[11] Because IV nurses function throughout the institution, it is essential that they present a professional image to both the patients and general staff. To operate an IV team successfully, it is important that the IV nurses function well independently, but

they must also have a commitment to the team model concept. IV nurses' responsibilities are directed toward positive patient outcomes, and a successful team must consider the tasks to be performed and the services offered using a team approach. Members of the team can find themselves tied up with various time-consuming or emergency procedures. It is imperative that there be communication with other members of the team, who must work together to assess the needs and staff resources available and determine how to complete the tasks that need to be performed effectively. The ability to meet care or access needs within a reasonable time frame is essential to avoid delays in therapy. The ability of the IV nurse to prioritize those needs and act on that judgment with clear communication with IV team and other health care team members is essential. By selecting nurses for the team who have demonstrated these qualities, the IV team's positive interactions with medical staff, other nurses, other departments, and patients is ensured, and the value of the individual professionals and the IV team as a whole to the organization is greatly enhanced.

Typical position descriptions for the IV nurse include clinical services with related responsibilities and relationships within the institution. The following is an example of a position description for the clinical IV nurse:

I. Purpose of the department and role of the position within the department: performs full range of responsibilities and duties of the IV therapy department as allowed by the Nurse Practice Act; provides direct patient care using nursing process and is accountable for own practice; participates as patient care advisor; initiates-participates in patient and staff education; demonstrates leadership skills.

II. Licenses, certificates, degrees, or credentials required to perform the duties assigned to the position: RN with at least 2 years' recent medical-surgical or critical care experience—BSN preferred, CRNI (Certified Registered Nurse, Intravenous) preferred, IV therapy experience preferred.

III. Functions

A. Assessment
  1. Make rounds on nursing units to monitor existing IV devices in use.
  2. Assess patients with regard to diagnosis and/or special conditions that have any bearing on IV therapy services.
  3. Recognize abnormal conditions or potential problems, take appropriate action, and notify appropriate personnel.

B. Planning
  1. Plan IV care for assigned patients.
  2. Build flexibility into daily routine to anticipate and handle unexpected situations.
  3. Integrate IV care with the nursing care plan.
  4. Develop teaching plans for individual patients.

C. Implementation
  1. Implement physician's orders according to needs and established nursing protocols.
  2. Implement standards of care identified at the unit level.
  3. Perform IV therapy procedures proficiently.
  4. Respond to calls for IV therapy services.
  5. Intervene in situations in which basic life support systems are threatened, untoward physiologic or

psychologic reactions are probable, or changes in normal behavior patterns have occurred.

    6. Document procedures, outcomes, and complications appropriately.

    7. Demonstrate skills and knowledge as applied to peripherally inserted central catheters.

D. Evaluation

    1. Evaluate patient response to care provided according to identified criteria.

    2. Participate in unit-based quality management activities, as indicated.

    3. Participate in product evaluation.

E. Communication

    1. Interact with health care team to keep them informed of changes in patient condition.

    2. Interact with others to promote and enhance positive relationships.

    3. Document interventions and evaluations accurately and promptly.

    4. Demonstrate understanding of policies and lines of communication within institution.

F. Leadership

    1. Identify problems in unit functions and either initiate solutions or inform appropriate persons.

    2. Participate in ensuring that the nursing care provided is safe and of high quality, and act as a role model to other staff members.

G. Professional development

    1. Participate in the evaluation of own performance by identifying strengths and weaknesses and developing a plan to improve weak areas.

    2. Work toward patient care competence in specialties common to IV therapy.

H. Education

    1. Identify and promote the level of clinical expertise required of staff to provide care to a specific patient population.

I. Research

    1. Participate in research projects in IV therapy.

    2. Demonstrate awareness of documented research involving nursing practice.

IV. Skills, knowledge, and abilities: the IV therapy nurse must have:

A. Ability to establish and maintain effective interpersonal relationships.

B. Ability to set priorities and organize work.

C. Ability to read, write, speak, and understand the English language and use medical terminology appropriately.

D. Ability to assist in moving patients and stand on feet over extended periods.

E. Ability to track clinical skills.

F. Knowledge of medications, indications, dosage ranges, side effects, and potential toxicity.

G. Knowledge of legal implications for clinical practice.

H. Skills to perform CPR.

I. Ability to work accurately and quickly under pressure.

J. Judgment skills to be able to make independent clinical decisions in routine patient care matters.

V. Physical characteristics of critical job functions to be performed: must have physical strength to assist in lifting patients; must see well enough to read charts and gauges, speak well enough to communicate over the phone, and hear well enough to take vital signs; must see well enough to start IVs.

VI. Special conditions of employment: must possess current RN license for the state; work overtime, weekends; must have graduated from an accredited school of nursing, and have 2 years' recent medical-surgical or critical care experience.

Position descriptions must include but are not limited to educational requirements, licensing requirements, certification requirements, general nursing or IV therapy–related experience, accountability, and specific areas of responsibility. Position descriptions should be congruent with state statutes, be measurable, and be used in the evaluation process.[3]

The IV nurse must provide an expert level of direct professional nursing care specific to IV therapy, establish standards and monitor the quality of nursing care, and provide consultation and serve as an educational resource for patients receiving IV therapy. There must be a clear understanding of the philosophy and standards of the institution, overall policies of the institution and department, functions of the department, and clinical and technical skill level requirements for their role.

Outpatient–Home Infusion IV Nurse

The IV nurse employed in outpatient or home infusion settings should meet all the requirements as outlined. Excellent technical skills, strong assessment skills, and the ability to act independently, with good judgment, are imperative for the IV nurse working in this environment to ensure delivery of quality services. Good communication skills are essential, and it has been found that a background in home health care is also helpful.

IV Team Manager

An IV therapy team should be managed by a currently licensed registered nurse. Five years of current experience in an acute care hospital setting is preferred, with a minimum of 2 years of experience in a nursing management role. Experience in budget preparation and management is desirable. National certification in intravenous therapy (CRNI) should be required, or a candidate should minimally meet the eligibility criteria for certification in the specialty of intravenous therapy. The individual must demonstrate good organizational and communication skills. To establish and maintain a successful IV team, the manager must have a high degree of interest and experience in the delivery of IV therapy. Maintaining skills and expertise in all aspects of the specialty is necessary for recognizing the need and implementing appropriate adjustments in services. Additional attributes that are desirable are dedication to the IV team concept, to IV nurses and, most importantly, to ensuring that patients receive quality IV care.[5] The IV nurse manager must also be well respected in the institution and be capable of dealing effectively with all hospital departments. The IV manager is held accountable for his or her own practice as well as work performed under his or her supervision. The title for this position (e.g., manager, director, supervisor, head nurse) may vary, depending on the department to which the team reports and the responsibilities of the position.

The IV therapy department manager's responsibilities are typically diverse and require good organizational and delegating skills. They center around writing and reviewing policies and procedures based on current recommendations and standards, keeping abreast of the latest developments in technology, budgeting, conducting performance evaluations, providing IV therapy–related orientation programs and continuing education programs within and often outside the institution, keeping the staff motivated, and developing and maintaining a quality management program. It is also crucial for the IV manager to serve on committees within the hospital related to IV therapy, such as pharmacy and therapeutics, infection control, product evaluation, nutritional support, safety, tumor board, and transfusion. Along with the clinical specialty rationales for membership on these committees, the participation of the IV therapy team in the evaluation, selection, standardization, and often servicing of IV-related equipment and supply items is important.

An IV therapy department manager must carefully design and implement an effective quality assurance and quality improvement program to ensure that acceptable care parameters are met. The program should address the delivery of necessary and appropriate care, achieving minimal complication rates and ensuring that all complications are investigated, and evaluate the results to determine whether they are attributable to such factors as nurse practice, procedural or systems issues, equipment failure, or supply defects. The IV team staff can provide the data from IV therapy monitoring and collect necessary data. The manager reports findings, assesses impact, and develops recommendations for corrective actions when necessary for improving outcomes. The following is an example of a position description for an IV therapy services manager. This formatting may be adapted to other positions.

I. Position summary: 24-hour administrative responsibility for the nursing and operational management of IV therapy services. The IV nurse manager reports directly to administration, physician, pharmacy, nursing, or blood bank. The IV nurse manager provides clinical supervision and administrative support for the members of the department. The IV nurse manager is responsible for coordinating services for patients, staff, and physicians according to approved hospital and departmental policies, procedures, and guidelines. The IV nurse manager maintains interdepartmental communication and relationships to ensure quality care, fiscal responsibility, optimal allocation of resources, and accurate, timely transmission of information. The IV nurse manager performs the duties of the IV nurse, as appropriate.

II. Duties and responsibilities

   A. Operational and administrative management

      1. Assume 24-hour responsibility for the clinical and administrative functions of IV therapy services.

      2. Develop and implement short- and long-term plans and goals for the department.

      3. Integrate IV therapy activities with other hospital departments to resolve identified problems, determine priorities, and provide direction relative to patient care issues.

      4. Interpret and ensure compliance of the department with standards of the JCAHO (Joint Commission on Accreditation of Healthcare Organizations) and federal and state regulatory agencies.

      5. Direct and coordinate activities of IV therapy personnel, recruit and interview prospective employees, counsel, evaluate, and provide in-service training to IV personnel, and evaluate employees with the participation of the assistant manager and/or educational coordinator of IV therapy services.

      6. Plan and develop the budget, monitor the revenue and usage, reimbursement, and departmental performance reports, and prepare monthly variance reports.

      7. Develop and revise philosophy, objectives, and policies and procedures based on the *Intravenous Nursing Standards of Practice.*[3]

      8. Evaluate new products and procure supplies related to the IV therapy specialty.

      9. Ensure safe, effective patient care through collaboration with nurses, physicians, and other health care providers.

      10. Develop and plan new programs for the department.

      11. Conduct IV therapy classes and in-service training with the assistance of the assistant manager and/or educational coordinator.

      12. Promote a climate conducive to high-quality service and harmonious working conditions.

      13. Develop and interpret job descriptions and performance appraisals.

      14. Develop and maintain a quality management program, interpret quality management monitors, and report to the appropriate institution committees.

      15. Review and respond to patient and family complaints, including those that may result in litigation, take appropriate actions, and report outcomes to risk management; also, investigate unusual events and ensure proper documentation.

      16. Maintain clinical competency in IV therapy, have delegated authority to certify others in the use of peripherally inserted catheters, and perform all the duties and responsibilities of an IV nurse as required by the departmental workload.

   B. Financial management

      1. Develop departmental budget objectives consistent with the overall goals of the institution.

      2. Prepare departmental budget, allocating financial resources to meet departmental objectives, and prepare specifications for capital equipment requests.

      3. Review financial reports and use such control figures as variances and productive hours to provide timely evaluations of department's conformance to budget, verify expenditures, monitor and evaluate staff productivity, and take action to meet budgeted productivity targeted.

   C. Personnel and resource management

      1. Develop workload standards to determine staffing requirements for the efficient use of personnel.

2. Evaluate performance and clinical competency of the staff.
3. Develop and revise job descriptions and performance standards, as necessary.
4. Develop and submit monthly work schedules for all department employees.
5. Monitor and direct corrective and disciplinary action as appropriate to ensure that standards of performance are met.
6. Respond to identified learning needs of staff and arrange for and/or provide educational programs.
7. Teach using in-service training, lectures, discussion, and written materials on both general and specialized topics.
8. Plan, organize, coordinate, and direct in-service education and clinical training programs for nursing staff in coordination with the education department.
9. Certify nursing personnel in specialized procedures related to IV therapy.

D. Professional development
1. Assume responsibility for personal professional development—continuously update clinical skills, maintain required certifications and keep abreast of current health care events.
2. Maintain association with professional and health-related associations and/or community groups.
3. Participate in professional seminars and workshops.
4. Maintain membership in professional organizations relevant to area of practice (Intravenous Nurses Society).

Job responsibilities for home infusion IV therapy managers typically include planning, organizing, coordinating, and evaluating the provision of nursing services and interfacing with home care agencies to ensure continuity of care. Many responsibilities for the home infusion manager are similar to those of the hospital-based manager. Additional responsibilities specific to a home infusion manager are as follows:

1. Coordinate nursing services relative to the delivery of IV therapy for patients at home or in the outpatient setting.
2. Supervise teaching of patients prior to discharge and/or at home.
3. Supervise in-service training of licensed personnel who perform services relative to therapies at home.
4. Develop policies and procedures for IV therapy for patients at home and in the outpatient setting.
5. Develop patient education materials for outpatient IV therapies.
6. Develop and participate in quality management programs.
7. Develop a marketing plan and actively participate in its execution.
8. Procure medical information relative to documentation for individual patients.
9. Oversee documentation process for charting.

A major and challenging responsibility for the IV manager is ensuring technical and clinical expertise and maintaining staff morale in an arena in which most activities are carried out independently. It is crucial to hold regular staff meetings so that participants can openly share problems, questions, and educational needs. Staff meetings also provide an excellent opportunity for in-servicing and reviewing procedures and equipment. Unit-based governing councils, which are part of a shared governance system, can also play an integral role in the success of the team and satisfaction of the staff. Governing councils allow for decision making and planning to take place at the staff level, and therefore provide for more ownership of the decisions as well as increase involvement and support regarding the implementation of new decisions and actions. The IV therapy manager must be aware of the aspects of this model that enhance the philosophy and meet the objectives of the IV team.

Assistant Manager

Larger and extremely active teams may require an assistant manager to assist with operational, clinical, and staff functions. The intravenous nursing specialist in this position could also serve in the role of educational coordinator, and share responsibility for staff development, competency reviews, and performance evaluation. The clinical qualifications for this role should be equal to those of the IV team manager, with some experience in nursing management functions desirable. Excellent communication skills are essential to this role, because this person is the primary liaison to nursing staff and other employees and departments within the facility.

Educational Coordinator

A strong supplement to be considered for inclusion in the IV therapy department is the educational coordinator. The educational coordinator's job description should include creating and maintaining an orientation program for new staff, providing continuing education and staff development programs and ongoing IV-related in-service training, acting as liaison to the medical and nursing staff, and encouraging the staff to attend outside educational meetings and to be active in their specialty organizations.

The educational coordinator should be responsible for teaching all clinical elements related to IV therapy practice. This individual either personally instructs or coordinates training classes or programs in such areas as management, supervision, consultation, technology, research, quality assurance, legal standards, communication, continuing education, patient education, clinical judgment, and practice and procedures. The educational coordinator is responsible for orienting and assessing the clinical skills of new IV team members and providing clinical guidance to all IV staff for the development of new skills. There may be responsibility for orienting and providing in-service programs to physicians and students, if that is seen as an organizational need. Encouraging IV nurses to participate in continuing education programs that are relevant to the specialty practice is an important aspect of the role. Additionally, the coordinator is responsible for assisting the manager with personnel-related matters, including performance appraisals. The role could include responsibility for data collection, review and revision of policies and procedures, and planning and implementation of IV therapy–related competency reviews.

Teams in large facilities may find it appropriate to incorporate IV nurse specialists within the team who are dedicated to specific subspecialty areas of the discipline. The role could be defined as that of clinical resource person. For example, a staff member may be dedicated to all the aspects of management of central venous catheters, nutritional support, or transfusion therapy, or may be the certifying agent for PICC insertion or chemotherapy administration. There may be an IV team specialist for all aspects of pediatric infusion therapy if there is a large and diverse pediatric population. It is important to recognize the specialist as a valuable resource available throughout the institution for consultation.

FUNCTIONS OF THE DEPARTMENT

When establishing the scope of the functions of the IV therapy department and the roles and functions of all the members of the IV team, it is important to evaluate the practice setting carefully, looking at current and potential demands for IV services. The scope of present services for IV therapies must be reviewed, the current demand for services and how that demand is being met must be ascertained, and the future demand for services must be carefully estimated. It is important to remember that as an IV therapy concept gains acceptance from the medical and nursing staffs, there is likely to be an increase in demands for existing services and requests for more sophisticated technologic procedures. Quality improvement needs must be carefully analyzed. Quality management data related to IV therapy are critical, providing valuable information for determining the essential functions needed to improve IV care. It is well known that IV teams deliver IV care with a higher level of expertise and have a positive impact on the quality of care, but it can be difficult to quantify the impact this has on the organization. Quality assurance data for evaluating the quality of IV care delivered are not consistently kept in hospitals without IV teams, but often must be estimated from random checks of individual units or obtained from other facilities of comparable size. Consideration also needs to be given to the scope of pharmacy services currently in place, as well as changes anticipated with the addition of the IV team. Once these have been determined, the desired team functions and service hours can be better defined.

The ideal IV therapy department should be staffed to provide the total spectrum of intravenous therapy services daily, for 24 hours a day. It has been documented that it takes the non-IV nurse up to three times longer than the IV nurse specialist to perform therapy. There is also the assurance of adherence to standards with the use of specialty nurses. The intravenous nurse should perform all functions connected with the administration of intravenous solutions, medications, chemotherapeutic agents, blood and blood components, and parenteral nutrition. The intravenous nursing team's responsibilities may include but are not limited to inserting intravenous cannulas, administering prescribed intravenous solutions, medications, and blood products, monitoring and maintaining intravenous peripheral and central access sites and systems, evaluating patient response to prescribed therapy, providing patient and family teaching and evaluating their comprehension and competency, documenting pertinent

information on the patient's record, and carrying out discharge planning. Compiling statistics to quantify and qualify intravenous therapy department services, productivity, and patient outcomes are an important function of the IV team staff. These are related to the quality of care and cost-justifying factors of the team's performance.[6]

In addition to providing a full spectrum of intravenous therapy services, the ideal team should provide these services to all areas of the hospital. If this is not possible, a realistic alternative is usually for critical care and emergency areas of the facility to provide their own IV-related care. However, it remains important for the IV team to be as involved as possible with these areas to provide whatever support is necessary and feasible. Service areas and responsibilities for the IV therapy services department are as follows:

I. Hours: The intravenous therapy department provides daily, 24-hour coverage, including holidays.
II. Service areas: All patient care areas are routinely serviced by the IV team. Note that if the IV team is not staffed to provide service to all areas of the hospital, limited service to some areas may be necessary. In this case, departments such as the emergency department, labor and delivery, presurgery preparation areas, and critical care units may be responsible for their own IV care. This is highly variable from facility to facility. It is important that the IV team still provide limited service and support intravenous care needs on request, and to the extent resources permit, to these areas and ancillary departments such as radiology, nuclear medicine, and cardiology.
III. Services (Note that possible services are listed, but any combination of services may be provided)
   A. Venipuncture (prn)
   B. Routine peripheral catheter site changes
   C. Initiation of blood components
   D. Assistance to physicians in central venous catheter (CVC) insertion
   E. Routine and prn CVC dressing care
   F. CVC blood withdrawals
   G. Daily peripheral site checks
   H. Implanted port access
   I. Declotting of CVCs
   J. Insertion and maintenance of PICCs
   K. Insertion and maintenance of long-arm peripheral catheters
   L. Consultation and teaching for long-term CVCs
   M. Preparation of selected large-volume parenteral solutions and intravenous medications
   N. Administration of intraspinal medications
   O. Care of intraspinal catheters
   P. Therapeutic phlebotomies
   Q. Member of code team
   R. Chemotherapy administration
   S. Arterial catheters, blood gases
   T. Administration of parenteral nutrition
   U. Evaluation of IV therapy–related equipment
   V. Data collection for IV-related statistics
   W. In coordination with the pharmacist, consultation on pharmacokinetic scheduling and compatibility issues
   X. Staff education through in-service training and orientation
   Y. Patient teaching for catheter care and home or outpatient infusion therapies

Z. Provision of outpatient IV therapies, patient monitoring, and education.

All the functions of an intravenous nursing team should be established in policy and procedure and should be based on the team objectives. The objectives should involve providing a systematic and consistent quality of IV therapy for the institution and its total patient population. Centralized responsibility and accountability should be built in for all IV services. Specific objectives for an IV team are as follows:

I. Philosophy
   A. The IV therapy department upholds the belief that each patient receiving intravenous therapy in a variety of settings should be provided with quality, individualized care.
   B. It is our belief that this is best accomplished by registered nurses who have acquired specialized knowledge and developed skills specific to the practice of intravenous nursing.
   C. The IV therapy department supports a holistic approach to the delivery of patient care.
   D. We believe our professional responsibility is to assist consumers in meeting their needs to achieve an individual level of wellness, including preventative, curative, and restorative measures.
   E. We strive for excellence through personalized, competent, and cost-effective care.
   F. We believe we have a responsibility to work with other hospital departments and other health care professionals and ancillary departments in coordinating and improving patient care services.
II. Objectives
   A. To provide standard, consistent, and progressive intravenous care to each patient receiving IV therapy by
      1. Establishing parameters of intravenous care and monitoring outcomes for all intravenous therapy department services.
      2. Developing, implementing, and adhering to IV therapy policies and procedures according to the *Intravenous Nursing Standards of Practice*,[3] with ongoing review.
      3. Evaluating intravenous therapy equipment for utilization that best serves the needs of the patient and the facility.
   B. To serve as role models, information resources, and consultants concerning all aspects of intravenous nursing by
      1. Providing intravenous therapy orientation and continuing education to appropriate health care personnel.
      2. Investigating, validating, and developing the intravenous nursing specialty through research.
      3. Actively participating in the utilization of new technologies.
      4. Conducting an ongoing evaluation of performance and competency of all IV nursing personnel.
      5. Using the nursing process through the collection of data, prioritization of problems and needs, development of a nursing care plan, and evaluation of patient outcomes.

An IV team's functions include some type of routine patient service rounds to designated areas of the institution. Rounds by the IV team or specific IV nurse, such as the central line nurse, may be made routinely, at specific intervals or a set number of times per shift or day. The system largely depends on such factors as the size of the facility, the workload type and volume, and staffing resources.

The IV team routinely reviews IV orders and maintains a patient profile, including IV solution and medication orders and the IV access device in place. Current patient information should be maintained on IV profile cards (Figs. 3–1 and 3–2). The intravenous nurse uses the nursing process, which includes assessment, problem identification or nursing diagnosis, implementation, and evaluation in the practice of intravenous therapy. A documented plan regarding routine and individual care needs is initiated and revised as needed. A system for communication must be established between the nursing units and other users and the IV team. If rounds are completed on a regular basis, messages can be left at designated areas for the IV nurse. When rounds are intermittent or infrequent, some type of paging system is needed to communicate with the IV nurse.

Nursing staff responsibilities in relation to intravenous therapy vary with the institution and revolve around the functions of the IV team. The IV nurse should be responsible for the selection, initiation, and routine evaluation of the appropriate access device and site. This includes initiation of solutions, tubings, and devices required to administer IV therapies ordered for patients. With 80 to 90% of patients receiving IV therapy at any given time, the IV nurse is an integral part of the nursing process for each patient. The IV nurse's role is no longer viewed as a technical position, but is one that consolidates the entire realm of knowledge regarding IV therapy and incorporates sound clinical assessment and intervention into the patient's care plan. It is essential that the IV nurse's role include time for thorough assessment regarding the patient's IV plan of care and input into this plan. If the IV team's staffing is limited, it may be necessary to designate some of the more routine technical portions of initiating and maintaining IV care to the staff nurse. For example, the staff nurse may be responsible for setting up IV equipment for the IV nurse. The nursing staff must be educated regarding the functions of the IV therapy department and be clear as to their own responsibilities regarding their patient's IV therapy needs. Regardless of functions performed by the IV team, every nurse is responsible for the routine, regular monitoring of a patient's IV site and infusions, and for ongoing patient assessment of the response to the therapies delivered. This monitoring, as described by INS, should be according to the patient's condition, age, and practice setting, and as established in IV therapy policy and procedure. An IV team's functions may include routine site checks performed on each shift or selected shifts, but site checks must be performed by the staff nurse in the interim, with appropriate nursing interventions as necessary.

Workload Standards

To allocate resources and validate productivity of the IV team appropriately, some type of workload management system must be used.[12] This must be specific for IV team activ-

IV PROFILE CARD

DX

ALLERGIES

ADDRESSOGRAPH

MD ORDERS

7175-50-1086 (12/91)

A

SITE 1								2nd SITE		REASON For 2nd Site
Date	Size	Date	Size	Date	Size	Date	Size	Date	Size	

COMMENTS:

RESTRICTIONS

NRSC

Date Requested

Date Obtained

CODE
Y   N

PALL
Y   N

B

Figure 3–1. IV profile card for peripheral catheters. *A*, Front. *B*, Back.

ities and applicable to the institution. These workload standards provide a means for measuring productivity of the IV team and also assist with estimating staffing needs. Workload standards can be supported and customized by time and motion studies or by using accepted, established standards. Some IV teams have been able to develop or modify existing systems to include the specialty area of intravenous therapy (Table 3–1 and Figs. 3–3, 3–4, and 3–5).

A patient classification system (PCS) may also be used to justify and measure the IV workload. This type of system allows for more accurate prediction of staffing requirements based on patient care needs, validation of the IV nursing team's productivity and cost effectiveness, prioritization of the IV nursing workload, and evaluation of the quality of IV nursing care.[13] The following summarizes the steps to follow for setting up a PCS for IV therapy,[14] and includes time values for IV therapy activities that may be used (Table 3–2):

1. Form a task force. Participation of experienced IV nurses, as well as nurse managers, is essential for the development and acceptance of an accurate, workable system.
2. Define IV therapy. The goals and objectives of IV therapy must be reviewed and the scope of practice and service defined to provide a basis for workload measurement.
3. Identify nursing activities. Nursing activities include

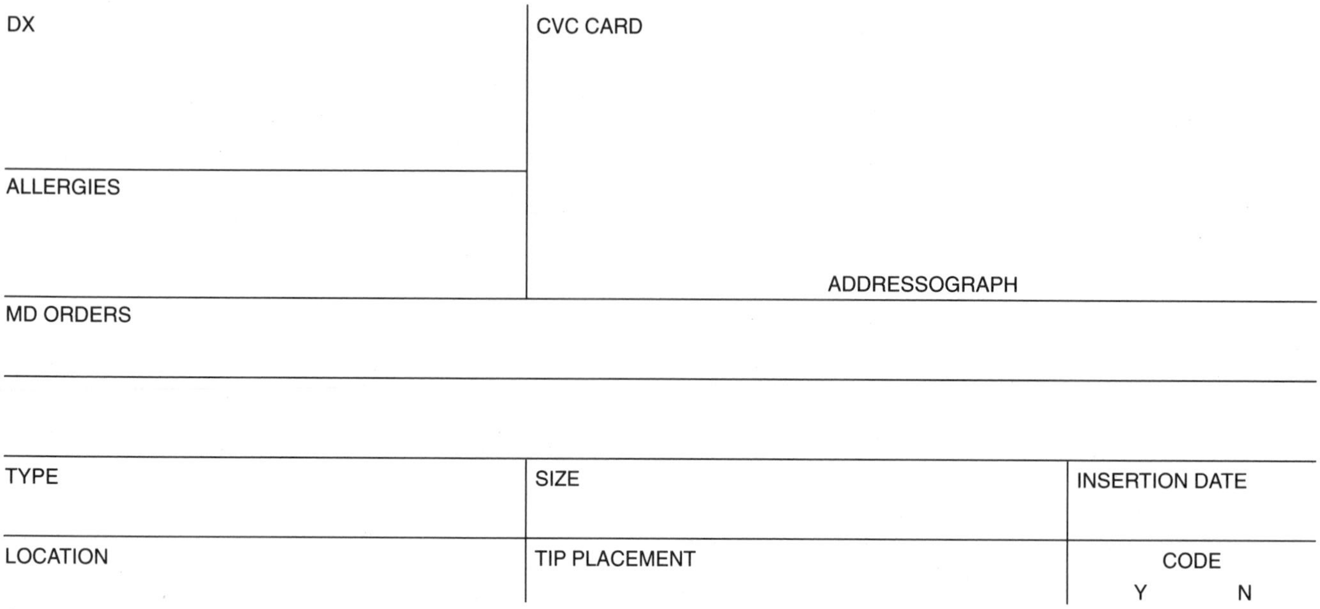

DX

CVC CARD

ALLERGIES

ADDRESSOGRAPH

MD ORDERS

TYPE	SIZE	INSERTION DATE
LOCATION	TIP PLACEMENT	CODE Y N

A

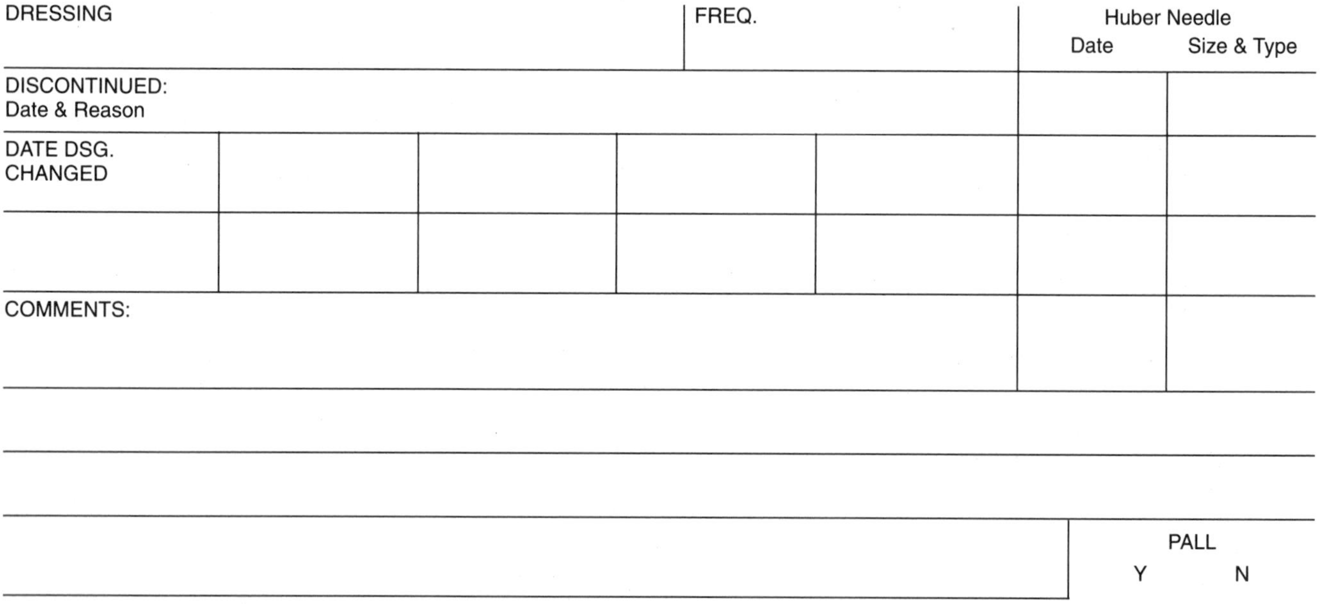

DRESSING   FREQ.   Huber Needle
                                                                                                                Date   Size & Type

DISCONTINUED:
Date & Reason

DATE DSG. CHANGED						

COMMENTS:

PALL
Y   N

B

Figure 3–2. IV profile card for central venous catheters. *A*, Front. *B*, Back.

both direct and nondirect care. Direct care encompasses all nursing interventions provided directly to the patient, whereas indirect care consists primarily of supportive measures. Each activity is categorized and defined as to the necessary requirements.

4. Develop time standards. A time standard is defined as the amount of time required to perform an individual activity based on the definition. For direct care activities, time standards are determined by using the consensus method or by performing time studies (see Table 3–2).

Indirect care activities are usually assigned a predetermined constant.

5. Establish the frequency of activities. Time and motion (frequency) studies provide a comprehensive database of activities performed, workload distribution, and staff utilization.

6. Determine primary indicators. Data from the frequency study are instrumental in establishing major care activities, which represent approximately 90% of the total direct care workload. Workload measurement is limited

Table 3-1

Inpatient IV Therapy Log Instructions

Activity or Procedure	Sample Log Entry With Comments	Approximate Time Spent (min)
New starts	# done. Simple start.	20
New starts (difficult)	# done. Difficult starts and/or 2 attempts.	45
Restart (RS)	# done. Simple restart.	20
RS (difficult)	# done. Difficult restart and/or 2 attempts.	45
Site check	# done. One for each patient. Includes site, bottle label and tubing labels, and "interventions."	10
IV push	# done. All meds pushed, including saline or heparin flushes.	5
Add-ons	# done. All solutions/piggybacks you hang. Does *not* include solution used for new start or blood product.	10
Blood products	Total # units. All blood products administered or delivered. Includes saline and tubing set-up.	
	Blood	45
	Up to 10 units platelets (list platelets and cryo separately).	60
CVC dressing/discontinue CVC	Total # done.	20
Peripheral dsg	Total # done.	10
Change tubing	Total # done. Incl. CVC ext.	10
DC IV	Total # done. DC, no restart	10
Troubleshoot	Total # of times spent checking tubing problems, pump alarms, etc.	5
Port access	Total # done. Includes dsg.	30
Blood draws	Total # done. Periph and CVC	15
CVC insert assist	Total # done. Dsg. not incl.	45
Long-arm cath insert	Total # done. Dsg. not incl.	60
PICC insert	Total # done. Includes assessment. Dsg. not incl.	120
Admixtures	Total # prepared.	15
Code Blue	# codes responded to only.	30
IV cards	Total # prepared.	5
Janitorial/batching	Total time spent cleaning carts, stocking shelves, batching, etc.	
In-service, assist with patient care, pt. ed., nursing instruction	Total time spent in these activities.	
Extra time	Time spent over the allotted time for procedures. Anything not listed above, such as incident reports, searching for equipment, etc., policies and procedures.	

to these primary indicators to offer an efficient, workable system. Time standards for these primary indicators are adjusted to compensate for excluded activities.

7. Select system options. IV therapy PCS can be based on prospective and/or retrospective data. Prospective data allow for the prediction of activities in determining staffing need, whereas retrospective data offer a comprehensive workload measurement for productivity analysis. Other options include determination of patient care hours per shift versus per day, use of IV nursing care need codes versus actual time requirements, and implementation of a manual versus a computerized system.

8. Develop an IV care plan. Based on the data determined by the previous steps, an IV care plan provides a format for recording data and calculating workload.

9. Conduct a pilot study. Testing the system on selected nursing units allows for the identification and correction of any deficiencies prior to widespread implementation.

10. Implement the system. Educate the staff and implement the system on all nursing units.

Staffing

To provide cost-effective patient care and reduce the incidence of complications related to intravenous therapy, an IV therapy team should provide full service with 24-hour-a-day coverage, 7 days a week.[3] The number of registered nurses comprising the team is determined by the number of hospital beds and/or number of patients served by the organization or agency, type and volume of the hands-on procedures performed, and intravenous therapies delivered. The ideal IV team is organized so that it is comprised of management, educational, and IV nurse staff full-time equivalents (FTEs) needed to provide optimum service levels to all patients receiving intravenous therapy.

Table 3-2

Example of Time Values

Activity	Adjusted Time (min)	Computer Time (min)	Kardex Points*
IV push	10.78	10.8	2
Site care	3.18	3.2	1
Piggyback	6.49	6.5	1
Venipuncture	16.08	16.1	3
Tubing change	7.08	7.1	1
TPN	5.24	5.2	1
CVC dressing	25.56	25.6	4
PCA	28.95	29.0	5
Chemotherapy	27.41	27.4	4
Blood	37.27	37.3	6
Indirect care	6.00	6.0	1

*1 point = 6 min.

	Date _____					Date _____					Date _____				
	Night	AM		PM		Night	AM		PM		Night	AM		PM	
		S	W	S	W		S	W	S	W		S	W	S	W
New starts (simple)															
N.S. (difficult)															
Restarts (simple)															
R.S. (difficult)															
Site checks															
I.V. push															
Add-ons															
Blood products															
CVC Dsg./DC CVC															
Peripheral dressing															
Change tubing															
DC IV's															
Troubleshoot															
Port access															
Blood draws															
CVC insert-assist															
Long arm cath insert															
PICC insert															
Admixtures															
Code blue															
IV cards															
Janitorial/batch															
Inserv/PT care/Ed.															
Extra time															
Initial															
# Central caths															
# PT on IV's															
# Peripheral caths															
Hospital census															
QUALITY MANAGEMENT LOG															
Phlebitis +1															
+2															
+3															
Infiltrated															
Clotted															

Figure 3–3. Example of an inpatient IV therapy log.

STATISTICS: IV THERAPY (Inpatient)

The following statistical information is submitted for _____ .

(month)   (year)

Inpatient IV Therapy	Actual Volume	Factor	Weighted Workload
a. New starts (simple)	_____	× 1.33	_____
b. New starts (difficult)	_____	× 3.00	_____
c. Restarts (simple)	_____	× 1.33	_____
d. Restarts (difficult)	_____	× 3.00	_____
e. Site checks	_____	× 0.66	_____
f. IV push	_____	× 0.33	_____
g. Add-ons	_____	× 0.66	_____
h. Blood products	_____	× 3.00	_____
i. Platelets	_____	× 4.00	_____
j. CVC Dsg./DC CVC	_____	× 1.33	_____
k. Peripheral Dsg.	_____	× 0.66	_____
l. Change tubing	_____	× 0.66	_____
m. DC IV	_____	× 0.66	_____
n. Troubleshoot	_____	× 0.33	_____
o. Port access	_____	× 2.00	_____
p. Blood draws	_____	× 1.00	_____
q. CVC insert-assist	_____	× 3.00	_____
r. Long arm cath insert...	_____	× 4.00	_____
s. PICC insertion	_____	× 8.00	_____
t. Admixtures	_____	× 1.00	_____
u. Code blue..	_____	× 2.00	_____
v. IV cards	_____	× 0.33	_____
w. Miscellaneous	_____	× 0.33	_____
x. Administrative hours	_____	× 4.00	_____

(Unit of service: 1.00 factor = 15 minutes)

Total weighted units of service (UOS)   = _____

Figure 3–4. Worksheet for determining weighted units of service for inpatient IV therapy.

In reality, FTEs for the IV therapy team are not always adequate to meet the ideal, and IV therapy department resources vary, depending on the organization. Most IV teams probably do not have the staffing resources available to provide all their specialty services as desired, and the related levels of care for their specialty. The choice must be made as to how best to use the expertise of the team within the facility. A good approach is the phasing in of team functions over time. Initial services should address the most immediate needs identified, and should be based on a realistic workload to establish the team on a firm, positive base. Once the team has been organized and is operating smoothly, successfully performing designated functions, additional services can be proposed as the need is recognized and resources allow. It is important to remember that additional expenditures needed to expand services must be justified by the incremental quality improvement that will be realized.[15]

When a full-service team cannot be justified, a limited service team, although not ideal, may be able to provide quality team services for some aspects of IV care. Determining the actual limited service hours is defined by budget considerations. Limited service teams can vary widely in the allocation of service hours. Typical options include covering day and evening hours, with no coverage during the night shift. Time studies related to workload volume help define the greatest hours of need. Some teams can flex their shift coverage into the late night and early morning hours, leaving only a 4- to 6-hour period without IV team coverage. This is obviously preferred when there are no resources for a full-service team, because it offers the least interruption of service. Other teams may only offer services during expanded day shift hours (i.e., early AM to early PM). This provides some consistent, quality care by IV nurses, but leaves primary responsibility related to IV care to the staff nurses during the hours when there is no IV team coverage. This may lead to inaccurate data collection and inconsistent quality in the care delivered. When a limited service IV team is in place, specific responsibility for IV functions during off-service hours must be defined and understood for the least interruption of therapy and the most efficient provision of care. Communication of those services performed by the general nursing staff is important to the clinical data collection for the facility and to the workload record management of the IV team.

Initially, to secure the hours needed for core or basic staffing, many of the nurses and nursing hours can be trans-

STATISTICS: IV THERAPY (Outpatient)

The following statistical information is submitted for _____ .
                                                        (month)   (year)

Outpatient IV Therapy	Actual Volume	Factor	Weighted Workload
a. Starts	_____	× 2.00	_____
b. Site check	_____	× 0.66	_____
c. IV push chemo	_____	× 2.00	_____
d. CVC dressing	_____	× 2.00	_____
e. CVC blood draw	_____	× 2.00	_____
f. Port access	_____	× 2.00	_____
g. Med. Admin. IVP/IM/SQ (other)	_____	× 0.66	_____
h. Amb. pump (setup/DC/CassChn)	_____	× 4.00	_____
i. Chemo infusion	_____	× 3.00	_____
j. PRBC transfusion	_____	× 8.00	_____
k. Platelet transfusion	_____	× 6.00	_____
l. Gamma globulin infusion	_____	× 5.00	_____
m. Phlebotomy	_____	× 4.00	_____
n. Peripheral blood draws	_____	× 1.00	_____
o. PIC or PICC insertion	_____	× 3.00	_____
p. Hydration therapy	_____	× 2.00	_____
q. Janitorial/stocking	_____	× 1.00	_____
r. Teaching	_____	× 2.00	_____
s. Observation time	_____	× 1.00	_____
t. Insurance verification	_____	× 1.00	_____
u. CVC insertion assist	_____	× 3.00	_____
v. Infusaid refill	_____	× 3.00	_____
w. Miscellaneous	_____	× 0.33	_____
x. Pharmacy compounding (UOS)			_____

(Unit of service: 1.00 factor = 15 minutes)

Total weighted units of service (UOS) = _____

Figure 3–5. Worksheet for determining weighted units of service for outpatient IV therapy.

ferred from the general nursing department and dedicated to IV therapy services. This eliminates the need for massive recruiting and hiring. There is a period of orientation and in-service training required during the initiation phase. Ongoing monitoring of staff and systems at this time is crucial to address any problems that might arise. To determine staffing requirements, time studies must be completed for each IV function, keeping in mind that productivity and efficiency improve after implementation. A time study should include collection of data on the average number of IV patients, IV functions performed on each shift, and admixtures prepared for each nursing unit. With the average time for each activity determined from current literature or for each facility, staffing needs can be estimated. Subsequently, the number of hours spent to perform IV therapy can be determined, as can the number of full-time equivalent personnel. After selecting the team members, additional departmental costs can be predicted.[4] Using time study estimates with estimated volume data defining distribution of the workload, staffing levels for each shift can be determined. For further accuracy, provisions for fatigue, delays, and travel time can be factored in. Orientation, vacation, holiday, and sick time relief can be estimated based on the benefited positions and on historical data for further staffing estimates.

IV teams that are also responsible for outpatient and home infusion therapies require additional staffing hours and may require travel adjustments to be included. Outpatient services may be provided in a dedicated room in the hospital setting or in an alternative setting. For smaller, hospital-based outpatient service operations, in-hospital IV nurses may be able to cover staffing needs, especially for those scheduled services. Ideally, an IV nurse should be assigned exclusively to cover outpatient and home settings. To be cost effective, all members of the IV team, whether in the hospital or an outpatient setting, should be able to function when needed in either environment. Twenty-four-hour service departments can also use their evening and night shifts in a cost-effective manner to cover off-hour calls from home infusion patients and outpatients. They can be a valuable resource for the home health staff in problem solving when they are managing the patient in the home setting, and for the staff in the skilled nursing facility (SNF). Coordination with the home health agency to make the necessary interventions in the home, when the patient cannot come in to the IV nurse, is an acceptable option. The initial contact and assessment for IV therapy–related issues best remain with the IV nurse specialist.

One problem encountered in staffing for the IV team is meeting emergency needs. How to cover that last-minute sick call or the extended illness of an employee is a dilemma that needs careful consideration by the IV team manager prior to the event. Staffing flexibility decreases with smaller team size, and the more specialized the services offered. The possibility for drawing staff from the general nursing population or even from agencies serving the area who have the necessary knowledge base and skills to perform on the IV team is not high. Thought must be given to maintaining reliable on-call resources of RNs. One solution is to cross-train interested nurses from the critical care specialty or the emergency department, where venipuncture skills are most likely to be maintained. The workload distribution might need to be adjusted temporarily to integrate the nonspecialist staff. For example, routine restarts should be assigned to the per diem staff and central line dressing care to the IV nurse specialist. In areas where there are a number of IV teams or home infusion organizations, and more IV nurse specialists might be available, those resources could be tapped and shared, providing a wide experience base for the IV nurse specialist and meeting the community needs. The possibility for establishing community-wide adherence to standards in infusion care becomes more realistic with large numbers of specialists involved in the practice.

Of course, for organizations with 24-hour IV team coverage, staffing problems are magnified. Without careful attention to maintaining resources, the cost in overtime and the decline in levels of quality or service could be detrimental to the objectives of the IV team. Smaller teams and home infusion companies also need to plan carefully for meeting staffing needs in many situations. Crisis staffing has a decidedly negative effect on the operations of the IV team.

MANAGEMENT CONSIDERATIONS

Management in health care has seen many changes in recent years. These changes have come about in part as a direct result of the changing health care scene. The recognition by hospital administrators of the need to approach fiscal management of their facilities in a way similar to that used by industry is evident. They have seen that finding managers who understand the business environment and hospital needs and attitudes is essential to maintaining and increasing effectiveness and efficiency.

To be successful, managers have to set objectives and organize, motivate, communicate, measure, and develop.[16] To be heard in an environment in which there are many managers with varying levels of skill in each of those areas, the development of communication skills that makes others more receptive and responsive to the written and spoken word is important. Success in management often results from learning how to listen to what others say. Managers who hear what other involved people have to say are at an advantage for making informed and appropriate decisions more easily. It is said that the two attributes most valued in managers are integrity and decisiveness.

The successes to be found in health care management, as in industry, stem from a philosophy of employee participation at every level. The shared governance model in nursing management embraces this concept. The results of greater retention and satisfaction of nurses in this practice environment have been documented. The manager who understands the benefits of allowing and encouraging employees to participate in the business decisions that affect them has led to success. Giving employees responsibility for their accomplishments, appraising and rewarding performance fairly, and motivating employees to work for the collective success are likely to contribute toward business success. This approach in the health care setting provides the structure for many health care professionals to "set the standards for their practice, to provide the education for that standard of practice that they set, and to evaluate the quality and consistency of that practice."[7] In specialty nursing practice, where there is already professional commitment to growth and excellence, this model has seen great acceptance and success.

The manager in the health care organization, a public service field, faces the same tasks as the manager in any other field: to perform the function for which the organization exists, to make the work productive, to help the worker achieve, to manage social impacts, and to carry out its social responsibilities. The attentions of the administration and each manager must be focused on objectives, goals, budgets, cost control, performance, and productivity. None of these areas is static, and strategies for management must be flexible and geared to change. The manager must have a clear vision of a desired result and the potential risks to obtain that result. The goals should always be attainable and the deadlines realistic, and the results must be worth the risks.

The most successful managers can deal competently with the sensitive matters of designing job descriptions, interviewing, appraising performance, and inspiring professional development. All this must be achieved within the framework of declining reimbursements and close scrutiny of productivity.

Managers must consider many innovative concepts, how they might improve some aspect of the functioning of the department and have an impact on productivity and the bottom line, and how the implementation of any one of those selected can meet short-term goals and influence long-term objectives. Some concepts to be considered are participative management, total quality improvement, and career planning.

Another area in which innovative concepts seem to arise weekly is information and communications technology. The possibilities for computerization in operations and information retrieval are astounding, and bring to the health care manager, especially the nurse manager, a different and often intimidating challenge. It is one that offers myriad opportunities for changing and improving operations and other aspects of management with the use of accurate reporting and tracking systems. This technology can help the IV team increase its value with improved productivity and streamlined operations. The ability to track and report results, review and track productivity, analyze expenditures, and access clinical information is enhanced with the exciting possibilities of computer technology.

Management of the IV Team

The IV team manager's role within an organization is defined according to the mission of the organization and the goals and objectives of the IV therapy department. The role depends to some extent on the reporting relationships. It is important that consideration be given to the mission of the organization in developing IV team goals. The manager can share information daily with all those using and affected by IV team services to see if goals and objectives are being met.

Administrative Responsibility

Once an IV team has been established, one of the most important functions of the manager is to address the team's objectives in regular reports to administration. This includes reports of progress toward meeting organizational goals, which gives administration a clear picture of the value of the IV team to the organization. It is also essential for the manager to identify departmental and personal goals that are distinct and separate from those of the organization, and address those also. There must be consideration given to identifying short-term and long-term goals with strategies devised for meeting them, including time lines. The manager must have a clear view of the results desired and a plan for achieving them.

The viability and value of the IV team depend on the ability of the manager to organize the structure under which it operates. This means selecting the type of organization that provides the desired efficiency, effectiveness, and productivity. Organization consists of describing each aspect of work to be done, setting the time frame for completion, and determining who is to do the work. An important aspect is the participation of the entire staff in the process of identifying departmental goals and establishing the plan for reaching them. Success depends on the collaborative efforts of the team, whether the goal is to increase productivity or select the team uniform. With the input of those on the staff who perform the functions, who have the most familiarity with daily operations, and whose performance and interactions are the key to the department's success, the development of realistic systems for the operation of the team is simplified for the manager.

It is the responsibility of the manager to provide the atmosphere and environment that is the most conducive for the staff to perform at their own personal best. The IV therapy department manager, as INS recommends, should be a registered nurse who meets all the criteria for the intravenous nurse specialty. The technical experience, skill, and knowledge are necessary, and are valuable in every aspect of managing the IV team. A clear understanding of the practice is essential.

Human Resources Management

Challenging aspects of managing the IV team include those associated with the selection, development, and retention of the staff. The importance of those who staff the IV team cannot be overemphasized. They are often the key ingredient for the success of an IV team. Each candidate must be viewed critically for the skills and qualities that are needed to enhance the department, organization, and profession. It is said that "effective managers . . . manage themselves and the people they work with so that both the organization and the people profit from their presence."[17] The

professionals who make up the successful IV team also fit that description.

INTERVIEW PROCESS

Determining the professional, social, and personal values that are shared by the manager and staff can provide the common bonds that make it easier to organize a team, design systems, budget appropriately, and move toward a common goal. The interview process provides an excellent opportunity to assess those values in each candidate. It is important to have an interview tool or technique that yields the information necessary to make the right choices for meeting the team's needs. Thought should also go into how the individual can fit within the organization. There are some interview models that involve a panel comprised of or including key staff members. These can be valuable when there are internal as well as external candidates to improve chances for making the best choice.

The interview process becomes important when considering a candidate for work in a setting in which he or she has never functioned. There is not always a clear picture of how the setting defines practice; for example, technical skills are important, but assessment and teaching skills are also essential and have a different focus in the outpatient or home infusion setting than in the acute care environment. It is important that the person fit the setting, as well as meet the requirements for a position. The following is an example of an interview tool to use for the IV nurse candidate.

These questions are suggested for use during interviews for IV nurse clinical staff. Because of the diverse and extensive level of knowledge required by the IV nursing professional, it is important to question the candidate thoroughly regarding IV-related experience and education. Throughout the interview it is also important to assess the candidate's personality and ability to work independently, yet still be a team player.

   I. Previous experience
     A. Experience and areas worked related to IV therapy
     B. Number of years in acute care
     C. Last day worked in acute care
     D. Home care experience
  II. Education and training
     A. Nursing degree achieved/Public Health Nurse Certificate
     B. National certification
     C. Advanced Cardiac Life Support/CPR
     D. IV-related education and training
     E. PICC certification
     F. Goals for certification or degree
 III. IV therapy–related technical and clinical experience
     A. Peripheral catheter insertion: number of insertions/ day
       1. Experience with pediatric and neonatal care
     B. Short-term central venous catheters
       1. Assistance with insertion
       2. Dressing changes
       3. Blood draws
       4. Patient education
     C. Long-term central venous catheters
       1. Assistance with insertion

  2. Dressing changes
  3. Patient education
  4. Blood draws
  5. Catheter repair and declotting
  6. Port access
 D. PICC catheters
  1. Experience with insertion
  2. Dressing changes
 E. Intraspinal catheters
  1. Dressing changes
  2. Medication administration
  3. Implanted pump refills
 F. Blood product administration
  1. Red cell products
  2. Platelets
  3. Fresh-frozen plasma
  4. Cryoprecipitate
  5. Use of microaggregate and leukocyte removal filters
 G. Admixtures
  1. Use of laminar flow hood
 H. Participation in Code Blues
  1. Familiarity with administering cardiac drugs
 I. Electronic monitoring device experience
  1. Pole-mounted infusion pumps
  2. Ambulatory infusion pumps
  3. PCA (patient-controlled analgesia)
 J. Experience working with chemotherapy agents
IV. Teaching
 A. Experience with patient teaching
  1. Do you enjoy it?
 B. Staff education experience
  1. In-service training received in, among other programs
  2. Interest level in providing in-service training to staff and other IV nurses
 V. Committee participation
 A. Previous committee participation
 B. Interest in committee participation
VI. Overall questions
 A. Why do you feel you would be the best person for this position?
VII. Daily situation questions
 A. It's the end of the shift and your relief is not here—what would you do?
 B. A co-worker consistently does something that drives you crazy, such as leaving the IV cart a mess. How would you handle it?
VIII. Work schedule
 A. Shifts and hours preferred
 B. Number of days and pay period preferred
 C. Availability on short notice
 D. Feelings about reduction in work hours due to low patient census or overtime related to very high patient census
 E. Willingness to attend meetings

When that perfect candidate is elusive, the next best thing is to hire the potentially perfect IV nurse who may lack the required skills but has the required nursing experience and a great interest in the intravenous nursing specialty. The potential can be realized through a staff development program designed to be flexible enough to meet the general needs, and that also addresses the individual areas of need identified for each new member of the team.

PERFORMANCE STANDARDS

It must be the clear expectation that each member of the team is accountable for his or her own practice and performance. A system for measuring performance must be established, with clearly defined criteria. It is valuable to have the participation of the IV team in defining the criteria.

The IV therapy team manager should be responsible for timely performance appraisals, required on an annual basis, but essential at intervals throughout the year, for coaching to higher levels of performance, and for submitting recommendations to strengthen performance. This can take place during more informal coaching sessions to enhance the potential for performance improvement and to recognize success. The following is an example of criteria-based performance standards to use for evaluating IV nursing clinical personnel. It is the responsibility of the manager to provide an equitable system for evaluating performance in relation to standards and expectations.

To facilitate objectivity and consistency in the evaluation process, each standard should be detailed with specific criteria for measuring the standard.

 I. Philosophy and standards
 A. Adheres to policies regarding
  1. Attendance, employee health, tardiness, parking, Occupational Safety and Health Administration (OSHA) requirements, licensure
 II. Patient care management
 A. Actively communicates with physician
 B. Reviews and interprets progress notes and appropriately implements physician orders
 C. Exhausts all options to obtain appropriate and timely physician response
 D. Maintains accurate diagnosis and current plan of care on IV therapy profile cards
 E. Concisely communicates plan of care in shift report
 F. Reviews patient tests, interprets results, and correlates this information with overall plan of care
 G. Identifies potential problems related to patient diagnosis
 H. Complies with current medication administration policies and procedures
 III. Nursing process
 A. Obtains an initial IV assessment; assesses patients with regard to diagnosis and/or special conditions that have any bearing on IV therapy
 B. Implements IV nursing measures to prevent potential problems related to patient's diagnosis and hospitalization
 C. Plans IV care for assigned patients; integrates IV care with the nursing care plan
 D. Communicates verbally with medical and nursing colleagues, patient, patient's family, and allied health disciplines
 E. Assesses psychosocial needs and makes appropriate referrals
 F. Participates in quality assessment activities

G. Fulfills the criteria for JCAHO and hospital nursing process requirements as evaluated by the process of five random chart audits

IV. Teamwork
   A. Uses problem resolution skills rather than complaining to improve unit environment
   B. Observes and reports unsafe practices using notification system and appropriate channels of communication
   C. Manages time to complete assignments within time allotted on shift; when not possible, informs manager of need for assistance
   D. Addresses patient and family complaints by active listening and endeavors to correct problem or refers to an appropriate authority
   E. Demonstrates flexibility as staffing needs change
   F. Assists, as requested, with orientation of staff members and teaching of students

V. Discharge planning
   A. Initiates referrals to IV therapy clinic, discharge planner, or home health to plan for potential post-hospital infusion care
   B. Implements patient education as related to outpatient IV therapy; develops teaching plans for individual patients

VI. Professionalism
   A. Shares new knowledge with co-workers after attending programs such as director-approved continuing education classes, seminars
   B. Identifies own learning needs and pursues appropriate education; must not be the same seminar as in section A, above
   C. Actively participates in evaluation of new products and equipment
   D. Reviews IV therapy policies and procedures during daily performance of duties
   E. Actively participates in new unit procedures and research projects
   F. Exhibits a positive attitude toward changes in the health care profession
   G. Participates in evaluation of own performance by identifying strengths and weaknesses and developing a plan to improve weak areas

VII. Environmental safety
   A. Demonstrates responsibility for patient safety by assessing need for safety precautions, instituting a safe plan of care, and providing a safe patient environment
   B. Demonstrates knowledge and application of infection control policies and procedures
   C. Demonstrates understanding of such emergency procedures as fire drills, evacuation measures, disaster policies

VIII. Technical skills
   A. Demonstrates competency in setting up, programming, and troubleshooting pumps, including
      1. PCA pumps
      2. Ambulatory pumps
      3. Syringe pumps
      4. Pole-mounted pumps

IX. Clinical skills
   A. Follows proper policy and procedures with venipunctures

B. Properly assesses IV sites and takes appropriate action to rectify any existing problems
C. Follows proper policy and procedure when caring for short- and long-term central venous catheters
D. Demonstrates proper policy and procedure and follows physician's orders in the administration of chemotherapeutic agents
E. Follows proper policy and procedure in the preparation of admixtures
F. Follows proper policy and procedure in the administration of blood products
G. Demonstrates necessary knowledge and follows proper procedure in responding to codes
H. Follows proper policy and procedure when caring for intraspinal catheters

CLINICAL LADDER PROGRAM

There are several models for rewarding clinical experience and expertise. The preferred programs are those that offer recognition of professional achievement and have a monetary incentive. The clinical ladder is a type of program that some facilities have designed and customized to meet their criteria. It is a means for encouraging nurses to develop and maintain a high level of clinical practice while rewarding and recognizing their accomplishments.[18] It is incentive and reward for the nurse who chooses to remain in a clinical role rather than move into management for advancement. Clinical ladder programs can be successfully implemented for IV nurses and can provide a system for recognizing and validating the expertise and higher clinical skill levels they have achieved. If the facility has a clinical ladder program in place it can be customized for the IV team, no matter where the team is in the organization, and whether the team is made up of RNs, LVNs, or both. Working with the human resources department for designing and implementing the program is essential. The evaluation tools used can and must be adjusted to the clinical ladder.

Several types of clinical ladder programs have been used; the most common have three to five levels. These can include education and experience levels only or can, when considering criteria for the IV nurse specialty, expand to include advanced skills, responsibilities, and certification. The following is an example of the basics of the clinical ladder levels:

I. Clinical nurse I: entry level nurse, or new graduate. RN with less than 1 year's experience.
II. Clinical nurse II
   A. At least 1 year's recent and relevant experience as an RN.
   B. Clinical nurse I may apply for the clinical nurse II level if employed as RN at this facility for a minimum of 1 year and has received a "meets standards" rating on current evaluation.
III. Clinical nurse III
   A. Clinical nurse II may apply for clinical nurse III level if a graduate of an accredited RN school of nursing, has worked a minimum of 1040 hours in each of the required years of experience specified in the following criteria, and meets one of the following criteria:

1. Baccalaureate degree in nursing with at least 3 years' RN experience in an acute care facility. Current evaluation at this facility must be above standards.
2. Baccalaureate degree in a field other than nursing with at least 4 years' RN experience in an acute care facility. Current full evaluation at this facility must be above standards.
3. Associate degree nurse or diploma program graduate with 10 years' experience in an acute care facility, 2 years of which must have been at this facility. Also, the last evaluation at this facility must be above standards.
4. Associate degree nurse or diploma program graduate with 8 years' RN experience at this facility, based on anniversary date. Current evaluation at this facility must be above standards.
5. Master's degree in nursing and at least 2 years' experience as an RN in an acute care facility. Current evaluation at this facility must be above standards.
6. Master's degree in a field other than nursing and at least 3 years' experience as an RN in an acute care facility. Current full evaluation at this facility must be above standards.

IV. Clinical nurse IV: a clinical nurse II or III is eligible to apply for the clinical nurse IV level if a graduate of an accredited RN school of nursing, has worked a minimum of 1040 hours in each of the required years of experience specified in the following criteria, and meets one of the following criteria:

A. Baccalaureate degree in nursing with at least 6 years' RN experience in an acute care facility, 3 years of which while practicing with a degree, and 1 year of the 3 as a clinical nurse III at this facility. Current evaluation at this facility must be above standards.
B. Baccalaureate degree in a field other than nursing with at least 7 years' RN experience in an acute care facility, 3 years of which while practicing with this degree, and 1 year of the 3 as a clinical nurse III at this facility. Current evaluation at this facility must be above standards.
C. Master's degree in nursing (MSN) with 3 years' RN experience in an acute care facility, 1 of which while practicing with MSN. Current evaluation at this facility must be above standards.
D. Master's degree in a field other than nursing with 4 years' RN experience in an acute care facility, 1 year of which while practicing with the MS degree. Current evaluation at this facility must be above standards.

It is obvious that, in this model, there would be no level I nurses on the IV team. It is necessary to define the skill levels and the productivity parameters that make an IV nurse eligible for moving to another level on the ladder. The criteria are specific to each practice and each facility. Attainment of national certification through the Intravenous Nurses Society, CRNI, should be integral in the design or added to the evaluation tool. Credentialing is one of the most essential ways for IV team staff to validate their competencies and lend credence to their specialty. It is important for the IV

nurse to achieve this competency in the specialty practice of IV therapy.

Another essential role for the IV therapy team manager is competency review and assessment for adherence to policies, procedures, and standards. This review might be an expectation for anyone who is responsible for managing IV access or administration. It is a necessary part of the orientation to a new procedure or piece of equipment. The observation of routine skills on a regular basis helps to ensure adherence to standards and enhances practice.

The clinical role the IV team manager assumes is service- and resource-dependent. It is critical for the manager to maintain skills and expertise in all aspects of IV therapy. Changes in the delivery of IV therapy are occurring at an astounding rate. The effective manager needs to remain abreast of all these developments to maintain credibility as a resource and to adjust services appropriately.

Policies and Procedures

The IV team manager is responsible for the development and continual revision of all IV therapy–related policies and procedures for the team and institution. Policies and procedures are the groundwork for departmental and clinical functions, serve as a guide to its operations, and provide the nursing staff with information they need to provide safe, quality IV care throughout the facility.

It is important to consider carefully the format and content of these written documents, which are used as guidelines for practice. The policies describe the course of action to be taken, and the purpose for that course of action should also be defined. This might be where the standard is described. There should be a detailed list of steps to be followed; the procedure, and the rationale for the action, the expected result of the action, and the steps to be followed when the expected result does not occur should also be presented. It is important to describe the products being used, including information on the effectiveness, safety, and risks of the product. It is helpful to evaluate the procedure format and content by testing whether someone unfamiliar with the practice could complete the procedure appropriately by following the instructions. Standards covering principles of care should be used to direct the end result or expected outcome. It is helpful and, in some facilities, required to list the references that support the policy. This can be determined to be a part of the document, or might be included in a separate section. The dates of approval and implementation must be documented and a record of the approving committee(s) must be made.

The manager is responsible for ensuring that the policies and procedures comply with state and federal laws and follow national guidelines, such as those from the *Intravenous Nursing Standards of Practice* (INS), Centers for Disease Control and Prevention (CDC), Joint Commission on Accreditation of Healthcare Organizations (JCAHO), Occupational Safety and Health Administration (OSHA), and American Association of Blood Banks (AABB). The home infusion industry has additional agencies and further requirements that must be addressed in policy and procedure.

IV therapy policies and procedures must be approved by the appropriate committees within the hospital and many, because of the invasive aspects, require physician approval. Once the procedures are devised and approved, they must be made available to the nursing staff as well as to members of the IV team. There must be documentation of the training and orientation programs used in the implementation, and records of who received that training must be kept, as applicable. The education department is an excellent adjunct to the education and implementation process. In fact, everyone involved in administering IV therapy must be familiar with the approved policy and procedure for each IV task. Annual review of policies and procedures is required, with appropriate updates as needed.

Quality Management

Increased positive patient outcomes enhance the rationale for using an IV therapy team to ensure the quality of the intravenous therapy care received by patients. From IV therapy monitoring, IV nurse specialists can provide the information for determining that the standards of care are being met. Criteria such as phlebitis, infection, clotted device, and infiltration rates are measurable indicators. The IV team manager assesses the impact, reports the findings, and makes recommendations for improving outcomes, as necessary.

The objective of a therapy audit is to evaluate the quality of IV nursing as reflected in the patient care records. Consequently, specific criteria or standards of care must be developed so that reviewers know precisely what constitutes quality IV nursing care. Evaluation standards and audit criteria can be developed on actual IV therapy practice and data retrieval methods implemented to assist in evaluating criteria. Criteria to evaluate include but are not limited to the following:

- Are needles disposed of in tamper-proof, leakproof, puncture-proof, disposable containers?
- Are the principles of asepsis followed in setting up equipment?
- Is the patency of intermittent infusion devices verified before medications are administered?
- Is adequate hand washing done before patient contact?
- Are gloves worn during venipuncture and discontinuing of intravenous catheters?
- Is approved skin preparation performed?
- Is the intravenous access device properly inserted?
- Is the IV nurse attempting venipuncture more than twice?
- Is the nurse pushing IV medications using proper procedure?
- Does the nurse flush with saline before and after the IV push administration?
- Is documentation accurate, complete, and legible?

In addition to assessing whether these steps are actually being followed, the therapy audit must also judge how well they are being completed. Does the degree to which the step is accomplished fall far below, meet, slightly exceed, or far exceed the standard? On a less frequent schedule, the IV audit should be expanded to assess the team's performance in more detail, considering questions such as the following:

- Is the IV solution container labeled with the patient's name and room number, type of solution and additives, time and date mixed, and IV bag or bottle number?

- Is the IV administration set labeled with the appropriate date and time?
- Has the IV access site been labeled with the type of device, gauge and length of device, date and time inserted, and initials of the person performing the insertion?
- Have all connections been secured?
- Is the documentation complete?

The data collection forms must include a mechanism for objective ratings and identification of problem areas, random data collection, and timely reporting. IV therapy audits must be conducted to ensure the quality of patient care services, reinforce accountability, and enhance learning. Exceptional performance and exceptional patient outcomes are criteria for the success of IV team services. The audit discloses not only areas where patient care could be improved, but also identifies areas where the team is performing exceptionally well. In addition, a properly conducted IV therapy audit improves communication among professionals and encourages better documentation.

Total quality management (TQM) is a system, strategy, and a philosophy being adopted by some organizations to meet current regulations and stay ahead of requirements.[19] This system is based on the involvement of the entire organization, from the top down, in the delivery of quality service and the commitment to quality improvement. Quality in health care is the customer's perception of the product or service provided, and the supplier's knowledge of customer requirements, variation among customers, and applicable standards of practice. The JCAHO embraces the concepts in its own ''Agenda for Change'' and in the development of indicators that focus on quality improvement.

The goal of any quality management program is to establish an organizational culture of service excellence that permeates administrative priorities, strategic planning, policies and procedures, physical design, and staff attitudes and behaviors.[4] It is possible that most IV teams already meet the objectives for this system. Actively soliciting customer feedback is a component that the IV team can easily add to its services, because personal contact is required for every service. It is essential that the results of that feedback, both negative and positive, be addressed. The immediate personal contact of the IV team manager with the customer and/or staff to respond to concerns, complaints, and compliments ensures implementation of the actions that lead to improvements, reinforcement and rewards for behaviors that result in satisfaction, and acceptable outcomes.

Financial Management

The financial profile of the IV therapy department can be efficiently recorded and analyzed by establishing it as a separate cost center. This allows the IV team manager, accounting, and administration to measure not only the department's current status but also to project its future impact on the institution's fiscal plan.

The budget is the fiscal or financial plan for a business. It is one tool that is necessary for examining the costs incurred for each department or service. It is one means for justifying the IV team. Costs include the supply component as well as the human resources component, and are calculated as direct or indirect expenses. The IV team manager or director is responsible for developing the budget, which must include personnel, operations, and capital expenditures. Consideration should be given to indirect departmental costs, such as those for electricity, telephone or FAX, computer and other equipment maintenance, food and office supplies, and personal protective equipment that might not be included in the operating budget. What is included in the budget is determined by the organization. The more input the department manager has in the process, the easier it is to calculate the budget or determine financial guidelines under which the department functions and by which it is judged.

For the operating budget, the calculations include all IV therapy department salaries, including those for managers, professional staff, and support staff, such as clerical workers. This is usually the highest cost item in the budget.

The cost items included for each employee are base salary with any estimated raises, shift differentials, and other differentials, such as credentialing, where applicable. Factored in are the individual benefit rate, including accrued vacation, holiday and sick time, insurance, retirement, tuition assistance, education, and other paid benefits. This total is calculated using projected productive hours for each employee or each position. Overtime calculations for each position, holiday coverage, and any standby hours or travel time anticipated for the department are estimated and determined based on the projected hours needed. Departmental productive hours, those needed for departmental functions, and nonproductive hours, such as education, sick time, and administrative hours, are totaled and calculated at the rate determined by the mix of employees to make up the final budget dollar amount.

The operating budget also includes all supply and equipment expenses necessary for the department to function, which might not include patient chargeable items. This figure might include expenses for such items as pharmaceuticals, instruments, medical-surgical supplies, miscellaneous office supplies and forms, travel, and education programs.

The operating budget may be projected in several ways, as determined by the finance department. Examining historical costs for IV-related expenses and calculating a cost per procedure, per work unit, or per patient day may be used for these projections. It is important to include projections for new programs in the budgeting process.

The capital expenditure budget reflects purchases of major equipment such as office furniture and equipment, electronic infusion instruments, IV carts, beepers, and computers. There is usually a cap, such as $500, which must be exceeded for equipment to be placed in the capital expenditures budget. Construction project budgeting may also be the responsibility of the department manager.

Any projections for revenue are included in the operating budget. It is sometimes possible for the IV team to charge for services as well as supplies. For example, charging for IV nurse placement of access devices or other specialized services may be possible, and must be investigated on an ongoing basis.

It is important that the staff be aware of and involved in the budget process, which is so important to its functions. With input in the decision making process, there is more acceptance of responsibility for the outcomes.

The budget is the guideline used to examine the financial performance of the IV team. The review and analysis of each component is necessary, at least on a monthly basis. It is the manager's responsibility to explain the deviations and implement actions for correcting, where necessary. It is also a chance to report successes in cost savings. If the department implements practices that result in savings, these should be recognized and reported, stating the dollars saved. With the IV team's selection and housewide implementation of needle safety devices for providing IV therapy, for example, the savings in needlestick costs can readily be identified; however, this may not be readily attributed to the IV team, unless reported.

JUSTIFICATION AND BENEFITS

The justification for an IV team centers largely around the benefits associated with delivering intravenous therapy by a team of specially educated nurses. Benefits inherent in the use of IV teams include standardization of equipment, improved productivity with better utilization of nursing resources, fewer patient complications, and improved risk management through the use of an expert's monitoring care. To demonstrate the justification of existing IV teams or for creating IV teams based on enhanced patient care and cost savings, IV supervisors and managers should build their case on a foundation that addresses environment, demand, costs, and benefits. Each area must be thoroughly researched and carefully analyzed, and the findings of this study must be skillfully presented to the institution's decision makers. The considerations given for initially establishing a team are crucial to remember, and should be reassessed as needed for continued justification of the team. A summary of the factors to consider when justifying a new team or maintaining an existing team is provided in Appendix I.

Evaluating the Environment

Both internal and external environmental factors must be considered in today's increasingly regulated and competitive hospital operating climate.[4] An analysis of internal factors should begin by identifying the institution's priorities and then showing how the IV team relates to those priorities. For example, if the facility has placed a high priority on improving the quality of IV care because of current deficiencies, the justification should focus on the advantages brought to the institution by the specialized knowledge and skill of the IV team. A complete internal analysis should also consider the institution's financial status and political structure, as well as the attitudes and perception of physicians, floor nurses, and patients. The external analysis should examine the effect of regulatory and demographic changes, third-party payer and competitor activities, human resources, and supply and technologic changes.

Assessing Demand

The demand for IV services should be assessed by using such figures as the number and type of IV services, number of patients receiving IV therapy, complexity of IV therapy procedures, materials used, and nurse time for each patient, department, and DRG. The potential for IV therapy use should be quantified for each DRG by the percentage of patients receiving IV therapy, average IV costs and charges per patient, and total and average patient days. The severity of the illness of hospital patients should also be assessed, because IV therapy needs increase with acuity as determined by secondary diagnoses, age, malnutrition, dehydration, and surgical versus medical stay.

Cost Considerations

The significant rise in hospital care costs over recent years has prompted much discussion and action about cost containment efforts directed toward maintaining the current cost of health care to the patient and third-party payers. Unfortunately, cost containment measures impose limitations on revenues without addressing the issue of expenses. This has made it more difficult than ever to justify new and existing specialized hospital services such as an IV team strictly on the basis of quality, cost, and revenue because it is difficult to increase patient charges to offset expenses.[20] It is essential for an IV team to be able to identify expenses and potential areas of savings through analysis of the costs and services entailed in delivering IV therapy. Cost justification is an obvious and critical element in maintaining and justifying an IV team. It is achieved through high productivity levels, decreased complications related to IV therapy, cost-effective product utilization, and the production of revenue.

Clinical data have demonstrated that intravenous teams are cost effective because of their efficient and effective use of equipment and because intravenous nurses practice at high productivity levels. Because it has already been demonstrated that an IV team can significantly improve patient care, the future of IV team services will be largely determined by the extent to which the team can support itself. The IV team can exist in the modern prospective reimbursement environment if it can become recognized as an important specialty, document the benefits it provides, and obtain patient and physician endorsement of its services. To justify, organize, and develop an IV team, it must be established that it is an important asset to a facility. It must also be shown that an IV team is well managed, has documented advantages, provides cost-effective services, and improves patient outcomes.

An IV therapy team controls costs by performing procedures efficiently. High productivity and thorough, accurate documentation have a positive impact on total costs. IV team managers must document the team's services so that the associated costs and benefits can be quantified. If IV nurses, through specialization, develop expertise and efficiency that save labor and material while decreasing the incidence of IV-related complications and the average length of stay, an administrator must be presented with irrefutable figures that demonstrate these facts.

Specialized IV nursing teams can be assets in any institution with their ability to reduce labor costs. Labor is the highest cost for most institutions and is obviously an area with tremendous potential for cost savings. In any given institution, a certain number of nurses must spend their time delivering IV therapy. Nurses might be spending two, three, or four times longer than an IV clinical specialist who is

delivering the same therapy. It stands to reason that substantial hours could be made available and redirected to other areas if an IV team were developed and made responsible for all IV-related aspects of patient care. Because labor represents the highest cost associated with IV therapy, it is important to show that labor can become more efficient through the use of IV specialists. An IV therapy team saves time and decreases costs by assuming responsibilities and tasks formerly performed by staff RNs. The time saved can be redirected to other patient care activities. Although the experience and statistics of IV teams in other hospitals may be used to support the justification of a team, the relative amount of labor required for IV services in the specific institution should be determined and considered independently.

IV teams can also have an impact on hospital costs through more efficient use of supplies and equipment. Supplies are frequently used ineffectively in hospitals. The IV nurse who uses IV therapy–related equipment is the best source for evaluating the particular needs of IV equipment in an institution. An IV therapy team lowers expenses by standardizing and controlling the use of IV-related materials and equipment and by controlling inventories of solutions and devices through a centralized system. The IV team should be responsible for purchasing products that are most suitable for that institution, considering the patient population and staff expertise, and standardizing the equipment as much as possible throughout the institution. Consideration must also be given to the amounts and types of products needed, product cost and quality comparisons, and the most cost-effective supply sources. When IV equipment is standardized throughout the institution, benefits result from cost savings available through manufacturer discounts for large-quantity purchases and the greater availability of equipment. The IV nurse should also actively participate with in-servicing of new equipment with the company representative, not only to provide credibility to the new product but to assess reactions of the nursing staff and answer questions related to the institution and its policies and procedures.

Over the last decade, DRGs and the PPS have resulted in substantial changes in the overall plan for justifying IV teams. The PPS produces a list of prices that Medicare pays for services delivered for each DRG. With the advent of changes in Medicare payment, the institution is accordingly reimbursed at a prospectively determined rate for treating a specific case, irrespective of the charges accumulated during the patient's stay. Use of the PPS negated one of the reasons most IV teams were organized during the period of Medicare cost reimbursement: to maximize hospital reimbursement by establishing IV therapy as an ancillary service. Under government PPS, hospital administrators view all ancillary departments such as IV teams as cost centers rather than as revenue centers. If an administrator determines that another cost center can deliver IV services more cost effectively, the IV team concept may be disregarded. Along with concise documentation on other potential and real cost savings, emphasis has been placed on maximizing potential and real revenue from other payers that might be generated by charging for services rendered by IV nurses. Services such as the insertion of access devices—for example, PICCs and midarm catheters, which require special knowledge and expertise that the intravenous nurse specialist is most likely to possess— may be reimbursed. Contracting to provide those services to alternative settings may be another revenue source. The time-proven strategy of depicting the teams as being exceptionally capable producers of revenue for the institution had to be redesigned to depict the teams as being exceptionally capable providers of cost-effective care.

Quality of Care

Another reason for organizing an IV team is to enhance quality of care through the use of competent intravenous therapy specialists. However, this can be difficult to prove objectively. The philosophy of the INS states that intravenous nursing teams should be used to minimize patient risk and to ensure quality services.[3] Because 80 to 90% of all hospitalized patients require intravenous therapy, it makes sense that the clinical expertise of an intravenous nursing team be used to meet the increasingly complex needs of these patients. Intravenous nursing teams provide high-quality patient care through more frequent monitoring of intravenous treatment modalities, thereby significantly decreasing the risk of complications related to intravenous therapy.[3] However, reports that IV teams improve the quality of care may be labeled subjective rather than objective because of the difficulty in quantifying this benefit.[4] Because IV therapy complications often are not well documented, and not all are preventable, an administrator can question whether an IV team minimizes the complications that occur from IV therapy. Reporting the decreased IV nosocomial infection and phlebitis rates is crucial when presenting the case for cost savings attributable to quality. The data needed to quantify these savings, however, are not easy to accumulate. Information may have to be obtained from medical records, infection control program reports, and IV incident reports. Additionally, a controlled study, either retrospective, concurrent, or prospective, may be necessary to provide more accurate documentation. From the study results, additional costs that may occur because of nosocomial infections and phlebitis can be obtained.

A prospective controlled trial conducted at one facility concluded that an IV team substantially reduced the iatrogenic complications related to IV catheters.[21] The results demonstrated that the rate of phlebitis is reduced from 32 to 15% by the institution of an IV team, and the incidence of cellulitis and suppurative phlebitis is reduced 10-fold, from 2.1 to 0.2%.[20] During the pilot project at another hospital, the IV team incidence of phlebitis was only 3.5%, 24.3% lower than the non–IV team incidence. The IV team's incidence of infiltration was a mere 5.1%, an astounding 71.3% below that of its non–IV team counterparts. Of the hospital's IV patients, 75% had infiltrations until the IV team was implemented.[20] A 30-month study of the impact of an IV team on the occurrence of phlebitis demonstrated a decreased volume and severity of phlebitis and a cost savings of approximately $17,000 annually.[22] The cost impact of complications associated with non–IV teams may be convincing if patients must stay in the hospital longer because of IV therapy complications such as phlebitis and infiltration.

Because of the difficulty in quantifying improvements in quality of care, it can be difficult for existing IV teams to continue to justify their existence in the face of increasing scrutiny during budget review. This presents a challenge to existing teams, and new IV teams will have more difficulty in becoming established. Therefore, it is necessary to implement a comprehensive IV team quality management program to justify the need for the specialty on a continual basis. Statistics provide ongoing justification, compared to national standards without teams. Areas that may be monitored include but are not limited to the following:

- Appropriate use of electronic infusion devices
- IV fluid administration
- Infection rates
- Vascular access device complications
- Blood and blood product administration
- IV medication administration
- Delays in therapy or extended lengths of stay attributable to lack of venous access or access complications

These criteria assess both the process and outcome variables of performance. If an institution determines that phlebitis rates are high, fluids are rarely on schedule, medication errors are high, filters and pumps are used incorrectly or inappropriately, IV sites are not rotated, tubing is not changed, documentation is poor, and no communication exists, then that institution is a prime candidate for IV team implementation. In some cases, the medical staff is the driving force for assessing the possibilities of implementing an IV team when the quality of patient care is threatened because of the lack of professional staff or a lack of expertise in the current staff.

Length of Stay

With the advent of DRGs and managed care, length of stay has become a critical measure of a hospital's success. Consequently, departments or systems that can reduce the number of days a patient has to stay in the hospital may determine whether the institution operates profitably. The use of an IV team ensures that therapy is consistently delivered as ordered by preventing delays because the IV couldn't be started or was interrupted by the development of an IV-related complication. A successful IV team also provides dedicated time for IV nurses to investigate physician orders, plan for therapy, and make recommendations for vascular access needs. This type of case management prevents the unnecessary continuation of IVs and ensures that the most appropriate type of infusion device is inserted for the reliable delivery of therapy. To determine how an IV team affects length of stay, the researcher should begin by identifying, for each DRG, patients with abnormally long stays and the reasons for those extended stays, such as severity of disease, nosocomial infection, medical complication, lack of IV placement and resultant interruption of therapy, delayed laboratory results, and failure to discontinue IV therapy. The next step is to determine a percentage of cost savings that is attributable to the IV team—for example, the number of patient days or supplies saved because of IV nurse intervention. It is also important to determine the number and percentage of patients discharged to home IV therapy services, the number of patients who could be discharged if outpatient or home IV services were available, the revenue potential (e.g., current reimbursement policy, payer mix), and the cost of providing these services. By deducting costs from revenues, the profitability of an IV team can be estimated and promoted.[4] With the facts available, the success of the marketing strategy becomes the deciding factor.

Risk Management and Liability

Risk management or liability issues for the institution are decreased with the use of an IV team. Intravenous therapy specialists who are monitoring and delivering IV care are more expert in anticipating and preventing potential patient complications than the general nurse. When IV therapy nurses manage or direct the use of advanced technologies and equipment for the delivery of care, safer product utilization results. Many lawsuits against hospitals are the results of complications that occur when equipment is used improperly or medications are administered incorrectly. The potential for intravenous therapy patient complications is greater with the lack of specialized skill in and knowledge of the various aspects of intravenous therapy.

The presence of an IV team establishes that the institution adheres to professional and court-recognized standards, such as the *Intravenous Nursing Standards of Practice*.[3] Intravenous therapy specialists operating in accordance with these and other national standards for intravenous therapy practice ensure that care is based on principles that have been established through expert development, review, and research. IV therapy–related complications lead to patient injury, increased hospital stays, and potential lawsuits. The ability to reduce these complications through the specialization provided by an IV team is a strong argument for approval of the concept. The first step in demonstrating that IV teams improve outcomes and decrease risks is to identify lawsuits that specifically involved IV complications. The total amount of legal fees, court costs, employee time, court awards, and settlements for these legal actions should be calculated. Plotting the frequency and costs of lawsuits may reveal trends that support the need for an IV team. Licensure allows and health care providers expect the staff nurse to initiate IV therapy and perform specialized IV functions, but knowledge and experience levels in this nursing specialty vary greatly and may be limited. In today's hospital climate, with the complex needs of acutely ill patients, it is becoming increasingly difficult for the staff nurse to remain or become proficient in all of these required skills.

Indispensability

Another strategy for maintaining an IV team is by delivering and taking responsibility for highly specialized services that increase the value of the IV team to the institution. In recent years, highly skilled procedures such as PICC insertions have become invaluable. The requirement for the development of specialized rather than general procedures gives the IV team additional responsibility and authority. If a hospital with a highly efficient, effective, and full-service IV team wanted to eliminate that IV team, it would have a difficult time providing these services, which have become standard. The IV team has become an important part of the institution by continually doing more and producing more.

Success, high productivity rates, and other measures of an IV team's importance to any institution must be tangible ones—there must be quantifiable data to support the assumptions.

Educational and In-Service Programs

Continuing educational and in-service programs related to IV therapy should be provided by IV nurse specialists. This is an important marketing tool for any IV team or infusion company, and establishes the importance of the IV nurse and his or her specific knowledge. When an IV nurse participates in the orientation of new staff nurses, a valuable opportunity is provided to discuss the benefits of the IV team to the institution and to their individual practice. Educational offerings provided by IV nurses also ensure that nurses in individual institutions and communities are being provided with the same knowledge base, and that the information provided is current and in accordance with established standards and guidelines.

Strength in Numbers

Continuing to justify the IV team requires the evaluation of the functions of other teams in the area and assessing how they are doing. Establishing a community standard that IV teams are the expectation rather than the exception provides tangible and immediate justification and support. It is also helpful for all IV team managers in a community to meet regularly to share clinical experiences, discuss practice issues, and evaluate technologies. An excellent example is the task force for IV teams established in one community.[23] The group is comprised of educators and IV nurses and provides a forum for new equipment review, sharing educational resources, and discussion of professional issues that affect practice. When several IV teams practice in a community, it is typical that one team is continually compared with another regarding services provided, staffing, cost effectiveness, and productivity. It is essential to keep the lines of communication open to share information and develop strategies for the continued success of the teams. When developing an IV team, it is important and helpful to use all resources for the specialty that are available. These can include those from nearby teams, as well as teams practicing outside the immediate area.

Positive Impact on Other Staff

An IV team can have a positive impact on the morale of other hospital staff, such as staff RNs or house officers previously responsible for IV-related duties. By relieving them of these duties, they experience fewer disruptions in their day and a decrease in associated frustrations. With 80 to 90% of patients receiving intravenous therapy, access challenges, and complex intravenous therapy administration, having the intravenous therapy specialist involved in the management and delivery of IV care relieves the staff nurse and/or house staff of the actual physical tasks required. It also provides the nurse or case manager with the security that the patient is receiving the safest and most cost-effective IV care available.

Marketing

Marketing is an essential component for the ongoing justification of IV services. The patient, our consumer, is a strong advocate for IV teams. The IV team has an important product to offer through our expertise, knowledge, and standardization. It is important to present the benefits that an IV team offers and build a good reputation. An IV team should be marketed as a potential source for referrals or admissions. This includes inpatient and outpatient services, such as education and IV services for home care patients and clinics.

It is not uncommon for patients to do some research on their own to satisfy their interest in having their health care needs delivered by institutions with a highly motivated and skilled professional staff. Patients' opinions about hospitals tend to be based on the care and responsiveness of the staff, because these are factors they believe they can judge, rather than medical procedures.[14] Consequently, the competence and skill of nurses on the hospital staff is crucial to any hospital marketing efforts. Consumer research shows that personal experience and word-of-mouth advertising create most of the image of a facility among consumers. It has been reported that satisfied customers tell between four and five others, whereas dissatisfied customers share that experience with between nine and ten others.[24]

Having a skilled IV team can be an important consideration that a patient evaluates. Patients are usually more afraid of having an IV started than of having various other procedures. Some patients are left with bruises and complications because inexperienced staff inserted or managed their peripheral access devices. When an experienced IV nurse delivers the therapy, however, the physical damage is minimized and patients normally find it less frightening. It is important to demonstrate that a particular hospital has a genuine concern for reducing an often distasteful aspect of hospitalization. Also, if the marketer can make potential patients aware of the significance of IV specialization, then that hospital stands an excellent chance of attracting the new patient it needs and wants. The advent of quality improvement parameters is also a function of quality measurement. Successful quality parameters are a result of patient-customer satisfaction. The presence of IV clinical nurse specialists can assist a facility in meeting patient-customer expectations and results in positive outcomes.

The future of IV teams continues to depend on the issues of quality care and allocation of resources. The challenge remains for those committed to the philosophy of the intravenous therapy specialty to provide rational and documentable justification for use of their specific product line.

The movement in the delivery of health care to all but the most acutely ill patient into alternative settings is underway. It has challenged specialists to bring their technology and expertise to the consumer safely and economically. We know that the delivery of intravenous therapy modalities can be adapted to most care settings, but nontraditional approaches and settings do not negate the need for clinical expertise. In fact, there seems to be a greater need for the specialist to provide clinical monitoring and reporting in alternative care settings.

The patient has become the customer for many specialty health care services in a wide variety of settings. Within the hospital, there is consolidation of clinically significant patient information in the medical record, which is readily retrievable. This defines the patient's needs, the care given, and the results of that care. All this information is necessary for assessing present needs and in planning for meeting future needs without repetition of services.

There is now a focus for meeting the demands for better access to essential clinical information in the form of a comprehensive database. The ability to retrieve clinical data from all external providers would give a complete medical picture each time a patient is seen by a physician, provide continuity, and make the process for providing care more efficient. Real managed care and its obvious advantages to the patient, as well as the health care delivery system, require that this issue be addressed.

The future role of the IV therapy department remains to be seen. There is an ever-increasing need for the expertise of specialists in infusion care and an ever-increasing demand for their services. It is the challenge of the intravenous nursing specialists to provide this expertise efficiently and cost effectively within a carefully managed health care system.

References

1. Gardner C. IV specialization: Current issues. JIN (suppl) 1989; 12:3–9.
2. Centers for Disease Control. Guidelines for Prevention of Intravenous Therapy Related Infections, Intravascular Infections: I.V. Therapy Related/October, 1981. Atlanta: Centers for Disease Control, 1981 (prepared by US Department of Health and Human Services).
3. Intravenous Nurses Society. Revised Intravenous Nursing Standards of Practice. JIN (suppl) 1990.
4. Burik D, Christina CW, Holtz JM. A workbook approach to justifying I.V. therapy teams under prospective payment. NITA 1984; 7:411–418.
5. Larkin M. Placement of I.V. teams in hospitals. NITA 1982; 5:80–81.
6. Thompson D. Guidelines for the proposal of an I.V. team. NITA 1982; 5:207–208.
7. Dugger B. Shared governance: Opportunities for intravenous nurses. JIN 1991; 14:41.
8. Gorski LA, Baldwin-Schmidt T. Home dobutamine therapy. In J Home Health Care Pract 1990; 2:11–20.
9. Baldwin R. Provision of intravenous therapy in a skilled nursing facility. JIN 1991; 14:366–370.
10. Wolfram C. The benefits of professional credentialling. JIN 1991; 14:363.
11. Plumer A. Organization of an intravenous department and guide to teaching. In Plumer A. Principles and Practices of Intravenous Therapy, 4th ed. Boston: Little, Brown and Co., 1987:15–30.
12. Baldwin DR. Workload management system for I.V. therapy. JIN 1988; 11:308–314.
13. Baldwin D. Patient classification system for I.V. therapy. JIN 1988; 12:313–320.
14. Kalafat J. A systematic health care quality service program. Hospital and Health Services Management 1991:571–587.
15. Seymour SB. Cost quality and staffing considerations for I.V. teams. NITA 1982; 5:325–326.
16. Drucker PF. Management Tasks, Responsibilities, Practices. New York: Harper & Row, 1974:400.
17. Blanchard K, Johnson S. The One-Minute Manager. New York: Berkley Books, 1985:18.
18. Speer EW. Clinical ladders for I.V. nurses? JIN 1988; 11:402–409.
19. Barger-Sailer L. Regulations: How to meet them, how to stay ahead of

them, how to anticipate future trends (abstract). Presented at the NAVAN Conference, San Francisco, 1991.

20. Baker JA. An approach to I.V. team development: Quality cost determinations. NITA 1978; 1:27.

21. Tomford JW, Hershey CO, McLaren CE, et al. Intravenous therapy team and peripheral venous catheter–associated complications: A prospective controlled study. Arch Intern Med 1984; 144:1191–1194.

22. Scalley RD, Van CS, Cochran RS. The impact of an I.V. team on the occurrence of intravenous-related phlebitis. JIN 1992; 15:100–109.

23. Marvin P, Acevedo M. Regional excellence in intravenous therapy: It all began with community intravenous therapy education. JIN 1991; 14:123–125.

24. Peterson K. Guest relations: Substance or fluff. Health Care Forum J 1988; Mar-Apr.:23–25.

I JUSTIFYING AND MAINTAINING INTRAVENOUS THERAPY TEAMS

• •

Justification for IV teams centers largely around the benefits associated with delivering intravenous therapy by a team of IV nurse specialists. The following guidelines may be considered for establishing an IV team or continuing justification of an established team.

FUNDAMENTAL CONSIDERATIONS

Justification

To justify the need for an IV team, the external environment, internal institution environment, demand for services, cost factors, and associated benefits should be thoroughly researched and carefully analyzed.

Maintenance. An established team may only have to research or analyze specific areas as needed for continual justification to maintain the IV team. However, at all times, an established team should be one step ahead and able to address all the factors used to justify a team.

I. ENVIRONMENTAL ANALYSIS[4]

To justify an IV team within an institution, first an analysis of both internal and external environmental factors must be performed to assess the demands on the institution that can offset its ability to support new services, financially and professionally. The data related to these factors may be obtained from administrators, financial managers, professional associations, and peer review organizations.

A. External environment
1. Impact of regulatory and demographic changes
2. Payer and competition activities
3. Worker supply changes
4. Technologic changes
5. Licensing changes
6. Other area institutions (Do other local hospitals have IV teams? If so, how do the functions, responsibilities, and coverage of the teams differ? If not, what is different about a non–IV team hospital so that they do not require an IV team?)

B. Internal environment
1. Identify priorities of the hospital management and the IV team, and then show how the IV team's strengths and weaknesses relate to those priorities. For example, point out how an IV team can control costs while maintaining a high quality of patient care.
2. Who are the decision makers of the institution, and who are those that influence the decision makers? Analyze the data from their perspective: what are their goals, what is important to them?
3. Examine the financial status of the hospital.
4. Consider the institution's internal power and political structure and overall climate for acceptance of services offered by the IV team by floor nurses, physicians, and patients.
5. What is the mission of the hospital?
6. How is the hospital performing financially with reimbursement considerations? What changes are being implemented?
7. In what way is the existing or proposed IV team compatible with the goals of the hospital (i.e., improved, cost-effective quality of care)?
8. What is the purpose of the IV team? Is this purpose recognized by administration?
9. What is the hospital's case mix? What are the implications for the IV team?

II. DEMAND FOR SERVICE ANALYSIS[4]

If the environmental analysis suggests that the IV team concept would receive support, the demand for services should be assessed to show the relative merits of an IV team to the institution. The following should be considered:

A. Evaluate the number and type of IV services that are being performed (starts, restarts, CVC maintenance procedures, tubing changes, infusion device manipulations, blood product administration).

B. Evaluate the number of patients receiving IV therapy and the intensity of IV therapy (e.g., days on therapy, procedures performed, materials and nurse time per patient, department, DRG).

C. The potential for IV therapy should be quantified for each DRG by the percentage of patients receiving IV treatment, average IV costs and charges per patient, and total and average patient days.

D. Assess severity of the illness of hospital patients. IV therapy increases with the severity of the illness, as determined by secondary diagnosis, age, malnutrition, dehydration, and surgical versus medical stay.

III. COST-BENEFIT ANALYSIS[4]

Once an analysis of the institution and demand for services has been done, the next strategy is to ''sell'' the concept of the IV team and its associated benefits. Major emphasis should be placed on the fact that IV teams can reduce hospital costs through savings in labor and materials.

A. Labor
  1. Labor is the largest element of cost associated with IV therapy. It is important to show that labor can become more efficient with the use of IV nurse specialists.
  2. Compare the workload unit requirements of IV specialists with those of non–IV specialists to demonstrate the efficiencies and salary differentials that provide savings. Fewer workload unit requirements are required by an IV team. Labor costs vary, depending on the salaries of the individuals providing IV therapy.
  3. Emphasize that time saved can be redirected to other patient care activities and that improved efficiency can result in decreased FTE requirements on the units.

B. Supplies
  1. Point out that IV teams can reduce material costs through more efficient use of supplies and standardization of IV-related materials and equipment.
  2. Evaluate the impact of an IV team in terms of total materials used and material usage efficiency. Compare this information with the materials that would be required without an IV team and then compare the total costs per procedure related to materials used with and without an IV team. It has been shown that an IV team can be associated with one-third the total material costs, as compared with a non–IV team.[4]

C. Improved quality of care
  1. Reports that IV teams improve quality of care may be regarded as subjective, rather than objective. It is important to define in quantitative ways the quality improvements offered by the IV team concept.
    a. Make a list of those items that define good or poor quality in IV care.
    b. Obtain information from medical records, infection control program reports, and IV incident reports. A controlled study—retrospective, concurrent, or prospective—may be necessary for more accurate documentation.
    c. Select two similar nursing units for a quality study. Using your list of quality measurements, perform random checks of IV patients and establish quality indices on both units; then, on one unit, implement a pilot study using the IV team concept. After implementation conduct a new study on both units and compare with previous results. Use statistical methods in your studies and use unbiased observers. Typically, phlebitis and infection rates are studied.
    d. Improved quality of care must provide clear cost savings.

  2. For maintaining an existing team, it is important to establish a continuing quality management program, conduct studies to demonstrate the improvements your team has accomplished, and identify problem areas.
    a. All members of the team should log in—on a daily, shift-by-shift basis—selected quality management data (e.g., number of patients with phlebitis, infiltrations, infections, clotted IVs). This can be best accomplished while documenting daily workload data (see Table 3–1).

D. Length of stay
  1. To determine how an IV team affects length of stay, identify patients with abnormally long stays and the reasons for those extended stays (e.g., severity of disease, nosocomial infection, medical complications, lack of IV placement and resultant interruption of therapy, delayed laboratory results, failure to discontinue IV therapy).
  2. After considering reasons for extended stays, examine a population or DRG on which an IV team would have a major impact.
  3. Specify the IV team's role in preventing extra patient days, and calculate the percentages of incremental preventable cost and incremental avoidable delays attributable to an IV team.
  4. For existing teams, all staff members should log in, at the end of their shift, any interventions that they have undertaken that would have an impact on length of stay or costs. This provides ongoing data for justification of the IV team. A simple method for collecting data would be to maintain a log book in the department for each IV nurse to note these interventions quickly. For example, there could be a column for the date, room number, patient's name, intervention, results, time required by the IV nurse, and signature of the person carrying out the intervention.

E. Risk management
  1. Plot the frequency and costs of lawsuits, which might disclose trends that support the need for an IV team.
  2. Identify lawsuits that specifically involved IV complications and then calculate the dollars spent for legal fees, court costs, employee time, court awards, and settlements for these suits against the hospital.

F. Marketing advantage
  1. Market an IV team as a potential source of referrals or admissions by being promoted as a time saver and more efficient source of IV therapy. This includes outpatient services, such as education and IV services for home care patients and outpatients.
  2. Emphasize the improved quality of care delivered by the institution with IV specialists providing care, based on national standards.
  3. Work with the hospital's marketing department to investigate strategies for marketing to the

community, as well as physicians and other staff.

IV. ORGANIZATION AND FUNCTIONS OF THE IV TEAM

Once the IV team concept has been proposed and accepted as a valuable service for the institution, there are several factors that must be considered when establishing the organization and functions of the team.

A. Identify the organizational structure that best benefits and enhances the team within the institution. Each organizational structure is associated with advantages and disadvantages, depending on the institutional environment. It is important to look for a structure that allows the team to meet its objectives, goals, and philosophy of care while remaining cost effective. Note that the INS recommends that the IV team be established as an independent department that reports directly to administration. Options include
1. Administration
2. Pharmacy
3. Blood bank
4. Nursing division
5. Medical director

V. ANALYZE CURRENT RESPONSIBILITIES
A. Compare current IV practice with proposed practice with an IV team. Consider
1. Admixture preparation
2. Venipuncture, maintenance, follow-up
3. CVC care
4. Blood product administration
5. IV-related activities performed by various classifications of employees
6. Current nursing policies regarding IV technique

VI. VOLUME OF IV THERAPY ACTIVITIES
A. Establish daily volumes of IV therapy activity for each nursing area. Sources of data include patient charts, pharmacy records, purchasing, and various documents maintained on the nursing units.
B. Establishing current volumes of IV therapy activities provides information for comparison of your institution with other hospitals, and establishes a baseline for comparison of growth and mix changes.

VII. ANALYZE HOSPITAL LAYOUT
A. Look at the layout in the facility, including unit location and size, and types of IV therapy services that are required.

VIII. RESOURCES AND STAFFING
A. What are the resources available for designing an IV team? What role is played by a group such as the nursing division or education department?
B. How many employees does the team need?
C. Is there a significant shortage of nurses? Is it difficult to staff and provide 24-hour coverage?
D. What role does an LVN/LPN play on your team?
E. What resources do you have to train your staff?

IX. FUNCTIONS OF THE IV TEAM
A. What are the services most needed by the institution? If unable to justify all the services it is desirable to provide, a good approach is to compromise

in the beginning and phase in functions over a period of time.
B. Is the team to be a 24-hour, 7-day-a-week team? (Remember that this is preferred for optimal functioning of the team.) What are the implications if it is not? If the team is part-time, who is responsible for IV functions during the other hours?
C. In what areas can the team provide services (e.g., general care areas, pediatrics-nursery, intensive care areas, emergency room, labor and delivery)?
D. Possible functions for the team include the following, but remember those services that cannot be provided as readily without a team. These should be emphasized, and provide the team with ongoing justification.
1. IV equipment selection and evaluation
2. Consulting
3. Patient instruction
4. Product defects, reporting to FDA
5. PICC and long-arm catheter insertion
6. Cytotoxic medication administration
7. Blood component administration
8. Plasmapheresis
9. Venipuncture
10. Medication administration
11. CVC care and maintenance
12. Therapeutic phlebotomy
13. Dialysis access
14. Arterial access
15. Blood draws
16. Code team member
17. Collection and documentation of infection control and quality assurance statistics
18. Extravasation management
19. Declotting catheters
20. Policy and procedure development and revision
21. Outpatient services
22. Home infusion services
23. Contracting services externally, skilled nursing facilities, etc.
E. Be specific regarding functions. For example, when doing a new IV start, is the IV team going to hang only the first solution, or will they hang subsequent bottles?

X. COSTS FOR THE IV TEAM (USE THE HOSPITAL ACCOUNTING DIVISION AS A RESOURCE)
A. What are the projected costs of the necessary staffing (include salary, benefits, sick leave, vacation)?
B. What are supply costs (projected or actual) for IV therapy activities?
C. What are the methods for charging? Are they part of general nursing care charges or are they special charges? What is included in the charge structure?

XI. ANALYZE REIMBURSEMENT AND REVENUE
A. Demonstrate how the IV team concept results in increased revenues—project potential increases. Check with other hospitals that have implemented teams for information.
B. Look at current reimbursement issues, such as fee for service, discounted fee for user, per diem rate, per case rates, and capitation.

XII. DEVELOP BUDGETARY GOALS
    A. Organizational goals
    B. Long-range objectives
    C. For established teams, forecast levels of activity for the coming year.
    D. Continually analyze how the team's role can expand, and re-evaluate services provided. Remember that with the continual changes in health care and technology, the primary functions of the team may be altered.

XIII. DEVELOPING UNITS OF SERVICE
    A. Develop units of service standards for labor hours needed to provide particular services. These standards provide productivity data. Determine units of service through time estimates, historical data averages, logging services, work sampling, predetermined accepted standards, and time and motion studies.
    B. Units of service need to be logged in by the IV staff daily on each shift. This can be accomplished efficiently through the use of computer and bar coding systems. Data can also be easily recorded manually with the use of daily tally sheets. Each nurse can log in procedures performed at the end of the shift and each procedure can then be converted to units of service.

XIV. PLAN OF CARE
    A. It is important to establish the IV team's role in patient assessment and plans of care specific to IV therapy. Establish a system for integrating the IV nursing plan of care into the overall plan of care.

XV. ADDITIONAL STRATEGIES FOR MAINTAINING AN IV TEAM
    A. Become indispensable
       1. Deliver and be responsible for highly specialized services such as PICC insertions.
    B. Educational and in-service programs
       1. Have members of the team be actively involved in nursing orientation, hospital-wide in-service training, and hospital and community educational programs.
    C. Continually evaluate the function and success of other IV teams in the area.
    D. Meet regularly with other IV team managers in the community.

CHAPTER 4 Quality Management

Donna R. Baldwin, MSN, CRNI

Quality management is the commitment to achieving excellence in health care. It is not a singular activity, but a ceaseless effort that seeks to improve outcomes by improving the processes involved in the delivery of patient care.[1] By means of ongoing monitoring, opportunities for improvement are identified, strategies for change are formulated, and planned actions are implemented. The approaches to quality management may vary, but the underlying goal is always the provision of effective and efficient patient care services that result in positive outcomes.[2]

Quality management in intravenous (IV) nursing seeks to ensure that the desired outcomes of IV therapy are achieved. Realistic objectives include the prevention of complications such as phlebitis, reduction of morbidity from IV-related infections, promotion of patient comfort during therapy, and provision of effective patient education. To achieve these goals, the IV nurse must understand and apply the basic principles of quality. This chapter therefore emphasizes the explanation of the concept of quality management as it relates to IV nursing.

Throughout the chapter there are numerous references to the Joint Commission on Accreditation of Healthcare Organizations (JCAHO). JCAHO was originally established as a voluntary, nongovernmental accrediting body for hospitals but has since expanded accreditation to all health care organizations. Quality management requirements have always been part of JCAHO's accreditation process, but introduction of the *Agenda for Change*, in 1986, shifted the focus from problem solving endeavors to continuous improvement of quality.[3] Because this transition is consistent with proven quality management techniques, JCAHO standards serve as the benchmark for quality in health care.

DEFINING QUALITY

There is an ever-greater emphasis on quality health care, but the concept is difficult to define. Quality has been broadly described as the comprehensive positive outcome to a product.[4] In health care, however, the product is multifaceted, which contributes to different perceptions of quality. A precise definition of quality health care acknowledges these differences and includes both the care and services delivered, as well as their perceived value to the consumer (Fig. 4–1).

Quality of Care

Quality of care has been defined as "the appropriate technical application of medical science to diagnose, treat, and cure disease."[5] It is the simplest description of quality, because it concentrates on the technical aspects of patient care.

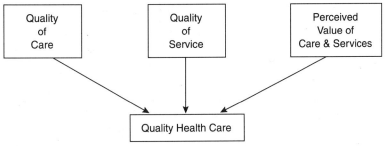

Figure 4–1. Scope of quality in health care.

Care is a product that can be observed, measured, tested, and controlled through statistical methodologies. For this reason, it is understandable that the National Association of Quality Assurance Professionals originally described quality as the levels of excellence produced and documented in the process of delivering patient care.[6]

The quality of IV nursing care relates to the technical aspects of care. IV nursing requires the performance of procedures based on established standards and compliance with procedure is relatively easy to observe, measure, and evaluate. An example is the performance of venipuncture, which requires appropriate selection of an insertion site and cannula, suitable preparation of the intended insertion site, correct insertion of the cannula, proper securing of the device, and accurate documentation of the procedure. If any steps of the procedure are omitted or inappropriate, quality IV nursing care has not been delivered.

One problem with an emphasis on the quality of care is the tendency to overlook outcomes. If, in the previous example, performance of the procedure was absolutely correct but the venipuncture was unsuccessful, the outcome was not achieved and quality care was not delivered. Therefore, quality of care requires both that the technical interventions are appropriate and that the intended results are achieved.

Quality of Service

Quality care is the major product delivered in health care, but service is the subjective aspect that influences the consumer's perception of quality.[5] The nursing procedure may be technically correct, but the patient judges the care according to how the service was delivered. In the case of IV nursing, services such as explanation of the venipuncture procedure before it is performed, consideration of the patient's desires in selection of the IV site, and timely restarting of the infusion following infiltration all influence the patient's perceptions of the quality of the IV nursing care.

Patient education is a major factor in providing quality service. The patient's opinion of quality remains fairly subjective, but the patient has a better understanding of what constitutes quality. For example, consider a patient with an IV infusion that becomes infiltrated. If the nurse has not instructed the patient about the signs and symptoms of infiltration, the patient may presume that there is something wrong with the way the cannula was inserted and that the infiltration is the result of poor-quality service. In contrast, if the possibility of infiltration had been discussed with the patient when the cannula was inserted, the patient could promptly alert the nurse if and when the signs of infiltration are noted. A timely restarting of the infusion then contributes to the patient's perception that quality service has been provided.

Perceived Value

Quality is also influenced by the perceived value of the care to the consumer. Consumers are now more conscious of the value of the care they receive, and expect the highest caliber care in relation to the cost. This is the basis of managed care, which attempts to create the perception of acceptable value in return for the cost of health care.[7]

Perceived value is sometimes a challenge in IV nursing. A nurse may routinely rotate the IV site on a pediatric patient (quality service) following the established procedure (quality care), but the child's parents may not perceive the value of this practice. In their eyes, the child is being subjected to an unnecessary painful experience. As with quality of service, the nurse must educate the parents about the value of routine site rotation and potential problems that may occur if this practice is eliminated.

Quality Health Care

The quest for a universal definition of quality health care continues, but the most accepted description has been offered by the Joint Commission on Accreditation of Healthcare Organizations (JCAHO). According to JCAHO, quality is "the degree to which patient care services increase the probability of desired outcomes and reduce the probability of undesired outcomes, given the current state of knowledge."[8] This definition represents the emphasis on outcomes that was introduced with JCAHO's *Agenda for Change*, and it encompasses all aspects of quality.

LEADERS IN QUALITY MANAGEMENT

Three names frequently mentioned in discussions of quality are Juran, Crosby, and Deming. These leaders defined, refined, and popularized the concept of quality in the business world, but their teachings serve as the groundwork for the quality initiative in health care.

J. M. Juran

Dr. Juran was among the first to recognize that product quality requires careful planning, control, and improvement. He conceptualized these basic managerial processes as the Juran trilogy. Although his teachings were initially applied to Japanese business, Juran's principles of quality planning, quality control, and quality improvement have since been used in American industry.[9]

Quality Planning. Quality does not occur by accident; it is the result of meticulous preparation. The major aspects of planning are the determination of customer needs and the development of products that meet those needs. The primary emphasis is on the external customers, who are the end users of the product, but consideration must also be given to the internal customers, who assist in product development.

Quality Control. The process of quality control requires that the actual product performance be evaluated and compared to the product goals so that actions are directed at resolving differences between performance and goals. To achieve quality control, all employees must be accountable and make use of the feedback loop.

Quality Improvement. Improving quality requires organized change to attain unprecedented levels of performance. It represents a transition from little q (narrow scope of quality limited to clients and products) to big Q (broad concept of quality that defines "customers" as all those who are affected and "products" as all goods and services). In addition, it exchanges the reactionary practices of "putting out fires" and "ready, fire, aim," for a proactive, systematic process that concentrates on improving all aspects of business. One of the best known methods for achieving quality improvement is by means of quality councils, also known as quality circles.

Philip B. Crosby

Crosby is a management consultant who worked his way up through the ranks of business. He introduced the philosophy of "do it right the first time," which conveys his belief that quality is free; it is the nonquality products that cost money, because they require rework. To explain the concept, Crosby used the phrase "zero defects." The expression emphasizes that compliance with defined standards and specifications is necessary to achieve quality; poor quality is the result of lack of compliance and nonconformance. However, it was also Crosby's contention that conformance requirements must be based on input from the worker who produces the product.[10]

W. Edwards Deming

Dr. Deming, the guru of quality, is best known for helping the Japanese achieve world-class quality in product manufacturing, but many American industries have since adopted his teachings. Like Crosby, Deming's philosophy of quality is based on the premise that problems with quality reside predominantly in an organization's systems, not in its employees.[11] Deming's strategy stresses continuous quality improvement and is based on the 14-point system for managing quality, as explained by the following:[12]

Deming's 14-Point System for Managing Quality

1. *Create consistency of purpose for product improvement.* The vision of the organization must be directed at continual refinement of the product. In order for an organization to become and remain competitive, there must be a strategy for the realization of continuous improvement.
2. *Adopt the new philosophy.* Mistakes and negativism cannot be tolerated. Instead, the philosophy of the organization must be dedicated to improvement of quality.
3. *Cease dependence on inspection.* Quality is the result of improved production processes, not the identification of defective products. Prevention reduces the need for inspection to produce a quality product.
4. *Avoid awarding business on price alone.* If the concentration is on quarterly dividends alone, quality and productivity suffer.
5. *Constantly improve.* Quality improvement is a continual

process, not a one-time activity. Improvement is the result of a never-ending pursuit to reduce waste and improve systems.
6. *Institute training.* Workers must be properly trained to perform effectively and efficiently. The organization must invest in training; failure to do so may be detrimental to survival of the organization.
7. *Institute leadership.* Management and leadership are different. Managers tell the worker what to do; leaders create a vision and guide the workers in achieving progressively improved outcomes.
8. *Drive out fear.* Fear inhibits innovation. If workers are fearful of expressing their ideas or asking questions, the job may continue to be done ineffectively or incorrectly.
9. *Break down barriers between staff areas.* Competition and rivalry between departments stem from conflicting goals. A unity in mission and promotion of teamwork within and among departments contribute to the identification of opportunities for improvement.
10. *Eliminate slogans, extortions, and targets for work force.* Quality is not a management-defined slogan and does not result from coercion of the workers to achieve optimal results. Workers must be involved in the identification of methods to improve quality and determination of how these expectations are communicated to others.
11. *Eliminate numerical quotas.* Quotas are counterproductive because they concentrate on numbers instead of the processes that can be improved.
12. *Remove barriers to pride of workmanship.* Workers need to be empowered to have pride in the quality of their work. To accomplish this, the organization must eliminate barriers, such as defective materials, that hinder the quality of the product.
13. *Institute vigorous program of education.* Quality improvement activities require that both managers and workers be educated about statistical techniques and team-building exercises.
14. *Take action to achieve transformation.* All workers must be involved in the change from quality control to quality improvement. The change must be led by a dedicated team of those in top management who have established a precise plan of action to improve quality.

From Walton M: Deming Management at Work. New York: Putnam, 1991.

APPROACHES TO QUALITY MANAGEMENT

With the increasing emphasis on quality in health care, organizations have initiated programs to control, assure, assess, improve, or manage quality. The focus of each program is quality, but the inherent strategies to promote quality care services are considerably different. As a result, the terms "quality control," "quality assurance," "quality assessment," "continuous quality improvement," and "total quality management" are not synonymous, and represent a paradigm shift in the approach to quality management.

It was once assumed that health care was of high quality, so the primary objective was to ensure that the level of care was maintained. When it was determined that the assumption of quality was inaccurate, health care began to adopt components of the industrial models of quality management. During the transition, quality programs in health care progressed from quality control to continuous quality improvement, and we are now embarking on an era of total quality management.[13]

Quality Control

Quality control (QC) is the evaluation of the production of quality goods or services by means of statistical methodologies. It was originally used for the inspection of equipment in the manufacturing industry and has been referred to as statistical quality control. The approach consists of retrospective inspection that compares a random sample of products with a predetermined, acceptable level of defects. Primary components of quality control include data collection and statistical analysis of data.[14]

The major disadvantages of quality control are the emphasis on statistical methods and the retrospective nature of the process. Data analysis should serve as the basis for decision making but, in quality control, there is a tendency for the statistical tools to become an end in and of themselves. Results are monitored and reported after the goods or services have been produced, without emphasis on improving outcomes. Hence, this tool-oriented approach is being replaced by problem-oriented and results-oriented techniques.[9]

An example of quality control in IV nursing might be the monitoring of phlebitis rates. Some organizations place great emphasis on collecting and analyzing data regarding the occurrence of phlebitis. However, once it is determined that the incidence of phlebitis is within the accepted range of 5% or less, no action is taken to further reduce the phlebitis rate.

Quality Assurance

Quality assurance (QA) may be defined as the determination of the degree of excellence through monitoring and evaluation to detect and resolve problems.[13] It is the most widely known of the approaches to quality because of the inclusion of QA requirements in the JCAHO standards since the 1950s. JCAHO accreditation is a voluntary process, but most states have now enacted mandatory QA requirements for licensure of health care facilities. In fact, in many states, the department responsible for licensure of health care facilities is titled the Quality Assurance Division.

Over the years, the QA activities required by JCAHO have evolved from performance of chart audits to problem-focused studies to ongoing monitoring and evaluation of patient care services. In 1986, JCAHO developed the *Agenda for Change*, which initiated the transition from QA to continuous quality improvement. The goal was to create outcome monitoring and evaluation processes to assist organizations in improving the quality of care provided.[15] Consistent with this change, JCAHO has since renamed their "Quality Assurance" standards "Quality Assessment and Improvement."[16, 17]

JCAHO has explained that the underlying rationale for the shift to assessing and improving quality is to overcome several weaknesses inherent in current QA practices. First, QA is frequently focused solely on the clinical aspects of care rather than the interrelated managerial, governance, support, and clinical processes that affect patient care outcomes. Sec-

ond, QA is typically discipline- or service-specific instead of concentrating on the interdisciplinary or cross-service nature of patient care. Third, QA is often individual or problem-oriented instead of examining the processes and systems involved in the delivery of patient care. Each of these tendencies inhibits the organization's ability to improve processes and thus improve patient care outcomes.[16, 17]

The term "quality assurance" may still be used, but it does not appropriately convey the intent of the current quality management programs. Quality cannot be assured; it can only be assessed, managed, or improved. Even the president of JCAHO, Dennis O'Leary, has admitted that, in retrospect, quality assurance was an "unfortunate semantic selection" because it does not accurately reflect JCAHO's vision of quality.[18] Table 4–1 lists the differences between quality assurance and quality improvement.

The clinical record reviews performed by some home health agencies serve as an example of QA. Such reviews consist of a retrospective chart audit that evaluates a random sample of documentation. The data collection tool is typically a checklist on which the presence or absence of the required elements of documentation is noted. The form is appropriate if the objective is to monitor documentation. However, it is of little value in the evaluation of care.

Additional disadvantages of this example of QA are the fact that it concentrates on the negative, it may be punitive, and it does not have an impact on patient care outcomes.[19] During the clinical record review, there is emphasis on the absence of documentation and identification of individuals responsible for the omissions. The collected data may then be used to address the deficiencies with the responsible individuals and evaluate their performance. Such practices promote the punitive nature of QA. If, on the other hand, the documentation is excellent, there is a perception that the individuals "passed the QA audit." In reality, the documentation, not the care, has been evaluated and the data are insufficient to induce improvements in patient care.

Quality Assessment

Quality assessment consists of monitoring, data collection, and data analysis to determine the level of quality of the care

Table 4–1	
Quality Assurance Versus Quality Improvement	
Quality Assurance	**Quality Improvement**
Problem-oriented	Results-oriented
Focuses on inspection	Focuses on prevention
Use of data to evaluate performance	Information trended to identify opportunities for improvement
Focuses on negative aspects of care	Focuses on positive aspects of care
Monitors nursing tasks	Monitors patient outcomes
Retrospective	Concurrent
Evaluates documentation	Evaluates care and services
Random monitoring	Planned, systematic monitoring
May be unrelated to standards	Based on standards
Fixed process	Dynamic process
Concentrates on compliance	Customer-driven
Reactionary	Proactive
Responsibility of QA coordinator/designee	Organization-wide commitment

and services provided. Because assessment is not directed at changing or improving outcomes, this activity is typically coupled with quality improvement. Quality improvement is the component necessary to initiate corrective actions or seize opportunities to improve the effectiveness and efficacy of services.[13]

The use of the initials "QA" for both quality assurance and quality assessment may be confusing. Quality assessment is an element of quality assurance; it is the measurement component. More often, quality assessment is combined with quality improvement to denote activities that both assess and improve the quality of patient care. To reduce the confusion with acronyms, it is the general consensus that "QA" stands for quality assurance, whereas quality assessment is typically linked with quality improvement and designated "QA/QI." Some organizations have further eliminated the confusion by substituting the term "continuous quality improvement" for QA/QI.

As nurses, we understand assessment; it is a basic component of the nursing process. Assessment requires observation and measurement of a problem or condition and, in quality assessment, we observe and measure the quality of nursing care. An example of quality assessment in IV nursing is the monitoring of phlebitis rates. Quality assessment is similar to quality control, but the merging of QA/QI ensures that assessment is not the only activity performed. QA/QI is a comprehensive process that identifies opportunities for improvement, initiates corrective actions, and evaluates the effectiveness of the corrective actions.[14] For example, if, during the QA/QI process, it was determined that the current incidence of phlebitis was 3%, activities would also include identification and implementation of methods to further reduce the phlebitis rate, and follow-up evaluation to determine whether a reduction has occurred.

Continuous Quality Improvement

Continuous quality improvement (CQI) is an approach to quality management that builds on the traditional quality assurance methods. An effective QA program provides a sound foundation for ongoing quality review in the transition to CQI. However, CQI broadens the focus from only the clinical aspects of care to all the facets of the organization that affect patient outcomes.[14] Inherent in this transition is a change in management philosophy and organizational culture, because there must be a visible commitment to CQI for the process to be effective. Current JCAHO standards emphasize that managers and leaders in the organization contribute to the CQI process by establishing expectations, providing necessary resources, and fostering communication and coordination of activities.[16, 17]

The scope of CQI is more extensive than the activities of quality assessment and improvement. CQI considers processes by determining how well they are performed, coordinated, and integrated and by developing strategies for further improvement; it recognizes both internal customers (i.e., all employees) and external customers (i.e., patients, physicians, third-party payers) and values their perceptions of the care and services delivered; and it promotes the pursuit of objective data to evaluate and improve patient outcomes.[20] An essential characteristic of CQI is that it is a continuous proc-

ess. Quality is not achieved and then discarded; quality is the result of long-term commitment to the ongoing evaluation and improvement of patient outcomes. CQI is based on the assumption that outcomes are never optimized but may be constantly improved.[21] This concept is best expressed by Dennis O'Leary's philosophy, "Even if it ain't broke, it can still be improved."[22]

Assuming that care can be continually improved, CQI may be applied to IV nursing. As with all aspects of clinical care, there are numerous procedures that are performed based on the rationale "we always do it that way." CQI encourages creativity in practice; however, nurses must be cognizant of the inherent risks in altering practice unless the innovations are based on valid research. Research is the foundation of IV nursing practice and has precipitated significant changes to improve patient outcomes. An example is the routine rotation of peripheral IV catheters based on research findings demonstrating an increased incidence of phlebitis when peripheral catheters made of Teflon are left in place longer than 48 to 72 hours. There is now controversy regarding the time frame for rotating peripheral catheters made of other polymers. In the quest to improve quality, valid research is needed to address this issue.

A distinctive feature of CQI is that it emphasizes improvement in the interdisciplinary processes involved in patient care delivery, not just individual activities. Application of this concept to IV nursing necessitates that all factors contributing to the quality of care be examined. An example is the process of IV medication administration. Steps involved in this process, in the hospital setting, include prescription of the medication by the physician, transcription of the order on the nursing unit, medication preparation and delivery by the pharmacy, and administration of the scheduled dose(s) by the nurse. Coordination of these various steps affects the quality of the desired outcome, which is efficient and effective IV medication administration. Therefore, with CQI, monitoring IV medication administration entails all functions contributing to the actual nursing procedure.

Total Quality Management

With the shift from QA to CQI, health care organizations have recognized that quality is not a fixed commodity defined by health care professionals but is a strategic mission that must be shared by the entire organization. As a result, several health care organizations have adopted a management system that fosters continuous improvement at all levels and for all functions by focusing on maximizing customer satisfaction. This system is aptly named "total quality management" (TQM).

Because both TQM and CQI are based on the teachings of the quality gurus Deming, Crosby, and Juran, the two approaches to quality management share several characteristics. First, both programs are customer-focused. The goal is to meet the expectations of both internal and external customers. Second, continuous process improvement is stressed. A culture conducive to ongoing quality improvement is the critical link between customer requirements and outcomes. Last, and most important, there must be total organizational involvement. Those in top management must be committed to the program and provide a clear vision for the organization; employees must be empowered to participate actively in the quality improvement process.[23]

Unlike CQI, TQM is not unique to health care. It has been successfully implemented as a strategic resource management system in various sectors of the service industry. Application of the system to health care has been prompted by the current regulated, cost-competitive environment of the health care industry. No longer can health care providers deliver just "acceptable" care and services. Health care affects patients' lives, so any outcome that is less than optimal may have serious ramifications.

Examples of Less than 100% Quality

If you settle for 99.9% quality, you get

- One hour per month of unsafe drinking water.
- 16,000 pieces of mail lost per hour.
- 20,000 wrong prescriptions per year.
- 500 incorrect surgical operations per week.
- 50 newborns dropped by the doctor per day.
- 22,000 checks deducted from the wrong account per hour.
- Two unsafe landings per day at O'Hare International Airport.
- 3200 missed heartbeats per person per year.

There are several distinctive characteristics of TQM. First, TQM contributes to a positive work environment by emphasizing horizontal cross-functional coordination and vertical integration. The clinical, managerial, and support staffs within the organization function as an interconnected network linked laterally, over time, in a collaborative culture. This is in contrast to the typical functional hierarchy in which the organization is a loose collection of separate individuals or departments. Second, TQM fosters collaboration by recognizing the underlying psychosocial principles affecting individuals and groups within the organization. There is a natural tendency for individuals to make judgments based on biases but, through careful and continual training, TQM overcomes these biases and creates an environment of trust. Third, TQM promotes teamwork as a means to break down barriers to communication and enhance interdepartmental collaboration. Active involvement and cooperation within the organization creates a common bond among team members by encouraging them to reach consensus on goals and collaborate on solutions.[24]

To realize total quality as a strategic management vision, the costs of quality must be acknowledged. The cost of quality has been depicted as an iceberg—on the surface are the visible costs of quality (e.g., quality management expenses, patient complaints, repeat work); the less obvious but larger costs (e.g., excessive employee turnover, lack of teamwork) are hidden below the surface. Application of the principles of TQM assists in uncovering and eliminating these hidden costs. The visible costs may then be delineated as either necessary or avoidable so that unnecessary expenditures are reduced.[25]

TQM is also effective, because it strengthens the customer-supplier chain. All employees are both customers and suppliers, linked in a chain that runs through the organization to the ultimate, external customer. Alignment and execution determine the strength of the chain. Alignment is defined as "doing the right thing," whereas the description of execution is "doing the thing right." When both alignment and execution are achieved throughout the chain, "right things are done right."[26]

As an integrated internal management system, TQM focuses on organizational improvement. The system is broader than the clinical aspects of IV nursing, but an organizational culture fostered by TQM facilitates improvements necessary to deliver quality IV nursing care.

Other Quality Acronyms

The programs implemented in the management of quality have been described as an alphabet soup—there are QC, QA, QA/QI, CQI, and TQM. However, additional acronyms may be used to describe many less known quality management programs. These include QRM (quality resource management), QAA (quality assessment and assurance), TQC (total quality care), QAI (quality assessment and improvement), and IQM (integrated quality management). The terminology differs, but the goal of all these programs is continuous improvement of processes, products, and services. Perhaps the confusion with the acronyms could be eliminated if health care organizations followed Crosby's suggestion simply to use the term "quality management."[27]

MEASURES OF QUALITY

Effective quality management is based on well-defined measures of quality. The measures are the criteria by which the levels of excellence are established, and they serve as a basis for quality improvement. However, establishing measures of quality in health care is a complex process. The delivery of patient care services does not result in a tangible product; the service is consumed as it is delivered. Traditional technical quality of conformance measures are therefore ineffective unless they are combined with behavioral norms that describe how the service is to be provided and criteria that outline the intended results of care.[23]

Measures of quality that integrate the technical features, behavioral aspects, and desired outcomes of health care are known as *standards*. Standards represent the agreed-on levels of excellence. They do not necessarily depict the optimum level of achievement but refer to the levels of achievement that are acceptable based on the realistic availability of resources and the current state of knowledge. Discrepancies between optimal and acceptable levels of performance serve as a catalyst for continual improvement. As a result, standards are dynamic and reflect progressively higher levels of acceptable achievement in the continual refinement of quality patient care.[13]

Standards have several distinguishing characteristics. First, they are predetermined. Levels of acceptable achievement are established prior to the delivery of care, not after the care is rendered. Second, standards are written. Accountability to standards requires written communication of the defined rules, actions, and conditions. Third, standards must be approved by an authority. Unless there is proper sanctioning by an entity empowered to enforce the standard and to which the individual is accountable, the standard may be ignored. Fourth, standards must be accepted by those individuals affected by the standards. Standards serve no purpose unless they represent an acceptable level of achievement. Fifth, in order for standards to be used as assessment tools, they must be measurable and achievable. Because of these characteristics, a standard is defined as an accepted written statement of predetermined rules, actions, and conditions that are measurable and achievable and that have been sanctioned by an authority.[19] (Additional information regarding standards is available in Chapter 5, Legal Aspects of Intravenous Nursing.)

Types of Standards

Standards determine whether the delivery of health care services is properly established, implemented, and/or evaluated. Properly established means that the structure of the organization is sufficient to support the acceptable levels of achievement, properly implemented signifies that the process by which the services are delivered reflects the established norm, and properly evaluated indicates that emphasis is placed on the outcomes of service.[28] Hence, standards may be divided according to the structures, processes, or outcomes that affect patient care.[29]

Structure

Structure standards refer to the conditions and mechanisms that provide support for the actual provision of care. They are the framework that facilitates patient care by defining the rules of the organization and its governance. Examples of structure standards are the mission, philosophy, and goals of the organization, which serve as a foundation for the commitment to quality.

Policies are a critical component of structure. They are the established rules that guide the organization in the delivery of patient care. A unique characteristic of policies is that they are not negotiable. This means that under no circumstances may a policy be modified.[19] If an organization's policy specifies that only registered nurses are permitted to administer IV medications, a licensed practical nurse may not perform the procedure.

Process

Process standards have been described as the ''working'' standards because they describe the functions performed by health care providers in the delivery of patient care. Structure standards specify what may be done, but process standards describe how it is done. As such, process standards focus on the practitioner and include job descriptions, performance standards, procedures, practice guidelines, and protocols.

A *job description* is a written record of the job qualifications, scope of responsibilities, and principal duties. It is a generic instrument that describes the basic functions of the position.[30] *Performance standards* evolve from the job description and define the level of performance required for the job.[28] For example, the job description for an IV nurse may

state that a basic function is performance of venipuncture, but the performance criteria specify that the IV nurse must adhere to aseptic technique, follow established policies and procedures, and demonstrate proficiency in the insertion of peripheral IV catheters.

Procedures involve psychomotor skills performed by health care providers in the delivery of patient care. Written procedures contain a series of precise steps that outline the recommended manner in which the skills should be performed.[30] Some organizations also have *practice guidelines*, which are based on the nursing process and further delineate care delivery. *Protocols* complement procedures and practice guidelines because they provide a basis for clinical decision making in specific patient care issues.[30] For example, the IV nurse follows the written procedure and practice guidelines for performance of the venipuncture, but complies with an established protocol for the use of a local anesthetic at the intended venipuncture site.

Although structure standards are non-negotiable, process standards may be modified based on the decision of the practitioner and as the situation demands.[19] For example, the written procedure specifies that the intended insertion site is to be prepared with povidone-iodine solution prior to venipuncture, but the patient is allergic to iodine. In such a situation, alcohol may be substituted to prepare the intended venipuncture site.

Outcome

Outcome standards concentrate on the end results of patient care. They are patient focused and reflect the desired goals of the care provided.[13] However, outcome standards are usually expressed in negative terms such as mortality rates, infection rates, phlebitis rates, and medication errors. To describe the desired outcomes accurately, positive criteria are preferable. Statements such as patient satisfaction, resolution of infection, control of pain, and maintenance of desired nutritional status better communicate the ultimate goal of patient care.

Because the outcome of care is typically a consequence of how the care was delivered, outcome standards are linked to process standards. For every process standard, there is an associated outcome; the process influences or determines the results to be achieved. For example, preparation of the insertion site, stabilization of the catheter, and rotation of peripheral catheters all influence the outcome of IV nursing care.

Health Care Standards

The delivery of patient care services encompasses three domains—clinical, professional, and administrative. There is a patient who receives the service (clinical domain), the nurse who delivers the service (professional domain), and organizational leaders who manage the service (administrative domain). These three domains parallel the types of standards (outcome, process, and structure). However, terminology that more appropriately describes the measures of quality in health care are standards of care, standards of practice, and standards of governance.[19]

Table 4–2

Examples of Standards of Care and Standards of Practice Regarding Fundamental Aspects of IV Therapy

Aspect of Care	Standard of Care	Standard of Practice
Plan of care	Patient has health care needs identified	Nursing care plan is established within 24 hours of completion of initial patient assessment
Initiation of infusion	Patient has infusion initiated for therapeutic or diagnostic purpose	Therapy is initiated on physician's order using the nursing process
Cannula site preparation	Patient is free of infection related to IV therapy	Peripheral insertion site is aseptically cleansed with antimicrobial solution prior to cannula insertion
Monitoring infusion	Patient receives infusions at prescribed flow rate	Patient assessments are performed at routine intervals and as required during the infusion
Disposal of sharps	Patient is safe from preventable hazards in the environment	Needles and stylets are disposed of in nonpermeable tamper-proof containers
Patient education	Patients have the right to receive information on all aspects of their care	Patients are informed of each treatment in clear, concise terminology

Standards of Care

The recipient of care, the patient, is the topic of the standards of care. The patient expects a predetermined level of care from the health care provider and standards of care describe these expectations and imply the expected outcomes. To measure quality based on expectations, JCAHO has indicated that standards of care must be developed within the organization. The standards may be either generic, addressing patient care throughout the organization, or they may be specific to the care delivered in or by a specialty area.[31] For example, a generic standard of care might state "patients can expect to acquire no infections resulting from nursing care"; a specific standard of care, relative to IV nursing, further stipulates that "patients can expect to receive IV therapy without complications of infection."

Standards of Practice

Standards of practice focus on the provider of care and represent acceptable levels of practice in patient care delivery. Like the standards of care, practice standards address the clinical aspects of patient care services and imply patient outcomes. However, standards of nursing practice define nursing accountability and provide a framework for evaluating professional competency in the delivery of patient care services. They are consistent with valid research findings, national norms, and legal guidelines, and they complement expectations of regulatory agencies. In Table 4–2, fundamental aspects of IV therapy are written as both standards of care and standards of practice.

Based on the premise that nurses, individually and collectively, are responsible and accountable for their practice, professional nursing associations have researched, developed, and published standards of nursing practice. These standardized methods reflect commitment to quality patient care and include both generic and specialty standards of practice.[32] Generic standards, such as the *Standards of Nursing Practice* from the American Nurses' Association, are universal for all types of nursing; specialty standards are applicable to a specific area of practice, such as the *Intravenous Nursing Standards of Practice* by the Intravenous Nurses Society.[33]

Because published standards of nursing practice define criteria relative to nursing accountability and professional competency, they may be adopted by health care organizations. This differs from standards of care, which must be developed and individualized by the organization in which the care is delivered.[13] For example, the *Intravenous Nursing Standards of Practice* defines the autonomy, accountability, and requirements of the specialty practice of IV nursing and are applicable to all practice settings where IV therapy is delivered.[33] The following is an example of the standard of practice relative to hand washing as presented in the 1990 revision of the *Intravenous Nursing Standards of Practice*:[33]

Standard of Practice for Hand Washing*

Principle. Hand washing is a routine infection control practice to decrease the potential risk of contamination and cross infection.

Standard. Hand washing shall be accomplished prior to and immediately after all clinical procedures.

Interpretation. Hand washing shall be a routine practice established in intravenous policy and procedure. Individuals may be carriers of pathogens. Touch contamination is a common cause of transmission of pathogens. The risk of contamination and cross infection is reduced by hand washing. Length of time, place, and method of hand washing shall be considered in achieving adequate infection control. Soap and water are adequate for hand washing; however, an antiseptic solution may be used. A bar of soap is not recommended for use, because it is a potential carrier of bacteria. Wall-mounted dispensers filled with liquid soap-antiseptic are recommended. These dispensers should be readily available and routinely inspected for signs of bacterial growth. Single-unit-of-use soap scrub packets are also recommended.

*From Intravenous Nurses Society: Intravenous Nursing Standards of Practice. Belmont, MA. The Intravenous Nursing Standards of Practice are under revision.

Standards of Governance

JCAHO is placing greater emphasis on the role of the health care organization's leaders in providing the necessary support and resources to improve patient care. Such expectations and responsibilities of managerial and other leaders can be established by means of standards of governance. Standards of governance define the administrative domain and establish parameters to measure the levels of excellence in leadership.[19] An example of a standard of governance is the statement ''organizational leaders will provide an environment that fosters the highest quality of patient care and employee satisfaction.''

MONITORING AND EVALUATING QUALITY: THE TEN-STEP MODEL

Quality cannot be improved unless it is measured and measurement cannot be accomplished unless there is a system to monitor and evaluate the services provided. Numerous monitoring and evaluation systems have been proposed, but most are based on fundamental problem solving techniques. The formats are similar to the nursing process in that they require assessment, planning, implementation, and evaluation.

The most widely accepted framework for quality management is the ten-step model developed by JCAHO. Although the model was originally introduced for traditional quality assurance, it has been expanded to incorporate the concept of continuous quality improvement. The scope of monitoring, evaluation, and problem solving activities now includes emphasis on the role of leadership in improving quality, appraisal of the flow of patient care services, identification of opportunities for improvement, and maintenance of improvements over time.[20] In the foreseeable future, it is expected that the ten-step model will continue to be the cornerstone for quality management in health care.[13] A comprehensive description of the ten steps follows, but the model is summarized in Table 4–3.

Step 1: Assign Responsibility

In the past, health care organizations managed quality by concentrating on the clinical aspects of care. With the transition to quality improvement, health care organizations began to realize that all processes that affect patient care services must be monitored and evaluated. Such organization-wide responsibility for quality management requires that the organization's leaders design an approach to continuous quality improvement that establishes strategic priorities and fosters both intradepartmental and interdepartmental commitment to the concept. Specific quality management activities may be delegated, but the leaders retain overall responsibility for quality improvement.[20]

In addition to the organizational responsibility for quality, there is responsibility for quality within and among the various departments of the organization. As a result, departmental leaders are responsible for the quality initiative within their respective areas and in collaboration with other managers. For example, the vice-president of patient care services is responsible for the continuous improvement of patient care services but must oversee and facilitate patient care activities affected by other departments.

Because there are a variety of patient care services in health care settings, the responsibility may be further delegated along services lines or the delegated responsibility may be unit-based. Examples in the hospital setting include the oncology service line director's responsibility for the care delivered to oncology patients and the responsibility of the director of IV therapy for quality IV nursing care. In both these cases, the delegated responsibility requires that monitoring activities include collaboration with other service lines and departments involved in that aspect of care.

Step 2: Delineate Scope of Care

Monitoring and evaluation of quality require that the elements that constitute care be identified. This determination of the scope of care and services may be based either on the identification of the activities performed in the delivery of care or on the recognition of key functions of the organization.[14]

Activities. Delineation of the scope of care according to the activities performed is the least complicated method. It is based on the who, what, when, and where of the care delivered. Specific components include types of patients served, conditions and diagnoses treated, services or treatments performed, types of practitioners providing care, sites of service, and times of service delivery.[34]

Because health care is typically organized according to department or service lines with this method, each department prepares a separate inventory of activities. For example, an IV therapy department could describe the scope of services as follows:

> The IV department provides intravenous nursing care to medical and surgical patients of all age groups. The primary procedures performed are venipuncture, IV medication administration, transfusion therapy, and maintenance of vascular access devices. Nursing care is provided by registered nurses on a 24-hour basis on nursing units using the services of the IV therapy department.

Key Functions. Key functions of the organization are the managerial, clinical, and support services that affect patient outcomes.[14] They have the greatest impact on the quality of care because they operate across service and departmental lines. JCAHO has stressed the importance of defining the primary functions of the organization because of the interdisciplinary nature of health care.[20]

Using the key function method, it may be established that clinical services such as pain management activities, patient

Table 4–3

JCAHO Ten-Step Model for Monitoring and Evaluation

Step	Description
1	Assign responsibility
2	Delineate scope of care and services
3	Identify important aspects of care and services
4	Determine indicators
5	Establish thresholds for evaluation
6	Collect and organize data
7	Initiate evaluation
8	Take action to improve care and services
9	Assess effectiveness of actions
10	Communicate results

education, and discharge planning are within the scope of services provided by the organization. Each of these functions influences patient outcomes and execution of the activity requires interdepartmental collaboration and coordination.

Step 3: Identify Important Aspects of Care

Activities or functions identified in the delineation of the scope of services serve as the basis for determining the important aspects of care. By prioritizing the aspects of care according to their level of importance to patient care outcomes, the significant aspects of care are identified. JCAHO has defined important aspects of care as those that occur frequently, affect large numbers of patients, produce problems, or place patients at risk. Risk is described as situations in which the care is not properly provided, not provided when indicated, or provided when not indicated.[16, 17] Cost may also be a consideration because of the escalating price of health care and changes in reimbursement.[19]

The four criteria used to determine important aspects of care are usually summarized as high volume, high risk, problem prone, or high cost. If the aspect of care meets three or more of the criteria, it is categorized as extremely important. Extremely important aspects are prioritized in the following order: (1) high risk, problem prone, high volume; (2) high risk, problem prone, high cost; and (3) high risk, high volume, high cost. Aspects of care that meet two of the four criteria are categorized as very important and range, in order of priority, from "high risk, problem prone" to "high volume, high cost."[19] Current JCAHO standards recommend that aspects of care be prioritized and that at least two high-priority aspects of care be selected for each service or major key function.[16, 17] Table 4–4 demonstrates application of the criteria for the prioritization of IV nursing care activities.

Step 4: Identify Indicators

An indicator is a quantitative measure that guides the monitoring and evaluation of important aspects of patient care.

Table 4–4

Example of Categorizing IV Nursing Care Activities*

IV Nursing Care Activities	High Volume	High Risk	Problem Prone	High Cost
Venipuncture	X	X		
Transfusion therapy		X	X	
Administration of antineoplastic agents		X		X
IV medication administration	X	X	X	
Infection control measures	X		X	
Patient education			X	
Monitoring infusions	X		X	
Parenteral nutrition			X	
Patient-controlled analgesia			X	
Epidural analgesia		X		

*Based on this example, two high-priority aspects of IV nursing care are IV medication administration and transfusion therapy.

Indicators do not directly measure quality but are numerical representations of the evaluation of care. As such, indicators serve as predictors of quality to reveal specific issues that warrant further investigation.[35]

Each indicator must be reasonably related to at least one important aspect of care.[16, 17] To accomplish this, representatives of the organization who are involved in the identified aspect of care work as a team of "experts" to develop pertinent indicators for monitoring. Drafted indicators are then evaluated to ensure that they possess five essential characteristics: reliability, validity, measurability, specificity, and relevancy.[19]

- *Reliability* denotes the ability to measure the variable regardless of who is gathering the data, when the data are collected, or from which source the data are obtained.
- *Validity* means that the indicator measures what it is intended to measure. A valid indicator identifies situations in which quality is lacking or confirms circumstances in which quality is present.
- *Measurability* is the ability to translate the important aspects of care into measurable, quantifiable terms to detect the level of quality.
- *Specificity* implies that indicators characterize a specific event. Each indicator must be precise and unique to the event to be measured.
- *Relevancy* requires that the indicator relates to and only to the critical aspect of care being measured.

Types of Indicators

In the monitoring and evaluation of patient care, different types of indicators may be appropriate. The type of indicator selected is determined by what is to be measured. Basically, indicators are characterized as to the type of event, seriousness of the event, or focus of the event.

Type of Event. There is a correlation between the type of event and the criteria that define patient care services. Hence, indicators may be classified as structure, process, or outcome.[35] *Structure indicators* pertain to the framework that provides support for the actual provision of care. For example, a structure indicator may specify "nurses delivering the IV nursing care will be certified IV nurses (CRNIs)." *Process indicators* describe components of the nursing process that are critical to patient outcomes. Pain management for terminal cancer patients is an example of a process indicator. *Outcome indicators* measure the results of the provider's activity in terms of the change that occurs in the patient's status, behavior, or knowledge. For example, patient knowledge may be used as an outcome indicator for patient education.

An outcome indicator required by JCAHO is patient satisfaction.[16, 17] The medical profession has questioned such an outcome measure as a valid means for measuring quality. It has been argued that health care quality involves what is best in the interest of the patient, not simply what the patient wants.[36] In contrast, nursing has endorsed the use of a satisfaction measure if it is comprised of four different functional perspectives. These include health status, knowledge function, skill function, and psychosocial function.[37] When a satisfaction survey includes each of these elements, it offers a comprehensive evaluation of how the care was delivered (processes) and the patient's perceptions of the results (outcomes).

Seriousness of Event. Indicators may be either sentinel or rate-based.[38] *Sentinel indicators* are serious, undesirable, yet unpredictable outcomes of care that require investigation each time the event occurs. An example of a sentinel event indicator is a broken, fractured, or ruptured peripherally inserted central venous catheter. In contrast, *rate-based indicators* pertain to events in which a certain proportion of events represent care. Intense review is only warranted if the rate exceeds the predetermined level or if there is a significant trend. Medication errors, nosocomial infections, and phlebitis rates are examples of rate-based indicators.

Focus of Event. Indicators may measure either the quality or the appropriateness of care.[19] *Quality indicators* are concerned with the effectiveness, efficiency, efficacy, continuity, consistency, and timeliness of care. However, the quality of care may be excellent, but the care may be inappropriate. For example, a total parenteral nutrition solution may be infused as prescribed and without complications, but the patient's nutritional status does not support the use of this therapy. *Appropriateness indicators*, therefore, measure whether the activity that is prescribed and/or performed is truly indicated based on the patient's condition.

Expressing Indicators

An effective indicator guides monitoring and evaluation activities because it signals issues that warrant further investigation. This requires that the indicator be expressed in a manner that quantifies the event. Various formats may be used to express indicators, but the two most frequent designs are indicator statements or ratios of events for a defined population and time frame.[39]

Indicator Statements. Both process and outcome indicators may be written as statements. A process indicator statement describes the nature and sequence of health care activities and may be expressed in terms of the appropriate nursing actions. For example, ''The patient with a newly inserted implanted infusion port will receive instruction regarding care and maintenance of the device prior to discharge from the hospital,'' or ''The nurse documents patient instruction regarding the implanted infusion port in the patient's medical record.'' In contrast, outcome indicator statements describe the results of the health care activities. Examples of outcome statements include ''Patient verbalizes understanding of care of implanted infusion port,'' or ''Patient/significant other demonstrates actions required to access the implanted infusion port prior to discharge.''

Each of the indicators presented in the preceding examples is desirable and represents a specific goal for patient care. However, they are not quantifiable unless every deviation from the stated indicator is fully investigated. An indicator statement is a quantifiable measure for sentinel events because, as a result of the seriousness of such events, each occurrence warrants intense investigation. The sentinel event indicator statement serves as an occurrence screen to trigger further investigation to identify ineffective processes or poor outcomes.[40] Examples of sentinel event indicator statements relative to IV nursing are as follows:

- Occurrence of a hemolytic transfusion reaction
- Home infusion therapy patient with unplanned readmission to the hospital
- Needlestick injury to health care worker
- Extravasation of a vesicant

Ratio of Events. Rate-based indicators may be written as statements. However, unless every deviation from the stated indicator is investigated, they must also be expressed as a quantifiable measure. Quantifying rate-based indicators may be accomplished by expressing them in the form of a ratio that compares the number of events to the defined population. This signifies that a certain proportion of the events are expected based on the current state of knowledge. In the ratio, a statement of the event being assessed is listed as the numerator and a statement of the total population being studied is written as the denominator:[35]

$$\text{Rate-based indicator} = \frac{\text{Number of events}}{\text{Total population}}$$

Expression of rate-based indicators requires that they be further defined as either performance or occurrence measures. Performance measures assess the processes involved in delivery of care. They are sometimes referred to as compliance measures, because they denote conformance with established practice.[35] Because performance measures relate to processes, they are typically labeled process indicators and are expressed as follows:

$$\text{Process indicator} = \frac{\begin{array}{c}\text{Number of times process}\\\text{successfully completed}\end{array}}{\begin{array}{c}\text{Total number of times}\\\text{process performed}\end{array}}$$

In contrast, the intent of occurrence measures is the identification of the consequences of care. The outcome of care is measured in terms of how frequently a particular desirable or undesirable event has occurred.[35] Occurrence measures are regarded as outcome indicators and are written as follows:

$$\text{Outcome indicator} = \frac{\text{Number of occurrences}}{\text{Total number of patients at risk}}$$

Current JCAHO standards specify that at least two relevant indicators be developed for the important aspects of care and service. The indicators need not measure outcomes directly; measures of structure or process may be used if the involved staff believe and can demonstrate that structure or process affects patient care outcomes.[16, 17] However, the simultaneous use of both process and outcome indicators provides a comprehensive evaluation of important aspects of care. Rate-based process indicators assess whether the predetermined level of performance was achieved, whereas rate-based outcome indicators ascertain whether the desired outcomes were realized. Examples of both types of indicators for IV nursing are presented in Table 4–5.

Step 5: Establish Thresholds for Evaluation

A threshold is the line of demarcation between compliance and noncompliance. Compliance indicates conformance to

Table 4-5

Examples of Rate-Based Process and Outcome Indicators

Aspect of Care	Indicator Statement	Type	Ratio of Events (Quantifiable Measure)
IV medication administration	Compliance with IV medication administration procedure	Process	No. of times IV medication procedure followed successfully
			Total no. of doses of IV medication administered
IV medication administration	Occurrence of medication errors	Outcome	No. of IV medication errors
			Total no. of doses of IV medications administered
Patient education	Compliance with patient education standards for long-term venous access devices (VADs)	Process	No. times standard of practice for patient education successfully followed
			Total no. of times standard of practice is used
Patient education	Occurrence of patients adequately prepared to care for VAD at discharge	Outcome	No. of patients who successfully completed VAD education
			Total number of patients who are discharged with long-term VADs

standards; all variables that can be controlled are controlled. Noncompliance signifies a lack of adherence to standards, or that variables cannot be controlled. The threshold for evaluation is a predetermined level of compliance or noncompliance that triggers the need for further investigation.[19] For example, the threshold of compliance in a sentinel event is 100%, because there is no tolerance for error. In a sentinel event, however, the threshold of noncompliance is 0%, meaning that each occurrence must be evaluated.

Thresholds for evaluation of rate-based events are more difficult to determine because they do not deal with the absolutes of 0 and 100%. Establishing the threshold depends on the seriousness of the event and the effect of the event on quality patient care, as well as customer expectations, published research, and baseline data.[13] Each of these factors is considered when determining the realistic level at which all manageable variables may be controlled. For example, if the nationally accepted phlebitis rate is 5% and historical information reveals that the incidence of phlebitis within the organization is between 4.45 and 5.35%, the threshold for evaluation could realistically be set at 5%.

JCAHO suggests that the thresholds for evaluation be written consistently to represent either the levels of compliance or noncompliance.[19] The preceding example illustrated a threshold of noncompliance. A threshold of compliance would concentrate on the absence, not the presence, of phlebitis. Hence, the threshold for evaluation would be set at 95% absence of phlebitis, or 95 out of every 100 patients with a peripheral IV catheter would demonstrate no evidence of phlebitis.

Practical use of thresholds for evaluation requires that they also be directional. Thresholds of noncompliance require further monitoring if the actual results are greater than the threshold. For example, the threshold for evaluation regarding the phlebitis rate would be set at greater than 5%. In contrast, for thresholds of compliance, subsequent monitoring is triggered if the actual results are less than the threshold. For example, if the absence of phlebitis is less than 95%, further investigation is warranted.

Thresholds for evaluation are not static but change as the quality of care continuously improves.[13] For example, if the threshold (of compliance) for evaluation for phlebitis is less than 90% but the actual compliance over the past year was between 94 and 95%, the threshold for evaluation may be increased to 95%. This is a positive approach to thresholds for evaluation because it represents a realistic determination of levels of compliance and demonstrates the ability to improve outcomes over time.

Thresholds are not the only mechanisms that identify levels, patterns, or trends requiring further evaluation. JCAHO has stated that any technique that determines inconsistencies with expected patterns or outcomes may be used. Examples of such techniques include benchmarking (comparison of the organization's performance with that of another organization or national norms), establishing specifications (ranges of acceptable performance), and calculating statistical parameters (mean and standard deviation).[13]

Step 6: Collect and Organize Data

Data must be collected to validate that standards are met, to identify opportunities for improvement, to provide a rationale for the utilization of resources, and to discern trends that warrant further evaluation.[16, 17] The collection is accomplished in a planned, organized, systematic, and ongoing manner so that the necessary information may be analyzed and evaluated efficiently. Typically, data collection forms are used to compile the necessary information. However, if used, such tools need to be simple to understand, expedite recording of the necessary data, and offer a standardized format that may be used for multiple indicators (Fig. 4-2).

Because data collection is a time-consuming effort, data collection tools are not the only method to obtain feedback for ongoing monitoring. JCAHO acknowledges that sources such as existing reports and survey documents may also be used.[20] Examples include patient satisfaction surveys and re-

By: _____	Codes:	Major aspects of care: Patient/family educational needs/interventions
Dates: From _____ to _____	Present/Yes = ✔	Patient outcome: The patient/family can expect to receive education specific to illness/hospitalization
Page _____ of _____ pages	Not present = –	
	Not applicable = NA	Threshold: 90%

Indicators:

1. Documentation reflects educational needs identified and lists interventions to be taken. (90%)
2. Patient/family receives teaching material as appropriate. (90%)
3. Patient/family response to teaching is documented. (90%)
4. Documentation reflects social service, home health or other referral has been requested as appropriate. (90%)
5. Prior to transfer/discharge, patient or significant other can demonstrate or verbalize treatment plan. (85%)
6. Special care needs are documented on careplan and/or interfacility transfer record. (90%)

Ref. No.	Patient I.D.	Demographic data		Indicators						Opportunities for improvement
		Nurse	Pt. room #	1	2	3	4	5	6	
1.										
2.										
3.										
4.										
5.										
6.										
7.										
8.										
9.										
10.										
11.										
12.										
13.										
14.										
15.										

NOTE: These criteria are for screening patient care. They do not constitute a standard of care.

Figure 4–2. Data collection tool.

ports of unusual occurrences, adverse drug reactions, and infection rates.

Prior to collecting the data, a decision must be made as to the frequency of the collection, sampling techniques, and sample size. It is generally recommended that the determination of frequency be based on how often the monitored event occurs, significance of the event, and potential problems associated with the aspect of care.[13] The ongoing nature of monitoring requires planning the collection efforts once the frequency is established. Calendars have proven to be an effective tool for scheduling both data collection and data analysis (Fig. 4–3).

Possible sampling techniques include both probability and nonprobability methods. The probability method is the most scientific because it involves random selection of the sample. By use of numerical tables, each case has an equal chance of selection for the review process. Nonprobability sampling reflects qualitative judgment and does not ensure selection based on chance. Convenience and quota sampling are examples of nonprobability methods.[41]

Sample size is a controversial issue. Because the sample must be representative of the total population under examination, application of the research process is the most accurate means to determine an appropriate sample size. However, some authors have offered general guidelines for sampling. They have suggested a sample size of 5%, or 20 cases (whichever is greater), for routine review, 10%, or 40 cases (whichever is greater), if the threshold for monitoring has been triggered, and 15%, or 60 cases (whichever is greater), for intensive review.[19] Because of the seriousness of a sentinel event, a 100% review is always required.

Data collection may involve either retrospective or concurrent review. Retrospective review entails collection of data after the care has been provided. In the past, such data collections were known as chart audits because they focused on the documentation of care after the patient was discharged. Retrospective reviews are the easiest to perform, but are the least effective in changing practice. In contrast, concurrent reviews are done while patients are still hospitalized or on service. Interviews and observations are examples of concurrent review, and the timeliness of such activities is instrumental in improving the quality of the care delivered.[14]

QUALITY IMPROVEMENT CALENDAR Infusion Monitoring Activities												
Major aspects of care (See abstract for indicators)	Jan	Feb	Mar	Apr	May	Jun	Jul	Aug	Sep	Oct	Nov	Dec
Discharge/transfer preparation	X	X	XO	X	X	XO	X	X	XO	X	X	XO
Patient educational needs/interactions	X	X	XO	X	X	XO	X	X	XO	X	X	XO
Patient safety (medication variances)	X	XO	XO	XO	XO	XO	XO	XO	XO	X	X	XO
Patient safety (falls)	XO	X	XO	X	X	XO	X	X	XO	X	X	XO
Infection control (universal precautions)			XO	O					XO	O		
Nursing process	X	X	XO	X	X	XO	X	X	XO	X	X	XO
Medication administration		XO			XO			XO	XO		XO	

Key   X = Data collection
      O = Data analysis/report to general manager

Figure 4–3. Calendar of quality improvement activities.

Step 7: Evaluate Care

Evaluation of care requires that the collected data be interpreted to determine trends or patterns, identify problems, and recognize opportunities for improvement. During this phase, the current practice is compared with pre-established standards and thresholds to identify variations. Variations are the differences in performance or outcomes related to an important aspect of care, and may be the result of controllable or uncontrollable factors. Controllable variances include system deficiencies, lack of knowledge, or limitations of equipment, and uncontrollable variances are the result of chance or unpredictable events.[19]

The scientific method is used to determine the underlying causes. It is a planned, organized, systematic approach directed at the identification of the causative factors, not the appraisal of individual performance.[13] As a result, there is a comprehensive analysis of the problem or opportunity, instead of reliance on "quick fixes," "knee-jerk" reactions, or "Band-Aid" tactics.

Variations identified during the evaluation of the data may be analyzed by statistical process control tools. These methods for decision making offer organized techniques to describe problems and plan solutions. Some of the techniques most commonly used are the run chart, cause-and-effect diagram, flow chart, and Pareto chart.[14]

Run Chart. A run chart displays the frequency of an event over a period of time. For example, the number of IV medication variances over the year may be documented on a run chart (Fig. 4–4).

Cause-and-Effect Diagram. The cause-and-effect diagram is used to examine all possible factors that may influence a given situation. For example, to solve the problem of delays

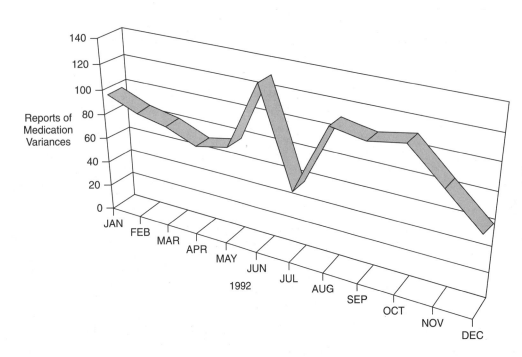

Figure 4–4. Run chart of medication variances for 1992.

in IV medication administration, a cause-and-effect diagram may be used (Fig. 4–5). As demonstrated in the example, the factors are grouped under the categories of management, manpower, materials, methods, and machines. Sometimes the diagram is referred to as a fishbone diagram because of its shape, or an Ishikawa diagram for its originator, Kaoru Ishikawa.

Flow Chart. A flow chart graphically displays the sequence of events required in a particular process. For example, the steps involved in the administration of a transfusion may be represented on a flow chart (Fig. 4–6).

Pareto Chart. On a Pareto chart, data is displayed in ranking order to determine priorities. For example, a Pareto chart may be used to identify and prioritize nursing activities performed by the IV team (Fig. 4–7).

Step 8: Take Action to Improve Care

Once the cause of the variance or opportunity for improvement has been identified, appropriate actions must be initiated. Improvements in quality require that the endeavors be carefully planned prior to initiation. This can be accomplished by the use of a written action plan that details the issue, desired outcome, target date, actions, projected completion dates, and responsible persons (Fig. 4–8). Such a document is effective because it documents what is expected,

who is responsible, what action is to be implemented, and when the actions are to be completed.[19]

Several rules must be followed in the development of action plans. First, there must be input from individuals responsible for the implementation. For example, when IV nursing activities are included in a nursing productivity system, the IV nurse must be involved in the project development. Second, the plan must be specific to the issue, but realistic and flexible. For example, if the issue is medication administration delay, specific steps must be identified to increase the timeliness of response, but the steps must be achievable and allow for alterations based on clinical judgment. Third, planned actions and outcomes must be timed, but the time span should not be excessive.[19] Establishing the target date as ''ongoing'' is never acceptable.

In health care, planned actions for quality improvement usually focus on four areas. The first area is education. Individuals responsible for assigned actions may require additional skills or knowledge to correct a problem or implement the innovation. However, it must be cautioned that education of the staff is not always the appropriate action. Often it is presumed that lack of compliance is the result of a knowledge deficit; in reality, the staff may be knowledgeable but chose not to conform to the established practice. For this reason, the second focus of planned action is employee development. If the cause of the problem is lack of compliance with established practice, actions must be taken to facilitate the growth and development of the individuals. The third area for emphasis is communication. Information regarding

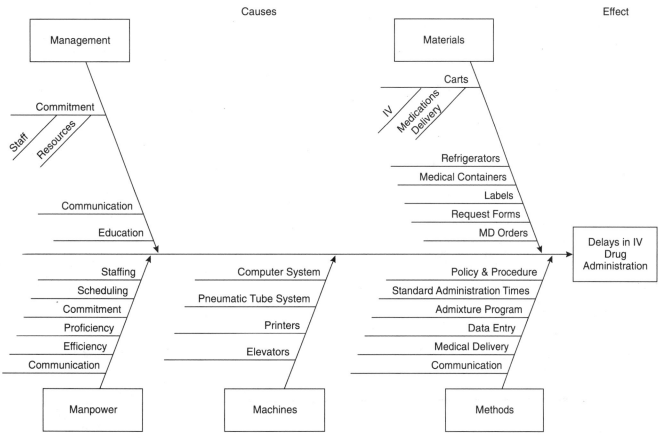

Figure 4–5. Cause-and-effect diagram of delays in IV drug administration in a hospital setting.

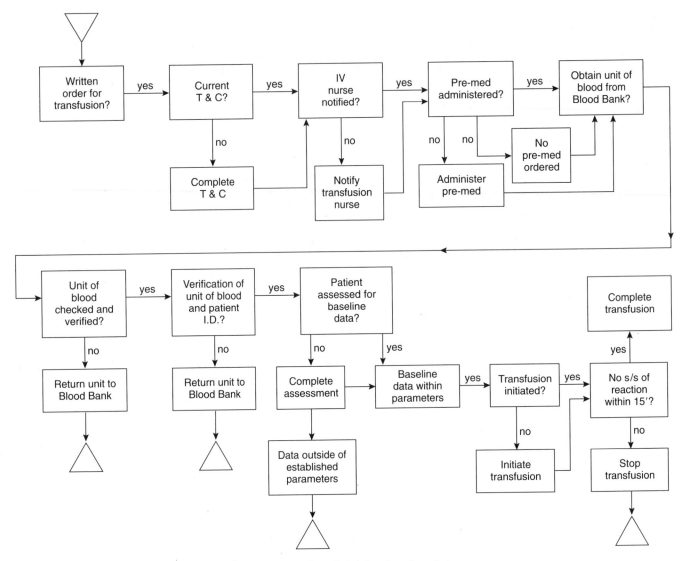

Figure 4–6. Flow chart of administration of transfusion.

monitoring and evaluation and the resultant action plan must be shared with all those involved in that aspect of care. Strategies for change are the final area that must be considered. The ultimate goal of an action plan is to effect the actual change.

Strategies for change need to be based on the change theory, and must recognize that individuals prefer the status quo to change. The change process consists of three stages known as unfreezing, moving, and, refreezing. The initial stage, unfreezing, requires that bonds that support the present system be weakened. The process of consciousness raising promotes dissatisfaction with the status quo and recognition of the need for change. In the second stage, moving, opposing forces create cognitive dissonance within the individuals affected by the change. There is a lack of agreement between the individuals' beliefs and their actions; the individual is performing as required by the change, yet continues to believe that the previous method is preferable. It is in the third stage, refreezing, that the actual change is incorporated into the individuals' belief system, and the actions representing the change then become the status quo.[42]

Change is difficult and can only be realized if there is a desire for change. Nurses involved in IV nursing prior to universal precautions had difficulty in adapting to the use of gloves for venipuncture and in learning not to recap needles. Changes in these practices occurred because there was a desire for change. Granted, the desire for change was stimulated by governmental regulations, but the change was the result of a conscious effort on the part of the nurses.

Step 9: Assess Actions and Document Improvement

The quality improvement plan may involve elaborate activities and the consumption of valuable resources, but this does not guarantee that the desired outcome will be achieved. Just as the nursing process relies on evaluation for continued revision of the plan of care, quality management requires that there be a determination of the effectiveness of the actions for further revision and refinement of the action plan.

Planned actions may be assessed either concurrently or

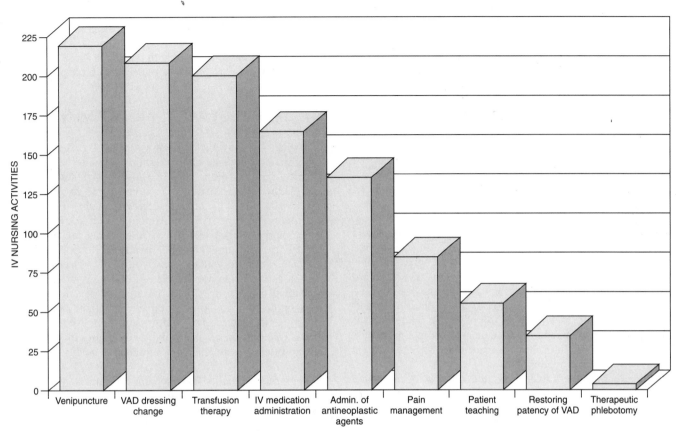

Figure 4–7. Pareto chart of IV nursing activities performed in 1992.

ISSUE	DESIRED OUTCOME	TARGET DATE	ACTIONS	COMPLETION DATE		RESPONSIBLE PERSON	ACTUAL OUTCOME
				PROJECTED	ACTUAL		

Figure 4–8. Action plan format.

retrospectively. Concurrent evaluation occurs during implementation of the plan to determine whether the interim objectives have been accomplished. In contrast, retrospective evaluation is performed following completion of the planned actions to ascertain whether the desired outcomes were realized.[14]

Retrospective evaluation of the action plan usually involves remonitoring the original indicator to determine the results. Because desired outcomes are not guaranteed, three different levels of achievement may have occurred. First, the desired results may be achieved. This can signify that the planned actions were successful, but monitoring is continued to ensure that the improvements are sustained over time. Second, the desired results may not be achieved, but there has been considerable progress. In this case, the problem, data, causes, actions, and target dates need to be re-evaluated and the action plan revised accordingly. Third, the desired results may not be attained, but achievement appears doubtful given the current state of circumstances. The standard may be unattainable, the thresholds for evaluation may be unrealistic, or the planned actions may be unachievable.[19] Examples include a standard of 0% phlebitis, a threshold of 100% for a patient education indicator, or an unexpected reduction in staff. In each case, there must be reassessment and revision of the action plan.

Regardless of the actual results, they must be documented. It has often been stated, ''If it's not documented, it's not done.'' This is as true for quality management as it is for nursing. Accreditation standards, legal requirements, and professional accountability necessitate that there be documented evidence of the intent of actions and the results. Therefore, a complete action plan contains evidence of the actual outcomes (see Fig. 4–8).

Step 10: Communicate Information

An effective quality management program is based on communication. Relevant information must be forwarded to the leaders of the organization who are ultimately responsible for quality improvement, and shared with all affected individuals. Current quality management literature offers no standardized format for reporting quality improvement activities, but two possible methods are written reports and organization-wide quality management committees.[13] The organizational leaders may receive the information by means of written reports. Each report needs to be a clear, concise description of the issue, relevant data, conclusions, recommendations, and evaluation of the effectiveness of the action plan.[19] Dissemination of information to the affected individuals can be accomplished through organization-wide quality management committees. Interaction of the committee members fosters interdisciplinary collaboration, reduces the possibility of duplication of monitoring efforts by other services, and encourages detection of additional opportunities for improvement.

Confidentiality is an issue that must be considered when planning how to communicate the relevant information. To safeguard the privacy of patients and the rights of health care workers, most organizations consider their quality management program confidential. Hence, communication regarding quality of service is limited to information pertinent to the maintenance of a general awareness of quality issues, prevention of similar quality problems in the future, and identification of opportunities for improvement. Specific information that identifies individuals is shared only with those responsible for direct action to resolve the identified problems.

INTEGRATED QUALITY MANAGEMENT

As quality management continues to evolve, the trend is to integrate monitoring and evaluation activities within the health care organization.[14] JCAHO hospital standards specify that infection control, utilization review, and risk management be included in the organization-wide quality assessment and improvement activities.[17] Although each activity has a distinct purpose, they all indicate trends that are useful in identifying opportunities for improvement. Infection control is directed at the surveillance and control of the transmission of disease, utilization review relates to the appropriate use of the patient care services, and risk management focuses on the identification and prevention of potential risks to the patient, health care worker, and organization. Merging these various functions under the umbrella of quality management services offers a comprehensive approach to quality improvement.

Integration of quality management activities is not new to IV nursing. Monitoring and evaluation of IV nursing care has always included trending of IV-related infections, determination of appropriateness of IV therapy, and prevention of IV-associated risks and complications. In fact, one of the pioneers of IV quality management, Cheryl Gardner, endorsed comprehensive monitoring as early as 1981. The current trend of integration of infection control, utilization review, risk management, and other quality management activities within health care organizations reduces the complexity of data collection and ensures that all aspects of quality IV nursing are evaluated.

Quality management integration also poses a challenge for IV nursing. As stated earlier, JCAHO advocates that quality assessment and improvement activities be interdisciplinary and cross-service rather than compartmentalized within departments or services. In the hospital setting, this means that the IV quality management program can no longer be limited to care provided by the IV team. Patients receive IV nursing care on units and in departments other than those serviced by the IV team. Examples include the critical care unit and emergency, surgery, and radiology departments. Integration of quality assessment and improvement activities requires that the IV team assume an active role in working with others to identify opportunities for improvements in IV nursing care throughout the organization.

Example of Integrated Quality Management for IV Nursing

Assign Responsibility. The executive for patient care services is responsible for all quality management activities relative to patient care but delegates the monitoring and evaluation of IV nursing care to the supervisor of the IV team.

Delineate Scope of Care. The IV supervisor and representatives from all areas delivering IV nursing care determine the scope of IV nursing services.

Identify Important Aspects of Care. It is determined that, because of the potential risks and complications associated with IV therapy, an important aspect of care is patient safety.

Identify Indicators. Insertion of peripheral IV cannulas is identified as a significant component of patient safety. To define the indicators further, the *Intravenous Nursing Standards of Practice* are reviewed and adopted as the standard for peripheral IV cannula insertion. The indicators, based on the standards, measure the incidence of phlebitis and levels of adherence to the infection control measures of adequate preparation of the site, stabilization of the catheter, and application of a sterile dressing.

Establish Thresholds for Evaluation. Because the nationally accepted phlebitis rate is 5% or less, this is accepted as the threshold of noncompliance. However, the thresholds need to be written in a positive manner, so the threshold (of compliance) for no evidence of phlebitis is set at 95%. Determination of the thresholds for evaluation regarding adherence to the infection control measures is more difficult because there are no data-driven percentages or ratios. Therefore, the threshold is based on the representative's knowledge and experience, and it is determined that compliance with infection control measures of less than 97% is the threshold for evaluation. The goal is still 100% compliance, but the indicator is realistic.

Collect and Organize Data. Data collection tools are developed, and the indicators are monitored for 1 month and compared with the predetermined thresholds. It is determined that the absence of phlebitis is 98%, but compliance with infection control measures is 94%. Because the variance in infection control measures is outside the established threshold, further evaluation is triggered.

Evaluate Care. Evaluation of the data indicates that the intent of the standards is met but opportunities for improvement are evident. First, there is a lack of consistency in the type of dressing applied to the IV site, and many of the dressings will not remain in place on diaphoretic patients. Second, the type of applicator used to prepare the intended site influences the selection of the prepping solution. Povidone-iodine is the preferred prepping solution, but swab stick applicators are only available on the nursing units; the other areas are using alcohol pads. Third, various taping techniques are used to secure IV cannulas, and some appear to be more effective than others.

Take Actions to Improve Care. The planned actions focus on the opportunities for improvement. Specific actions include standardization of IV dressings that are effective for all types of patients, selection of cost-effective, user-friendly prepping solution applicators for use by all staff inserting peripheral IV cannulas, and consensus on acceptable taping techniques. Once these decisions are reached, education of the staff is initiated regarding application of the selected dressings, site preparation using the preferred applicator, and established taping techniques.

Assess Effectiveness of Actions. Monitoring of the outcome indicator (phlebitis) and the process indicator (compliance with infection control measures) continues. The data demonstrate a decline in phlebitis rates and higher compliance with standards of practice.

Communicate Results. Ongoing reports of monitoring and evaluation are prepared and forwarded to the patient care executive and the hospital quality management council.

Longitudinal Review

The major settings for IV nursing care have expanded from the hospital to a variety of alternate practice sites including ambulatory care, home health, and extended care. IV nursing care may be limited to any one of these settings but, more typically, patients continue to receive IV therapy as they move across the continuum of health care. For example, a 68-year-old patient is admitted to the hospital for cellulitis of the foot and is prescribed a 21-day course of IV antibiotics. On the fourth day of therapy, it is determined that he no longer requires acute care. Because the administration of IV antibiotics is considered skilled care, the patient is transferred to a skilled nursing facility until the course of therapy is completed. After 2 weeks, the patient decides he can function independently and returns home. Arrangements are made for a home health agency to administer the remaining doses of the antibiotic.

In this scenario, the patient received IV nursing care in three different practice settings. As he progressed from one level of care to the next, he had the same IV nursing care needs, but delivery of services may have varied and decisions made at one level had an impact on the next. Evaluation of the quality of care, in this situation, warrants evaluation of care across the continuum, a process known as longitudinal review.[13] In such a review, quality management is directed at the integration of health care services required by the patient. The quality indicators would therefore focus on the selection of an IV cannula appropriate for the duration of therapy, professional IV nursing collaboration as the patient progresses from one level of care to the next, and the ultimate outcome of the therapy.

Because of the continuum of care, an influential governmental report has suggested that, to ensure excellence in health care, episodes of illness be evaluated regardless of when or where the care was provided.[43] Quality is not site-specific; it requires integration and collaboration among practice settings. Therefore, quality management continues to evolve, and longitudinal reviews may emerge as the next phase in the quality improvement process.

References

1. Freeland B. Moving toward continuous quality improvement. JIN 1992; 15:278–282.
2. Ives JR. Quality initiates in health care. Boston Nurse News 1993; 2:5–6.
3. Roberts JS, Coale JG, Redman RR. A history of the Joint Commission on Accreditation of Hospitals. JAMA 1989; 238:936–940.
4. Graham NO. Quality assurance in hospitals: Strategies for assessment and implementation. Rockville, MD: Aspen, 1990.
5. Bradford L. Total quality management: Doing it wrong the first time. Med Interface 1992; 4:61–66.
6. Kibbie P. The National Association of Quality Assurance Professionals,

Utilization Review and Risk Management: A Study Guide and Primer. Chicago: National Association of Quality Assurance Professionals, 1986.

7. Gillen TR. Deming's 14 points and hospital quality: Responding to the consumers' demand for the best value health care. J Nurs Qual Assur 1988; 2:70–78.

8. Joint Commission on Accreditation of Healthcare Organizations (JCAHO). 1991 Accreditation Manual for Hospitals. Chicago: JCAHO, 1990.

9. Juran JM. Juran on Leadership for Quality. New York: Free Press, 1989.

10. Crosby PB. Quality Is Free: The Art of Making Quality Certain. New York: New American Library, 1979.

11. Deming WE. Out of Crisis. Cambridge, MA: MIT Center for Advanced Engineering Study, 1989.

12. Walton M. Deming Management at Work. New York: Putnam, 1990.

13. Meisenheimer CG. Improving Quality: A Guide to Effective Programs. Gaithersburg, MD: Aspen, 1992.

14. Koch MW, Fairly TM. Integrated Quality Management. St. Louis: C. V. Mosby, 1993.

15. Joint Commission on Accreditation of Healthcare Organizations. Agenda for Change. Chicago: JCAHO, 1990.

16. Joint Commission on Accreditation of Healthcare Organizations. Accreditation Manual for Home Care, 1993. Chicago: JCAHO, 1992.

17. Joint Commission on Accreditation of Healthcare Organizations. Accreditation Manual for Hospitals, 1992. Chicago: JCAHO, 1991.

18. O'Leary DS. CQI: A step beyond QA. Qual Rev Bull 1991; 17:4–5.

19. Katz J, Green E. Managing Quality: A Guide to Monitoring and Evaluating Nursing Services. St. Louis: C. V. Mosby, 1992.

20. Joint Commission on Accreditation of Healthcare Organizations. Transitions: From QA to CQI. Chicago: JCAHO, 1992.

21. Berwick DM. Continuous improvement as an ideal in health care. N Engl J Med 1989; 320:53–57.

22. O'Leary D, Ripple H. Responding to harsh criticism of the JCAHO. Nurs Econ 1989; 7:126–128.

23. Milakovich ME. Creating a total quality health care environment. Health Care Manage Rev 1991; 16:9–20.

24. Milakovich ME. Total quality management for public service productivity improvement. Public Productivity Manage Rev 1990; 14:19–32.

25. Labovich GH. Managing Quality and Productivity in Healthcare. Burlington, MA: Organizational Dynamics, 1988.

26. Labovich GH. Keeping your internal customers satisfied. Wall Street J; July 6, 1987.

27. Crosby PB. Let's Talk Quality. New York: McGraw-Hill, 1990.

28. Marker CG. The Marker Model for nursing standards: Implications for nursing administration. Nurs Admin Q 1988; 12:4–12.

29. Donabedian A. Structure, process, and outcome standards. Am J Public Health 1969; 59:1833.

30. Gillies DA. Nursing Management: A Systems Approach, 2nd ed. Philadelphia: W. B. Saunders, 1989.

31. Joint Commission on Accreditation of Healthcare Organizations. Implementation of the Revised Standards to Nursing Care, 1990, Workshop Materials. Chicago: JCAHO, 1990.

32. Thompson MW, Hylka SC, Shaw CF. Systematic monitoring of generic standards of patient care. J Nurs Qual Assur 1988; 2:9–15.

33. Intravenous Nurses Society. Intravenous Nursing Standards of Practice. Belmont, MA: Intravenous Nurses Society, 1990.

34. Joint Commission on Accreditation of Healthcare Organizations. The Joint Commission Guide to Quality Assurance. Chicago: JCAHO, 1988.

35. Williams AD. Development and application of clinical indicators in nursing. J Nurs Care Qual 1991; 6:1–5.

36. Donabedian A. Continuity and change in the quest for quality. Clin Perform Qual Health Care 1993; 1:9–16.

37. Wilson AA, Hartnett M, Ferrari R. Outcome measurement from the functional status perspective. Home Health Care Nurse 1992; 10:32–46.

38. Joint Commission on Accreditation of Healthcare Organizations. Characteristics of clinical indicators. Qual Rev Bull 1989; 15:333.

39. Schroeder P. Process and outcome integrated in care of MI patients. Nurs Quality Connect 1991; 8:6.

40. Tan MW. Occurrence screens: A risk and quality control tool for intravenous nurses. JIN 1990; 13:308–311.

41. Polit DF, Hungler BP. Nursing Research: Principles and Methods, 4th ed. New York: J. B. Lippincott, 1991.

42. Bennis W. The Planning of Change. New York: Holt, Rinehart & Winston, 1969.

43. General Accounting Office. Quality Assurance: A Comprehensive National Strategy for Health Care Is Needed. Washington, DC: GAO/PEMD-90-14BR, 1990.

CHAPTER 5 Legal Aspects of Intravenous Nursing

Donna R. Baldwin, MSN, CRNI
Donna Lee Mantel, Esq., BSN, RN, JD

Nowhere in professional nursing has the role of the nurse grown as fast, as effectively, and as favorably as in intravenous (IV) nursing. The development of IV nursing reflects a general trend in the nursing profession. Nurses today monitor complex physiologic data, operate sophisticated life-saving equipment, and coordinate the delivery of a patient's health care services. More importantly, nurses now have responsibility for exercising discriminating judgment. No longer do nurses blindly follow physicians' orders but they collaborate with the physician to ensure that their patients receive the highest quality of care.

The expanding responsibility of IV nurses has advantages as well as disadvantages. The nurse's emerging role offers rewards such as intellectual stimulation and professional satisfaction. However, the heightened status also means increased legal risks for the nurse and the added potential for liability. It is therefore the intent of this chapter to broaden awareness of the legal aspects of IV nursing. Four major topics are discussed: the legal standard of care, legal terminology, principles of the legal process, and risk management strategies.

LEGAL STANDARD OF CARE

Nurses have a duty to provide reasonable, prudent patient care as required by the situation. The care delivered by the nurse must comply with what is expected, given the set of circumstances in which the care is provided. This is known as the legal standard of care.

The legal standard of care is used to evaluate the quality of nursing conduct and has several important characteristics.[1] First, the standard of care is a reasonable expectation of the nursing care. This means that it represents the typical performance of a professional nurse who has special knowledge and skill beyond that of an ordinary person. For example, an IV nurse would be expected to calculate the flow rate for an IV infusion. Second, the standard of care is measurable. The care can be evaluated based on what a similarly prepared nurse would do in the same situation. As an example, all nurses who have earned the credentials "CRNI" would be evaluated by the same standard as a result of the successful completion of the IV nursing certification examination. Third, the standard of care is valid based on where the care was delivered. There is variability based on the state where the care is delivered, thus influencing the established standard by which the care may be evaluated. An illustration of such variability is the insertion of a peripherally inserted central catheter (PICC). Until recently, some states did not consider this procedure within the realm of nursing practice, whereas other states allowed it to be performed by professional nurses. Fourth, the standard of care must be applicable based on the current state of knowledge. Standards evolve with increasing knowledge and experience, so the care must be evaluated within the historical context of when the care was delivered. For example, the 1990 revision of the *Intravenous Nursing Standards of Practice* is applicable only to IV nursing care delivered since this document was published.

Standards can be voluntary, such as those promulgated by professional groups, or they may be mandated legislatively. Nursing, like most other professions, is regulated by these dual controls, both of which are aimed at providing quality patient care. Professional standards are the forerunners of legal standards. What has become the customary, usual nursing practice, as defined by the profession, later translates into the legal duty the nurse owes to the patient.

The nurse must demonstrate a familiarity with standards to deliver safe, competent nursing care. However, in IV nursing, a myriad of standards are applicable, depending on the facts and issues involved in the situation. The location where the care is provided, the qualifications of the nurse, the procedure performed, and the type of product involved all influence the applicability of the standard. As a guideline, the legal standards of care for IV nursing are derived from four sources: federal statutes, state statutes, professional standards, and institutional standards. A summary of the sources of the legal standards of care is presented in Table 5–1.

Federal Statutes

Federal statutes are laws that have been enacted by Congress and are published in the *Federal Register*. The most applicable federal statutes, relative to IV nursing, concern occupational safety and health, infection control, environmental hazards, medical device safety, control of drug abuse, federally funded insurance programs, and patient self-determination.

Table 5–1

Legal Standards of Care Relative to IV Nursing
. . . .

Source	Agency	Example
Federal statutes	OSHA	Hazard Communication Standard
		Work-Practice Guidelines for Personnel Dealing with Cytotoxic Drugs
		Occupational Safe Exposure to Bloodborne Pathogens: Final Rule
	FDA	Safe Medical Device Act of 1990
	DEA	Controlled Substance Act
State statutes	Department of Health	Licensure of health care facilities
	Board of Nursing	Nurse Practice Act
Professional standards	JCAHO	*Accreditation Manual for Hospitals*
		Accreditation Manual for Home Care
	ANA	*Standards of Nursing Practice*
	INS	*Intravenous Nursing Standards of Practice*
	AABB	*Technical Manual*
	ECRI	*Health Devices* (journal)
Institutional standards	Department of Nursing	Nursing policies
		Nursing procedures

Occupational Safety and Health. By law, the Occupational Safety and Health Administration (OSHA) has the authority both to establish and enforce regulations to promote job safety and protect the health of workers. This has resulted in the Hazard Communication Standard or ''right to know'' law, which requires that all employees be informed of the hazardous potential of chemicals encountered in the work place.[2] Hence, IV nurses must be trained as to warning labels on hazardous chemical containers used within the health care organization and the use of material safety data sheets (MSDSs).

In 1986, OSHA addressed the hazardous potential of cytotoxic drugs with the *Work-Practice Guidelines for Personnel Dealing With Cytotoxic Drugs.*[3] Cytotoxic drugs, including many of the antineoplastic agents, have genotoxic, mutagenic, or teratogenic potential. Because such drugs may be potentially harmful to the health care worker, protective equipment is required to prevent skin exposure and aerosolization of the drug. OSHA recommendations include the use of a biologic safety cabinet to prepare cytotoxic drugs, the use of surgical latex gloves and a lint-free, long-sleeved, cuffed, nonpermeable gown for drug administration, and special procedures in the event of a drug spill.[3]

To protect health care workers from human immunodeficiency virus (HIV) infection OSHA, in 1987, expanded the interpretation of its ''general duty clause.'' OSHA originally used precautions issued by the Centers for Disease Control and Prevention (CDC) as the basis for compliance interpretation. As a result, IV nurses were required to comply with universal precautions to prevent exposure to HIV. In 1991, OSHA established the standard entitled *Occupational Safe Exposure to Bloodborne Pathogens,* which expands on universal precautions and addresses the risk of occupational exposure to bloodborne pathogens, including both HIV and hepatitis B virus (HBV). The standard specifies that all body secretions can be potentially infectious and that personnel having contact with patients must adhere to strict guidelines.[5] These precautions are a combination of engineering and work practice controls, and compliance with the guidelines are subject to comprehensive enforcement procedures.[4] The following summarizes the rules the IV nurse must follow to minimize or eliminate the risk of exposure to bloodborne pathogens:

Regulations Regarding Occupational Exposure to Bloodborne Pathogens[4]

Universal Precautions. Universal precautions are based on the premise that blood and certain body fluids (e.g., mucus, saliva, urine, feces, drainage) are considered potentially infectious. Training must be conducted in a manner appropriate to the employees' educational backgrounds so that they understand this concept.

Hepatitis B Vaccinations. If an employee is exposed to blood on the average of at least once per month, the employer must offer hepatitis B vaccine to the employee free of charge.

Sharps Disposal. Contaminated needles and sharps must be disposed of in puncture-resistant, leak-proof containers that are easily accessible and appropriately labeled.

Gloves. Vinyl or latex gloves must be worn if exposure to blood or body fluids is anticipated. The gloves must be of appropriate quality for the procedure to be performed and of appropriate size for the health care worker. If the employee is allergic to standard gloves, hypoallergenic gloves must be provided by the employer.

Protective Equipment. Equipment such as gowns, masks, and eye protectors must be available and used if exposure to skin, eyes, mouth, or clothing is anticipated.

Hazard Communication. Infectious waste must be labeled ''Biohazard'' to prevent accidental injury or exposure.

Infection Control. The CDC was established in 1946, under the Public Health Service (PHS), to prevent disease by means of surveillance, research, and demonstration projects.[5] Although the purpose of this agency is not to regulate health, the CDC is responsible for providing guidance in the form of recommendations, which are considered voluntary standards. An example was the issuance of guidelines for the prevention of intravascular infections in 1978. Sometimes the voluntary guidelines issued by the CDC may be adopted by a federal agency and, in effect, become regulations. Such was the case when OSHA adopted the universal precautions developed by the CDC for compliance interpretation.

Environmental Protection. The Environmental Protection Agency (EPA) is a federal regulatory agency responsible for overseeing the enforcement of laws enacted to protect the environment. There are five federal laws administered by the EPA that have particular importance in health care: (1) Toxic Substance Control Act (TSCA), which grants EPA control over chemical hazards; (2) Resource Conservation and Recovery Act (RCRA), whereby the EPA tracks the movement of hazardous waste from creation to disposal, or "cradle to grave"; (3) Medical Waste Tracking Act (MWTA), which grants the EPA authority to establish practices for the handling and disposal of infectious waste; (4) Comprehensive Environmental Response, Comprehension and Liability Act (CERCLA), whereby the EPA has the authority to implement and finance the cleanup of hazardous waste; and (5) Superfund Amendments and Reauthorization Act (SARA III), which focuses on the community's "right to know" regarding hazardous materials.[6–8]

Medical Device Safety. Since 1938, the Food and Drug Administration (FDA) has been responsible for the regulation of products, such as food, cosmetics, prescription and over-the-counter medications, biologic agents, and medical devices to ensure that they are safe and effective for their intended purposes.[9] With enactment of the Safe Medical Device Act of 1990, hospitals, ambulatory surgical facilities, nursing homes, and outpatient treatment facilities are legally required to report to the FDA whether a medical device may have contributed to the serious injury, serious illness, or death of a patient in the facility. The term "device" is broadly defined and may include IV-related equipment such as catheters, solution containers, and electronic infusion devices.[10] Home health care is currently excluded, but the FDA may expand interpretation of this standard in the future. However, it is the IV nurse's professional responsibility, regardless of the practice setting, to inspect product integrity prior to use and report any suggested or potential medical device problems. Guidelines for reporting product problems to the FDA are listed in Table 5–2.

Control of Drug Abuse. The Comprehensive Drug Abuse Prevention and Control Act, also known as the Controlled Substances Act, was passed in 1970. The purpose of the act was to provide for the control of drug abuse and the enforcement of its provisions by the FDA and the Drug Enforcement Agency (DEA) of the Department of Justice. By law, controlled substances are classified according to five schedules based on the potential for abuse, accepted medical uses, and potential for physical or psychologic dependence. The DEA, however, has the authority to reschedule drugs, schedule a previously unlisted drug, or remove a drug from the schedule.[11] IV nurses must be aware of the schedules and subsequent revisions because of the stringent requirements regarding the handling, storage, and documentation of controlled drugs.

Federally Funded Insurance Programs. The Health Care Financing Administration (HCFA) is a federal agency that was created in 1977 to administer the Medicare program and the federal portion of the Medicaid program. Because the HCFA is responsible for ensuring the quality of health care for beneficiaries participating in these federally funded health insurance programs, the agency sets standards for health care providers receiving Medicare-Medicaid reimbursement. Nurses employed by such providers must be aware of, and comply with, the applicable standards, which are commonly referred to as HCFA regulations.

Patient Self-Determination. The Patient Self-Determination Act of 1990 requires that all health care providers ac-

Table 5–2
Product Problem Reporting Program

When to report?
Problems with medical devices should be reported if the event observed involves, or has the potential to cause, a death, serious injury, or life-threatening malfunction. This includes problems such as

- User error is the cause (the design of the device or unclear/incomplete labeling may have contributed to the problem).
- A decision is made to no longer use the device because of a malfunction that has occurred.
- Repeated repairs fail to solve the problem.
- Design or repair changes by the manufacturer have adversely affected the performance, safety, or efficacy of the device.
- The problem was the result of incompatibility between devices of different manufacturers and labeling failed to warn the user of this potential for problems.
- The malfunction results in prolonged hospitalization, readmission, or repeated surgical procedures.

What to report?
A complete description of the problem and information regarding the device needs to be submitted, including

- Product name.
- Manufacturer's name and address.
- Identification numbers of the device (lot number, model number, serial number, expiration date).
- Problem noted (including any actual or potential adverse effects).
- Name, title, and practice specialty of the user of the device.

How to report?
Problems are reported to the Medical Device and Laboratory Product Problem Reporting Program (PRP), which is administered by the United States Pharmacopeial Convention, Inc. (USP) under contract between the USP and the FDA. Reports are accepted by USP via a toll-free telephone call to (800) 638-6725; in Maryland, call collect, (301) 881-0256. Reports may also be submitted in writing, using the PRP form, and mailed to

United States Pharmacopeia
12601 Twinbrook Parkway
Rockville, MD 20853

cepting Medicare and Medicaid payments provide written information regarding advance directives. An advance directive is a document by which an adult patient may legally decide about future medical treatment. The information is provided at the time of admission to the facility, and it recognizes the patient's rights as a competent adult to decide about the use of do-not-resuscitate (DNR) orders and the withdrawal of life-sustaining equipment.[12]

State Statutes

A *jurisdiction* is a legally established geographic area, such as a state. Variations exist among state statutes because each state government may enact laws specific for that geographic area. A state cannot enact a law that conflicts with federal laws, but it may pass additional regulations.[13] The primary types of state statutes that affect the delivery of IV nursing care are the Nurse Practice Acts, requirements for licensure of nurses, joint policy statements, and licensing of health care facilities.

Nurse Practice Acts. The Nurse Practice Act defines the practice of professional and licensed practical nursing within the state. Although each state has a Nurse Practice Act that describes the nurse's role and function, the definition of nursing is typically generalized. This allows the employer to delineate additional functions and activities that the nurse may perform during employment.

Relative to IV nursing, a state Nurse Practice Act may offer specific guidelines. Some states publish standards in a general language; the subsequent evaluation and approval of specific criteria for nursing behavior is provided in bulletins or newsletters.

Requirements for Nurse Licensure. Each Nurse Practice Act specifies that the nurse must be licensed to practice nursing within the state. The minimum requirements for licensure are established by the State Board of Nursing. The State Board of Nursing is also empowered to suspend or revoke the license of any nurse for violation of the specified norms of conduct for that state. For example, the nurse must meet the minimum requirements to be licensed as a registered nurse in the state of New York, but the license may be revoked if the nurse fails to comply with New York's established rules of conduct.

Joint Policy Statements. When questions arise regarding the professional responsibility of nurses to perform specific therapeutic procedures and the questions cannot be answered by existing state statutes, a joint policy statement may be issued. Sponsors of joint policy statements include the state nursing association, the medical society, and the state hospital association.[14]

Licensing of Health Care Facilities. Each state has a Department of Health that sets standards for the licensing of health care facilities within the state. Although these standards are generally directed toward the physical facilities, qualifications of employees, and maintenance of records, they are interrelated with the nursing process. For example, the state health department may mandate how and where medications are to be stored, and the nurse's conduct must not violate these standards.

Professional Standards

Professional standards are not merely the minimum criteria enacted by the legislature but represent an attempt by a peer group to establish a level of competency that is expected by the profession.[15] (Additional information on professional standards is provided in Chapter 4, Quality Management.)

In health care, the professional standards may apply to the entire industry, or they may pertain only to a specific profession or specialty. The accreditation standards published by the Joint Commission on Accreditation of Healthcare Organizations (JCAHO) exemplify national health care industry standards. In contrast, specific standards that affect IV nursing have been developed by the American Nurses Association (ANA), the Intravenous Nurses Society (INS), the American Association of Blood Banks (AABB), and the American Society of Hospital Pharmacists (ASHP). Criteria developed by the Association for the Advancement of Medical Instrumentation (AAMI) and the Emergency Care Research Institute (ECRI) also influence professional standards for intravenous nursing.

Joint Commission on Accreditation of Healthcare Organizations. JCAHO is a nongovernmental accrediting body that defines optimal, achievable standards for health care organizations such as hospitals, home care, nursing homes, and ambulatory care centers. The intent of the standards is to improve the quality of health care provided to the public by stimulating health care organizations to meet or exceed the standards through accreditation.[16]

American Nurses Association. The ANA has published generic standards for nursing practice that focus on the delivery of nursing care related to the five steps of the nursing process: assessment, diagnosis, planning, implementation, and evaluation.[17] As such, they may be considered the foundation for nursing practice.

Intravenous Nurses Society. INS, formerly known as the National Intravenous Therapy Association (NITA), introduced the first standards for IV nursing in 1980. The standards are reviewed annually, and subsequent revision of the standards reflects changes in practice and technologic advances. The *Intravenous Nursing Standards of Practice* are specific to the specialty practice of IV nursing, but are applicable to all practice settings in which IV therapy is delivered.[18]

American Association of Blood Banks. The AABB publishes standards regarding the professional practice of blood donation, blood processing, and transfusion therapy.[19] These standards address the safe and effective replacement of blood and blood components. Criteria from the AABB standards that relate to IV nursing are included in the *Intravenous Nursing Standards of Practice*.

American Society of Hospital Pharmacists. The ASHP is the national professional association that represents pharmacists in organized health care settings. Based on published research, ASHP has offered guidelines that affect IV nursing. An example is the guidelines concerning the handling of cytotoxic drugs that were published in 1990.[20] As with the AABB standards, the ASHP standards relative to IV nursing are reflected in the *Intravenous Nursing Standards of Practice*.

Association for the Advancement of Medical Instrumentation. The AAMI is a professional organization that promotes interdisciplinary interaction regarding the use of medical devices. By generating information, services, and forums, AAMI assists in determining criteria for the selection and utilization of medical instruments such as electronic infusion devices.

ECRI. This independent nonprofit agency, formerly known as the Emergency Care Research Institute, is dedicated to improving the safety, efficacy, and cost effectiveness of health care technology. ECRI publishes a monthly journal, *Health Devices*, which provides comparative evaluations of medical devices, including infusion devices.[21]

Institutional Standards

In addition to governmental and professional standards, each institution or agency also specifies its own standards in a policy and procedure manual. *Policies* are guidelines or general statements as to when a particular procedure, method, or action is to be employed. In contrast, *procedures* are a step-by-step outline of how the action or method is to be

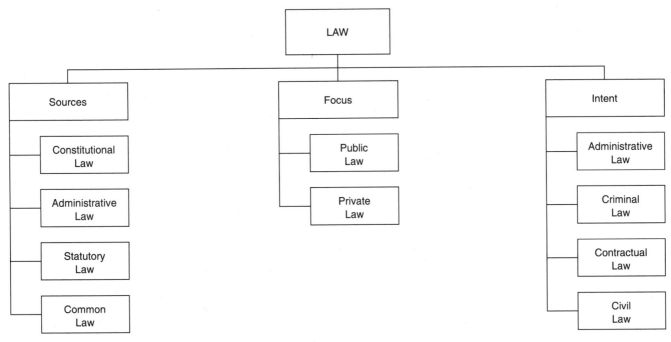

Figure 5–1. Types of laws.

performed.[22] The following is an example of a policy and the corresponding procedure:

Example of a Policy and Corresponding Procedure: Changing of IV Administration Set

Policy

IV administration sets will be changed every 24 to 48 hours (including in-line filters, extension tubing, volume-control sets, and secondary piggyback administration sets) and as required. Every effort will be made to perform the set change at the time a new IV solution container is hung.

Procedure

1. Prepare new solution container.
2. Close flow control clamp on new administration set.
3. Remove protective cover from spike and insert spike of new administration set into new solution container.
4. Fill drip chamber half-full and prime tubing.
5. Close flow control clamp on old administration set.
6. Remove tape securing old administration set.
7. Disconnect old administration set from cannula and insert new set.
8. Secure new administration set with tape.
9. Adjust flow rate as prescribed.
10. Discard contaminated equipment.

Note that, for clarity, nursing actions generic to all procedures (i.e., identify patient, assemble equipment, wash hands, glove, and document) have been omitted from this example.

LEGAL TERMINOLOGY

In an age that greatly emphasizes the legal rights of people, nurses have a responsibility to understand the basic pre-

cepts of law. Our society is founded on a legal system of principles and processes by which individuals may resolve problems and disputes without resorting to physical force. To comprehend this legal system and apply the principles to the practice of IV nursing, the nurse must be cognizant of the terminology commonly used in discussions of legal matters.

Origins of Law

The term "law" has been broadly defined as those standards of human conduct that are established and enforced by the authority of an organized society through its government. In the United States, there are four sources of law: constitutions, legislation, regulations, and judicial opinions.[23] The federal constitution is the highest form of law and is considered "organic law" because it defines the organization of our government. The constitution provides the framework of government by establishing the legislative, executive, and judicial branches that are responsible for the other three sources of law.

In addition to the federal government, every state has a constitution and the three branches of government. The powers of the state government are subject to the limitations on states as written in the federal constitution, the stipulations of the state constitution, and restrictions necessary for the operation of the federal systems. Local governments are created by the state and may only exercise those powers conferred on them by the state government.

Categories of Law

There are numerous types of laws and various methods by which they are categorized (Fig. 5–1). Frequently, laws are categorized as to the four sources from which they originate. Using this method, laws may be categorized as the following: (1) *constitutional law*, originating from the federal and state constitutions; (2) *statutory law*, enacted by the legislative branch of government; (3) *administrative law*, issued by administrative agencies that have been established by the legislature or appointed by the executive branch; and (4) *common law*, which results from interpretation of the laws by the judicial system.[24] Some texts also classify law as public and private law. Constitutional, statutory, and administrative laws are considered *public law* because they deal with public welfare. In contrast, *private law* is concerned with the rights, duties, and legal relations involving private individuals. Contractual law and laws regarding negligence and malpractice are components of private law.[23]

Laws may also be categorized as to their intent. Such a classification emphasizes how the law affects the nurse and which laws are applicable to practice. Therefore, the categories of law relative to IV nursing include administrative law, criminal law, contractual law, and civil law.

Administrative Law. Statutes are laws that are enacted by the legislature and are known as statutory law. When the legislature enacts statutes to regulate business or confer benefits on its citizens, it may be difficult to foresee variations necessary for proper execution of the law. As a means to provide for this eventuality, the legislature may establish an administrative agency empowered to make rules and regulations that have the force of laws.[23] Examples of such federal administrative agencies are the Occupational Safety and Health Administration (OSHA), the Food and Drug Administration (FDA), and the Health Care Financing Administration (HCFA). Regulations from each of these agencies affect the practice of IV nursing. Rules issued by OSHA focus on protection of the health care worker, FDA regulations emphasize product safety, and HCFA guidelines affect providers participating in the Medicare program.

States may also have administrative agencies that are created by the legislature. The primary example is the State Board of Nursing, also referred to as the Board of Nurse Examiners, Nurse Licensing Board, or Nursing Board. These boards set requirements for, and grant approval to, nursing schools, conduct licensing examinations, and issue and renew licenses for nurses. In addition, they are empowered to revoke or annul a nurse's license if there is evidence of incompetence, fraud, or deceit in securing the license, unprofessional conduct, practicing while impaired, criminal acts, or gross negligence.[13]

Criminal Law. Laws relating to an offense against the general public that results in a harmful effect against society as a whole are classified as criminal law. The primary emphasis of criminal law is defining behaviors that are prohibited or controlled by society. Criminal offenses are prosecuted by a governmental authority and punishment may result in fines and/or imprisonment. Performance of IV nursing procedures in an unlawful manner that violates the Nurse Practice Act or the Medical Practice Act are examples of criminal offenses.[23]

There are two types of criminal actions, misdemeanors and felonies. *Misdemeanor* is a general name for every sort of criminal offense that does not amount to a felony. In contrast, a *felony* typically denotes an offense of considerable gravity and includes all offenses that are punishable by death, by imprisonment for 1 year or longer, or by fines in excess of $1000. If the damage exceeds $1000, then the criminal action is considered a felony. Other examples of felonies include murder, manslaughter, theft, and larceny.[25]

Contractual Law. A contract is an agreement between two or more persons that creates, changes, or eliminates a legal right or obligation. Most nurses do not have an employment contract but enter into a general, flexible arrangement with the employer. However, even if the employing agency has no written contract, there is still a binding legal commitment based on a mutual understanding. The nurse has a duty to perform the nursing assignment in accordance with the standards of professional nursing practice; the employer's duty is to provide a safe work place and properly trained and qualified co-workers.[23]

As more and more IV nurses become entrepreneurs, there is an increasing need for nurses to understand how to negotiate written contracts for their services. Consideration must also be given as to how the contract may be terminated. If the nurse fails to perform the obligations required by the contract, a breach of contract may be committed and the nurse may be required to pay damages. *Damages* is a term generally referring to a sum of money awarded to one person because another person has disregarded that person's rights.[29]

Civil Law. The legal rights and obligations of private citizens are the focus of civil law. This category is commonly referred to as case law because it is decided by a judge and/or jury. By law, individuals or groups of individuals are protected from harm and, if an injury occurs, may take civil action to be awarded damages. If the civil offense is a private wrong against another's person or property, it is referred to as a *tort*. Torts are the result of a private act or omission, and may be further classified as intentional, unintentional, or quasi-intentional.[1]

Intentional Torts. An intentional tort involves the purposeful invasion of some legal right of a person. The two best known intentional torts are assault and battery. Although the two terms are frequently linked, they have separate and distinct meanings. *Assault* is the unjustifiable attempt to touch another person or the threat to do so in such a way as to cause the person to believe it will be done.[23] For example, if a competent adult patient refuses to have a venipuncture performed, but the nurse proceeds to assemble the venipuncture equipment and to prepare to perform the procedure, the patient has been assaulted. *Battery* is defined as the unlawful carrying out of threatened physical harm.[23] If, in the previous example, the nurse proceeded to apply the tourniquet and actually performed the venipuncture, the action would be considered battery.

The term "coercion" is frequently used to explain assault and battery. *Coercion* is the forcing of another person to act in a certain manner by means of threats or intimidation. Hence, coercion of a rational adult patient to perform venipuncture constitutes assault and battery.[14]

Another example of intentional tort is *false imprisonment*, which involves the act of placing individuals in a confined area against their will.[23] In the practice of IV nursing, it is sometimes necessary to restrain a patient's extremity to stabilize and secure the IV cannula. In such situations, the nurse must follow policies and procedures governing the use of restraints and only resort to restraints when the patient's safety is in jeopardy. Failure to follow these guidelines may result in allegations of false imprisonment.

Unintentional Torts. The inadvertent act, or the failure to act, that results in injury or harm to a person is an unintentional tort. Unintentional torts may involve an action that is unreasonable and inappropriate or the lack of an action that is reasonable and appropriate. Two types of unintentional torts are negligence and professional malpractice.

Negligence is defined as not doing something that a reasonable layperson would do given the situation. For example, if a person drives through a red light and causes an accident, the conduct is deemed to be negligent. However, the opposite also constitutes negligence, because a person is negligent if something is done that a reasonable person would not do in similar circumstances.[24]

When negligent conduct occurs on the part of a member of a profession, it is considered *malpractice*. Medical malpractice has been further defined as deviation from the professional standard of practice that a qualified health care provider of the same specialty would follow given similar circumstances. In this context, malpractice may be considered synonymous with professional negligence, because the failure to act in a reasonable and prudent manner, as defined by the profession, may result in harm to the patient.[24] For example, death of a patient as a result of the administration of 1000 ml of 3% sodium chloride infusion, instead of the prescribed 1000 ml of 5% dextrose in 0.33% sodium chloride, may be ruled as malpractice.

Although malpractice implies the failure to act in a reasonable and prudent manner, it also denotes stepping beyond one's authority. Each state has a Nurse Practice Act that defines the scope of nursing practice. If the nurse performs a procedure outside the boundaries of nursing practice, it may be ruled an illegal "practice of medicine" in violation of the Medical Practice Act for that state.[23] For example, insertion of a peripherally inserted central catheter (PICC) in a state that does not permit nurses to insert such devices could be considered malpractice.

Quasi-Intentional Torts. The categories of civil wrongs that involve a person's reputation or peace of mind are considered quasi-intentional torts. *Defamation* damages a person's reputation through the use of false and malicious statements. If the statements are written they are known as libel; slander consists of verbal or spoken statements. A person's peace of mind may be violated through *invasion of privacy* or by a *breach of confidentiality*. Patients are vulnerable to unauthorized release of private and confidential information concerning their diagnosis, prognosis, treatment, and plan of care.[23] Hence, nurses have a legal duty and professional responsibility to ensure that these civil rights of patients are not violated.

Legal Processes

In our legal system there are three forums in which legal disputes are settled, and each has unique rules of procedure and rules of evidence. Violation of the regulations set by an administrative agency and disciplinary disputes are determined within the administrative law forum. For example,

State Board of Nursing decisions are governed by the state administrative laws. Criminal charges are heard in a criminal law forum. An example is the use of criminal laws to try a nurse charged with a criminal offense. Tort disputes, such as negligence or malpractice, are referred to a civil law forum, which is always a court. In such a civil action, the person who has been wronged seeks compensation for the harm or injury suffered. This differs from criminal or administrative law, which seeks to punish the wrongdoer.[23]

Two basic legal rights are paramount in the legal process. First, as Americans, we have a right to access courts for dispute settlement. There are two sides to the dispute, the plaintiff and the defendant, and both have the right to use the legal system to settle the conflict. In a case questioning the nurse's care, the *plaintiff* may be the injured patient (who initiated a civil suit) or the state agency or prosecutor (if the offense involves an administrative or criminal action). The *defendant* is the person accused of violating the standard of care (civil law), acting unprofessionally (administrative law), or committing a criminal offense (criminal law).[24]

The second basic liberty is the right to due process. This means that certain principles must be followed within a fair and just forum, including provision of proper notice, arrangement of an opportunity to be heard, presentation of evidence, and cross-examination of witnesses.

LEGAL PRINCIPLES

As a result of the growth and increasing complexity of IV nursing, the greatest legal risk for nurses practicing this specialty is negligence, also known as negligent conduct or malpractice. The plaintiff may believe the nurse was negligent, but legal action cannot be initiated unless several rules are followed.

Elements of Negligence

If a patient (plaintiff) believes that an act performed by a nurse, or the nurse's failure to act, has resulted in injury or harm, the legal process begins once he or she selects a lawyer to represent his or her interests. The counsel for the plaintiff (the allegedly injured patient or heirs) must then determine whether there is a basis for the lawsuit. This involves a review of the medical record, data collection, interviews, and review of the case by an expert. Because the plaintiff has the burden of proof, counsel must determine whether there is evidence of the elements of negligence.

In a lawsuit, the plaintiff (patient) must present evidence that the defendant (nurse) failed to use the degree of skill and judgment commensurate with the nurse's education, experience, and position. In other words, there must be evidence of failure to conform to what a reasonably prudent nurse would have done, or would not have done, if placed in the same situation. The four elements necessary to prove negligence are duty of care, breach of duty, causation, and type of injury compensable by law.[24]

Duty of Care. The first element that must be proven by the plaintiff is that the defendant owed a duty of care. This means that the nurse was in some way responsible for the patient. For example, if the nurse is performing venipuncture on a patient to initiate an infusion, there is a duty of care to the patient. However, if the mother of the patient becomes faint during the venipuncture procedure and falls, injuring her wrist, the duty of care to the patient's mother is questionable. The nurse owed a duty of care to the patient but not to the patient's mother, unless there was a prior realistic agreement to do so. Hence, the mother (as a defendant) will probably not be successful in proving duty of care.

Breach of Duty. The second critical element that must be proven is that the defendant violated, or breached, the duty of care owed to the patient. The breach of duty may be the result of a failure to act (omission) or performance of an act (commission). For example, necrosis and tissue sloughing resulting from infiltration of a peripheral infusion of 10% dextrose in water may be the result of failure to monitor a peripheral IV site (omission), but injury caused by initiation of an infusion without the order of a physician (commission) may also be considered a breach of duty. Other examples of breach of duty relative to IV nursing are as follows:

1. *Delay in drug administration.* A lidocaine infusion has been prescribed for a patient experiencing ventricular tachycardia. Although the infusion is to be initiated immediately, the order is not communicated to the IV nurse and there is a 3-hour delay until the infusion is initiated.
2. *Failure to administer infusion at the prescribed rate.* A dehydrated patient is to receive an IV infusion at 150 ml/hour, but the drop rate is incorrectly calculated and the solution infuses at 50 ml/hour.
3. *Inappropriate administration of a drug.* Phenytoin is administered at a rate of 100 mg/min and the patient experiences a severe adverse reaction.
4. *Failure to provide patient education.* A patient is discharged home with a long-term central venous catheter. No arrangements are made for home health care and the patient is not instructed regarding care of the catheter.

Breach of duty may also result from barriers to the delivery of patient care. In home infusion therapy, obstacles such as a patient who refuses to follow the treatment regimen may affect the agency's ability to manage the patient's care. However, termination of care without reasonable notice and adequate time for the patient to secure additional care may be interpreted as patient abandonment. When an agency contracts to provide services to the patient, there is a duty owed to the patient. Regardless of the reasons, termination of care without adequate notice or provision represents a breach of duty.

In the case of a private citizen, such as a landlord, the jury can generally comprehend what a "reasonably prudent" landlord would have done based on the circumstances. In this case, the law allows for the jurors themselves to use their common sense in reaching a verdict. A nursing negligence case, however, is far more complex because the allegation is that the nurse breached the standard of "reasonable nursing care." Because the law recognizes that the average juror does not understand medical terminology, the nursing process, nor the legal standard of nursing care, it is mandated that the jury be educated by qualified witnesses as to the circumstances of the case. This is the role of the expert witness. An *expert witness* is a health care provider who is called on to educate the judge and jury regarding the appropriate standard of care and to identify the deviation from the established standard. Typically, the expert witness is of the same profession, has similar experience as the defendant, and has demonstrated expertise in the specialty practice.[29] For example, a CRNI with extensive experience in home infusion therapy would be qualified to offer expert testimony if the case involved the actions of a home care IV nurse.

In offering the expert testimony, the witness may rely on personal knowledge and experience, professional articles, published standards of practice, and nursing documentation contained in the patient's medical record to educate the jury as to the allegations in the case. Once the jury understands the applicable standard of care for the situation involved in the case, the expert may then offer an opinion as to whether the defendant deviated from the established standard. Because nursing negligence is a complex issue, expert witnesses may be used to testify both for and against the defendant. The plaintiff's expert witness will attempt to convince the jury that the defendant (nurse) deviated from the accepted nursing standards; expert testimony for the defense will support that the defendant's actions represented "reasonable nursing care." The jury, however, is not governed by the opinion(s) of the expert(s) and can reject either or both testimonies.[26]

Causation. The third element that must be proven is causation or proximate cause. By law, the injury to the plaintiff must be the result of negligent conduct on the part of the defendant. Patients may be injured because of the conduct of the nurse but, if the nurse was performing in a reasonable, safe manner, the nurse is not responsible for the harm. For example, if a nurse administers penicillin IV to a patient and an allergic reaction ensues, the nurse is only responsible if he or she failed to check for possible allergies prior to administration of the drug. However, if the patient had no known allergies, there is no liability on the part of the nurse.

An important criterion in establishing proximate cause is foreseeability. In retrospect, it is often easier to determine what "should" have been done in a given situation. *Foreseeability* requires that the defendant's actions be judged based on the facts known at the time of the occurrence.[26]

Legally Compensable Injury. The final element of negligence is that the patient suffered some type of injury, and the injury must be of a type for which the law allows compensation. Because the plaintiff must prove that the negligent conduct was actually responsible for some harm or injury, it is common to have severe negligence without a lawsuit. For example, the nurse performs venipuncture to initiate an infusion of 5% dextrose in 0.225% sodium chloride, but 5% dextrose in 0.45% sodium chloride was prescribed. If the nurse discovers the error prior to initiating the infusion and no harm has come to the patient, then there can be no lawsuit. Often, potential clients contact malpractice attorneys and relate how they were "almost" injured by a nurse or physician. However, the common reply to these individuals is that, by law, "almost doesn't count"; if there is no injury, there can be no lawsuit.

Common Areas of Nursing Negligence

To avoid the risks of negligence, the nurse needs to be aware of those areas most commonly associated with negligent conduct and institute actions to prevent liability. Areas of negligence specific to IV nursing include medication administration, equipment use, failure to act, lack of communication, and negligent conduct of another.[23]

Medication Administration. The actions of nurses relating to the administration of medications have been the subject of more lawsuits than any other area of nursing. Examples include the failure to verify the medication label, failure to follow the physician's orders, administration of an overdose, or drug administration at an unspecified or erroneous time. If the nurse fails to meet the professional expectations relative to medication administration and the failure results in injury to the patient, the nurse is liable. Many cases involving medication errors are settled prior to jury trial because the health care organization's records furnish ample proof of the error.

Equipment Use. Protection of the patient from equipment hazards is a responsibility the nurse assumes when using items such as IV cannulas, solution containers, administration sets, and electronic infusion devices. The nurse has the duty to reasonably inspect, maintain, use, and supervise equipment to prevent obvious harm to the patient. Nurses have been held responsible for not properly using and disposing of equipment, for not supervising the use of equipment, and for leaving equipment in an inappropriate area. In cases in which the patient cannot prove when, where, or by whom he or she was injured, courts have found nurses responsible through the application of a doctrine called *res ipsa loquitur*. This doctrine means that the injury is so obvious that it "speaks for itself."[26] For example, when an unconscious patient sustains injury from a hematoma caused by an unsuccessful venipuncture attempt, he or she certainly is unable to testify as to how or by whom the injury occurred. In this situation, the law allows the patient to prove, by virtue of the obviousness of the situation, that it was the negligence of the nurse performing the venipuncture that caused the injury.

If, however, the nurse can prove that ordinary precautions were taken to protect the patient from danger, the nurse is not liable, even though the patient was subsequently injured. Such may be the case when a peripheral IV catheter breaks off and harms the patient during an IV infusion. If the nurse has inspected the catheter prior to insertion and detected no visible defect, the nurse is not responsible for the manufacturer's defective product.

Failure to Act. Affirmative nursing actions are the subject of most lawsuits, but the failure to act, on the part of the nurse, may also cause injury to the patient. An example of negligent failure to act might occur if the nurse receives an order to administer a potassium infusion to a patient experiencing cardiac dysrhythmia but fails to respond to the order. If, because of the failure to act, the dysrhythmia becomes life-threatening and subsequently results in death, the nurse is liable for the patient's demise.

Lack of Communication. Although failure to communicate is closely related to the failure to act, it may be the sole specific cause of injury. Examples of nursing negligence resulting from lack of communication are the failure to inform the physician of abnormal findings noted during the nursing assessment or the failure to notify the physician of a patient's deteriorating condition. Clearly, nurses have an obligation to communicate significant data and exercise sound clinical judgment as to what is significant regarding the patient's status.

Negligent Conduct of Another. Along with the person who is primarily responsible, a nurse may be liable for allowing or aiding the negligence of that other person. For example, if a physician fails to specify the route of administration for a drug, and the nurse administers the drug without checking the route with the prescribing physician, both the nurse and physician are jointly responsible if an injury occurs. However, if the nurse did attempt to contact the physician, it is insufficient simply to document the attempts to contact the physician. If there is a lack of action by the physician, the nurse is required to advise authorities within the organization so that intervention on behalf of the patient is ensured.[27]

Time Constraints

The statute of limitations is often referred to as a *rule of repose* because each case must be filed within a certain time frame or it is automatically rejected by the courts.[26] Although all citizens are allowed their "day in court," plaintiffs cannot abuse this right and hold the defendant in suspense long after an incident occurs. The reason for the time constraint is fairness to all parties. If a plaintiff waits beyond the legal time limit to file a lawsuit, the defendant may be unable to locate co-workers or witnesses who can testify on his or her behalf, critical records may have been destroyed, memories of the incident may have faded, and justice cannot be served.

Time limits differ according to the type of lawsuit and the state in which the suit is filed. For example, in New Jersey, lawsuits regarding nursing negligence must be filed in court within 2 years of the injury, but clients have 6 years in which to file attorney malpractice cases. Because a patient may not be aware of the negligence until a delayed injury manifests itself, an exception to rigid time frames is mandated by the "discovery statute."[29] This means just what it implies; the statutory time only begins once the injury is discovered.

Tools of Discovery

Once the complaint is filed in court and served on the defendant, the discovery phase of litigation begins. Two tools of discovery that are frequently used are interrogatories and depositions. The first step in discovery is *interrogatories*, which are written questions to be answered by the defendant. Although the questions encompass more than the issue of the specific case, interrogatories uncover relevant facts regarding the dispute. The following is a list of sample questions that may be contained in an interrogatory:

1. State fully: (a) your full name, (b) date of birth, (c) residence, (d) professional address, (e) area of specialization, if any, and (f) board-certified specialty, if any.
2. State your professional nursing training, qualifications, and experience in detail, including: (a) each university or college attended by you, (b) each degree awarded to you and the date(s) of same, (c) each hospital with which you have been affiliated at any time up to the present, includ-

ing the nature of such affiliation and inclusive dates, (d) each nursing society or association of which you have ever been a member and the inclusive dates of membership, and (e) bibliography of all your publications, including titles, dates, and publishers.

3. State the date upon which and place where you first saw the patient, Ms. O, and indicate: (a) a detailed account of the nursing, physical, or other history you received about the plaintiff, (b) a description of the nature and scope of any and all examinations or procedures performed by you on this occasion of the plaintiff's first treatment, (c) your observations regarding the plaintiff's condition, (d) a description of all treatments and/or therapy, medication, or instructions rendered by you on June 25, 1990, and (e) nursing diagnoses rendered as to the nature of Ms. O's condition.

4. State in chronological order each and every date when you thereafter saw the patient and indicate: (a) a description of all examinations or procedures performed by you on each such visit, (b) a description of all treatments and/or therapy, medication, or instructions rendered by you on each such visit, and (c) a nursing diagnosis rendered as to the nature and/or cause of any disease, bodily impairment, disabilities, conditions, or symptoms.

5. State the names and addresses of any and all persons who have knowledge of any facts relative to the issues in this case and for each such person so named, state to the best of your knowledge the substance of all information or knowledge known about this case.

6. State in full and complete detail what you contend the cause or causes of the injuries as mentioned in Ms. O's complaint were, identifying each person responsible for any cause.

In contrast, a *deposition* is a statement taken from the witness under oath but outside the courtroom. This is a formal procedure in which the opposing party's attorney asks questions of the witness and the entire exchange is recorded by a court reporter.[29]

The following are excerpts taken from the deposition of a nurse who was the defendant in an IV-related lawsuit. The plaintiff was the father of an infant whose right foot had been severely damaged due to infiltration of the IV infusion. The nurse was charged with negligence because of her failure to appropriately monitor the infusion. During the deposition, the questions were asked by the plaintiff's (father's) attorney; the answers were supplied by the defendant (nurse).

Q. Do you have any memory of what IV solution the patient was receiving on April 10, 1990?

A. Dextrose in water 10%.

Q. 10% dextrose in water, is that the same concentration as in the blood?

A. No, that's hypertonic solution.

Q. By hypertonic, do you mean that the solution going into the patient's vein was stronger chemically than what he already had in his body?

A. Yes.

Q. Is it fair to say that this is a reason why it could be very irritating to the patient's veins and tissues?

A. Yes.

Q. So then, it's fair to say that the tonicity would be one reason why you wouldn't want that concentrated solution to get out into his body tissues?

A. Right.

Q. On April 10, 1990, who was responsible for observing the IV on the patient?

A. If you mean on the 7–3 shift, I was assigned to the patient.

Q. That means, as the nurse assigned to the patient, you were responsible for observing that the IV was infusing correctly.

A. Yes.

A key component of the discovery phase is the use of written standards of care. Interrogatories and depositions of the defendant concentrate on the extent of the nurse's familiarity with professional standards of practice. A lack of familiarity with applicable standards seriously detracts from the defendant's credibility as a witness. Conversely, a well-prepared defendant can take advantage of the opposing attorney's questions. By effectively communicating familiarity with the standards cited, the nurse may retaliate against any inference of negligence, and point out how the nursing actions met or exceeded the written guidelines.

Responsibility for the Nurse's Actions

Liability denotes that a person has a legal responsibility to fulfill an obligation. Because nurses are responsible for delivering reasonable, prudent nursing care, they are liable for deviations from the established standard and any resultant wrongdoing. This is known as the *rule of personal liability*.[28] For example, the nurse administers a prescribed medication but rapid injection of the drug results in harm to the patient. In this situation, the physician who prescribed the medication is not responsible for the nurse's negligence in administering the drug; the harm was the result of the nurse's actions, not the physician's.

Although the nurse is responsible for the nursing actions, in select circumstances the physician may be held jointly accountable for the negligence of a nurse. This primarily concerns the operating room, where the nurse is considered the ''borrowed servant'' of the physician. This legal principle is derived from agency law and it places the responsibility on the person who is clearly in charge of the situation and who has the greatest control over all present. It is often referred to as the ''captain of the ship'' doctrine because it analogizes the surgeon to a ''captain'' who is the master of all the ''crew'' present in the operating room while the surgery is performed. Outside the operating room setting, physicians have rarely been found to be responsible for nurses' negligence.[26]

Another concept that must be considered in determining responsibility is the doctrine of *respondeat superior*, or ''let the master answer.'' According to this legal principle, an employer is liable for damages caused by a wrongful act of his or her servant within the scope of his or her employment. As a result, the nurse is held liable for negligence, but the employer may also be held responsible for the nurse's actions. The doctrine does not absolve the nurse from responsibility for the actions but allows both the nurse and the employer to be named in the lawsuit. Application of this legal principle is most common in cases in which a nurse does not have liability insurance and the plaintiff must rely on the employer's insurance to cover the injury.[26]

Locality Rule in Nursing Litigation

The courts have, at times, imposed on medical malpractice cases a uniform definition of reasonable conduct. This is known as the *locality rule*. The rule is a uniquely American legal doctrine and is specific to the medical profession. Based on the rule, the conduct of members of the medical profession may only be measured against the conduct of other medical professionals in that locality. The underlying rationale is that physicians practicing in smaller towns and rural areas may possess adequate theoretic knowledge but are not afforded the exposure to sophisticated techniques. Currently, the theory has come under serious attack because of the wide circulation of medical information, such as professional journals and postgraduate courses, which serves to establish national standards for medical care. In the past, the locality rule was occasionally applied to nurses practicing in rural areas; however, the rule is no longer applicable to nurses because of national standardized testing for licensure.

Reasons for Being Named Defendant When No Negligence Exists

The fact that a nurse is named as a defendant in a negligence case does not necessarily mean that the nurse was negligent. Indeed, the nurse may be an "innocent victim" who is sued even though not directly involved in the care of the patient who filed the lawsuit. There are legal complexities that play a hidden role in the lawyer's decision to name a nurse as a defendant, and they involve more than if the nurse had done something "wrong." The lawyer for the plaintiff has a similar responsibility to the client as the nurse to the patient; there is a responsibility to do everything possible to obtain the best results for the client according to accepted standards of professional practice. To accomplish this, three legal technicalities may be employed.

Statute of Limitations. As previously stated, there is a time frame within which a plaintiff may file a lawsuit or lose the chance to have a day in court. If the plaintiff does not contact an attorney until shortly before the statute of limitations expires, there may be insufficient time to investigate the facts of the case fully. To protect the client's interests, the attorney may name every person who could possibly be responsible for the injury. For example, if a patient dies as a result of an overdose of heparin and four different nurses administered the medication to the patient during the last 2 days of the patient's life, the attorney may name all four nurses as defendants. Those nurses who are subsequently determined to be fault free are then removed from the lawsuit prior to the trial.

Fear of the "Empty Chair" Defense. In the so-called "empty chair" defense, the defendant claims that someone not named in the lawsuit was responsible for the injury. To prevent this type of defense strategy, the attorney for the plaintiff may name other nurses involved in the patient's care in the lawsuit. There are overlapping responsibilities in health care, and often, no one person is solely responsible for what happens to the patient.

Charitable Immunity Statute. A third reason a nurse may be named as defendant is an immunity statute that has been enacted by many states to protect charitable institutions. This statute protects such institutions from excessive liability by setting limits on the amount of compensation for which they are responsible in a negligence lawsuit.[26] For example, in New Jersey, the immunity statute places the limit on awards against charitable institutions at $250,000. Unfortunately, no such limit applies to the nurse defendant. Because the institution may be liable for damages if a nurse employed by the institution harms the patient through negligent conduct *(respondeat superior)*, the plaintiff's attorney can name the nurse as a defendant to override the limits set on the institution's liability.

RISK MANAGEMENT

Risk management is a system used by health care organizations to identify, analyze, and implement strategies for eliminating, minimizing, and coping with liabilities.[29] Although the discipline of health care risk management did not emerge until the mid-1970s, several states now mandate such programs for health care facilities, and JCAHO standards require risk management activities for hospital accreditation.

Concepts

The initial phase of risk management is the identification of the organization's exposures to loss. The four areas that expose an organization to loss are liability, property, personnel, and net income. In health care, liability is the greatest concern because of the risk of medical malpractice and negligence. However, the organization must also consider property exposures caused by physical damage to the facility and the equipment contained within it, personnel exposures related to employee injuries and occupational diseases, and net income exposures resulting from theft or embezzlement.[30]

The second step in risk management is evaluation of the potential loss based on the exposures. By means of a series of complex determinations, the likelihood and potential severity of loss from the liability, property, personnel, and net income exposures may be calculated. The most appropriate strategy is then selected to manage each potential risk.

The primary emphasis of risk management is the actual managing of the exposures. This is the third step in the process of reducing and/or preventing unplanned loss, and may require either risk financing or risk control. *Risk financing* is based on transferring the risk of financial loss from the organization to others through agreements, contracts, or insurance. Purchasing of commercial insurance and establishing a self-insurance fund are examples of risk financing. In contrast, *risk control* focuses on activities within the organization that can reduce or eliminate the risk. Risk control activities include exposure avoidance, risk shifting, loss prevention, and loss reduction.[31]

Because an exposure that has been completely avoided cannot produce a loss, *exposure avoidance* is an effective risk control technique. However, in health care, it may not be a viable option. For example, if a hospital determined that IV medication administration posed the greatest threat of nursing negligence, elimination of this practice would exemplify risk avoidance, even though such an action would be neither possible nor realistic.

A more feasible method of controlling risk is by *risk transfer*, which shifts the responsibility and liability by means of a contractual agreement. Instead of the organization providing the services that subject it to risk exposure, the services may be contracted from another organization that accepts responsibility for the potential exposure to loss. For example, a nursing home may contract professional nurses from an outside agency to administer IV medications within the facility. As part of the agreement, the agency would assume responsibility for the nurses' actions.

Although the first two methods of controlling risks are directed at eliminating the risk exposure, the third technique focuses on preventing the exposure to loss. *Loss prevention* is therefore any measure that reduces the probability or frequency of a particular type of loss. Identification of trends (e.g., the incidence of phlebitis) and interventions (e.g., measures to reduce the current rate of phlebitis further) are two examples of preventative programs that may be used to avert a loss-producing event.

The final method, *loss reduction*, is comprised of measures to reduce the severity of losses. Loss prevention reduces the frequency of the loss but does not completely eliminate any chance of a loss occurring. Therefore, loss reduction measures are designed to lessen the size or extent of a loss. If a patient develops an IV-related complication, loss reduction measures include appropriate care following the injury, safeguarding the patient from further injury, and courteous treatment of the patient as a potential claimant.

Strategies

In practice, risk management strategies combine the elements of both loss reduction and loss prevention. Through a series of reactive and proactive activities, the potential for risk exposure is managed. The following are examples of risk management strategies that may decrease the risk of potential liability.[1]

Patient Rights

A critical responsibility of nurses is the duty not to violate patient rights. State and federal regulations governing health care mandate that every patient receiving health care be afforded certain rights. Hence, nursing care should be delivered in a manner that honors the rights of the patient. The five major topics pertaining to these rights are informed consent, refusal of treatment, discharge planning, freedom from restraints, and confidentiality. All these issues are based on a professional obligation to the patient, but also carry with them legal consequences.

Informed consent is one of the most effective proactive risk management strategies. Patients must be provided with sufficient information to enable them to decide rationally whether to undergo treatment. In order for the consent to be valid, the patient must receive sufficient information to make an informed decision, be capable of granting consent, and must not be coerced.[32]

An example of informed consent could involve the insertion of a PICC. The nurse must provide accurate and complete information including a description of the procedure, potential benefits of such a catheter, possible risks associated with the procedure, and available alternatives. This information must be provided in a language understood by the patient, and there must be an opportunity for dialogue between the patient and nurse regarding the information. Only after the patient has considered all options can consent be obtained, and it must reflect the patient's voluntary agreement to the procedure.

Although consent may be obtained verbally, a written agreement may also be required. Such may be the case with specialized procedures such as PICC insertion. Documentation of the consent generally consists of evidence that the patient has received the necessary information and that the patient has agreed to the proposed procedure. Because such documentation may protect both the patient and the nurse, consent forms are used as a risk management tool. However, the patient's signature on the form does not necessarily imply understanding of the informed consent.

Refusal of treatment refers to the right of every competent adult patient to decline the therapy. Because the patient's wishes are paramount to any decision regarding health care, health care professionals are legally required to honor the patient's decisions and any advance directives. For example, a patient has the right to refuse a transfusion. However, the patient must be informed of the consequences of such a decision and should be required to sign forms documenting receipt of the information and confirmation of the decision.

Refusing care may also take the form of leaving the health care facility against medical advice (AMA). Unless patients pose a danger to themselves or others that necessitates emergency detention for observation or psychiatric care, patients cannot be held against their will. However, patients must be informed of the consequences of leaving, provided with adequate discharge instructions, and requested to sign forms confirming that they are leaving the facility against medical advice.

Discharge planning concentrates on preparing the patient for eventual discharge from the health care facility. Because patients are discharged when care is no longer medically necessary, governmental regulations mandate that patients be informed of and prepared for their date of discharge.

Preparation of the patient for discharge begins at the time of admission to the facility and continues throughout the patient's stay. For example, if a patient is admitted for insertion of an implanted port, instructions regarding care of the port should be initiated at the time of admission and continued until discharge. By doing so, the patient may be adequately prepared to care for the port, and discharge does not need to be postponed until patient teaching has been completed.

Freedom from restraints is a basic right of every patient. The only exceptions are in emergency situations or if the patient's safety is in jeopardy. If such a situation exists, the restraints must be ordered by a physician, the patient must be closely monitored, and the need to continue the use of restraints must be documented. For example, a restraint may be required to stabilize and secure an IV cannula, but the restraint must be prescribed by the physician for this specific purpose and for a definite period of time. In addition, because of the potential risks associated with the use of restraints, the patient's extremity must be closely monitored.

VARIANCE REPORT
HOME INFUSION THERAPY

A. STAFF MOST CLOSELY INVOLVED (circle one) 1. Attending physician 2. RN 3. LPN 4. Pharmacist 5. Pharmacy technician 6. IV nurse 7. Delivery technician	**B. I.V. VARIANCE** (circle one) 1. Incorrect compounding 2. I.V. not checked properly 3. Incorrect rate 4. Infiltration 5. Phlebitis +1 6. Phlebitis +2 7. Phlebitis +3 8. Phlebitis +4
C. DELIVERY VARIANCE (circle one) 1. Nondelivery 2. Delivery off schedule 3. Incomplete delivery 4. Wrong product delivery 5. Product damaged	**D. MEDICATION VARIANCE** (circle one) 1. Adverse effect 2. Omission 3. Duplication 4. Incorrect time 5. Incorrect route 6. Incorrect medication 7. Incorrect patient 8. Incorrect dose 9. Documentation incorrect

Figure 5–2. Example of categorizing IV-related variances on an unusual occurrence report form.

Confidentiality denotes that information about the patient must be kept private and should not be released without the patient's permission. This includes information contained in the patient's medical record and details regarding the patient's diagnosis, treatment, and expected length of stay.

Because of the risk of exposure to bloodborne pathogens, IV nurses may be concerned if a patient is HIV-positive. If the results of HIV screening are available on the patient's medical record, the nurse must ensure that this information is kept confidential. Unauthorized disclosure carries fines and, if the disclosure results in economic, bodily, or psychologic harm, the person who disclosed the information may be liable for damages.

Unusual Occurrence Reports

Documentation of an unusual occurrence is a reactive risk management strategy that provides the facts concerning an event that may result in risk exposure. It is an internal reporting mechanism that notifies the organization that an event has occurred and provides an opportunity to investigate the situation while the circumstances are still clear.[29] Such documents were once referred to as "incident reports" but, because of the negative connotation, the terminology has been replaced with "reports of an unusual occurrence" or "variance reports."

A report of an unusual occurrence can be a strategy crucial to the organization's risk management program if several key principles are followed when preparing the report. First, the report must be an objective account of the event. The purpose of the report is to record the facts; personal opinions should never be included in the document. To ensure that the reports are factual and nonjudgmental, some organizations have con-verted to a checklist format to record the information (Fig. 5–2). Second, the type of occurrence must be noted. This assists in trending analysis to monitor patterns of occurrences. Third, the report must include an assessment of the patient's condition prior to the occurrence and the results of the occurrence or injury. This aids in determining the extent of the injury or severity of the risk exposure. Fourth, no reference to the report should appear in the patient's medical record. Unusual occurrence reports are confidential internal reporting mechanisms. If the patient's medical record contains evidence of a report and the patient later files a lawsuit, the report must be presented in court.[23]

Documentation

Accurate documentation in the medical record objectively describes the care rendered and the patient's response. Because the lawsuit may be filed years after the event occurred, the documentation in the medical record is often the only factual information available to determine whether there was a deviation from the standard of care. However, the reliability of the medical record may be discredited if there are a lack of consistency, contradictory entries, unexplained time gaps, alterations and obliterations, omissions, or illegibility.[29]

Nurses know that documentation in the medical record must be objective, legible, timely, complete, and accurate. Therefore, the problem with documentation is often the result of a lack of compliance, not a lack of education. As nurses deliver patient care, they often become frustrated with the amount of "paperwork" required by their jobs. However, the documentation may be the only evidence demonstrating that the nursing actions met the legal standard of care. (For additional information, refer to Chapter 26, Documentation.)

Professional Liability Insurance

Insurance is a risk management strategy whereby the nurse may transfer to an insurer the financial risk resulting from a nursing action that harms a patient. Because of the doctrine of *respondeat superior*, health care facilities and agencies usually carry insurance for negligent acts of their employees performed within the scope of their job responsibilities. However, many nurses also carry their own individual professional liability insurance.

The decision to purchase liability insurance is a personal one, and many factors must be considered. First, without insurance, the nurse may be required to use personal assets to compensate for a patient's injuries. However, if the actions were within the scope of employment, the damages may be covered by the employer's insurance policy. Second, the potential risks must be evaluated. If there is a significant risk of personal liability because of the practice setting and nursing interventions employed, the purchasing of individual insurance may be warranted. Third, purchasing of insurance requires that the nurse enter a contract with the insurer. As part of the contract, the nurse agrees to pay premiums and the insurer agrees to compensate the patient if the nurse is found guilty of malpractice. The nurse must evaluate the price of the premiums and understand that compensation is limited to the terms set in the insurance policy. Because insurance can be complex, the nurse must consider all benefits and risks prior to purchasing professional liability insurance.

Patient Relations

It has been stated that it is easier to sue an enemy than a friend. A patient who perceives the nurse as an impersonal, aloof person who is unconcerned with the patient's welfare is more apt to initiate legal activity against the nurse if an injury occurs. However, if the lines of communication are open between the nurse and the patient and expressions of anger, fear, and complaints by the patient are promptly investigated and resolved, claims of negligence may be avoided.[14]

Quality Management

Quality management is the continuous effort to improve patient care. It serves as a risk management strategy because it is a proactive approach to identify opportunities for improvement. Not only are problems identified and resolved, but outcomes are improved by enhancing the processes involved in patient care. (For additional information, see Chapter 4, Quality Management.)

In today's increasingly cost-conscious and litigious health care environment, IV nurses must provide quality IV nursing care. Excellent nursing care is the best method of preventing liability. If the care is rendered appropriately, the patient is adequately monitored, the actions are accurately documented, and the physician is informed of changes in the patient's condition, patient injury and litigation may be avoided.

References

1. Beare PG, Myers JL. Principles and Practice of Adult Health Nursing. St. Louis: C. V. Mosby, 1990.
2. Myers CE. Pharmacy implications of the revised OSHA Hazard Communication Standard. Am J Hosp Pharm 1989; 46:990–1001.
3. OSHA. OSHA work-practice guidelines for personnel dealing with cytotoxic (antineoplastic) drugs. Am J Hosp Pharm 1986; 43:1193.
4. Miramontes H. Progress in establishing safety protocols based on CDC and OSHA recommendations. Infect Control Hosp Epidemiol 1990; 11:561–562.
5. OSHA. Occupational safe exposure to bloodborne pathogens: Final rule. Washington, DC: Department of Labor, Docket No. H-370, Dec. 6, 1991.
6. Goode LD. Flowing by the waste-side: The emerging national policy on medical waste. Acad Med 1989; 64:514–515.
7. Nemeth JC. Organizations must be aware of hazardous regulations. Occup Health Saf 1985; 54:30–48.
8. Gough AR, Markus K. Hazardous materials protections in ED practice: Laws and logistics. J Emerg Nurs 1989; 15:477–480.
9. Scott WL. Medical-device complication reporting: A quality assurance mechanism. JIN 1990; 13:178–182.
10. Safe Medical Devices Act of 1990 (Public Law 101–629).
11. Shlafer M, Marieb EN. The Nurse, Pharmacology, and Drug Therapy. Redwood City, CA: Addison-Wesley, 1989.
12. Fletcher JC. The patient self-determination act. Hastings Center Rep 1990; 20:33–35.
13. Rhodes AM, Miller RD. Nursing and the Law, 4th ed. Rockville, MD: Aspen, 1984.
14. Plumer A, Cosentino F. Principles and Practices of Intravenous Nursing, 4th ed. Boston: Little, Brown and Co., 1987.
15. Katz J, Green E. Managing Quality: A Guide to Monitoring and Evaluating Nursing Services. St. Louis: C. V. Mosby, 1992.
16. Joint Commission on Accreditation of Healthcare Organizations. First Annual Invitational Forum for Liaison Network Organizations, Workshop Materials. Chicago: JCAHO, 1993.
17. American Nurses Association. Standards of Nursing Practice. Kansas City, MO: American Nurses Association, 1973.
18. Intravenous Nurses Society. Intravenous Nursing Standards of Practice. Belmont, MA: Intravenous Nurses Society, 1990.
19. American Association of Blood Banks. AABB Technical Manual, 10th ed. Philadelphia: J. B. Lippincott, 1990.
20. American Society of Hospital Pharmacists. ASHP technical assistance bulletin on handling cytotoxic hazardous drugs. Am J Hosp Pharm 1990; 47:1033–1048.
21. Ritter HT. Evaluating and selecting general-purpose infusion pumps. JIN 1990; 13:156–161.
22. Gillies DA. Nursing Management: A Systems Approach, 2nd ed. Philadelphia: W. B. Saunders, 1989.
23. Creighton H. Law Every Nurse Should Know, 5th ed. Philadelphia: W. B. Saunders, 1986.
24. Fiesta J. The Law and Liability: A Guide for Nurses, 2nd ed. New York: John Wiley & Sons, 1987.
25. Nurse's Legal Handbook. Springhouse, PA: Springhouse Corp, 1985.
26. Fiesta J. Nurse's role as an expert witness. Nurs Manage 1991; 22:28–29.
27. Lumsden DJ. Legal risks in a changing practice environment. JIN 1990; 13:59–67.
28. Bernzweig EP. Nurse's Liability for Malpractice, 3rd ed. New York: McGraw-Hill, 1981.
29. Goldman TA. Risk management concepts and strategies. JIN 1991; 14:199–204.
30. Kraus GP. Health Care Risk Management. Owings Mills, MD: Rynd Communications, 1986.
31. Head GL, Horn S. Essentials of Risk Management, Vol II. Malvern, PA: Insurance Institute of America, 1991.
32. Hogue E. What you should know about informed consent. Nursing 1986; 6:47–48.

PHYSIOLOGIC CONSIDERATIONS

CHAPTER 6 Anatomy and Physiology

Lynn C. Hadaway, BS, RNC, CRNI

Related to Intravenous Therapy

• •

▬▬▬ **Integument and Connective Tissue**
    Structure
    Effects of Aging
    Role in Infection Control
    Wound Healing
    Neurologic System
    Functional Divisions
    Anatomic Divisions
    The Thoracic Cavity
    Bony Thorax
    Respiratory System
    The Heart
    Peripheral Vascular System
    Blood Vessel Structure
    Location of Important Arteries
    Location of Important Veins
    Systemic Blood Flow
    Blood Volume and Distribution
    Physical Properties of Blood
    Pressure and Resistance to Flow
    Velocity and Types of Blood Flow
    Nursing Diagnoses

• •

Knowledge of the anatomy and physiology of the skin, peripheral vasculature, and cardiopulmonary and neurologic systems is crucial for the safe administration of any parenteral therapy. Many factors relating to these body functions can encumber or increase the success of infusions. Conversely, parenteral therapy administration can have a detrimental effect on the anatomy and physiologic function of all body systems. Our goal is to consider all pertinent factors in an effort to manage the risk of parenteral therapy and ensure a positive outcome for the patient.

When any IV device is inserted, the skin is the first organ affected. Skin serves several functions, including acting as a mechanical barrier to microorganisms and radiation, sensory and temperature regulation, and aiding in fluid and electrolyte balance. Breaking this natural barrier increases the risk of infection. The use of antiseptic solutions, ointment, and dressing materials can affect the skin's natural composition of bacteria, oils, and sweat. Factors such as age, chronic disease, and the environment can produce changes in the skin, making entry through the skin a difficult process.

Vascular anatomy is of primary importance when locating and cannulating veins or arteries. Both the insertion site and location of the cannula tip are important considerations. Extreme variations in pH, osmolality, volume, and rate can alter the risk of complications if consideration is not given to the size of the vessel lumen and the amount and type of blood flow. Fluid volume status and general cardiopulmonary condition can limit the volume and rate of infusion and lead to a negative patient outcome when not monitored closely.

The neurologic system affects all other systems and can influence the success or failure of any parenteral therapy. The sensory receptors in the skin, the innervation of the walls of veins and arteries, the systemic responses evoked by emotion and pain, and the use of the epidural space for infusions necessitate the need for knowledge of the central nervous system.

Finally, variation in personal technique used for insertion, infusion, injection, and withdrawal is another vital component affecting anatomy and physiology. The impact of differences in cannula types and components and solution composition can be evaluated and monitored more easily than the nuances of individual technique. A thorough working knowledge of the anatomy and physiology of multiple body systems, combined with a carefully crafted expertise, are necessary to ensure a positive patient outcome.

INTEGUMENT AND CONNECTIVE TISSUE

The integument, or skin, is a highly specialized organ that protects the body from its environment. It ranges in thickness from 1.5 to 4.0 mm, with the thickest skin appearing on the palms of the hands and plantar aspect of the feet.[1] Skin is divided into two layers, the epidermis and the dermis. Lying immediately under the dermis is the hypodermis, which is composed of adipose tissue. This layer cushions and protects the underlying structures and acts as insulation for the body (Fig. 6–1).

Loose connective tissue lies under the skin and is composed of several types of fibers and cells. Its primary functions include providing structure and defense. Superficial veins for venipuncture lie in this layer of loose tissue.

Structure

Epidermis

The epidermis is composed of five layers, or strata, of squamous cells. These layers represent different stages of the maturation process. Individual cells are constantly maturing, moving upward to the surface and being replaced by new cells from the base. These cells, or keratinocytes, contain keratin, a protective protein found in epithelial tissue that is subject to drying and other mechanical stresses. The maturation process for the cells results in a ''mass of chemically inert, mechanically resistant parallel fibers embedded in a dense matrix.''[1] Stressful agents such as prolonged exposure to sunlight, habitual pressure, and abrasion may cause thickening of the keratin layer. This may explain difficult venipunctures in some patients, especially those who are manual laborers or others whose life style involves excessive exposure to sunlight.

Two additional types of cells can be found in the epidermis, Langerhans' cells and melanocytes. Langerhans' cells function in cellular defense by detecting antigens and bringing them in contact with T lymphocytes. This process may be clinically responsible for skin reactions such as allergic contact dermatitis or graft rejection. Patients with some types of skin diseases and those exposed to ultraviolet radiation may have a reduced number of Langerhans cells, or the cells may be functionally impaired.[2] Melanocytes contain the pigment that imparts color to the skin. Variation in color depends on the number and composition of melanocytes, as well as on genetic, hormonal, and environmental factors.

Between the epidermis and dermis is a basement membrane, or lamina. This membrane has a mechanical function, providing additional support and flexibility to the skin. It contains adhesive materials that help anchor the epidermis to the dermis. Other cellular activities, such as antigen-antibody complex development and the filtration of other large molecules, occur in this membrane.

Dermis

The dermis, the thickest layer of the skin, is soft connective tissue with varying amounts of elastin fibers, collagen

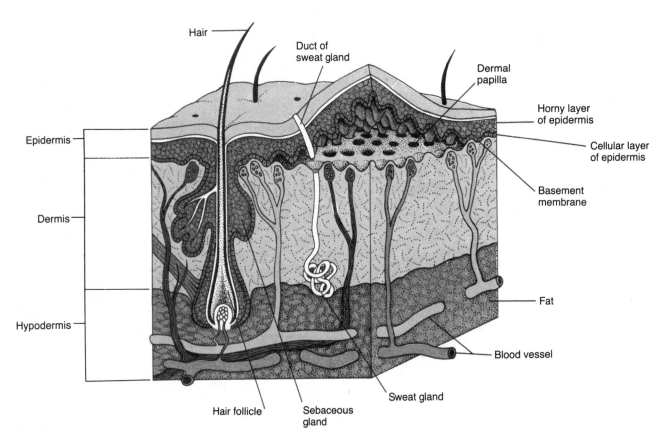

Figure 6–1. Anatomy of the skin. (From Ignatavicius DD, Bayne MV. Medical-Surgical Nursing: A Nursing Process Approach. Philadelphia: W.B. Saunders, 1991:1134.)

fibers, blood, and lymphatic vessels. Collagen is arranged in bundles and is the largest component of the dermis. Sebaceous glands, sweat glands and ducts, hair follicles, and arrector pili muscles surrounding the follicles are also located in the dermis (see Fig. 6–1).

Two layers of dermis can be identified. The papillary layer is immediately under the epidermis and serves to anchor the epidermis mechanically and support it metabolically. Finger-like projections extend into the base of the epidermis to enhance the bond between the two layers. The reticular layer is the deepest and is characterized by dense, irregular, connective tissue. This type of connective tissue is formed by strong collagen fiber bundles arranged in a multilayered network, providing the ability to stretch. Elastin fibers are usually thinner and have almost perfect recoil.

The hair bulb, responsible for generating the growth of hair, is located in the dermis and is surrounded by the hair follicle. Arrector pili muscles extend at an angle from the follicle into the dermis. When these muscles are stimulated by cold or emotion, the hair shaft is pulled upward and the skin appears dimpled. Sebaceous glands are located in the angle between the muscle and follicle and the muscular action expresses sebum, the secretion from the sebaceous glands. Sebum passes through a duct, into the hair follicle, and onto the skin surface. The complete function of sebum, composed of glycerides, cholesterol, and wax esters, is not known, but it is believed that it lubricates and protects the hair and skin and contributes to individual body odor.

Sweat glands and ducts arise from the dermis and communicate with the skin surface. These glands secrete a clear, odorless fluid containing urea, lactate, amino acids, and ions such as sodium, chloride, calcium, and bicarbonate. Secretion is stimulated by temperature elevation and emotional stimulation.

Subcutaneous Tissue

Continuing downward to the next layer, the superficial fascia is a layer of loose connective tissue (Fig. 6–2). This layer contains the same collagen and elastin fibers as the dermis. Adipose tissue or fat cells are located in this layer, where they serve as energy stores and thermal insulation. A large variety of defensive cells similar to those found in the blood are found in this tissue. Among all these important components lies the superficial veins used for peripheral venipuncture.

Defense cells include fibroblasts, macrophages, lymphocytes, and mast cells. Fibroblasts, the most abundant, are involved with the synthesis of proteins and help create a fibrous matrix that forms granulation tissue during wound healing. Macrophages play a key role in defense mechanisms of the immune system by attacking and engulfing foreign substances. These cells can be mobile or attached to other fibers and are similar in action to circulating monocytes and Langerhans' cells in the epidermis. Macrophages are responsible for bringing antigens in contact with lymphocytes.

Lymphocytes are present in loose connective tissue, but their number can increase greatly during pathologic states. They synthesize and secrete antibodies after stimulation from an antigen. There are two types of lymphocytes, B and T. B lymphocytes originate in the bone marrow, and travel to various locations through the lymph. They mainly produce antibodies or immunoglobulins when stimulated by an antigen. T lymphocytes are formed in the bone marrow and then migrate to the thymus gland before moving into the lymphatic system. Their function is not completely known, but, they do destroy viruses, fungi, and tumor cells.

Mast cells, also originating in the bone marrow, are similar to basophils in the blood and are another means of protection in the skin and loose connective tissue. The mean number of mast cells in the skin ranges from 7,000 to 12,000/mm³.[2] They can be found in large numbers around blood vessels and nerves.

The granular components of mast cells include heparin, histamine, leukotrienes (slow-reacting substances of anaphylaxis), and many types of enzymes. Mechanical or physical stimuli such as light, heat, cold, trauma, vibration, and pressure can cause mast cells to release their contents. These cells also respond to chemical or immunologic stimulation, such as contact with antigens to which the body has been exposed in the past. This contact initiates the antigen-antibody complex. The clinical picture of mast cell stimulation includes urticaria and angioedema. Urticaria is defined as limited areas of raised erythema and pruritis involving the superficial portion of the dermis. Angioedema indicates that the edema has extended to the subcutaneous layers, which may explain why urticarial rings occur around the venipuncture sites of some patients. Generalized reactions have also been documented to occur from mast cell stimulation with the release of large amounts of histamine into the circulation. Increased capillary permeability, smooth muscle contraction, and alterations in clotting have been attributed to mast cell stimulation.

Blood is supplied to the skin through small arteries that penetrate from the superficial fascia to the reticular layer of the dermis and then branch into a sheet-like plexus. Arterioles supply sweat and sebaceous glands and hair follicles with another plexus that is formed as arterioles pass through the reticular and papillary layers of the dermis. Capillaries loop upward to the base of the epidermis and venules pass back through the dermis to join small veins in the superficial fascia.[1] The skin is also served by a large number of small lymphatic vessels with numerous anastomoses at all levels.

The nerve supply to the skin is extensive and acts as a sensory organ and as a regulator of response to thermal stimuli. Sensory receptors in the form of free nerve endings provide needed information about the external environment. Encapsulated mechanoreceptors are found in the deep dermal layer and respond to weight, pressure, and vibrations.

Effects of Aging

The normal aging process can have a distinct affect on the appearance and performance of the skin. Another source of skin changes is habitual sun exposure, called photoaging or dermatoheliosis.[2]

Changes in the appearance of skin attributed to age include wrinkling, dryness, and looseness. These effects can be found in all layers and cells of the skin (Table 6–1). Such changes indicate that the skin has a continually decreasing capability to respond to forces and strain, becoming more rigid and inflexible. The frequent clinical picture of these problems as related to parenteral therapy includes bleeding from veni-

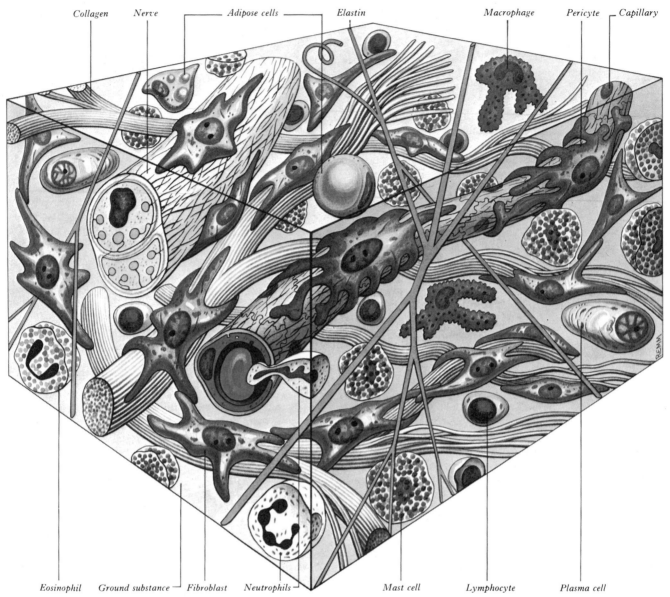

Collagen   Nerve   Adipose cells   Elastin   Macrophage   Pericyte   Capillary

Eosinophil   Ground substance   Fibroblast   Neutrophils   Mast cell   Lymphocyte   Plasma cell

Figure 6–2. Schematic reconstruction of loose connective tissue showing the characteristic cell types, fiber, and intercellular spaces. (From Williams PL, Warwick R, Dyson M, Bannister LH [eds]. Gray's Anatomy, 37th ed. New York: Churchill Livingstone, 1989:59.)

puncture sites, shearing of skin layers when tape or dressing materials are removed, and excessive skin dryness with the use of alcohol and other antiseptic agents.

Photoaging as a result of exposure to the sun differs with the length of exposure, gender, and individual differences in the skin. However, the same problems are seen as those that occur with the normal aging process.

Role in Infection Control

The three most important factors in infection control are immunocompetence, nutritional status, and the maintenance of an intact integument. Therefore, careful attention must be given to the condition of the skin under dressings, the individual's response to various antiseptic solutions and dressing

materials, and the number of venous, arterial, or epidural cannulations with the necessary break in the skin.

The skin's primary function in the control of infection is as a mechanical barrier to the invasion of pathogenic organisms. Other factors pertaining to the skin's role in providing a chemical barrier remain under investigation; these include the presence of an antibacterial substance in sebaceous secretions, the role of circulating immunoglobulins, cellular immunity and delayed hypersensitivity, and the low pH of the skin. At birth, the skin of the infant is sterile. However, over the first week of life, the skin is colonized with Staphylococcus aureus, and the pH of the skin drops from 7.0 to 5.5.[2] All these factors influence which organisms can colonize normal skin.

Skin flora has been labeled according to its ability to survive and multiply. Resident flora are those organisms that can live on skin, whereas transient flora are deposited on the

Table 6–1

Anatomic and Physiologic Changes Related to Aging

Location	Change(s)
Epidermis	Flattening of projections between the two layers; widening space between keratinocytes; slower maturation of keratinocytes; decreased thickness of layer
Dermis	Decreased thickness of layer; thicker and calcified elastin fibers, sometimes with complete fragmentation; decrease in total amount of collagen; reduction in vascular network around hair follicles and glands; decreased number of blood vessels and shorter capillary loops; decreased amount of mucopolysaccharides, resulting in changes in turgor; decreased number of nerve endings; decreased number of sweat glands and sweat production
Cells	Decreased number of melanocytes, resulting in decreased protection from ultraviolet light; decreased number of mast cells and reduction in histamine release

skin from the environment. It is difficult to categorize all organisms that may be found on the skin in this manner. The number and type of organisms differ on each area of the body and at various times of the day.

Resident flora primarily consists of Propionibacterium acnes, aerobic diphtheroids, Staphylococcus epidermis, and gram-negative bacilli in moist areas such as the axilla and groin. Transient flora include aerobic spore-forming organisms, streptococci of several groups, Neisseria, and Staphylococcus aureus.

Wound Healing

Because initiating any parenteral therapy requires breaking the skin, it is appropriate to consider the process necessary for the healing of that wound. The anatomy of skin has been presented from the outer surface inward. However, to understand the process of restoring the dermis and epidermis after injury, it is necessary to discuss the repair of the dermis and then the regeneration of the epidermis.

Immediately after any wound, the initial phase is one of inflammation when platelets and mast cells have been stimulated (Fig. 6–3). Bleeding is controlled by activation of the complex clotting cascade and the activation of platelets. The permeability of local blood vessels increases and causes plasma proteins to leak into the wound, forming an extravascular clot. Neutrophils, which control bacteria, and monocytes enter the wound. Monocytes become macrophages and have a phagocytic action, as well as releasing chemicals necessary for granulation.

The second phase, proliferation or granulation, is characterized by the formation of a large number of capillaries. These are embedded in a thick matrix of fibronectin, a glycoprotein that acts like a glue. Macrophages are present in this stage and act to débride the wound. Collagen is synthesized, which adds more strength to the tissue.

Two factors may inhibit the healing process at this point. The presence of anti-inflammatory steroids prevents macrophages from entering the wound, thus slowing the formation

of granulation tissue. A lack of ascorbic acid (vitamin C) can interfere with the production of collagen.

The final stage of dermal repair is remodeling. Granulation tissue, containing a large number of cells and blood vessels, is gradually replaced with scar tissue, which contains fewer cells and vessels. Fibronectin is removed and replaced with randomly cross-linked collagen fibers. Over time, these fibers become more organized, and the tensile strength of the new tissue improves. This entire process usually occurs over several months.

Within a few hours after injury, the epidermis begins to regenerate new epithelial cells. Keratinocytes use a "leap-frog" action, moving over each other to reach the bed of the wound. They then stop moving and begin to divide, forming new epidermal cells.

NEUROLOGIC SYSTEM

The human nervous system acts as an information loop. When changes in the environment are picked up by the sensory organs of the body, information is fed back to the controlling organ, or brain, which coordinates this with numerous other pieces of information, decides what response to make, and then communicates that response back to the body.

The system can be studied in many ways. Distinct functional divisions of the nervous system include the following: (1) the sensory ability to transmit information from tactile, visual, and auditory receptors; (2) the motor functions, controlling all skeletal and smooth muscles; and (3) the autonomic system, which controls glands and smooth muscles. Anatomic divisions are the central system, composed of the brain and spinal cord, and the peripheral system, composed of 12 cranial and 31 spinal nerves.

Functional Divisions

Sensory Receptors

There are five types of sensory receptors (mechanoreceptors, thermoreceptors, nociceptors, electromagnetic receptors, and chemoreceptors), with corresponding stimuli for each (Table 6–2). Except for electromagnetic receptors, all have an affect on parenteral therapy. Many types of stimulation, such as heat, light, cold, pressure, and sound, must be processed appropriately. All these variations in modalities of sensation are transmitted along different afferent fibers, ending at a specific point in the central nervous system. This is called the "labeled line" principle,[3] and means that pain receptors transmit a painful response regardless of whether it is caused by puncture, crushing, or electricity. The sensation of touch is transmitted along the same path, no matter how the stimulation occurs.

The sensation of pain can have a profound impact on parenteral therapy. Pain can be felt quickly (fast pain) or slowly (slow pain). Fast pain is felt within 0.1 second after stimuli but slow pain takes seconds to be felt, and may increase over minutes.[3] All pain receptors in skin, subcutaneous tissue, and vessel walls are free nerve endings. Fast pain is associated with skin punctures, cuts, or electrical

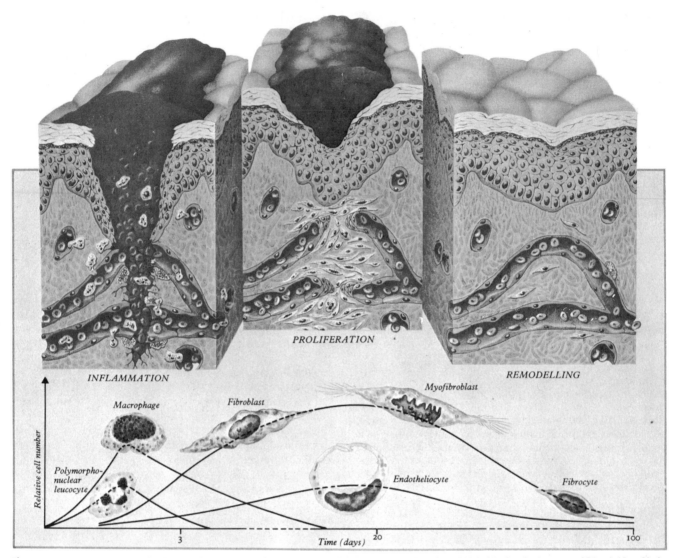

INFLAMMATION

PROLIFERATION

REMODELLING

Macrophage

Fibroblast

Myofibroblast

Polymorpho-nuclear leucocyte

Endotheliocyte

Fibrocyte

Relative cell number

3   *Time (days)*   20   100

Figure 6–3. Normal response of skin to incision. (From Williams PL, Warwick R, Dyson M, Bannister LH [eds]. Gray's Anatomy, 37th ed. New York: Churchill Livingstone, 1989:85.)

shock. Slow pain occurs more slowly but is more intense, occurring over a prolonged period, and is usually associated with tissue destruction. Mechanical, thermal, and chemical stimuli can activate pain receptors. Fast pain is evoked primarily by mechanical and thermal means, whereas slow pain is associated with all three. Histamine, bradykinin, potassium ions, serotonin, and various acids are chemicals that can stimulate pain receptors, and these are all found in damaged tissue.

Bradykinin appears to be of the greatest importance in producing pain, especially when the pain is caused by tissue damage.[3] Bradykinin is produced by a series of enzymatic activities initiated by tissue damage. Procedures such as difficult vessel puncture, rapid or improper methods of cannula advancement, and the inadvertent subcutaneous infusion of chemically irritating medications can produce tissue damage. In addition to stimulating pain receptors, bradykinin also has potent effects on the dilation of arterioles and increased capillary permeability. Small amounts of bradykinin injected intradermally can cause a large amount of edema in the area because of a dramatic increase in the size of the openings in the capillary wall.[3]

Motor Function

Information controlling muscular and secretory functions is sent from the central nervous system along efferent nerve fibers. These motor functions are controlled by specific areas of the cerebral cortex and brain stem. The pyramidal tract or corticospinal tract is the principal pathway for the transmission of impulses from the motor cortex through the brain stem and down the spinal cord. Other pathways for impulses include the mesencephalon (midbrain) and the cerebellum. The term "extrapyramidal motor system" has been used clinically to describe those motor functions outside the pyramidal system. There are many functions and pathways included in this term, and it is difficult to use it for physiologic purposes. However, the term "extrapyramidal side effects" is used to describe uncoordinated motor movements of the neck, jaw, and extremities that are associated with the administration of some types of medications.

Autonomic Nervous System

The autonomic system regulates the body's internal organs and controls such functions as glandular secretions, arterial

Table 6–2		
Sensory Receptors and Related Parenteral Therapy Procedures		
Type of Receptor	**Sensation**	**Effect of Parenteral Therapy**
Mechanoreceptor	Skin tactile sensibilities	Palpation for veins and arteries; application of antiseptic solutions and dressings; removal of tape and dressings
	Deep tissue sensibilities	Puncture of vein or artery; tight or constricting dressing
	Arterial pressure control through the baroceptor or pressure receptor system in all large arteries	Excessive infusion of intravenous fluid, increasing circulating blood volume, and activating pressure receptors
	Hearing	
	Equilibrium	
Thermoreceptor	Cold, warmth	Application of heat or cold to treat phlebitis and/or infiltration
Nociceptor	Pain	Puncture of vein or artery for insertion of any cannula; puncture of lumbar area for epidural catheter insertion; removal of dressings; infusion of irritating medications subcutaneously; application of extreme heat or cold
Electromagnetic receptor	Vision	None
Chemoreceptor	Decreased arterial pressure stimulates receptors in aorta and carotid arteries to respond to low oxygen levels and increased carbon dioxide levels	Inadequate amount of solution infused, resulting in decreased circulating blood volume
	Osmotic changes in blood	Infusion of extremely hypertonic or hypotonic solutions
	Taste	
	Smell	

blood pressure, sweating, and body temperature. Perhaps the most astonishing factor about this system is the speed with which changes occur. The heart rate can be doubled within 3 to 5 seconds, the blood pressure can drop enough to cause fainting within 4 to 5 seconds, and sweating can occur within seconds.[3] The two major divisions of this system are the sympathetic and parasympathetic (Fig. 6–4). The vagus nerve contains about 75% of all parasympathetic nerve fibers.

It is difficult to generalize about the effects of each of these systems on an individual organ. Sympathetic stimulation may cause excitation in some organs but have an inhibitory effect on another. The same can be said for the parasympathetic system. Also, the two systems may work in a reciprocal arrangement, with one causing excitation and the other producing inhibition. For example, sympathetic stimulation increases the rate and force of heart contraction, and parasympathetic stimulation has the opposite effect. Systemic blood vessels, especially in the skin of extremities, are constricted by sympathetic stimulation, and thus increase the difficulty in performing peripheral venipuncture. Parasympathetic stimulation has no effect on blood vessels except those in the face that react in the form of a blush.[3]

Anatomic Divisions

Central Nervous System

The spinal cord extends from the medulla oblongata and occupies about two-thirds of the length of the vertebral column. In most adults, the cord terminates between the first and second lumbar vertebrae. The cord is enclosed within three protective layers. The pia mater is the most proximal to the cord, the arachnoid mater is next, and the dura mater is the most distal. Between the pia and arachnoid mater is the subarachnoid space, which contains cerebrospinal fluid. The subdural space lies between the arachnoid and dura mater and does not contain fluid. This space, below the level of the cord, can be used for the epidural infusions of medication, such as for pain management.

Peripheral Nervous System

Twelve pairs of cranial nerves and 31 pairs of spinal nerves compose this system. Cranial nerves originate at the base of the brain and have four functions—motor, somatic sensory, special senses, and parasympathetic.

Of primary importance for parenteral therapy is the vagus nerve, which has the longest course of any cranial nerve. Numerous branches extend to the pharynx, larynx, heart, lungs, esophagus, stomach, liver, pancreas, spleen, small intestines, and kidneys. The heart is innervated by six branches of the vagus nerve. Stimulation leads to a depressant effect on the cardiac muscle, with clinical symptoms of bradycardia and hypotension. This syndrome is known as vasovagal syncope, and it may be preceded by weakness, nausea, vomiting, and pallor. The nervous and cardiovascular systems react together, but the exact physiologic mechanisms are unknown. This reaction could be triggered by pain, fear of pain, emotional stress, or the Valsalva maneuver.

The brachial plexus arises from cervical and thoracic spinal nerves, passing posteriorly to the clavicle in close proximity to the subclavian artery and veins. There are two large branches of this plexus, the supraclavicular and infraclavicular (Fig. 6–5). These branches bifurcate into smaller nerves that serve the muscles and cutaneous areas of the

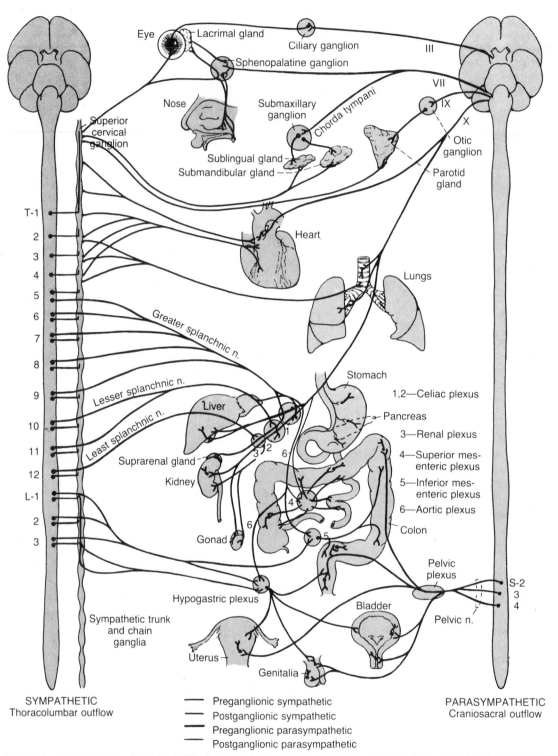

Figure 6–4. Autonomic nervous system. (From Jacob SW, Francone CA. Elements of Anatomy and Physiology, 2nd ed. Philadelphia: W.B. Saunders, 1989:129.)

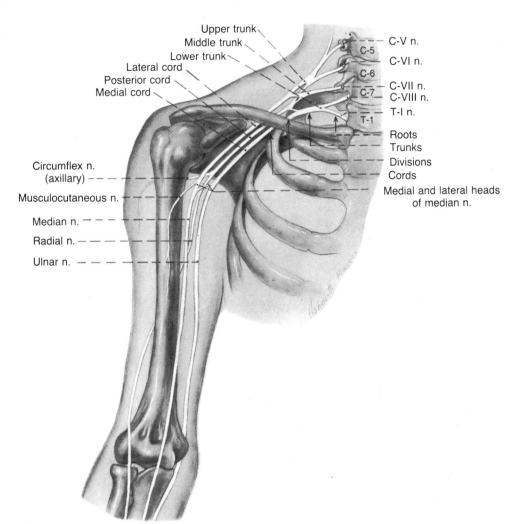

Upper trunk
Middle trunk
Lower trunk
Lateral cord
Posterior cord
Medial cord

C-5
C-6
C-7
T-1

C-V n.
C-VI n.
C-VII n.
C-VIII n.
T-I n.

Roots
Trunks
Divisions
Cords
Medial and lateral heads
of median n.

Circumflex n.
(axillary)
Musculocutaneous n.
Median n.
Radial n.
Ulnar n.

Figure 6–5. Brachial plexus and its skeletal relations. (From Jacob SW, Francone CA. Elements of Anatomy and Physiology, 2nd ed. Philadelphia: W.B. Saunders, 1989:126.)

shoulder, chest, and upper and lower arm. The close proximity of this group of nerves to the puncture site(s) of the subclavian vein make damage to the nerves and ultimately the areas served by that nerve a real possibility.

The median, ulnar, and radial nerves are all branches of the brachial plexus. The median nerve passes laterally to the brachial artery and then crosses the artery, descending medially into the antecubital fossa and then into the forearm and palm of the hand. Branches of the median nerve can be superficial in the volar aspect or palm side of the wrist (Fig. 6–6). Veins in this area appear to be good for cannulation, but venipuncture is usually painful in this area because of the close proximity of the nerve.

In the lower extremity, the sacral plexus arises from the sacral vertebrae and descends the leg in much the same manner as the brachial plexus in the arm. Of particular importance is the medial plantar nerve, which passes on the medial aspect of the foot near the ankle. The saphenous nerve passes close to the saphenous vein on the anterior aspect of the foot. When the foot of an infant is used for venipuncture, with subsequent immobilization of the joint, the nerves can be damaged if adequate padding and range of motion exercises are not used.

THE THORACIC CAVITY

The borders and boundaries of the thorax help determine the optimal locations for cannula insertion and cannula tip placement. The presence of any cannula and the solutions infused can affect the physiology of the heart and lungs, in addition to the anatomy of the vessels.

Bony Thorax

The first rib curves from the first thoracic vertebra to the upper border of the sternum. This junction is difficult to palpate because the clavicle joins the sternum immediately in front of and superior to it (Fig. 6–7). The costoclavicular ligament connects the first rib with the lower border of the clavicle close to the sternum. Motion of the sternoclavicular joint is involved with all shoulder movement. The first rib moves with respiration.

Subclavian vein cannulation in the medial aspect or close to the junction of the clavicle and first rib can have a negative outcome. The scissor-like action of these bones can sever the cannula, causing a catheter emboli.[4, 5] Positioning the patient

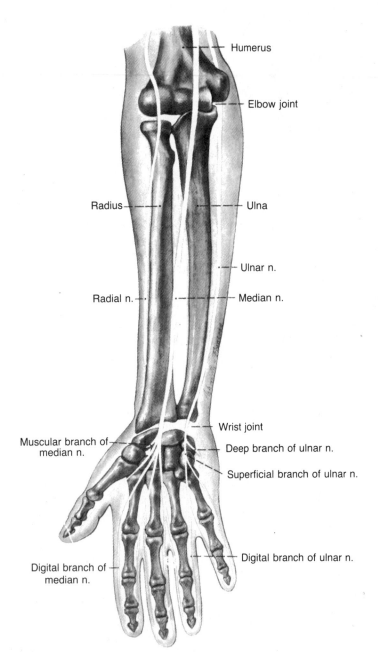

Humerus

Elbow joint

Radius

Ulna

Ulnar n.

Radial n.

Median n.

Wrist joint

Muscular branch of median n.

Deep branch of ulnar n.

Superficial branch of ulnar n.

Digital branch of ulnar n.

Digital branch of median n.

Figure 6–6. Nerves of the right forearm and hand (palmar view). (From Jacob SW, Francone CA. Elements of Anatomy and Physiology, 2nd ed. Philadelphia: W.B. Saunders, 1989:127.)

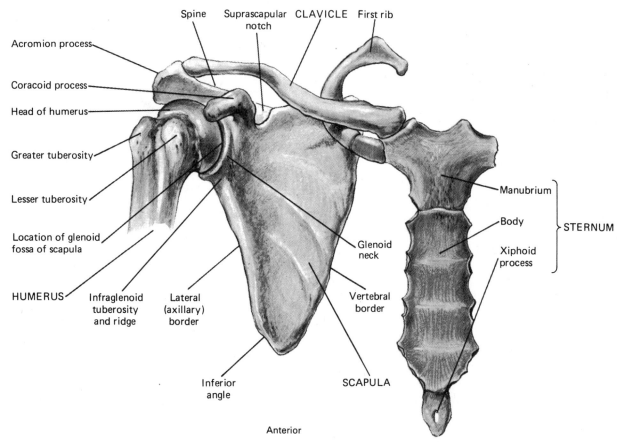

Figure 6–7. Anterior view of the scapula, sternum, and shoulder girdle. (From Solomon EP, Phillips GA. Understanding Human Anatomy and Physiology. Philadelphia: W.B. Saunders, 1989:87.)

in the Trendelenburg position with a rolled towel or sheet between the scapulas helps open the angle of these bones. When the patient is moved from this position, the angle is closed. The minimal clinical problem is compression of the cannula, causing difficult infusion. Irritation to the tunica intima of the vein could compound the problem, with the possibility of a thrombosis developing. This can be eliminated by making the venipuncture in a more lateral location, at the axillary vein, and then advancing into the central system.

Whereas venous cannulas may be a causative or contributing factor in some patients, compression of the axillosubclavian veins with or without subsequent thrombosis can be documented in patients with no invasive procedures such as cannulation. Alterations in the normal anatomy of the soft tissue around these veins can lead to venous compression during heavy lifting or during sleeping or working with the arm elevated.[6] Venous cannulation can increase the risk of thrombosis in these patients.

The kidney-shaped opening formed by the first rib, sternum, and vertebra is the thoracic inlet. It measures about 5 cm from front to back, and about 10 cm from side to side, and it is angled downward toward the anterior side.[1] This small opening must accommodate many important structures, including the subclavian arteries and veins, carotid arteries, internal jugular vein, thymus gland and its muscles and nerves, trachea and esophagus, part of the brachial nerve plexus and vagus nerve, and upper part of the pleura and apex of the lungs. Venous cannulas inserted, terminating, or passing through the veins in this area could lead to complications affecting all these structures.

Respiratory System

Anatomically, the primary components of this system with regard to parenteral therapy include the trachea, bronchi, and lungs. Functionally, our purpose here is to examine the exchange of air between the environment and the lungs, the diffusion of oxygen and carbon dioxide between the lungs and the blood, and the movement of gases into and out of the various cells of the body.

Pulmonary Anatomy

The top of the lung, or apex, arches upward into the thoracic inlet and extends about 3 to 4 cm above the first costal cartilage and 2.5 cm above the medial aspect of the clavicle.[1] This is extremely close to the subclavian vein, thus creating the risk of pneumothorax with puncture of the subclavian vein. The base of the lungs is immediately above the diaphragm, which separates the thoracic cavity from the abdominal cavity.

The blood flows into the lungs through the pulmonary arteries, which carry deoxygenated blood. Pulmonary arteries and arterioles are short segments of vessels with large diameters. They have thin walls and are capable of distention, thus allowing for a large blood volume capacity. They follow the path of the bronchi, branching into smaller arterioles with the network of capillaries surrounding each alveoli. The venous side of this same pathway, carrying oxygenated blood, follows the path of bronchioles, and becomes larger as it returns to the pulmonary veins. These veins are short and their ability to distend is about the same as the veins in the systemic circulation.

Intravenous solutions contain many types of particulate matter. Undissolved drug particles, precipitate from incompatible drugs, rubber cores of vials or solution containers, glass particles from ampules, and plastic particles from administration sets make up this particulate matter. The most likely place for these particles to stop during intravenous infusion is the microcirculation of the lungs. One study has provided information about the examination of autopsied lung tissue from 11 patients who had lengthy stays in an intensive care unit.[7] Samples of lung tissue were taken from 12 locations in each patient, mainly from the apex, base, and close to the pulmonary hila. The study used a scanning electron microscope and was the first to demonstrate particles as small as 0.8 μm. Embolism of the microcirculation, damage to the capillary endothelium, and the formation of thrombi and granulomas around these particles were noted. More acutely ill patients, immunocompromised patients, and those with a prolonged need for intravenous infusion can benefit by final filtration of solutions. Avoiding respiratory complications can lead to a more positive patient outcome.

Physiology of Respiration

Because the lungs can expand and contract like balloons, pressures inside the chest are of great importance. The negative pressure in the pleural space becomes more negative during inspiration. Alveolar pressure, or the pressure inside the alveoli, is equal to atmospheric pressure when no air is moving in or out and the glottis is open. When the alveolar pressure falls, inspiration occurs. With about 500 ml of air inside, the pressure rises above atmospheric pressure and expiration occurs. The Valsalva maneuver increases the chest pressure by holding air in the lungs against a closed glottis.

To prevent an air embolus, positive pressure in the chest is necessary when manipulating the line of a cannula whose tip lies within the thorax. Cannula insertion, changing administration tubing, inadvertent disconnection of the tubing, and cannula removal can place the patient at risk for an air embolus.

Gases, such as oxygen, carbon dioxide, and nitrogen, dissolved in water or body fluids exert the same pressure and movement as in the gaseous state. Gas molecules in the alveoli are still in the gaseous state, whereas gas molecules in the blood are dissolved. Transfer of the molecules occurs because of the partial pressure exerted by each gas. The partial pressure of oxygen in its gaseous state inside the alveoli is greater than the partial pressure of oxygen in the blood, so this pressure forces oxygen to move into the pulmonary membrane and into the capillary. The same is true for carbon dioxide—its partial pressure is greater in the blood so the transfer is in the opposite direction, from the blood across the membrane and into the alveolar sac.

The respiratory membrane is extremely thin but is composed of several layers (Fig. 6–8). The capillary is so small that a red blood cell must squeeze through the wall, with the

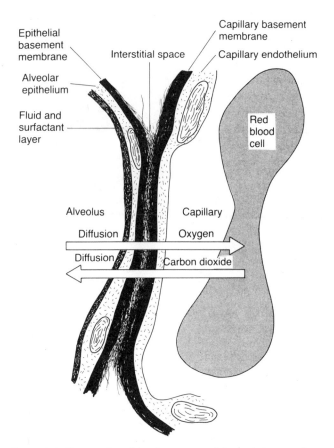

Figure 6–8. Cross section of the ultrastructure of the respiratory membrane. (From Guyton AC. Textbook of Medical Physiology, 8th ed. Philadelphia: W.B. Saunders, 1991:429.)

gases diffusing directly into and out of each red cell without passing through plasma. Although this individual unit is extremely small, there are about 300 million alveoli in both lungs, with the surface area of the respiratory membrane covering about 50 to 100 m² in a normal adult.[3] With gaseous exchange over such a large area, the speed of diffusion is understandable.

The Heart

Heart Wall

The heart is enclosed in a protective sac, called the pericardium, which extends between the second and sixth costal cartilages. The great vessels leading away from and into the heart are also enclosed in the pericardium (Fig. 6–9).

The pericardium has two layers, an outer fibrous layer and an inner serous layer. The fibrous layer is composed of strong collagen fibers and covers the aorta, superior vena cava, right and left pulmonary arteries, and the four pulmonary veins. The serous layer is further divided into the parietal and visceral layers, with the latter also being known as the epicardium. Between these two layers is a thin film of fluid that allows the heart to move. Vascular access devices within the great vessels and heart inside the pericardium have the potential to erode through the wall. Two clinical conditions can occur: (1) pericardial effusion, with fluid leaking between the

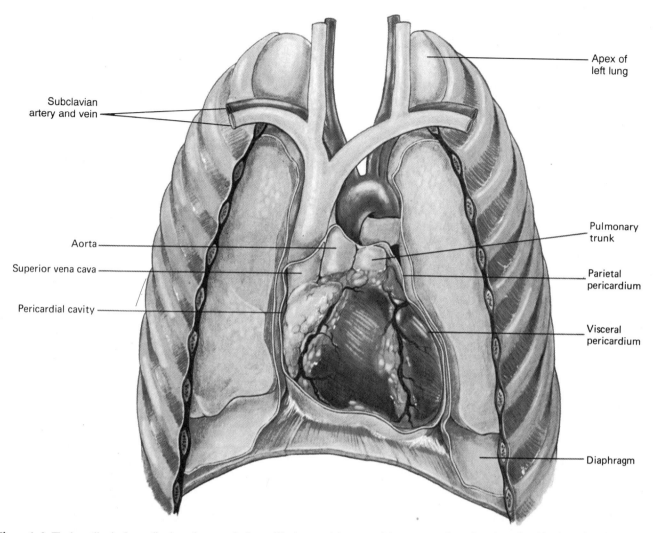

Figure 6–9. The heart lies in the mediastinum between the lungs. The heart and the roots of the great vessels are loosely enclosed by the pericardium. (From Solomon EP, Phillips GA. Understanding Human Anatomy and Physiology. Philadelphia: W.B. Saunders, 1987:210.)

layers of the pericardium; or (2) cardiac tamponade, with the blood and fluid exerting pressure on the heart.

The endocardium is the innermost layer of the heart and is comprised of a single layer of endothelial cells. This is a continuation of the same endothelial layer as that found on the internal surface of all arteries and veins.

Right Heart

The superior and inferior vena cava join the atrium of the right heart on the posterior aspect. The superior vena cava returns blood from the upper part of the body and has no valve. The inferior vena cava returns blood from the lower part of the body, is larger than the superior vena cava, and has a semilunar valve near the opening into the atrium. The atrium acts as a reservoir but has only enough pumping ability to move blood through the triscupid valve into the right ventricle.

Cardiac Function

Cardiac output, the quantity of blood pumped into the aorta each minute, is regulated by changes in the volume of blood flowing into the heart and control of the heart by the autonomic nervous system. Venous return is defined as the amount of blood flowing into the right atrium each minute. The heart has a unique ability to pump out all that is returned, avoiding any pooling of blood in the veins. This is known as the Frank-Starling mechanism. For this reason, the heart can adapt easily to normal changes such as increased activity of exercise. The force of the contractions increases as the heart chambers stretch to accommodate larger volumes. Stretching the right atrium also stretches the sinoatrial node, which signals an increase in the rate. It also initiates a nervous reflex that passes to the brain and back to the heart through the sympathetic nerves and the vagi to increase the rate.

PERIPHERAL VASCULAR SYSTEM

In order for oxygen and carbon dioxide to be transferred at the cellular level, blood must reach all tissues of the body through an immense network of interconnecting tubes. Anatomic names for these tubes, based on size and structure, include arteries, arterioles, capillaries, venules, and veins.

They may also be described in functional terms as vessels of distribution (arteries), resistance (arterioles), exchange (capillaries), and capacitance, or reservoir (veins). Small venules act as exchange vessels and larger venules act as a reservoir.

Blood Vessel Structure

The walls of all arteries and veins are arranged in three layers—the tunica intima (innermost layer), tunica media (middle layer) and tunica adventitia (outer layer) (Fig. 6–10). These layers have structural differences determined by the location and function of each vessel (Table 6–3).

The tunica intima is composed of a single layer of smooth flat endothelial cells that lie along the length of each vessel, subendothelial connective tissue, and a basal lamina or basement membrane. The tunica media contains smooth muscle and other fibrous tissue and is arranged around the circumference of the vessel. The tunica adventitia is connective tissue whose fibers are arranged along the length of the vessel. There is much variation in these tunics, depending on the type of vessel.

All blood vessels, lymphatic vessels, and the heart are lined with endothelium, which is a single layer of flat, smooth cells arranged along the length of the vessel. This layer of cells rests on a basement membrane to provide additional support. Each cell is linked together to form occluding or tight junctions, which prevent the leakage of fluids and cells from the vessel. Capillary walls are characterized by a thin endothelial structure, the presence of more junctions between cells, and fenestrations or openings in the cells, which allow for the rapid transfer of fluid and other substances (Fig. 6–11). Biochemical mediators such as histamine, serotonin, leukotrienes, prostaglandins, and bradykinin alter vascular permeability by creating a separation of these cells.

Endothelial cells have a negative charge that repels other negatively charged cells such as platelets, thus controlling clot formation. Arterial endothelial cells store the von Willebrand clotting factor.[1] Many other metabolic and enzyme systems are found in the endothelial cells of blood vessels and are currently under further study. Damage to these cells is the beginning of the inflammation process of phlebitis and of the clotting process that can cause thrombosis. The endothelial cells of veins and arteries can be damaged by the following:

1. Rapid cannula advancement
2. Cannula advancement without anchoring skin and vein by holding traction on skin
3. Insertion of cannula too large for lumen of vein
4. Insertion of cannula close to area of joint flexion without adequate support from hand boards
5. Inadequate taping, allowing for motion of cannula
6. Inadequate skin preparation, allowing for invasion of microorganisms
7. Nonocclusive, dirty, or wet dressing, allowing for invasion of microorganisms
8. Location of cannula tip that causes impingement of tip on vein wall
9. Infusion of particulate matter
10. Infusion of hypertonic or hypotonic fluids
11. Infusion of solution with an extremely high or low pH
12. Rapid infusion of quantities too large for vessel lumen to accommodate

Smooth muscle in the tunica media is composed of long, tapered spindles of muscle fibers. These spindles are arranged in bundles or layers around the circumference of the vessel and contract together as a single unit. Each bundle is closely arranged so that their cell membranes adhere in numerous places. The action potential for each bundle stimulates the remaining ones by communicating gap junctions through which ions flow freely. Smooth muscles of blood vessels are capable of maintaining contraction or a state of tension for lengthy periods. Several other differences exist between the function of smooth muscles and skeletal mus-

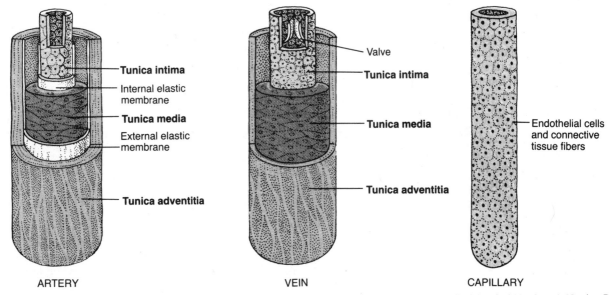

ARTERY — Tunica intima / Internal elastic membrane / Tunica media / External elastic membrane / Tunica adventitia

VEIN — Valve / Tunica intima / Tunica media / Tunica adventitia

CAPILLARY — Endothelial cells and connective tissue fibers

Figure 6–10. Microscopic anatomy of an artery, vein, and capillary. (From Ignatavicius DD, Bayne MV. Medical-Surgical Nursing: A Nursing Process Approach. Philadelphia: W.B. Saunders, 1991:2083.)

Structural Differences in Blood Vessels in Arterial and Venous Walls

Layer	Arteries	Arterioles (lumen diameter, <0.5 mm)	Capillaries	Venules	Veins
			Blood Vessels		
Tunica intima	Elastic arteries—elongated endothelial cells, multiple layer subendothelial tissue, and fenestrated elastic membrane; thicken with age and fatty deposits; contain baroreceptors and chemoreceptors Muscular arteries—thinner, allowing diffusion of metabolites; contain other afferent nerve fibers	Thin layer of endothelial cells with basal lamina	Single cell layer of endothelium and thin basal lamina	Endothelial layer and basal lamina	Endothelial layer of shorter, broader cells and basal lamina
Tunica media	Elastic arteries—thicker with more elastic and fibrous tissue arranged in circular bands; responds to pumping action of heart Muscular arteries—smooth muscle fibers controlling constriction and relaxation	Decreasing amounts of elastin; muscle cells form communicating (gap) junctions, allowing diffusion of ions and electrical stimulation	No middle layer	Small venules— no middle layer Larger venules— thin layer of smooth muscle	Thick layer of connective tissue with elastin fibers and smooth muscle fibers, although thinner than same layer in arteries
Tunica adventitia	Elastic arteries—thin layer of collagen fibers Muscular arteries—contain collagen and elastin; contain vasa vasorum, lymphatic channels, and both efferent and afferent nerve fibers	Fine collagen fibers; contain vasa vasorum, lymphatic channels, and efferent nerve fibers	Thin reticular tissue with occasional fibroblasts and mast cells	Thin fibrous tissue	Loose connective tissue, with elastin fibers; contain vasa vasorum, afferent and sympathetic nerves

cles. The force of contraction is greater in smooth muscles and less energy is required to maintain contraction. Also, smooth muscles can shorten by two-thirds their length during contraction, thus allowing the vessel lumen to change from very large to extremely small.

The stress-relaxation phenomenon of smooth muscles is another important aspect of blood vessel physiology. When a tourniquet is placed on the extremity to distend peripheral veins, the muscle fibers elongate to accommodate the increased volume collecting in the veins. The pressure in-

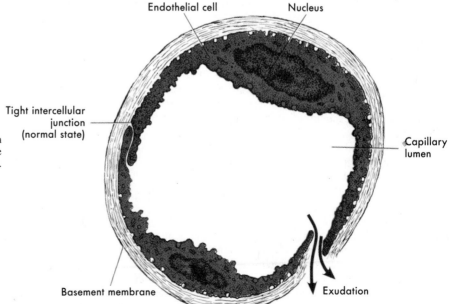

Figure 6–11. Cross section of a capillary. (From McCance KL, Huether SE. Pathophysiology: The Basis for Disease in Adults and Children. St. Louis: C.V. Mosby, 1990:219.)

creases quickly and then, within a few seconds, falls back toward the normal level, even with the increased volume. When the tourniquet is removed, the volume and pressure suddenly fall and, within several minutes, the normal pressure is re-established. Knowledge of this process is crucial when timing the removal of a tourniquet and the advancement of long cannulas into the vein. Obstruction may be encountered if not enough time has elapsed to allow equilibrium to return.

Another characteristic of smooth muscles is excitation by stretch. When smooth muscles have been excessively stretched, the muscles contract and automatically contract to resist that stretch. This explains what happens when a tourniquet has been left in place for an extended period and the veins can no longer be palpated.

Stimulation of the tunica media by trauma or changes in temperature and pressure can lead to vascular spasm. If an artery is affected, the result is an interruption in the flow of blood to the area served by that artery, with possible necrosis of that tissue. When this occurs in a vein, the outcome is not as negative, but the patient experiences pain at the site from a change in the blood flow.

The aorta, its major branches, and the pulmonary arteries are elastic arteries because the flow of blood is rapid and under high pressure, so these vessels need to be composed of a large amount of elastic tissue. This allows for a high degree of distensibility, especially during ventricular systole when blood is forced out into these arteries. Medium and small arteries are muscular arteries, containing more muscular tissue, and are capable of controlling blood flow by constriction and dilation. Distention and recoil keep blood flowing during diastole in a smooth yet pulsatile manner.

As arteries branch and become smaller in diameter, they are known as arterioles. They further subdivide into terminal arterioles and metarterioles. All are considered to be resistance vessels. On the capillary end of each metarteriole is a precapillary sphincter, which controls the flow of blood through the capillary bed (Fig. 6–12).

The venous side of the circulation is known for its compliance or the ability to increase in volume with a given increase in pressure. The amount of elastic tissue found in the wall of the vessel is the primary reason for the difference in compliance or capacitance. About three times more of the circulating volume of blood is located on the venous side than the arterial side. Combined with the ability of the venous walls to distend about six to ten times more than the arterial walls, a small increase in pressure results in a much larger quantity of blood in any vein. The same pressure increase in a corresponding artery would not result in a volume increase.

Blood is supplied to the vessel walls by the vasa vasorum, a dense capillary network within the tunica adventitia of each vessel. These capillaries may be a branch of the artery it serves or may be from a distant artery. In veins, this network may penetrate to the tunica media.

Sympathetic nerves are located in the adventitia of large arteries and veins. A steady flow of impulses are sent from the vasomotor center in the medulla and pons of the brain to maintain the vasomotor tone, which is a partial state of contraction of all vessels. Norepinephrine, the neurotransmitter at the synapse of these sympathetic nerves, acts on the α-adrenergic receptors of the smooth muscles in the vessels to

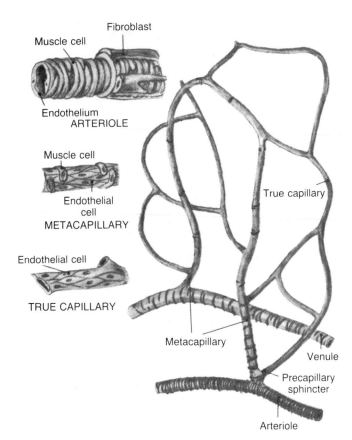

Figure 6–12. Diagrammatic representation of a portion of a capillary bed typical of many tissues. Precapillary sphincters regulate the flow of blood from the metacapillary into true capillaries. (From Jacob SW, Francone CA. Elements of Anatomy and Physiology, 2nd ed. Philadelphia: W.B. Saunders, 1989:184.)

cause contraction. This state of contraction supports the arterial pressure and keeps blood moving back to the heart. There are no nerve endings in vessels that directly cause vasodilation. Instead, a decrease in the impulses causing vasomotor tone leads to vasodilation. Also located in the intima and adventitia of systemic arteries are afferent peripheral nerves. Some of these may carry pain impulses, whereas others are baroreceptors and chemoreceptors (see Table 6–2).

Valves are found in veins, but not in arteries. Valves are semilunar folds, extending from the tunica intima into the lumen of the vein (see Fig. 6–11). They are composed of collagen and elastin fibers covered with endothelial cells. Usually, valves are arranged in pairs, but there can be three folds or leaflets together as well as a single leaflet at other locations. Valves can be found in most veins, except for extremely small and large ones. They can be found at bifurcations or where two veins unite. However, there is little or no documentation about any specific locations for valves within the superficial veins used for venipuncture, probably because of the great variations among individuals. On the proximal side of each valve the vein wall expands, creating a sinus above each valve. When veins are distended, such as with the application of a tourniquet, blood flow is temporarily stopped. This creates a pooling of blood in these sinuses and yields a "knotted" appearance externally.

The purpose of valves is to keep blood moving toward the

heart by way of the muscle pump, sometimes called the venous pump (Fig. 6–13). With the contraction of each muscle during movement pressure is applied to the vein, forcing blood back toward the heart. This pumping action opens the proximal valve and closes the distal valve, preventing a backward flow. Venous blood flow in all extremities is against gravity, resulting in a great rise in venous pressure if this pumping system fails. When valves become damaged or incompetent, pressure rises in the distal end of the extremity. The pooling of blood in capillaries causes fluid to leak outside the circulatory system, resulting in edema and a decreased blood volume.[3, 8] This muscle pump may have an impact on cannulas made of soft, flexible material, causing these cannulas to migrate out of the vein. This may occur more frequently with patients in the home care setting who are engaged in normal activities of daily living.

The normal pattern of blood flow is through the aorta, which branches into smaller arteries, but there are some deviations from that pattern. Rather than ending in an arteriole,

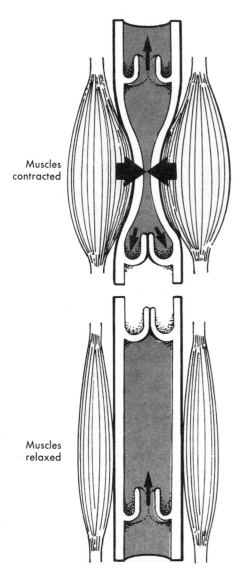

Figure 6–13. The muscle pump. (From McCance KL, Huether SE. Pathophysiology: The Basis for Disease in Adults and Children. St. Louis: C.V. Mosby, 1990:889.)

Muscles contracted

Muscles relaxed

two arteries may anastomose and bypass the capillary bed. This occurs in some arteries in the brain, intestines, and joints. An arteriovenous anastomosis is a small artery and vein connected together. These may be found in mucous membranes and deep in the dermis of the hands and feet. The venous side is affected by the higher pressure from the arterial side, and may result in unsuccessful venipuncture attempts in this area.[1, 9]

Location of Important Arteries

The axillary artery extends from the first rib to the lateral edge of the chest in the axilla. The axillary sheath is a neurovascular bundle containing the axillary artery, axillary vein, and parts of the brachial nerve plexus controlling the arm (Fig. 6–14). The continuation of the axillary artery is the brachial artery, which moves down the arm to immediately below the elbow. There it divides into the ulnar artery, on the medial side of the arm, and the radial artery, on the lateral side of the arm (see Fig. 6–14).

Although the radial artery is smaller than the ulnar artery, it is preferred for arterial puncture for blood withdrawal and cannula insertion because it is more superficial and can be stabilized for easier entry. It is imperative that the Allen test be performed to assess the collateral circulation. This is done by locating and compressing both arteries and noting the blanching that occurs. When only the ulnar artery is released color should return to the entire hand, indicating the ability of this artery to supply blood to the whole hand. If this positive assessment cannot be made, another site should be chosen.

Location of Important Veins

Systemic veins can be divided into two types, superficial and deep. Deep veins accompany arteries, usually of the same name, and both are enclosed in a protective sheath of connective tissue, known as venae comitantes. Superficial veins, best suited for venipuncture, lie in loose connective tissue under the skin. This location allows for easy movement of these veins. Therefore, during any attempt to cannulate a vein, some method must be used to anchor the vein. Without securing the vein, puncture and advancement of the cannula result in unnecessary damage to the endothelium of the vein and could lead to phlebitis. The use of one hand to hold traction on the skin over the vein during complete cannula advancement secures the vein, as needed (Fig. 6–15).

Superficial veins in the hand and forearm are the primary ones for the initiation of intravenous therapy, but both upper extremities should be carefully assessed (Table 6–4). Small digital veins line the borders of the fingers and unite on the back of the hand to form the dorsal venous network (Fig. 6–16). On the lateral aspect of the wrist, proximal to the thumb, the cephalic vein rises from the dorsal veins. Close to this area are perforating veins, which pierce the deep fascia and connect the superficial veins with the deeper veins of the hand. The cephalic vein at this location is large enough for the insertion of a cannula, but there are several points to consider. The motion of the wrist may increase the patient's

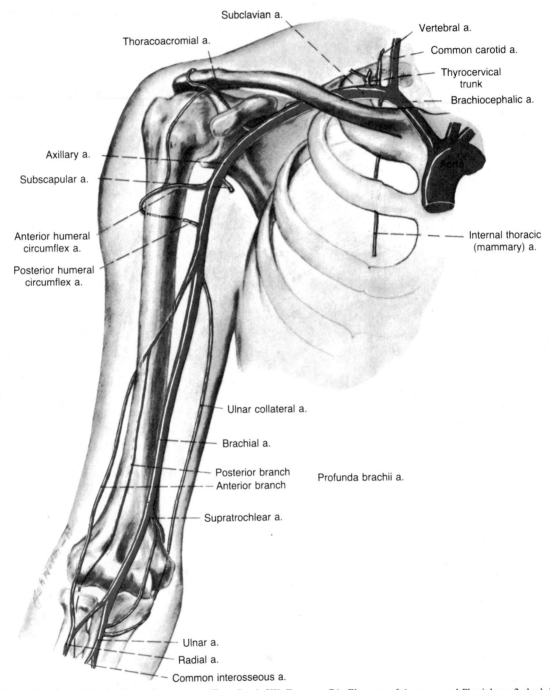

Figure 6–14. Arteries of the right shoulder and upper arm. (From Jacob SW, Francone CA. Elements of Anatomy and Physiology, 2nd ed. Philadelphia: W.B. Saunders, 1989:191.)

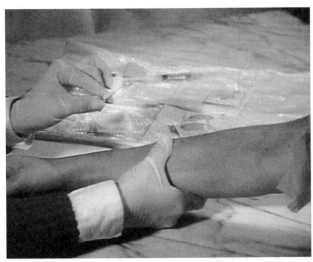

Figure 6–15. Holding traction on the skin over a vein during complete cannula advancement will secure the vein and prevent damage to the endothelium of the vein.

general discomfort, and irritation to the tunica intima results from movement of the cannula. Also, there are three long tendons that control the motion of the thumb. Although the vein is superficial to these tendons, slight movement of the thumb during the venipuncture procedure could easily obscure the vein.

The cephalic vein moves up the lateral aspect of the arm into the antecubital fossa. There may also be a network of veins on the lateral forearm that forms an accessory cephalic, joining the cephalic vein at or above the antecubital fossa (Fig. 6–17).

Moving medially across the palmar side of the forearm, the median vein ascends from the superficial palmar veins. In the wrist, these veins may appear to be suitable for venipuncture, but are usually situated between two branches of the median nerve. This results in extremely painful venipuncture and should be avoided (see Fig. 6–17).

The basilic vein is on the posterior-medial aspect of the forearm. Although it is usually a large vein, it may have been overlooked, and venipuncture may be awkward. This vein can be easily palpated and punctured when the patient's arm is placed across the chest, with the nurse on the opposite side of the patient from the arm being examined (Fig. 6–18).

The radial and ulnar veins parallel the arteries of the same name in the venae comitantes. There is communication between the deep and superficial veins, and the muscle pump can be used to distend the superficial ones. By instructing the patient to open and close the hand, the muscle action helps force blood from the deep veins into the superficial ones, thus distending them for easier palpation and puncture.

The median vein joins the basilic vein slightly below the antecubital fossa on the medial aspect (see Fig. 6–17). The basilic vein at this level is the best insertion site for antecubital catheters. However, on some patients, this vein may be located too far to the posterior aspect of the elbow, making venipuncture difficult. Palpation of this vein should begin on

Table 6–4		
Short Peripheral Cannula Insertion Sites for Children and Adults		
Site	**Advantages**	**Disadvantages**
Dorsal venous network of hand	Most distal site, allowing successive sites in a proximal location; can be visualized and palpated easily; easily accessible	Should be stabilized on hand board; smaller than veins in forearm; diminished skin turgor and loss of subcutaneous tissue in geriatric patients; excessive subcutaneous fat in infants; limited ability to use hand may present problems for patients at home
Cephalic vein	Large vein; easy to stabilize; easily accessible for caregiver and patient; may be palpated above antecubital fossa	May be obscured by tendons controlling thumb; puncture sites directly in wrist and antecubital fossa can increase complications because of joint motion
Accessory cephalic	Medium to large vein(s); easy to stabilize; can be palpated easily	Valves at junction of cephalic may prohibit cannula advancement; length of vein may be too short for cannula; may not be located on children
Median	Medium vein; easy to stabilize; easily accessible for caregiver and patient	Puncture in wrist may be excessively painful because of close proximity of nerve; may be slightly more difficult to palpate and visualize
Basilic	Large vein; can be palpated easily; may be available after other sites have been exhausted	More difficult to access because of location; may be difficult for patient to access and observe site; puncture site directly in antecubital fossa may result in increased complications because of joint motion; cannot be palpated above antecubital fossa
External jugular	Large vein; easily accessible for emergency situations	Increased complications because of motion of neck; occlusive dressing difficult to maintain
Dorsal venous network on foot	Easily accessible	May not be easily palpated because of age or disease-related changes; higher incidence of complications related to impaired circulation; difficult to stabilize joint; greatly limits ability to walk
Medial and lateral marginal veins of foot	May be large; usually easy to palpate and visualize	Higher incidence of complications related to impaired circulation; difficult to stabilize joint; greatly limits ability to walk
Great and small saphenous	Large veins; usually easy to palpate and visualize	Higher incidence of complications related to impaired circulation; located close to perforating veins connecting to deep veins of the leg

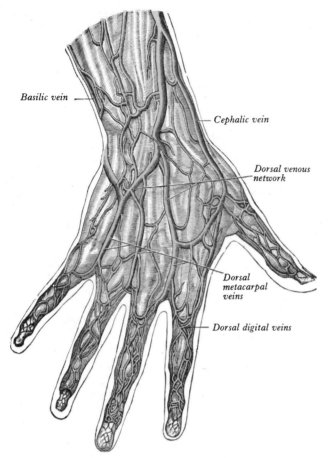

Figure 6–16. Superficial veins of the hand. (From Williams PL, Warwick R, Dyson M, Bannister LH [eds]. Gray's Anatomy, 37th ed. New York: Churchill Livingstone, 1989:806.)

the distal end in the forearm and the course of the vein followed to evaluate its location.

In the antecubital fossa, the cephalic vein communicates with the basilic vein by the median cubital vein (see Fig. 6–17). There is also communication with the deep veins where the median cubital vein enters the basilic vein. Variations in the median cubital vein may be seen. Some patients may have two branches of this vein, one angling toward the basilic, known as the median basilic, and the second one angling from the center of the fossa toward the cephalic, known as the median cephalic vein. Because of variations, careful evaluation and assessment of each patient is important when insertion of an antecubital cannula is planned (Table 6–5).

The upper part of the arm has three veins of importance. The cephalic vein continues upward lateral to the biceps muscle. The basilic vein is medial to the biceps and extends to the superior axilla, where it becomes the axillary vein (see Fig. 6–17). Also in the upper arm is the brachial vein, located deep in the arm as a vena comitans in the sheath with the brachial artery.

The distal end of the axillary vein can be considered as the beginning of the veins in the shoulder area. The axillary vein is classified as a deep vein; it extends from the lateral aspect of the chest in the axilla to the lateral border of the first rib. The axillary vein receives the brachial vein at its

midpoint and the cephalic vein near the border of the rib. The cephalic vein can also have variations in its path. It may only join the axillary vein, only connect with the external jugular in the neck, or branch into two smaller veins connecting with the axillary and external jugular veins (Fig. 6–19). There are three suprascapular veins and several other veins joining the axillary vein in this area, and as many as 40 valves can be documented in this region.[10] For this reason,

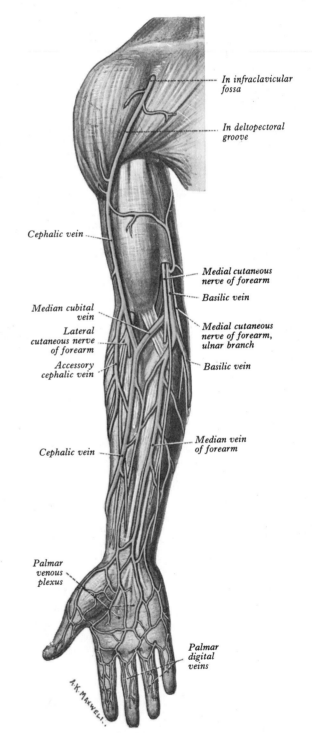

Figure 6–17. Superficial veins of the right upper extremity. (From Williams PL, Warwick R, Dyson M, Bannister LH [eds]. Gray's Anatomy, 37th ed. New York: Churchill Livingstone, 1989:806.)

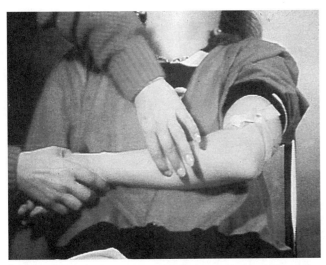

Figure 6–18. The basilic vein is easily palpated and punctured by placing the patient's arm across the chest toward the nurse, who is positioned on the side opposite the intended site.

antecubital catheters can take several wayward paths, and the actual tip location can only be confirmed by chest radiography.

There are four jugular veins draining the head and face, with three of them located superficially (Fig. 6–20). The external jugular vein is on the outer border of the neck. The posterior external jugular vein drains the occipital region and the anterior jugular vein drains the face, with both joining the external jugular at the base of the neck. The external jugular joins the subclavian vein at its midpoint. The internal jugular vein is a deep vein covered by the muscles of the neck. It joins the subclavian vein at its proximal end.

From the lateral edge of the first rib to the sternal edge of the clavicle, the continuation of the axillary vein is the subclavian vein. The vein angles upward as it arches over the first rib and passes under the clavicle, forming a narrow passage for the vein (see Fig. 6–8). The apex of the lungs is also extremely close to the location of the subclavian vein, increasing the potential for pneumothorax when puncture of

the subclavian is performed (see Fig. 6–8). Table 6–6 lists central venous cannulation locations.

At the top of the thoracic inlet, the internal jugular and subclavian veins join to create the brachiocephalic vein, also called the innominate vein. At this junction is the location of the last venous valve before the heart. The left brachiocephalic vein, which is approximately 6 cm in length, is about twice as long as the right (Fig. 6–21).

There is another structure at this location, the thoracic duct, which is a large, deep lymphatic vessel that receives a large quantity of lymph from the entire body (Fig. 6–22). Damage to this large vessel may occur during puncture of the large blood vessels in this area. Lymph is composed of various fluids and cells draining from capillary beds. Lymphatic vessels follow the path of other blood vessels throughout the body. The flow of fluid is aided by valves inside the vessels, and is the result of muscular contraction and compression from the pulsation of neighboring arteries.

The two brachiocephalic veins unite at the lower border of the first rib to form the superior vena cava. About 7 cm long and 2 cm wide, it descends to the level of the third costal cartilage, where it joins the right atrium of the heart. On chest radiography, its location is seen in the right mediastinal border. At the second costal cartilage, the fibrous pericardium of the heart begins and encompasses the lower half of the superior vena cava.

Other tributaries unite with the great thoracic veins and have been documented as aberrant locations for central venous cannulas.[11] The internal thoracic (mammary) vein joins the superior vena cava at the superior end. The left and right inferior thyroid veins join the respective brachiocephalic veins, draining the esophageal, tracheal, and laryngeal areas. The left superior intercostal vein joins the left brachiocephalic vein. The azygos vein drains the spinal column, and enters the posterior side of the superior vena cava immediately above the beginning of the pericardium (Fig. 6–23).

In the lower extremity, the pattern of vascular distribution is similar to that of the upper extremity, with the superficial veins in the subcutaneous fascia and the deep veins accompanying the deeper arteries. The greatest difference is the presence of more valves in the lower extremity. The dorsal metatarsal veins form a network across the top of the foot.

Table 6–5		
Antecubital Cannula Insertion Sites for Children and Adults		
Site	**Advantages**	**Disadvantages**
Basilic	Largest vein; straight pathway in upper arm and thorax	May be located too far to the posterior side for sterile procedure and routine care; may only be able to palpate a short segment
Median	Communicates with larger basilic; easily accessible for insertion and routine care	
Median cubital		
Median basilic	Joins with larger basilic; easily accessible for insertion and routine care	Valve may be located at junction with basilic, causing obstruction to cannula advancement
Median cephalic	Easily accessible	Valve may be located at junction with basilic, causing obstruction to cannula advancement; terminates in smaller cephalic; may not be present in some patients
Accessory cephalic	Easily accessible for insertion and routine care	Valve may be located at junction with cephalic, causing obstruction to cannula advancement; terminates in smaller cephalic; may not be present in some patients
Cephalic	Easily accessible for insertion and routine care; easy palpation and visualization above and below antecubital fossa	Smaller than basilic; pathway in upper arm and thorax is variable and unknown

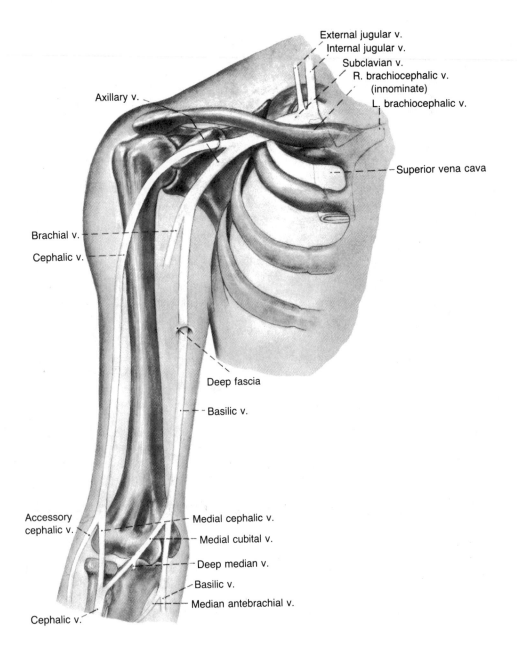

Axillary v.

Brachial v.

Cephalic v.

External jugular v.

Internal jugular v.

Subclavian v.

R. brachiocephalic v.
(innominate)

L. brachiocephalic v.

Superior vena cava

Deep fascia

Basilic v.

Accessory
cephalic v.

Medial cephalic v.

Medial cubital v.

Deep median v.

Basilic v.

Median antebrachial v.

Cephalic v.

Figure 6–19. Veins of the right shoulder and upper arm. (From Jacob SW, Francone CA. Elements of Anatomy and Physiology, 2nd ed. Philadelphia: W.B. Saunders, 1989:192.)

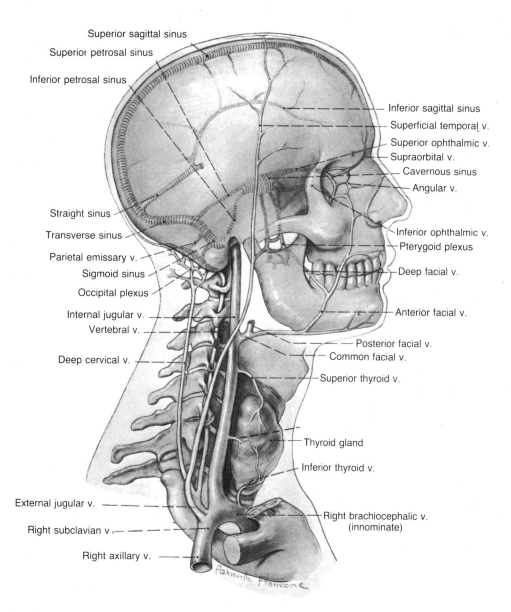

Superior sagittal sinus
Superior petrosal sinus
Inferior petrosal sinus
Inferior sagittal sinus
Superficial temporal v.
Superior ophthalmic v.
Supraorbital v.
Cavernous sinus
Angular v.
Straight sinus
Transverse sinus
Inferior ophthalmic v.
Pterygoid plexus
Parietal emissary v.
Sigmoid sinus
Deep facial v.
Occipital plexus
Internal jugular v.
Anterior facial v.
Vertebral v.
Posterior facial v.
Common facial v.
Deep cervical v.
Superior thyroid v.
Thyroid gland
Inferior thyroid v.
External jugular v.
Right brachiocephalic v.
(innominate)
Right subclavian v
Right axillary v.

Figure 6–20. Venous drainage of the head and neck. (From Jacob SW, Francone CA. Elements of Anatomy and Physiology, 2nd ed. Philadelphia: W.B. Saunders, 1989:186.)

Table 6–6

Central Venous Insertion Sites in Children and Adults

Site	Advantages	Disadvantages
Subclavian		
Infraclavicular	Easily accessible for insertion; flatter surface to maintain occlusive dressing; more published studies using this site; some believe this site has better anatomic landmarks; preferred for children	Longer needle may be necessary to pass through skin and muscle compression of vein and cannula with possible fracture of cannula if insertion is made in a medial site
Supraclavicular	Shorter distance from skin to vein; easily accessible	Occlusive dressing may be difficult to achieve in hollow contour above clavicle
		Both sites associated with pneumothorax, hemothorax, hydrothorax, brachial nerve plexus injury, thoracic duct injury, and injury to other superior mediastinal structures
Jugular		
Internal	Larger vein diameter; multiple insertion sites; easily accessible; straighter path to superior vena cava	May damage carotid arteries
External	Superficial vein, usually visible and easy to palpate	Cannula tip location in superior vena cava not always as successful as internal jugular
	Both sites are associated with fewer complications than subclavian	Maintaining occlusive dressing on either is extremely difficult because of movement of neck and beard on male patients
Femoral	Alternative site in emergencies; tip location in large inferior vena cava	Occlusive dressing is extremely difficult with high infection rates associated with this site; associated with higher incidence of thrombosis and other serious complications

On the border of each foot lie the medial and lateral marginal veins. The great saphenous vein extends from the medial marginal vein in the foot up the medial aspect of the leg to the femoral vein in the inguinal area. It is also the longest vein in the body. The small saphenous vein arises from the lateral marginal vein at the ankle to above the knee, where it joins the popliteal vein (Fig. 6–24).

The superficial veins are connected to the deep veins by perforating veins at the ankle, distal calf, and around the knee. These perforating veins have valves that prevent blood from flowing from the deep veins to the superficial veins. Muscular action pumps blood toward the heart. However, if the valves are not functioning properly, or during periods of muscle relaxation or atrophy, blood can move into the superficial veins. The increased pressure in the superficial veins causes fluid to leak into the subcutaneous tissue, with edema

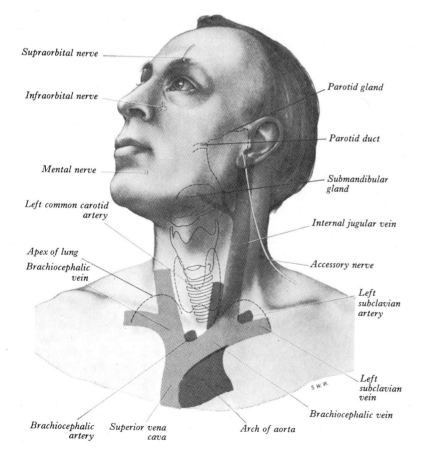

Supraorbital nerve

Infraorbital nerve

Mental nerve

Left common carotid artery

Apex of lung
Brachiocephalic vein

Parotid gland

Parotid duct

Submandibular gland

Internal jugular vein

Accessory nerve

Left subclavian artery

Left subclavian vein

Brachiocephalic vein

Brachiocephalic artery   Superior vena cava   Arch of aorta

Figure 6–21. Surface projections of some important structures in the face, neck, and upper part of the thorax. (From Williams PL, Warwick R, Dyson M, Bannister LH [eds]. Gray's Anatomy, 37th ed. New York: Churchill Livingstone, 1989:808.)

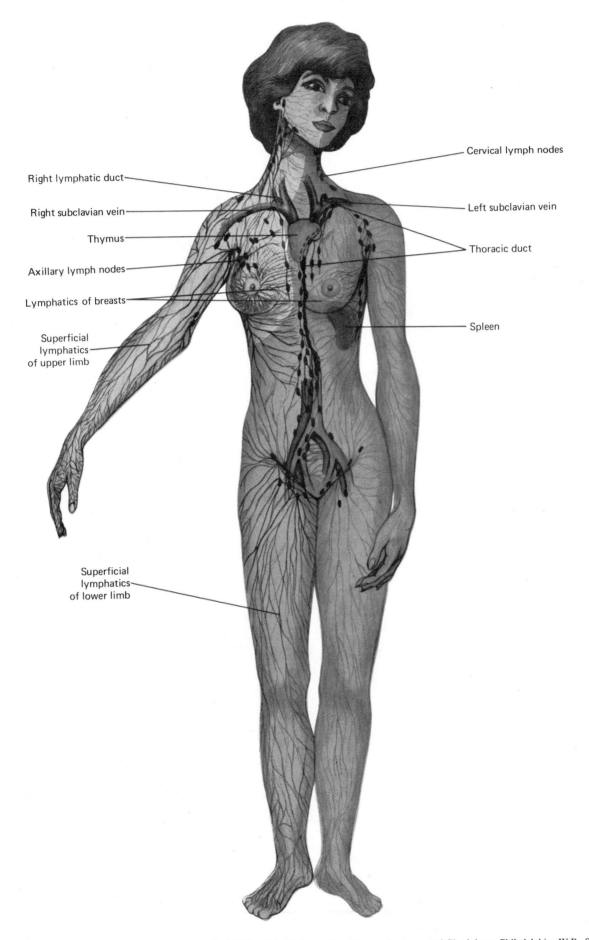

Figure 6–22. The lymphatic system. (From Solomon EP, Phillips GA. Understanding Human Anatomy and Physiology. Philadelphia: W.B. Saunders, 1989:240.)

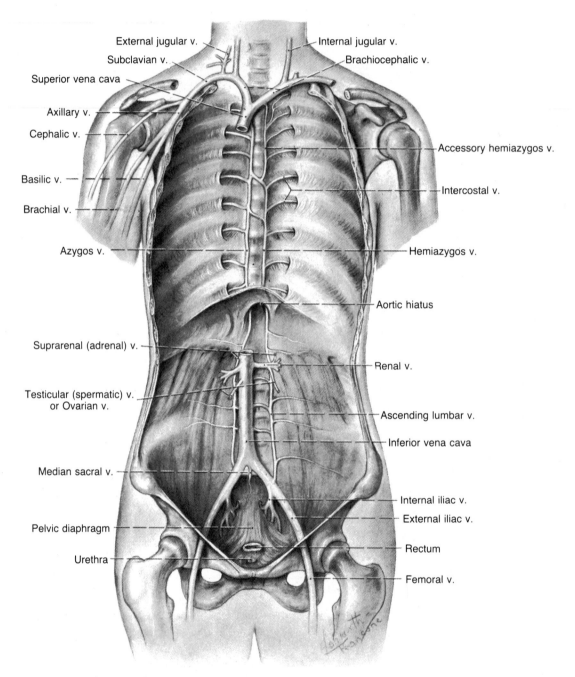

Figure 6–23. Vena cava and tributaries. (From Jacob SW, Francone CA. Elements of Anatomy and Physiology, 2nd ed. Philadelphia: W.B. Saunders, 1989:189.)

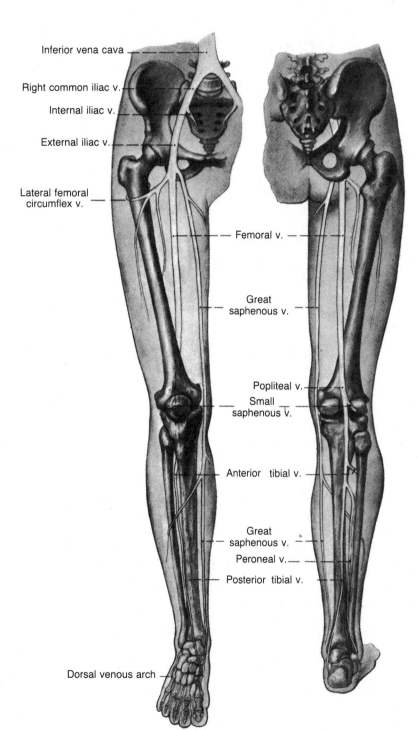

Figure 6–24. Veins of the right pelvis and leg. (From Jacob SW, Francone CA. Elements of Anatomy and Physiology, 2nd ed. Philadelphia: W.B. Saunders, 1989:196.)

Inferior vena cava

Right common iliac v.

Internal iliac v.

External iliac v.

Lateral femoral circumflex v.

Femoral v.

Great saphenous v.

Popliteal v.

Small saphenous v.

Anterior tibial v.

Great saphenous v.

Peroneal v.

Posterior tibial v.

Dorsal venous arch

seen on examination. This increased pressure leads to blood stagnation and results in enlarged and tortuous superficial veins called varicosities. Ulcerations can result from the damaged tissue and lack of circulation. Because of this process, the use of veins in the feet and ankles for the routine delivery of any intravenous therapy is not recommended.

SYSTEMIC BLOOD FLOW

Flow of any fluid is the amount of fluid that can pass a given point in a given period of time. For instance, the cardiac output of blood in an average resting adult is about 5 L/min. The circulation of blood is in a closed system and depends on more factors than the amount of blood pumped by the heart. These factors are the same as those for fluid flowing through any other closed system—the volume and properties of the fluid, the pressures within the system and the resistance to those pressures, the velocity or speed of flow, the type of flow, and the ability of the system to comply with changes in demand.

Blood Volume and Distribution

Precise regulation of the blood volume is the result of a complex interaction between cardiac output, excretion of excessive amount of fluids, and electrolytes by the kidneys, and hormonal and nervous system factors. Inability of the heart to pump strongly enough to perfuse the kidneys, an increase in red cell production (polycythemia), and the creation of additional space for blood, such as pregnancy and large varicose veins, can increase the total volume of the system.

Physical Properties of Blood

The viscosity of any fluid is defined as the degree of resistance to flow when pressure is applied. Two components of blood create its viscosity, the hematocrit, or the percentage of cells in blood, and the plasma proteins. However, the effect of the hematocrit is far greater than that of the plasma proteins. Friction from a high concentration of cells increases viscosity. Generally, the hematocrit ranges from 38 to 42%; its viscosity is about 3, the viscosity of plasma proteins is about 1.5, and that of water is about 1.[3] Many disease states, injuries, and fluid and nutritional imbalances can alter this normal value, with a corresponding increase in viscosity.

Viscosity is affected by vessel diameter. The most rapid flow in large vessels is found in the center of the vessel, with the flow closest to the vessel intima being the slowest. As the velocity of flow decreases the viscosity increases, so blood flowing through small vessels and capillaries has a higher viscosity. Red blood cells can adhere to each other or to the vessel walls and form stacks, called rouleaux. Cells can become lodged in constricted places within small vessels as well. Offsetting these factors that increase viscosity is the fact that, in capillaries and small vessels, cells line up and pass through in a single file, decreasing the viscous properties of many cells moving randomly together. This is called the Fahraeus-Lindqvist effect, and it is found in vessels smaller than 1.5 mm in diameter.[3] Because of these contradicting

factors, it is difficult to assess the total effect of the hematocrit on viscosity in small vessels and capillaries.

The presence of cannulas in vessels with a small lumen might have the same effect on the viscosity of blood. Therefore, it is important to use the smallest cannula in the largest possible vessel. This allows room for blood to flow adequately between the wall of the vein and the wall of the cannula. Knowledge of the patient's hematocrit and careful attention to adequate hydration are also important.

Pressure and Resistance to Flow

The greatest pressure, about 100 mm Hg, is found in the aorta because of the pumping action of the heart. From this point the pressure gradually decreases until it reaches the junction of the vena cavae and the right atrium, where it measures 0 mm Hg. In the capillary bed, the pressure ranges from 35 mm Hg on the arterial side to 100 mm Hg on the venous side, with a functional pressure in the capillary of about 17 mm Hg.[3] It is the difference in pressure that causes the flow of blood.

Flow through a single vessel is most affected by the diameter of the vessel (Fig. 6–25). When the diameter doubles, the flow rate increases 16 times and, with a four-fold increase in lumen diameter, the flow rate dramatically increases 256 times.

Force from this pressure is met by resistance from the vessel wall or vasomotor tone. Resistance is controlled by the vasomotor center in the brain stem that sends impulses to the sympathetic nerve endings located in all vessels except the metarterioles, precapillary sphincters, and capillaries.

Blood flow through the capillary bed is not constant, as in other vessels, but is intermittent, based on the needs of the tissue served. When the oxygen level in the tissue decreases the precapillary sphincter opens, allowing flow to proceed. The primary purpose of the thin capillary membrane is allowing diffusion of substances through the membrane. Two opposing forces control the amount of molecular movement across the membrane, hydrostatic pressure and colloid osmotic pressure.

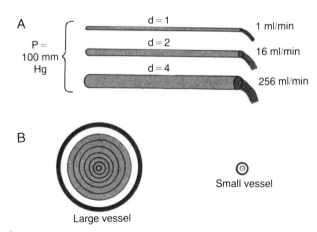

Figure 6–25. *A,* Demonstration of the effect of vessel diameter (d) on blood flow. *B,* Concentric rings of blood flowing at different velocities; the farther away from the vessel wall, the faster the flow. (From Guyton AC. Textbook of Medical Physiology, 8th ed. Philadelphia: W.B. Saunders, 1991:156.)

Hydrostatic pressure is created by the presence of fluid in the vessel and the interstitial space. Colloid osmotic pressure is the opposing force exerted by the presence of plasma proteins. Proteins do not pass through the capillary membrane easily, which results in a difference in protein concentration between the plasma and interstitial fluid, and this difference remains steady. The concentration of plasma proteins is normally about 7 g/dL with the interstitial protein level about 2 to 3 g/dL.[3] Colloid osmotic pressure is also called oncotic pressure to distinguish it from the osmotic pressure of fluid moving from the interstitial space into each individual cell.

As blood enters the arterial side of the capillary the hydrostatic pressure is greater, forcing fluid to move into the interstitial space. The smaller amount of fluid in the capillary decreases the hydrostatic pressure, causing the colloid osmotic pressure to force fluids back into the venous side.

Pressure in the peripheral veins is directly related to the pressure in the right atrium and to the heart's ability to pump blood out of the right atrium.

Normally, the right atrial pressure is 0 mm Hg, or about equal to the atmospheric pressure around the body. In a variety of clinical conditions, this can range from as high as 30 mm Hg during cardiac failure or the transfusion of massive amounts of blood, to as low as -5 mm Hg when the blood flow to the heart has been altered by hemorrhage or some other severe impediment.

Velocity and Types of Blood Flow

Velocity is the distance blood moves in a specific period of time. Normally, blood moves through the aorta at a rate of 33 cm/sec but, in capillaries, the velocity drops to 0.3 mm/sec.[3]

Flow can be in two types or patterns, laminar or turbulent. In laminar flow, the blood moves in layers or concentric circles through the vessels (see Fig. 6–25). As blood moves through the vessels, the layer touching the vessel wall is slowed because of adherence to the wall. The next layer slides easily over the outer one, and the innermost layer moves easiest.

Turbulent flow is in all directions, flowing crosswise and lengthwise along the vessel (see Fig. 6–25). This type of flow is created when the vessel's inner surface is rough, there is an obstruction or a sharp turn in the vessel, or the amount of flow has increased greatly.

▶ NURSING DIAGNOSES

Nursing diagnoses related to the physiologic systems discussed in this chapter can be found in human response patterns I and IX from NANDA's *Taxonomy I*. Pattern I is exchanging, which ''involves mutual giving and receiving and is used to classify many of the physiologic processes within the body,'' and pattern IX is feeling, which ''involves the subjective awareness of information.''[12]

A partial list of appropriate nursing diagnoses is given by the following.

Potential for Infection

This is related to the effects of medications (antibiotics, steroids) and to the presence of invasive lines.

Expected Outcomes

1. The patient will not develop any signs or symptoms of infection during the administration of prescribed medications or use of invasive lines.
2. The patient and significant other(s) will demonstrate understanding of the causes and risks associated with infection and practice precautionary measures.

Altered Renal Tissue Perfusion

This is related to exchange problems, as in the infusion of nephrotoxic antibiotics (aminoglycosides, vancomycin, antifungal agents), hypovolemia, and hypervolemia.

Expected Outcomes

1. The patient will have good fluid and electrolyte balance as evidenced by adequate urinary output and serum electrolyte results.
2. The patient will maintain safe serum levels of medications as evidenced by serum drug monitoring.
3. The patient will regain normal blood levels of nitrogenous waste products as evidenced by normal BUN and serum creatinine levels.

Altered Peripheral Tissue Perfusion

This is related to trauma to arteries from puncture for cannula insertion or blood sample withdrawal, interruption in venous flow, as in thrombosis or thrombophlebitis development, and decreased venous flow, as in the insertion of a large-gauge cannula in a vein.

Expected Outcomes

1. The patient will regain warm, dry skin.
2. The patient will have absence of palpable venous cords and pain.
3. The patient will have absence of peripheral edema distal to cannula placement.

Potential Impaired Skin Integrity

This is related to age, mechanical factors of dressing material or tape and antiseptic solutions, decreased nutritional intake, and medications (steroids, hormones).

Expected Outcomes

1. The patient will have skin integrity maintained by the use of appropriate types of dressing materials and appropriate application and removal techniques.
2. The patient will maintain good hydration and nutritional status.

Impaired Skin Integrity

This is related to age, mechanical factors of dressing material or tape and antiseptic solutions, decreased nutritional intake, and medications (steroids).

Expected Outcome

1. The patient will have healing of skin lesions with return to intact skin.

Pain

This is related to injury by chemical agents (vesicant medications, solutions with extreme tonicity and pH ranges) and physical agents (insertion of any parenteral cannula).

Expected Outcome

1. The patient will have an increasing comfort level as evidenced by decreasing complaints of pain, use of improved coping mechanisms, employment of pain relief measures, and decreased focus on pain.

References

1. Williams PL, Warwick R, Dyson M, Bannister LH. Gray's Anatomy, 37th ed. London: Churchill Livingstone, 1989.
2. Fitzpatrick TB, et al. Dermatology in General Medicine, 3rd ed. New York: McGraw-Hill, 1987.
3. Guyton AC. Textbook of Medical Physiology, 8th ed. Philadelphia: W. B. Saunders, 1991.
4. Aitken DR, Minton JP. The "pinch-off sign": A warning of impending problems with permanent subclavian catheters. Am J Surg 1984; 148:633–636.
5. Rubenstein RB, et al. Hickman catheter separation. J Parent Enteral Nutr 1985; 9:754–757.
6. Roos DB. Thoracic outlet syndromes: Update 1987. Am J Surg 1987; 154:568–573.
7. Walpot H. Particulate contamination of intravenous solutions and drug additives during long-term intensive care. Anaesthetist 1989; 38:544–548.
8. McCance KL, Huether SE. Pathophysiology: The Biologic Basis for Disease in Adults and Children. St. Louis: C.V. Mosby, 1990.
9. Plumer AL. Principles and Practices of Intravenous Therapy, 4th ed. Boston: Little, Brown and Company, 1987.
10. Agur AMR. Grant's Atlas of Anatomy, 9th ed. Baltimore: Williams & Wilkins, 1991.
11. Lum PS, Soski M. Management of malpositioned central venous catheters. JIN 1989; 12:356–365.
12. Neal MC, Paquette M, Mirch M, et al. Nursing Diagnosis Care Plans for DRGs. Venice, CA: General Medical Publishers, 1990.

CHAPTER 7 Fluids and Electrolytes

Rose Anne Lonsway, MA, CRNI
Judy Terry, BSN, CRNI

- -

- -

The study of fluids and electrolytes can be an intimidating challenge. With all its intricacies, the body relies on water, one of the simplest elemental forms that we have for existence. Water makes up almost two-thirds of an adult's body weight. The relationship and balance of water with electrolytes and the compartments found within the body determine the human health and well-being.

The continuous biochemical processes of the body work to maintain the body at a state of equilibrium. Water moves between various spaces and compartments. This movement depends on the types and amounts of solutes within the body. On a daily basis, the body strives to match excretion to intake. Any alteration in intake or excretion results in an imbalance. Recognition and prevention of, or interventions to correct, these imbalances are some of the most important roles the nurse has when caring for the patient requiring intravenous therapy. It is important to understand the purpose that water serves in the human body. Its various functions include provision of a medium for cellular metabolism, assistance in the transportation of materials into and out of the cells, action as a solvent in which many of the solutes available for cell function are dissolved, assistance in the regulation of body temperature, maintenance of the physical and chemical consistency of intracellular and extracellular fluids, help in the digestion of food through hydrolysis, and provision of a medium for the excretion of waste from the body.

It is estimated that a normal healthy person needs approximately 2600 ml of fluids daily to meet the body's water requirements. It has also been estimated that the absolute minimum amount of water required in that same healthy person is approximately 1500 ml daily. These facts make it possible to see the importance of water in the functioning of the human body to prevent breakdown of the homeostatic regulating mechanisms. It is also important to realize that an alteration in the body's normal fluid and electrolyte balance affects not only functions within the fluid compartments, but can eventually affect every system of the body. Therefore, it is vital to understand how water and electrolytes work within the homeostatic framework.

Illness or disease states easily cause a disruption of the delicate balance of the body fluid and its solutes. The treatment of these imbalances might lead to further complications. With proper knowledge of the intravenous fluids and electrolytes that are administered on a daily basis, it is possible to prevent further complications. It is therefore imperative that the nurse responsible for delivering fluids, electrolytes, and other medications has a thorough working knowledge of the normal fluid and electrolyte balances and movements within the body. Understanding the physiologic effects of intravenous fluids and electrolytes in the presence of an imbalance is an important aspect of infusion therapy.

TRANSPORT MECHANISMS

Understanding fluid and electrolyte therapy begins with understanding the intake, output, and utilization of water and electrolytes. Regulating mechanisms include osmosis, diffusion, and filtration, which all affect the movement of water and electrolytes within the body. All cells in the body are surrounded by a membrane, which is selectively permeable to some substances depending on the construction of the cell membrane itself and the ionic charge of particles or solutes attempting to move through the membrane.

Regulating Mechanisms

Osmosis

Osmosis is the movement of fluid through a semipermeable membrane. During osmosis, fluid moves in relation to the concentration of solutes. It involves the movement of fluid through a membrane from an area of low solute concentration to an area of high solute concentration. This process continues to occur until the solutions on both sides of the membrane are of equal concentration. The force of this movement depends on the concentration gradient—that is, the difference in concentration on either side of the membrane. The process of osmosis depends on how much of the membrane is involved and on certain characteristics of the solution—the temperature, solute solubility, and particularly the concentration.[1, 2]

The number of solutes in a solution is expressed by a unit of measurement called the osmol. Osmolality describes the number of osmols per kilogram of water. The liter is the usual unit of measure for water volume. Osmolality can be expressed as a total volume of 1 liter of water plus a small volume occupied by the solutes in that liter of fluid. Osmolarity refers to the number of osmols per liter of solution. Osmolality is expressed as Osm/kg water; osmolarity is expressed as Osm/liter. Usually there is little difference between these two measurements when expressed in clinical practice. The important thing to remember is that osmolality reflects the potential for water movement and water distribution between and within body fluid compartments.

Diffusion

Diffusion is the random movement of molecules and ions from an area of higher concentration to an area of lower concentration in a solution. There are several factors that influence how diffusion occurs: membrane permeability, the size of the diffusing molecule or ion, differences in electrical potential of the ions involved, and pressure gradients on either side of the membrane. An example of diffusion is the exchange of oxygen and carbon dioxide between the alveoli and capillaries in the lungs.

Filtration

Filtration is the movement of solutes and water through selectively permeable membranes. The solutes and water move from an area of higher pressure to an area of lower pressure. Filtration involves both solutes and water and their movement in relation to hydrostatic pressure. It differs from diffusion and osmosis in that diffusion and osmosis are a response to concentrations, and filtration is a response to pressure.

The pressure during filtration is hydrostatic. Hydrostatic pressure is generated by the pumping action of the heart and is opposed by oncotic pressure. Oncotic pressure is exerted mainly by plasma proteins, specifically albumin. The Gibbs-Donnan equilibrium is important to understanding oncotic pressure. This principle states that electrolytes separated by a semipermeable membrane behave in predictable ways.[3, 4] For example, if solutions containing different amounts of sodium and chloride are separated by a semipermeable membrane, the water, sodium, and chloride move across the membrane until equilibrium exists on both sides of that membrane (diffusion). If a protein that is not diffusible is added to one side of the membrane, it changes the equilibrium because of the presence of the protein. Equilibrium occurs but, if the protein is an anion, the concentration of cations is higher on the side of the membrane containing the protein (anion). This accounts for the difference in osmotic pressure between the two sides of the membrane, and is called oncotic pressure (Fig. 7–1).[5]

The movement of fluid into or out of the capillaries depends on the balance between opposing forces. These forces are referred to as Starling forces when they relate to the movement of water and solutes through capillaries. Again, it is oncotic pressure that opposes capillary hydrostatic pressure.

The arteriolar side of a capillary has a hydrostatic pressure of approximately 32 mm Hg. This generally exceeds the plasma oncotic pressure, resulting in filtration or the movement of fluid out of the capillary and into the interstitium.[3]

The venous (venule) side of the capillary has a pressure of approximately 15 mm Hg, and as such is lower than the plasma oncotic pressure (approximately 22 mm Hg). In other words, the plasma oncotic pressure is greater than the hydrostatic pressure, resulting in fluid being pulled from the interstitium into the plasma in the vessel. This process is also known as absorption.

Both capillary hydrostatic pressure and plasma oncotic pressure are influenced by tissue hydrostatic pressure and tissue osmotic pressure. The net effect of tissue and capillary hydrostatic and oncotic pressures determines movement between capillaries and the interstitium.

Interstitial fluid is formed at the arteriolar side of the capillary bed and plasma fluid is formed at the venule side of the capillary bed. This fluid formation is constantly occurring to maintain homeostasis. Alterations in equilibrium between these fluids can occur without noticeable changes to the total volume of extracellular fluid.[5]

Examples of filtration are glomerular filtration in the kidney and the movement of fluids and electrolytes between the interstitium and capillary beds.

Active Transport

Another way in which solutes and fluids move in the body is active transport, whereby molecules or ions move through a selectively permeable cell membrane. The movement is against the way these molecules would naturally flow, or against the concentration gradient. As previously stated, in diffusion the movement of any substance occurs from the area of higher concentration to that of lower concentration without any expenditure of energy. It requires energy to move a molecule against its natural concentration gradient. Energy comes from processes (chemical reactions) carried on within the cell. The process of active transport requires a pump, such as a sodium-potassium pump.

The sodium-potassium pump is present in all cell membranes of the body and is fueled by adenosine triphosphate (ATP). Both sodium and potassium ions can diffuse through cell membranes in small amounts. When this happens, sodium and potassium concentrations eventually become equal inside and outside the cell over a period of time. The sodium-potassium pump is responsible for moving sodium to the outside of the cell and moving potassium back to the inside of the cell against a concentration gradient. The sodium-potassium pump is especially important to nerve and muscle fibers for the transmission of impulses. It also has an effect on the glands, allowing the secretion of substances, and in all body cells to assist in preventing cellular swelling. The importance of this active transport process can be seen when the metabolism of the cell stops and ATP is no longer available to keep the sodium-potassium pump working. In this event, the cell immediately begins to swell and can eventually burst.

Ionization

An important factor in the movement of fluid in the body is the electrical charge of the particles or solutes that are components of a particular fluid. Solutes are chemical compounds that act in one of two ways when in solution—they either remain as a whole or develop an electrical charge when dissolved. Compounds that develop an electrical charge break up into separate particles, called ions, in a process called ionization, and such chemical compounds are commonly known as electrolytes. Some electrolytes may have a positive charge when placed in water, whereas others develop a negative charge. Ions are dissociated particles of an electrolyte that carry either a positive charge (a cation) or a

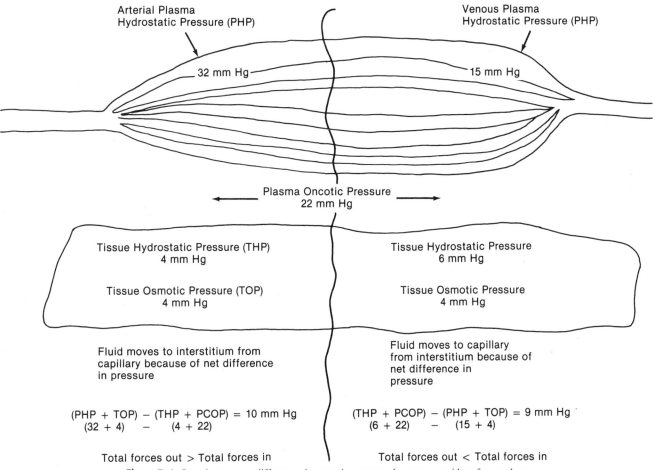

Figure 7–1. Oncotic pressure: differences in osmotic pressures between two sides of a membrane.

negative charge (an anion). Cations are electrolytes such as sodium, potassium, calcium, and magnesium. Anions, the negatively charged particles, are chloride, bicarbonate, phosphate, and sulfate.

The number of electrically charged ions in a defined amount of fluid is measured as milliequivalents per liter (mEq/liter); milliequivalent refers to the chemical activity of an element. To achieve electrical balance, the amount of cations and anions in a solution (expressed in milliequivalents) must always equal one another. Milliequivalents are used as the measure of ions rather than milligrams, because milligrams only measure the weight of the electrolyte. Weight gives us no indication of the number of ions or the number of electrical charges contained in the ion. Therefore, mEq is the more descriptive measure to use as a patient's electrolyte status is monitored (Table 7–1).[6]

Other substances important in the homeostasis of fluids and electrolytes are glucose, protein, organic acids, oxygen, and carbon dioxide. Although these are not necessarily considered charged particles, they are important in the body's state of balance.

Homeostatic Mechanisms

There are many homeostatic mechanisms that help keep the volume and composition of body fluids within the narrow range that the body regards as normal. Before discussing the regulating organs, there are two principles that are helpful to remember when considering homeostasis in the body.

The first principle states that the overall amount and composition of fluid within each compartment must remain stable, and that electrical neutrality must exist within each compartment. In other words, the ions must be balanced between anions and cations. There should be no net electrical charge within any compartment at any given time. The basic composition and basic amount of fluids within each compartment

Table 7–1			
Electrolyte Composition of Extracellular and Intracellular Fluid			
	Fluid Concentration (mEq/liter)		
Electrolyte	**Intra-cellular**	**Extracellular (Intravascular)**	**Extracellular (Interstitial)**
Cation			
Na^+	10	142	145
K^+	141	5	4
Ca^{2+}	2	5	3
Mg^{2+}	27	2	3
Anion			
Cl^-	1	104	116
HCO_3	10	27	30
HPO_4	100	2	2

should remain the same. In addition to maintaining balance, the compartments are constantly exchanging and replacing individual ions. The amount of work required to maintain this balance can use up to 20% of the body's ATP stores.

The second principle is osmolality, which states that the osmolality among the intracellular, interstitial and intravascular compartments needs to be equal. In osmosis, if there is a difference in the total number of active particles, the water moves into the compartment that contains the higher number of particles. A solution of higher osmolality has a lower water concentration (or higher particle concentration) than a solution of lesser osmolality.

Regulatory Organs

Many organs are normally associated with maintaining the body's homeostasis, such as the kidneys, heart and blood vessels, lungs, skin, adrenal glands, hypothalamus, pituitary gland, parathyroid gland, and gastrointestinal tract.

The kidneys are considered to be the primary force in homeostasis, because the kidneys' major function is to adjust the amount of water and electrolytes that leave the body so as to equal the amount that enters the body. The kidneys selectively excrete or maintain electrolytes as they monitor the body's feedback mechanisms. This allows the kidneys to play a role in maintaining acid-base balance as well as fluid balance. Kidneys excrete waste and remove foreign substances from the blood that have been absorbed from elsewhere in the body. They produce bicarbonate to maintain the acid-base balance and also erythropoietin, a hormone that stimulates the bone marrow to accelerate the production of red blood cells. The kidneys' role in acid-base balance is seen in the regulation of the pH of extracellular fluid. The kidneys selectively retain or excrete hydrogen ions, which assist in maintaining the pH of the extracellular fluid.

There are many hormonal and enzymatic influences on the kidney that assist in homeostasis. Renin is both produced and secreted in the juxtaglomerular apparatus (JGA) of the kidney. Renin is a proteolytic enzyme that triggers the release of angiotensin I, angiotensin II, and thereby aldosterone. The renin-angiotensin-aldosterone system regulates sodium reabsorption in the renal tubules. Homeostasis depends on an appropriate circulating volume, and renin assists in this process. The kallikrein-kinin system works to stimulate renin and prostoglandin production in the kidneys. The kinins also work to achieve renal vasodilatation and increase sodium excretion from the kidneys.[5]

Natriuretic factor, also known as atriopeptin, has only recently been identified and is classified as a hormone. The mechanism of action of natriuretic factor, however, has not yet been precisely defined. Currently, it is believed that it influences fluid loss, electrolyte loss, and vascular tone changes. This factor can cause renal vasodilatation and increased excretion of sodium. It is thought that it can interfere with the secretion of aldosterone and thereby interfere with sodium reabsorption in the kidney, specifically the distal tubules and collecting ducts. Although natriuretic factor has been found in the plasma and the heart, it is secreted in the atria when increased blood volume and increased central venous and right atrial pressures exist.[3, 5] All these influences work together to balance the excretion and reabsorption of

fluids and electrolytes through and within the kidney. It is obvious why alterations in kidney function have a devastating effect on the system as a whole.

The heart and blood vessels play a major role in fluid balance. The action of the heart and the resulting circulation through the blood vessels allow blood flow to reach the kidneys in sufficient volume to regulate water and electrolytes. The pumping action of the heart provides this circulation of blood through the kidneys, which then allows urine to form. When renal perfusion is adequate, it provides for adequate renal function. Additionally, there are special stretch receptors in the blood vessels and atrium of the heart. Their purpose is to react to hypovolemic states by stimulating fluid retention.

The lungs assist in achieving homeostasis through the ventilatory process. The lungs are under the control of the medulla oblongata. Based on responses to hydrogen level changes in the blood, the lungs act rapidly to correct metabolic acid-base disturbances. The lungs also regulate oxygen and carbon dioxide levels.

The pituitary gland stores antidiuretic hormone (ADH). ADH is manufactured in the hypothalamus and causes the body to retain water. This water-conserving function has several effects. One is the maintenance of osmotic pressure by controlling water retention or excretion by the kidneys. ADH also plays a small role in the control of blood volume. When blood volume is decreased, the ADH level increases, resulting in the retention of water. When the blood volume is increased, ADH secretion is decreased, and water is excreted through the kidneys.

The adrenal glands, positioned above the kidneys, consist of two different sections, the adrenal cortex and the adrenal medulla. The adrenal cortex secretes aldosterone, a mineralocorticoid hormone. Aldosterone acts on the kidney tubular cells, is active in the reabsorption of sodium and water, and can decrease potassium excretion. An increase in the level of aldosterone results in the retention of sodium and the loss of potassium. When sodium is retained, water is also retained. A decreased secretion of aldosterone results in the excretion of sodium and water and the retention of potassium. Cortisol is also secreted by the adrenal cortex. Among its many functions, cortisol assists in blood pressure regulation by regulating the amount of vasoconstriction necessary to maintain a normal blood pressure. Aldosterone is thought to be the more powerful of the two hormones, but when cortisol is secreted in large quantities it can have an effect on sodium and fluid retention and potassium excretion. Cortisol is classified as a mineralocorticoid.

The parathyroid glands are attached to the lateral lobes of the thyroid gland. There usually are four to five glands, but the number varies among individuals. Parathyroid hormone is secreted from the parathyroid glands. Parathyroid hormone has an effect on calcium and phosphate concentrations, and influences the reabsorption of calcium. An increase in the parathyroid hormone level increases the serum calcium concentration and lowers the serum phosphate concentration. The reverse is also true. A decreased secretion of parathyroid hormone lowers the serum calcium and elevates the serum phosphate concentrations. Decreased serum calcium levels stimulate the release of parathyroid hormones, which in turn increase the serum calcium level. The thyroid gland, which secretes calcitonin, also has an effect on calcium levels in the body. If there is an increase in the serum calcium level, this causes an increased secretion of calcitonin. The effect of calcitonin on calcium can be viewed as having the opposite effect as parathyroid hormone on calcium levels.

Other organs that affect fluid and electrolyte balance in the body are the skin and the gastrointestinal (GI) tract. Because the skin communicates with our environment, it allows the escape of water from the body through perspiration. The GI tract also plays a role in water absorption and reabsorption.

All the organs of homeostasis can be likened to a symphony. To make music, each participant needs to play its role and interact with all the other participants. When they play together, beautiful music can be made. So it is with the organs of homeostasis. Through their interdependencies and interactions they all work together to meet a common goal: the maintenance of a balanced state in the human body.

FLUID AND WATER MOVEMENT

Fluid Compartments

The internal environment of the human body is largely composed of fluid, with water being the most abundant component. Approximately 60% of body weight in an adult is water (Fig. 7–2). The amount of total body water, as it relates to body weight, varies among individuals because of the difference in the amount of adipose tissue, which contains little water.

Body water is distributed between defined compartments, the intracellular compartment, extracellular compartment, and transcellular compartment. Intracellular fluid is the fluid content of all the cells in the body, and represents about two-thirds of total body weight. Extracellular fluid comprises about one-third of total body weight. The extracellular fluid compartment is divided into two separate areas. Fluid found in tissue spaces between blood vessels and cells of the body is referred to as interstitial fluid, and includes lymph fluid. The other component of the extracellular fluid is plasma, which accounts for approximately 5% of total body weight. Extracellular fluid serves two functions in the body. First, it provides a relatively constant environment for the cells and second, it aids in transporting substances to and from the cells. Plasma, sometimes referred to as vessel fluid, is a highly specialized fluid in the body, and contains red blood cells and protein in large amounts. Protein helps retain the special nature of plasma because it provides osmotic pull and preserves vessel water composition. The protein content is what makes plasma highly specialized, because protein is generally found only in a particular space or vessel. Any particle confined to a particular space pulls water into that space.[2, 6]

Transcellular fluid is considered to be a component of the extracellular fluid compartment. The fluid that is contained in the transcellular areas is specialized and is composed of cerebrospinal, pleural, peritoneal, or synovial fluid. It is separated from the blood but, unlike the other fluid compartments, it is separated by capillary endothelial cells and epithelial tissue; therefore, it is compartmentalized fluid.

In addition to understanding where fluid is contained in the body, it is important to consider the composition of various fluids and how this affects the movement of water; transcellular fluid, however, is not usually considered when talking about fluid and electrolyte balance. When transcellular fluid is lost it produces symptomatology because of the special attributes of the fluid in the transcellular spaces. Gastrointestinal tract fluid is regarded as transcellular fluid.

Although the intracellular and extracellular fluids contain the same types of anions and cations, the amounts in which they are found vary between the two compartments. The principal cation in the intracellular fluid is potassium. Found in lesser amounts are magnesium, sodium, and calcium. Major anions in the intracellular fluid are phosphate, and bicarbonate and chloride in lesser amounts. The fluid cation found in most abundance in the extracellular fluid is sodium; present in much smaller amounts are potassium, calcium, and magnesium. The principal anion of the extracellular fluid is chloride, and bicarbonate and phosphate are found in smaller amounts.

The major electrolytes in extracellular fluid, therefore, are sodium as a cation and chloride as an anion. Sodium, chloride, and bicarbonate represent more than 90% of the total amount of solutes found in the extracellular space. Potassium is the major cation within the cells, and magnesium is also found in high concentration. The anions in the intracellular compartment are phosphate, sulfate, bicarbonate, and proteinate (Fig. 7–3).

Movement of Fluids and Electrolytes

It is now time to discuss how fluid and electrolytes move within the body. One way that water moves in the body is through osmotic pressure. The distribution of water in the body depends on electrolyte balance and on the distribution of electrolytes and fluids within the intracellular and extracellular compartments. Osmotic gradients are established and maintained by solutes. Water is largely unconfined within the respective compartments; however, as previously stated, electrolytes are usually confined to their respective compartments.

Effects of Body Fluid Concentration

If there is no water movement through a membrane because of an osmotic balance, the solutions on either side of

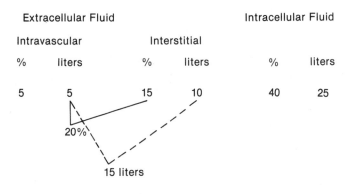

Extracellular Fluid				Intracellular Fluid	
Intravascular		Interstitial			
%	liters	%	liters	%	liters
5	5	15	10	40	25

20%

15 liters

Total body fluid = 60%
(average adult)

Figure 7–2. Distribution and amount of body fluids in an "average" adult.

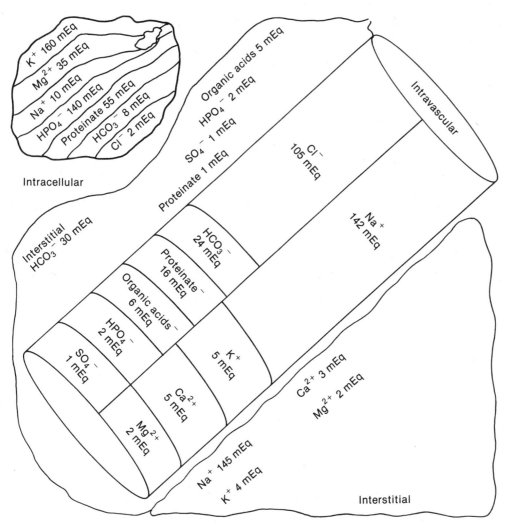

Figure 7–3. Anions and cations of intracellular, interstitial, and intravascular fluids.

the membrane are isotonic. That is, they each exert the same amount of osmotic pressure on both sides of the membrane, and contain the same amount of osmotically active solutes. Isotonic osmolality is considered to be approximately 300 mOsm/liter.[7] Fluid containing a large number of solutes is considered hypertonic when compared with water containing no solute particles. Conversely, water is considered hypotonic when compared to a fluid containing many solute particles. Osmotic pressure refers to how strongly water can be pulled across a membrane; the strength or pressure of that pull depends on the amount of solutes or molecules in the solution.

Colloids. Electrolytes and other low-molecular-weight substances exert a normal osmotic pressure. Colloids, such as protein and albumin, are nondiffusible substances that have a higher molecular weight. Therefore, they exert a higher osmotic pressure, the colloid osmotic or oncotic pressure, which causes water to be pulled into the intravascular space.

Cystalloids. Diffusible substances are referred to as crystalloids. They are important in fluid balance because they can pass through capillary walls, which are the barriers between plasma and interstitial fluid. Crystalloids can expand both the intravascular and interstitial spaces. Usually, only about 25% of crystalloids administered remain in the intravascular space, with the rest moving to the interstitial space. Examples of crystalloids are dextrose in water, electrolytes in water, and sodium chloride solutions.

Plasma. The plasma component of the extracellular fluid responds in a special way to fluid balance because of the protein component of the plasma. Proteins pull water into the intravascular space.

Sodium. Fluid balance is also regulated by the sodium concentration in the plasma, with some influence from glucose and urea within the plasma. Sodium contributes more than 90% of extracellular fluid solutes. The osmotic pressure produced by sodium determines the state of cellular hydration. Osmosis occurs when the extracellular fluid contains an electrolyte content lower or higher than normal. For example, if plain water with no electrolyte content were injected into the bloodstream, the red blood cells in the plasma would absorb the water. This would cause the cells to swell and burst. If a solution with a high sodium content were injected into the body, the red blood cells would lose water to the salt and result in the cells shrinking.

Solute Concentration. Solute concentration and the associated osmotic force affect body water distribution. As stated earlier, water moves from an area of lower solute concentration to an area of greater solute concentration, or an area of high osmolality. A change in the osmolality of one compartment always alters the osmolality of the other compartment or, stated another way, a change in extracellular fluid compartment osmolality dictates a change in the osmolality of the intracellular fluids. The body is striving for homeostasis, and there is water movement until the osmolality values of both compartments are relatively equal.

Fluid Pressure

To understand the movement of fluids and solutes within the body, fluid pressures and the amounts of solutes and water in the various compartments must be considered. As water moves to achieve a state of equilibrium, so do pressures exerted on the fluids move to reach a state of equilibrium. There are four pressures to be considered when studying water exchange between plasma and interstitial fluid. Movement is determined by blood hydrostatic and colloid osmotic pressures on one side of the capillary membrane, and by interstitial fluid hydrostatic and colloid osmotic pressures on the other side. Blood hydrostatic pressure forces fluid out of the capillaries into the interstitial fluid on one side; however, blood colloid osmotic pressure draws it back into the capillaries. Interstitial fluid hydrostatic pressure forces fluids out of the interstitial space into the capillaries, and interstitial fluid colloid osmotic pressure moves fluid back out of the capillaries. The net effect is that two of these pressures exert a force in one direction, and two exert pressure in the opposite direction. The difference between these two sets of opposing pressures represents the net or effective filtration pressure. An increase in plasma volume causes an increase in hydrostatic pressure of the blood, which then affects the pressure gradient and the movement of fluid. This results in a condition known as edema.

Hydrostatic pressure is comparable to the principle of filtration, which is the transfer of water-soluble substances from an area of high pressure to an area of low pressure. Fluid and water-soluble substances are moved by hydrostatic pressure in the vessels. Hydrostatic pressure can be exerted by the pumping action of the heart. The difference in arterial and venous pressure also plays a role in the movement of fluids. Hydrostatic pressure is greater than colloid osmotic pressure at the arterial end of a capillary, which causes fluids to move out of the vessel. Conversely, the osmotic force is greater than the hydrostatic pressure on the venous end of a capillary, enabling fluid to re-enter a capillary on the venous end.[2]

Vascular Effects

In order for the body to function correctly, there must be enough circulating fluid to allow for osmosis, diffusion, and filtration. Baroreceptors, or stretch receptors, located in the carotid sinuses and the aortic arch, respond to the amount of stretch in the vessel wall. The stretch depends on the volume of blood flowing through it. If there is a drop in arterial pressure, these baroreceptors generate fewer impulses, which in turn cause an accelerated heart rate and an increase in blood pressure. The mechanism controlling water movement between fluid compartments is a rapid response system. Its primary action is to maintain a normal blood volume, even

at the expense of interstitial fluid volume. The interstitial space may expand by several liters over a long period without major changes in the intravascular or intracellular compartments.

Body Fluid Volume and Composition

Age, gender, and the amount of adipose tissue all affect the amount of fluids in the human body. Women have less body fluid than men because men have less body fat. This gender difference in fluid amount is not seen until adolescence, but remains throughout life. A newborn has 70 to 80% of body weight as fluid. Premature infants have an even higher percentage of fluid, approximately 90% of their body weight. Infants are more susceptible to fluid volume deficit, because their bodies have a higher fluid percentage and they have more extracellular fluid. More than half of the newborn's body fluid is extracellular fluid. In the adult, extracellular fluid accounts for only one-third of body fluid. Extracellular fluid is more readily lost from the body. By the end of the second year of life, the infant's total body fluid approaches that of the adult, or approximately 60%—36% cellular fluid and 24% extracellular fluid. The adult body composition of 40% cellular and 20% extracellular is reached by puberty. After the age of 40 years, the total fluid percentage of body weight begins to decrease for both men and women. After 60 years of age, the percentages decrease even more, because with aging there is a decrease of lean body mass and an increase in fat content. Therefore, the body holds less water. The fluid composition for the various ages is shown in Table 7–2.[8]

Water Regulation

INTAKE AND OUTPUT

There are various ways to achieve intake and output of fluids and electrolytes. Water is taken into the body by food or drink. The liquid that is ingested is measured as part of intake. Liquid is also taken into the body through food. Water is formed by oxidation when food is broken down into energy by the body. Oxidation releases water for use in metabolism; approximately 350 ml of water comes from the oxidation process daily. Thirst is controlled by osmoreceptors found in the hypothalamus and by intravascular volume. ADH plays an important role in preventing dehydration and

Table 7-2

Body Fluid Volume and Composition

	Approximate Percentage by Gender		
Age	Male	Female	Both
Premature infant			90
Full-term newborn			70–80
1 year			64
Puberty–39 years	60	52	
	(40 cellular, 20 extracellular)		
40–60 years	55	47	
Over 60 years	52	46	

Adapted from Metheny NM. Fluid and Electrolyte Balance: Nursing Considerations, 2nd ed. Philadelphia: J. B. Lippincott, 1992:5.

therefore hypertonicity of body fluids. Thirst is an even more important mechanism in supplying endogenous water to the body, and is activated when the total body water content is decreased by about 2%. The kidneys, in addition to excreting urine, can adjust the amount of water and electrolytes that leave the body so that it equals the amount of water and electrolytes that enter the body. They have a vital role in fluid and electrolyte balance and in acid-base balance. On average, the kidneys filter approximately 170 liters of water in a 24-hour period. This amount varies according to the fluid intake. The usual amount of fluid output through the kidney is approximately 1 ml of urine/kg of body weight/hour in all age groups.

Antidiuretic Hormone. The release of antidiuretic hormone (ADH) in response to osmotic dehydration is affected by plasma osmolality. Osmoreceptors can detect very small changes in the plasma concentration of sodium and other solutes. With a normal plasma osmolality, the secretion of ADH is low enough to permit maximum urinary output. If plasma becomes hyperosmolar, the ADH system responds to maintain maximum kidney water retention while solutes continue to be lost in an effort to bring osmolality back to normal. The reverse is also true: in a hypo-osmolar state, ADH secretion is diminished, allowing the excretion of water while solutes are retained by the kidney. This process acts to return the plasma to a more normal osmolality.

Thirst Mechanism. The thirst mechanism is activated when stimulated by osmoreceptors in the anterior hypothalamus. Plasma osmolality and sodium concentrations are usually kept within a narrow range. The upper limit of this range is determined by the osmotic threshold for thirst referred to as the tripping mechanism.[2] When the sodium concentration increases by about 2 mEq/liter above the normal level, the physical desire for water intake increases. Thirst is tripped, so that the extracellular fluid level returns toward normal.[2]

Perspiration. Water and electrolytes can be lost through the skin: these are referred to as sensible losses. Sensible losses, or perspiration, can account for up to 6 liters of fluid lost in 24 hours under hot, dry conditions, with the average being 1.5 liters in 24 hours. Perspiration is considered to be a hypotonic solution; it contains chiefly sodium and potassium. Losses by perspiration vary according to the environmental temperature. Body temperature and ambient room temperature affect the amount of perspiration losses. The skin also loses water by evaporation, which can be up to 600 ml/day. Evaporation is considered to be an insensible loss.

Respiration. Approximately 300 ml of water are lost through the lungs in any 24-hour period. This 300 ml of water is considered insensible water loss, and the amount lost varies according to the rate and depth of respiration. In addition, the lungs play a role in homeostasis because of their ability to eliminate about 13,000 mEq of hydrogen ions in 24 hours, which is significantly more than the kidneys excrete.

Gastrointestinal Tract. The GI tract is responsible for 100 to 200 ml of fluid loss daily. Even though this amount is lost on a daily basis, the GI tract can filter up to as much as 8 liters of fluid in 24 hours. Much of this fluid is reabsorbed through the small intestine. Greater losses can occur from adverse conditions such as diarrhea, vomiting, or fistula development.

Other Mechanisms. Water and electrolytes can be lost through other mechanisms, such as tears from the eyes and in feces. Abnormal losses can occur from the use of strong diuretics, which deplete body fluids and electrolytes, or through wound drainage, fever, hyperventilation, mechanical ventilation, and gastrointestinal tubes.

Intake Requirements. The goal is to maintain a state of equilibrium between fluid compartments and between the body's daily fluid intake and output. The average healthy adult requires from 2000 to 2800 ml of fluid/day. Usually, 1000 to 1500 ml of this total are taken into the body in liquid form. Another 800 to 1000 ml come from food eaten during the day. Oxidation in body tissues accounts for another 350 ml. Fluid loss amounts to approximately 2500 ml/day. When the body is functioning correctly, the intake is balanced by the output.

Effects of Age on Intake and Output

When considering the intake of fluid into the body and the output of that fluid and associated electrolytes, the effect of age on homeostatic mechanisms should be considered. The elderly may experience up to a 50% reduction in kidney function, which results from a decrease in blood flow to the kidneys. There is also an inability to concentrate urine when the fluid intake is reduced, so the glomerular filtration rate (GFR) is also decreased. This indicates that the elderly are more susceptible to drug toxicities because of decreased renal function. Cardiac output and stroke volume of the heart are lowered in the elderly. Glands may atrophy, which reduces the ability to eliminate fluid through perspiration and causes some control of body temperature to be lost. There is sometimes a loss of muscle tone of the intestinal tract. Thirst mechanisms may be diminished in the aging person, so the attempt to reach homeostasis based on thirst is then compromised.

There is proportionately more water in the extracellular compartment of an infant than an adult. Therefore, the infant is more vulnerable to fluid volume deficit. The infant may turn over half of its extracellular fluid daily, whereas adults may change only one-sixth of their extracellular volume in the same 24-hour period. This means that the infant has less body fluid in reserve. Infants have a large amount of metabolic waste to excrete because their daily fluid exchange is up to two times greater per unit of body weight than that of an adult. Large volumes of urine are formed each day to excrete all the waste products. Infants have a proportionally higher body surface area than adults, so they have a greater fluid loss potential through their skin. Infants can also suffer greater losses from the GI tract in a relatively shorter period of time than adults.

Fluid Disorders

Homeostatic mechanisms of the body are complex and delicate. Generally, this system has the ability to maintain equilibrium, but sometimes these mechanisms fail and the body can be in a state of fluid deficit or excess.

Fluid Volume Excess

An increase in the extracellular fluid volume is known as fluid volume excess, or hypervolemia. The increased volume may occur with the intravascular or interstitial fluids. Hypervolemia is generally the result of an increase in the body sodium concentration, which in turn causes water retention. Because both the sodium and water are retained, the relative serum sodium concentrations remain essentially normal.[8] Once an imbalance develops, the body attempts to compensate. This occurs through the release of atrial natriuretic factor, which causes the kidney to increase the rate of filtration and excretion of sodium and water. There is also a decrease in the aldosterone and ADH levels.

Cause. The cause of fluid volume excess is related to an increase in sodium, water, or a combination of the two, which can be caused by regulatory mechanisms.[8] The kidneys, which help regulate sodium and water, may be diseased, leading to sodium and water retention. This is particularly true in the presence of a decreased output. An increased release of ADH and aldosterone results in fluid retention.

Another major organ that is a part of the normal regulatory system is the heart. In conditions such as congestive heart failure, the diseased heart cannot circulate the intravascular fluids adequately. This pseudointravascular deficit signals the kidneys to conserve sodium and water, leading to a fluid volume excess.

A malfunctioning liver (e.g., as in cirrhosis) could lead to excessive fluid retention. In cirrhosis, the retention is related to a decreased serum albumin level, which facilitates the loss of intravascular fluids into the interstitial space. Additional fluid may be lost into the peritoneal cavity because of hepatic venous obstruction. Again, this decreased intravascular volume signals the kidney to release more renin, which leads to an increase in the aldosterone level and results in sodium and water retention.

Hypervolemia may occur as a result of an excessive sodium and fluid intake. This is generally caused by the excessive administration of IV fluids, particularly those that contain sodium. Also, the excessive ingestion of sodium contained in food or medications may lead to fluid volume excess; this is especially true in those with a heart or kidney abnormality.

Other potential causes of hypervolemia include the administration of excessive doses of steroids or fluid volume shifts within the body. In the case of steroids, the increased fluid volume is related to sodium and water retention. A shift of interstitial fluid to plasma may occur with the treatment of burns. Often, initial burn treatment includes the administration of large amounts of IV fluids because of a fluid volume deficit. Several days later there is a shift of fluid from the interstitial space back into the intravascular space which could then lead to hypervolemia.

Assessment. The signs and symptoms of hypervolemia are related to the location and degree of fluid volume excess, and to the rate of onset. A sudden, rapid onset results in more pronounced problems.

Probably the most visible characteristic is edema, which is increased fluid volume in the interstitial space. When edema is present, it is usually most visible in dependent areas, as well as around the eyes. The degree of edema may be determined by applying finger pressure around the ankle and sacral areas. Removing the finger leaves a small indention or pit as the fluid excess becomes more severe.

Weight gain usually accompanies the increased fluid volume. This would not occur, however, if the increase were a shift from another compartment. Weight gain occurring over a short time frame is considered to be a mild fluid excess if the increase is 2%; a moderate excess is 5%, and a severe excess is 8%.[8]

Fluid may shift to another cavity in the body, primarily the abdominal cavity. The accumulation in the abdominal cavity is known as ascites, and is frequently seen in those with advanced renal or hepatic disease. It is noted by shortness of breath or decreased cardiac output caused by the increased pressure of the excessive fluid volume.

Other characteristics of hypervolemia may include pulmonary edema, which can lead to moist rales, shortness of breath, and wheezing. There may be an increase in blood pressure, distention of the neck veins, slower emptying of the peripheral veins, and a more rapid and bounding pulse rate. Polyuria is present if the kidneys are functioning normally.

Laboratory findings reveal a decreased hematocrit resulting from hemodilution. If the excessive volume is caused by water retention, the serum sodium level and osmolality decrease. In most cases, the urine-specific gravity also decreases. Pulmonary congestion may be revealed on chest x-ray. Because of a decrease in oxygen transport capabilities with pulmonary edema, the arterial blood gases may show a decreased PaO_2 and $PaCO_2$ and an increased pH.

Correction. Treatment of fluid volume excess includes determining the cause and treating accordingly. When this is not possible or effective, it is necessary to treat the disorder symptomatically. This generally includes sodium restriction, fluid restriction, bedrest, and/or diuretic administration. There may be special requirements for some patients, such as paracentesis in the case of ascites. Dialysis may also be indicated in the presence of renal disease.

The sodium restriction may extend to the diet and to medications, particularly those containing a sodium salt. There are also a variety of over-the-counter preparations that contain sodium.

The use of diuretics is not always the answer but is helpful in most cases of edema. Severe hypervolemia may necessitate the administration of diuretics by the intravenous route.

Nursing interventions should include monitoring vital signs and body weight. Any continued presence of edema should be noted. Intake and output records, as well as electrolyte levels, should be monitored, particularly following diuretic administration.

Observations should be clearly documented, including the response to diuretics. All abnormal observations should be communicated to the physician.

Fluid Volume Deficit

Fluid volume deficit, or hypovolemia, occurs as a result of excessive but relatively equal fluid and electrolyte depletion in the extracellular compartment. The body attempts to compensate for the losses through an increase in thirst and heart rate, and the release of ADH and aldosterone. If the deficit is severe and not corrected in a timely manner, it could lead to renal failure and death.

Cause. Hypovolemia may result from an abnormal loss of body fluids or an inadequate fluid intake, which affects the fluid and electrolyte content. Fluid deficit may be caused by the loss of gastrointestinal fluids. This may occur through vomiting, diarrhea, suctioning, and fistulas.

The skin is another mechanism for fluid loss. Under normal conditions, fluid is lost through the skin as a means of regulating body temperature. In the presence of a fever, however, there are abnormal, insensible fluid losses. Any type of trauma related to the skin, such as burns and cuts, also facilitates the abnormal loss of fluids.

Excessive loss takes place through the renal system. This may be caused by polyuria related to administering osmotic diuretics or concentrated IV solutions and tube feedings. Polyuria may also occur with hyperglycemia and some renal disorders.

Trauma, surgery, and bleeding disorders may result in hemorrhage, which rapidly decreases the intravascular fluid volume. There may also be a decrease in the circulating volume because of third spacing. With this phenomenon, there is a shift of fluid from the circulating volume into a space where it cannot be easily exchanged with fluid in the extracellular space. Because third spacing is only a shifting of fluid, there is really no actual fluid loss. The fluid deficit in this case is the result of the decreased circulating volume.

Finally, hypovolemia may occur because of a decreased fluid intake, particularly in the infant and older adult population. Infants have a larger body surface area and tend to lose more fluid than adults. Additionally, they depend on others to provide oral fluids. Older adults have a decreased sense of thirst and therefore are less likely to seek fluid replacement. The ability to replace fluid may be further complicated by decreased mobility. Also, patients who cannot respond to thirst (e.g., are confused or comatose) are subject to fluid volume depletion.

Assessment. As with fluid volume excess, the signs and symptoms of hypovolemia are related to the degree of the deficit and how fast it occurs. There is a loss of weight as the fluid volume decreases, except in the case of third spacing.

Assessment reveals a decreased central venous pressure, flattened jugular vein while in the supine position, and slow filling of the hand veins. The lower circulating volume leads to a decreased blood pressure and possibly to postural hypotension. With less volume present, there is decreased tissue perfusion, which creates a variety of problems including muscle weakness, dizziness, lethargy, and confusion. As the body tries to maintain an adequate intravascular volume, the pulse rate increases and becomes weaker. The kidneys try to conserve fluid, so there is a decreased urinary output.

Skin turgor should be checked by pinching the skin, which slowly returns to the normal position in the presence of hypovolemia. The tongue, which normally has one furrow, has several small furrows. The eyes appear sunken and the face has a pinched expression.

As the fluid loss becomes more severe, the patient may go into shock. The extremities become cool and clammy, diaphoresis occurs, urinary output drops sharply, and the patient may become comatose.

Laboratory findings reveal an increased blood urea nitrogen (BUN) level. This is the result of the kidneys conserving water and urea, which follows the water. The hematocrit also increases except when the deficit is caused by hemorrhage. With blood loss, red blood cells and serum are lost in equal amounts. However, as the body attempts to compensate for the fluid deficit, interstitial fluid shifts into the intravascular space and the hematocrit decreases. There is an increase in the urinary specific gravity and osmolality. The electrolyte levels, serum osmolality, and acid-base balance vary according to the type of fluid lost and the causative factor.

Treatment. The treatment of hypovolemia includes correcting the cause of the deficit and returning the extracellular fluid to a normal level. If the deficit cannot be replaced by oral fluids, IV therapy should be initiated based on physician orders, patient assessment, and established procedures. An isotonic electrolyte solution (e.g., lactated Ringer's) is generally used to initiate therapy for hypovolemia. The severity of the deficit generally dictates the administration rate. As the fluid is replaced, the IV solution may be changed to one that provides free water. This assists the kidneys to excrete wastes.

If the deficit is severe enough, oliguria may be present. In this case, it is important to determine whether the cause is fluid volume deficit or renal disease. This may be accomplished through a fluid challenge test, in which the patient is monitored closely as IV solutions are administered. If the kidneys respond by producing urine, then the oliguria is probably the result of fluid volume deficit. With no increase in urinary output, the cause of the oliguria is most likely related to renal failure or decreased cardiac function.

During treatment for fluid volume deficit, it is important that the patient be monitored closely. This includes the urinary output, vital signs, hemodynamic pressures, and body weight. Monitoring laboratory test results can help maintain normal fluid and electrolyte levels. The rate of administration for IV solutions should be monitored to prevent fluid overload. The assessment findings need to be clearly documented and the physician notified of abnormal parameters.

ACID-BASE BALANCE

The complexity and delicate balance required and carried out by the body continues to be seen in the principles of acid-base balance. It is imperative that this balance be maintained within a very narrow range, with a pH between 7.35 and 7.45. Any excess in either direction, without correction or intervention, can result in death. It is interesting to note that most byproducts of metabolism, or waste products, tend to be acidic. Therefore, the body functions so as to excrete and balance acidic waste products. Again, following the rules of homeostasis, the body attempts to excrete acidic substances in a way that balances the amount of acidic products generated through metabolism.

pH

Understanding pH requires understanding the function of hydrogen and what constitutes an acid and a base. Certain characteristics of a solution are measured by its pH, which is the hydrogen ion concentration of the solution. Because this concentration is very small, it is generally expressed as a logarithm. For example, water has a pH of 7, which can be expressed as a negative logarithm, or 0.0000001 (10^{-7}). The use of the logarithm makes it much easier to work with and conceptualize the pH value.

The concentration of hydrogen ions in a solution determines its acidity or alkalinity. If a solution is acidic, it has a low pH. If a solution is alkaline, it has a high pH. The normal pH range is 1 to 14, with 7 being approximately neutral. Water, with its pH of 7, is considered to be neutral because of the balance between the concentration of hydrogen ions (H^+) and hydroxyl (OH^-) ions. Hydroxyl ions are released when a base breaks apart in water, and hydrogen ions are released when an acid dissociates in water.

Acid

An acid is a chemical substance that dissociates and donates hydrogen ions to a solution or in combination with another substance. Acids can be classified as strong or weak. Strong acids (e.g., hydrochloric acid, HCl), release hydrogen ions into solution and tend to remain dissociated in that solution. Weak acids (e.g., carbonic acid, H_2CO_3) also give up hydrogen ions in solution but not completely, as does the strong acid. Weak acids are only partially dissociated in acidic solutions.

Volatile acids are acids that can form a gas and are eliminated from the body as a gas, so they therefore are excreted from the lungs. An example of a volatile acid is carbonic acid, which is a combination of carbon dioxide (CO_2) and water (H_2O). Nonvolatile or fixed acids cannot be converted into gas form. They are excreted by the kidneys in the urine and in small amounts in feces. Nonvolatile acids result from various metabolic processes within the body. Some are produced in the form of uric acid, which is an organic acid. Some may be in the form of sulfuric and phosphoric acids. Nonvolatile acids and the hydrogen they release are eliminated by the kidneys. It is important to remember that any discussion of acids is basically a discussion of hydrogen ion concentration. To summarize, nonvolatile hydrogen ions are excreted through the renal system or the kidneys, and volatile hydrogen or acids are excreted through the lungs or respiratory system.[4]

Respiratory System Influences

Most of the carbonic acid available in the body is found in conjunction with carbon dioxide gas. Therefore, the pH of body fluids is affected by changes in the carbon dioxide concentration. When the concentration of carbon dioxide gas in body fluids is increased, the pH decreases. Conversely, when the concentration of carbon dioxide gas is decreased, the pH increases. The rate of alveolar ventilation is a major factor in the regulation of carbon dioxide concentration in the body. Alveolar hyperventilation causes carbon dioxide to be blown off through the lungs. In turn, the release of carbon dioxide through the lungs decreases the concentration of carbon dioxide in body fluids and increases the pH. On the other hand, alveolar hypoventilation causes the retention of carbon dioxide, and a decreased pH results.

When the hydrogen ion concentration is affected, the pH is affected. Therefore, the rate of ventilation changes in conjunction with alterations in the rate and depth of breathing. The peripheral and central chemoreceptors found in the body respond to changes in the carbon dioxide and hydrogen ion concentrations. The peripheral chemoreceptors found in the carotid and aortic bodies respond to the carbon dioxide and hydrogen ion concentrations in circulating blood by stimulating networks in the medulla oblongata. Respiration increases or decreases relative to the carbon dioxide and hydrogen ion concentrations in the circulating blood.

The central chemoreceptors in the medulla monitor hydrogen ion concentrations in the cerebral blood flow and brain interstitial fluid. They then signal the medulla to change the rate and depth of alveolar ventilation. An increase in hydrogen ion concentration and the drop in pH that follows decrease the rate of alveolar ventilation. This feedback mechanism does have a limitation, however, in that the control of hydrogen ion concentration through the respiratory feedback system cannot always return the hydrogen ion concentration to its normal value. This is because, as the pH moves toward 7.4, the stimulus to increase or decrease ventilation is removed. Carbon dioxide gas exchange occurs through the lungs and excretes the bulk of acid formed in the body. More than 99.5% of the normal daily acid load and 100% of the CO_2 that result from metabolism are eliminated through the lungs.

The respiratory feedback system is a rapid response system that can respond to changes in the pH within minutes to several hours to begin the correction of the pH. Therefore, it is necessary for a second system to take over when the respiratory feedback mechanisms are not sufficient by themselves.

Bases

A base is a chemical substance that, when dissociated in solution, can combine with a hydrogen ion. When the base takes on a hydrogen ion, it in effect removes the hydrogen from a solution. Examples of bases are bicarbonate and protein. Proteins can function as bases because they act as anions and easily bind or accept hydrogen ions. Bases may be strong or weak, just like acids. A strong base easily accepts hydrogen and removes it from solution. Hydroxyl ions (OH^{2-}) are strong bases. Weak bases do not have the same affinity for hydrogen ions as a strong base, and are only partially dissociated in alkaline solutions. Bicarbonate is considered a weak base.

In the human body, most of the acids and bases required for life are weak acids and weak bases. Strong acids and strong bases would allow sudden and dangerous changes in the pH of body fluids. The presence of weak acids and weak bases allows for a greater degree of stabilization of pH within the body's systems. Weak acids or bases can act to neutralize strong acids or bases.

For example, consider the following equation:

$$NaHCO_3 + HCL \longrightarrow H_2CO_3 + NaCl$$

| Sodium bicarbonate (weak base) | Hydrochloric acid (strong acid) | (yields) | Carbonic acid (weak acid) | Sodium chloride (salt) |

By adding hydrochloric acid, which is a strong acid, to sodium bicarbonate, which is a weak base, they dissociate and combine to yield carbonic acid, which is a weak acid, and sodium chloride. By reacting this way, the weak base minimizes the change in pH by neutralizing the strong acid.

The same can be seen with a weak acid used to neutralize a strong base. For example,

$$H_2CO_3 \quad + \quad NaOH \quad \longrightarrow \quad NaHCO_3 \quad + \quad H_2O$$

| Carbonic acid (weak acid) | Sodium hydroxide (strong base) | (yields) | Sodium bicarbonate (weak base) | Water |

When carbonic acid (weak acid) is added to sodium hydroxide (strong base), the chemical dissociation and combination yields sodium bicarbonate, which is a weak base, and water. Again, this minimizes a precipitous change in body pH. A strong acid or a strong base in each of these examples has been buffered by the addition of a weak acid or a weak base.

Renal System Influences

The renal system responds to changes in hydrogen ion concentration, as does the respiratory system. However, the renal system responds more slowly. It may take up to several days for the renal system to achieve its purpose fully in pH correction. The kidneys work to regulate bicarbonate concentration in extracellular fluid and to excrete the acidic results of metabolism that the lungs cannot eliminate.

Metabolic or nonrespiratory acid-base imbalances may result from the excessive accumulation of or loss of fixed or nonvolatile acids and their buffers. There are several major processes involved in the renal system's regulation of hydrogen. Hydrogen is secreted through the kidneys. There is a relationship between the amount of hydrogen secreted and the concentration of carbon dioxide in the extracellular fluid. When there is a higher concentration of carbon dioxide in the extracellular fluid, more hydrogen ions are secreted. Conversely, the lower the amount of carbon dioxide in extracellular fluid, the fewer hydrogen ions are secreted.

Because the respiratory system is responsible for the excretion of the majority of hydrogen ions, there is only a small degree of hydrogen ion elimination through the kidneys. The kidneys, however, reabsorb bicarbonate in an amount that equals the remaining excess hydrogen ions. When hydrogen moves from the cells and tubules of the kidneys into the urine formed in the tubules, it can then be exchanged for sodium ions, and the hydrogen is excreted. Sodium ions are usually paired up with an anion, which preserves electrical neutrality between the positively and negatively charged ions. The sodium ions that are reabsorbed move into the plasma and then combine with HCO_3^- (bicarbonate ion) to form sodium bicarbonate. As a result of hydrogen-sodium exchange, bicarbonate is produced to maintain homeostasis.

The amount of exchange between hydrogen and sodium can be influenced by a deficiency in chloride, an increase in the level of plasma carbon dioxide, and also aldosterone secretion, which alters the retention of sodium. These all accelerate the exchange process, which can be slowed by a decrease in the carbon dioxide level or a decrease in aldosterone secretion. There is also an influence on the exchange by the urine pH. When the urine pH reaches a value between 4.0 and 4.5, this halts the secretion of hydrogen. This, in turn, stops the exchange of hydrogen and sodium.

Hydrogen can also combine with ammonia (NH_3) in the distal tubules of the kidneys. When the NH_3 moves from the cells into the urine, it attaches to hydrogen in the urine and forms the ammonium ion (NH_4^+). Ammonium then combines with an anion (either chloride or sulfate), and they all are excreted in the urine. The purpose of this mechanism, again, is to increase the amount of bicarbonate and to balance the carbonic acid:sodium bicarbonate ratio by the regulation and excretion of hydrogen ions. Ammonium ions are substituted for the bicarbonate ions, resulting in the excretion of ammonia. This allows for the preservation of bicarbonate, the excretion of excess hydrogen ions, and the maintenance of neutrality between positive and negative ions.

It is also possible for phosphates to combine with hydrogen ions, allowing the hydrogen to be excreted with the phosphate in urine. If all these mechanisms fail to restore the acid-base balance, it is also possible for potassium and extracellular fluid volume alterations to work to achieve this balance.[3]

Buffers

In addition to respiratory and renal system influences, there is a system of buffers that works to maintain acid-base balance. In the presence of an acid-base disturbance there are three main mechanisms to regain homeostasis, and we have already discussed two of these. One is the increase in alveolar ventilation. This depends on the lungs and chemoreceptors, and acts to reverse an alteration within 1 or 2 minutes. The second defense mechanism is hydrogen ion elimination coupled with increased bicarbonate reabsorption. This occurs in the kidneys and provides the strongest defense against acid-base disturbances. However, it takes several hours to several days for the renal system to try to re-establish equilibrium. The third defense is a system of buffers. The buffer system begins immediately to equilibrate the hydrogen ion concentration.

A buffer acts to protect the body against hydrogen ion concentration fluctuations. Buffers can inactivate excess hydrogen ions and hydroxyl ions. By doing so, they can maintain the pH of the body within the normal range.

CARBONIC ACID–SODIUM BICARBONATE BUFFER SYSTEM

Carbonic acid (H_2CO_3) and sodium bicarbonate ($NaCO_3$) work together as a buffer system. Because this system is composed of carbonic acid and sodium bicarbonate, it is affected both by the lungs and the kidneys. The lungs excrete or retain carbonic acid or its component, carbon dioxide, and the kidneys excrete or retain sodium bicarbonate. This is the most important buffering system in the extracellular fluid. It can buffer up to 90% of the hydrogen ions contained in extracellular fluid, and has little effect on the cells.

Because of the effects of carbonic acid or sodium bicarbonate, the buffering must occur through the lungs or kidneys. This means that the pH can be moved up or down by the renal system, the respiratory system, or both, acting together. Carbonic acid and sodium bicarbonate are measured by their relative concentrations. The ratio between the two is

1:20, or 20 parts of sodium bicarbonate to every 1 part of carbonic acid. When monitoring acid-base balance, it is important to monitor this ratio. When it is disturbed, the hydrogen balance in the body is also disturbed.

PHOSPHATE BUFFER SYSTEM

The phosphate buffer system operates at a slightly different pH than the carbonic acid-sodium bicarbonate buffer system. Phosphate buffer is more abundant within the cell, so its role is more cellular than extracellular. It works mainly in the tubular fluid of the kidneys. This system can buffer strong acids and strong bases into weak acids and weak bases, so that the weakened state of the acids or bases has little effect on the pH of the blood.

PROTEIN BUFFER SYSTEM

Proteins can act as both intracellular and extracellular buffers, and as acids or bases, a property referred to as amphoteric. Their ability to behave as an acid or base depends on the pH of the solution, and makes proteins a powerful buffering system. Proteins tend to buffer carbon dioxide quickly and buffer bicarbonate more slowly, over a period of up to several hours.

In addition, hemoglobin and oxyhemoglobin can act as a buffer system. This system works because there is a reaction that occurs between hemoglobin and hydrogen ions within the red blood cells. The red blood cell is permeable to bicarbonate ions. Therefore, when a hydrogen ion is bound by hemoglobin, a bicarbonate ion diffuses out of the red blood cell into the plasma. The bicarbonate ion is then exchanged for a chloride ion to maintain electrical neutrality.

Compensatory Mechanisms

Compensatory mechanisms are activated in the presence of a hydrogen imbalance. There are three basic compensatory mechanisms. The first is the dilution of hydrogen in the extracellular fluid and the buffering systems discussed earlier. The second compensatory mechanism is the respiratory system, and the third is the renal system.

The goal of compensation is to bring the pH toward normal without overcompensating or correcting the pH past the point of normal to the opposite alteration. The normal parameters for pH are 7.35 to 7.45. The absolute normal value is considered to be 7.4. By definition, acidemia is a condition in which the hydrogen ion concentration is elevated in the blood. Stated another way, the blood could have an acid excess or a base deficit, reflected by a pH of less than 7.35. Alkalemia is a condition in which the hydrogen ion concentration of the blood is decreased. Stated differently, the blood could have an acid deficit or a base excess, indicated by a pH greater than 7.45. Acidosis and alkalosis are the processes that result in acidemia or alkalemia. These terms may be used interchangeably.

Blood Values: Measurement and Interpretation

The evaluation of acid-base balance is based on various blood gas values. In addition to acid-base balance, they are used to determine the level of oxygenation within the patient's body, both extracellularly and intracellularly. Usually, blood gases are measured from arterial blood, which provides information about the oxygenation status of the blood passing through the lungs. Occasionally, mixed venous blood is used rather than arterial blood to determine the status of the oxygen in the tissues. If the tissues are receiving adequate oxygen, this can mean that both the ventilation and circulation within the body are adequate to meet the patient's needs and establish acid-base balance.

The three parameters monitored most frequently are the pH, $PaCO_2$, and bicarbonate levels. As stated earlier, pH measures the level of hydrogen ions present, which determines the alkalinity or acidity of the blood.

The $PaCO_2$, or PCO_2 as it is sometimes called, is a measure of the tension exerted by carbon dioxide in its gas form. The "P" represents the pressure or tension exerted by the carbon dioxide gas. The "a" designates arterial blood. If it were a venous sample, the letter "v" would be substituted for "a." When there is no "P" preceding the CO_2 level, it refers to the total CO_2 rather than the amount of carbon dioxide in the blood as a gas. The total CO_2 content is the amount of CO_2 gas that can be obtained from plasma when a strong acid is added in a laboratory setting. The total CO_2 content consists of bicarbonate, carbonic acid, and dissolved carbon dioxide gas.

Because the total CO_2 content measures the sum of bicarbonate, carbonic acid, and dissolved CO_2, an elevation of the plasma CO_2 content indicates alkalosis. A decrease in plasma CO_2 content indicates acidosis.

By measuring the $PaCO_2$, the partial pressure of carbon dioxide in arterial blood, the presence of alkalosis and acidosis may be determined. When this value is lower than 35 mm Hg, hypocapnia is present, and indicates respiratory alkalosis. Conversely, when this value is greater than 45 mm Hg, hypercapnia is said to be present, and indicates respiratory acidosis.

When discussing blood gases, consideration must be given to the CO_2 and the oxygen (O_2) concentrations in the blood. PaO_2 is the amount of pressure exerted by oxygen dissolved in arterial blood. Most oxygen carried by the blood is carried by hemoglobin. A small amount of oxygen is dissolved in plasma. Therefore, there are three ways to measure oxygen in the blood. The first is oxygen content, defined as the number of milliliters of oxygen carried in 100 ml of blood. The PO_2, or the pressure exerted by oxygen dissolved in plasma, is the second measurement. The third is the oxygen saturation of hemoglobin.

Oxygen saturation is a measure of the percentage of oxygen that is carried on the hemoglobin in relation to the total amount of oxygen that the hemoglobin is able to carry. Oxygen saturation provides the closest estimate of the total amount of oxygen carried in the blood. The PO_2 is only the pressure exerted by the small amount of oxygen that is dissolved within the plasma. A relationship exists between the PO_2 and the O_2 saturation of hemoglobin. An oxyhemoglobin dissociation curve shows this relationship. When the PO_2 in plasma is low, hemoglobin carries less oxygen. Conversely, when the PO_2 in plasma is high, the hemoglobin carries a great deal of oxygen.

The hemoglobin molecule has room to carry four molecules of oxygen. If all four oxygen receptor sites on the

Table 7-3

Normal Blood Gas Values*

. . . .

Parameter	Arterial	Venous (Mixed)
pH	7.35–7.45	7.33–7.43
O_2 saturation	95% or higher	70–75%
PaO_2	80–100 mm Hg	35–40 mm Hg
$PaCO_2$	35–45 mm Hg	41–51 mm Hg ($PvCO_2$)
HCO_3	22–26 mEq/liter	24–28 mEq/liter
Base excess	−2 to +2	0 to +4

*May vary slightly with the institution and geographic location.

hemoglobin are filled, then 100% O_2 saturation has been reached. If three oxygen receptor sites are filled and one is not, then 75% O_2 saturation has been reached. When measuring the arterial oxygen content, it is the sum of the oxygen chemically bound to hemoglobin and the oxygen dissolved in plasma that equals the PO_2. A normal O_2 saturation level is considered to be 95% or higher. The normal PaO_2 level is from 80 to 100 mm Hg in arterial blood.

The bicarbonate level is the concentration of bicarbonate in plasma that has been specially manipulated with oxygen at a $PaCO_2$ of 40 mm Hg. This is done in a laboratory to saturate the hemoglobin fully, and is called the standard bicarbonate measure. When this equilibration is performed, any abnormality that continues to exist in the standard bicarbonate level is known to have a metabolic cause. A normal bicarbonate level is between 22 and 26 mEq/liter. Other parameters used to evaluate the blood gas status are base excess and anion gap (see later).

The interpretation of blood gas results begins with three basic steps (see Table 7–3 for a list of normal blood gas values). The first step in the process is to look at the value of the pH. As stated earlier, 7.35 to 7.45 is a normal pH, with 7.4 being a midpoint. It therefore follows that if the pH is lower than 7.35, an acidotic state exists in the body. If the pH is greater than 7.45, an alkalotic state exists in the body. The second parameter to assess is the $PaCO_2$, which has a normal value between 35 and 45 mm Hg. If the value of $PaCO_2$ is below 35 mm Hg, a state of respiratory alkalosis exists. If the value is greater than 45 mm Hg, a respiratory acidosis exists. This is known to be true because the $PaCO_2$ is considered to be a respiratory parameter, and CO_2 is considered to act as an acid.

The third parameter to examine is the bicarbonate level. Again, the normal bicarbonate level is 22 to 26 mEq/liter. A value lower than 22 mEq/liter indicates a metabolic acidosis, and a value higher than 26 mEq/liter indicates a metabolic alkalosis. The bicarbonate level reflects the metabolic status, which can also be referred to as nonrespiratory or renal.

There are several helpful hints to remember when interpreting blood gas values. Although it has already been stated, it should be noted that if a change in pH is mainly caused by a change in the bicarbonate level, the cause of the alteration is nonrespiratory or metabolic. If the change in pH is caused by changes in the PCO_2, the driving force behind the alteration is respiratory in nature. When the pH and PCO_2 move in opposite directions, the primary effect on the acid-base imbalance is the respiratory system. If the change in pH and PCO_2 are in the same direction, there is a nonrespiratory or metabolic cause. The following may be useful in making these determinations:

Aid to Interpreting Blood Gas Values

Respiratory Alterations:

- pH up PCO_2 down
- pH down PCO_2 up

Metabolic Alterations:

- pH up PCO_2 up
- pH down PCO_2 down

The body always tries to keep the ratio of bicarbonate to PCO_2 at 20:1. This indicates a ratio of alkali (bicarbonate) to acid (CO_2). When it remains at 20:1, the pH remains unchanged, or around the normal level. If the bicarbonate increases, there is an alkalosis, which causes the pH to rise. If the bicarbonate (base) falls, there is an acidotic state and the pH falls. The change in this ratio is described as base excess.

Base excess is most descriptive of the concentration of bicarbonate in the blood, and is generally only affected by metabolic processes. The normal base excess is between +2 and −2. A positive base excess value signifies that there is too much base present and not enough acid. A negative value indicates too little base and too much acid. Therefore, a positive base excess value reflects a metabolic alkalosis and a negative value indicates metabolic acidosis. The plasma proteins and hemoglobin may also be considered bases and can influence the presence of a base excess to a smaller degree.

Acid-Base Alterations

Respiratory Acidosis

Respiratory acidemia occurs when an event causes the $PaCO_2$ to rise above 45 mm Hg. This event is usually associated with a decreased ventilatory exchange, which results in the CO_2 of the blood increasing because of an increase in the hydrogen ion concentration. The pH of the blood then decreases to below 7.35. As a result of alveolar hypoventilation, CO_2 is not eliminated through the lungs. Various disease states and alterations can cause this acidotic state:

Causes of Respiratory Acidosis

Depression of the respiratory center (medulla)
Drug overdose
Any medication or condition that causes respiratory depression
Guillain-Barré syndrome
Myasthenia gravis
Chronic bronchitis
Emphysema
Pneumothorax
Hemothorax
Pulmonary fibrosis
Acute alcoholism
Burns of the respiratory tract
Congestive heart failure
Adult respiratory distress syndrome

The causes of respiratory acidosis may be acute or chronic. The differentiation between acute and chronic states of acidosis is usually attributed to how long the carbon dioxide retention has lasted. In the chronic state, $PaCO_2$ levels can increase slowly or may remain stable over time, but at a level that is considered to be elevated. In the acute state, there is a rapid or sudden rise in the CO_2 level with a previously normal-acid base balance. Generally, chronicity results from a disease or condition that in some way decreases or prevents the gaseous exchange that normally occurs between the blood and alveolar air, or that causes obstruction. Obstruction prevents the exhalation of carbon dioxide by decreasing the surface area of the lung.

Findings on Assessment. Patients experiencing respiratory acidosis may exhibit headache, fatigue, or drowsiness resulting from CNS (central nervous system) depression. Confusion, disorientation, or coma may result, as well as fatigue, weakness, tremors, dyspnea, hypoventilation, cardiac dysrhythmias, and possibly cyanosis. It is important to recognize that the clinical presentation between acute and chronic respiratory acidosis is slightly different. This is particularly noticeable in patients with chronic obstructive pulmonary disease (COPD).

Compensatory Response. Patients with COPD gradually accumulate carbon dioxide over time. Because the alteration occurs gradually, compensatory changes have already occurred when the $PaCO_2$ level moves above 50 mm Hg. The respiratory center and the medulla no longer use carbon dioxide to stimulate respiration. Hypoxia then becomes the major respiratory drive in place of the increased CO_2. In this chronic state, if a patient receives too much oxygen, the stimulus for respiration is then removed. The patient develops carbon dioxide narcosis because the lack of oxygen as the stimulus to breathe is compensated for by the delivery of oxygen from an external source. Additionally, because of the compensated state of a chronic respiratory acidosis, the bicarbonate level in a patient with chronic alterations is elevated on measurement of blood gases. When a state of respiratory acidosis exists, the body responds in various ways (Table 7–4). The initial response includes the initiation of buffering by noncarbonate buffers. In other words, hemoglobin and proteins in the extracellular fluid and phosphates, proteins, and lactate in the intracellular fluid are activated in an attempt to regulate and overcome the increase in hydrogen ions. The respiratory rate increases to try to "blow off" excess hydrogen ions as a byproduct of the breakdown of carbonic acid into water and CO_2. If the alteration is not corrected by this mechanism, other buffer systems go into

effect. The kidneys secrete hydrogen ions and increase the retention of bicarbonate. Sodium is reabsorbed to maintain ionic balance within the body. The buffer also increases the chloride shift in the blood, because red blood cells give up a greater number of chloride ions and exchange them for bicarbonate. This results in excess carbonic acid being neutralized, and the normal 20:1 ratio between sodium bicarbonate and carbonic acid is reinstated.

▶ NURSING DIAGNOSIS

Nursing Assessment Parameters

In the patient with respiratory acidosis, the following are areas for assessment and monitoring:

- Vital signs
- Skin color
- Skin temperature
- Moistness of mucous membranes
- Muscle strength
- Level of consciousness
- Monitoring of ordered laboratory results

High-Risk Nursing Diagnosis

- Ineffective airway clearance
- Ineffective breathing pattern: hypoventilation
- High risk for electrolyte imbalance
- Impaired gas exchange
- High risk for injury, cardiac dysrhythmia
- Sensory-perceptual alteration, altered level of consciousness
- Alteration in thought process

Potential Outcomes

- Patient demonstrates improved blood gas values and vital signs.
- Patient has minimal or no signs/symptoms of impaired gas exchange
- Patient demonstrates methods necessary to improve breathing pattern.

Respiratory Alkalosis

Any disease process that reduces carbon dioxide in the blood or $PaCO_2$ results in a respiratory alkalemia. The hydrogen ion concentration is decreased, which causes a rise in the pH to a level above 7.45. Because the problem is respiratory in nature, the $PaCO_2$ is lower than 35 mm Hg. The respiratory alkalosis is caused by hyperventilation, which comes from the alveolar level. The hyperventilation acts to decrease the hydrogen ion concentration and this results in the increased pH. Respiratory alkalosis can arise from several disorders, and may be classified as acute or chronic:

Table 7–4

Blood Gas Alterations in Respiratory Acidosis*

Parameter	Direction of Change
pH	Down (<7.35)
$PaCO_2$	Up (>45 mm Hg)
HCO_3	Normal or up (>26 mEq/liter)
Na^+	Normal (usually)
Cl^-	Down in compensation
K^+	Up

*Breathing pattern—hypoventilation.

Causes of Respiratory Alkalosis

Hyperventilation syndrome
Trauma
Infection, particularly encephalitis or meningitis
Brain tumors (tumors may be malignant or nonmalignant)
CVA (cerebrovascular accident)
Pharmacologic agents (salicylate poisoning, nicotine, aminophylline-type drugs, some catecholamines)
Heat stroke
Fever
Gram-negative septicemia
Exercise beyond the person's normal capabilities
Carbon monoxide poisoning
Hypotension
Severe anemia
Pneumonia
Pulmonary edema
Pulmonary emboli
Mechanical overventilation
Chronic respiratory alkalosis
Trauma
Recovery phase of CVA
Recovery phase of central nervous system infections
Central nervous system malignancies
Severe ongoing anemia
Heart conditions that cause cyanotic conditions
Pregnancy
Hepatic disease
Treatment for metabolic acidosis

Findings on Assessment. The patient with respiratory alkalosis presents with hyperventilation and dyspnea, and may sigh frequently. Tachycardia, atrial dysrhythmia, and possibly severe ventricular dysrhythmia may follow respiratory alkalosis. Palpitations, syncope, substernal chest pain, and seizures have occurred following mechanical overventilation. Carpal-pedal spasm, paresthesia, tingling in the fingers and toes, and circumoral numbness may also be seen. Patients may state that they are lightheaded, complain of weakness and muscle cramps, and exhibit hyperactive deep tendon reflexes. They may possibly convulse if hypocalcemia is present.

Compensatory Response. When the pH of the extracellular fluid reaches a level above 7.45, there is a release of hydrogen ions from the intracellular compartment (Table 7–5). These ions are usually exchanged for potassium. Lactate and

Table 7–5

Blood Gas Alterations in Respiratory Alkalosis*

Parameter	Direction of Change
pH	Up (>7.45)
$PaCO_2$	Down (<35 mm Hg)
HCO_3	Normal until compensation
Na^+	Normal
Cl^-	Up with compensation
K^+	Down
Ca^{2+}	Down

*Breathing pattern—hyperventilation.

other metabolic acid production is increased to compensate for the alkalotic state. The body then begins to move into other compensatory actions. The same three compensatory mechanisms discussed earlier for respiratory acidosis are activated.

The buffer system works in the plasma by increasing the plasma content of organic acids. These acids then combine with excess bicarbonate ions to provide neutralization and maintain the 1:20 ratio between carbonic acid and sodium bicarbonate.

The pulmonary system decreases the rate and depth of respiration to achieve an increase in the carbon dioxide level. This continues until the carbon dioxide reaches a level that again stimulates respiration in the medullary centers and the baroreceptors. The change in respiration also causes hydrogen ions to be secreted in excess to compensate for the decrease of carbonic acid in the plasma.

Hydrogen ions secreted above the needs of the compensatory mechanisms are excreted through the kidney. This also decreases the amount of ammonia that is produced, which allows for the retention of hydrogen ions until the 1:20 ratio of carbonic acid:sodium bicarbonate is reinstated.

Nursing interventions center around assistance to alleviate the underlying cause of hyperventilation. Monitoring the cardiac, pulmonary and neurologic systems, as well as the fluid and electrolyte status, is necessary.

▶ NURSING DIAGNOSIS

Potential Nursing Diagnosis

- Anxiety
- Ineffective breathing pattern
- Hyperventilation
- High risk for electrolyte imbalance
- Knowledge deficit regarding the role of inducing altered breathing pattern
- High risk for injury, seizure activity, cardiac dysrhythmia
- Sensory perceptual alteration, altered level of consciousness, impaired gas exchange
- Self-care deficit: bathing, hygiene, toileting

Potential Outcomes

- Patient demonstrates improved blood gas values and vital signs.
- Patient demonstrates effective breathing patterns as evidenced by blood gas values within normal limits, with no evidence of cyanosis.
- Patient verbalizes less fatigue and weakness by increased participation in self-care activities.

Metabolic Acid-Base Alterations

Metabolic acid-base alterations include any acid-base disturbance that is not caused by an alteration in the carbon dioxide level in the extracellular fluid. These metabolic alterations basically involve bicarbonate levels and base excesses. When metabolic processes lead to a buildup of acids or loss of bicarbonate, the bicarbonate values drop below the normal range, resulting in a negative base excess value. Conversely, when there is a loss of acid or an accumulation of excess bicarbonate, the bicarbonate levels rise, resulting in a positive base excess value. As stated earlier, base excess refers to bicarbonate. It may also include other bases in the blood such as plasma, protein, or hemoglobin. Metabolic alterations include metabolic alkalosis and metabolic acidosis.

METABOLIC ACIDOSIS

Metabolic acidosis results from an accumulation of metabolic acids. These are also referred to as fixed acids and include all acids except carbonic acid, which is a respiratory acid. Metabolic acidemia results when there is a decrease of bicarbonate concentration in the extracellular fluid to less than 22 mEq/liter. A base deficit exists, and the pH is below 7.35. These parameters result from an increase in metabolic (fixed) acids (Table 7–6).

When discussing metabolic acidosis, it is important to understand the concept of an anion gap. An anion is a substance with a negative charge. Body fluids are essentially electrically neutral. The number of cations or positively charged ions equals the number of negatively charged ions or anions. Because sodium accounts for approximately 90% of the cations in extracellular fluid, it represents a large amount of the positively charged ions. To compensate, the sum of the chloride and bicarbonate ions matches the sodium ions.

This total is made more equal when minor ions such as sulfate, phosphate, and organic acids are included in the measurement. Because of the amounts found in the blood, sodium, chloride, and bicarbonate are easily measured, and are referred to as measured anions. Minor ions are difficult to account for and are referred to as unmeasured ions, or the anion gap. Metabolic acidemia can result from an increase of unmeasurable anions as well as from conditions with no increase in unmeasurable ions. Therefore, it is important to understand the difference to allow proper monitoring of the patient and anticipate potential problems.

There is a formula available to help determine the amount of anion gap, which indicates which process is occurring. The anion gap is calculated by using the values of the serum sodium, chloride, and bicarbonate levels. The serum chloride and bicarbonate ion concentrations are added together and subtracted from the serum sodium concentration: $[Na^+] - ([Cl^-] + [HCO_3^-])$. If this difference is greater than 15 mEq/liter, there is an increase in unmeasured ions or an anion gap. The normal range for the anion gap is 10 to 14 mEq/liter.[4, 5]

There are three major mechanisms that allow metabolic acidosis to occur: loss of base from the body through the GI tract; loss of base from the body through urine; or an increase in metabolic acid production. If there is an increase in acid production, this acid production may overwhelm body buffer systems and pulmonary and renal mechanisms. This is considered an extrarenal cause of metabolic acidemia. A renal source of metabolic acidemia could result from a problem in the renal tubules, which would cause retention of acid.

Causes of metabolic acidemia with an increased anion gap (greater than 15 mEq/liter) include normal chloremic ketoacidosis, diabetes, alcoholism, starvation, uremia, lactic acidosis, and toxins found in salicylate, methanol, or ethylene glycol poisoning. Metabolic acidemia associated with a nor-

mal anion gap (10 to 14 mEq/liter) is associated with hyperchloremia and potassium loss caused by diarrhea, renal tubular acidosis, nephritis, early renal failure, or urinary tract obstruction. It can also be drug-induced; amphotericin B or the infusion of hydrochloric acid can cause metabolic acidemia.

It is believed that diarrhea is probably the most common cause of normal anion gap metabolic acidemia. With diarrhea, it is possible to lose large amounts of bicarbonate through the intestines. ''A general guide for the possible development of nonrespiratory acidosis with no increase in immeasurable anions is the presence of any drainage tube (except a Foley catheter) below the umbilicus. This includes the drainage of pancreatic juices, ureterosigmoidostomy and any other drainage tubes in use.''[9]

Findings on Assessment. Patients with an alteration toward metabolic acidosis have tachypnea, hyperpnea, Kussmaul respiration (particularly when acidosis is severe), fatigue, weakness, malaise, nausea, vomiting, abdominal pain, stupor, and coma. Sometimes headache, drowsiness, confusion, cardiac dysrhythmia, hypotension, shock, and pulmonary edema are also present.

Compensatory Response. Hemoglobin and phosphate buffers are predominant in the compensation for metabolic acidemia, because bicarbonate ions are used in decreasing hydrogen ion concentration. The lungs compensate by increasing alveolar ventilation—blowing off carbon dioxide to reduce hydrogen ion levels. Because the cause of the alteration is nonrespiratory, the lungs respond because of the increased hydrogen ion concentration in the cerebral fluid. Because the lungs cannot excrete fixed acids, the kidneys are the primary compensatory mechanism for correcting the alteration. The urinary buffers of ammonia and ammonium and the phosphate buffer system are called on, but it may be 24 hours before the renal system can begin to move the pH in the proper direction. It is estimated that 4 or 5 days may be needed for the entire acid load to be excreted.

Monitoring Parameters. Monitoring parameters include the assessment of vital signs, intake and output, weight, skin color, temperature, GI function, muscle strength, and the monitoring of laboratory values. It may be necessary to institute seizure precautions and maintain bedrest if the acidosis is severe. The patient may need assistance in maintaining conscious orientation.

▶ NURSING DIAGNOSIS

Potential Nursing Diagnoses

- High risk for electrolyte imbalance
- High risk for infection
- High risk for injury: altered level of consciousness or cardiac dysrhythmias, compromised protective reflexes
- Sensory perception alteration, altered level of consciousness
- Alteration in thought process

Potential Outcomes

- Patient is oriented to time, place, and person, or has a measurable decrease in signs and symptoms of an impaired thought process.

T a b l e 7 – 6

Blood Gas Alterations in Metabolic Acidosis

Parameter	Direction of Change
pH	Down (<7.35)
$PaCO_2$	Normal, until compensation occurs
HCO_3	Down (<20 mEq/liter)
Na^+	Normal (unless diuresis)
K^+	Up or normal
Cl^-	Up, down, or normal

- The patient does not develop an infection, as evidenced by normal temperature and vital signs.
- The patient has no incidence of injury.
- The patient returns to acid-base balance as evidenced by a mental status usual or normal for the patient.
- Respirations are unlabored (between 16 and 20 respirations per minute).
- Headache, nausea, and vomiting are absent.
- Blood gas values return to the normal range for the patient.

METABOLIC ALKALOSIS

A metabolic alkalemic state results from some process that increases the bicarbonate ion concentration or decreases the hydrogen ion concentration. The result of this alteration increases the pH to a level greater than 7.45. Metabolic alkalosis tends to occur less frequently than metabolic acidosis. The exception to this is the patient with nasogastric suctioning or fluid loss from the upper gastrointestinal tract, such as vomiting. The bicarbonate concentration can increase either because of loss of hydrogen ions from the extracellular fluid or by addition of bicarbonate to the extracellular fluid.

A metabolic alkalosis can develop from diuretic therapy, excessive ingestion of alkaline drugs, corticosteroid therapy, severe hypocalcemia and, as previously stated, in the patient with vomiting or continuous nasogastric suction without proper electrolyte replacement. These alterations result in hydrogen ion loss and excess sodium bicarbonate, which affects the 1:20 ratio between carbonic acid and sodium bicarbonate and causes a base alteration.

Findings on Assessment. The patient may exhibit signs of confusion, irritability, disorientation, muscle cramps, hyperactive tendon reflexes, tetany, carpal-pedal spasms, polyuria, polydipsia, nausea, vomiting, diarrhea, or hypoventilation. A laboratory examination reveals decreases in the serum potassium and serum chloride levels, although the sodium level generally remains unchanged (Table 7–7).

Compensatory Responses. Intracellular phosphates and proteins shift to the extracellular compartment. The phosphate and protein buffering systems provide hydrogen ions, which buffer excess bicarbonate ions. Alveolar hypoventilation occurs in an effort to retain carbon dioxide, thereby increasing the $PaCO_2$. During compensatory efforts, a secondary respiratory acidosis may occur because of the retention of carbon dioxide and decreased oxygen intake. This results in hypoxia. The $PaCO_2$ attempts to rise in relation to the increase in pH. This is necessary to re-establish the 20:1 ratio, enabling the pH to move back toward the normal range. The kidneys can excrete bicarbonate rapidly and therefore attempt to restore normal bicarbonate levels in the extracellular fluid. If chloride ions are unavailable, the bicarbonate may be reabsorbed. This is because sodium reabsorption requires a negatively charged ion, either chloride or bicarbonate. When there is not enough chloride, the kidney reabsorbs bicarbonate in its place.

▶ NURSING DIAGNOSIS

Monitoring Parameters

The patient should be monitored on an ongoing basis for vital signs, intake and output, weight, level of consciousness, muscle strength, and ongoing laboratory values. Losses from the upper GI tract should be monitored, such as gastric suctioning or vomiting.

Potential Nursing Diagnoses

These can include

- Electrolyte imbalance—high risk for hypochloremia, hypokalemia, hypocalcemia
- High risk for injury—altered level of consciousness, cardiac dysrhythmia, neuromuscular irritability, seizure activity, tetany, sensory-perceptual alteration

Potential Outcomes

- Patient can verbalize fewer problems with sensory perception alteration deficit.
- Patient experiences no injury related to neuromuscular irritability, seizure activity, or tetany.

Mixed Acid-Base Alterations

The preceding acid-base alterations are considered to be primary acid-base alterations. It is possible for patients to undergo single imbalances, but there are clinical conditions in which a patient may exhibit two primary acid-base disturbances concurrently. When a patient presents with an acid-base alteration it is important to realize that, as compensation occurs, more than one acid-base alteration may occur simultaneously. Mixed acid-base disorders are a combination of respiratory acidosis, respiratory alkalosis, metabolic acidosis, and metabolic alkalosis. When the normal compensatory responses to one of these alterations fail, a mixed disturbance can occur. Mixed disturbances can also occur in various clinical circumstances. When dealing with mixed alterations,

T a b l e 7 – 7

Blood Gas Alterations in Metabolic Alkalosis

Parameter	Direction of Change
pH	Up (>7.45)
$PaCO_2$	Normal (up when compensation occurs)
HCO_3	Up (>26–30 mEq/liter)
Na^+	Normal
K^+	Down
Cl^-	Down

the arterial pH alone cannot give the total picture of the underlying pathophysiology. The pH only provides information on the current status of the hydrogen ion.

An example of a mixed acid-base alteration is metabolic acidosis and respiratory alkalosis. This condition can be associated with cardiac and pulmonary arrest, severe pulmonary edema, or poisoning. With this alteration the patient can exhibit a high, low, or normal blood pH. The pH level depends on the severity of the two primary disorders. The bicarbonate and $PaCO_2$ values are usually low. Metabolic acidosis and metabolic alkalosis is another condition in which there is little change in the blood pH. Conditions that may lead to metabolic acidosis and metabolic alkalosis are salicylate intoxication, sepsis, and severe liver disease. Metabolic alkalosis and respiratory acidosis is usually evidenced by a high bicarbonate level and a high $PaCO_2$. Conditions associated with this alteration are generally chronic pulmonary diseases such as COPD, particularly in a patient with chronic respiratory acidosis who has suddenly experienced improved ventilation.

Metabolic alkalosis and respiratory alkalosis can result in a severe alkalemia, which is associated with critical illness. Contributory conditions include severe liver disease coupled with vomiting, gastric suction, overinfusion of Ringer's lactate and bicarbonate, diuretics, steroids, and massive transfusion of citrated blood.

It may be difficult to recognize these mixed acid-base alterations without a systematic examination of the patient and laboratory data. It is helpful to follow the steps given earlier to evaluate blood gas results systematically. In mixed alterations, it is extremely important to apply the anion gap calculation and base excess parameters to understand both the primary and complicated disturbances.

Degree of Compensation

The last factor to consider in acid-base balance alterations is the degree of compensation present. Acid-base alterations can be uncompensated, compensated, fully compensated, or partially compensated. They can also sometimes be considered to be corrected. An acid-base alteration is considered to be corrected when all the acid-base parameters (usually pH, $PaCO_2$, bicarbonate) return to normal. This is done by effecting a change in the acid-base component that is primarily affected (Table 7–8). Compensation occurs when the alteration in pH is returned toward normal by resolution of the component not primarily affected by the alteration. In other words, if the primary alteration is of respiratory origin, the compensatory system is metabolic.

An acid-base alteration is acutely uncompensated when there is an abnormal pH and a change in one blood parame-

ter, either the respiratory or metabolic parameter. In partial compensation, the pH has moved toward normal but has not yet achieved normality. All three values (pH, $PaCO_2$, and bicarbonate) remain abnormal. Compensation occurs more slowly than changes credited to the buffering process. When an acid-base alteration is corrected, all parameters return to normal.[3]

Reaching an understanding of alterations in acid-base balance is complex and sometimes confusing. The material presented in this section is an overview. For more in-depth information, it is recommended that further study be undertaken to understand the more complex principles and their applications fully.

PRINCIPLES OF ELECTROLYTE THERAPY

Electrolytes

As noted earlier, chemical compounds known as electrolytes dissociate in water to positive ions (cations) or negative ions (anions). Disorders of electrolytes can have profound effects on the body.

Sodium

Sodium is found mainly in the extracellular fluid and has a positive charge (cation). The normal value for the serum sodium level is 135 to 145 mEq/liter. The major role of sodium is in controlling water distribution and maintaining the extracellular fluid volume. This control is accomplished through the kidneys' excretion and conservation of sodium, which is primarily determined by water metabolism. Excess sodium triggers the thirst mechanism and the resulting fluid intake stimulates ADH secretion, leading to fluid retention and normalization of the serum sodium concentration. On the other hand, a decreased serum sodium level inhibits the secretion of ADH and allows for water diuresis, which results in equalization of the water and sodium levels. When the intake and output do not balance, or the internal control mechanism is not functioning properly, imbalances occur.[8]

HYPONATREMIA

Once the serum sodium level falls below 135 mEq/liter, homeostasis no longer exists. The sodium deficit is classified as hyponatremia.

Cause. Sodium deficit, or hyponatremia, may be related to excessive losses but is primarily the result of a disproportion-

---

Table 7–8

Direction of Compensation in Acid-Base Alterations

Disturbance	Primary Effect	Compensation	pH
Metabolic acidosis	Low HCO_3	Low $PaCO_2$	Toward high alkaline
Metabolic alkalosis	High HCO_3	High $PaCO_2$	Toward low alkaline
Respiratory acidosis	High $PaCO_2$	High HCO_3	Toward high alkaline
Respiratory alkalosis	Low $PaCO_2$	Low HCO_3	Toward low acid

ate excess of water. Usually, when losses occur, there is an approximately equal proportion of water and sodium or a slightly larger amount of water lost. However, because deficits lead to thirst and greater intake, the amount of water may exceed the sodium. Also, the continued use of certain diuretics, particularly those classified as thiazides, may lead to excessive losses.

Hyponatremia may be caused by an increased extracellular fluid volume. The increase may be related to increased production of ADH, as found in the syndrome of inappropriate antidiuretic hormone (SIADH). The SIADH may be the result of neoplasms, central nervous system disorders, medications, and pulmonary disease. As water is retained, the serum sodium is diluted. Psychogenic polydipsia, a psychiatric disorder, may occasionally initiate an excessive intake of fluids that the normal kidney may not be able to excrete. Edema may lead to dilution of the sodium content. Sodium deficits resulting from water gain may be caused by continued or excessive hypotonic or sodium-free IV solutions.

Finally, the laboratory may report an artificial hyponatremia. This occurs in the presence of hyperlipidemia or hyperproteinemia in which lipids or protein, which are sodium-free, occupy more than the normal volume of the blood sample.[10] This type of hyponatremia has no clinical significance, because the sodium-water content remains normal.

Assessment. Assessment findings vary according to the degree of the deficit and the rate of onset; a more rapid onset results in more severe symptoms. Gastrointestinal symptoms include anorexia, nausea, and vomiting. Many of these are caused by the low serum sodium concentration, which allows water to be pulled into the cells. The major impact of this fluid shift is seen in the form of neurologic effects, including muscular weakness and spasms, personality changes, irritability, and possibly eventual seizures and coma.

When the cause of hyponatremia is a decreased extracellular fluid volume, the symptoms are those of fluid volume deficit (e.g., elevated pulse rate, postural hypotension, decreased blood pressure). On the opposite side, when the causative factor is increased extracellular volume, the signs and symptoms are those of fluid volume excess (e.g., increased blood pressure, edema, weight gain, distended neck veins).

Laboratory findings reveal decreased serum and urine sodium levels and serum osmolality.

Correction. Correction of hyponatremia is accomplished by replacing the sodium, preferably by oral replacement. Sodium may also be replaced through gastric tube feedings and intravenous solutions (e.g., 0.9% sodium chloride solution).

Deficits related to fluid gain may be treated with diuretics to help excrete the excess fluid. With severe hyponatremia, hypertonic saline solutions (3 or 5% sodium chloride) may be used in addition to loop diuretics. Caution must be exercised when hypertonic saline solutions are being administered to prevent intravascular fluid overload.

The treatment plan for hyponatremia resulting from SIADH involves removing the cause. If this is not possible, fluids need to be restricted and diuretics administered. Additional medications to inhibit the action of ADH may be used for patients requiring long-term therapy.

HYPERNATREMIA

Sodium excess, or hypernatremia, occurs when the serum sodium level exceeds 145 mEq/liter.

Cause. Excessive amounts of sodium and an abnormal loss of water are causative factors for sodium excess. The excessive volume may be the result of an increased intake or decreased loss of sodium. As the sodium level increases, thirst also increases and results in fluid intake that normalizes the concentration. This mechanism generally prevents hypernatremia. However, there are some situations in which this process fails and the hypernatremia is caused by an inability to respond to thirst. Included are infants, older adults, and comatose patients who cannot obtain replacement fluids. It may also result from the administration of medications and sodium-containing IV solutions, particularly hypertonic saline.

Water loss may occur in a variety of ways and for a number of reasons. Increased losses may occur through the skin because of fever or burns, in the lungs because of infections, and in the kidneys because of osmotic diuresis. Water may also be lost because of a lack of ADH or the kidneys' inability to respond to ADH, as in diabetes insipidus.

Assessment. Assessment of hypernatremia reveals thirst, dry and sticky mucous membranes, and a decrease in tears and saliva. The temperature is elevated and the skin appears flushed. There may be problems with speech because the tongue is rough, red, dry, and swollen. The fluid status depends on the cause; water loss leads to symptoms of fluid volume deficit and sodium gain leads to those of fluid volume excess.

Many of the symptoms are related to alterations in intracellular volume as fluid is drawn from the cells in an attempt to decrease the intravascular sodium concentration. Restlessness, weakness, and fatigue are early signs of a moderate sodium imbalance. As the imbalance becomes more severe, with the cells becoming more dehydrated, the signs become more apparent. Dehydration of brain cells leads to agitation, seizures, and coma.

Laboratory findings show an elevated serum sodium level and serum osmolality. If the hypernatremia is the result of fluid loss, the central venous pressure is low. There is also an increased urine specific gravity and osmolality with the exception of diabetes insipidus or osmotic diuresis, in which there is a decrease.

Correction. Correction of hypernatremia depends on the cause and is directed toward decreasing the sodium to normal levels. When the excess levels are caused by sodium gain, initial treatment is restricting sodium intake.

An excess in sodium resulting from fluid loss necessitates the restoration of the fluid volume through oral or intravenous fluids. Dextrose 5% in water or hypotonic saline may be given to correct the sodium imbalance. Caution must be exercised to prevent overcorrection, which might cause a shift of fluid into the cells, particularly the brain cells. Diuretics may be used in conjunction with IV solution administration to decrease the potential for overcorrection.

Treatment of diabetes insipidus depends on the type and primary problem. Measures include replacement of the ADH, use of diuretics, and sodium restriction.

Nursing interventions vary according to the cause and may

include restricting sodium intake or initiating IV therapy to improve the fluid volume deficit. Monitoring includes observation of neurologic signs and providing a safe environment in the presence of confusion, delirium, and seizures. During fluid replacement, any signs of cerebral edema should be reported immediately to the physician.

Potassium

Potassium is the main cation in the intracellular compartment. There are approximately 2500 to 3000 mEq of potassium in the body, and all but approximately 2% are located within the cells.[10] The normal serum potassium level is 3.5 to 5.0 mEq/liter. It is important in influencing neuromuscular function and in cell metabolism. Potassium is continually moving into and out of the cells. The potassium-sodium pump assists in keeping most of the potassium in the cell and the sodium outside the cell. Acid-base balance also plays a role in maintaining potassium levels. Potassium tends to be pulled out of cells in the presence of acidosis and shifted back into cells with alkalosis.

The majority of potassium is excreted through the kidneys. The initial depletion of potassium occurs at a more rapid rate until it reaches 2 mEq/liter, at which point the loss occurs more slowly and may reflect a wider deficit range.[10]

HYPOKALEMIA

Hypokalemia, or potassium deficit, occurs when the serum potassium level falls below 3.5 mEq/liter.

Cause. The major cause of hypokalemia is potassium loss, which may occur for various reasons. The primary site for potassium loss is the renal system, and it is often associated with the use of diuretics. Gastrointestinal disorders such as vomiting and diarrhea account for some of the depletion. Gastric suctioning and fistulas are also factors in developing potassium deficits. Losses may be excessive because of increased aldosterone levels, magnesium depletion, increased sweating, and osmotic diuresis.

The cause may stem from an inadequate intake. As long as oral intake is not a problem, potassium levels are maintained easily through ingestion of a variety of foods. However, when intake by mouth is limited or not possible, the deficit can result from inadequate replacement in parenteral or total parenteral nutrition solutions.

The increased release of aldosterone and epinephrine may be triggered by physical or emotional stress. Aldosterone increases urinary excretion, taking potassium at the same time. Serum levels are decreased by additional epinephrine production, which increases the shift of potassium into the cells.

The temporary shifting of potassium from the extracellular compartment into the cells may also be related to alkalosis, increased glucose, insulin, and the process of tissue repair from burns and trauma.

Assessment. Minimal potassium deficits are often asymptomatic. Symptoms are generally focused on neuromuscular changes. With more severe deficits, there is a slowing of impulses required for the muscles and nerves to transmit signals. As a result, there may be fatigue, muscle weakness, leg cramps, paresthesias, and diminished deep tendon reflexes. There is decreased bowel motility, along with nausea and vomiting.

Cardiac abnormalities are common in the presence of hypokalemia. Various atrial and ventricular dysrhythmias may occur. Electrocardiogram changes may include flattened and inverted T waves, enlarged U waves, and ST segment depression. With potassium deficits, patients become more sensitive to cardiac toxicity in the presence of digitalis preparations.[11]

Laboratory findings reveal a serum potassium level below 3.5 mEq/liter. Frequently, the arterial blood gas values show a metabolic alkalosis. Potassium is found in urine samples, with the amount varying with the cause of the deficit. The electrocardiogram shows abnormal tracings, as described earlier.

Correction. The goal of treatment is to replace the potassium. Diet or potassium supplements may be used to treat mild to moderate deficits. If oral intake is not possible or the deficit is severe, the potassium is replaced through the intravenous route. Intravenous preparations of potassium include potassium acetate, potassium phosphate, and potassium chloride, with the latter being the most frequently used. Because potassium is excreted by the kidneys, a non-potassium–containing solution may be used to provide hydration and to determine renal function prior to administering any potassium preparations. Potassium must not be given by IV push, and must be diluted and thoroughly mixed throughout the IV solution prior to administration. The final IV concentration generally should not exceed 40 mEq/liter, with a flow rate not to exceed 20 mEq/hour except in cases of severe depletion, in which initial concentrations of 60 to 80 mEq/liter may be used.[12] Caution should be exercised when administering high concentrations because of the potential for cardiac side effects. In these situations, cardiac monitoring is recommended. An IV solution containing additional potassium may prove to cause pain in the area where it first enters the vein. This may necessitate decreasing the concentration or the flow rate.

Nursing interventions include establishing IV access and administering a properly diluted potassium admixture, as ordered. Questionable orders or laboratory findings should be referred to the physician prior to initiating therapy. During the administration of potassium-containing solutions, the patient should be observed for possible vascular intolerance. Electrocardiogram readings and serum potassium levels should be monitored on an ongoing basis. All procedures and assessments should be properly documented.

HYPERKALEMIA

Hyperkalemia, or potassium excess, occurs when the serum potassium level exceeds 5.0 mEq/liter.

Cause. The cause of hyperkalemia is primarily related to decreased excretion, increased intake, or shift of potassium from the cells. It is most often associated with renal disease leading to inadequate excretion. Also, potassium-sparing diuretics may lead to excessive fluid loss, leaving high potassium levels. Adrenal insufficiency and any condition causing a decreased aldosterone level may increase fluid excretion, leading to hyperkalemia. The potassium excess may also result from the administration of certain medications, such as nonsteroidal anti-inflammatory agents or β-adrenergic blockers.[10]

The administration of inappropriate amounts of potassium may lead to excesses. This may occur through oral intake as well as inadequate dilution or rapid infusion of potassium-containing solutions. Normally, the body can adapt to influxes of potassium, but factors affecting absorption or excretion may inhibit normalization of the levels.

Hyperkalemia may be caused by potassium shifting from the cells. This may result from cell breakdown, as in trauma, burns, or hemolysis, because as much as 80 mEq of potassium may be contained in 1 kg of tissue.[10] The conditions associated with cell breakdown often occur in conjunction with acidosis. Metabolic acidosis also enhances the movement of potassium from the cells as the positively charged hydrogen ion enters the cells. Hyperglycemia resulting from insulin deficiency may pull potassium from the cells as water moves out of the cells in an attempt to dilute the excessive intravascular glucose content. Because insulin acts to force potassium into the cells, any deficiency in insulin may lead to hyperkalemia.

When laboratory tests indicate a high serum potassium level without any clinical indicators, consideration should be given to the method of collecting the blood sample. Inaccurate high levels may occur because of the tourniquet being in place too long, hemolysis of blood cells, delayed separation of serum and cells, or drawing blood samples in close proximity to an infusing IV solution containing potassium.

Assessment. Assessment for hyperkalemia usually reveals altered cardiac or neuromuscular activity. Cardiac dysrhythmias are probably the most prominent characteristics. With excessive levels, initially there are high, peaked T waves, especially in the precordial leads. Progressively, there is a prolonged PR interval, ventricular dysrhythmias, widened QRS complex, merger of the T wave and QRS complex, ventricular fibrillation and, finally, possible cardiac standstill.

Excessive potassium levels alter the impulses needed to send messages to the nerves and muscles. This leads to paresthesias (of the face, tongue, hands, and feet), irritability, and gastrointestinal hyperactivity, resulting in nausea, diarrhea, and abdominal cramping.

Diagnostic findings reveal a serum potassium level above 5.0 mEq/liter. Values indicative of metabolic acidosis are often seen with arterial blood gas studies. Electrocardiograms indicate the abnormal findings described earlier.

Correction. The treatment goal for hyperkalemia is to eliminate the cause of the excess and return the potassium level to within normal limits. Mild excesses may be treated by eliminating the cause. Moderate excesses may include the use of hypertonic glucose IV infusions and insulin (particularly for insulin-deficient patients) to shift potassium into the cells. The insulin aids in moving the potassium into the cells, whereas the glucose helps prevent hypoglycemia. The effect lasts for several hours. Also, shifting potassium back into the cells may be accomplished by administering sodium bicarbonate intravenously. This usually takes effect in approximately 1 hour and lasts for several hours. Both these therapies are only temporary measures, because they do not actually remove any of the excess potassium from the body. Slower but more permanent forms of treatment include cation exchange resins, hemodialysis, and peritoneal dialysis. With

excessively high levels, more immediate forms of treatment should be used in conjunction with these methods. Severe potassium excess is treated with an IV infusion of calcium gluconate. Again, the calcium is only a temporary measure, but it also helps counteract the adverse effects of the potassium on the neuromuscular membranes.

Nursing interventions include monitoring the serum potassium level, cardiac function, intake and output, and signs and symptoms. Initiation of IV access may be needed to administer solutions and medications (see earlier). When sodium- or calcium-containing medications are used, it is also important to observe for imbalances of these electrolytes. Patients receiving digitalis should be monitored for digitalis toxicity if calcium gluconate is the treatment of choice.

Calcium

The normal serum levels of total calcium are 4.3 to 5.3 mEq/liter, or 8.5 to 10.5 mg/dL. The electrolyte, calcium, is important in the formation of teeth and bones. It is also necessary for muscle contraction and neural function, where it regulates contractions and transmission of nerve impulses, and has a sedative effect on nerve cells. It is important for normal blood coagulation. Calcium is available in ionized and nonionized forms. The ionized component is considered to be free calcium and makes up slightly less than half of the total serum calcium. The majority of the remaining nonionized calcium is bound to protein with a small percentage chelated to nonprotein anions, including phosphate, citrate, and carbonate.

Calcium is regulated by the parathyroid hormone, which is released by the parathyroid gland, and calcitonin from the thyroid gland. The parathyroid hormone is responsible for promoting the transfer of calcium from bone to plasma.

The action of shifting calcium from plasma to bone is produced by calcitonin. Calcium is eliminated through urine, the gastrointestinal tract, bone deposition, and sweat. It has a reciprocal relationship with phosphorus.

HYPOCALCEMIA

A calcium deficit, or hypocalcemia, occurs as the serum calcium level drops below 4.5 mEq/liter (8.5 mg/dL).

Cause. Calcium deficits may be related to reduced intestinal absorption, increased loss, altered regulation, and albumin, phosphorus, or magnesium imbalances.

The decreased intestinal absorption of calcium may be related to vitamin D deficiency, small bowel disease (in which most of the dietary calcium is absorbed), and decreased intake. Also, intestinal surgery affects calcium absorption.

Excessive losses of calcium may be caused by renal disease or the use of loop diuretics. Calcium may also be lost through fistulas or damaged skin, as might occur with burns.

Because the parathyroid glands produce parathyroid hormone, any damage to or surgical removal of these glands may lead to hypocalcemia. With slightly less than half of the ionized calcium bound primarily to albumin, any decrease in these albumin levels has an effect on the calcium levels. Also, alkalosis may increase the amount of calcium bound to albumin. Medications that might alter the hepatic metabolism of vitamin D, such as phenytoin and phenobarbital, can affect calcium levels.[11]

Other electrolytes play a role in maintaining balanced calcium levels. Because of the reciprocal relationship of calcium and phosphorus, as the serum level for one goes up the other level goes down. Therefore, excessive phosphorus levels result in deficient calcium levels. This may occur with extensive tissue damage, hypothermia, or cell destruction caused by cancer chemotherapy. Hypomagnesemia is also associated with calcium deficits. This is the result of impaired parathyroid hormone secretion and decreased response to the hormone.

Assessment. Many of the symptoms associated with hypocalcemia are related to neuromuscular activity, such as numbness and tingling of the extremities (fingers and toes) and of the circumoral region, as well as tetany and convulsions. There may be muscle cramps and hyperactive deep tendon reflexes. Chvostek's sign is positive and is presented as unilateral twitching of the facial muscles by tapping the facial nerve just in front of the ear. Trousseau's sign is also positive and is apparent through the development of carpal spasm following inflation of a blood pressure cuff that has been placed on the upper arm. Mental changes may include depression and confusion. As the deficits increase in severity, there may be respiratory effects, including dyspnea and laryngeal muscle spasms. Cardiovascular findings may show dysrhythmias and a prolonged QT interval.

Hypocalcemia may cause dry skin, brittle nails, and dry hair. It has also been reported that chronic deficits may lead to retarded growth and lower IQ scores in children.[8]

Laboratory test results show a decreased serum calcium level. There may also be other electrolyte imbalances, including excessively high phosphorus and abnormally low magnesium levels.

Correction. The goal of the treatment plan should be to eliminate the cause of the deficit and return the serum calcium level to within the normal range. Acute symptomatic hypocalcemia requires immediate treatment.

Calcium deficits necessitate the use of oral or, in emergency situations, intravenous administration of calcium. Calcium chloride (2 to 10% solution) and calcium gluconate (10% solution) may be used, with the latter being preferable. The initial calcium dose is 7 to 14 mEq for adults and 1 to 7 mEq for children, with additional doses as dictated by serum levels.[12]

Calcium chloride ionizes more readily and is therefore more potent and irritating to tissues than calcium gluconate. The IV infusion of both medications should be given slowly to prevent sensations of heat, hypotension, bradycardia, and cardiac arrest.[13] Also, both calcium preparations may cause tissue irritation and burning, and there may be necrosis and sloughing of tissue if IV extravasation occurs. A more diluted concentration of calcium gluconate is preferred to a direct IV injection because of the potential side effects.

Nursing interventions need to include ongoing monitoring of the signs and symptoms, laboratory tests results, and electrocardiogram readings. Precautions related to respiratory problems and tetany should be exercised. If required, an IV line should be established according to the INS *Nursing Standards of Practice*.[14] Also, because of potential problems related to extravasation, the site should be carefully monitored.

HYPERCALCEMIA

Hypercalcemia, or calcium excess, occurs when the serum calcium level exceeds 5.5 mEq/liter.

Cause. The most common causes of hypercalcemia are malignancy and hyperparathyroidism, with others accounting for only approximately 10% of the hypercalcemia-related cases.[10] Malignancy-related excesses are usually produced by secretion of the parathyroid hormone or related substances from the tissue affected by the cancer, medications such as androgens, estrogen, or theophylline, or bone metastasis.

When hyperparathyroidism is present, there is an increase in the parathyroid hormone level. This higher concentration causes an excessive amount of calcium to shift from the bone, an increase in retention of calcium by the renal system, and increased gastrointestinal absorption.

Other causes include excessive administration of IV calcium and oral intake of calcium through milk and antacids. There may be a decrease in urinary excretion because of thiazide diuretics or renal failure. Hypercalcemia may follow prolonged immobilization as a result of the lack of bone stress (weight-bearing), which is important for bone resorption and deposition.[11] Finally, there may be an increase in the ionized portion of the calcium because of acidosis.

Assessment. Assessment findings of hypercalcemia vary according to serum levels and rate of development. Symptoms are related to the effects of calcium on neuromuscular excitability and cell membrane permeability. This sedative action results in fatigue, muscular weakness, and depressed deep tendon reflexes. The neuromuscular effect also carries over to the gastrointestinal tract, where there may be anorexia, nausea, vomiting, or constipation.

Excessive calcium levels can alter the kidneys' ability to concentrate urine, resulting in polyuria and fluid volume depletion. These adverse effects may lead to acute or chronic renal failure.

Hypercalcemia can produce mental changes, including confusion, depression, memory impairment and, if not corrected, acute psychosis.

Laboratory findings reveal an increased serum calcium level. The electrocardiogram demonstrates a shortened QT interval and ST segment, a widened and rounded T wave, and a slightly widened QRS and PR interval.

Correction. As with all imbalances, the treatment goal is directed at eliminating the cause and returning the calcium level to within normal limits. Mild hypercalcemia may be treated by decreasing or eliminating medications that might contribute to the excess, encourage mobilization, and increase fluid intake.

Hypercalcemia may become life-threatening and require immediate treatment. This can include the IV administration of saline solutions, because sodium helps inhibit calcium reabsorption. Patients with normal renal and cardiac function initially receive a 0.9% sodium chloride solution. The solution is given rapidly to provide sodium and intravascular volume, because frequently patients also have a fluid volume deficit. The saline solution helps dilute the calcium concentration and facilitates calcium excretion. Furosemide (Lasix) is usually given in conjunction with the saline infusions to help prevent fluid overload and to increase calcium excretion further. Once adequate fluid volume has been attained, slower infusions of 0.9% and/or 0.45% sodium chloride solution(s) may be given to increase calcium elimination.

Other measures include the administration of calcitonin, intravenous phosphate, and diphosphates, as well as peritoneal dialysis or hemodialysis. Mithramycin (Plicamycin), a cytotoxic antibiotic, may be used to decrease bone resorption. Corticosteroids may be used to reduce intestinal calcium absorption and to decrease reabsorption by the renal system. However, the long-term side effects of glucocorticoid therapy need to be considered.

Nursing interventions include ongoing monitoring of serum calcium levels, electrocardiograms, and renal function. Following emergency treatment, caution should be taken to observe for signs of calcium, potassium, and magnesium deficits. The patient should be monitored for signs of fluid volume overload when large volumes of IV saline are being administered. All information should be documented clearly and precisely, and the physician notified of any abnormal findings.

Magnesium

Magnesium is a cation that is located primarily in the bones and teeth. The remainder of the magnesium in the body is located within the cells, where it is one of the major electrolytes, and approximately 1% is found in the extracellular fluid. Normal serum levels are 1.5 to 2.5 mEq/liter. Like calcium, the serum levels do not accurately reflect the total amount of magnesium in the body. Because part of the magnesium is bound to protein, serum albumin levels should be considered when making decisions related to imbalances. Calcium is controlled mainly through renal excretion and distal small bowel absorption.

The role of magnesium is multifaceted, and includes the activation of enzymes related to carbohydrate and protein metabolism. It is important in activating the sodium-potassium pump. Magnesium acts directly on the myoneural junction, affecting neuromuscular irritability and contractility. It acts on the skeletal muscle by depressing acetylcholine release at the synaptic junction. The cardiovascular system is affected through a peripheral action that produces vasodilation.[8] Magnesium levels and activity are interdependent with those of calcium and potassium.

HYPOMAGNESEMIA

Hypomagnesemia, or magnesium deficit, occurs when the serum magnesium level falls below 1.5 mEq/liter. The deficit is often found in the critically ill patient and may be mistaken for hypokalemia.

Cause. Magnesium deficit may result from a decreased intake, abnormal absorption, or an increased output, as well as chronic alcoholism. A decreased intake may be related to prolonged malnutrition, prolonged administration of magnesium-deficient IV or hyperalimentation solutions, and occasionally to a diet deficient in magnesium.

A decreased uptake of magnesium may occur with any problems related to the lower gastrointestinal tract, because this is where most of the absorption takes place. This may occur in the presence of inflammatory bowel disease or following surgical procedures involving the lower gastrointestinal tract.

Many consider the most common cause of hypomagnesemia in the United States to be chronic alcoholism.[8] Individuals suffering from alcoholism frequently suffer from semistarvation, leading to reduced intake of magnesium-containing foods. There may also be impaired renal function, allowing for increased losses, as well as intestinal malabsorption, which decreases the utilization of the electrolyte. Additionally, there may be intermittent diarrhea, which increases the losses.

Other causes include refeeding following prolonged malnutrition caused by magnesium being pulled from the intravascular fluid and deposited into new cells. Some medications, such as diuretics, laxatives, aminoglycosides, and cisplatin (Platinol) may cause deficits. Increased elimination through prolonged diarrhea, intestinal fistulas, vomiting, and nasogastric suctioning may lead to magnesium deficits.

Assessment. Symptoms related to hypomagnesemia are most often manifested through neuromuscular changes, and the degree is related to the level of the deficit. Included are increased reflexes, tremors, convulsions, and tetany. Chvostek's and Trousseau's signs are positive. There may be paresthesias present, and possibly painfully cold sensations in the hands and feet. Increased nerve transmission may lead to mood changes, ranging from apathy and depression to extreme agitation and hallucinations.

Hypomagnesemia may result in various cardiac dysrhythmias, such as ventricular tachycardia and fibrillation. This deficit may increase the potential for cardiac toxicity.

Correction. The goal of the treatment plan is to eliminate the cause and correct the deficit. The aggressiveness of the treatment is directly related to its severity. Mild deficiencies may be treated with diet or oral supplements, whereas more severe deficits may necessitate the intramuscular or intravenous administration of magnesium.

Magnesium sulfate is usually the drug of choice, particularly for more severe deficits. The onset of action is immediate and the duration of action is approximately 30 minutes. Caution should be exercised because of the potential for overdose and for hypermagnesemia, which may lead to respiratory paralysis. Prior to administering magnesium, the knee jerk reflexes should be checked. If these are absent, the dose should be withheld and the physician notified. Prior to the IV administration of magnesium sulfate, the respiration rate should be at least 16 and the urinary output 100 ml over the 4 hours preceding the scheduled dose. The dosage varies according to the severity of the deficit. It may be given intramuscularly or intravenously. The suggested IV dose is 5 g in 5% dextrose in water or 5% dextrose in saline, to be infused over 3 hours.[12]

Nursing interventions should include monitoring of serum magnesium laboratory findings and urinary output, because magnesium is eliminated by the kidneys. There should be periodic checks of the knee jerk reflexes, because these disappear prior to depressed respirations. Vital signs should be monitored and preparations made to counteract depressed respirations in case of magnesium excess, including artificial ventilation and IV calcium administration. Seizure precautions should also be exercised. All procedures and responses to therapy should be clearly and precisely documented.

HYPERMAGNESEMIA

Hypermagnesemia, or magnesium excess, usually occurs when the serum magnesium level exceeds 2.5 mEq/liter.

Cause. Hypermagnesemia usually occurs from a decreased output or an increased intake. The major cause of the decreased output is renal disease. However, even in these situations, it is often associated with additional intake, such as magnesium-containing medications or IV solutions. Excesses may be present with endocrine disturbances such as hypothyroidism or hyperparathyroidism.

Antacids and laxatives are examples of medications that, if used excessively, may lead to hypermagnesemia. Also, the use of enemas and continuous or large doses of magnesium to treat eclampsia may increase the levels.

Assessment. Clinical indicators, which are primarily related to the nervous and cardiovascular systems, usually do not appear until severe levels are reached. A review of current literature reveals no consistency in the relationship of magnesium levels to clinical indicators. However, it is known that once the magnesium ions are excessive, they interfere with the transmission of neuromuscular impulses. This may lead to increased muscle weakness, paralysis, and depressed deep tendon reflexes. Respiratory muscles may be depressed, leading to respiratory arrest in the presence of excessively high levels.

As the serum levels increase, so do the cardiovascular indicators. Lower serum levels may result in flushing and a sensation of skin warmth caused by peripheral vasodilatation. With more severe high levels, the pulse rate may decrease, which could lead to complete heart block.

Laboratory findings reveal an increased serum magnesium level. Electrocardiogram readings may show prolonged PR, QT, and QRS intervals. Tracings in the presence of excessively high levels may indicate heart block and, finally, cardiac arrest.

Correction. The treatment plan should be directed at eliminating the cause and returning the magnesium levels to within normal limits. Magnesium-containing foods and medications should be eliminated, if possible. More moderate levels may be treated by the intravenous administration of 0.45% sodium chloride solution and diuretics to help the kidneys excrete the excess magnesium. The kidneys need to be functioning properly prior to initiating this form of therapy.

For more severe excesses, calcium gluconate may be administered intravenously. This antagonizes the action of the magnesium but is only a temporary measure. Dialysis may be indicated in the presence of renal impairment.

Nursing interventions include monitoring of the serum magnesium laboratory values. Precautions should be exercised, including having equipment and medication available in the event of respiratory or cardiac arrest. Patients and families should be instructed in regard to the excessive use of over-the-counter magnesium-containing medications. All procedures, including the administration of IV solutions and medications, and observations, particularly those related to the deep tendon reflexes and respirations, should be accurately documented.

Phosphorus

Phosphorus is found in the intracellular and extracellular fluids but is the primary anion in the intracellular compartment. Most of the phosphorus is located in the teeth and bones. Like calcium and magnesium, the serum levels do not necessarily reflect the true levels of the total body content. Most of the phosphorus is found in the form of phosphate, and the two terms are frequently used interchangeably. Normal serum phosphorus levels range from 1.8 to 2.6 mEq/liter, or 2.5 to 4.5 mg/dL. The levels vary according to gender, age, and diet.

The metabolism and homeostasis of phosphorus are related to those of calcium. They have an inversely proportional relationship, and both are controlled by the parathyroid glands. Both electrolytes need vitamin D for absorption from the gastrointestinal tract.

Phosphorus is important in carbohydrate, protein, and fat metabolism. It is necessary for nerve and muscle function and for the maintenance of the acid-base balance, in which it is the primary urinary buffer. Phosphorus is used in the formation of energy-storing substances such as ATP.[11] It is also essential in the functioning of red blood cells, utilization of vitamin B, and transmission of hereditary traits.

HYPOPHOSPHATEMIA

Hypophosphatemia, or phosphorus deficit, results when the serum phosphorus level falls below 1.8 mEq/liter.

Causes. Hypophosphatemia may result from increased losses or utilization, decreased intestinal absorption, or intracellular shifts. The increased losses may be the result of glycosuria, hypokalemia, or hypomagnesemia. The use of diuretics (thiazides) increases the elimination of phosphorus.

Problems related to the gastrointestinal tract, such as diarrhea, vomiting, vitamin D deficits, and lack of absorption, lead to phosphorus deficits. Also, the continuous use of antacids leads to phosphorus binding.

Transient intracellular shifts play a major role in phosphorus deficits. The administration of concentrated glucose solutions increases insulin production, which causes the phosphorus to shift into the cells. Shifts may also be related to an increased intracellular pH, as with respiratory alkalosis.

Patients suffering from malnutrition may develop phosphorus deficits as calories are provided for nourishment. Because of poor nourishment and gastrointestinal problems, such as diarrhea and vomiting, the alcoholic patient may also experience hypophosphatemia.

Assessment. As with most electrolyte imbalances, symptoms related to hypophosphatemia are related to the severity of the deficit and whether it is acute (sudden decrease) or chronic (gradual decrease). Included are those related to the neurologic system, such as confusion, seizures, coma, paresthesias, weakness, numbness, and ataxia. Weakness may lead to difficulties in speaking and breathing.

Cardiovascular findings are related to decreased respiratory function and include myocardial dysfunction and chest pain. If prolonged, dysrhythmias may develop. Hematologically, the phosphorus deficit affects the structure and function of blood cells, which may lead to hemolytic anemia.[11] Platelet dysfunction may result in bruising and bleeding.

Hypophosphatemia may lead to decreased motility of the gastrointestinal tract. This is evidenced by nausea and vomiting and may lead to other problems, such as intestinal ileus.

Diagnostic findings show a decreased serum phosphorus level. There may also be decreased serum potassium and magnesium levels. Other problems may be noted, such as those related to the endocrine system, depending on the cause of the deficit.

Correction. The treatment goal is to eliminate the cause of the deficit and help return the phophorus level to within normal range. The best treatment is prevention of the imbalance through such measures as not using phosphorus-binding antacids, particularly if there is increased potential for phosphorus deficits.

Mild to moderate deficits may be treated through diet and oral supplements. More severe deficits may require intravenous supplements, such as sodium phosphate or potassium phosphate.

HYPERPHOSPHATEMIA

Hyperphosphatemia, or phosphorus excess, occurs when the serum phosphorus level exceeds 2.6 mEq/liter.

Cause. Hyperphosphatemia is most often related to renal disease (acute and chronic). It might also be caused by increased intake, destruction of cells, excessive losses from nonrenal causes, and shifts from cells to the extracellular fluid.

In renal failure, the diseased kidney cannot excrete phosphorus, which leads to excessive levels. An increased intake may be the result of laxatives containing phosphate, vitamin D excess, or phosphorus supplements.

Shifts may occur from cells being damaged and releasing phosphorus. Respiratory acidosis may also be responsible for an intracellular to extracellular shift.

Assessment. There are no direct symptoms related to phosphorus excess, but most are related to hypocalcemia. When excess levels of phosphorus are sustained for prolonged periods, precipitation of calcium phosphate may occur in areas other than the bones.

Laboratory findings reveal an increased serum phosphate level, above 2.6 mEq/liter. Other tests may be performed to help determine the cause (e.g., determination of creatinine and parathyroid hormone levels).

Nursing interventions include monitoring the serum phosphorus and calcium levels. Patient and family education is directed at avoiding foods and medications that contain high phosphorus levels. Precautions should be exercised in event of hypocalcemic tetany, such as monitoring for seizures, confusion, and laryngeal muscle spasms.

Application of Principles to the Postoperative Patient

Preparation to prevent or minimize complications related to fluids and electrolytes should begin, if possible, prior to surgery. A thorough history and physical may indicate pre-existing conditions, such as diabetes mellitus, renal disease, and/or cardiovascular disease. These may also indicate that the patient has been unable to eat properly or has experienced prolonged nausea and vomiting. The history clarifies what medications the patient is or has been receiving. Of particular importance are corticosteroids, which could alter the response to surgery. Diagnostic tests reveal the fluid and electrolyte status. Physical assessment also provides helpful information related to such characteristics as edema, dry skin and membranes, and abnormal vital signs.

It is much easier to deal with many of these issues prior to surgery rather than during surgery or postoperatively. Intravenous solutions may be given to correct fluid volume deficits and, depending on the type of solution, calories and electrolytes may also be provided. Diuretics may be given to eliminate excessive fluid volume. If known far enough in advance, the patient's nutritional state can be improved through the use of total parenteral nutrition solutions.

During surgery, there is always the danger of excessive loss of blood, resulting in fluid volume deficit. Depending on the volume lost, replacement may include the administration of IV fluids and/or blood and blood products. There may be third spacing of fluids, which could create a fluid volume deficit.

Postoperatively, there are imbalances in fluid volume, including fluid volume excess and fluid volume deficit. In addition to the neuroendocrine response from the anesthetic, there is also the stress related to the pain and trauma of surgery. The response is an increased release of ADH and adrenocorticotropic hormone (ACTH). ADH leads to the retention of fluid and ACTH increases the release of aldosterone and hydrocortisone, resulting in the retention of water and sodium and the elimination of potassium. The net result is increased fluid volume. The period of fluid retention lasts approximately 48 to 72 hours following surgery.[11] Other factors that may predispose the patient to excessive fluid volume include medications, possible fluid shifts, tissue catabolism, and the excessive administration of IV fluids.

Other factors may affect output that are not related to the stress response of surgery. These may include hypovolemia caused by the presurgery fluid status or loss of fluid during the surgical procedure. Also, altered cardiovascular functions or renal failure may stimulate the body to retain water and sodium.

The surgical process may precipitate electrolyte imbalances. Electrolyte dilution may occur along with the fluid volume excess discussed earlier. A potassium deficit is the most common imbalance noted. However, caution should be exercised in administering supplements, because some potassium is released because of surgical trauma to the cells. If indicated by laboratory tests, potassium may be replaced after the first 24 hours.[8] A sodium deficit may also occur; this might be related to fluid volume excess, surgery-related stress, and medications received before and during surgery. Treatment is not generally indicated but caution should be exercised to eliminate unnecessary free water to prevent water intoxication.

Electrolyte excess may occur in the presence of fluid volume deficit. Also, hyperkalemia may result from the release of potassium from the cells during the surgical process.

There may be alterations in the acid-base balance. Pain, anesthetics, and narcotics may be responsible for shallow respirations. These in turn could cause respiratory acidosis. Patients who are on ventilators or hyperventilate for any reason may develop respiratory alkalosis. Metabolic acidosis may occur as a result of excess lactic acid in patients who are hypotensive.

Other Disease States

Syndrome of Inappropriate Antidiuretic Hormone

The syndrome of inappropriate ADH occurs when there is excessive release of ADH or a similar substance. Predisposing factors include medications, including nonsteroidal anti-inflammatory drugs; tumors, especially oat cell carcinoma; and central nervous system disorders. Excessive ADH decreases the excretion of water. As this occurs, the serum sodium level and osmolality decrease. The increased fluid volume increases glomerular filtration and decreases aldosterone release, resulting in the increased elimination of sodium. Because the intracellular concentration is greater, extracellular fluid is pulled into the cells. This can be life-threatening, particularly if water is drawn into the brain cells.

Assessment reveals findings related to fluid volume excess with edema, as well as to intake exceeding output. Depending on the severity of the sodium deficit, there may be neurologic indicators, such as lethargy, headaches, seizures, and finally, coma. Laboratory results reveal decreased serum sodium, BUN, and creatinine levels. Urine test findings show a low sodium level and an increased specific gravity and osmolality.

The treatment goal is directed at correcting the cause. If this is not possible, treatment depends on the severity of the imbalance, ranging from fluid restriction to the IV administration of concentrated saline solutions and diuretics.

Burns

The skin is the largest organ of the body and serves a variety of functions. These include acting as a protective barrier, regulation of body temperature, and housing of sensory receptors. The skin is composed of the epidermis, the outer layer; the dermis, the inner layer; and a subcutaneous layer that binds the skin to underlying organs. The severity of the burns depends on the total area involved, depth, patient's age, location, and any other injuries or pre-existing medical problems. They may be classified as first-, second-, or third-degree burns.

Burns damage the skin, which then no longer acts as a protective barrier and sets the stage for fluid and electrolyte imbalances. The first phase is classified as the fluid accumulation phase, and starts almost immediately following the burn. The injury to the cells and vascular system allows fluid to shift from the plasma into the interstitial space, a process that continues for 36 to 48 hours.[8] It may result in fluid volume deficit and, depending on the level of severity, possible renal damage.

Proteins and electrolytes are lost at the same time that water is being lost. Cell damage releases potassium. This, in conjunction with hypovolemia and renal damage, leads to hyperkalemia. There are also abnormal losses of sodium, calcium, and phosphorus. Depending on the degree of pain, there may be hyperventilation, leading to respiratory alkalosis. The damaged cells may release acids, or there may be hypovolemia-induced lactic acid production, resulting in metabolic acidosis.

It is important to maintain fluid volume. Moderate to severe burns require IV fluid replacement. It is important that fluids be delivered only at a rate high enough to maintain the desired intravascular volume and urinary output. Usually, after the first 24 hours, the damaged capillaries start to seal and the fluid loss decreases. Caution needs to be exercised at this time to prevent fluid volume overload.

Fluid replacement therapy varies among physicians and according to the type of fluid and volume. Some regimens include lactated Ringer's solution, which is a balanced electrolyte solution that approximates components found in plasma. Others use 0.9% sodium chloride, but this may create an imbalance because of an excessive amount of chlorides. Some physicians advocate the use of colloids to replace plasma. Nursing interventions should include initiating an IV line to deliver fluid replacement, monitoring the administration process, and evaluating vital signs. Equally important is checking output. Laboratory findings to be monitored include serum electrolyte and blood gas levels. Pre-existing conditions or other injuries may necessitate other laboratory tests. All information needs to be documented and the physician notified of any abnormal findings.

Diabetes

There are two forms of diabetes that affect fluid and electrolyte balance, diabetes insipidus and diabetes mellitus.

DIABETES INSIPIDUS

Diabetes insipidus is a disorder related to water imbalance caused by a lack of ADH or by failure of the kidney to respond to the ADH. The excessive water loss through the kidneys results in a decreased volume in the extracellular fluid compartment. Without proper treatment, dehydration (intracellular and extracellular), hypotension, and hypovolemic shock can occur.[11] Characteristics of diabetes insipidus include an intense thirst, weight loss, excessive urinary output, and neurologic symptoms, such as confusion, irritability, and seizures. Laboratory findings reveal an increased serum sodium level and osmolality. The urine osmolality is decreased. It is important to determine the cause of the polyuria, which can be accomplished by vasopressin administration.

Diabetes insipidus is treated by ADH replacement (vasopressin). Initially, the fluid volume losses may need to be replaced by IV solutions. Caution should be exercised during fluid replacement to prevent water intoxication.

Nursing interventions include monitoring intake and output, body weight, and serum sodium levels. An IV may need to be initiated to provide fluid replacement. Also, during vasopressin administration, the patient needs to be monitored for other complications, particularly water intoxication.

DIABETES MELLITUS

Diabetes mellitus is a disease resulting from a lack of insulin, which leads to an increased blood sugar level and urinary output. Diabetes mellitus is related to decreased glucose utilization, increased fat mobilization, and protein utilization. It is characterized by glycosuria, water and electrolyte imbalances, ketoacidosis, and coma. The process begins with insulin deficiency, which decreases glucose utilization by the cells and results in an increased blood glucose level and glucose production by the liver. As this process continues, the serum osmolality increases, thus pulling fluid from the cells into the extracellular fluid. This results in cellular dehydration and polyuria and, when prolonged, leads to fluid volume deficit.

As the fluid shifts, electrolytes also shift, leading to electrolyte imbalances. Initially, there is an excess serum potassium level that results from the potassium being pulled from the cells, metabolic acidosis, and decreased intravascular fluid volume.

Once treatment has been initiated, hypokalemia develops as a result of potassium returning to the cells, dilution related to an increased intravascular volume (from IV fluids), increased urinary excretion, and correction of acidosis.[8] In addition to potassium, there are usually deficits in the serum phosphorus and sodium levels.

The absence of insulin decreases the use of glucose. Therefore, the body must search for other sources of fuel. Fat stores are mobilized, leading to an increased serum lipid level. The increased fat metabolism increases ketone formation and causes a decrease in the pH of body fluids (metabolic acidosis). The ketones may spill over into the urine and may be excreted by the lungs. In addition to the increased breakdown in fats, there is increased protein mobilization.

Characteristics of diabetic ketoacidosis include polyuria, polydipsia, nausea, vomiting, and hyperventilation with acetone odor respirations. Because there is the potential for fluid volume deficit, characteristics ranging from weight loss to postural hypotension may be present. There may also be a variety of signs and symptoms related to electrolyte imbalances caused by electrolyte excesses or deficits.

Laboratory findings reveal hyperglycemia and an increase in the serum osmolality, BUN and creatinine levels, hemoglobin, hematocrit, and total protein. The serum bicarbonate level and pH decrease. Serum electrolyte imbalances, including those involving potassium, sodium, and phosphorus, may involve excesses or deficits, depending on the severity of the ketoacidosis and the treatment status.

Treatment includes fluid replacement, initially with a 0.9% sodium chloride solution; a 0.45% sodium chloride solution may be used depending on pre-existing conditions related to fluid retention. Subsequent infusions may be changed to 0.45% sodium chloride solution to provide free water, which facilitates renal excretion and the normalization of serum osmolality. As intravascular dilution occurs, the serum glucose level drops, which may necessitate the use of a glucose-containing IV solution. Insulin may be given to help correct the high glucose levels. An initial bolus may be given, and then additional insulin may be added to an IV solution and given on a continuing basis. Only regular insulin should be given by the intravenous route.

Nursing interventions include initiating and monitoring an IV line to help maintain homeostasis. Laboratory data, particularly serum glucose and electrolyte levels, need to be monitored on a continuing basis. The patient should be observed for symptoms related to fluid volume deficit and electrolyte imbalances. Close monitoring should include observation for signs and symptoms of hypoglycemia if the imbalance is overcorrected. All procedures and responses to therapy should be properly documented.

Homeostasis, or a state of equilibrium, is maintained by the body under normal conditions. This balanced state is achieved through various checks and balances. The preceding information describes this delicate process and the imbalances that may occur when the body cannot function properly. Correction of the imbalance may be as simple as eliminating the cause or as complex as initiating life support measures, including the use of intravenous fluids and medications.

Part of the homeostatic mechanism involves the maintenance of fluid balance. As mentioned earlier, water travels throughout the various body compartments. Fluid shifts are an attempt to balance fluid intake and output and are affected by the solutes contained within the various compartments, pre-existing medical conditions, intake volume, and the environment. The crucial role of water has been discussed in detail throughout this chapter. Alterations in this role can lead to imbalances and complications. The fluid volume also affects the concentration of the solutes, and any imbalances may also precipitate various side effects.

Equally important to fluid balance is electrolyte balance. Electrolytes have a direct impact on the movement of fluid, and thus on the maintenance of fluid balance. These ions affect the functioning of all major systems, including the cardiovascular, renal, and neurologic systems. The body generally maintains the proper types and concentrations of electrolytes to ensure normal activity. Abnormal concentrations can lead to ill effects, with severe excesses and deficits possibly leading to death.

As stated at the beginning of this chapter, it is important that the nurse be knowledgeable about normal fluid and electrolyte levels and their importance to the overall maintenance of homeostasis. It is also important to recognize abnormal findings and to understand their impact on the body. Most imbalances resolve, if recognized and alleviated or treated promptly, and the body returns to a normal state.

The nurse also needs to be familiar with proper treatment modalities, which helps ensure that appropriate equipment and supplies are available. It allows the nurse to be able to question possible incorrect treatment orders or laboratory findings. Knowledge of normal and abnormal findings related to fluid and electrolyte balance, along with expertise in IV therapy, help ensure prompt, quality patient care.

References

1. Ignatavicius DD, Bayne MV. Medical Surgical Nursing: A Nursing Process Approach. Philadelphia: W. B. Saunders, 1991:231.
2. Guyton AC. Textbook of Medical Physiology. Philadelphia: W. B. Saunders, 1991:179, 278, 315.
3. Dolan JT. Critical Care Nursing. Philadelphia: F. A. Davis, 1991:411–412, 594–595, 598–599, 744–745.
4. Smith E, Kinsey M. Fluids and Electrolytes: A Conceptual Approach, 2nd ed. New York: Churchill Livingston, 1991:20–21, 84–88, 96–118.
5. Kokko JP, Tannen RL. Fluids and Electrolytes. Philadelphia: W. B. Saunders, 1986:65–67, 76, 248.
6. Corbett JV. Laboratory Tests and Diagnostic Procedures With Nursing Diagnosis, 3rd ed. Norwalk, CT: Appleton and Lange, 1992:109–110, 229.
7. Smeltzer SC, Bare BG. Brunner and Suddarth's Textbook of Medical-Surgical Nursing. 7th ed. Philadelphia: J. B. Lippincott, 1992:125.

8. Metheny NM. Fluid and Electrolyte Balance: Nursing Considerations, 2nd ed. Philadelphia: J. B. Lippincott, 1992:5, 21, 48–49, 56–69, 100, 112, 209, 287, 305.

9. Ahrens T. Critical Care, 2nd ed. Norwalk, CT: Appleton and Lange, 1991:115.

10. Braunwald E, ed. Harrison's Principles of Internal Medicine, 11th ed. New York: McGraw-Hill, 1987:202–204, 207, 1870.

11. Horne MM, Heitz UE, Swearingen PL, et al. Fluid Electrolyte and Acid-Base Balance: A Case Study Approach. St. Louis: Mosby–Year Book, 1991:173, 195, 202, 211–216, 382, 397.

12. McEvoy GK. AHFS Drug Information 94. Bethesda, MD: American Society of Hospital Pharmacists, 1994:1374, 1664–1665.

13. Govoni LE, Hayes JE. Drugs and Nursing Implications, 5th ed. East Norwalk, CT: Appleton-Century-Crofts, 1985:190.

14. Intravenous Nurses Society. Revised Intravenous Nursing Standards of Practice. JIN (Suppl.), 1990.

CHAPTER 8 Infection Control

Roxanne Perucca, BSN, CRNI
Carolyn Hedrick, BSN, CRNI
Judy Terry, BSN, CRNI
Jim Johnson, Pharm D, BCPS

The administration of intravenous therapy increases the risk of a patient developing an infectious complication. It is estimated that annually more than 50,000 hospital patients in the United States develop a nosocomial, intravascular device-related bloodstream infection, 90% of which originate from various types of central venous catheters.[1] The actual number of device-related infections is probably greater because the intravascular device or infusate is often not cultured. Intravascular device-related infection is largely preventable.[2] The occurrence of a device-related infection greatly increases treatment costs and the patient's morbidity rate.

Nurses involved in the maintenance of vascular access devices must have the knowledge base and competency to initiate appropriate central venous catheter (CVC) care protocols, implement nursing actions that prevent the occurrence of complications, and make appropriate nursing interventions, if complications occur. The principles of infection control provide the foundation for the delivery of intravenous therapy. Prevention begins with being knowledgeable about the risk factors that can predispose a patient to an intravascular device-related infection.

To understand the principles of infection control it is important to understand some key concepts. The following infection control terms are briefly defined here and are discussed in greater detail later in this chapter:

1. A nosocomial infection is hospital-acquired and was not present or incubating at the time of admission.
2. Colonization is the growth of microorganisms in a host without overt clinical expression or detected immune reaction. Microorganisms frequently colonize on the surface or in the inner lumens of intravascular devices. Colonization also refers to the persistent presence of microorganisms at a particular site. Certain species of bacteria form colonies on the surface of the skin or on certain regions of the body. For example, the colonization of Staphylococcus aureus in the nares or on the epidermal surface of the skin is considered normal.

3. A bacteremia is a bloodstream infection that is identified by positive blood cultures. Although there are many types of bacteremias, most are commonly classified as primary and secondary. A primary bacteremia has no identified underlying source, but is usually associated with the use of IV devices. A secondary bacteremia arises from an existing infectious source. For example, a patient with an intra-abdominal wound infection or a burn patient is at risk for developing a secondary bacteremia. Signs and symptoms of a bacteremia may include fever, chills, hypotension, and a positive blood culture.
4. Sepsis, or septicemia, is a systemic infection in the circulating blood caused by the presence of pathogenic microorganisms or their toxins in the body. Septicemia can occur when microorganisms migrate into the bloodstream and a profound systemic reaction results. Signs and symptoms of septicemia are described later in this chapter.

IMMUNE SYSTEM AND SUSCEPTIBILITY TO INFECTION

When a venipuncture is performed the body's first line of defense, the transcutaneous barrier, is broken. Breaking the skin barrier provides an avenue for the entry of many microorganisms such as fungi, bacteria, and viruses. Because the immune system is a complex network of cells and organs, only an overview is provided here. Leukocytes (white blood cells) are an important component of the immune system. There are three different types of leukocytes—granulocytes, monocytes, and lymphocytes. Granulocytes are divided into three groups, neutrophils, eosinophils, and basophils. The normal white blood cell count (WBC) ranges from 5,000 to 10,000/mm³.[3] Neutrophils and lymphocytes compose 80 to 90% of the total WBC. A differential WBC count provides more specific information related to infections and disease processes (Table 8–1).[4]

Table 8–1

Leukocytes*
• •

Cell Type	Normal Range (cells/mm³)
Granulocytes	
Neutrophils (total)	2,500–7,000
Segments	2,500–6,500
Bands	0–500
Eosinophils	100–300
Basophils	4–100
Agranular (mononuclear)	
Lymphocytes	1,700–3,500
Monocytes	200–600

*Normal range, 5,000 to 10,000 cells/mm³.

Granulocytes and monocytes are the foundation of the body's nonspecific immune response. Neutrophils (bands and segments) are frequently referred to as polymorphonuclear leukocytes, and form the body's first line of defense against infection. Segments are mature neutrophils. Bands are a less mature cell of a neutrophil, but these cells are capable of fighting infection. Polymorphonuclear leukocytes can destroy invading bacteria and viruses and have a circulation half-life of 6 to 8 hours.[5] Neutrophils are the first cells to appear in large numbers within exudates in the initial inflammation stages. Neutropenia refers to a decrease in the absolute neutrophil count. An absolute neutrophil count of less than 1000/mm³ predisposes the individual to infection; counts under 500/mm³ predispose to serious, life-threatening infections.[6]

The second line of defense is formed by monocytes, cells that are also referred to as macrophages. Neutrophils and monocytes (macrophages) both engulf and partially digest or phagocytize invading antigens. Monocytes are stronger than neutrophils, ingest larger particles of debris, respond late during the acute phase of infection, the inflammatory process, and continue to function during the chronic phase of phagocytosis. The B and T lymphocytes form the specific immune response system. Lymphocytes have specific antigen recognition and can neutralize toxins and phagocytize invading bacteria and viruses.[7] An increase in the number of lymphocytes (lymphocytosis) occurs in chronic and viral infections.

Eosinophils and basophils are other types of WBCs. During allergic reactions and parasitic conditions, the number of eosinophils increases. However, an increase in steroids, during stress or by parenteral administration, decreases the number of eosinophils and basophils. During the healing process, basophils are increased.

Although the immune system is a complex, dynamic system, its components are interdependent. One missing element can cause the entire immune system to be ineffective. Frequently, patients who require vascular access devices have a severe underlying illness, receive multiple infusions of solutions and medications, have extended hospitalization, and may be immunosuppressed. Patients who are immunocompromised are at greater risk for developing an intravascular device-related infection.

Many risk factors have been identified as increasing a patient's susceptibility to developing an IV-related infection.[8] Because a patient's related risk factors cannot be altered, it is important to implement catheter care protocols that decrease the risk factors for developing an IV-related infection. The following are factors that influence host defense:

Leukopenia
Diminished granulocyte function
Immunosuppression and immunodeficiency
Burns
Presence of concurrent infection
Severe underlying illness
Age (younger than 1 year or older than 60 years)

IV-RELATED INFECTIONS AND COMPLICATIONS

Source of Microorganisms

Despite improved catheter technology, antibiotic-impregnated catheters, cuffs, and dressing materials, catheter-related infections continue to occur. IV-related infections can result when the intravenous infusion system becomes contaminated. Contamination can occur by intrinsic or extrinsic means. Microorganisms may be introduced into the intravenous system by IV fluids or additives, intravenous tubing, ointment, and intravenous cannulas or catheters. Contaminates can be introduced during container and tubing changes or while medications are added to the infusion system. Contamination can also occur because of inadequate hand washing, using improper aseptic technique while inserting an intravenous cannula or catheter, prepping the insertion site incorrectly, or allowing a damp, soiled, or no longer intact dressing to remain on the insertion site.

IV-related infection can result from an endogenous or exogenous source of microorganisms. An endogenous infection is caused by the patient's own flora. For example, a central venous access device inserted into the subclavian or jugular vein of an intubated patient may become colonized by the microorganisms from endotracheal secretions. Exogenous infection is an infection resulting from the transmission of organisms from a source other than the patient. Inadequate hand washing by health care personnel can spread transient flora from patient to patient, and cause an exogenous infection.

Contamination of any of the following can lead to the growth of microorganisms: the infusate, the administration equipment, the insertion site, or the intravenous catheter.

Fluid-Related Contamination

Infections related to IV therapy vary from local to systemic, with outcomes ranging from localized pain to death. Fluid-related contamination is one of the main causative factors of IV-related infections and may have intrinsic or extrinsic causes. The fluids given by the intravenous route include basic fluids, medications, blood, and blood products. Epidemics of infusion-associated sepsis are most often related to contaminated infusate.[9] In addition to the IV equipment and fluids, there may be infections caused by contaminated or unreliable antiseptic solutions.

The following are causative organisms of fluid-related contamination[2]: Family Enterobacteriaceae (Enterobacter [Aerobacter] cloacae, E. agglomerans, Serratia marcescens, and Klebsiella spp.); Pseudomonas cepacia, P. acidovorans, and P. pickettii; Xanthomonas maltophilia; Citrobacter freundii; and Flavobacterium and Candida spp.

Fluid-related microorganisms may be present in large numbers and still not be visible to the naked eye. Therefore, close scrutiny of the product container for cracks or leakage of the fluid, for color and clarity, and of the patient are vital. Introduction of the microorganisms may occur prior to arrival at the health care facility (intrinsic) or during the course of clinical use (extrinsic).

INTRINSIC CONTAMINATION

Intravenous products can become contaminated prior to reaching the health care facility, and many articles have described worldwide occurrences. Probably the most well-known incident occurred in the United States between 1970 and 1971. It involved intravenous products manufactured by one company after changing the lining of the screw cap closures. This change resulted in 378 patients in 25 hospitals developing Enterobacter (Aerobacter) cloacae or E. agglomerans septicemia, which contributed to the deaths of 40 patients.[2]

IV fluids can become contaminated at any time during the sterilization process. After the product has been sterilized, any damage to the IV fluid container provides an entry point for microorganisms. This may be in the form of a damaged port seal, a crack in a bottle, or a hole in a plastic IV bag. Damage and contamination of the IV container can occur at the manufacturing site or at any point during storage or delivery to the health care facility. A defect in the fluid container may occur during the manufacturing or sterilization process. For example, if no seal is placed or if a seal is mispositioned on the port of an IV bag, fluid contamination may result.

Intrinsic contamination occurs on an infrequent basis. However, when it does occur, there may be far-reaching effects because of the large volumes of product that are produced and processed at one time. Also, if a contaminant is introduced into the fluid at the manufacturing level, there is more time for the microorganism to proliferate before it actually reaches the patient.

Prevention is the best form of therapy. Close inspection of IV fluids and their containers is imperative. Bottles should be checked for cracks; this includes looking at the bottle under the label. The neck of the bottle should be checked to ensure that all the closure components are intact. IV bags should be checked for puncture holes by squeezing the container and rotating the bag. Fluid containers should be observed for droplet formation on the bag surface. All protective coverings and seals for entry ports should be inspected to ensure proper fit. The clarity of the solution should be inspected and the manufacturer's expiration date should be noted. If there is any question about the sterility of the IV product, it should not be used. If intrinsic contamination is suspected, the IV nursing supervisor, pharmacist, manufacturer, and Food and Drug Administration (FDA) should be notified immediately. Samples of the affected product with the same lot number should be made available for inspection and analysis.

Blood and blood products may also be contaminated at the collection site. The collection bag may have been contaminated during the manufacturing process or during transportation and storage of the product. The port may have been contaminated during the actual collection process or, in the case of components, during the separation process. The storage time and temperature are directly proportional to the increased growth level of microorganisms. The resulting transfusion reaction is most often related to the endotoxins produced by psychrophilic, gram-negative bacteria. The following endotoxins are associated with transfusion reactions: Pseudomonas spp., Citrobacter freundii, Escherichia coli, and Yersinia enterocolitica.

Just as with IV fluids and medications, blood and blood products should be inspected carefully. The blood collection container needs to be checked for possible damage. The contaminated blood may appear normal, have a purple color, or show signs of hemolysis. In any case, it should not be used if the integrity of the product is suspect.

A transfusion reaction related to contaminated blood can have a number of signs and symptoms, including high fever, diarrhea, vomiting, hemoglobinuria, renal failure, shock, generalized muscle pain, and disseminated intravascular coagulation. Even though contamination is rare, it can be fatal. Treatment should be initiated immediately and include IV antibiotics and vasopressor medications or steroids. However, the best treatment is prevention through adherence to aseptic technique, administration of blood immediately after being removed from controlled refrigeration, infusing within 4 hours, and replacing IV tubing following administration of the product.

EXTRINSIC CONTAMINATION

Extrinsic contamination occurs in the health care facility or in the patient's home. IV fluids or medications may be contaminated during the admixture procedure, which can result from the improper use of laminar flow hoods or by using hoods that are malfunctioning. Incorrect use of admixing equipment, such as needles, syringes, or calibrating devices, may lead to contaminated products. Because products are prepared in large numbers in IV admixture programs, the potential for patient exposure to contamination is high. Admixed fluids that are not refrigerated for long periods have an increased rate of proliferation of microorganisms, thus increasing the risk and severity of infection. Fluid admixtures should be used within 6 hours of admixing or should be refrigerated immediately.[2] Intravenous products, whether in the hospital or at home, may also be contaminated while adding medications to fluid containers already in use. Damage may occur during delivery and storage of the product, which allows microorganisms to enter the sterile container. Finally, the IV fluid may become contaminated by the use of improper technique while administering intermittent medications, or by the failure to maintain a sterile, closed infusion system.

Clinical indications of extrinsically contaminated IV fluids occur infrequently. However, when there is a resulting septicemia, the signs and symptoms are undistinguishable from those of septicemia with an intrinsic cause.

Early detection and treatment are extremely important if the outcome is to be positive. The treatment of an extrinsically induced septicemia is the same as for an intrinsic infection. As with all infections, prevention is certainly preferable. Maintaining aseptic technique is important. This includes proper hand washing, correct use of sterile admixing equipment and supplies and, when applicable, correct use of laminar flow hoods. Staff members involved in this process should have to demonstrate admixture competencies on a routine basis, particularly those individuals staffing admixture programs.

Equipment-Related Contamination

The equipment used in the administration of IV fluids, medications, or blood products needs to provide a sterile pathway from the container to the patient. Equipment may become contaminated during the manufacturing process, when therapy is initiated, or during therapy.

INTRINSIC CONTAMINATION

On the manufacturing level, the product may become contaminated during the sterilization process or while in storage.

Also, the product may be made improperly—for example, an IV set port cover may be missing or may not fit correctly. Finally, the equipment may become contaminated during delivery from the manufacturer to the health care facility.

EXTRINSIC CONTAMINATION

Extrinsic contamination may occur as therapy is initiated or during the course of administration. Contamination of the IV line may occur as the administration set is being added to the fluid container if the spike of the set comes in contact with the outside of the port. Equipment may become contaminated as auxiliary sets are added (e.g., filters, extension sets). Finally, the sterile pathway may become contaminated as the administration set is added to a peripheral intravenous cannula or a central venous access device.

The venipuncture procedure offers ample opportunity for the contamination of equipment. Improper site preparation, touch contamination of the cannula, and improper application of the dressing are some of the primary means whereby contamination can occur.

During the course of therapy, the IV pathway may become contaminated at any point along the line. This may occur as additional solutions or medications are connected or when air is removed from the line. Contamination may occur when there is accidental separation of the line at any connection. If flushing is necessary, as with intermittent infusions, the line may become contaminated. Some equipment, such as a line for intermittent medication administration or a stopcock tends to be more susceptible to contamination. Soiled or damp dressings left in place are also a source of contamination. Tubing that is left in place too long, including blood sets, provides a source for microorganisms to proliferate. Suppurative phlebitis and an intravascular thrombus can yield a large number of microorganisms that can circulate throughout the body.

Many extrinsic sources exist, all of which can contaminate the intravenous system. Many catheter-related infections are caused by the extrinsic contamination of the insertion site and of the intravenous catheter. Both are considered crucial areas for the prevention of IV-related infections.

Contamination at the Insertion Site

An important potential source of infection is the tract created by the intravenous cannula through the normal cutaneous barrier. The colonization of organisms at the insertion site is associated with the highest incidence of catheter-related infections.[1, 10] The vast majority of IV-related bloodstream infections are caused by microorganisms that colonize on the skin.[2]

The microorganisms of the skin are classified as two types of flora, resident and transient. Resident flora are also referred to as colonizing flora.[11] These microorganisms are considered to be permanent residents of the skin and are not readily removed by mechanical friction. Some examples of resident skin flora are Staphylococcus epidermidis, S. aureus, Corynebacterium (diphtheroids or coryneforms), Propionibacterium and Acinetobacter spp., and the Klebsiella-Enterobacter group.

Transient flora (also referred to as contaminating or noncolonizing flora) are organisms that are not consistently present in most people. Escherichia coli survives poorly on the skin and is classified as a noncolonizing flora.[11] Transient flora are loosely attached to the skin, vary daily in quantity, and can be readily transmitted on the hands of health care workers. When hands are properly washed with soap and water using mechanical friction, transient flora are removed.

Other important properties of the skin are temperature and moisture. The skin on the upper and lower extremities has a lower temperature than that on the trunk and neck. The higher the skin temperature, the greater the occurrence of microbial growth. Most central venous catheters are inserted into the trunk, which has a higher temperature and thus a greater potential for microbial growth. Skin surface moisture is another important property of infection control. Superhydrated skin supports an increased growth of microorganisms.[12] Much controversy exists over what type of dressing material should be used with a central venous catheter (CVC). Technology related to transparent semipermeable (TSM) dressings is evolving. Newer types of TSMs are available that allow for improved moisture vapor transmission and reduced microbial colonization by antiseptic bonding. Studies have concluded that the collection of moisture enhances the proliferation of microorganisms, so it is essential to maintain a dry, sterile, and intact IV site dressing.

Catheter-Related Contamination

The intravenous catheter is an extrinsic source for potential contamination of the intravenous system. Maki has reported that the lowest infection rates occur with the use of small peripheral intravenous steel needles, Teflon, or polyurethane catheters.[1] CVCs are associated with an increased risk of catheter-related infection. The comparison and interpretation of studies reporting catheter-related sepsis rates is difficult because of the variance among different patient populations and their severity of illness, differences in catheter use and length of catheterization, and poorly defined criteria for determining catheter-related infections.[13]

Catheter design and composition contribute to the risk of infectious complications. Catheter size has an obvious impact. The larger the catheter, the larger the venipuncture site through the skin and vessel; therefore, greater injury is caused in the tissues. With a larger catheter it is more difficult to stabilize and maintain an intact dressing. It is recommended that the smallest gauge cannula of the shortest length possible be used to administer the prescribed therapy.

The relationship between the number of catheter lumens and the risk of a cannula-related infection is uncertain. Frequently, patients who require multilumen catheters are critically ill, require total parenteral nutrition, may be immunocompromised, and have extended hospitalizations. It is important to reduce the number of cannula manipulations as much as possible, to adhere to strict aseptic technique, and to designate each lumen of a multilumen catheter for a specific purpose. Current data are inconclusive about the catheter hub as a potential source of contamination. Some investigators have suggested that the colonization of microorganisms on the catheter hub increases the risk for developing a catheter-related infection.[14, 15]

Catheter composition has also been suggested as a possible factor in the occurrence of IV-related infections. Currently, most CVCs are composed of polyvinylchloride or a silicone elastomer. Both materials are soft and flexible. Polyvinyl-chloride catheters have been reported to have a higher incidence of coagulase-negative Staphylococcus colonization than Teflon catheters.[16] Polyurethane and silicone elastomer catheters have been associated with much less thrombogenicity.[17] Although polyurethane and silicone elastomer catheter materials are less thrombogenic, most authorities believe that all intravenous catheters become coated with a fibrin sheath several hours after insertion.[10] This fibrin sheath may promote bacterial adherence and increase bacterial replication around the intravascular portion of the catheter.[18]

Microscopic examination of infected CVCs has shown microorganisms primarily on the external surface.[9] Staphylococci, normal residents of the skin flora, cause about two-thirds of IV-related infections.[8] Staphylococcus aureus is the most common gram-positive organism causing bacteremia.[19] Numerous studies have noted the ability of coagulase-negative staphylococci to grow and proliferate on the inner and outer surfaces of intravascular catheters in the absence of any other externally supplied nutrients.[20] Following attachment to the catheter surface, coagulase-negative staphylococci produce a glycocalyx solution referred to as slime. This polysaccharide slime protects coagulase-negative staphylococci by providing resistance to the natural immune mechanisms and even to the prolonged administration of high-dose bactericidal drugs.[19]

New CVC technology focuses on the prevention of catheter-related infections. Catheters are now available that are bonded with antimicrobial substances such as chlorhexidine and silver sulfadiazine to prevent bacterial colonization.[21] In an attempt to decrease the formation of fibrin sheaths, catheters can be coated with heparin and hydromere. A collagen cuff impregnated with antimicrobial silver ions can be attached to the catheter at the time of insertion, and is also available preattached to the CVC. The cuff acts as a mechanical barrier to prevent the migration of microorganisms along the transcutaneous catheter tract.[22]

Other strategies being investigated are the prophylactic use of antibiotics, such as locking catheters with vancomycin (Vancocin).[23] The prophylactic use of urokinase to decrease the formation of a fibrin sheath is currently being studied,[24] and research is underway to determine the relationship between the formation of a fibrin sheath and the bacterial colonization rate. Thus, much technology and research are now focused on the intravascular catheter as the source of many IV-related infections.

HEMATOGENOUS DISSEMINATION

Another causative factor of IV-catheter-related infections is hematogenous seeding from a distant site of infection. Central venous and arterial catheters can be colonized from remote, unrelated sites of infection. Current studies suggest, however, that the occurrence is infrequent.[1] Most yeast vascular access infections appear to be the result of hematogenous seeding from another site of infection. Research is being conducted on the ability of microorganisms to translocate across the gastrointestinal tract to normally sterile tissues such as the mesenteric lymph nodes, spleen, liver, and blood.[25] Examples of bacteria associated with gut translocation include Escherichia coli, Klebsiella pneumoniae, Pseudomonas aeruginosa, Candida albicans, Staphylococcus epidermidis, and enterococci.

E. coli is the most common gram-negative bacillus isolated from septic patients.[19] Bacteria can translocate in patients who are not fed enterally and, as a result, intravascular catheter sepsis and multiple system organ failure can occur. The translocation of endotoxins or bacteria across an ischemic or malnourished intestinal mucosa has been reported as a possible pathway for the migration of bacteria into the lymph nodes or liver.[26]

Phlebitis

One of the most common complications associated with intravenous therapy is phlebitis. This condition can be defined as an inflammation of the vein and it can have many causes, such as host factors (inclusive of the patient's history and present condition), cannula insertion technique, cannula site location, condition of the cannulated vein, cannula material, length and gauge of the cannula, stabilization of the cannula, duration of cannulation, compatibility of solutions, type and pH of medication or solution, skin preparation, frequency of dressing change, and ineffective filtration. Signs and symptoms of phlebitis can include pain, tenderness, redness (erythema), elevated skin temperature at the insertion site, palpable cord along the affected vein, reduction in the infusion rate, and elevated body temperature as the phlebitis progresses.[27]

The three major types of phlebitis are related to the causative factors—mechanical, chemical, or bacterial. Mechanical phlebitis is caused when the vein becomes irritated from the use of a cannula too large for the size of the vein, movement of the cannula within the vein, or frequent manipulation of the catheter. Unnecessary irritation to the vein can be avoided when the smallest gauge and shortest length cannula is used to administer the prescribed therapy. Proper cannula stabilization and adequate taping can eliminate any movement of the cannula within the vein. When manipulation of the cannula is reduced, the potential for venous irritation is decreased.

Chemical phlebitis can occur when acidic or alkaline solutions and/or medications are infused. The lower or higher the pH of a solution or medication, the greater the risk of developing phlebitis. Any additive that increases the tonicity of the solution increases the phlebitis risk. Particulate matter is another factor related to the development of chemical phlebitis. Particulates can be found in solutions, especially those containing medications. These particles may occlude capillaries and are irritating to the tunica intima of the vein.[27]

The *Intravenous Nursing Standards of Practice* has recommended that a phlebitis scale be used to rate phlebitis according to the signs and symptoms exhibited.[28] This scale should be established in the institution's policy and procedure to provide a uniform measurement of the degree of phlebitis. (See Chapter 24, Intravenous Complications, for a phlebitis scale.) The following are most important for decreasing the incidence of phlebitis through prevention:

1. Use aseptic technique for fluid preparation and cannula insertion.
2. Infuse hypertonic solutions through larger veins or central venous catheters.

3. Rotate cannula sites according to the *Intravenous Nursing Standards of Practice*.[28]
4. Select the smallest gauge cannula to administer the prescribed therapy.
5. Use proper taping technique for maximum catheter stabilization.
6. Use a 0.2-μ filter for the removal of particulate matter.

Close monitoring of the insertion site and prompt intervention can prevent the occurrence of peripheral thrombophlebitis. This condition not only involves inflammation of the vein, but also the formation of a blood clot within the vein. Signs and symptoms include a decreasing flow rate, tenderness along the vein, progressively cord-like vein, limb edema, redness above the venipuncture site, and warmth along the vein.[27] Thrombophlebitis can cause an embolism if left untreated or undetected. The treatment of choice is removal of the IV catheter, administration set, and fluid container. The infusion should be restarted in the opposite extremity using totally new equipment.

Bacterial phlebitis occurs when the intravenous infusate becomes contaminated, thus allowing bacteria to enter into the solution and proliferate. Bacterial contamination of the infusion system can occur because of compromise of aseptic technique during the admixture of fluids, inadequate skin preparation, failure to inspect containers for cracks or leaks, and improper cleansing of injection sites prior to the administration of medications. Bacterial phlebitis is also referred to as septic phlebitis, and can predispose a patient to septicemia.[27]

Phlebitis may also be suppurative. This term is used when purulent drainage (pus) can be expressed from the cannula insertion site. Suppurative phlebitis increases the risk of developing a systemic infection. Infrequently, suppurative phlebitis appears with peripheral IV cannulas. It occurs more commonly with the use of central venous catheters.[2]

Sepsis

Septicemia, or sepsis, can occur when pathogenic microorganisms or their toxins migrate into the bloodstream and cause a systemic infection. The most frequent life-threatening complication of vascular access devices is septicemia.[29] Sepsis can result from any of the following conditions: localized infection at the insertion or exit site, catheter tunnel, or portal pocket; infusion of contaminated fluids; colonization of the patient's own cutaneous flora through the cutaneous tract when the catheter is inserted; and inadvertent contamination introduced during catheter manipulation. Intravascular device-related septicemia is frequently caused by staphylococci (especially coagulase-negative staphylococci), Trichophyton beiglii, or Corynebacterium, Bacillus, Candida, Fusarium, or Malassezia (Pityrosporon) spp.[2]

Catheter-related fungal infections are frequently associated with the administration of total parenteral nutrition and the long-term administration of broad-spectrum antibiotics. Although Candida is usually the cause, studies have reported the occurrence of fungemia caused by Malassezia furfur in newborn infants receiving lipid infusions.[30]

A localized catheter-related infection is usually evidenced by the presence of redness, edema, or purulent drainage at the insertion or exit site, tunnel, or portal pocket, an elevated temperature, and elevated white blood cell counts. Signs and symptoms of an intravascular device-related septicemia include fever, chills, tremors, nausea, vomiting, abdominal pain, diarrhea, confusion, seizures, hyperventilation, respiratory failure, shock, vascular collapse, and death. The identification of septicemia in critically ill patients can be difficult. Nurses must be aware of the patient's history, possible risk factors, and the clinical signs and symptoms associated with septicemia, and must implement prompt interventions if septicemia is suspected.

APPROPRIATE ANTIMICROBIAL THERAPY FOR INFECTION

It is helpful to view therapy for infectious diseases, especially in hospitalized patients, in terms of three stages as described by Quintiliani and colleagues.[31] When an infection is diagnosed or suspected, broad-spectrum therapy, usually intravenous, is initiated and directed at the majority of possible offending organisms. This "stage 1" therapy may be guided by a report of sample microscopy (e.g., morphology: bacilli, cocci, or other forms; Gram's stain: positive or negative). Stage 1 patients are usually unstable from the standpoint of their infectious process. Attempts to isolate causative organisms by sampling suspected sites of infection are generally made prior to the initiation of antibiotics. Antimicrobials active against several nosocomial pathogens are listed in Table 8–2.

Table 8–2

Antimicrobial Agents Effective Against Some Nosocomial Pathogens

Organism	Antimicrobial Agents
Gram-positive	
Staphylococci (methicillin-sensitive)	First-generation cephalosporin, nafcillin
Staphylococci (methicillin-resistant)	Vancomycin
Enterococci	Ampicillin or vancomycin with or without aminoglycoside
Clostridium difficile (diarrhea, colitis)	Oral vancomycin, oral metronidazole
Gram-negative	
Klebsiella spp.	Cephalosporin, quinolone (e.g., ciprofloxacin)
Escherichia coli	
Enteric bacilli (Enterobacter, Citrobacter, Serratia)	Imipenem or third-generation cephalosporin (not Enterobacter), with or without aminoglycoside
Pseudomonas aeruginosa	Ceftazidime, aztreonam, or extended spectrum penicillin (e.g., piperacillin) with or without aminoglycoside, ciprofloxacin
Acinetobacter spp.	Imipenem, ciprofloxacin
Legionella spp.	Erythromycin with or without rifampin
Other	
Candida spp.	Amphotericin B, fluconazole, ketoconazole
Aspergillus spp.	Amphotericin B, itraconazole
Anerobes	Clindamycin, metronidazole, ticarcillin/clavulanate, ampicillin/sulbactam

In stage 2, therapy is adjusted to antimicrobials active against the isolated organisms. Results of antibiotic sensitivity testing are used to guide therapy, when available. The use of antimicrobials with a narrower spectrum of activity minimizes their effect on institutional and normal host bacterial flora, and is often less expensive as well. A final stage is reached when the patient shows signs of successful treatment and is converted to oral therapy prior to discharge.

Selection of antibiotics at any stage of therapy involves several considerations in addition to an assessment of the likely pathogens involved. Patient factors such as underlying disease states, renal and hepatic function, sites of infection, age, and immune status are considered. In general, patients with compromised immune systems require more aggressive antimicrobial therapy and monitoring. Drug factors include toxicity, drug interactions and compatibilities, cost, and pharmacokinetics. Pharmacokinetics describes how the body processes drugs physiologically and includes absorption (not a factor with intravenous medications), distribution within the body, metabolism, and excretion. Dose, route, and frequency of administration are chosen with these factors in mind.

Monitoring antimicrobial therapy involves continued consideration of patient factors (signs and symptoms of infection), pathogen factors (isolation and testing of infecting organisms), and drug factors (dosage adjustment and toxicity monitoring).

Patient Factors

Body temperature is maintained within narrow limits by the hypothalamic temperature regulatory centers in the brain. Fever (core body temperature elevated above normal) is often a sign of infection. When proper antibiotic therapy combines with host defenses to eradicate an infection effectively, fever usually resolves and can be followed as a measure of response to antibiotic therapy. Exogenous chemicals, including antimicrobials and other medications, can sometimes be a cause of fever. Concurrent corticosteroids, acetaminophen, aspirin, or other nonsteroidal anti-inflammatory drugs act as antipyretics. Thus, they may mask a fever and can complicate the monitoring of antimicrobial therapy. The predictability of fever as a response to infection in the elderly has also been questioned.[32]

Another indicator of infection and response to antimicrobial therapy is the peripheral leukocyte count (also called the white blood cell count, WBC). The WBC is typically elevated in response to an acute bacterial infection and, because of the short life span in the blood of many of these cells, usually drops rapidly during successful treatment. Patients with low leukocyte counts (neutropenia) may respond poorly to therapy for infection. Similarly, patients with other defects in humoral or cellular immunity may have impaired neutrophil function and be at risk for bacterial and fungal infections in spite of normal leukocyte counts. Noninfectious causes of elevated leukocyte counts include myeloproliferative disorders, trauma, acute myocardial infarction, and corticosteroid or lithium therapy. The presence of immature granulocytes (band neutrophils) is an indicator of bone marrow response to the presence and treatment of infection. These are reported as ''bands,'' ''stab cells,'' or a ''left shift.''

Pathogen Factors

Culturing offending pathogens for identification and in vitro susceptibility testing is an important facet of monitoring antimicrobial therapy. Many microorganisms are identified in the laboratory by growth pattern or biologic substrate usage. An increasing number of organisms are identified using immunologic or genetic tests, some of which are rapid because they do not require the organism to grow for the purpose of the test (e.g., direct antigen tests for diagnosis of group A streptococcus).

If the intravenous catheter is in any way implicated, it should be cultured. The recommended method for culturing a catheter, according to the *Intravenous Nursing Standards of Practice,* is the semiquantitative culture technique.[28] To perform a semiquantitative culture, the area around the insertion site is thoroughly cleansed with 70% alcohol and permitted to air-dry. Alcohol is recommended because the residual antimicrobial activity of iodine-containing solutions may kill organisms on the catheter when it is removed. After the catheter is withdrawn, at least 5 cm of the tip and the catheter segment, beginning 1 to 2 mm inside the skin-catheter junction point, is clipped off with sterile scissors into a sterile specimen tube or cup. If present, purulent drainage should be cultured prior to cleaning the site. A positive, semiquanative culture of 15 or more colony-forming units (CFUs) confirms a local cannula infection.[2] The semiquantitative culture technique may fail to detect bacteremia and significant colonization of the internal lumen of the catheter tips.[33] Another disadvantage of the semiquantitative culture method is that the catheter must be removed, even though the catheter may not be colonized or may not be the source of infection.

The use of quantitative blood cultures drawn through a peripheral vein and through the intravenous cannula can be a helpful alternative. The two blood culture results are compared. If the results of the catheter blood samples are greater than or equal to five times the peripheral blood sample, a catheter-related infection is suspected and the catheter should be removed. If a catheter has been replaced over a guide wire, the new catheter should be removed to prevent recurrence of the organism.

Once isolated and identified, organisms are tested for susceptibility against antimicrobial agents. Several testing methods have been developed and standardized. The multiple tube dilution method involves growing the organisms in broth containing serial dilutions of the antibiotic being tested to determine the minimum inhibitory concentration (MIC). The MIC is the dilution that inhibits growth and is used as a measure of susceptibility. In the agar plate disk diffusion test (Kirby-Bauer), antibiotic-impregnated disks are placed on a surface on which the organism grows. After incubation for several hours, a zone of inhibition, in which no organism grows because of the presence of antibiotic, is evident around each disk. The size of this zone defines susceptibility for that antibiotic agent. The broth dilution test has been automated through the use of microtube methods. Many automated systems combine identification of the organism with susceptibility testing, thus decreasing the time needed to make this information available to clinicians. In addition, slow-growing organisms or those difficult to culture may be tested for certain characteristics predictive of antimicrobial susceptibility. For example, Hemophilus influenzae is tested for the

Major Toxicities of Some Intravenous Antimicrobial Agents

Drug Class	Dose/Infusion-Related Toxicity	Other Toxicity
Penicillins	Phlebitis, CNS (seizures)	Hypersensitivity
Cephalosporins	Phlebitis	Hypersensitivity, bleeding, hypoprothrombinemia
Imipenem/cilastatin	Phlebitis	Seizures
Erythromycin	Phlebitis, ototoxicity	
Tetracyclines	Nephrotoxicity, ototoxicity	
Vancomycin	Infusion-related histamine reaction—"red man syndrome" (rash, hypotension)	Additive nephrotoxicity with aminoglycosides
Amphotericin B	Phlebitis, hyperkalemia, renal dysfunction, infusion-related fever, shaking chills	Anemia, electrolyte disturbances
Acyclovir	Phlebitis, obstructive renal toxicity	
Fluconazole		Hepatotoxicity
Ciprofloxacin, ofloxacin	CNS toxicity (?)	
Metronidazole	Neuropathy	
Cotrimoxazole (Septra, Bactrim)	Bone marrow depression	Hypersensitivity

production of β-lactamase enzyme, rendering it resistant to ampicillin sodium.

In addition, assessment of patient responses to anti-infective therapy involves monitoring for resolution of the physical signs of infection, whether directly by physical examination or indirectly through the use of imaging techniques (i.e., chest radiograph for pneumonia).

Drug Factors

For therapy to be successful, antimicrobial agents must reach sites of infection in concentrations sufficient to inhibit or kill the pathogen. Distribution volume, tissue penetration, plasma protein binding, elimination, and other pharmacokinetic characteristics determine the quantity of drug reaching the infected tissue. When given by intermittent infusion or injection, blood concentrations fluctuate. Maximum levels ("peaks") are achieved just following a dose; the lowest levels or nadir ("trough") concentrations are determined just prior to administering a dose. The extent of bacterial killing for some agents (aminoglycosides, quinolones) depends on how high the peak level is above the MIC (concentration-dependent killing), whereas for others (penicillins, cephalosporins) the factor determining success appears to be the amount of time the drug concentrations remain above the MIC (time-dependent killing).[34]

Several antimicrobial agents require blood concentration monitoring and dosage adjustment to minimize toxicity while maintaining efficacy. Individual patients handle drugs differently, so a standardized dose might produce subtherapeutic levels in one patient and toxic concentrations in another. Pharmacokinetic principles are used to adjust dosing regimens to achieve desired blood concentrations. Routinely monitored antibiotics include aminoglycosides (gentamicin sulfate, tobramycin sulfate, amikacin sulfate, netilmicin sulfate), vancomycin hydrochloride, chloramphenicol sodium succinate, and flucytosine.

Formerly, the treatment of infections with intravenous antibiotics involved serious risks, with the potential of adverse reactions. This is less true today with the availability of infusion rate control devices and safer antibiotics. However, monitoring for toxicity remains an important component of

successful antibiotic therapy. The toxicity of some commonly used intravenous antibiotics is shown in Table 8–3.

Persistent infection during antimicrobial therapy may have several causes. Organisms may be resistant to the antimicrobial being used. Alternatively, the antimicrobial may not be reaching the site of infection because of noncompliance, inadequate dose, or persistence of the infection in a site not penetrated by the drug (e.g., abscess, empyema). The antibiotics themselves may be a cause of fever (see earlier). Compromised host immune systems, as in the case of neutropenia after cytotoxic chemotherapy, may be a cause of poor response to antimicrobial pharmacotherapy. Resistant organisms and "drug fever" may be treated by changing antibiotics. Peripheral septic thrombophlebitis may require surgical resection of the vein, with or without continued antibiotic therapy. Septic thrombosis of the central veins requires removal of the catheter and high-dose bactericidal antimicrobial therapy for at least 4 to 6 weeks and, if there are no contraindications, the patient should be heparinized.[9]

CONTROL MEASURES

Principles of Asepsis

The risk of catheter-related infection can be decreased by adhering to the principles of aseptic technique. Asepsis begins with the proper use of topical antimicrobial agents. Topical antiseptics are used for washing the hands, preparing and maintaining the insertion site, and disinfecting equipment.

There is universal agreement regarding the value and importance of proper hand-washing technique. Although most health care personnel are aware of the importance of hand washing, the recommendations are often ignored. It is unknown whether hand washing with an antiseptic soap or with plain soap and water is more beneficial. A definitive double-blinded clinical trial of the effects of hand washing with an antiseptic on nosocomial infection rates has not been done.[11]

Prior to the application of an antimicrobial solution, any excess hair may be removed by clipping. Shaving is not recommended because of the increased potential for microabrasions. Clippers with disposable heads for single-patient use are suggested. The four antimicrobial solutions recommended by the *Intravenous Nursing Society Standards of Practice* for cannula site preparation are 70% isopropyl alcohol, tincture of iodine, 1 to 2% iodophors, or chlorhexidine gluconate.[28] All site preps are applied with friction, working outward from the insertion site in a circular pattern. An area equal to the size of the dressing that is applied should be prepped. Most catheter care protocols begin with the application of 70% isopropyl alcohol, which rapidly reduces microbial counts on the skin. Isopropyl alcohol 70% has instant kill by denaturing protein. After the alcohol preparation has been allowed to air-dry, if the patient is not allergic to iodine, an application of tincture of iodine (1 to 2% iodine and potassium iodine in 70% alcohol) or povidone-iodine is applied. Tincture of iodine has the combined effect of isopropyl alcohol and iodine and can cause skin irritation.

Povidone-iodine solutions are referred to as iodophors, and consist of iodine and a carrier substance. The amount of free iodine is decreased but the antimicrobial effects are similar to those of iodine. As a result, less skin irritation occurs. Iodine and iodophors penetrate the cell wall and replace the microbial contents with free iodine. Iodophors require approximately 2 minutes of skin contact time to allow for the release of free iodine.[11] Povidone-iodine has the capability to kill gram-negative and gram-positive organisms, fungi, and yeast. However, povidone-iodine is rapidly neutralized in the presence of blood, serum, and other protein-rich materials.

Chlorhexidine-gluconate (Hibiclens) has been used for years as a hand-washing agent and is now being promoted for use as a skin antiseptic. Unlike povidone-iodine or alcohol, application of a 2% chlorhexidine solution to the skin leads to a residual antibacterial activity that persists for 6 hours after application. Chlorhexidine bonds chemically to the protein in the bacterial cell wall. A study conducted by Maki concluded that a 2% chlorhexidine solution used for site preparation before insertion and for postinsertion site care could substantially reduce the incidence of device-related infection.[35] Commercially prepared, single-use packages of chlorhexidine are not currently available in the United States.

In the past, acetone was used to remove fatty acids and microorganisms that were harbored on the skin. A study done by Maki showed that cleansing with acetone increased the local inflammation at the exit site, produced skin irritation, and did not improve microbial removal or reduce the incidence of catheter-related infection.[36]

Clinical trials conducted on the efficacy of antimicrobial ointments have not been conclusive. One large randomized trial found no benefit against infection with the application of topical povidone-iodine ointment to CVC insertion sites.[37] The *Intravenous Nursing Standards of Practice* recommends the application of an antimicrobial ointment as indicated by institutional policy.[28] Practice recommendations suggest that, if an antimicrobial ointment is used, the dressing should be changed every 48 hours.

There has been considerable controversy about the level of barrier precautions necessary for the insertion of a CVC. Maki's study concluded that the use of maximal barrier protection (sterile gloves, long-sleeved sterile gown, surgical mask, and large sterile sheet drape) resulted in less risk of catheter sepsis because touch contamination was decreased.[1]

Prevention

Catheter-Related Infections

Catheter-related infections can be decreased by the development of policies and procedures that establish catheter care protocols. The administration of intravenous therapy should be based on established, professional, nursing standards of practice. Standardization of care is a critical component. Studies have validated that specialized nurses are most likely to maintain aseptic technique in the delivery of intravenous care and, as a result, the rate of catheter-related infections is substantially lower.[1, 24]

The preventative strategy to reduce catheter-related infection begins with routine inspection of the insertion site. Early detection and treatment are extremely important. The policies and procedures of an institution should state the method and frequency for monitoring and administering site care as determined by the following: age of the patient, condition of the patient, therapy prescribed, and practice setting. The information obtained from site inspections allows the nurse to implement immediate interventions if any signs or symptoms of a catheter-related infection become evident. As a result, early nursing interventions minimize the severity of local complications and prevent the occurrence of systemic complications.[38]

Intrinsic and extrinsic equipment contamination can best be prevented by careful inspection of all equipment prior to use and through meticulous technique while performing procedures. Routine peripheral site changes also reduce the risk of developing phlebitis. The *Intravenous Nursing Standards of Practice* recommends that peripheral sites be rotated every 48 hours or immediately if contamination is suspected.[28] Ideally, at the time of recannulation, the administration set and the solution container should be routinely changed. If the cannula is removed because of the development of a complication, the administration set and fluid container should be discarded and a new system implemented. The new infusion system should be restarted in the opposite extremity, if possible.

Maintenance of a closed system also decreases the incidence of catheter-related complications and infection. The number of tubing connections is directly proportional to the potential for contamination. Therefore, fewer junctions within the infusion system lessen the risk of contamination. Administration sets with preattached in-line filters are recommended. If connections are necessary, Luer-Lok fittings are preferable. If this is not possible, the junctions should be secured. All add-on devices should be changed according to the institution's tubing change policy and standards.

Quality control measures should be used to ensure the best possible intravenous care. Admixed solutions should be prepared using aseptic technique under a laminar flow hood. A pharmacy-directed admixture program is recommended in the *Intravenous Nursing Standards of Practice*.[28] A program for sterility testing can be used in the admixing process to monitor aseptic technique and ensure product integrity.

Prior to initiation of therapy, all solution containers should be visually inspected for problems such as precipitate and cloudiness. Glass bottles should be free from cracks. Bags should be squeezed to ensure that there are no defects in the seams or tiny holes present. The expiration date should be verified before the infusion is begun.

All administration sets and extensions should be examined prior to use. This inspection should include observation of the entire set and making sure that the protective coverings over the spike (proximal end) and distal end are intact. If the product or package integrity is compromised or not sealed, the product should not be used. Visual inspection of the venipuncture device also helps prevent the use of a defective product.

Guidelines are important in the selection and purchase of IV-related equipment. IV nurses should actively participate in the selection of these products. Before new products are considered, there should be an evaluation of the product to see whether it falls within the standards of care and allows for the safe administration of IV therapy. Criteria to be considered include the following: connections need to withstand normal pressures of electronic infusion devices; catheters should be radiopaque in case of catheter breakage; and the equipment must be accurate and facilitate the prevention of inadvertent contamination. When selecting equipment, it is important to remember that closed systems that do not require air decrease the chance for contamination.

Quality assurance programs can significantly decrease the incidence of catheter-related complications. These tools evaluate the adherence to departmental policies and procedures. A quality control evaluation tool can be used to ensure that proper procedures are being followed when performing venipunctures or delivering site care. A checklist can be used for peer review of the process and should include the following: universal precautions, selection of equipment, priming of the administration set, vein selection, prepping procedure, venipuncture technique, taping of the catheter, dressing procedure, and labelling of the site and set. A surveillance system is essential for all nursing personnel who maintain vascular access devices. Establishing a collaborative relationship with the epidemiology department can be an excellent resource for monitoring the delivery of quality intravenous care, determining culture reports on vascular access devices, identifying nursing units or areas that need education or interventions to improve the delivery of IV care, and acquiring the latest research and information regarding the practice of infection control.

Blood-Borne Pathogen Transmission

The Centers for Disease Control (CDC), the Occupational Safety and Health Administration (OSHA), and the American Hospital Association recommend the application of universal precautions by health care workers at all times to prevent the transmission of bloodborne pathogens. OSHA's standard makes universal precautions an enforceable legal requirement and delineates what inspectors survey.[39] These rules instruct health care workers to use protective barriers such as gloves, mask, protective eyewear, and fluid-impervious gowns when a potential for exposure to blood or body fluids exists. Health care workers must treat the blood and body fluids from all patients as being potentially infected with hepatitis B virus (HBV), human immunodeficiency virus (HIV), and other bloodborne pathogens.

Gloves can reduce the IV nurse's risk of infection, but little protection is offered from needle stick injuries. For this reason, the use of needleless devices, safety syringes, and cannulas is recommended. To prevent needle stick injuries, needles should never be recapped, bent, or broken. After use, needles and syringes should be disposed of in an impervious, puncture-proof container located as close as possible to the patient's care area.

The employer has a responsibility to provide education regarding universal precautions, to identify the existence of hazardous waste, to supply personal protective equipment (PPE) such as goggles, gloves, needleless devices, and safety syringes, and to monitor workers' adherence to the protection measures. It is the employee's responsibility to recognize hazardous wastes, to read information on material safety data sheets (MSDS), and to follow recommendations for the safe handling and disposal of hazardous materials.

Infection Control in the Home

Increasingly, vascular access devices are being cared for in the home. The same basic principles for infection control and standards of practice also apply in the home or in an alternative care setting. Because home IV therapy is a rather recent development, few studies are available about vascular access device infection rates or catheter care protocols in alternative care settings. However, it is generally believed that the at-home risk factors should be somewhat reduced for developing a catheter-related infection. Future research and study are needed to describe infection risks and the nursing management of vascular access devices in the home and in alternative care settings.

In all health care environments, patient teaching is an important component for preventing catheter-related complications. In the home or alternative care setting, thorough patient teaching regarding vascular access management is even more crucial. Information regarding catheter management should be individualized to meet the patient's needs but remain consistent with the established policies and procedures of the infusion care company and with the *Intravenous Nurses Society Standards of Practice*. Patient education regarding home IV therapy should address infection control principles such as hand washing, aseptic technique, sterility, and the proper method of handling equipment. Information regarding dressing changes, site assessments, and recognizing signs and symptoms of possible complications should also be provided. It is essential that the patient and family be provided adequate nursing support and follow-up to prevent the occurrence of catheter-related complications.

▶ NURSING DIAGNOSIS

Potential Nursing Diagnosis

- High risk for infection
- Impaired skin integrity
- Anxiety
- Pain
- Knowledge deficit related to IV complications

Patient-Client Outcomes

- No evidence (signs or symptoms) of infections throughout hospitalization

- Patient experiences minimal anxiety related to intravenous therapy as evidenced by verbalization of concerns, lack of restlessness, normal vital signs, and appropriate sleep patterns
- Patient experiences minimal pain as evidenced by responses of 1 on a pain scale of 1 to 5, with 1 being mild pain and 5 being severe pain
- After initial teaching session, patient lists signs and symptoms to report to nurse and identifies ways to prevent infection of catheter site

References

1. Maki DG. Infection caused by intravascular devices: Pathogenesis, strategies for prevention. In Maki DG (ed). Improving Catheter Site Care. New York: Royal Society of Medicine Services, 1991:3–27.
2. Bennet JV, Brachman PS, eds. Hospital Infections. Boston: Little, Brown, and Co., 1992:849–898.
3. Goodner B. Nurse's Survival Guide. El Paso, TX: Skidmore-Roth, 1992:133.
4. Kee LJ. Laboratory and Diagnostic Tests with Nursing Implications, 3rd ed. Norwalk, CT: Appleton & Lange, 1991:311–313.
5. Frey AM. The immune system and intravenous administration of immune globulin. JIN 1991; 14:315–330.
6. Price SA, Wilson LM. Pathophysiology: Clinical Concepts of Disease Processes. St. Louis: C.V. Mosby, 1992:194–195.
7. DiJulio J. Hematopoiesis: An overview. Oncol Nurs Forum 1991; 18:3–6.
8. Nafziger DA, Wenzel RP. Catheter-related infections: Reducing the risk—and the consequences. J Crit Illness. 1990; 5(8)857–863.
9. Bisno AL, Waldvogel FA. Infections Associated with Indwelling Medical Devices. Washington DC: American Society for Microbiology, 1989:161–177.
10. Henderson DK. Intravascular device-associated infection: Current concepts and controversies. Infect Surg 1988; 7(6):365–399.
11. Larson E. Guidelines for use of topical antimicrobial agents. Am J Infect Control 1988; 16:253–266.
12. Aly A, Shirley C, Cunico B, et al. Effect of prolonged occlusion on the microbial flora, pH, carbon dioxide and transepidermal water loss on human skin. J Invest Dermatol 1978:378–381.
13. Wickham RS. Advances in venous access devices and nursing management strategies. Nurs Clin North Am 1990; 25:345–364.
14. Sitges-Serra A, Linares J, Perez JL, et al. A randomized trial on the effect of tubing changes on hub contamination and catheter sepsis during parenteral nutrition. J Parenteral Enteral Nutrition. 1985;9:322–325.
15. Rose SG, Pitsch RJ, Karrer FW, et al. Subclavian catheter infections. JPEN J Parenter Enteral Nutr 1988; 12:511–512.
16. Sheth NK, Franson TR, Rose HD, et al. Colonization of bacteria on polyvinyl chloride and Teflon intravascular catheters in hospitalized patients. Am Soc Microbiol 1983; 18:1061–1063.
17. Linder LE, Cuelaru I, Gustavsson B, et al. Material thrombogenicity in central venous catheterization: A comparison between soft, antebrachial catheters of silicone elastomer and polyurethane. JPEN J Parenter Enteral Nutr 1984; 8:399–406.
18. Vaudaux P, Pittet D, Haeberli A, et al. Host factors selectively increase staphylococcal adherence on inserted catheters: A role for fibronectin and fibrinogen or fibrin. J Infect Dis 1989; 160:865–875.
19. Murray PR, Drew WL, Kobayashi GS, et al. Medical Microbiology. St. Louis: C.V. Mosby, 1990:52,59,107.
20. Peters G, Locci R, Pulverer G. Adherence and growth of coagulase-negative staphylococci on surfaces of intravenous catheters. J Infect Dis 1982; 146:479–482.
21. Modak SM, Sampath L. Development and evaluation of a new polyurethane central venous antiseptic catheter: Reducing central venous catheter infections. Infect Med 1992; 9(6):23–24.
22. Flowers RH, Schwenzer KJ, Kopel RF, et al. Efficacy of an attachable subcutaneous cuff for the prevention of intravascular catheter-related infection. JAMA 1989; 261:878–883.
23. Cowan CE. Antibiotic lock technique. JIN 1992; 15:283–287.
24. Fraschini G. Prevention of infections in VADS using declotting agents. JVAN 1993; 3:19–20.
25. Alexander JW. Nutrition and Translocation. JPEN J Parenter Enteral Nutr 1990; 14:170–174.
26. Kinney JM. Clinical Biochemistry: Implications for nutritional support. JPEN J Parenter Enteral Nutr 1990; 14:148–156.
27. Phillips LD. Manual of I.V. Therapeutics. Philadelphia: F.A. Davis, 1993:233–237.
28. Intravenous Nurses Society Intravenous Nursing Standards of Practice. Belmont MA: Intravenous Nurses Society, 1990:35, 42, 43, 45, 46, 48.
29. Maki DG, Cobb L, Garman JK, et al. An attachable silver-impregnated cuff for the prevention of infection with central venous catheters: A prospective randomized multicenter trial. Am J Med 1988; 85:307–314.
30. Dickinson GM, Bisno AL. Infections associated with indwelling devices: Concepts of pathogenesis; infections associated with intravascular devices. Antimicrob Agents Chemother 1989; 33:597–601.
31. Quintiliani R, Cooper BN, Briceland LL, et al. Economic impact of streamlining antibiotic administration. Am J Med 1987; 82(suppl A):391–394.
32. Wasserman M, Levinstein M, Keller E, et al. Utility of fever, white blood cells, and differential count in predicting bacterial infections in the elderly. J Am Geriatr Soc 1989; 37:537–543.
33. Brun-Bruisson C, Abrouk F, Legrand P. Diagnosis of central venous catheter-related sepsis. Arch Intern Med 1987; 147:873–877.
34. Vogelman B, Craig WA. Kinetics of antimicrobial activity. J Pediatr 1986; 108:835–840.
35. Maki DG, Ringer M, Alvarado C. Prospective randomised trial of povidone-iodine, alcohol, and chlorhexidine for prevention of infection associated with central venous and arterial catheters. Lancet 1991; 338:339–343.
36. Maki DG, McCormack KN. Defatting catheter insertion sites in total parenteral nutrition is of no value as an infection control measure. Am J Med 1987; 83:833–840.
37. Prager RL, Silva J. Colonization of central venous catheters. South Med J 1984; 1:458–461.
38. Puntis JWL, Holden CE, Smallman S, et al. Staff training: A key factor in reducing intravascular catheter sepsis. Arch Dis Child 1990; 65:335–337.
39. Occupational Safety and Health Administration. Washington, DC: Occupational safe exposure to bloodborne pathogens: Final rule. Washington, DC: Department of Labor, Docket No. H-370, Dec. 6, 1991.

INTRAVENOUS AGENTS

CHAPTER 9 Parenteral Fluids

Judy Terry, BSN, CRNI
Carolyn Hedrick, BSN, CRNI

Fluids and electrolytes play an important role in maintaining homeostasis. When imbalances occur, parenteral fluids are the most common intravenous agents employed for correction. Intravenous solutions are also used to provide nutrients or act as a vehicle for medication administration.

This form of therapy should be performed in a safe manner that includes awareness of the patient's physical status and clinical picture as well as legal implications. Determination of the type of fluid needed is based on the nursing assessment, laboratory findings, and the purpose for which it is being prescribed. To act properly on the physician's order, the nurse must be familiar with the various IV solutions, including their uses, components, and potential complications.

The preceding information should be incorporated into a nursing care plan. This plan should also include applicable nursing diagnoses with measurable outcomes. Through careful planning and a strong database, the delivery of intravenous therapy should be a safe and effective treatment modality.

PATIENT SAFETY

The determination that a patient's treatment plan should include IV therapy brings with it the responsibility for patient safety. This includes being cognizant of the patient's physical status, individual clinical considerations, and legal implications.

One of the first considerations should be the physical status of the patient. This includes knowing the age and the respective fluid and electrolyte requirements. The infant, adult, and older adult all have different body compositions and means of monitoring homeostasis. The infant has a higher rate of extracellular fluid exchange, a higher metabolic rate, and a higher fluid loss than the average adult. There are also variables in the adult population, such as gender—women have a lower percentage of body fluid than men. Obese patients also have a lower percentage of fluid.

The percentage of body fluid generally continues to decrease as the age increases because of an increase in fat content. In the older adult, changes related to the renal system often result in a decreased concentrating ability, so fluid loss may increase. Respiratory changes can result in a decreased ability to remove secretions. Neurologic changes often lead to a lessened sense of thirst, which is an indicator of fluid needs. The ability to perspire may be diminished because of skin changes, so it is more difficult to use the standard test of skin turgor to determine fluid status.

All body systems are affected at some point and can influence the fluid and electrolyte status. This must be considered during the planning and therapy phases of care to prevent dehydration or fluid overload.

Clinical considerations are important aspects of patient safety; these include the appropriate route of administration, product, and administration rate. In determining the proper route of administration, the concentration of the IV solution should be considered. Fluids with higher osmolality, such as total parenteral solutions, need to be given through a central line.

Sensory deficits of the patient should be assessed. Special planning on an individual basis may be necessary to prevent physical injury and provide accurate treatment, particularly for those patients with sight or hearing impairment. For example, the plan could include a special visual alarm on a pump for someone who has a hearing impairment.

The mobility of the patient should be considered when

planning IV fluid therapy. Site selection in the nondominant extremity may ensure better compliance. Otherwise, as the patient moves about, there may be difficulty in maintaining a viable IV line, which affects the ability to deliver IV therapy. Specific problems include the patient removing the venipuncture device, the tubing being pulled apart, and dislodging the IV set from the IV solution container.

Site selection is equally important for the immobile patient. Extremities may require elevation or exercises to prevent stasis during fluid administration. Placement of the catheter should receive special consideration for those patients who require assistance for turning and getting out of bed. Advanced planning can eliminate the interruption of IV solution administration. The patient's orientation should be assessed. Caution should be exercised for those who are confused, disoriented, or agitated to prevent accidental dislodging of the venipuncture device and IV tubing. Control clamps should be placed out of reach, if possible, or mechanical infusion devices used to prevent deviation of the IV solution flow rate.

Ensuring that the correct product is provided to the patient is an area in which the potential for errors is high. Prior to administering an IV solution, it should be checked carefully with the order on the patient's chart. The physician should be contacted if there is any doubt about what has been ordered. Frequently, the IV solution is used as the vehicle for administering IV medication. Caution should be taken to ensure stability and compatibility. Pharmacists can be helpful in making this determination when questions arise. Verification of the product's expiration date is also an important component of providing a correct and safe IV solution. The potential for errors can be eliminated by comparing the type of solution, any additives, and the volume with the original order. The actual administration date should be verified.

The correct flow rate should also be determined during the order check. This is another situation in which errors frequently occur. The correct administration rate is important to provide successful parenteral fluid therapy. Delivering a highly concentrated solution too rapidly could lead to fluid overload. Incorrect flow rates for electrolyte-containing solutions may lead to excesses or deficits in the body's electrolyte content.

Another area related to patient safety concerns the patient's legal rights. Prior to instituting treatment, the patient has the right to refuse or consent to the planned course of therapy unless decided otherwise by the courts. This is based on the patient's freedom of religion and the right of privacy,[1] including invasion of bodily integrity. The patient should be fully informed about the IV solution and any medication(s) to be administered, in addition to the process of delivering the fluids. Information related to possible complications or side effects should be provided to the patient prior to instituting treatment.

In addition to the freedom of choice, the patient has the right to expect that IV solutions and all related supplies and equipment are safe for use. IV solution containers should be checked for defects such as holes in a bag or cracks in a bottle. Clarity of the solution and the absence of particulate matter should be verified.

Proper aseptic technique should be employed while admixtures are being prepared in laminar flow hoods by properly trained personnel. Venipuncture devices, IV tubing, and other related materials should be sterile and function as designed without undue harm to the patient.

IV SOLUTION ADMINISTRATION AND MONITORING: NURSE QUALIFICATIONS

It is important that not only the products for IV solution administration but also the personnel involved meet required standards. Responsibilities related to IV solution administration may be delegated to the registered nurse (RN) or the licensed practical/vocational nurse (LPN/LVN). In some health care facilities, basic venipuncture procedures and monitoring may be shared by the RN and LPN/LVN, whereas the more specialized procedures are relegated only to the RN. This varies from one state to the next. However, a basic requirement is meeting state board standards, including licensure. The license granted by the State Board of Nursing signifies that a nurse has met the requirements for entry into practice.

Once a nurse has been hired to administer or monitor IV solutions, the health care agency has the responsibility to see that the employee is properly oriented. Continuing education programs should be provided on a regular basis to review basic material and to provide information about new IV solutions and techniques for their delivery.

Today, with an increased emphasis on IV therapy and more sophisticated technology, nurses are choosing to become certified in the specialty of IV therapy. This certification requires that a nurse master knowledge related to all areas of IV therapy, including IV solutions, as well as the skills necessary to practice in the clinical setting. This process leads to continued competency through the educational programs required to maintain the certification credentials, thus offering additional protection to the public.

Quality patient care in the specialty of IV therapy requires that a nurse be knowledgeable about IV solutions and the medications administered in those solutions. First, the nurse needs to understand how the IV solution is to be used. It may be needed to provide free water, replace or maintain electrolytes, deliver medications, or supply calories. IV solutions can be used to decrease or eliminate certain electrolytes or fluids.

After determining how the solution is to be used, it is helpful to know the action of the solution. The IV solution may be used to dilute and therefore decrease the level of an electrolyte in the body. Some IV solutions containing one electrolyte may be used to counteract the action of another electrolyte. Knowledge of how the solution or electrolyte is eliminated is useful. For example, before giving potassium to a patient with a renal disease, it is important to know that this electrolyte is eliminated by the kidneys. Knowing how an IV solution works, its contents, and how it is used help determine whether the product is indicated to treat a specific disease or condition. If the IV solution contains potassium, then it would not be indicated for use in treating hyperkalemia.

The nurse also needs to be familiar with contraindications, side effects, and adverse reactions of IV solutions or medications. The body maintains a delicate balance of fluids and electrolytes. Whenever IV solutions are administered, there is always the possibility that a fluid deficit or excess may occur. Therefore, it is important to know the signs and symptoms of these imbalances. Other products, such as 10% dextran, may produce an anaphylactoid reaction. Colloidal solutions, such as hetastarch, may interfere with platelet function because of hemodilution. A competent nurse who administers IV solutions should be aware that side effects exist and should alert other health care workers to potential problems and how they might be detected. There are times when a solution may be contraindicated because of an existing problem or condition. Because a side effect of 10% dextran is bleeding, this IV solution would not be indicated for patients with severe bleeding disorders. The side effects and contraindications are presented in more detail later in this chapter as specific IV solutions are discussed.

The nurse should be adept at completing accurate physical assessments prior to initiating treatment. This is beneficial to the physician in determining the need for intravenous therapy. The need for physical assessment does not stop at this point. These skills should be used on a continuing basis while monitoring therapy. The findings should be shared in a timely manner with the physician and other appropriate health care workers.

The nurse is the final link that pulls all the pieces together and is therefore one of the best patient advocates for patient safety and well-being. This requires that the nurse have the skills to use information from the patient history, physical assessment, and laboratory findings, and have a knowledge base related to intravenous solutions. With all these pieces in place, a determination about the appropriateness of the order can be made. The nurse should contact the physician if there are any discrepancies. Only in this way can the patient be assured of receiving appropriate intravenous therapy.

DETERMINATION OF FLUID NEEDS

Clinical Status

Fluid and electrolyte balance is a complex subject but is the basis for parenteral fluid administration. This delicate balance (or homeostasis) is easily affected by normal changes (e.g., aging) and abnormal changes (e.g., disease processes) within the body. Chapter 7, Fluids and Electrolytes, presents more information on clinical status, including nursing assessment and monitoring.

Laboratory Findings

The next important aspect of determining fluid needs is the review and interpretation of a patient's laboratory findings. The two systems that have the most direct impact on fluid and electrolyte balance are the renal system and the cardiovascular system. Therefore, the tests that reflect the proper functioning of these organs (kidneys and heart) require consistent and close scrutiny.

Renal function tests start with determination of the blood urea nitrogen (BUN) level. Elevated levels are primarily caused by kidney disease or urinary tract obstructions. Variations above normal can also be caused by fluid volume deficit, protein intake in excess of body needs, or a catabol-

istic state (e.g., starvation). A decreased BUN level may mean decreased protein metabolism or overhydration.

Creatinine is the next indicator to evaluate. In all kidney diseases in which greater than 50% of the nephrons are destroyed, the creatinine level is elevated.[2] The higher the level, the greater the percentage of nephron loss. Severe fluid volume depletion may be indicated by a creatinine level that is slightly elevated.

Because both the BUN and creatinine levels indicate renal function, they should be evaluated together. In volume depletion, the BUN level is elevated, whereas the creatinine level is normal or slightly elevated.

The urine specific gravity is a test that measures the urine concentration. In fluid volume deficit, the specific gravity is elevated because of water loss from such processes as third spacing of body fluid, burns, and gastrointestinal fluid loss. In fluid volume excess, the specific gravity is decreased, as with renal disease.

The urine osmolality is the final test to be evaluated when determining renal function. Fluid volume deficit elevates the urine osmolality, whereas fluid volume excess decreases it. Urine osmolality should be evaluated in conjunction with serum osmolality, and the specimens should be collected simultaneously.

Cardiovascular tests begin with an electrocardiogram (ECG). Fluid and electrolyte imbalances can often be detected and even diagnosed by the significant changes they cause in the P, Q, R, S, and T waves of the tracing.

The next determination is made on the serum electrolytes, including potassium, sodium, calcium, magnesium, chloride, and phosphorus. Each individual electrolyte has a normal range. Deviation from normal indicates specific conditions related to deficits and excesses in body fluid and in one or more of the electrolytes. (For further information on individual electrolytes, see Chap. 7.)

The complete blood count (CBC) should be evaluated. This screening test includes the following measurements: hemoglobin, hematocrit, red blood cell count (RBC), white blood cell count (WBC), differential red and white blood cell count, and a red cell examination with stain. Abnormalities in fluid and electrolyte balance cause these results to be increased or decreased. For example, severe dehydration caused by nausea, vomiting, and diarrhea results in an elevated hematocrit, whereas rapid administration of excessive amounts of intravenous fluid decreases the hematocrit.

Blood gases are important indicators because they determine the patient's acid-base status. These tests measure the hydrogen ion concentration, the partial pressure of oxygen, and the partial pressure of carbon dioxide in arterial blood. Acid-base disturbances may be caused by fluid- and electrolyte-related problems, such as vomiting, diarrhea, and kidney disorders.

Abnormal clotting test results indicate fluid needs. The partial thromboplastin time (PTT) detects deficiencies in almost all the clotting factors. In acute hemorrhage, this indicator is decreased. The prothrombin time (PT) screens for defects in other areas of the clotting mechanism. Causes of a prolonged PT include medications, vitamin K deficiency, hepatic disease, and obstructive jaundice. Plasma volume expanders, such as hetastarch and crystalloid solutions, may cause the PTT and PT to be prolonged. These fluids may be indicated in cases of fluid imbalance (e.g., burns, fluid removal caused by ascites).

Serum amylase is another laboratory test to be considered. This measures the enzyme amylase that is produced by the pancreas and salivary glands and helps with the digestion of carbohydrates. An elevation of this enzyme level is most commonly seen in pancreatitis. Fluid and electrolyte imbalances and infections are seen with the acute form of pancreatitis.

The serum glucose level should also be monitored. If this level is greatly elevated, osmotic diuresis occurs, resulting in a fluid volume deficit.

The bilirubin determination is important because it indicates disease processes such as anemias, cirrhosis, hepatitis, and biliary tree obstruction. Bilirubin results from the destruction of old cells and produces an orange-yellow or jaundice color. The diseases associated with abnormal bilirubin levels each have the potential for causing fluid and/or electrolyte disturbances.

Lactate dehydrogenase (LDH) is another cellular enzyme that is associated with carbohydrate metabolism. Tissue injury causes release of this enzyme, which is found in body organs, skeletal muscles, and red blood cells. This test is especially useful in determining myocardial damage after an infarction, damage that could lead to fluid and electrolyte problems.

The last laboratory parameter to review is osmolality, which denotes the concentration of dissolved particles per unit of water. This can be measured in both serum and urine. Dehydration causes an increase in osmolality (both serum and urine), whereas water excess results in a decreased osmolality. The ratio of urine osmolality to serum osmolality after fasting for 14 hours is usually 3:1.[2]

Fluid Requirements

When determining fluid needs, it is important to know the purpose for administering intravenous solutions. For example, is this fluid needed for replacement or maintenance? The reason for knowing the purpose is that it affects the type and amount of fluid that is ordered.

Replacement therapy has a two-fold rationale. The first is restoration of pre-existing fluid losses, which occurs when the previous output has been more than the intake. After kidney status has been considered, a hydrating solution (e.g., 5% dextrose in 0.2% sodium chloride) is administered. This restores an adequate output of urine and then allows electrolytes to be replaced. The other rationale for replacement therapy is restoration of present fluid and electrolyte losses, such as loss of intestinal fluid through continuing diarrhea. A solution such as lactated Ringer's injection can be used to replace this type of loss. Replacement of continuing losses prevents the problems of acidosis and alkalosis.

Maintenance therapy provides the ongoing nutrient needs of the patient. These include water, electrolytes, dextrose, protein, and vitamins. Water is necessary for adequate kidney function and the replacement of insensible losses. Because distilled water is hypotonic and causes hemolysis, glucose is added to make it isotonic; therefore, it can be administered intravenously. The addition of salt to distilled water also makes it isotonic and renders it parenterally acceptable.[2]

Water and electrolyte requirements can be provided by the administration of balanced solutions that contain daily electrolyte needs. Increased needs for particular electrolytes should be monitored through laboratory tests and strict measurement of intake and output. These parameters should be considered according to the patient's history, present condition, and ongoing nursing assessments. Electrolytes (e.g., sodium, potassium, calcium) can be added to the intravenous solutions when deficiencies are identified. Solutions containing no electrolytes can be used when excesses exist.

Glucose (dextrose) improves liver function by being converted into glycogen, supplies calories for energy, thus sparing protein, and decreases the development of ketosis caused by the burning of fat stores for energy. Because of these vital functions, it is an important nutrient for body maintenance. Glucose can be provided by peripheral intravenous infusions in 5 and 10% concentrations. Total parenteral nutrition solutions provide glucose in 25% concentrations.

Protein is also a necessary nutrient for maintenance. This nutrient is required when an illness extends over a long period. The body normally uses protein for cell repair, enzyme and vitamin synthesis, and wound healing. Amino acid solutions provide intravenous protein and are calculated at 1 g/kg of body weight as the daily requirement for a healthy adult.[3]

Vitamins are necessary so that the body can use other nutrients. Vitamin B complex is needed to metabolize carbohydrates and to maintain gastrointestinal function. Vitamin C is used to promote wound healing. These vitamins are the ones most frequently administered intravenously because they are water-soluble and excreted in the urine. Therefore, replacement is necessary. The body retains fat-soluble vitamins, and thus it is not necessary to provide them in maintenance therapy.

Calculating Fluid Needs

Having discussed the areas for consideration when determining fluid needs, the next step is to review basic calculations necessary for proper administration.

Body surface area (BSA) is a patient-specific measurement used to calculate fluid or fluid maintenance requirements. This is determined in square meters (m²) obtained by using a nomogram to correlate weight (in kilograms) and height (in inches). Because 1500 ml of fluid are required for each square meter of BSA, then

$$m^2 \times 1500 = \text{maintenance requirements}[4]$$

Weight is an important indicator of fluid balance. A 1-kg weight loss or gain is approximately equal to a 1-liter loss or gain of fluid. For the sake of consistency, the patient should be weighed at the same time every day, using the same scale and wearing the same amount of clothing. A history of recent weight gain or loss is extremely helpful in determining the type and severity of fluid imbalances. The following can be used to determine fluid volume excess or deficit severity in acute gains or losses of body weight: 2 to 5%, mild; 5 to 10%, moderate; 10 to 15%, severe; 15 to 20%, fatal.[5]

An important point to remember is that there may be no change in body weight when third spacing is occurring. However, a severe volume deficit may be present because of this loss of usable body fluid.

Ongoing monitoring is vital to the well-being of the patient with potential fluid and electrolyte imbalances. The nursing physical assessment covering all areas previously discussed should be performed regularly and consistently. The intake and output record should be a standard nursing order on these patients. Accuracy is of utmost importance. Therefore, all liquids (intake or output) should be carefully measured and, when unmeasurable, the volume should be estimated. Laboratory tests should be repeated frequently and the results evaluated in view of the patient's clinical status.

Caloric needs is another parameter that might be required when administering parenteral fluids. Maintenance requirements in a healthy individual may be calculated by using a basal metabolic rate (BMR) chart. The relevant value is found on the chart and is multiplied by the body surface area (obtained from a nomogram) of the patient:

$$BMR \times body\ surface\ area\ (BSA) =$$
$$maintenance\ requirements$$

Indirect calorimetry is another method used to measure caloric expenditure, and is more individualized. Specialized equipment is used to measure oxygen consumption and carbon dioxide production in the patient's expired air. This method is based on the principle that these gases are directly related to energy production in the body when it is at a steady state. The results are converted into the energy expenditure by using a mathematical calculation and projecting the results for a 24-hour period.[6]

As stated earlier, osmolality is the measurement of the concentration of solutes in a solution (body fluid). Changes in osmolality affect water movement into and out of the cell. An increase in extracellular osmolality causes cells to shrink or shrivel, whereas a decrease causes cells to swell and burst. Therefore, intravenous preparations have a narrow osmolality range. Extracellular osmolality is primarily determined by the sodium level because it is the main solute found in extracellular fluid. A rough estimation of extracellular osmolality can be made by multiplying the plasma sodium concentration by 2. A more accurate estimate also takes into consideration glucose and urea. After dividing the weight per liter of glucose and urea by the molecular weight of each, the result is the osmolality concentration. This allows the equation to be expanded, and is a more accurate estimate. The formula for determining the osmolality of extracellular fluid (ECF) is as follows[7]:

$$Osmolality\ of\ ECF = 2\ [plasma\ Na^+] + \frac{plasma\ glucose}{18} + \frac{BUN}{2.8}$$

where 18 and 2.8 are the molecular weights of the glucose and BUN.

For example,

$$Osmolality\ of\ ECF = 2\ (135) + \frac{90}{18} + \frac{28}{2.8}$$
$$= 270 + 5 + 10$$
$$= 285$$

Fluid Order and Preparation

The initiation of parenteral fluids begins with the fluid order. This order, written by the patient's physician, contains the instructions necessary for the nurse to administer the solutions and medications required.

Fluid Type and Amount

The first component of the order is the fluid type and amount. The physician identifies the specific solution needed to treat the patient's condition. In doing this, the physician takes into consideration the present diagnosis, other existing conditions, the length of the current illness, body size and weight, the physical assessment findings, and laboratory data. The amount of the solution may be written as part of the order (e.g., 5% dextrose in water, 1000 ml) or may be determined by the rate prescribed (e.g., 200 ml/hour).

Medications and Dosage

The second order component is any necessary medication(s) and the dosage(s). These are determined by the patient's condition. In parenteral therapy, the medication may be anything from an electrolyte to replace losses to a chemical or drug for treating a specific problem. The dosage is tailored to the patient's age, size, and acuity level. If the pharmacy preparing the medication is allowed by the physician to use substitutions (a generically equivalent product), this is also noted on the original order. Some institutions have standing order agreements with their medical community regarding medication substitutions.

Flow Rate

The next vital component of the order is the flow rate. This must be specified, and the nurse is responsible for calculating this rate if the doctor orders an amount of solution to be infused over a certain period of time. The nurse is also responsible for recognizing signs and symptoms that may indicate an infusion rate that is either too fast or too slow.

A fluid order that specifies a keep vein open (KVO) flow rate is incomplete, and the physician should be consulted for a definite hourly rate. (The exception to this is an institutional policy agreed on by the medical and surgical staffs as to the definition of a KVO rate [e.g., KVO = 20 ml/hour].) Otherwise, this notation for a rate is the decision of each nurse caring for the patient and has legal implications, in that each nurse's definition of KVO might be different and difficult to defend.

The physician also orders the date and time for the infusion to be initiated. This may be stated as a definite time (e.g., 10:00 PM) or may be indicated by the date and time the order is written.

Route of Administration

Another component of the order is the route of administration. Parenteral fluids may be introduced into the body in several ways (e.g., intravenously, intra-arterially, subcutaneously, or intraosseously). Factors such as the patient's disease process, vein condition, degree of hydration, and medications required for treatment play important roles in determining the best and most effective route.

Infusion Device

The last component of the order may be an infusion device. Many institutions have protocols for the use of such devices, whereas other facilities have policies that allow for the routine use of infusion devices on all patients. In the latter case, the device would not need to be addressed in the order. Patients who are to be discharged on home IV therapy require orders for any type of ambulatory device that may be necessary.

Solution Preparation and Labeling

After the order is written, the solution must be prepared. The fluid may be plain (containing no additives), premixed (medication is added during the manufacturing process), or admixed (medication is added by the institution using the product). Aseptic technique should be strictly followed when preparing all solutions, and they should be prepared in a laminar flow hood. Possible solution and medication incompatibilities should also be investigated. These precautions help ensure the most sterile product possible for delivery into the vascular system.

All solutions should be properly labeled for the patient. This label should contain the patient's name and room number, date and time needed, medication name and amount, fluid name and amount, initials of the person performing the admixture, initials of the person who verifies the preparation to be correct, and expiration date. Any substitutions or special instructions should be noted. The prescribed flow rate may also be seen on the label.

Order Verification

The nurse administering the solution is responsible for verification of the order. The original and complete physician's order should be read and the solution compared to be certain that the fluid is correct.

Patient Identification

Patient identification is the next step in the process. Not only should the patient's name be stated by the nurse, but the arm band should also be checked. If there is any question concerning any component of the order or the type of solution ordered in regard to the patient's condition, the physician should be contacted before therapy is initiated.

Appropriateness of Order

The last responsibility of the nurse to be considered is the appropriateness of the solution prescribed for the patient's condition. Many disease processes influence the fluid and electrolyte balance. Thus, renal function, cardiac function, clinical status, and maintenance requirements must be examined. A physical assessment and chart review provide valuable information for making this determination. They also assure the nurse that the fluid ordered, if delivered correctly, will not further complicate the patient's clinical condition.

CHARACTERISTICS AND TYPES OF IV FLUIDS

There are various intravenous solutions available for use. The solutions are made up of multiple components with individualized amounts of each. These components and their characteristics must be considered when selecting the appropriate intravenous solution (Table 9–1).

Tonicity

Fluids within the body are continually moving from one compartment to another in an attempt to maintain homeostasis. This is accomplished through several processes, including osmosis, in which water moves from a less concentrated fluid to one that is more concentrated. This is controlled by the osmotic pressure. In describing solutions, the term ''tonicity'' is often used in place of osmotic pressure or tension, and it is usually related to the number of particles found in blood.

Osmolality is a term also used in relation to particle content. It represents the number of particles (solute) per kilogram of solvent (water) and is expressed as milliosmoles (mOsm). As the particle count increases, the concentration increases, resulting in changes in chemical behavior. The osmolality of body fluids is approximately 310 mOsm/liter.[8]

Isotonic Solution

A solution that is isotonic has the same tonicity as plasma. This means that the osmotic pressure is the same on the inside and outside of a living cell that is in contact with a solution. Therefore, water neither enters nor leaves the cell. Examples of isotonic IV solutions include 0.9% sodium chloride, 5% dextrose in water, and lactated Ringer's. These solutions are used to expand the extracellular fluid and do not cause movement of fluid from or into the blood cells. The approximate osmolality of isotonic IV solutions is 240 to 340 mOsm/liter.[9]

Hypotonic Solution

Solutions that are considered to be hypotonic have an osmolality of less than 240 mOsm/liter. Therefore, these solutions exert less osmotic pressure than the fluid in the extracellular compartment. This allows water to be drawn from the extracellular fluid. If blood cells are placed into a hypotonic solution, water is drawn from the solution into the blood cells. Depending on the degree of hypotonicity, the volume of fluid being pulled into the blood cells may cause them to swell and burst. An example of a hypotonic IV solution is 0.45% sodium chloride. Patients should be monitored closely when receiving hypotonic solutions. Sterile distilled water should never be used without the presence of additives because of the degree of hypotonicity, which can cause hemolysis.

Hypertonic Solution

The osmolality of hypertonic solutions is greater than 340 mOsm/kg, so these solutions exert more osmotic pressure

Table 9 – 1

Characteristics of Intravenous Solutions

Manufacturer(s)/IV Solution*	Tonicity	Osmolarity (mOsm/liter)	Approximate pH†	Na⁺	K⁺	Ca⁺	Mg²⁺	Cl⁻	HCO_3^-	Lactate	Acetate	Citrate
Dextrose/saline solutions												
A,B,M/dextrose 2.5% and 0.45% sodium chloride	Isotonic	280	4.5 [4.0]	77				77				
M/dextrose 5% and 0.11% sodium chloride	Isotonic	290	4.3	19				19				
A,B,M/dextrose 5% and 0.2% sodium chloride	Hypertonic	320	4.4 [4.0]	34				34				
A,B,M/dextrose 5% and 0.3% sodium chloride	Hypertonic	365	4.4 [4.0]	56				56				
A,B,M/dextrose 5% and 0.45% sodium chloride	Hypertonic	405	4.4 [4.0]	77				77				
A,B,M/dextrose 5% and 0.9% sodium chloride	Hypertonic	560	4.4 [4.0]	154				154				
M/dextrose 10% and 0.2% sodium chloride	Hypertonic	575	4.3	34				34				
M/dextrose 10% and 0.45% sodium chloride	Hypertonic	660	4.3	77				77				
A,B,M/dextrose 10% and 0.9% sodium chloride	Hypertonic	815	4.3 [4.0]	154				154				
Saline solutions												
A,B,M/0.45% sodium chloride	Hypotonic	155	5.6 [5.0]	77				77				
A,B,M/0.9% sodium chloride	Isotonic	308	5.7 [5.0]	154				154				
B,M/3% sodium chloride	Hypertonic	1030	5.0 [5.0]	513				513				
A,B,M/5% sodium chloride	Hypertonic	1710	5.8 [5.0]	855				855				
Dextrose solutions												
A,B,M/5% dextrose and water	Isotonic	253	5.0 [4.5]									
A,B,M/10% dextrose and water	Hypertonic	505	4.3 [4.5]									
A,B,M/50% dextrose and water	Hypertonic	2526	4.2 [4.0]									
Electrolyte solutions												
A/Normosol R	Isotonic	295	6.6	140	5		3	98	23‡		27	
B/Plasmalyte A	Isotonic	294	7.4	140	5		3	98	23‡		27	
B/Plasmalyte R	Isotonic	312	4.0–6.5	140	10	5	3	103		8	47	
M/Isolyte E	Isotonic	315	6.0	140	10	5	3	103			49	8
A,B,M/Ringer's	Isotonic	310	5.8 [5.5]	147	4	4		155				
A,B,M/lactated Ringer's	Isotonic	275	6.6 [6.5]	130	4	3		109		28		
Dextrose/electrolyte solutions												
A,B,M/dextrose 5% in Ringer's	Hypertonic	562	4.3²	147	4	4.5		156				
A,B,M/dextrose 5% in lactated Ringer's	Hypertonic	527	4.9³	130	4	2.7		109		28		
A,B,M/dextrose 2.5% in half-strength lactated Ringer's	Isotonic	263	5.0	65.5	2	1.4		54		14		
Miscellaneous solutions												
A,B/dextrose 5% and 5% alcohol	Hypertonic	1114	4.5 [3.5–6.5]									
A,B,M/5% sodium bicarbonate injection	Hypertonic	1190	8.0 [7.0–8.5]	595					595			
A,B,M/sodium lactate injection (1/6 M sodium lactate)	Hypertonic	335	6.5	167						167		
A,B/10% mannitol injection	Hypertonic	549	5.7 [4.0]									
A,B/15% mannitol injection	Hypertonic	823	5.7 [4.0]									
A,B/20% mannitol injection	Hypertonic	1098	5.7 [4.0]									
A,B/6% dextran and 0.9% sodium chloride	Isotonic	308	4.5 [4.0]	154				154				
A,B/10% dextran and 0.9% sodium chloride	Isotonic	252	4.5 [4.0]	154				154				
A,B/10% dextran and 5% dextrose injection	Slightly hypotonic		4.0					154				

*A, Abbott; B, Baxter; M, McGaw.

†Value given in brackets repesents approximate pH of Baxter product.

‡Gluconate.

157

than the extracellular fluid. Thus, when these solutions are used, fluid is pulled into the vascular system. Blood cells placed into a hypertonic solution cause water to be drawn out of the cell, causing it to shrink. Patients receiving hypertonic solutions should be monitored to prevent fluid overload, particularly if the solutions are extremely concentrated and are being given at a rapid rate. Examples of hypertonic solutions include 3 and 5% sodium chloride, 20% dextrose, 50% dextrose in water, and 5% dextrose in lactated Ringer's.

Types of Intravenous Solutions

Various types of intravenous solutions may be administered for a number of indications. Their use also includes the possibility of adverse side effects, so precautionary measures should be followed (Table 9–2).

Dextrose Intravenous Solutions

Parenteral dextrose solutions are available in various concentrations, including 2.5, 5, 10, 20, 30, 40, 50, 60, and 70%. Dextrose is also available in combination with other types of solutions (e.g., 5% dextrose in lactated Ringer's, 5% dextrose in 0.9% sodium chloride). The 5 and 10% solutions can be given peripherally. Those concentrations higher than 10% are diluted or given through central veins. A general exception is the administration of limited amounts of 50% dextrose given slowly through a peripheral vein as emergency treatment of hypoglycemia.

Intravenous dextrose solutions contain water and dextrose, which is a monosaccharide (simple sugar) that is freely soluble in water. Dextrose provides calories and increases the level of glucose in the blood. The 5% dextrose in water solution provides 5 g of dextrose/100 ml (170 cal/liter). The osmolality of this solution (253 mOsm/kg) is slightly less than normal range, but is still generally considered to be isotonic.

In addition to providing calories, 5% dextrose in water also provides free water. The dextrose is metabolized quickly to carbon dioxide and water. This leaves only water, which can cross all membranes and be distributed as needed in the appropriate fluid compartment.[10]

More concentrated dextrose solutions, 20 to 70%, are hypertonic, and range from 505 to 3530 mOsm/liter. When these solutions are being administered, consideration should be given to the possibility that tolerance to glucose may be compromised by sepsis, stress, hepatic, and renal failure, as well as the use of some medications such as steroids or diuretics.

Major Uses. The major use of dextrose solutions is as a source for hydration and calories, particularly the more concentrated solutions. These are usually added to amino acid solutions and are given through a central line to help provide total parenteral nutrition. Hypertonic dextrose solutions, mainly 50%, are used to correct blood glucose levels related to hypoglycemia. These solutions may also be used as the solvent for IV medication administration. Drug information should be reviewed to ensure compatibility between the IV fluid and medication.

Complications. There may be complications related to administering the dextrose solutions intravenously. Vein irritation may occur because of the slightly acidic pH (3.4 to 4.0) of the solution. The use of 5% dextrose in water for hydration should be monitored closely, particularly if used past the initial stage of treatment. This solution does not contain electrolytes. Therefore, continual administration may dilute the body's normal store of electrolytes and can lead to water excess or water intoxication. This may be signaled by changes in behavior, rapid weight gain, and abnormal neuromuscular activity. If not corrected, this could lead to permanent brain damage and possibly death.[11] Dextrose solutions should not be used in the same IV line with blood because of possible agglomeration (clustering).

There are other problems associated with the use of hypertonic dextrose solutions. If given rapidly, these solutions may cause hyperglycemia, which can lead to osmotic diuresis and result in a loss of fluids and electrolytes and possibly hyperosmolar coma. Excessive amounts of hypertonic dextrose may place a sudden demand for an increase in insulin production (hyperinsulinism) causing weakness, diaphoresis, and confusion.[7] There may be a need to add insulin to total parenteral nutrition solutions containing dextrose to prevent adverse affects related to insulin production. Unless hypertonic solutions are diluted prior to peripheral administration, vein irritation, vein damage, and thrombosis may result. Hypertonic solutions are contraindicated for patients with preexisting conditions such as anuria, delirium tremens, diabetic coma, and glucose-galactose malabsorption syndrome.

Prior to any medication being added to a dextrose solution, compatibility information should be checked. Dextrose may also affect the stability of admixtures (e.g., ampicillin sodium). A pharmacist should be contacted for additional information about questionable admixtures.

Sodium-Containing Intravenous Solutions

Major Uses. The replacement of sodium losses is important because sodium is the major cation found in the extracellular fluid, and it controls water distribution. There are various intravenous solutions available to supplement sodium intake, with a pH ranging from 4.5 to 7. Their concentrations vary from 0.45 to 5%. The 0.45% sodium chloride solution is hypotonic, with 1000 ml containing 77 mEq of sodium and 77 mEq of chloride. It provides sodium, chloride, and free water and is used primarily as a hydrating solution. It may also be used to treat hyperosmolar diabetes.

Sodium chloride also comes as an isotonic solution containing 154 mEq of sodium and 154 mEq of chloride per liter. This 0.9% sodium chloride solution closely approximates the osmotic pressure of body fluids but does contain slightly more sodium and chloride than is found in the plasma.[7] It does not enter the intracellular fluid compartment but does expand the extracellular fluid.

Continuous infusion of 0.45% sodium chloride may lead to dilution and depletion of electrolytes. Because of the small amount of sodium in this solution, continuous use or excessive amounts may result in hyponatremia. Another complication that should be monitored is calorie depletion, because there is no source of calories in the solution.

The 0.9% sodium chloride solution is used to replace

Table 9–2

Summary of IV Solutions

IV Solution	Potential Uses	Side Effects and Precautions
Dextrose	Provides calories; provides free water; diluent for IV medication administration	Tolerance to glucose may be compromised by stress, sepsis, hepatic and renal failure, steroids, and diuretics; vein irritation; water intoxication; possible agglomeration; hypertonic solutions: hyperglycemia, osmotic diuresis, hyperosmolar coma, hyperinsulinism
Electrolytes		
Sodium	Sodium replacement; chloride replacement; treats hyperosmolar diabetes; metabolic alkalosis (with Na depletion and fluid loss); diluent for IV medication administration; initiation and discontinuation of blood transfusions	Hyponatremia (with continuous or excessive use of 0.45% NaCl); calorie depletion; hypernatremia; peripheral edema; depletion of other electrolytes; hyperchloremia
Multiple electrolytes	Provides calories (if contains dextrose); provides electrolytes; provides free water	Excessive electrolytes (with rapid administration/solution type); electrolyte deficit (with same solutions where there are abnormal losses or no intake); calorie deficit (if contains no dextrose); fluid overload (related to Na content); IV solution content should be considered in relation to pre-existing conditions; metabolic alkalosis (excessive administration of lactated Ringer's)
Other electrolyte solutions	Same as above	Same as above
Plasma expanders		
Dextran	Shock/anticipated shock related to trauma, surgery, burns, or hemorrhage; prevention of venous thrombosis and pulmonary embolism prophylactically during surgery	Anaphylactoid reactions; GI disturbances; interferes with laboratory testing: decreased hematocrit and plasma protein, temporary extended bleeding time; hypervolemia: electrolyte imbalances, tissue dehydration; pre-existing conditions should be considered (e.g., renal or cardiac disease); use caution in presence of active hemorrhage
Mannitol	Promotes diuresis and excretion of toxic substances; for intracranial pressure and cerebral edema; reduces intraocular pressure	Hypervolemia: electrolyte imbalances, tissue dehydration; extravasation may lead to skin irritation and tissue necrosis; interferes with laboratory testing; pre-existing conditions should be considered (e.g., renal or cardiac disease); use caution because of possible crystal formation
Hetastarch	Shock related to trauma, burns, hemorrhage, and surgery; increase granulocyte yield during leukapheresis	Hypervolemia: electrolyte imbalances, tissue dehydration; anaphylactoid reactions; interferes with laboratory testing: may increase bleeding times, platelet function, decreased hematocrit and plasma protein; pre-existing conditions should be considered (e.g., renal or cardiac disease); hypervolemia: electrolyte imbalances, tissue dehydration
Albumin	Shock/impending shock caused by hypovolemia; provide protein (hypoproteinemia); hyperbilirubinemia; erythroblastosis fetalis	Pre-existing conditions should be considered (e.g., renal or cardiac disease); hypervolemia: electrolyte imbalances, tissue dehydration; interferes with laboratory testing: decreased hematocrit and plasma protein; anaphylactoid reactions; bleeding postoperatively and post-trauma
Plasma protein fraction	Shock related to burns, surgery, hemorrhage, etc; provides protein (on temporary basis)	Cardiac and GI symptoms; chills, fever, urticaria; back pain; hypervolemia; hypernatremia; bleeding postoperatively and post-trauma; pre-existing conditions should be considered (e.g., cardiac or renal disease)
Sodium bicarbonate	Metabolic acidosis; severe hyperkalemia	Possible metabolic alkalosis, hypocalcemia, and hypokalemia (with rapid administration); hypernatremia; pre-existing conditions should be considered (e.g., cardiac or renal disease); hypervolemia: electrolyte imbalances; extravasation may lead to skin irritation and tissue necrosis
Sodium lactate	Mild to moderate metabolic acidosis	Hypernatremia; hypervolemia: electrolyte imbalances; metabolic alkalosis and/or hypokalemia (with rapid administration); pre-existing conditions should be considered (e.g., cardiac or renal disease)
Alcohol	Provides calories (if contains dextrose), provides free water	Pre-existing conditions should be considered (e.g., hepatic or renal impairment, shock); hypervolemia: electrolyte imbalances, acid-base imbalances; intoxication; extravasation may lead to phlebitis and tissue necrosis
Premixed solutions	Vary according to medication added	Vary according to medication added

losses of sodium and chloride. It is used to treat metabolic alkalosis accompanied by sodium depletion and fluid loss.[10] This solution is often used to initiate or discontinue blood transfusions, because it does not hemolyze erythrocytes. Some medications require this isotonic solution as a diluent to ensure stability.

There are two hypertonic sodium-containing solutions (3 and 5%). The 3% sodium chloride solution contains 513 mEq/liter of sodium and the same amount of chloride, and has an osmolarity of approximately 1025 mOsm/liter. The 5% solution has 855 mEq/liter of sodium and an equal amount of chloride, and has an approximate osmolarity of 1710 mOsm/liter.

Hypertonic sodium chloride solutions are used to treat hyponatremia that can occur for various reasons (e.g., excessive sweating, vomiting, renal impairment, excessive water intake). These solutions are generally reserved to treat severe deficits or to be used in situations in which the patient is symptomatic because of hyponatremia.

Complications. The use of an isotonic saline solution may result in complications. Rapid infusion rates or continuous administration of only 0.9% sodium chloride solutions may lead to hypernatremia and fluid overload, potentially leading to all the problems associated with these conditions, including peripheral edema and electrolyte dilution. Other electrolytes may be depleted as a result of continuous infusion of isotonic sodium chloride. Because there is no calorie source, there may be problems related to the nutritional status.

In addition, the rapid or continuous use of hypertonic 3 or 5% sodium chloride intravenous solutions may result in hyperchloremia or hypernatremia. Close monitoring of the flow rate and laboratory test results can eliminate many of the complications.

Multiple Electrolyte Intravenous Solutions

A number of formulations are available to provide electrolytes. Some of them contain a source of calories. The signs, symptoms, and laboratory test results of the patient should be used to determine the correct formulation. The electrolyte content of a specific solution varies among manufacturers.

RINGER'S INJECTION

Ringer's injection is an isotonic solution with a pH of 5.4 to 6. The electrolyte content includes sodium, 147 mEq/liter, potassium, 4 mEq/liter, calcium, 4 mEq/liter, and chloride, 155 mEq/liter, which approximates that found in the plasma.

Major Uses. Ringer's injection is used to replace electrolytes and acts as a water source for hydration. The solution is often used to replace extracellular fluid losses.

Complications. Even though the content is similar to that of plasma, continual delivery of only Ringer's injection may lead to complications. The solution contains potassium and calcium, but the amount is not adequate for maintenance or replacement if there is no intake or abnormal losses are present. Rapid administration may lead to excessive amounts of electrolytes. Administration of only this type of fluid could result in a calorie deficit. These solutions may also cause fluid overload, which could result in diluting the electrolytes.

As with any type of fluid, this could also cause a congestive disorder or pulmonary edema. Because Ringer's injection contains electrolytes, there is always the danger of delivering an excessive amount of one or all of the components.

Ringer's injection also is available with dextrose added (5% dextrose in lactated Ringer's). It provides the same electrolytes as well as 5 g of dextrose and 170 calories. The osmolality is 561 mOsm per liter, making it a hypertonic solution, and the pH is approximately 5.8. It has the same applications as Ringer's injection, plus the ability to provide calories.

Prior to using Ringer's injections, each component should be considered. For example, because the solution contains potassium, precautions need to be exercised when treating patients with cardiac or renal disorders. If the solution contains dextrose, then caution should be exercised if diabetes mellitus is present.

LACTATED RINGER'S SOLUTION

Another solution classified as containing multiple electrolytes is lactated Ringer's. The electrolyte content is similar to that found in plasma and includes sodium, potassium, calcium, and chloride. An extra ingredient, lactate, has been added as a buffer and is metabolized to produce bicarbonate, which is normally found in the extracellular fluid.[7] It is an isotonic solution with a pH of about 6.6.

Major Uses. Lactated Ringer's solution (Hartmann's solution) provides electrolytes and is used to treat hypovolemia. When oral intake is limited or absent, or losses are abnormally high, lactated Ringer's does not provide adequate electrolytes for maintenance therapy. There is no magnesium provided, so it may have to be supplemented.

Complications. The same complications as those produced by Ringer's injection are applicable for lactated Ringer's solutions. These include overhydration, electrolyte excess (particularly sodium), electrolyte dilution, and calorie depletion. Excessive administration may lead to metabolic alkalosis.

Lactated Ringer's solution is contraindicated in patients with hepatic disorders because lactate is metabolized in the liver. A different solution should be considered in the presence of lactic acidosis, because the body's buffering system can be overloaded.

Some calories (170 cal/liter) may be provided in addition to electrolytes by using 5% dextrose in lactated Ringer's. The inclusion of dextrose changes the concentration and makes it a hypertonic solution (527 mOsm/liter) with a pH of about 4.9.

The same problems and contraindications are applicable for 5% dextrose in lactated Ringer's. Additionally, consideration should be given to conditions and diseases affected by dextrose.

Other Electrolyte Solutions

There are other electrolyte solutions available in addition to the group of Ringer's and lactated Ringer's solutions. The names and formulations differ, depending on the manufacturer (See Table 9–1). The use of the various electrolyte combinations often depends on the experience of the physician and on solution availability. The patient's clinical picture, including laboratory test results, should be assessed when selecting the appropriate solution. Electrolyte solutions are generally isotonic until dextrose is added and they become hypertonic. However, this may vary, depending on the electrolyte content. All formulations contain sodium, potassium, and chloride. Others may contain calcium, magnesium phosphate, and buffers, with the latter being provided as bicarbonate, gluconate, lactate, and acetate. As mentioned earlier, lactate is metabolized to produce bicarbonate. In cases of hepatic disease, acetate, which is metabolized by the muscles and other peripheral tissues, is substituted for lactate, because it is converted in the liver.[7]

These solutions may be used for maintenance or replacement of electrolytes. Solutions containing dextrose provide calories. Depending on the formulation, the fluids may be used to treat hypovolemia and to provide free water.

Before any electrolyte solutions are used, the patient's history and physical and laboratory findings should be assessed. The solution should then be selected to meet the individual's electrolyte, caloric, and hydration needs.

Complications include fluid overload, electrolyte depletion, electrolyte dilution, and calorie depletion. Complications result from the administration rate, intravenous formulation, pre-existing conditions and diseases, and current illness.

Plasma Expanders

Solutions used to expand the intravascular space are known as colloids, or plasma expanders. The increase in volume is accomplished by these solutions pulling fluid from the interstitial spaces. These fluids include dextran, mannitol, hetastarch, and albumin.

DEXTRAN

Dextran solutions have effects similar to those of human albumin for expanding intravascular volume. There are two types of dextran, high molecular weight and low molecular weight.

High molecular weight dextrans are available with average molecular weights of 70,000 and 75,000. These 6% solutions are diluted in either 5% dextrose injection or 0.9% sodium chloride solution. The intravascular volume is increased in excess of the volume infused. The increased volume depends on the amount of solution administered, the preadministration fluid status, and the renal status. The maximum effect occurs approximately 1 hour after administration and the increased volume lasts about 24 hours. During this time, the large dextran molecules are slowly broken down to glucose, which is then metabolized to carbon dioxide and water.[10]

Major Uses. High molecular weight dextran is used for treating shock or anticipated shock related to trauma, surgery, burns, or hemorrhage.[12] Dextran solutions should not be used as substitutes for blood and blood products. However, they may be used on short notice if there is no time for crossmatching or if blood or blood products are unavailable.

Complications. Some complications are related to the use of high molecular weight dextran. It may cause severe anaphylactoid reactions, wheezing, tightness in the chest, and gastrointestinal disturbances, including nausea and vomiting. Blood samples for typing and crossmatching should be drawn prior to dextran administration, since dextran may interfere with laboratory testing. Because fluid is being drawn into the vascular system, patients should be monitored for circulatory overload. The increased fluid volume may result in a lowered hematocrit and plasma protein level. The hydration status needs to be monitored closely because overhydration leads to dilution of electrolytes, and lack of adequate fluids may result in tissue dehydration. When larger volumes of dextran are administered, the bleeding time may be temporarily extended.

Dextran is contraindicated for patients with renal diseases, congestive cardiac failure, and bleeding disorders. It should not be used for patients with known hypersensitivity to dextran.

Low molecular weight dextran is a polymer of glucose that has an average molecular weight of about 40,000. The 10% dextran is available in 5% dextrose injection and 0.9% sodium chloride solution. The maximum volume expansion is attained shortly following completion of administration and is affected by the volume delivered, the pre-existing fluid status, and the excretion rate. Most of the dextran is excreted by the renal system within 24 hours. The fluid expansion improves the circulatory status, including microcirculation, even though the exact mechanism is unknown.

Major Uses. Low molecular weight is used to treat shock related to vascular volume loss such as that produced by burns, hemorrhage, surgery, and trauma. Because of its action in preventing sludging of blood, low molecular weight dextran is used to help prevent venous thrombosis and pulmonary embolism during surgical procedures.

Complications. An anaphylactoid reaction is rare but may be fatal. The hydration status is important, because limited intake may result in depletion of tissue fluids, or excessive fluids may cause dilution of electrolytes. Circulatory overload may occur, leading to various congestive states. Dextran can have an adverse effect on hepatic function. Higher doses may increase bleeding times. Because of the expansion of vascular volume, there may be dilution of the hematocrit and plasma protein. Blood should be drawn prior to dextran administration, because dextran may interfere with laboratory testing.

This solution should not be given to patients with cardiac or renal disease caused by possible overload problems, and is contraindicated in the presence of thrombocytopenia, hypofibrinogenemia, and hypersensitivity. Dehydrated patients should receive fluids prior to dextran infusion. Caution should be used where active hemorrhage is present.

MANNITOL

Mannitol is a sugar alcohol substance that is available in a variety of concentrations, from 5 to 25%. This solution is limited to the extracellular space, where it draws fluid from the cells and eventually ends up in the plasma. A small percentage of the mannitol is reabsorbed, and most of it is excreted within 3 hours by the kidney. It ranges from 274 to 1098 mOsm/liter, depending on the concentration, and has a pH of 4.5 to 7.

Major Uses. This colloid is used to promote diuresis in the oliguric phase of acute renal failure and to help promote excretion of toxic substances in the body. The treatment of intracranial pressure and cerebral edema may include the use of mannitol. Reduction of excess cerebrospinal fluid may occur within 15 minutes of initiating the solution and lasts for 3 to 8 hours after the solution is discontinued. When other forms of treatment have been unsuccessful, mannitol may be used to reduce high intraocular pressure. It does not penetrate the eye but does reduce high intraocular pressure by pulling fluid from the anterior chamber of the eye.[10] This usually occurs within 30 to 60 minutes of administration, and the effects last from 4 to 6 hours.

Complications. Fluid and electrolyte imbalances are the most frequent and severe complications encountered with mannitol administration. Fluid is drawn from the cells into the vascular system, which may lead to cell dehydration or fluid overload. The excess fluid may cause an increased loss of electrolytes or have a dilutional effect on the electrolytes, leaving a deficit. If dehydration occurs, there may be an electrolyte excess, with the greatest effect being on the sodium and potassium levels. It may have an adverse effect on the nervous system, including toxicity and interference with maintaining cerebrospinal fluid pH. Extravasation of mannitol may lead to skin irritation and tissue necrosis. There may be interference with laboratory test results related to electrolytes and with blood ethylene glycol concentration.

Mannitol should be used cautiously for patients with an impaired cardiac or renal system. It is contraindicated in the presence of anuria, severe pulmonary and cardiac congestion, severe dehydration, pregnancy, and intracranial bleeding, if it is present other than during a craniotomy.

Caution should also be exercised in monitoring the product for the presence of crystal formation. The use of an in-line filter is recommended during the administration of mannitol.

HETASTARCH

Hetastarch is a synthetic polymer with colloidal properties similar to those of human albumin. It is available in a 6% concentration in 0.9% sodium chloride. The colloidal osmotic effect pulls fluid from the cells into the intravascular space, thus increasing the volume in this area. Maximum volume expansion occurs shortly after completion of the infusion. The duration of effect depends on the preadministration fluid status, distribution of the hetastarch, and renal function status. The molecules within this solution vary in size. The smaller hetastarch molecules (hydroxyethylated glucose) are excreted rapidly, but it may take 2 weeks or longer for the larger molecules (starch) to be degraded sufficiently for elimination. It does not interfere with blood typing and crossmatching, as do other colloidal solutions.

Major Uses. This solution is used for fluid replacement to treat shock related to a decreased circulating volume resulting from trauma, burns, hemorrhage, and surgery. It is also used with leukapheresis to help increase the yield of granulocytes.

Complications. The administration of hetastarch may produce a severe anaphylactoid reaction. It may interfere with platelet function and increase bleeding times. As with any volume expander, the danger of fluid overload is always a possibility. This may lead to disorders related to congestion, dilution, or depletion of electrolytes, dehydration of peripheral tissue, electrolyte excess, and a decrease in the hematocrit and plasma protein levels.

Hetastarch is contraindicated in the presence of severe cardiac and renal disorders, particularly when oliguria or anuria is present. It also should not be used in the presence of bleeding disorders.

ALBUMIN

Albumin is a natural plasma protein prepared from human blood and blood-related products, and is available in 5 and 25% concentrations. It plays an important role in the regulation of plasma volume and tissue fluid balance. The administration of albumin causes fluid to be pulled from the interstitial space into the intravascular space. Because it is a plasma protein, there may be a slight increase in the plasma protein volume. The 5% solution is isotonic. The 25% solution is hypertonic, and 25 g of albumin provides plasma protein equivalent to that in 500 ml of plasma, or two units of whole blood.[12]

Major Uses. Albumin is used for plasma volume expansion in treating shock or impending shock related to a circulatory volume deficit. It is used temporarily to provide protein when hypoproteinemia is present. Because of its bilirubin-binding capability, albumin 25% may be used in treating hyperbilirubinemia or erythroblastosis fetalis. The 5% solution is generally used to treat hypovolemia, and the 25% solution is usually reserved for treatment when there are fluid and sodium restrictions.

Complications. The potential for complications should be considered if cardiac, hepatic, or renal disease is present. These systems may be unable to handle the increased intravascular volume if they are impaired. The increased circulating volume may result in fluid overload and lead to further complications. Anemia may occur if large volumes of albumin alone are used to replace blood loss. The rapid influx and excretion of fluid may dilute or deplete electrolytes. The serum protein concentration and hematocrit should be monitored, because these levels may be decreased. Symptoms of allergic reactions may be present. Bleeding may occur post-operatively or post-traumatically as the intravascular volume and pressure increase. Albumin may alter laboratory findings. Its use is contraindicated for patients with severe anemia, cardiac failure, or known hypersensitivity.

PLASMA PROTEIN FRACTION

Plasma protein fraction (PPF) is isotonic and is similar in action to human albumin in expanding the intravascular volume. It is a 5% solution containing proteins, with approximately 83 to 90% being albumin derived from pooled blood, plasma, and serum. It is not blood group or Rh-specific and contains no clotting factors. It is a transparent, nearly colorless to slightly brownish solution that contains 130 to 160 mEq of sodium/liter and no more than 2 mEq of potassium/liter.

Major Uses. PPF is used to expand the plasma volume and acts by causing fluid to shift from the interstitial spaces into the circulatory system. It is used to treat shock related to burns, surgery, hemorrhage, or any condition resulting in a volume deficit. When treating hypovolemia-related conditions, the initial dose is 250 to 500 ml (12.5 to 25 g of protein). Thereafter, the dose is related to the patient's condition and response. The flow rate should be adjusted according to the patient's response but should not exceed 10 ml/min.[10] This solution is not a substitute when whole blood, red blood cells, or albumin is indicated.

It may also be used temporarily to provide protein in cases of hypoproteinemia. The recommended daily dose for adults is 1000 to 1500 ml, which contains 50 to 75 g of protein.

Complications. Adverse side effects include tachycardia, flushing, erythema, nausea, vomiting, headache, chills, fever, urticaria, back pain, and hypersalivation. These side effects occur on an infrequent basis.

Just as with any solution used for volume expansion, caution should be exercised to prevent vascular overload. Patients should be monitored for signs of hypervolemia, such as pulmonary edema. Because of the sodium content, sodium levels should be monitored. The patient should be observed for signs of bleeding as the intravascular volume and blood pressure increase. Caution should also be exercised in the presence of hepatic or renal failure. The use of PPF is contraindicated with cardiopulmonary bypass procedures and may be contraindicated with severe anemia or cardiac failure.

Alkalizing Solutions

SODIUM BICARBONATE

Sodium bicarbonate solution is an alkalizing agent and a sodium salt. The 5% sodium bicarbonate solution dissociates to provide the bicarbonate ion, which is the principal buffer in the extracellular fluid. Bicarbonate helps maintain osmotic pressure and acid-base balance. The administration of sodium bicarbonate increases the plasma bicarbonate concentration and may increase the plasma pH until the body compensates and returns the level to a normal value.

Major Uses. Sodium bicarbonate is used in the treatment of metabolic acidosis associated with many diseases, including severe renal disease and cardiac arrest. It is administered in the treatment of severe hyperkalemia, in which it alkalinizes the plasma and results in a temporary shift of potassium into the cells. The sodium in the solution also antagonizes the cardiac effects of the potassium.

Complications. Metabolic alkalosis, hypocalcemia, and hypokalemia may occur following the rapid or excessive administration of sodium bicarbonate. There may be water and sodium retention leading to hypernatremia, particularly when there is a pre-existing condition such as renal or cardiac disease. The fluid overload may lead to electrolyte imbalances. Extravasation may cause chemical cellulitis, necrosis, ulceration, and/or sloughing.

Patients with metabolic and respiratory alkalosis are not generally candidates for sodium bicarbonate therapy. It is also contraindicated in the presence of hypocalcemia or hypochloremia. Caution should be exercised when cardiac or renal problems exist.[10]

SODIUM LACTATE

Sodium lactate (one-sixth M lactate) is an alkalizing agent that is oxidized in the liver to bicarbonate and glycogen. Approximately 1 to 2 hours are required to complete the conversion of lactate to bicarbonate.

Major Uses. When the normal production and utilization of lactic acid are in place, sodium lactate is used to treat mild to moderate metabolic acidosis. Because the conversion of lactate to bicarbonate requires 1 to 2 hours, it is not recommended for use in treating severe acidosis.

The sodium contained in the solution may lead to hypernatremia and hypervolemia. There may also be deficits or excesses of other electrolytes. Excessive amounts or rapid administration may lead to metabolic alkalosis or hypokalemia.

Complications. Caution should be taken when using sodium lactate for patients with hypervolemia, congestive heart failure, or renal disorders causing oliguria or anuria. It should not be used for patients having excessive lactate levels or impaired lactate utilization. Sodium lactate should not be used in the treatment of lactic acidosis or in the presence of hypernatremia or respiratory alkalosis.

Alcohol Solutions

Alcohol solutions contain ethyl alcohol (5%) and are diluted in 5% dextrose injection. The body can metabolize the alcohol in a 5% solution at a rate of 200 to 400 ml/hour. The metabolism rate may vary depending on the patient's weight and tolerance, and is lowered with starvation and increased by insulin. The alcohol is metabolized primarily in the liver to acetaldehyde or acetate.[13] Alcohol solutions provide a source of water and carbohydrates. The 5% alcohol in 5% dextrose injection contains 450 cal/liter and has an average pH of 4.3.[13]

Alcohol in dextrose solutions are used to replace water and to provide calories. The 10% alcohol solution has been used to decrease uterine activity during labor, but has now been largely replaced with other types of therapy.

These solutions should be used with caution in the presence of hepatic and renal impairment, shock, and actual or anticipated postpartum hemorrhage, and following cranial surgery. Because of its effect on blood sugar, alcohol solutions should be used carefully in patients with diabetes mellitus. Continuous or rapid administration may lead to hypervolemia, intoxication, congested states, pulmonary edema, dilution of electrolytes, and acid-base imbalances. Care should be taken to avoid extravasation, because these hypertonic solutions may cause phlebitis and tissue necrosis.

The use of alcohol and dextrose solutions is contraindicated in patients with diabetic coma, urinary tract infection, and epilepsy. The patient's history should be checked carefully for alcoholism, in which case this solution should not be used.

Premixed IV Solutions

There are a large number of premixed intravenous solutions available for use. These solutions have many advantages over the use of manually prepared admixtures. Premixed solutions have been sterilized after the admixture procedure and therefore have a longer shelf life. There is no difficulty in the proper selection of the correct diluent, and the pH has been adjusted to improve stability. Finally, the correct amount of medication has been added to the proper volume and type of IV solution. Premixed solutions decrease the amount of time needed to get the fluid to the patient, which is particularly important in emergency situations. There are also disadvantages in using premixed intravenous solutions. The wrong amount of medication may be used if a particular admixture comes in more than one dosage, or if there are multiple types that are premixed and the wrong medication or solution is used. There may be an increased cost associated with the use of premixed IV solutions.

The number of medications now available in the premixed form is increasing. Potassium chloride comes in several concentrations, as well as in various IV solutions. The use of each of these depends on the patient's history, physical assessment, and laboratory findings. Before any of the potassium-containing solutions are administered, it is important to establish good renal function. Complications are related to the content of the particular fluid. Rapid infusion or continual administration may lead to hypervolemia, electrolyte excess (particularly potassium), and/or electrolyte dilution. The use of only one type of solution over an extended period may result in electrolyte depletion or, if no source of nutrients is available, calorie depletion. The patient should be monitored carefully for electrolyte imbalances during the course of treatment.

Other medications premixed in IV solutions include heparin sodium, theophylline, lidocaine, and dopamine hydrochloride. There are also some antibiotics available premixed in small volumes of intravenous solutions. Just as for premixed potassium solutions, it is important to review the patient's history, physical assessment, and laboratory findings. The nurse should be familiar with complications related to the particular medication and the base IV solution to which it has been added. The pharmacy department should be contacted if information is unclear or unfamiliar.

In regard to the complications of intravenous fluid administration, there are metabolic and physical concerns. The metabolic issues have been discussed in detail as related to each solution. There are also physical complications involved with IV fluid administration. These include vascular tolerance, which depends on the patient's general health status, the condition of the veins, pH of the intravenous solution or medication, and the concentration. Acidic solutions and hypertonic solutions may be irritating to the lining of the vessel and may become painful for the patient. The infiltration of hypertonic solutions may cause irritation and subsequent necrosis and sloughing of subcutaneous tissue. Most complications can be corrected by slowing the infusion rate or by discontinuing the solution or admixture.

►NURSING DIAGNOSIS

Parenteral fluid administration, as already discussed, has many facets, and is not without its complexities and compli-

cations. All these concerns make it challenging for the nurse who is caring for the patient with potential imbalances. Because of this, there are nursing considerations and applicable nursing diagnoses that can be made concerning these patients.

Potential Nursing Diagnosis

- Fluid volume excess
- Fluid volume deficit
- High risk for fluid volume deficit
- High risk for infection
- Knowledge deficit concerning intravenous therapy and the procedures involved

Patient-Client Outcomes

- The patient returns to a state of fluid and electrolyte equilibrium, as evidenced by normal laboratory values, urinary output, and stable weights.
- The patient does not develop an infection, as evidenced by normal vital signs and absence of signs indicative of inflammation.
- By the end of the first teaching session the patient can verbalize the reason(s) for the necessity of parenteral fluids, describe the initiation procedure (briefly), and list two signs or symptoms that should be reported to the patient's nurse.

References

1. Miller RD. Problems in Hospital Law, 6th ed. Rockville, MD: Aspen, 1990:251–254.
2. Metheny NM. Use Considerations, 2nd ed. Philadelphia: J.B. Lippincott, 1992:32–34, 171.
3. Plummer A. Principles and Practices of Intravenous Therapy, 4th ed. Boston: Little, Brown, & Co., 1987:84.
4. Metheny NM. Quick Reference to Fluid Balance. Philadelphia: J.B. Lippincott, 1984:58.
5. Horne MM, Swearingen PL. Pocket Guide to Fluids and Electrolytes. St. Louis: C.V. Mosby, 1989:103.
6. Davis J, Sherer K. Applied Nutrition and Diet Therapy for Nurses, 2nd ed. Philadelphia: W.B. Saunders, 1994:267.
7. Horne MM, Heitz UE, Swearingen PL, et al. Fluid, Electrolyte, and Acid-Base Balance: A Case Study Approach. St. Louis: Mosby–Year Book, 1991:42, 135–137.
8. Mathewson KM. Pharmacotherapeutics: A Nursing Process Approach. Philadelphia: F.A. Davis, 1994:249.
9. Philips LD. Manual of I.V. Therapeutics. Philadelphia: F.A. Davis, 1993:112.
10. McEvoy GK. AHFS Drug Information 92. Bethesda, MD: American Society of Hospital Pharmacists, 1993:814, 1561, 1577, 1588, 1601, 1634.
11. Metheny NM. Fluid and Electrolyte Balance: Nursing Considerations, 2nd ed. Philadelphia: J.B. Lippincott, 1992:58, 209.
12. Gahart BL. Intravenous Medications, 9th ed. St. Louis: Mosby–Year Book, 1993:189, 498.
13. Abbott Laboratories. Manufacturer's package insert (5% alcohol in 5% dextrose). North Chicago: Abbott Laboratories, 1989.

Blood Component Therapy

Jane A. Weir, BA, BSN, CRNI

This chapter on blood component therapy is presented as a foundation on which to construct a broader understanding of the more encompassing subject of transfusion therapy. The topics addressed are neither intended to be all-inclusive of the discipline of transfusion therapy nor are they offered as a "how-to" manual. They are intended to establish a firm theoretic footing and a practical framework on which the practitioner may build within the practice setting.

It was less than 200 years ago that James Blundell performed the first blood transfusion to save a life. Since that time, because of incredible advances in knowledge and technology that have been made in blood group identification, collection, fractionation, storage, and transmissible disease testing, transfusion medicine has evolved into a specialty all its own. This specialty has made advances in new surgical procedures possible and has been the support for the ever-changing approaches to cancer chemotherapy.

Blood component therapy has advanced so far and so fast, and is so commonplace in current medicine, that there could

be a tendency to approach this familiar therapy with some complacency. Therefore, it is of benefit to be reminded that this is a "living transplant" that carries with it significant risks, only a few of which are avoidable. Consequently, this effective and readily accessible therapy should be prudently employed with the potential for benefit always outweighing the potential for harm. Furthermore, it is the duty of the practitioner in transfusion therapy to be knowledgeable in the application of this therapy, and to be familiar with possible untoward effects and their appropriate interventions.

DONOR TESTING

All blood donated for the purpose of homologous transfusion, as well as autologous donations that are "crossed over" to the homologous pool, if not used by the donor, must be subjected to a number of tests (Table 10–1).

ABO and Rh Typing (Red Cell Antigens)

1. ABO forward typing is the process in which red blood cells are mixed with a known antibody (anti-A or anti-B). This process identifies the antigen(s) present on the red cells by visually apparent agglutination of the cells when antibody combines with corresponding antigen (e.g., anti-A with antigen A).
2. ABO reverse typing is the testing of serum for the presence of predicted ABO antibodies by adding red blood cells of a known ABO type to it.

Table 10–1

Testing of Donor Blood

Test	Parameter Indicates by Results
ABO: forward typing	Presence of antigen A or B on RBC
ABO: reverse typing	Presence of antibody A or antibody B in plasma
Rh typing:	
With anti-D sera	Presence of D antigen on RBC
With anti-D sera, indirect antiglobulin test (IAT)	Presence of weak D
Screen for unexpected antibodies	Presence of antibodies other than anti-A and anti-B
Screen for transmissible disease:	
Serologic test for syphilis (STS)	Treponema infection
Hepatitis B surface antigen (HBsAg)	Infectivity for hepatitis B
Hepatitis C (anti-HCV)	Infectivity for hepatitis C
Hepatitis B core antibody (anti-HBc)	Surrogate test for non-A, non-B hepatitis
Alanine aminotransferase (ALT)	Surrogate test for non-A, non-B hepatitis
Human immunodeficiency virus (HIV)	Presence of antibody to HIV-1 and HIV-2
Human T-cell leukemia-lymphoma virus (HTLV-I)	Presence of antibody to HTLV-I/II

I would like to recognize the assistance of Denise M. Dreher, CRNI, in preparing the section of this chapter entitled Autologous Transfusion. Ms. Dreher's broad knowledge of the topic in general as well as her extensive experience within the practice of intraoperative autologous transfusion were of immeasurable value.

3. Rh typing is accomplished by testing the red cells against anti-D serum. If agglutination occurs, the red cells possess the D antigen and the blood is Rh-positive. However, if no agglutination is apparent, the red cells must be tested further to rule out the presence of the weakly expressed D antigen called weak D (formerly referred to as D^u). This antigen can be identified most reliably by indirect antiglobulin testing (IAT) after incubating the red blood cells with anti-D sera. Red cells that possess the weak D are given to Rh-positive recipients.
4. Additional testing for red cell antigens is not recommended or encouraged by the American Association of Blood Banks (AABB).

Screening for Unexpected Antibodies

Unexpected antibodies are those other than anti-A or anti-B. Many if not most blood banks screen all donated units for clinically significant antibodies rather than limiting their search to the donor group most likely to harbor them (e.g., donors with a history of pregnancy or previous transfusion). In general, clinically significant antibodies are those known to have caused hemolytic disease of the newborn (HDN), a frank hemolytic transfusion reaction, or unacceptably short survival of transfused red blood cells.[1]

Screening for Transmissible Disease

All donor blood must be tested to detect units that might transmit disease. Components and whole blood units must not be used for transfusion unless all tests are nonreactive, negative, or have values within normal limits.

1. Test for syphilis using the serologic test for syphilis (STS), as required by the Food and Drug Administration (FDA).
2. Test for the presence of the hepatitis B surface antigen (HBsAg) to identify hepatitis B infectivity.
3. Test for the presence of the antibody to the hepatitis C virus (HCV), which is an identified member of the non-A, non-B hepatitis viruses.
4. Test for the presence of the hepatitis B core antibody (anti-HBc), which is part of the surrogate testing to identify the possibility of non-A, non-B hepatitis infectivity. Additionally, anti-HBc can be part of the screening for hepatitis B.
5. Test for the alanine aminotransaminase (ALT) level, a serum enzyme level, that, if elevated can signal liver malfunction. It is included as surrogate testing for the possible presence of non-A, non-B hepatitis, because of its specificity for liver disease.
6. Test for the presence of the antibody to human immunodeficiency viruses 1 and 2 (anti-HIV–1/2). A positive result using standard screening methods requires a repeat standard screen and then a confirmatory screen using a more specific assay.
7. Test for the presence of the antibody to the human T-cell lymphotropic virus I (anti-HTLV–I/II). See later, Adverse Effects.

BLOOD STORAGE AND PRESERVATION

Because blood is a living tissue at the time of its harvest from a donor and must remain healthy during its storage, substances are added to this donated blood to meet two conditions necessary for successful shelf life:

1. A food source must be provided to maintain adequate nutrition to the stored cells.
2. Anticoagulation must be achieved to ensure that the blood remains in its liquid cellular state for the duration of the storage period.

There are several anticoagulants-preservatives from which to choose. All provide the aforementioned necessary conditions for shelf life, but differ in the length of storage time that they provide (Table 10–2).

CPD (citrate-phosphate-dextrose) and CPDA-1 (citrate-phosphate-dextrose-adenine) differ in composition by just one substance, adenine. However, the addition of adenine prolongs the shelf life by 14 days and is of great significance to a blood transfusion service whose concern revolves around adequate blood reserves and their ability to supply on demand. CPDA-1 is currently considered the anticoagulant-preservative of choice for whole blood, but it is also used when the donated unit may be processed into separate components.

The additive systems approved by the FDA for the extended storage of red blood cells (not for whole blood, plasma components, or platelets) differ in composition. They may contain varying combinations of dextrose, adenine, phosphate, and citrate, as well as other substances such as saline or mannitol. The additive systems are secondary or "add-on" solutions because they are used only with red blood cells that were harvested in a primary anticoagulant-preservative such as CPD.

Anticoagulants and Preservatives

The following is a brief summary of the substances that participate in blood preservation and their functions within the process.

Citrate. Sodium citrate by itself or sometimes in combination with citric acid achieves anticoagulation by inhibiting several calcium-dependent steps in the coagulation cascade. It also slows the process of glycolysis, which is the conversion of glucose to lactic acid and ATP through various metabolic pathways (Embden-Meyerhof, Kreb's cycle, and the electron transport system). By slowing this process, adequate

Table 10–2		
Anticoagulants-Preservatives		
Anticoagulant-Preservative	**Composition**	**Shelf Life Provided (days)**
CPD	Citrate, phosphate, dextrose	21
CPDA-1	CPD plus adenine	35
Additive systems	CPD plus various preservative combinations	35–42

T a b l e   1 0 – 3

Biochemical Changes During Blood Storage

Parameter	CPD (Whole Blood)		CPDA-1 (PRBC)		AS-3* (PRBC)	
			Anticoagulant-Preservative Used			
Storage (days)	0	21	0	35	0	42
pH	7.20	6.34	7.55	6.71	7.27	6.47
ATP (% of initial value)	100	86	—	45	—	56
2,3-DPG (% of initial value)	100	44	—	2.6	—	4.1
Survival 24 hours after transfusion (%)	100	80	100	71	—	82

*AS-3 is available from Nutricel, Cutter Biological, Berkley, CA.

amounts of ATP continue to be produced while the limited supply of sugar in the stored cells is protected from being depleted.

Phosphate. Inorganic phosphate acts as a buffer that helps maintain the pH.

Dextrose. When sugars were first investigated as possible participants in blood preservation, red blood cells were thought to be impermeable to them. Therefore, it was theorized that the sugar would act as a colloid to protect the cells against hemolysis. It was soon recognized that cells were permeable to dextrose, and that this was an excellent food source for the stored cells.[2] Dextrose is a deterrent to hemolysis but not as a result of a colloidal action. It supplies the food source from which adenosine triphosphate (ATP), the principal intracellular energy storage compound, is formed. Adequate supplies of ATP are necessary for the continued integrity of the cell.

Adenine. Although there appear to be other factors involved, the ATP content of stored red blood cells can generally be equated with their viability (i.e., their capability of surviving in the recipient's circulation after transfusion). In the 1950s, it was shown that the ATP content of stored cells could be restored with the addition of adenosine.[2, 3] However, because of its toxicity, adenosine was never employed in transfusion practice. Later, it was discovered that the addition of adenine, which in conjunction with the 5-carbon sugar ribose makes up the adenosine molecule, accomplishes the same positive result of restoring ATP levels in stored red cells.[2]

Mannitol. This participant in blood preservation is seen in at least one of the additive systems. Mannitol appears to reduce hemolysis by its effect as an osmotic stabilizer. In a study comparing an additive system that uses mannitol to one that does not, it was found that the level of hemolysis in the mannitol system is lower than in the system without that additive. However, in both cases, the level of hemolysis was within acceptable limits.[4]

Biochemical Changes in Stored Blood

In addition to the decline in ATP levels seen during blood storage, there are many other biochemical parameters that are changing. Plasma levels of potassium and hemoglobin rise, whereas plasma sodium, pH, and intracellular levels of 2,3-diphosphoglycerate (2,3-DPG) decline. The decline in pH and 2,3-DPG is the result of glucose metabolism. As the red cells use glucose to produce ATP, hydrogen ions accumulate and the pH falls. This decrease in pH has a direct effect on the level of red blood cell 2,3-DPG, which declines in an environment of declining pH.

The role of 2,3-DPG in red blood cell function is one of facilitator. This organic phosphate influences the dissociation of oxygen from its hemoglobin transport at the tissue level. When the levels of 2,3-DPG are high, oxygen is readily released at any given partial pressure (PO_2). However, when 2,3-DPG levels are low, the affinity of hemoglobin for oxygen is enhanced and less oxygen is released at the same PO_2.

Blood is stored at 1 to 6 C, which contributes to its preservation in two ways. Lowered temperatures retard bacterial proliferation and slow the glycolytic cycle. Table 10–3 lists biochemical changes that occur when blood is stored at 1 to 6 C.[1, 4, 5] These changes are known as the ''storage lesion'' of blood and some are fully corrected in vivo after transfusion. Because the recipient's compensatory homeostatic mechanisms can correct the red blood cell storage lesion, these changes are rarely of any clinical significance. Both ATP and 2,3-DPG levels are restored in donor cells following transfusion. Volunteer donors, whose blood was stored for 35 days in CPDA-1 and two different additive solutions, showed an increase in 2,3-DPG levels to 50% of normal within seven hours and 95% of normal within 72 hours after transfusion.[6] In theory, stored red cells whose 2,3-DPG levels are low should not be capable of providing immediate improvement in tissue oxygen levels in the face of severe trauma or complicated surgery. However, even in massive transfusion, the adverse effects of the red blood cell lesion are usually inconsequential unless the recipient is already severely compromised.[1]

Rejuvenation of Red Cells

Red cells stored up to three days beyond their expiration date can be incubated (at 37 C for one hour) in FDA-approved solutions containing inosine, pyruvate, phosphate, adenine, and sometimes glucose, which increase the cellular levels of ATP and 2,3-DPG. These ''rejuvenated cells'' may be washed and used within 24 hours, or may be glycerolized and frozen for extended storage.[1, 7]

Table 10-4

ABO Blood Groups

Possible Genotypes	Phenotype	Blood Group	RBC Antigen	Plasma Antibody
OO	O	O	Neither A nor B	A and B
AA or AO	A	A	A	B
BB or BO	B	B	B	A
AB	AB	AB	A and B	Neither A nor B

IMMUNOHEMATOLOGY

Immunology is the scientific discipline that deals with the immune system and the immune response (i.e., the antibody response to antigenic stimulus). It is the discipline that narrows the view of immunology to focus specifically on the antigens and antibodies of the blood.

The antigens of the blood are called agglutinogens. They are found as integrated parts of the red cell membrane, as components of the white cells, and as soluble substances in the plasma. The largest group of these agglutinogens, which numbers more than 400 and belongs to 24 known systems, is associated with the red cells.

The first set of red cell antigens, the ABO system, was discovered by Landsteiner at the turn of the twentieth century. This system has been revealed to be the most important of the known systems and is the foundation for determining compatibilities in transfusion therapy.

ABO System

There are four blood types in the ABO system, A, B, AB, and O. The name of the blood type is determined by the name of the antigen on the red cell. The type of antigen present on the red cell is an inherited characteristic, with the A and B genes being equally dominant, and the O gene being recessive (Table 10–4).

The A and B genes determine the presence of the A and B antigenic determinant sites, respectively. Although the O gene is inactive and does not code for any erythrocyte alloantigens, blood group O erythrocytes do exhibit an antigenic glycoprotein on their surface, the H antigen. This glycoprotein is not the product of the O gene, as evidenced by its presence on red blood cells of all types.

The A, B, and H antigens are related to each other in the following way. During the synthesis of the blood group molecules, the H antigen is synthesized first. Thus, the H antigen is present on all red cells. If the A gene is present, it codes for a transferase (enzyme), which facilitates the attachment of the sugar N-acetylgalactosamine to the H antigen. This chemical complex is the antigenic determinant for blood group A. Similarly, the B gene codes for a different transferase, which allows for the attachment of an alternate sugar group, D-galactose; this completes the antigenic determinant for blood type B. Group O individuals do not possess either enzyme system, and thus group O erythrocytes possess only the unmodified H antigen on their surface.[1,8]

The antibodies of the ABO system occur naturally (i.e., without direct antigenic stimulation) and are called isohemagglutinins. They are complete and, in the presence of red cells that exhibit the corresponding antigen, can cause agglutination in a saline medium. The antibody that agglutinates type A is called antibody A (anti-A) and the corresponding antibody for antigen B is antibody B (anti-B).

It is this adversarial relationship between antigen and corresponding antibody that is the basis for understanding compatibilities within the ABO system. The antigens are located on the cells and the antibodies reside in the plasma. Therefore, if a unit of red cells is to be administered, this unit should be thought of as an antigen and should be given only to a recipient who does not exhibit the corresponding antibody. In other words, corresponding antigens and antibodies should be kept separate. Red cells should not be given to individuals who carry the matching antibody in their plasma. Conversely, plasma should not be given to an individual who possesses the matching antigen (Table 10–5).

Rh System

The Rh system is complex and extensive. With almost 50 Rh antigens having been identified, a complete discussion of this system is not included here. Sufficient for the topic of routine transfusion therapy are the unmodified terms of Rh+ (Rh-positive) and Rh− (Rh-negative), which refer to the presence or absence of the red cell antigen D, respectively.

The blood recipient who carries the antigen D (Rh-positive) may receive products that are either Rh+ or Rh−. However, if a recipient is Rh-negative, that individual should receive blood products that are Rh-negative. This is espe-

Table 10-5

Summary of ABO System Compatibilities

Component	Donor	Recipient
Whole blood	Give type specific only	
Packed red cells (stored, washed, or frozen and washed)	O	O, A, B, AB
	A	A, AB
	B	B, AB
	AB	AB
Plasma (FFP)	O	O
	A	A, O
	B	B, O
	AB	AB, B, A, O
Platelets: RBC—ABO and Rh-compatible preferred	O	O, A, B, AB
	A	A, AB
	B	B, AB
	AB	AB
Cryoprecipitate: plasma—ABO-compatible preferred	O	O
	A	A, O
	B	B, O
	AB	AB, B, A, O

cially true for Rh-negative women of childbearing age who might become sensitized to the D antigen, which could raise the potential for complications in subsequent pregnancies.[1]

PREPARATION AND CLINICAL APPLICATION OF BLOOD COMPONENTS

Whole Blood

Whole blood requires no further processing beyond collection into an anticoagulated closed collection system and testing. It is stored at 1 to 6 C with the satellite pack attached. If packed cells are needed at any time during the shelf life of the blood, this satellite pack allows for their separation within a closed system. However, because whole blood transfusions are rarely used beyond the situation of massive blood loss, most homologous donations are not stored as whole blood but are "split" into components soon after donation. Autologous donations, which are planned to be transfused back to the donor within the shelf life period for refrigerated blood, are stored whole. These units are often given as whole blood. They can be spun down and given as packed cells, however, if the donor or recipient does not need or cannot tolerate the additional volume that the plasma represents.

Clinical applications for the administration of whole blood include the following:

- Increased oxygen-carrying capacity *and* volume expansion necessary
- Active bleeding (25 to 30% blood volume loss)
- Multiple trauma, hemorrhagic shock

Packed Red Blood Cells

Packed cells are prepared by separating the plasma from the cellular portion of a unit of whole blood. This can be done at any time up to the date of expiration of the whole blood. Separation can be accomplished either by

1. Causing a rapid separation of cells and plasma with centrifugation, or
2. Allowing the separation to happen by sedimentation (store the blood in an upright position; cells settle at the bottom and plasma concentrates on the top).

Once separation has occurred, 200 to 250 ml of plasma can be manually expressed into the attached satellite bag.

The shelf life of a unit of packed red cells (PRBCs) is the same as that of a unit of the whole blood from which it was obtained. An exception to this would be if an additive system were mixed with the cells at the time of their separation (see earlier, Anticoagulants and Preservatives). These additive systems, which must be used within 72 hours of the blood donation, extend the shelf life of the packed cells from 35 to 42 days.

PRBCs are used to increase the oxygen-carrying capacity (i.e., red blood cell mass) in patients with symptomatic anemia that is not treatable with iron or other hemoglobin supplements.

Modified Packed Red Blood Cells

PRBCs can be modified during processing or infusion.

Modified During Processing

Saline-Washed RBCs. Saline washing of red blood cells is carried out in the blood bank using automated or semiautomated equipment designed for this purpose. The washed cells are then suspended in sterile normal saline, and the processed product has a hematocrit of 70 to 80%. This process removes platelets and cellular debris, diminishes plasma to trace levels, and reduces the number of leukocytes. The leukocytes are not eliminated, so this component does contain viable lymphocytes and can precipitate the graft-versus-host response (see later). Washed packed cells may be made from stored packed cells at any time during the shelf life. However, once the cells have been washed, which is an open system, their shelf life at 1 to 6 C is 24 hours. This limited shelf life is imposed because of concerns for bacterial contamination. Washed red cells can still transmit infectious diseases, including hepatitis.[9]

Washed packed cells are used for patients with recurrent or severe allergic reactions thought to be related to one or more plasma proteins, and for neonatal and intrauterine transfusions.

Frozen-Deglycerolized Packed Cells. The once numerous reasons for freezing blood that existed two decades ago have dissipated over time because of advanced technologies. Today, blood is frozen for one reason—long-term storage. For autologous blood, this extended storage capability means that blood can be "stockpiled" well beyond the 42-day shelf life afforded by refrigeration. This allows for the scheduling of elective surgical procedures beyond the immediate future while still offering the safety of autologous transfusion during the procedure or postoperatively.

In addition to its application in autologous transfusion, freezing of blood is used to maintain stores of rare blood types. The AABB *Standards*[7] allows frozen blood storage intended for routine transfusion for up to 10 years. For blood of rare phenotypes, this 10-year frame may be extended at the discretion of the blood bank director.

Blood that is to be frozen may be collected in CPD or CPDA-1 and stored as whole blood, or it may be stored as packed cells with or without an additive system. Usually, blood is glycerolized and frozen within the first 6 days after donation. Glycerol is added to the cells before freezing because it is a cryoprotective agent that prevents cell dehydration and mechanical damage from ice formation. Although the first 6 days is the usual window in which to freeze blood, red cells nearing the end of their shelf life may be rejuvenated for up to 3 days post-expiration and then frozen. This option helps eliminate unnecessary waste of valuable blood stores. Frozen blood is maintained at −65 C or below.[1]

When a unit of frozen blood is needed, it is first thawed in a water bath (37 C) or a dry warmer (37 C). It is then washed to remove the glycerol, which is hypertonic to the blood. The washing process used to deglycerolize red cells is the same as that used to process washed red cells.

The same concerns for bacterial contamination that exist for saline-washed packed cells exist for frozen-deglycerolized cells. This product must be infused within 24 hours of processing. Also, as is true with washed packed cells, frozen-deglycerolized cells can transmit infectious disease and have been shown to contain viable lymphocytes.[9]

Clinical applications for frozen-deglycerolized red blood cells are the same as those for washed packed red blood cells.

Modified During Infusion: Leukocyte-Filtered Red Blood Cells

This modified product is indicated for patients who have experienced repeated febrile non-hemolytic reactions associated with the transfusion of red cells or platelets (see later, Adverse Effects: Immediate). In addition, leukocyte-filtered red cells and platelets should be used as prophylaxis against alloimmunization in selected patients who are expected to receive long-term blood component therapy.

Leukocyte-reduced packed cells can be prepared in the blood bank by centrifugation and filtration, as well as by automated saline washing of liquid or previously frozen blood. Until rather recently, frozen and washed packed cells, which have a 95 to 99% reduction in leukocytes, were considered the components of choice when white blood cell reduction was indicated. However, the new generation of in-line leukocyte filters used during transfusion, is more efficient and less costly. These filters eliminate 99 to 99.9% of leukocytes from red cell or platelet suspensions.[10–12]

Clinical applications for leukocyte-filtered red blood cells include the following:

● Patients with repeated, febrile, nonhemolytic transfusion reactions
● Patients at risk for HLA alloimmunization who may face future hemotherapy
● Patients at risk for post-transfusion cytomegalovirus infection

Fresh-Frozen Plasma

Fresh-frozen plasma (FFP) is prepared by removing the plasma from a unit of whole blood and freezing it within 6 hours of collection. The storage time for FFP is 1 year at −18 C or below. This component, if kept frozen and then thawed in a warm water bath (30 to 37 C) just before use, is an excellent source of all clotting factors, including the labile factors V and VIII, as well as fibrinogen. The activity of these labile factors is lost when plasma is stored in the non-frozen state.[1]

Fresh-frozen plasma is indicated when clotting factors are needed for which a concentrate is not available, in the presence of severe liver disease in which limited synthesis of plasma coagulation factors may be suspected, and if needed to counteract the effects of warfarin therapy.

Clinical applications for fresh-frozen plasma include the following:

● For patients with active bleeding who have multiple coagulation factor deficiencies secondary to liver disease
● For patients with disseminated intravascular coagulation (DIC) and evidence of demonstrated dilutional coagulopathy from large-volume replacement

● For patients with congenital factor deficiencies for which there are no concentrates (e.g., factors V and XI)
● For warfarin reversal

Platelet Concentrates

Platelet concentrates can be prepared by two methods; as single units from multiple donors or as multiple units from a single donor.

Multiple Donors, Single Units

1. A freshly donated unit of whole blood less than 6 hours old and kept at room temperature is centrifuged to separate off the platelet-rich plasma.
2. The platelet-rich plasma is then centrifuged at 20 C to separate off all except 50 to 70 ml of the now platelet-poor plasma.
3. After this second centrifugation, that which remains is a single unit of random-donor platelets suspended in plasma. These 50 to 70 ml of plasma ensure that the platelets are kept at a pH of 6 or higher to maintain their viability during the 5-day storage period at 20 to 24 C.

Single Donor, Multiple Units

Plateletpheresis is the harvesting of multiple units of platelets from a single volunteer donor. The quantity taken from a single donor is approximately equal to six units of random-donor platelets. This can be accomplished through the use of automated machines called cell separators. There are two types of cell separators, intermittent flow and continuous flow. Each system has its advantages and disadvantages, but they both accomplish the same objective. Cell separators isolate blood components so that the desired component may be harvested as a concentrate, and those components not needed are returned to the donor.

Although plateletpheresis is an efficient way to obtain supplies of platelets, there are two reasons why this method is not used exclusively to obtain this component. There are risks to the donor, including but not limited to allergic reactions, chills, syncope, and citrate toxicity. The citrate toxicity is related to the anticoagulation of the donor blood that is necessary before it is processed through the cell separator.[2] This anticoagulant, in varying amounts, is ultimately infused along with the returned components to the donor. The second reason that plateletpheresis is limited in use is that there continues to be significant controversy over its cost-versus-benefit ratio.

Single-donor platelets have been used for patients who need repeated platelet infusions and are at risk for alloimmunization to foreign leukocyte antigens (HLAs) that are present on leukocytes and platelets. It has been widely accepted that the risk for alloimmunization increases with the increasing number of donors to whom the recipient is exposed. Therefore, for those at risk, the single-donor option reduces the recipient's donor exposures from six to one with the use of each single-donor unit. However, there is an increasing amount of evidence that appears to support the idea that it is not the number of donor exposures, but rather the number of allogenic donor leukocytes, which plays the major role in HLA alloimmunization and platelet refractoriness.[1, 13]

Refractoriness is the state of being unresponsive to platelet transfusions. The post-transfusion platelet count shows little improvement, if any, because previously acquired HLA antibodies immediately destroy the infused platelets. This situation creates significant obstacles to the successful treatment of thrombocytopenia. Therefore, refractoriness needs to be avoided because, once it is established, it is not easily circumvented. It appears that the route to avoiding this problem is to diminish the risk for alloimmunization.[2] This could be accomplished to a great degree if future technology provides for leukocyte-eliminating filters or techniques.

The most suitable single-donor platelet preparation is the HLA-matched product that is obtained by plateletpheresis from a volunteer donor who is HLA-matched to a specific recipient. Although this is a limited match (i.e., donor and recipient have only some HLA antigens in common), HLA-matched platelets may be considered for individuals who demonstrate unresponsiveness to random-donor and single-donor unmatched concentrates.

In a comparison study of the platelet products relating to post-transfusion nonhemolytic febrile reactions, Chambers and colleagues[14] found a 21.4% post-transfusion febrile reaction rate when multi-donor platelets were given, an 8.4% reaction rate with unmatched single-donor platelets, and a 4.9% reaction rate with an HLA-matched single-donor product (Table 10–6). This study concluded that there is little doubt that single-donor products are superior to the random-donor concentrates in limiting post-transfusion immunologic responses. However, the narrow margin of reaction rates between the matched and unmatched single-donor preparations favor using single-donor unmatched platelets as the component of choice unless the refractory state has been reached and HLA matching might be unavoidable.

In practice, probably because of the increased cost of the single-donor preparations, random-donor pooled platelets are used until unresponsiveness to transfusion becomes apparent.

Cryoprecipitate

Cryoprecipitated antihemolytic factor is prepared by slowly thawing a unit of fresh-frozen plasma at 4 to 6 C and recovering the cold precipitated protein by centrifugation. Once harvested, the cryoprecipitate can be refrozen at − 18 C or below and stored for 1 year. This component is a rich source of the entire factor VIII complex (Table 10–7), factor XIII, and fibrinogen. It is the only source of concentrated fibrinogen.

Cryoprecipitate is used in the treatment of hemophilia A, von Willebrand's disease, hypofibrinogenemia, and factor XIII deficiency.

Table 10-6

Postplatelet Transfusion Febrile Reaction Rates

Platelet Preparation	Reaction Rate (%)
Random-donor, pooled	21.4
Single-donor, unmatched	8.4
Single-donor, HLA-matched	4.9

Table 10-7

Factor VIII Complex

Factor	Activity
VIII:C	Procoagulant
VIII:Ag	Immune reactant antigen
VIII:vWF	Von Willebrand's factor— required for normal platelet function

Hemophilia A (Classic Hemophilia). This sex-linked inherited disorder is manifest in males but is transmitted by female carriers. The clotting factor deficiency in classic hemophilia is factor VIII:C. In addition to using cryoprecipitate to correct this deficiency, commercial factor VIII concentrates also provide factor VIII:C.

Von Willebrand's Disease. This condition, the most common of the inherited coagulopathies (Table 10–8), is not sex-linked and affects both sexes. All three of the measurable activities of the factor VIII complex are deficient in von Willebrand's disease. However, it is the deficiency of factor VIII:vWF that is responsible for the capillary defect seen in this coagulopathy. Von Willebrand's factor is necessary for normal platelet function, and thus a diminished level of this factor results in platelet dysfunction characterized by capillary defect.

Most of the commercial factor VIII concentrates contain relatively small amounts of von Willebrand's factor and are therefore not effective in treating this disease. However, some newer concentrates are being used in the treatment of von Willebrand's syndrome.[2, 8, 15]

Hypofibrinogenemia. This deficiency may be inherited or may be acquired as part of the DIC syndrome.[1] Cryoprecipitate is the only source presently available for concentrated fibrinogen, so it is necessary if intervention is indicated to correct this deficiency.

Factor XIII Deficiency. This condition can have consequences that are as serious as those of hemophilia A or hemophilia B. It can be treated with cryoprecipitate or with pasteurized factor XIII concentrate prepared from plasma or placenta.[2, 16, 17]

ADMINISTRATION OF BLOOD COMPONENTS

Administering a blood component is the last step in the process of matching a donor component with a recipient in need. Remembering that the most common causes of fatal

Table 10-8

Inherited Coagulopathies

Type	Factor Deficiency
Hemophilia A (classic hemophilia)	VIII: C
Hemophilia B (Christmas disease)	IX
Von Willebrand's disease (vascular hemophilia, angiohemophilia)	VIII: C, VIII: Ag, VIII: vWF

transfusion reactions are an improperly labeled blood sample, a mislabeled component unit, and a misidentified recipient-patient, it is clear that the majority of errors that result in fatality surrounding transfusion are clerical rather than laboratory failures. The transfusionist is in the position of being the last person in the chain with the opportunity to discover a clerical error, and should be attentive to every detail of the administration procedure and guard against the relaxed posture that so often accompanies familiarity.

The policies and procedures for the administration of blood components vary greatly among providers of this therapy. However, the purpose for all policies and procedures, which is to ensure precision and safety, is universal. Therefore, those who administer transfusion therapy should be knowledgeable of policy and adhere strictly to the procedures embraced by their particular institution or home care provider.

Basic Guidelines for Blood Administration

1. Gloves should be worn when handling blood products.
2. Blood should not be out of controlled refrigeration for longer than 30 minutes without being initiated as a transfusion.
3. Blood should not be stored in nonblood bank refrigerators because they are subject to vast fluctuations in temperature.
4. No intravenous solution other than isotonic saline (0.9%) should be added to or administered simultaneously with blood.
5. A blood administration set should not be affixed ("piggybacked") into a main line that has been used for any solution other than isotonic saline.
6. All blood components must be filtered using in-line or add-on filters that are appropriate for the component or specifically requested by a physician's order.
7. A new administration set and filter should be used for each transfusion. A blood filter should not be used for more than 4 hours.[1]

Table 10–9 presents a detailed summary of blood components, including their preparation, indications for use, blood type compatibility, administration, and special considerations.

SPECIAL EQUIPMENT

Blood Warmers

Blood warming during transfusion is recommended in limited situations. This can be accomplished by using any one of several commercial instruments that were designed for this purpose. Most of these instruments consist of dry heating blocks or controlled water baths that surround a portion of the infusion tubing downstream from the blood supply and immediately prior to the infusion site.

Blood warming should not be attempted by using uncontrolled measures such as holding the unit of blood under hot water or subjecting it to warming in a microwave oven. Such

severe treatment of the blood cells can result in hemolysis and/or severe reactions. The AABB recommends that blood not be heated beyond 38 C (104 F).[7]

All blood warmers are designed to help transfer heat. The efficiency of this heat transfer depends on several factors:

1. The temperature of the heating element (flat bed or water bath)
2. The surface area of the heating element
3. The diameter and surface area of the tubing being used to deliver the blood
4. The length of time the blood being infused remains in contact with the heat source

If any of these factors (temperature, surface area, or duration of contact) are changed, the efficiency of the heat transfer is altered. Therefore, in cases in which rapid infusion is necessary, a speeding up of the infusion rate reduces the time the blood is in contact with the heating element, and the efficiency of the heat transfer is also reduced.

Indications for Blood Warming

Multiple Trauma-Massive Blood Loss. Hypothermia is a serious threat for the patient who has lost large quantities of blood and requires multiple transfusions of refrigerated blood. A decrease in the body temperature at the SA node to 86 F (30 C) can precipitate cardiac arrhythmia and cardiac arrest.[1] Therefore, when large quantities are to be infused rapidly, blood warming is indicated. This is especially true if the infusion is through a central catheter. However, the present generation of blood warmers has been criticized for slow heat transfer and suboptimal flow rates in this setting. This has led to the evaluation of newer technologies that use increased temperatures to accomplish the delivery of adequate volume and warming of the blood.[18] Additionally, another technique called rapid admixture has been reported.[19] This involves keeping a normal saline IV solution stored in a clinical incubator at 70 C. When needed, the warmed bag of saline (250 ml) is connected directly to the unit of packed cells to be infused and the saline is squeezed into the blood bag. This warms the blood to 37 C in less than one minute.

Cold Agglutinin Disease. These cold-loving autoantibodies correspond to the carbohydrate antigens I and i, which are found on human red blood cells.[8] Many otherwise normal individuals have some anti-I in their serum, which can be demonstrated when tests are done at 4 C. This antibody, if present, is usually found at low titers and does not cause hemolysis. However, cold agglutinin hemolysis occurs both as a self-limited syndrome in association with certain infectious diseases and as a chronic illness, often without cause. Sometimes, however, it is seen to accompany lymphoma and other reticuloendothelial malignancies. The anti-I titers seen in cases of hemolysis are high and red cell destruction can occur either extravascularly, within the phagocytic cells or intravascularly, leading to hemoglobinemia.

The trigger for the activation of the anti-I to bind with the antigen on the red blood cell, and thus cause hemolysis, is exposure to cold temperatures. Therefore, individuals who may need a blood transfusion and who are known to carry a significant titer of anti-I should be transfused using an in-line blood warmer.

Summary of Blood Components[1, 20, 132]

Component	Preparation and Composition	Use and Indications	ABO-Rh Compatibility		Administration	Special Considerations
			Donor	**Recipient**		
Whole blood	RBCs, white blood cells (WBCs), plasma, platelets (WBCs, platelets, and some clotting factors not viable after 24 hours of storage)	Increases red blood cell mass, increases volume	O A B AB Rh+ Rh−	O A B AB Rh+ Rh−, Rh+	Transfuse through blood filter; infuse within 4 hours	One unit of whole blood increases hemotocrit (Hct) by 3%; increases hemoglobin (Hgb) by 1 g/dL; availability of packed red cells has made use of whole blood obsolete in most cases; never infuse blood with anything except 0.9% saline
			Donor	**Recipient**		
Packed red blood cells (PRBCs)	RBCs, WBCs, platelets, minimal plasma	Increase red blood cell mass and oxygen-carrying capacity	O A B AB Rh+ Rh−	O, A, B, AB A, AB B, AB AB Rh+ Rh−, Rh+	Transfuse through blood filter; infuse within 4 hours	Hct of product is 60–80%; one unit of RBCs increases Hct by 3%; increases Hgb by 1 g/dL; never infuse PRBCs with anything except 0.9% saline
Red blood cells (RBCs) Leukocyte-reduced	RBCs, negligible WBCs, minimal plasma and platelets	Same as PRBCs plus: decreases risk for alloimmunization (HLA) and disease transmission (CMV)	Same as PRBCs		If not processed in blood bank, use in-line or add-on leukocyte reduction filter	Leukocyte reduction filter for RBCs *not* interchangeable with leukocyte reduction filter for platelets; other considerations are same as above for PRBCs
Red blood cells Saline-washed	RBCs, minimal WBCs, no plasma, no platelets	Same as for PRBCs plus decrease risk for alloimmunization to leukocyte or HLA antigens, reduce incidence of urticarial and anaphylactic reactions to plasma proteins	Same as PRBCs		Same as PRBCs	Unit must be given within 24 hours of saline washing; never infuse RBCs with any IV fluid or medications except 0.9% saline; Hct of product is 70–80%; contains viable lymphocytes and can induce GVHD
Red blood cells Frozen-deglycerolized	Same as washed red blood cells	Same as PRBCs plus prolonged blood storage of autologous blood and rare blood types	Same as RBCs		Same as PRBCs	Blood may be frozen up to 10 years; once blood has been thawed and deglycerolized, must be transfused within 24 hours; Hct of product is 70–80%
			Donor	**Recipient**		
Fresh-frozen plasma (FFP)	Plasma, all clotting factors	Treatment of some coagulation disorders; reversal of warfarin in patients who require emergency invasive procedures	O A B AB Rh+ Rh−	O A, O B, O AB, O, A, B Rh+, Rh− Rh−, Rh+	Transfuse through blood filter	Must be infused within 24 hours of thawing, may be stored for up to 1 year at −18 C
Platelets Random donor	Platelets, plasma, small numbers of RBCs and WBCs	To control or prevent bleeding associated with deficiencies in platelet number or function; not usually effective in conditions of rapid platelet destruction (e.g., ITP and DIC)	ABO-Rh compatibility is preferred (because of RBCs in product), but not mandatory; an Rh− female in childbearing years should receive Rh− platelets—if she receives Rh+ platelets, titers should be monitored and/or consideration given for administration of Rh immune globulin		Transfuse through blood filter; once individual units are pooled, should be infused within 6 hours; concentrates may be infused individually, or pooled immediately before administration	Prophylactic pretransfusion medications (e.g., antihistamine and/or acetaminophen) may be given to patient to decrease incidence of chills, fever, and allergic reactions; repeated transfusions may lead to alloimmunization to HLA and other antigens and result in development of a "refractory" state manifested by unresponsiveness to platelet transfusion; leukocyte reduction filter for platelets may be used; one unit of platelets should increase platelet count of 70-kg adult by 5000/μl
Apheresed	Platelets (one unit equivalent to six random-donor units), some RBCs, WBCs, and plasma	Same as random-donor platelets; may be used in nonrefractory patients to limit multiple random donor exposures, especially in long-term chemotherapy	Same as random-donor platelets	Same as random-donor platelets	Prophylactic pretransfusion medications may be given; leukocyte reduction filter for platelets may be used
HLA-matched	Same as apheresed platelets, but with some donor HLA antigens in common with recipient	Same as random-donor platelets; used for patients unresponsive to random-donor platelet concentrates because of HLA alloimmunization; may be used in patients being considered for future transplantation	Same as random-donor platelets	Same as random-donor platelets	Prophylactic pretransfusion medications may be given; leukocyte reduction filter for platelets may be used; advance scheduling to obtain HLA-matched platelets usually required; blood sample for HLA typing should be drawn before immunosuppressive therapy is started—leukopenia can make HLA typing difficult

Table continued on following page

173

Table 10-9

Summary of Blood Components[1, 20, 132] *Continued*

Component	Preparation and Composition	Use and Indications	ABO-Rh Compatibility		Administration	Special Considerations
			Donor	Recipient		
Granulocytes	Granulocytes, varying amounts of lymphocytes, RBCs, platelets; all of these are suspended in 200–300 ml of plasma	Treatment of patients with neutropenia or WBC dysfunction with a serious infection unresponsive to conventional antibiotic therapy	O A B AB Rh+ Rh−	O, A, B, AB A, AB B, AB AB Rh+ Rh−, Rh+	Transfuse through blood filter; should be administered ASAP after collection, within 24 hours of collection	Use of prophylactic pretransfusion medications strongly urged (e.g., antihistamines, acetaminophen, steroids, meperidine); slow infusion over 4 hours recommended
			Donor	Recipient		
Cryoprecipitate	Factor VIII, von Willebrand's factor, factor XIII, fibrinogen (suspended in plasma and frozen)	Treatment of deficiencies of factor VIII (hemophilia A), factor XIII, and fibrinogen; treatment of von Willebrand's disease	O A B AB Rh+ Rh−	O A, O B, O AB, O, A, B Rh+, Rh− Rh−, Rh+	Transfuse through blood filter; may be infused as single units or pooled	Saline 0.9% may need to be added to each bag of cryoprecipitate to facilitate recovery of product (only 10–15 ml of cryoprecipitate/plasma in each bag); must be infused within 6 hours of thawing or 4 hours of pooling
Factor VIII concentrate	Lyophilized concentration of factor VIII, trace amount of other plasma proteins	Factor VIII deficiency (hemophilia A); some of the newer concentrates can be used in von Willebrand's disease	Not required		Quantity of factor VIII present in each vial noted as international units (IU); reconstituted with sterile diluent; IV injected using filter needle or given by intravenous IV drip using a component recipient set	May be used prophylactically before therapeutic procedures; risk of transmission of infectious disease is reduced, but not eliminated by processing[17]
Factor IX concentrate	Lyophilized concentration of factor IX	Factor IX deficiency (hemophilia B), also known as Christmas disease	Not required		Quantity of factor IX present in each vial noted as activity units; reconstituted with sterile diluent; IV injected using filter needle or given as IV drip using component recipient set	Risk of transmission of infectious disease reduced but not eliminated by processing
Albumin	96% albumin; 4% globulin and other plasma proteins; available as 5% or 25% solution	Volume expansion when crystalloid solutions are not adequate; treatment of hypoproteinemia	Not required		5% solution is isotonic; 25% solution is hypertonic, increases circulating volume by 4–5 times infused volume; infuse *slowly*	Does not transmit viral diseases because of extended heating period during processing
Immune serum globulin: nonspecific	IgG antibodies	Provides passive immune protection; treatment of hypogammaglobulinemia	Not required		May be given IM or IV, but various preparations are route-of-administration-specific	Intramuscular injections may be painful, warm compresses may alleviate discomfort; possibility of hypersensitivity and anaphylactic reactions
Rh immune globulin	IgG anti-D	Administered to Rh− patients who have been exposed to Rh (D) antigens through transfusions; administered to Rh− women who have been exposed to Rh (D) antigens through pregnancy—prevents hemolytic disease of the newborn in a subsequent pregnancy	Same as for nonspecific immune serum globulin		Same as for nonspecific immune serum globulin	Should be given within 72 hours of exposure for maximum effect; intramuscular injections may be painful—warm compresses may alleviate discomfort
Hepatitis B immune globulin	High titers of hepatitis B antibody	Provides passive immunity following exposure to hepatitis B virus	Not required		Same as for nonspecific immune serum globulin	Should be given within 72 hours of exposure for maximum effect; intramuscular injections may be painful—warm compresses may alleviate discomfort

In addition, exchange transfusions in infants and rapid transfusion in children (over 15 ml/kg/hour)[20] are situations that warrant the use of blood warmers.

Specialized Blood Filters

Blood filters are generally used to eliminate blood clots and cellular debris of storage from the infusing blood component. The size of the particles being filtered out is determined by the micron pore size of the filter. A standard blood filter of 170 μ traps particles that are 170 μ or larger. However, microaggregates, which are composed of degenerating platelets, leukocytes, and fibrin strands, range in size from 20 to 160 μ.[1] Some of these microaggregates, which form in blood after five days or more of storage, can pass through standard blood filters without difficulty. Therefore, when it is deemed medically necessary to eliminate debris smaller than 80 to 170 μ, specialized filters have to be used.

Microaggregate Filters. These filters eliminate debris as small as 20 to 40 μ or larger. They are used routinely during cardiopulmonary bypass[1] and often during large-volume replacement in massive trauma. The use of these specialized filters is not considered warranted in routine transfusion therapy.

Leukocyte Reduction Filters. These filters were first developed in Europe in the 1970s. The original filter material was cotton wool, which was later replaced by cellulose acetate fibers. Today, the most widely used leukocyte reduction filters are a flatbed, multilayered design using polyester fibers to provide the filter network. This latest generation is reported to remove 99 to 99.9% of WBCs from red cells or platelet suspensions.[10, 21]

There are widely recognized reasons for the use of leukocyte reduction filters:

1. To circumvent or prevent HLA alloimmunization. The minimum dose of WBCs capable of stimulating antibody production is unknown. Although using leukocyte-filtered components may reduce but not completely eliminate the risk for alloimmunization,[11] the filtered product carries the lowest level of residual leukocytes.
2. To reduce the risk for cytomegalovirus (CMV) transmission. Transfusion-associated CMV (TACMV) infections have been linked to the transfused peripheral blood leukocytes in which the virus establishes latent infection.[22, 23] In addition to reducing the risk for CMV transmission, WBC filters have been linked in theory to reductions in another post-transfusion viral infection, human T-cell leukemia-lymphoma virus type I (HTLV-I).[24–26]

Prestorage filtration to reduce leukocytes has been advocated for the following:

1. Reducing the risk for transfusion-associated Yersina enterocolitica transmission[27]
2. Extending platelet life (disintegrating WBCs during storage may release hydrolytic enzymes, which can damage platelet membranes)[28]
3. Producing a superior quality of packed cells that are WBC-reduced and microaggregate-free[29]

ADVERSE EFFECTS

From the standpoint of disease transmission, blood component therapy has never been safer than it is today. With the new technologies in filtration, cell separation, and cell salvaging for autotransfusion, never have so many options been available for hemotherapy. It is, however, a double-edged sword. Blood component therapy has the potential to deliver great therapeutic benefit while at the same time it is known to carry significant risks, only some of which are preventable. The balance of these two, risk versus benefit, should always be weighted toward the therapeutic benefit.

The adverse effects of blood transfusion can be classified as immunologic or nonimmunologic depending on whether there is a triggering of the immune system. Additionally, they may be divided into categories of immediate and delayed effects. Immediate effects are those that occur within the first 48 hours of transfusion. Delayed effects are those that can appear at any time beyond the immediate time frame.

Immediate Effects

Immediate adverse effects of blood transfusion can be immunologic or nonimmunologic (Table 10–10).

Immunologic Classification

Intravascular Hemolysis. The cause of this potentially fatal reaction is ABO incompatibility. The ABO antibodies fix complement efficiently, and this undesirable event proceeds quickly. Because mortality has been associated with intravascular hemolysis, its rapid recognition and immediate intervention can avoid the need for dialysis in the face of renal failure (see Table 10–10 for signs and symptoms).

The most common causes for ABO incompatibility are an improperly labeled pretransfusion blood sample for type and crossmatching, an improperly identified donor unit, *or* an improperly identified recipient. Unfortunately, these are all avoidable errors, and the intravascular hemolytic reaction, which is the primary cause of transfusion-associated death,[30] is also the most preventable. The following steps should be taken if a hemolytic reaction is suspected:[1, 20]

Procedure to Follow if Hemolytic Reaction Is Suspected

1. **STOP TRANSFUSION.** Take down the blood and all tubing involved. Attach a new bag of saline using all new administration equipment to the IV catheter and *keep the IV open.*
2. Notify the physician and the blood bank immediately.
3. Check the blood bag compatibility tag, label, and patient identification for clerical errors.
4. Send anticoagulated and clotted blood samples, a blood transfusion reaction form (if applicable), and blood bag to the blood bank. The blood bank may also request a freshly collected urine sample.
5. The physician may order blood urea nitrogen (BUN), creatinine, and coagulation studies.

Table 10–10

Immediate Transfusion Reactions

Reaction	Cause	Signs and Symptoms	Treatment
Intravascular hemolysis	ABO incompatibility	Fever, low back pain, pain at IV site, hypotension, renal failure	Support blood pressure, maintain urine output, dialyze for renal failure
Extravascular hemolysis	Non-ABO incompatibility (e.g., Rh, Kidd, Kell)	Fever, anemia, increased bilirubin, positive DAT	Geared to signs and symptoms, which can resemble those of intravascular hemolysis but seldom as severe
Febrile nonhemolytic (FNH)	WBC antigen-antibody reaction	Fever, chills, rigors	Antipyretics; with history of FNH, pretreat with antipyretics
Transfusion-related acute lung injury (TRALI)	Anti-HLA antibodies	Acute respiratory insufficiency, chills, fever, cyanosis, hypotension	Respiratory support; IV steroids
Allergic	Antibodies against foreign plasma protein	Urticaria	Oral or IM antihistamines
Secondary response—anaphylaxis	Absent IgA and high-titer anti-IgA antibodies	Flushing, dyspnea, hypotension	Blood pressure support; epinephrine
Bacterial contamination	Most severe: gram-negative psychrophilic organisms (endotoxin-producing)	Fever, shock, DIC, renal failure	High-dose antibiotics; blood pressure support; steroids

Extravascular Hemolysis. This hemolytic event is caused by the presence of antibodies to blood group systems other than ABO, such as Rh, Kidd, Kell, or Duffy. The antibodies do not cause immediate hemolysis within the vascular tree but bind with the corresponding antigen-carrying red cells. These cells are then seen as ''defective'' by the body and destroyed extravascularly. This hemolysis is not as rapid as that seen in ABO incompatibility, and the signs and symptoms are usually less dramatic. The post-transfusion direct antiglobulin test is positive because of the coating of the red cells with antibodies in vivo.

Febrile Nonhemolytic Reaction. A febrile nonhemolytic reaction (FNH) is defined as a temperature rise of 1 C or more occurring in association with transfusion and without any other explanation.[1] A common cause for this event is an antigen-antibody response involving HLA-antigens on donor white cells in conflict with antibodies in the recipient. The outward appearance of this reaction, which can include significant temperature rise often accompanied by rigors, can be dramatic and be unnerving to the blood recipient. However, the signs and symptoms of this reaction are usually self-limiting.

FNH reactions are usually seen in recipients who have a history of multiple transfusions or multiple pregnancies and have developed a significant HLA antibody titer. For individuals who have experienced two or more of these reactions, leukocyte-filtered products should be considered for future transfusions.

Transfusion-Related Acute Lung Injury (TRALI). This is the most severe transfusion reaction caused by leukocyte antibodies, and probably occurs more frequently than is reported. The offending antibodies can be found in recipient plasma but, in almost 90% of cases, the antibodies that precipitate this event are found in the donor plasma.[31] The donor group with the highest potential for harboring leukocyte antibodies is multiparous women.

Although not completely understood, there appear to be two mechanisms by which this immune response precipitates

symptoms of acute respiratory insufficiency without evidence of heart failure:

1. The leukocyte antigen-antibody reaction produces white cell aggregates large enough to be trapped in the pulmonary microvasculature, producing transient changes in the vascular permeability, with resultant pulmonary edema.[1, 32]
2. The immune response may activate complement, which results in the release of histamine and serotonin. Both these substances, which participate in smooth muscle constriction and increased vascular permeability, could be active contributors to respiratory distress and pulmonary edema.

In most cases, if TRALI is recognized early and is treated promptly with vigorous respiratory support, this potentially disastrous post-transfusion event recedes within 48 to 96 hours.[31, 33] TRALI is accompanied by a mortality rate of approximately 5%.[31, 34] Table 10–10 presents the signs, symptoms, and appropriate interventions.

TRALI is not often recurrent. If it does occur more than once in the same person, it should be assumed that the antibodies are in the recipient and the precipitating factor is the donor leukocytes. In these cases, future transfusions should be leukocyte-filtered.[8]

Urticaria. This immediate type of hypersensitivity reaction is usually seen following a transfusion with plasma or blood components that is accompanied by a large volume of plasma (e.g., whole blood or platelet concentrates). The cause of this reaction is thought to be a foreign plasma protein to which the recipient responds with an allergic display.

If the signs and symptoms do not broaden beyond simple urticaria, the physician may opt to interrupt the transfusion long enough to administer an antihistamine by intravenous injection, wait for the symptoms to recede, and proceed slowly with the transfusion. Seldom does the clinical picture of an urticarial reaction warrant the termination of the transfusion. If a patient has a history of multiple allergic reactions to transfusion, pretreatment with an antihistamine may be considered appropriate.

Secondary Response: Anaphylaxis. The secondary or anamnestic response almost always occurs in individuals who have been sensitized (i.e., carry an antibody titer) to a foreign protein. The anaphylactic reaction occurs quickly and can quickly proceed to life-threatening shock.

The following features of the anaphylactic reaction distinguish it from other immediate responses:

1. Occurs after the infusion of only a few milliliters of blood or plasma
2. Occurs in the absence of fever

The array of symptoms that may accompany the secondary response are respiratory distress, bronchospasm, abdominal cramps, nausea, vomiting, diarrhea, shock, and loss of consciousness.[1]

Some of these reactions occur in IgA-deficient individuals who, through previous transfusion or pregnancy, have developed an anti-IgA titer. When these individuals are given blood products that contain IgA, the secondary response may be precipitated. It is possible to obtain blood components from donors who are IgA-deficient. However, most authorities recommend that these components be reserved for individuals in whom anti-IgA has been identified and who have had previous documented anaphylactic reactions.[1]

Nonimmunologic Classification

Marked Fever With Shock. This complication of transfusion therapy is caused by bacterial contamination of donated blood, which can occur at any time during the harvesting and processing.[35, 36] Mesophilic (warm-loving) organisms proliferate best in components that are stored at room temperature, whereas psychrophils (cold-loving) multiply best at refrigerator temperature. It is the gram-negative psychrophils that are responsible for the most clinically dramatic and life-threatening septicemic transfusion reactions. These severe reactions are characterized by high fever, hypotension, DIC, and renal failure. To avert a fatal outcome, these reactions require immediate intervention with high-dose intravenous antibiotics combined with therapy for shock, including steroids and vasopressors.[1]

Nonimmune Hemolysis. Most cases of this category of hemolysis are related to improper handling of the blood product during processing, storage, or administration. Nonimmune hemolysis can result from the following:

1. Red cell exposure to nonisotonic IV solutions
2. Improper storage: nonglycerolized freezing or overheating
3. Mechanical stress: small-bore infusion catheter, roller pump (cardiac bypass), improper PSI pressure infusion pump, blood bag pressure cuff

Miscellaneous Adverse Effects

Circulatory Overload. Post-transfusion congestive heart failure is usually seen in individuals who are already cardiac or pulmonary decompensated. However, high infusion rates or large-volume replacement can precipitate decompensation in those who are borderline unstable.

Air Embolism. This rarely seen event can occur with improper manipulation of administration equipment during transfusion through a central access. If an administration set is disconnected from a central line without that line being clamped or the Valsalva maneuver being used, atmospheric pressure that supersedes central venous pressure can be responsible for the introduction of air into the central circulation. This can also occur when improper technique or equipment is used to infuse blood under manual or mechanical pressure.

Hypothermia. This complication is seen with rapid infusion of large volumes of refrigerated blood. (See later for a description of the potential consequences, Specialized Equipment: Blood Warmers.)

Citrate Overload: Hypocalcemia. Citrate is metabolized by the liver, and blood recipients with liver impairment may be unable to handle the high citrate load that accompanies large-volume transfusion. As the plasma level of citrate rises, it binds with free calcium and a secondary hypocalcemia results. Depending on the severity of the calcium deficit, the calcium may be replaced by oral supplement or intravenous infusion.

Hyperkalemia. When red cells are stored in the cold, the potassium content of the cells decreases and that of the plasma increases. This is caused by cellular disintegration, with resultant potassium release. Therefore, the longer the blood is stored, the higher is the extracellular level of potassium. In red cell concentrates prepared from CPDA-1 whole blood, the plasma potassium level rises from 5.1 to 78.5 mmol/liter within the 35-day storage period.

Potassium toxicity that causes ventricular fibrillation is a rare complication of transfusion. It depends on the number of units given and their storage age, as well as on the pretransfusion potassium status of the recipient. In practice, apart from special circumstances in which large amounts of blood are infused rapidly, potassium toxicity needs be considered only when transfusing patients whose plasma potassium concentration is already elevated (e.g., anuric patients with extensive wounds involving muscle).[2]

Delayed Effects

Delayed adverse effects of blood transfusion can be immunologic or nonimmunologic.

Immunologic Classification

Graft-Versus-Host Disease. Graft-versus-host disease (GVHD) is a well recognized but rare complication of transfusion therapy. It is most frequently caused by the infusion of immunocompetent lymphocytes into a severely immunosuppressed recipient. Historically, those who have been viewed at highest risk for GVHD are those whose immune systems are suppressed for one of the following reasons:

1. Congenital immunodeficiency
2. Human immunodeficiency virus (HIV) infection
3. Premature birth

4. Immune suppression secondary to aggressive chemotherapy or radiation therapy in ongoing cancer treatments or intentional immune suppression in transplantation

Once infused, the immunocompetent lymphocytes engraft, multiply, and turn against the "foreign tissues" of the recipient-host. The resulting clinical picture of this immune response is dramatic, including fever, hepatitis, bone marrow suppression, and overwhelming infection progressing to an often fatal outcome. It has been reported that 75 to 90% of cases of transfusion-associated graft-versus-host disease (TA-GVHD) involve serious morbidity[37] and most reported cases have ended in mortality.[38] This is in contrast to the 10 to 15% mortality rate for GVHD following bone marrow transplantation.[39]

TA-GVHD can be prevented by pretransfusion irradiation of all blood products containing lymphocytes.[40] This radiation does not kill the donor lymphocytes but renders them incapable of replication in the recipient, thus eliminating an essential step in the graft-versus-host response. The minimum dose of radiation as set forth in the *Standards*[7] of the American Association of Blood Banks is 1500 cGy. However a broad range of dosages (1500 to 5000 cGy) are actually used at blood centers nationwide.[41, 42] Of sites surveyed by the Transfusion Practice Committee of the AABB, 74% used dosages of 1500 to 2500 cGy.[43]

When irradiation of red blood cells is needed, it is usually carried out as close to the time of transfusion as possible. Any unit of cells that is properly typed and crossmatched to the recipient is appropriate for this purpose without regard for its length of time in storage. Mature red blood cells are seen as relatively resistant to radiation damage at dosages less than 5000 cGy, and have a normal in vivo survival rate.[44] However, RBCs that are irradiated and subsequently stored at 4 C for 21 to 28 days show significant changes,[45] which can include the following:

1. Increased potassium (k^+) levels
2. Decreased red blood cell ATP levels
3. Decreased in vivo survival

Prestorage irradiation of packed cells has never been seen as optimal but has been recognized as necessary in situations in which immediate pretransfusion irradiation is not an option. There are two ways to accomplish the irradiation of PRBCs and their subsequent storage to meet the need for delayed infusion:

1. The cells can be irradiated and stored in their liquid state at 4 C. It is not recommended, however, that they be stored longer than 28 days because of their significantly lower post-transfusion cell recovery rates as compared to those in controls.[46]
2. The red cells may be irradiated immediately after donation, stored in the liquid state for up to 6 days, and then frozen for future use. A study by Drobyski and colleagues[47] demonstrated that exposure of red cells to irradiation before frozen storage does not significantly affect the in vitro or in vivo parameters of red cell function measured after deglycerolization. Additionally, the post-deglycerolization red cell recovery and the 24-hour in vivo survival of irradiated cells did not differ from those cells that were not irradiated.

A small number of cases of TA-GVHD have now been recognized in immunocompetent patients who received directed donation transfusions from first-degree relatives.[48, 49] The cause of this immune response seems to be the similar genetics shared by the donor and recipient. The donor lymphocytes are sufficiently similar not to be recognized as "foreign" by the recipient. However, with engraftment and proliferation of these donor cells, which are sufficiently dissimilar not to recognize the recipient as "self," the immune system is triggered and the natural cascade of events leads to the graft-versus-host response.[50]

Since 1989, the AABB has recommended the irradiation of all directed donations from first-degree relatives.[51] In addition, there are published data to support the position that this genetic mismatch form of TA-GVHD is a greater risk with second-degree relative donations.[52] Therefore, there is support for the irradiation of all directed donations from blood relatives of any degree.

Post-transfusion Purpura. Post-transfusion thrombocytopenic purpura[1] is a rare event related to the presence of a platelet-specific antibody. It is seen almost exclusively in multiparous women. The development of this antibody probably results from the sensitization during pregnancy of an antibody-negative woman, producing in a discernible antibody titer. Post-transfusion purpura is not a common occurrence, because 98% of the population already carries the precipitating antigen, leaving only 2% of the population at risk.

When an antibody-positive individual is transfused with antigen-positive platelets, the donor platelets are destroyed. In some recipients, their own antigen-negative platelets are destroyed, also leading to a clinical picture of severe thrombocytopenia. Although this condition is usually self-limiting, it can be severe enough to warrant exchange plasmapheresis. Continued infusion of platelets appears to be ineffective as a treatment, because the transfused platelets are destroyed as rapidly as they are given.

Nonimmunologic Classification: Transmitted Diseases

A blood transfusion is not a benign procedure. Although warnings concerning the "cookbook" approach of prescribing transfusions routinely for all patients exhibiting a hematocrit below a predetermined level dates back in the literature to at least the 1950s,[53] it is only rather recently that a significant reduction in the numbers of transfusions being given has been seen. In the present atmosphere of heightened awareness surrounding the adverse effects of hemotherapy, this trend comes as no surprise. It is interesting, however, that bloodborne diseases that have always carried with them significant morbidity and mortality were well known prior to the recognition of AIDS. Therefore, it seems that the precipitating factor for real change had to be something as potentially devastating as the risk for a disease that now appears to carry an eventual 100% mortality rate.

Diseases transmitted through blood transfusion are not limited to those with a viral cause, although viruses seem to be the center of attention. Diseases caused by bacteria and protozoa are well known as post-transfusion entities.

BACTERIAL INFECTIONS

Bacterial contamination of a donated unit of blood can have several causes: (1) pre-existing donor infection; (2)

contamination during the phlebotomy procedure; or (3) contamination during the processing of the donation. An estimated 13 million units of blood are collected annually in the United States. It is not known exactly how frequently the transfusion of one of these bloods endangers a life because of bacterial contamination. Because only fatality reports are mandated by the FDA, serious adverse effects resulting from a transfusion that was contaminated may not receive the attention they deserve unless a fatality occurs.[30]

During the years 1986 to 1991, 182 transfusion-related fatalities were reported to the FDA. Of these, 29 (15.9%) were caused by bacterial contamination. Of the 29 deaths, 8 were associated with red cell components and 7 of those 8 were attributed to the gram-negative coccobacillus Yersinia enterocolitica.[54, 55] Y. enterocolitica infection usually presents as gastrointestinal distress, including diarrhea, fever, and abdominal pain. However, infection with this organism can present a clinical picture that ranges from mild or nonexistent features to a severe scenario, including ulceration of the terminal ileum and septicemia that can mimic appendicitis.[56] There is no concern that a person in the acute phase of this infection would likely be a blood donor. However, because most cases of Y. enterocolitica resolve quickly, it is believed that this bacillus, having been phagocytized but not fully destroyed by the potential donor's white cells, are harbored in and transmitted by the donor white cells to the future recipient.

Another opportunity for contamination exists during the acquisition of the donor unit. An estimated 1 to 2% of percutaneously acquired blood samples are contaminated, primarily with components of the normal skin flora.[57] These organisms belong to a group called mesophiles, which exhibit an optimal growth temperature range of 30 to 44 C. They do not survive refrigerator temperature (4 to 6 C) well and are therefore not associated with post-transfusion bacteremias traceable to a component that was stored under refrigeration.

Platelets are stored at room temperature and thus pose a high risk for harboring and transmitting mesophiles. Although few in number, there are documented cases of post-transfusion septicemia resulting from platelet concentrates contaminated with organisms of the normal skin flora (most frequently Staphylococcus epidermidis and diphtheroid bacilli).[36, 58] These are the most frequent isolates from platelet concentrates, but many other organisms have been linked to postplatelet transfusion septic incidents.[59–61] Estimates of platelet concentrate contamination range from 1.6 to 2.5% for individual platelet units to 7.4 to 10.9% for fresh platelet pools.[62, 63] However, bacterial counts are usually low in the contaminated units and clinically recognized septicemia caused by platelet transfusion is rare.[62, 64] The duration of platelet storage seems to be the key factor in the risk of sepsis. Multidonor platelets stored for 5 days pose a five times greater risk for transfusion-associated sepsis than platelets stored for 4 days or less.[64] The frequency of concomitant antibiotic therapy that exists in the patient population requiring platelet infusions may contribute to the low incidence of reported clinical events.[36]

Psychrophiles are the opposite of mesophiles. These organisms have optimal growth temperatures around 29 C. However, they tolerate low temperatures and proliferate at a substantial rate, even at 0 C. The psychrophilic grouping of organisms includes predominantly pseudomonads and therefore presents a challenge to blood banking and transfusion therapy. In addition to their ability to survive refrigerator temperatures, pseudomonads can use citrate as their carbon source. The combination of the citrate-based anticoagulations preservative system and the refrigerator temperatures under which blood is stored provides a suitable environment in which these gram-negative organisms can flourish.

Transfusion-associated gram-negative sepsis, although extremely rare, has a potentially fatal outcome. The rapidly progressing clinical picture usually includes high fever, shock, DIC, and renal failure that requires immediate intervention. Treatment may include high-dose antibiotics and therapy to combat shock, including high-dose steroids and vasopressors.[1] In addition to Y. enterocolitica and the pseudomonads, other gram-negative organisms associated with post-transfusion septic shock have been Escherichia coli[59] and Salmonella.[60]

At one time, because syphilis is a bloodborne as well as a sexually transmitted disease, it was a notable post-transfusion complication. However, syphilis is now rarely seen secondary to blood transfusion for two major reasons:

1. All donated units are serologically tested for syphilis (mandated by the FDA).
2. Treponema pallidum is not likely to survive at 4 to 6 C for more than 72 hours. Therefore, only blood components stored at room temperature carry any risk of infection.[65]

PROTOZOAL INFECTIONS

Malaria. There are four species of malarial plasmodia in humans—Plasmodium vivax, P. ovale, P. malariae, and P. falciparum. The clinical presentation of the disease produced and the incubation periods differ by species. However, all share a life cycle stage in which the parasite resides within the host erythrocytes. It is during this erythrocytic cycle that the potential exists for transmission of the disease through blood transfusion.

The occurrence of post-transfusion malaria is uncommon, but it has risen over the past few decades because of increased world travel and immigration. However, because there is no practical screening test for malaria, exclusion of donors at high risk for harboring the parasite seems to be the only effective measure for prevention.[1] The estimated risk of acquiring malaria through a blood transfusion is 1:1,000,000/unit.[66]

Babesiosis. As in malaria, the causative agent of babesiosis is a protozoan, Babesia microti. This parasite, which is found mostly on the northeast coast of the United States with a concentration on Cape Cod and the islands of Massachusetts, has the northern deer tick as its vector. The clinical picture resulting from this infection can range from the mild febrile event seen in most cases to a severe and even fatal outcome, which has occurred when the infection is superimposed on immunosuppression or splenectomy.

Although not a frequent occurrence, babesiosis can be transmitted through blood transfusion for two reasons:

1. B. microti has an intraerythrocytic phase in its life cycle.
2. An individual infected with this parasite could be asymptomatic and donate blood.

The present risk for acquiring Babesiosis through a blood transfusion is 1:1,000,000/unit.[66]

Toxoplasmosis. Toxoplasmosis is found worldwide and is caused by the protozoan Toxoplasma gondii. Theoretically, this organism could be a concern in transfusion therapy for several reasons:

1. The parasitemia can persist beyond the acute illness in the asymptomatic, chronically infected individual[67] who could be a blood donor.
2. The organisms are infectious for most cells of warm-blooded animals, except the non-nucleated red blood cells.
3. These parasites can survive for many weeks in blood stored at 4 to 6 C.[67]

However, the only reported cases of post-transfusion toxoplasmosis have involved leukocyte concentrates administered to patients with malignancies and immunosuppression.[67, 68]

Chagas' Disease. Chagas' disease, or South American trypanosomiasis, is a life-threatening cardiac disease that is being seen with increasing frequency in the United States, particularly in states bordering Mexico. The agent of Chagas' disease is the protozoan Trypanosoma cruzi, which is a flagellate transmitted by blood-sucking insects. This parasite invades the macrophages of the host and is ultimately spread throughout the body. A small percentage of those infected develop symptoms of an acute illness, but most infected individuals remain asymptomatic. Chagas' disease is considered to be life-threatening throughout its three phases: acute, latent, and chronic. In the acute phase, mortality is most often secondary to congestive heart failure and meningoencephalitis. In the chronic phase of the disease, death has also frequently been seen as a result of lethal arrhythmia or thromboembolic complications.[69]

The characteristic of Chagas' disease that makes it a concern for transmission by blood transfusion is its high incidence of asymptomatic infection. This disturbing lack of symptoms is seen during the acute and latent phases of the illness. However, in reality, post-transfusion Chagas' disease is a rare event. Currently, the estimated risk for transfusion-acquired Chagas' disease is 1:1,000,000/unit.[66] This low risk can be maintained by continued diligence toward mandatory testing of donors from endemic areas as well as travelers to those areas.[70]

VIRAL INFECTIONS

With the identification of the human immunodeficiency virus (HIV) and the recognition of its impact on hemotherapy comes a renewed interest in post-transfusion disease of viral cause. The three virus groups of greatest concern in blood component therapy are the primary hepatic viruses, the herpesviruses, and the human T-cell lymphotropic viruses.

Primary Hepatic Viruses. Post-transfusion disease whose cause can be linked to the primary hepatic viruses has not been eradicated. However, its incidence has been significantly reduced because of the following changes and additions to procedures for blood acquisition and screening:

1. Routine serologic testing of donor units for hepatitis B viral markers (by federal mandate, 1972)
2. Routine testing for surrogate markers for possible non-A, non-B hepatitis—alanine aminotransferase and hepatitis B core antibody (AABB mandate, 1987)
3. Routine testing for antibodies to the hepatitis C virus (1990)
4. Moving to an all-volunteer blood donor force; paid donor groups were shown to be associated with a seven-fold higher incidence of post-transfusion hepatitis (PTH)[8]

With the additions to screening procedures and the more restrictive policies regarding blood donation, the current risk of post-transfusion hepatitis is about 3% for each unit transfused.[66, 71] This is in sharp contrast to the 33% incidence of PTH seen in the days of paid donors and prior to the introduction of testing for HBsAg, anti-HCV, and surrogate markers.[72]

The hepatitis virus family consists of five identified human pathogens—hepatitis A (HAV), hepatitis B (HBV), hepatitis C (HCV), hepatitis D (HDV, or delta agent), and hepatitis E (HEV). Not all members of this family are associated with post-transfusion hepatitis. However, a brief description of each is included here for completeness.

Hepatitis A. Hepatitis A is a single-stranded RNA virus. It was previously known as "infectious hepatitis" and is recognized as the most common type of hepatitis, with worldwide distribution. It is primarily spread by the fecal-oral route and is common in areas where sanitation is poor, especially in underdeveloped countries. There is, however, a significant incidence in the West. More than 90% of the people in underdeveloped countries have hepatitis A during their first 20 years of life, and at least 50% of urban-dwelling adults in developed countries such as the United States exhibit serologic evidence of prior HAV infection.[73]

Although the primary mode of transmission for HAV is the fecal-oral route, the virus has been reported on rare occasions to be the causative agent in cases of post-transfusion disease.[74, 75] Post-transfusion HAV infection is rare because HAV viremia is short-lived, hepatitis A does not progress to a chronic hepatitis and has no long-term carrier state, and immunity to HAV is lifelong after symptomatic or asymptomatic infection.[76]

Hepatitis B. The hepatitis B virus belongs to a group of viral agents called the hepadnaviruses, which are DNA viruses that attack liver cells. This intact virion has three areas of antigenic capability: (1) hepatitis B surface antigen (HBsAg), which is incorporated into the outer shell or envelope; (2) hepatitis B core antigen (HBcAg), which is the protein of the nucleocapsid; and (3) the less well understood hepatitis B core-related antigen (HBeAg), which is thought to be part of the virion core. Hepatitis B virus is synthesized in the hepatocytes only. HBcAg is formed in the nucleus of the hepatocyte and the HBsAg is synthesized in the cytoplasm. HBcAg leaves the nucleus and is coated with HBsAg as it passes through the cytoplasm.[76] The surface antigen produced is markedly greater than the amount required for assembly of the complete virus. This explains why HBsAg circulates in amounts 10^6 to 10^7 times greater than the complete virus in acute infection.[77] The host response to each hepatitis antigen is to produce specific and distinct antibodies to each.

Hepatitis acquired after exposure to infected blood during a transfusion or from infected needles or equipment is sometimes associated with hepatitis B. However, post-transfusion hepatitis B, which was once a frequent and greatly feared event with potentially fatal consequences, has been significantly reduced, but not eliminated. The CDC has estimated that the current post-transfusion risk for hepatitis B is 1:50,000 transfusion recipients and 1:200,000 transfused units.[1, 78] The incidence of hepatitis B in blood recipients is essentially equal to the incidence of clinical hepatitis B in those who have not received blood.[66]

Hepatitis C (non-A, non-B). The broad category of non-A, non-B (NANB) hepatitis has long been known as a cause of transfusion-associated disease. Prospective studies done in the 1970s and early 1980s estimated that the risk for post-transfusion NANB hepatitis is between 5 and 18%.[71, 79–81] At that time, the causative agents were unknown. However, they were suspected to be multiple and probably of viral origin.

Lacking a specific test for non-A, non-B hepatitis, in 1987 the AABB mandated the surrogate testing of all donated blood for elevated levels of the liver enzyme alanine aminotransferase (ALT) and for the presence of antibody to the hepatitis B core antigen (anti-HBcAg). These tests appear to detect different populations of donors potentially capable of transmitting NANB hepatitis,[1] and were added in an attempt to decrease the risk for hepatitis transmission.[82] Subsequent studies have shown that there was a decrease in transfusion-associated hepatitis after the implementation of surrogate testing.[1, 83]

The discovery that has had the greatest impact on lowering the incidence of PTH has been the identification of the hepatitis C virus (HCV). HCV is the predominant member of the broader category called non-A, non-B. Although there may still remain unknown entities that cause non-A, non-B hepatitis (called non-A, non-B, non-C), studies have indicated that at least 80% of cases of non-A, non-B hepatitis can be attributed to HCV.[71, 84]

Clinically, HCV infection usually presents a significantly less dramatic picture than HBV. Many of these infections are asymptomatic and can be detected only with liver function studies. However, 50% of cases of PT-HCV become chronic with evidence of moderate to severe liver disease, including cirrhosis. Fortunately, the frequency of this severe picture does not appear to be high, but hepatoma, liver failure, and death have been reported.[66]

In combination, surrogate testing and screening for antibodies to HCV have been reported to have reduced the risk of HCV seroconversion to 0.03%, or 3:10,000 units transfused.[71]

Hepatitis D (delta agent). The hepatitis D virus, also known as the delta agent, is a defective RNA virus that requires the hepatitis B coat to replicate. HDV consists of a single-stranded RNA core surrounded by an antigen protein (HDAg), all of which are enclosed in an outer shell of HBsAg. The RNA core and antigenic protein layer are transmissible as an independent agent but the delta virus can only infect and cause illness in the presence of HBV infection.[85] The clinical picture of HBV-HDV infection is almost always more severe than the presentation of hepatitis B alone. Additionally, the severity of the illness seems to depend on whether hepatitis B precedes the delta infection.[86]

Prevention of hepatitis D is an attainable goal in those individuals who are not hepatitis B carriers. The hepatitis B vaccine prevents the acquision of HBV infection and thereby indirectly prevents infection by hepatitis D.[77, 87] Health care workers should be encouraged to seek this protective route. Unfortunately for those who already harbor HBV, there is no easy pathway to ensure protection from a superinfection of HDV.

Hepatitis D can be transmitted by parenteral exposure. However, post-transfusion hepatitis D is not a common event.

Hepatitis E. The hepatitis E virus has been identified as the causative agent of a short-incubation, epidemic, enteric form of disease seen in individuals who have been exposed to fecally contaminated water. It is endemic to southwest Asia and Africa. It is usually a mild disease, except where the infection presents in the third trimester of pregnancy. In those cases, there has been a high mortality rate.[88]

Although HEV is spread by the fecal-oral route, this virus does not exhibit similar morphology to that of HAV. No carrier state or chronic liver disease has been associated with hepatitis E infection, and it is not a concern in transfusion therapy.

Herpesviruses. The human herpesvirus family includes herpes simplex virus (HSV) 1 and 2, varicella-zoster virus (VZV), cytomegalovirus (CMV), and Epstein-Barr virus (EBV). All members of this family are large, enveloped DNA viruses that are known to establish latent infections with the potential for reactivation after varying periods.[26] Latent, slow, and chronic infections are the three categories of persistence. The ability to establish persistence is the hallmark of most transfusion-transmitted viruses.[89] However, although all members of this family show persistence, not all present a risk for post-transfusion infection.

Herpes Simplex Virus (HSV). Neither HSV-1 or HSV-2 has been associated with post-transfusion infection. The primary infection with either of these viruses is a local event that does not usually extend beyond the neighboring lymph nodes that drain the eruption site. HSV viremia is seen during primary infections, which usually occur in childhood. Most adults carry the antibody to HSV, and adult primary infection is uncommon. Therefore, the viremia that would be necessary for this infection to be transmitted through a blood transfusion rarely occurs. The exception to this would be in patients with pre-existing immune suppression. It is unlikely that such a picture would coincide with blood donation.[89]

Varicella-Zoster Virus (VZV). Infection with VZV is an experience that most people have had before reaching adulthood. Primary infection produces the disease varicella (chickenpox), a common and generally benign childhood illness. Adults and individuals of any age who are immunosuppressed form a small group at risk for more serious illness. Persons who have had varicella may later develop zoster (''shingles''), which is the illness produced by the reactivation of the latent VZV.[26]

Varicella-zoster virus is not a complication of transfusion therapy for several reasons:

1. Viremia is accompanied by overt clinical illness and therefore a viremic individual would not likely be a blood donor.
2. VZV's site of latency is neural tissue, which is not involved in blood transfusion.
3. Most people are infected with VZV at an early age, which produces lasting immunity to exogenous reinfection.[89]

Cytomegalovirus (CMV). This member of the herpesvirus family has worldwide distribution, as evidenced by world antibody prevalence studies that have shown variations ranging from 40 to 100%.[90] Although most CMV infections are asymptomatic, this virus is known to be a common cause of congenital viral infection,[91] a causative agent for a mononucleosis-like syndrome, and a significant pathogen in bone marrow,[26, 92] liver,[93] and heart[94] transplantation patients.

CMV is known to be one of the infectious agents most frequently transmitted by blood transfusion. This is probably attributable to the fact that prospective blood donors can be infected with CMV and are infectious without apparent disease because of the following:

1. Infections, both primary and recurrent, are largely asymptomatic.
2. Viremia occurs in both primary and recurrent infections.
3. Most importantly, sites of latency for this virus include one or more of the peripheral blood leukocytes.[89, 95]

In spite of CMV's high potential for involvement in post-transfusion infection, the transfusion of blood from a seropositive donor to a seronegative recipient does not automatically result in a post-transfusion infection. Studies of the transmissibility of CMV by blood transfusion have consistently shown that only a subset of seropositive donors transmits the virus.[22] It has been estimated that the rate of infectivity among blood donors ranges from 0.14 to 12% and the transmission rate of CMV to seronegative recipients from seropositive donors ranges from 0.9 to 17%.[96]

Asymptomatic infection with no known sequelae is the outcome of the majority of transfusion-associated CMV (TA-CMV) infections. Therefore, blood with a reduced risk for transmitting CMV is not necessary in the immunocompetent recipient. The one exception to this would be that if a seronegative expectant mother requires a transfusion, CMV-negative blood should be chosen because this agent can be transmitted perinatally.[97] About 10% of infants infected with CMV in utero develop congenital abnormalities, including but not limited to central nervous system damage resulting in seizures, deafness, and mental retardation.[98]

The immunocompromised individual is at much greater risk for significant morbidity and even mortality from TA-CMV infection. Those individuals include premature infants,[99] tissue and organ transplant recipients,[100] and oncology patients.[101] Therefore, when transfusion is indicated for these patients, blood and blood components with a reduced risk of transmitting CMV should be chosen. Methods appropriate to achieve this end include the following:

1. The use of blood and blood components from CMV-negative donors
2. The use of a leukocyte filter for the administration of all blood and components[102]

Epstein-Barr Virus (EBV). Epstein-Barr virus, like other members of the herpesvirus family, is a common cause of infection worldwide. In most countries, more than 90% of blood donors have neutralizing anti-EBV that coexists with latent virus in peripheral blood and lymph nodes.[2]

Asymptomatic infection with EBV is common in young children but, in the adolescent and young adult, this infection is usually manifest as infectious mononucleosis. As is true with cytomegalovirus, Epstein-Barr develops into a persistent, latent infection after the primary episode with its accompanying period of viral shedding. One site for EBV latency is the B lymphocyte.

Epstein-Barr virus can be transmitted through blood transfusion. Cases have been reported in which investigators traced the origin of the post-transfusion illness back to donors who were incubating infectious mononucleosis but were asymptomatic at the time of donation.[103] This is the only scenario that has a major role in transfusion-associated EBV infection, but this is an uncommon event.

Human T-Cell Lymphotropic Virus (HTLV). This group of viruses is comprised of the human retroviruses, and all can cause persistent, permanent infection.[104] There are four types of human T-cell lymphotropic viruses.

HTLV-I
- Isolated in 1978 by Gallo and associates from an American man with T-cell leukemia
- Can be transmitted through blood transfusion
- Known causative agent in adult T-cell leukemia-lymphoma (ATL)[104–107]
- Linked with neurologic diseases: tropical spastic paraparesis (TSP); HTLV-I–associated myelopathy (HAM)
- Endemic in intravenous drug abusers in some US urban areas[104, 108, 109]
- Seroprevalence in US blood donors between 0.025 and 0.10%[110, 111]
- Risk of transmission decreases with increasing storage time[112]
- Transmission linked to cellular components only[24]
- Routine screening began in 1988 for anti–HTLV-I[2] (Note: retrospective studies have shown that infectivity almost always aligned with seropositivity.[113])

HTLV-II
- Isolated in 1982 from a patient with hairy cell leukemia[26]
- Serologic surveys suggest that HTLV-II infection occurs in selected subpopulations of intraveous drug abusers and hemophiliacs[108]
- Routine screening for HTLV-I also detects HTLV-II
- Has not yet been linked to human disease[98]

HIV (HTLV-III)
- Isolated in 1983–1984 by Montagnier and associates (France); named lymphadenopathy virus I (LAV-I)[26]
- Isolated in 1984 by Gallo and associates (United States); named human T-cell leukemia-lymphoma virus III (HTLV-III)[26]
- Routine blood bank screening for antibody to HIV begun in 1985
- Conclusively shown to cause acquired immunodeficiency syndrome (AIDS)[116, 117]
- 1986 international committee recommended common name of human immunodeficiency virus (HIV)[118]

- Has been conclusively shown to be transfusion-transmitted[119, 121]
- Transmission associated with whole blood, cellular components, plasma, and clotting factors[2]
- Known to have at least two strains, HIV-1 and HIV-2
- Infectivity rate is 90% for recipients of antibody-positive blood[122]
- Of the HIV-positive US population, 2% of adults and 9% of children are thought to have acquired the infection through blood or blood components[123]
- Current risk of transfusion-associated HIV infection estimated at 1:150,000/unit[124]

HTLV-IV
- Most recent isolate of this family
- Isolated from healthy people in Senegal, West Africa[114]
- Shown to have growth characteristics, affinity for CD4-positive T cells, and major viral proteins similar to those of simian T-cell lymphotropic virus (STLV), which causes immune deficiency in monkeys[115]
- No human disease yet associated with this virus[26, 104]

All the HTLVs appear to target the T lymphocyte and therefore, whether these infections are active or latent, they could be candidates for transmission by blood transfusion. Two members of this group of viruses have been positively linked to human diseases, HTLV-I and HIV. Of these two, the one that has seized the greatest amount of attention, both from the scientific community and the public at large, is HIV. Probably not since the early revelations about syphilis has a medical-scientific problem been surrounded by so many emotionally charged issues, and probably not since the heightened sense of urgency displayed during the polio epidemic in the 1950s has a disease entity been so vigorously pursued.

AUTOLOGOUS BLOOD TRANSFUSION

Autotransfusion (also known as autologous blood transfusion) is the collection and reinfusion of the patient's own blood for the purpose of intravascular volume replacement.[125] This procedure's historical roots can be traced to 1818, when an Englishman, Blundell, salvaged vaginal blood from patients with postpartum hemorrhage. By swabbing the blood from the bleeding site and rinsing the swabs with saline, he found that he could reinfuse the result of the washings. This unsophisticated method resulted in a 75% mortality rate, but marked the start of autologous blood transfusion.[126] The early 1900s saw others try autotransfusion (during limb amputations, ruptured ectopic pregnancies, splenectomies, and neurosurgery) with varying degrees of success. The interest in autotransfusion dwindled during World War II because there was a large pool of donors. After the war, blood testing, typing, and crossmatching techniques were improved, making blood banks the answer to the increased demand for blood.[126] In 1970, Klebanoff brought modern credibility to the concept of autotransfusion with his report of a roller pump system for retrieval of blood that was used successfully in Vietnam.[127]

The National Blood Policy, published in 1974, provided the impetus for the increased use of autotransfusion throughout the country. Its four goals were to maintain the following: (1) an adequate blood supply; (2) availability of blood to all people; (3) efficient utilization of blood; and (4) the highest standards of transfusion therapy with the safest blood.[126] In response to increasing public and professional awareness and concern about the potential infectious disease complications of homologous blood transfusion, interest in alternative transfusion programs of all forms mushroomed in the early 1980s.[128]

Autologous blood represents the safest possible blood for transfusion. Eliminated is the risk of exposure to bloodborne infectious agents such as human immunodeficiency virus (HIV), hepatitis, and malaria.[127] Autologous blood also provides a ready resource for patients with rare blood types or antibodies to minor antigens. Because there are more than 50 identifiable blood factors, there is a decreased risk with autotransfusion of hemolytic or febrile reactions that can result from isosensitization to leukocytes, platelets, and red cell antigens.[125]

There are currently four types of autotransfusion: (1) preoperative autologous blood donation; (2) perioperative isovolemic (normovolemic) hemodilution; (3) intraoperative cell salvage; and (4) postoperative blood salvage.

Preoperative Autologous Blood Donation

The most widely available form of the autologous options is the preoperative collection, storage, and reinfusion of donated blood, sometimes referred to as predeposit donation. Patients scheduled for elective surgical procedures anticipated to require blood replacement should be considered as candidates for this option. Consents for predeposit donation are required from the donor-patient's physician, the blood bank physician, and the donor.[7] If the donor-patient is a minor, the parent or guardian must give consent.

Hospital blood banks have a maximum surgical blood order schedule (MSBOS), which is a list of surgeries with the number of units of blood to be made available for each procedure. The number of units listed in the MSBOS is the number of units that should be donated before surgery, if time and the patient's hemoglobin level allow.[129]

The ideal donor-patient is in good health, afebrile, and has four to six weeks until surgery. The hemoglobin concentration should be no less than 110 g/liter (11g/dL). The packed cell volume, if substituted, should be no less than 0.33 (33%).[7] Patients with active infection or who may be bacteremic are not eligible, because bacteria may proliferate while the collected blood is stored.

There are no age limits for autologous transfusion procedures.[7] Although it has been shown that older donors have neither more nor different blood donation reactions than younger donors, some donor centers administer intravenous fluid, usually 0.9% normal saline, during or after the phlebotomy to prevent hypovolemia, which may occur in elderly, cardiac, and underweight patients. Underweight donors should have proportionately smaller units withdrawn.[129]

An important aspect of patient management for those participating in predeposit programs is iron replacement. Several studies have indicated that near-maximal erythropoiesis (approximately three to four times normal red cell production) can effectively be achieved after two to three weekly phlebotomies, provided the patient is taking an iron supplement. The recommended oral dose of iron (ferrous sulfate) is 300 mg three times daily, if tolerated. Patients should begin oral iron supplements as soon as surgery is scheduled.[128]

The risks of preoperative autologous blood donation include vasovagal reactions, most often in the form of self-limited lightheadedness caused by transient hypotension and bradycardia. Such reactions occur during 2 to 5% of all blood donations, whether autologous or homologous.[130] Pallor, sweating, dizziness, nausea, and a drop in heart rate and blood pressure during the donation suggest a vasovagal reaction, which can progress to a sudden loss of consciousness and vasomotor collapse. This reaction, often brought on by stress or apprehension, is most common among first-time donors.

The preferred phlebotomy schedule is weekly, with the last unit drawn no less than 72 hours before surgery. The donated blood is usually stored in the liquid state at 1 to 6 C for 35 to 42 days, depending on the anticoagulant-preservative system used. If a longer storage period is necessary, the blood may be frozen. In addition, autologous blood that was not frozen at the time of donation can be rejuvenated and subsequently frozen when it reaches its expiration date. This practice prevents autologous blood from being discarded when surgery is delayed.

The AABB *Standards*[7] require only ABO and Rh testing for autologous donations. Some collection facilities perform testing for HIV, HTLV-I, hepatitis B and C, surrogate markers, and syphilis. If these additional tests are not done, the blood must be labeled for autologous use only. This additional testing facilitates the ''crossing over'' of unused autologous blood into the homologous inventory, because the blood has been predetermined to meet AABB testing requirements for volunteer homologous donations. This practice varies among facilities.

Perioperative Isovolemic (Normovolemic) Hemodilution

Hemodilution is an option for patients who can tolerate rapid withdrawal of blood before surgery. This procedure involves collecting one or two units of blood in CPD or CPDA-1 immediately prior to a surgical procedure, usually after anesthesia has been induced, and replacing the blood with a sufficient volume of crystalloid or colloid solution to attain normovolemic hemodilution. The blood collected at the start of the procedure is stored at room temperature in the operating room. Because the blood is fresh and kept at room temperature, the platelets and clotting factors remain viable.

The rationale for hemodilution is based on studies done in the early 1970s that demonstrated that isovolemic hemodilution, using dextran and crystalloid leads to lowered blood viscosity, and that maximum oxygen delivery is attainable when the hematocrit is lower than 30%. It appeared, based on their work, that the viscosity-lowering effect of hemodilution leads to a sufficient increase in cardiac output and perfusion to more than compensate for the diminished oxygen-carrying capacity of the red blood cell reduction.[128]

The application of this option has obvious limitations.

First, the patient on whom this procedure is done must be able to tolerate a significant blood loss before surgery is begun. Second, because the amount of blood that can be safely drawn off is limited, it may not be adequate to meet the volume replacement required. In such cases, homologous blood would have to be used as a supplement. Therefore, this option, as for predeposit autologous transfusion, may reduce but often does not eliminate the need for homologous blood use.

Intraoperative Autotransfusion-Cell Salvage

Intraoperative autotransfusion (also known as IAT) is the collection of shed blood from the surgical field and its subsequent reinfusion to the patient. It can be used in cardiac, vascular, and selected trauma surgeries, as well as liver transplants and orthopedic procedures. Intraoperative salvage is often appropriate for procedures in which the anticipated blood loss is approximately 20% of the patient's estimated blood volume.[131] IAT is especially useful when preoperative donation is impossible or inadequate. The rule of thumb in IAT is that a return of three units using this method makes it cost-effective. However, many argue that any cost using this method is offset by the reduced risk of autologous versus homologous transfusion.

There are numerous blood collection and cell processing machines available. The objective is the same for all: collect, in some cases process, and return. If processing machinery is used, the blood shed from the surgical field is suctioned off and anticoagulated through a dual-lumen catheter, which terminates in a collection reservoir. When the volume in this reservoir reaches the optimal level for processing, the blood is washed, spun, and returned.

There are situations in which IAT should not be used. Because neither filtration nor washing can completely remove bacteria from blood, salvage is not attempted during procedures that involve spilled intestinal contents, bacterial peritonitis, intra-abdominal abscesses, or osteomyelitis.[130] Additionally, IAT is not usually used if a collagen hemostatic agent has been placed in the wound. These powdered agents, which activate the clotting cascade when in contact with red blood cells, have a molecular size similar to that of red cells, and may not be eliminated by cell washing. Also, because malignant cells cannot be removed from salvaged blood, IAT is usually contraindicated in cancer resections. Returning salvaged blood could result in the seeding of malignant cells to other areas.

The contraindications to blood salvage are relative, and must be weighed against the alternatives. For example, in the patient with penetrating trauma of the abdomen resulting in disruption of the gut and massive bleeding, it might be considered better to salvage and reinfuse the shed blood than to allow the patient to exsanguinate if homologous blood is not available in sufficient quantities.[131]

Postoperative Blood Salvage

Postoperative salvage is the collection of shed blood from the postoperative surgical wound for reinfusion to the patient.

Continuous and intermittent techniques and equipment are available for salvaging blood lost after surgery. These methods are usually used to collect blood lost from chest tubes or joint cavities. Because anticoagulation is not employed, this blood is defibrinated and contains high titers of fibrinogen-fibrin degradation products. Such collections may be processed using cell washing techniques before reinfusion, or they may be reinfused without processing. In either case they must be filtered, and microaggregate filtration is preferred when cell washing has not been used. AABB recommends that shed blood collected under postoperative or post-traumatic conditions be reinfused within 6 hours of initiation of the collection.[7]

References

1. Walker RH, ed. Technical Manual, 11th ed. Bethesda: American Association of Blood Banks, 1993.
2. Mollison PL, Engelfriet CP, Contreras M. Blood Transfusion in Clinical Medicine, 9th ed. London: Blackwell Scientific, 1993.
3. Gabrio BW, Donohue DM, Finch CA. Relationship between chemical changes and viability of stored blood treated with adenosine. J Clin Invest 1955; 34:1509.
4. Simon TL, Marcus CS, Myhre BA, Nelson EJ. Effects of AS-3 nutrient-additive solution on 42 and 49 days of storage of red cells. Transfusion 1981; 21:178–181.
5. Moore GL, Peck CC, Sohmer PR, Zuck TF. Some properties of blood stored in anticoagulant CPDA-1 solution, a brief summary. Transfusion 1981; 21:135–137.
6. Heaton A, Keegan A, Holme S. In vivo regeneration of red cell 2,3-diphosphoglycerate following transfusion of DPG-depleted AS-1, AS-3 and CPDA-1 red cells. Br J Haematol 1989; 71:131–136.
7. Widmann FK, ed. Standards for Blood Banks and Transfusion Services, 14th ed. Arlington, VA: American Association of Blood Banks, 1991.
8. Kruskall MS. Blood transfusion. In Robinson SH, Reich PR, eds. Hematology, 3rd ed. Boston: Little, Brown and Co., 1993.
9. Haugen RK. Hepatitis after transfusion of frozen red cells and washed red cells. N Engl J Med 1979; 301:393–395.
10. Callaerts AJ, Gielis ML, Spengers ED, Muylle L. The mechanism of white cell reduction by synthetic fiber cell filters. Transfusion 1993; 33:134–138.
11. Bock M, Wagner M, Knupple W, et al. Preparation of white cell-depleted blood: Comparison of two bedside filter systems. Transfusion 1990; 30:26–28.
12. Sirchia G, Wenz B, Rebulla P, et al. Removal of white cells from red cells by transfusion through a new filter. Transfusion 1990; 30:30–33.
13. Meryman HT. Transfusion-inducer alloimmunization and immunosuppression and the effect of leukocyte depletion. Transfus Med Rev 1989; 3:180–193.
14. Chambers LA, Kruskall MS, Pacini DG, Donovan LM. Febrile reactions after platelet transfusion: The effect of single versus multiple donors. Transfusion 1990; 30:219–221.
15. Cohen H, Kernoff PBA. Plasma, plasma products and indications for their use. Br Med J 1990; 330:803–806.
16. Smith JK. Trends in the production and use of coagulation factor concentrates. In Developments in Hematology and Immunology, Vol 26. London: Kluwer Academic Publishers, 1990.
17. Mannucci PM, Schimpf K, Abe T, et al. Low risk of viral infection after administration of vapor-heated factor VIII concentrate. Transfusion 1992; 32:134–137.
18. Kruskall MS, Pacini DG, Malynn ER, Button LN. Evaluation of a blood warmer that utilizes a 40 C heat exchanger.
19. Judkins D, Iserson KV. Blood warming: Avoid hypothermia. J Emerg Nurs 1991; 17:146–151.
20. Pisciotto PT, ed. Blood Transfusion Therapy: A Physician's Handbook, 3rd ed. Arlington, VA: American Association of Blood Banks, 1989.
21. Steneker I, Van Luyn MJA, Van Wachem PB, Biewenga J. Electron-microscopic examination of white cell reduction by four white-cell reduction filters. Transfusion 1992; 32:450–457.
22. Lamberson HV, Dock NL. Prevention of transfusion-transmitted cytomegalovirus infection. Transfusion 1992; 32:196–198.
23. Sayers MH, Anderson KC, Goodnough LT, et al. Reducing the risk for transfusion-transmitted cytomegalovirus infection. Ann Intern Med 1992; 116:55–62.
24. Herr V, Ambruso D, Fairfax M, et al. Transfusion-associated transmission of human T-lymphotropic viruses type I and II: Experience of a regional blood center. Transfusion 1993; 33:208–211.
25. Okochi K, Sato H, Hinuma Y. A retrospective study on transmission of adult T-cell leukemia virus by blood transfusion: Seroconversion in recipients. Vox Sang 1984; 46:245–253.
26. Joklik WK. Virology. Norwalk, CT: Appleton and Lange, 1988.
27. Kim DM, Brecher ME, Bland LA, et al. Prestorage removal of Yersinia enterocolitica from red cells with white-cell reduction filters. Transfusion 1992; 32:658–661.
28. Sloand EM, Klein HG. Effect of white cells on platelet storage. Transfusion 1990; 30:333–337.
29. Davey RJ, Carmen RA, Simon TL, et al. Preparation of white cell-depleted red cells for 42-day storage using an integral in-line filter. Transfusion 1989; 29:496–498.
30. Hoppe PA. Interim measures for detection of bacterially contaminated red cell components. Transfusion 1992; 32:199–201.
31. Popvsky MA, Chaplin HC Jr, Moore SB. Transfusion-related acute lung injury: A neglected, serious complication of hemotherapy. Transfusion 1992; 32:589–591.
32. Latson TW, Kickler TS, Baumgartner WA. Pulmonary hypertension and noncardiogenic pulmonary edema following cardiopulmonary bypass associated with an antigranulocyte antibody. Anesthesiology 1986; 64:106–111.
33. Popovsky MA, Moore SB. Diagnostic and pathogenetic considerations in transfusion-related acute lung injury. Transfusion 1985; 25:573–577.
34. Wolf CFW, Canale VC. Fatal pulmonary hypersensitivity reaction to HLA incompatible blood transfusion: Report of a case and review of the literature. Transfusion 1976; 16:135–140.
35. Heltberg O, Skov F, Gertner-Smidt P, et al. Nosocomial epidemic of Serratia marcescens septicemia ascribed to contaminated blood transfusion bags. Transfusion 1993; 33:221–227.
36. Muder RR, Yee YC, Rihs JD, Bunker M. Staphylococcus epidermidis bacteremia from transfusion of contaminated platelets: Application of bacterial DNA analysis. Transfusion 1992; 32:771–773.
37. Moroff G, Luban NL. Prevention of transfusion-associated graft-versus-host disease. Transfusion 1992; 32:102–103.
38. Akahoshi M, Takanashi M, Masuda M, et al. A case of transfusion-associated graft-versus-host disease not prevented by white-cell reduction filters. Transfusion 1992; 13:169–172.
39. Hayakawa S, Chishima F, Sakata H, et al. A rapid molecular diagnosis of post-transfusion graft-versus-host disease by polymerase chain reaction. Transfusion 1993; 33:413–417.
40. Anderson K, Weinstein HJ. Irradiation of blood components to prevent graft-versus-host disease. In Kurtz SR, Baldwin ML, Sirchia G, eds. Controversies in Transfusion Medicine: Immune Complications and Cytomegalovirus Transmission. Arlington, VA: American Association of Blood Banks, 1990.
41. Pelszynski M, Moroff G, Luban N, et al. Dose-dependent lymphocyte inactivation in red blood cell units with gamma radiation (abstract). Transfusion (suppl) 1991; 31:17S.
42. Rosen NR, Weidner JG, Boldt HD, Rosen DS. Prevention of transfusion-associated graft-versus-host disease: Selection of an adequate dose of gamma radiation. Transfusion 1993; 33:125–127.
43. Anderson KC, Goodnough LT, Sayers M, et al. Variations in blood component irradiation practice: Implications for prevention of transfusion-associated graft-versus-host disease. Blood 1991; 77:2096–2102.
44. Button LN, DeWolf WC, Newberger PE, et al. The effects of radiation on blood components. Transfusion 1981; 21:419–426.
45. Davey RJ, McCoy NC, Yu M, et al. The effect of prestorage irradiation on posttransfusion red cell survival. Transfusion 1992; 32:525–527.
46. Friedman KD, McDonough WC, Cimino DF. The effect of prestorage gamma irradiation on post-transfusion red blood cell recovery (abstract). Transfusion (suppl) 1991; 31:50S.
47. Suda BA, Leitman SF, Davey RJ. Characteristics of red cells irradiated and subsequently frozen for long-term storage. Transfusion 1993; 33:389–392.
48. Thaler M, Shamiss A, Orgad S, et al. The role of blood from HLA-homozygous donors in fatal transfusion-associated graft-versus-host disease after open-heart surgery. N Engl J Med 1989; 321:25–28.

49. Capon SM, DePond WD, Tyan DB, et al. Transfusion-associated graft-versus-host disease in an immunocompetent patient. Ann Intern Med 1991; 114:1025–1026.

50. Otsuka S, Kunieda K, Kitamura F, et al. The critical role of blood from HLA-homozygous donors in fatal transfusion-associated graft-versus-host disease in immunocompetent patients. Transfusion 1991; 31:260–264.

51. AABB makes recommendations regarding direct donations and graft-versus-host disease. AABB News Briefs 1989; 12:1–2.

52. Kanter MH. Transfusion-associated graft-versus-host disease: Do transfusions from second-degree relatives pose a greater risk than those from first-degree relatives? Transfusion 1992; 32:323–327.

53. Crosby WH. Misuse of blood transfusion. Blood 1958; 13:1198–1200.

54. Tipple MA, Bland LA, Murphy JJ, et al. Sepsis associated with transfusion of red blood cells contaminated with Yersinia enterocolitica. Transfusion 1990; 30:207–213.

55. Update: Yersinia enterocolitica bacteremia and endotoxin shock associated with red blood cell transfusions—United States 1991. MMWR 1991; 40:176–178.

56. Anderson JD. The Enterobacteriaceae. In McLean DM, Smith JA, eds. Medical Microbiology Synopsis. Philadelphia: Lea & Febiger, 1991.

57. Rutman RC, Miller WV. Transfusion Therapy: Principles and Practices. Rockville, MD: Aspen, 1985.

58. Shayegani M, Parsons LM, Waring AL, et al. Molecular relatedness of Staphylococcus epidermidis isolates obtained during a platelet transfusion-associated episode of sepsis. J Clin Microbiol 1991; 29:2768–2773.

59. Arnow PM, Weiss LM, Weil D, Rosen NR. Escherichia coli sepsis from contaminated platelet transfusion. Arch Intern Med 1986; 146:321–324.

60. Heal JM, Jones ME, Forey J, et al. Fatal Salmonella septicema after platelet transfusion. Transfusion 1987; 27:2–7.

61. Braine HG, Kickler TS, Charache P, et al. Bacterial sepsis secondary to platelet transfusion: An adverse effect of extended storage at room temperature. Transfusion 1986; 26:391–393.

62. Buckholz DH, Young VM, Friedman NR, et al. Detection and quantitation of bacteria in platelet products stored at room temperatures. Transfusion 1973; 13:268–275.

63. Buckholz DH, Young VM, Friedman NR, et al. Bacterial proliferation in platelet products stored at room temperature. N Engl J Med 1971; 285:429–433.

64. Morrow JF, Braine HG, Kickler TS, et al. Septic reactions to platelet transfusions: A persistent problem. JAMA 1991; 266:555–558.

65. Churchill WH, Kurtz SR, eds. Transfusion Medicine. Boston: Blackwell Scientific, 1988:124–125.

66. Dodd RY. The risk of transfusion-transmitted infection. N Engl J Med 1992; 327:419–420.

67. Barker LF, Dodd RY. Viral hepatitis, acquired immunodeficiency syndrome, and other infections transmitted by transfusion. In Pelz LD, Swisher SN, eds. Clinical Practice of Transfusion Medicine, 2nd ed. New York: Churchill Livingstone, 1989.

68. Wolfe MS. Parasites other than malaria, transmissible by blood transfusion. In Greenwalt TS, Jamieson GA, eds. Transmissible Diseases and Blood Transfusion. New York: Grune and Stratton, 1975:

69. Estes MEZ. Chagas' disease. Crit Care Nurs 1989; 9:48–64.

70. Appleman MD, Shulman IA, et al. Use of questionnaire to identify potential blood donors at risk for infection with Trypanosoma cruzi. Transfusion 1993; 33:61–64.

71. Donahue JG, Munoz A, Ness PM, et al. The declining risk of posttransfusion hepatitis C virus infection. N Engl J Med 1992; 327:369–373.

72. Alter HJ. Posttransfusion hepatitis: Clinical features, risks and donor testing. In Dodd RY, Baker LF eds. Infection, Immunity and Blood Transfusion. New York: A. R. Liss, 1985.

73. Szmuness W, Dienstag JL, Purcell RH, et al. Distribution of antibody to hepatitis A antigen in urban and adult populations. N Engl J Med 1976; 295:755–759.

74. Hollinger FB, Khan NC, Oefinger PE, et al. Posttransfusion hepatitis type A. JAMA 1983; 250:2313–2317.

75. Noble RC, Kane MA, Reeves SA, et al. Posttransfusion hepatitis A in a neonatal intensive care unit. JAMA 1984; 252:2711–2715.

76. Saver DK. Hepatitis in clinical practice. Postgrad Med 1986; 79:194–214, 218–230.

77. Aach RD. Primary hepatic viruses: Hepatitis A, hepatitis B, delta hepatitis and non-A, non-B hepatitis. In Insalco SJ, Menitove JE, eds. Transfusion-Transmitted Viruses: Epidemiology and Pathology. Arlington, VA: American Association of Blood Banks, 1987.

78. Public Health Service Interagency guidelines for screening blood donors of blood, plasma, organs, tissues and semen for evidence of hepatitis B and hepatitis C. MMWR 1991; 40:1–17.

79. Alter HJ, Purcell RH, Holland PV, et al. Donor transaminase and recipient hepatitis. JAMA 1981; 246:630–634.

80. Stevens CE, Aach RD, Hollinger FB, et al. Hepatitis B virus antibody in blood donors and the occurrence of non-A, non-B hepatitis in transfusion recipients: An analysis of the Transfusion-Transmitted Virus Study. Ann Intern Med 1984; 101:733–778.

81. Aach RD, Lander JJ, Sherman LA, et al. Transfusion-transmitted viruses: Interim analysis of hepatitis among transfused and nontransfused patients. In Vygas GN, Cohen SN, Schmid R, eds. Viral Hepatitis. Philadelphia: Franklin Institute Press, 1978:383–396.

82. Menitove JE. Rationale for surrogate testing to detect non-A, non-B hepatitis. Transfus Med Rev 1988; 2:65–67.

83. Chambers LA, Popovsky MA. Decrease in reported posttransfusion hepatitis: Contributions of donor screening for alanine aminotransferase and antibodies to hepatitis B core antigen and changes in the general population. Arch Intern Med 1991; 151:2445–2448.

84. Aach RD, Stevens CE, Hollinger FB, et al. Hepatitis virus infection in post-transfusion hepatitis—an analysis with first- and second-generation tests. N Engl J Med 1991; 325:1325–1329.

85. Delta hepatitis—Massachusetts. MMWR 1984; 33:493–494.

86. Smedile A, Farci P, Giorgio V, et al. Influence of delta infection on severity of hepatitis B. Lancet 1982; 2:945–947.

87. Hadler SC, DeMonzon M, Ponzetto A, et al. Delta viral infection and severe hepatitis: An epidemic in Yucpa Indians of Venezuela. Ann Intern Med 1984; 100:339–344.

88. Polesky HF, Hanson MR. Transfusion-associated hepatitis C (non-A, non-B) infection. Arch Pathol Lab Med 1989; 113:232–235.

89. Tegtmeier GE. The role of blood transfusion in the transmission of herpes viruses. In Insalco SJ, Menitove JE, eds. Transfusion-Transmitted Viruses: Epidemiology and Pathology. Arlington, VA: American Association of Blood Banks, 1987.

90. Krech U. Complement-fixing antibodies against cytomegalovirus in different parts of the world. Bull WHO 1973; 49:103–106.

91. Brett WJ, Pass RF, Stagno S, Alford CA. Pediatric cytomegalovirus infection. Transplant Proc (suppl 3) 1991; 23:115–117.

92. Forman SJ. Bone marrow transplantation. Transplantation Proc (suppl 3) 1991; 23:110–114.

93. Arnold JC, O'Grady JG, Otto G, et al. CMV reinfection/reactivation after liver transplantation. Transplant Proc 1991; 23:2632–2633.

94. Anthuber M, Sudhoff F, Schuetz A, Kemkes, BM. Donor-transmitted infections in heart transplantation—HIV, CMV, and toxoplasmosis. Transplant Proc 1991; 23:2634–2635.

95. Dulbecco R, Ginsberg HS. Virology, 2nd ed. Philadelphia: J. B. Lippincott, 1988.

96. Tegtmeier GE. Posttransfusion cytomegalovirus infections. Arch Pathol Med 1989; 113:236–245.

97. Stagno S, Pass RF, Cloud G, et al. Primary cytomegalovirus infection in pregnancy: Incidence, transmission to fetus and clinical outcome. JAMA 1986; 256:1904.

98. Volk WA, Benjamin DC, Kadner RJ, Parsons JT. Essentials of Medical Microbiology, 4th ed. Philadelphia: J. B. Lippincott, 1991.

99. Preiksaitis JK, Brown L, McKenzie M. Transfusion-acquired cytomegalovirus infection in neonates. Transfusion 1988; 28:205–208.

100. Ho M. Cytomegalovirus infection and indirect sequelae in the immunocompromised transplant patient. Transplant Proc (suppl 1) 1991; 23:2–7.

101. Ho M. Cytomegalovirus: Biology and Infection. New York: Plenum Press, 1982.

102. Gilbert GL, Hayes K, Hudson IL, et al. Prevention of transfusion-acquired cytomegalovirus infection in infants by blood filtration to remove leukocytes. Lancet 1989; 2:1228–1231.

103. Turner AR, McDonald RN, Cooper BA. Transmission of infectious mononucleosis by transfusion of pre-illness blood. Ann Intern Med 1972; 77:751–753.

104. Looney DH, Redfield RR. HTLV retroviruses and transfusion-transmitted disease. In Insalco SJ, Menitove JE, eds. Transfusion-Transmitted Viruses: Epidemiology and Pathology. Arlington, VA: American Association of Blood Banks, 1987.

105. Poiesz BJ, Ruscetti FW, Gazdar AF, et al. Detection and isolation of type C retrovirus particles from fresh and cultured lymphocytes of a patient with cutaneous T-cell lymphoma. Proc Natl Acad Sci USA 1980; 77:7415.

106. Vchiyama T, Yadoi J, Sagawa K, et al. Adult T-cell leukemia: Clinical and hematological features of 16 cases. Blood 1977; 50:481–492.

107. Gallo RC, Blattner WA, Reitz MS, Ito Y. HTLV: The virus of adult T-cell leukemia in Japan and elsewhere. Lancet 1982; 1:683.

108. Robert-Guroff M, Weiss SH, Giron J, et al. Prevalence of antibodies to HTLV-I, II, and III in intravenous drug abusers from an AIDS epidemic region. JAMA 1986; 255:3133–3137.

109. Sandler SG. HTLV-I and II. New risks for recipients of blood transfusions? JAMA 1986; 256:2245–2246.

110. Donegan E, Pell P, Lee H, et al. Transmission of T-lymphotropic virus type I by blood components from a donor lacking anti-p24: A case report. Transfusion 1992; 32:68–71.

111. Williams AE, Fang CT, Slamon DJ, et al. Seroprevalence and epidemiological correlates of HTLV-I infection in U.S. blood donors. Science 1988; 240:643–646.

112. Donegan E. Transfusion-transmitted HTLV-I and -II: Infectivity and clinical consequences in donor and recipients (abstract). Transfusion (suppl) 1991; 31:41S.

113. Inaba S, Sato H, Okochi K, et al. Prevention of transmission of human T-lymphotropic virus type I (HTLV-I) through transfusion, by donor screening with antibody to the virus. Transfusion 1989; 29:7–10.

114. Barin F, Denis F, Allan JS, et al. Serologic evidence for virus related to simian T-lymphotropic retrovirus-III in residents of West Africa. Lancet 1985; 2:1387.

115. Kanki PJ, Barin F, Boups S, et al. New human lymphotropic retroviruses related to simian T-lymphotropic virus-III (STLV-III). Science 1986; 232:238.

116. Gallo RC, Wong-Staal F. A human T-lymphotropic retrovirus (HTLV-III) as the cause of the acquired immunodeficiency syndrome. Ann Intern Med 1985; 103:679–689.

117. Sarngadharan MG, Popovic M, Bruch L, et al. Antibodies reactive with human T-lymphotropic retroviruses (HTLV-III) in serum of patients with AIDS. Science 1986; 224:506–508.

118. Coffin J, Haase A, Levy JA, et al. Human immunodeficiency viruses. Science 1986; 232:697.

119. Feorino PM, Jaffe HW, Palmer E, et al. Transfusion-associated acquired immunodeficiency syndrome. N Engl J Med 1985; 312:1293–1296.

120. Evatt BL, Ramsey RB, Lawrence DN, et al. Acquired immunodeficiency syndrome in hemophiliac patients. Ann Intern Med 1984; 100:499.

121. Curran JW, Lawrence DN, Jaffe H, Kaplan JE, et al. Acquired immunodeficiency syndrome (AIDS) associated with transfusion. N Engl J Med 1984; 310:69.

122. Donegan E, Stuart M, Niland JC, et al. Infection with human immunodeficiency virus type I (HIV-1) among recipients of antibody-positive blood donations. Ann Intern Med 1990; 113:733–739.

123. Centers for Disease Control: HIV/AIDS Surveillance Report. Atlanta: Centers for Disease Control, 1991:1–18.

124. Phillips LD. Manual of I.V. Therapeutics. Philadelphia: F. A. Davis, 1993.

125. Martin E, Harris A, Johnson N. Autotransfusion Systems (ATS). Crit Care Nurs 1989; 9(7):65–73.

126. Nicholson E. Autologous blood transfusion. Nurs Times 1988; 84(2):33–35.

127. Peterson K. Nursing management of autologous blood transfusion. J Intraveno Nurs 1992; 15(3):128–134.

128. Silvergleid A. Clinical Practice of Transfusion Medicine, 2nd ed. New York: Churchill Livingstone, 1989.

129. Drago A. Banking on your own blood. AJN 1992; 92(3):61–64.

130. Autologous Transfusion. AJN 1991; 91(6):47–48.

131. Stehling L, ed. Perioperative Autologous Transfusion: Transcribed Proceedings of a National Conference. American Association of Blood Banks, Arlington, VA, 1991; 11–12, 23–37.

132. Transfusion Therapy Guidelines for Nurses. NIH Publication No. 90-2668, Sept 1990.

CHAPTER 11 Pharmacology

Donna R. Baldwin, MSN, CRNI

The intravenous (IV) route is rapidly becoming a common route of parenteral drug administration in many health care settings.[1] Intravenous drugs were once reserved for emergency situations or critically ill patients. They are now routinely used throughout the hospital, as well as in outpatient and home care settings. With the dramatic increase in the use of the IV route for drug delivery, nurses have assumed increased responsibility. Nurses administer the IV drugs, monitor the patients' responses to pharmacologic agents, and instruct patients regarding the prescribed drug therapy. Therefore, nurses must have a thorough understanding of the principles of IV drug administration. This knowledge is necessary both for the safety of the patient and to ensure quality patient outcomes.

It is the intent of this chapter to broaden the nurse's knowledge regarding IV drug therapy. Because of the breadth of the subject, the chapter has been divided into three sections. In the first, the nurse's role in IV drug administration is reviewed. Specific consideration is given to legal aspects of IV drug administration and application of the nursing process. The second section discusses the various aspects of IV drug delivery. Commonly used equipment is described, as well as the different modes of IV drug administration. The greatest emphasis is placed on the final section. Here, the different classifications of IV drugs are presented and the drug most representative of each classification is examined in detail.

CONSIDERATIONS FOR INTRAVENOUS DRUG ADMINISTRATION

As nurses assume greater responsibility for IV drug administration, they require increased knowledge. Although nursing students are usually restricted from administering IV drugs (except under the close supervision of their instructor), nursing education has begun to place more emphasis on the pharmacology and administration of drugs by the IV route. Health care facilities supplement this educational base by providing specialized courses for nurses assigned to IV teams and critical care. However, the typical staff nurse in the hospital and home care settings may only receive limited orientation to IV therapy. This is unfortunate, because the responsibility for IV drug administration and patient monitoring frequently rests with the staff nurse.

Nursing Responsibilities

The determination of who may administer IV drugs is based on Nurse Practice Acts. Each state has such an act, but most only broadly define the scope of professional nursing responsibilities. This differs for a licensed practical nurse (LPN) in that several states have established boundaries in which the LPN may practice. These boundaries may include specific educational programs that the LPN must complete prior to administering IV drugs and restrictions on the drug administration procedures that may be performed.[2]

In addition to Nurse Practice Acts, health care facilities have established policies regarding nursing responsibilities. Although these policies cannot exceed the limits established by the Nurse Practice Act, they may clarify or place further restrictions on nursing functions. For example, institutional guidelines for IV drug administration define who may administer certain drugs.[3] Some hospitals also place specific restrictions on drugs administered by direct IV injection with the use of "IV push lists."[4]

A third set of guidelines regarding IV drug administration is contained in the *Intravenous Nursing Standards of Practice*.[5] This document provides criteria to measure the quality of IV nursing care, including IV drug administration. Because the standards are meant to protect the public and define nursing accountability, they serve as the basis for the development of IV policies in all practice settings in which IV drugs are administered.

Legal Considerations

To legally administer an IV drug, or any drug, the medication must be prescribed by a physician or appropriate licensed professional. However, it is the nurse's responsibility to ensure that the order is complete, correct, appropriate, and valid. A complete order must contain the name of the drug, dosage, route of administration and frequency or time of administration, date and time the order was written, and signature of the prescribing physician. Problems arise when any of these components are missing or unclear.

A correct and appropriate order is one that is indicated and proper for the patient's condition. Indications for each drug classification and specific drugs are discussed later in this chapter. Determination of the appropriateness of the order is based on the nursing assessment of the patient and requires knowledge of both pharmacokinetics and pharmacodynamics. Pharmacokinetics focuses on the effects of the body on the drug; pharmacodynamics involves the effects of the drug on the body.

A valid medication order requires that the order be written and signed by the physician or some other authorized health care professional. Although verbal orders are acceptable in some situations, the order is not legally finalized until countersigned by a licensed physician or appropriate licensed professional.[6]

There are additional legal considerations regarding controlled substances. These are prescription drugs that, because of their high potential for drug dependence and/or abuse, are covered by the Controlled Substances Act of 1970. The act established five categories of controlled substances, known as schedules, based on their potential for abuse, the medical indications, and the potential dependence of the drug. Many of the IV drugs administered for pain control are Schedule II drugs that have specific prescription and record keeping requirements.[7]

A third area that has legal implications is the administration of investigational drugs. Informed consent must be obtained from all patients and/or families participating in clinical drug trials. This means that the patient must be supplied information by the principal investigator regarding the risks, benefits, expected effects on the disease process, and alternatives to the investigational therapy prior to consenting to participate in the trial. In addition, the clinical trial must be approved by the appropriate institutional committee and drug information must be readily available for the nurse administering the drug.[8]

Legal consideration must also be given to the occurrence of medication errors. Errors may be associated with prescribing and dispensing the drug, but they more commonly occur because of failure to follow safe administration procedures. The five rights of medication administration specify that the *right* dose of the *right* drug must be administered to the *right* patient at the *right* time and by the *right* route. Errors have resulted because of the ''look alike'' generic names of the cephalosporin antibiotics, failure to identify the patient appropriately, administration of the drug by an incorrect route, and the route not being specified by the physician. Documentation of errors, as part of a risk management program, can aid in the identification of trends and the correction of such problems.[9] Such documentation should be initiated by the person discovering the error.

Nursing Process

The administration of IV drugs requires proper application of the nursing process. The patient must be assessed, the drug therapy must be planned and implemented, the patient outcomes must be evaluated, and the plan of care must be reviewed and revised based on the evaluation. These basic steps are interrelated and are essential to ensure that drug therapy results in the desired patient outcomes.

Assessment

Patient assessment begins with a review of the patient's health history. Pertinent questions to ask are the following:

''What is the current disease?''
''What other drugs are currently being used?''
''What medications were used in the past?''
''Did the previous medications have any unexpected effect?''

During the questioning, it is particularly important to obtain information about known allergies to drugs, foods, and environmental factors. There are cross-sensitivities between many drugs, so that an allergy to one may result in similar effects with another. A primary example is the possible cross-sensitivity between penicillins and cephalosporins.

A second area to be assessed is the patient's life style and resources. This is particularly important in home care and should include the family as well as the patient. Specific factors to consider are the patient's and family's daily schedule and the physical and human resources available. How will the drug therapy schedule affect the daily schedule? Will the caregiver be available at the scheduled administration times? Are there material resources available to enable safe and appropriate use of the drug and equipment required for administration?

The third area to assess is the patient's and family's knowledge level and desire for information. This may significantly influence adherence with the drug regimen. Because the desire for information and the ability to comprehend it vary among patients, assessment of these factors aids in allotting adequate time for patient and family education.

The last area to be assessed is patient-related factors that may alter the patient's response to the drug. These include genetic factors, pre-existing conditions, and age. Genetic factors, such as the absence of a specific enzyme, may affect the drug's action within the body. Renal, liver, and cardiovascular disease may be pre-existing conditions that impair the metabolism or elimination of the drug. Age is also a predictor of drug response. For example, children do not have the mature physiologic mechanisms needed for adult dosages, whereas physiologic changes in older adults tend to extend the effects of drugs within the body. In addition, drug interactions and incompatibilities with other medications the patient is receiving, and body fat content, may negatively affect the drug response.

Planning

A comprehensive assessment aids in identifying the nursing diagnosis specific to the patient and the drug therapy. Examples of nursing diagnoses are ''potential for injury related to altered electrolyte balance resulting from furosemide administration'' and ''knowledge deficit related to IV administration of cefazolin.''[10] Although nursing diagnoses may be difficult to master, they are instrumental in defining and communicating patient problems relative to the drug therapy. There are several textbooks available to assist the nurse in determining the appropriate nursing diagnoses.

Once the pertinent nursing diagnoses have been identified, the patient's plan of care may be established. The care plan should include both short-term and long-term goals, and focus on actions to achieve the desired patient outcomes.[11]

An important feature to consider when planning care for the patient is the time response aspects of drug action. Although the drug may be administered as a single dose, it is

Table 11–1

Untoward Drug Responses
∙ ∙

Response	Effects	Example
Tolerance	Increasing amounts of drug needed to produce same therapeutic response	Patient receiving morphine infusion over 2 weeks has decreasing relief from pain
Tachyphylaxis	A rapidly developing tolerance occurring after very few doses have been given	Has been reported with sodium nitroprusside
Accumulation	Administration of a drug at rate faster than can be metabolized	May occur when the usual adult dosage of gentamicin is administered to a patient with renal impairment
Idiosyncrasy	Unpredictable response that differs in quality from expected response but not caused by hypersensitivity	Aplastic anemia develops in 1 in 40,000 patients who receive chloramphenicol
Drug allergy	Adverse response to a drug resulting from previous exposure to that or a related drug and mediated by an antigen-antibody reaction; hypersensitivity	Reaction that occurs when penicillin is given to patient with penicillin allergy
Dependence	Continued administration of the drug required to prevent withdrawal syndrome	Patient receiving hydromorphone for cancer pain has visible tremors, restlessness, and profuse perspiration when a dose is withheld

more common for it to be administered repeatedly. The repeated administration of the drug at regular intervals causes the plasma concentration of most drugs to reach a constant concentration in the blood. This is known as the "plateau principle."[12] If plans are not made to administer the drug at the scheduled times, the plateau may not be reached, seriously affecting the effectiveness of the drug therapy.

Another time response factor to consider when planning the patient's care is the therapeutic drug concentration range. Whereas a plateau is achieved with a fixed dosing schedule, there are still peaks and troughs in the drug plasma concentration. The peak concentration occurs immediately following intravenous administration of the drug, and the trough level is the minimum concentration present immediately prior to administration of the next scheduled dose. Several drugs have a relatively narrow margin of safety, indicating that there is a close range between concentrations that produce therapeutic responses and those that cause serious adverse effects.[13] When such drugs are prescribed, arrangements must be made to determine whether the drug levels are within a therapeutic range. The most important aspect of this planning is ensuring that blood samples are drawn appropriately in conjunction with a scheduled dose. An example would be peak-trough levels for gentamicin, which require that a trough specimen be drawn 30 minutes prior to the scheduled dose, the dose infused over 30 minutes, and the peak specimen drawn 30 minutes following completion of the gentamicin infusion.

A third time response aspect to consider is the plasma half-life of the drug. Half-life refers to the amount of time required for the elimination processes to reduce the blood concentration of the drug by 50%.[14] For example, many IV drugs are eliminated by the kidneys. Because renal impairment may increase the half-life of such drugs, planning should include verification that reduced dosages have been prescribed.

Implementation

The three key areas involved in implementation are patient education, drug administration, and documentation. Because of differences among health care settings, these three areas

may not receive equal attention. In home care, greater emphasis is placed on patient education to prepare the patient for the self-administration of medication. This differs from the hospital setting, in which IV drugs are usually administered by the nurse. Regardless of the setting, documentation plays a vital role, because it validates that the actions have been implemented.

Evaluation

Evaluation of the drug therapy determines the effectiveness of the drug and may require modification of the patient's plan of care. A therapeutic response is desired because it signifies that the intended effects of the drug have been produced. However, there may be an ineffective or toxic response. An ineffective response may indicate that less than the minimum required dose has been administered, or that other factors have interfered with the action of the drug.[15] An example of an ineffective response is when a patient has only slight relief from pain following the administration of morphine. In contrast, a toxic response is an exaggeration of the usual pharmacologic actions of the drug or the appearance of signs and symptoms related to drug toxicity. For example, the toxic response to digoxin is typically evidenced by the clinical symptoms of anorexia, nausea, and vomiting.

The patient should also be evaluated for unexpected and undesired effects from the drug. Although these responses are often called side effects, this term is misleading. Side effects are therapeutically undesirable but are a consequence of the normal action of the drug. An example is the loss of potassium from the body following the administration of furosemide. Untoward drug responses, also known as adverse effects, are undesired and unexpected responses.[15] Table 11–1 describes several potential untoward drug responses.

Untoward effects may be caused by the interaction of the drug with other drugs within the body. The two major types of drug interaction are antagonism and synergism. Antagonism occurs when one drug inhibits the action of the other. An example of antagonism is the effect of morphine on metoclopramide. Synergism refers to an interaction in which the combined effect of the two drugs is greater than that of either drug alone, and may result in either summation or potentiation. When the combined effect is equal to the sum of the effects of both drugs, it is known as summation. In contrast, potentiation occurs when the combined effects of the drugs exceeds the sum of their separate actions.[15] The combined antibacterial effects of penicillin and chloramphenicol are an example of summation; ototoxicity is the result of potentiation when gentamicin and ethacrynic acid are administered concurrently.

DRUG ADMINISTRATION

The nurse's role in IV drug administration may include preparation of the drug, drug delivery, and preparing the patient to self-administer the drug. The extent of these responsibilities is determined by the health care setting. In the inpatient setting, the nurse may have responsibility for drug preparation and/or administration, whereas home care usually requires that the patient and/or family be educated in self-administration techniques.

Drug Preparation

Generally, IV drugs and admixtures are prepared in a centralized pharmacy, in which there is greater assurance of accuracy and sterility in the preparation of drugs. Although a pharmacist typically prepares the admixtures, this may be done by nurses employed by the pharmacy and working under the direction of the pharmacist. Nurses may also prepare IV drugs in emergency situations or when preparation must be done immediately prior to administration.

Laminar Flow Hood

When IV drugs are prepared in the pharmacy setting, it is usually done under a laminar flow hood. The design of the laminar flow hood prevents airborne contaminants from entering the IV solution. Air enters the back of the hood and is circulated through filters before it is directed out into the work area in uniform, parallel streams. Either a horizontal or vertical laminar flow hood may be used; however, vertical models are recommended for the preparation of cytotoxic agents.[16]

Drug Containers

IV drugs are available in various containers, including ampules, vials, partially filled solution containers, additive piggyback vials, and premixed admixtures. Ampules pose the greatest risk because of the possibility of particulate contamination. Glass fragments may enter the ampule when it is broken open, but this risk is reduced when the drug is drawn up with a filter needle. Vials are another potential risk of particulate contamination because of the risk of "coring." When the needle is introduced through the rubber stopper of the vial, the needle bevel may cut away fragments of the rubber seal.[15]

Partially filled containers and additive piggyback vials, often referred to as "minibags" or "minibottles," may be a potential source of particulate matter. This may be the result of incomplete reconstitution of the powdered drug or precip-

itates formed by the physical incompatibility of the admixture. Partially filled containers of 50 to 100 ml of 0.9% sodium chloride or dextrose 5% in water require that a liquid form of the drug be added to the container. With an additive piggyback vial, the drug contained in the vial is in powdered form, which must be reconstituted with a small volume of diluent. Because these containers are used to infuse the drug into the patient, an in-line filter should be used to remove any particulate matter present following preparation.

Premixed admixtures are prepared by the manufacturer and require no further preparation. However, they are sometimes available in frozen form, which must be restored to room temperature prior to administration. An example of an admixture available in frozen form is penicillin G. It is generally recommended that frozen admixtures not be warmed by placing them in a water bath or exposing them to microwave radiation.[17] The preferred method is to allow the admixture to thaw at room temperature.

Diluents

Another consideration for the preparation of IV drugs is the diluent used for reconstitution of the drug. Diluents with bacteriostatic properties, such as bacteriostatic sodium chloride, contain benzyl alcohol as a preservative. Although this bacteriostatic agent is desirable in most situations, it is contraindicated for neonates and for the administration of intraspinal or epidural drugs.[17] In addition, certain drugs such as amphotericin B are incompatible with preservatives and must be reconstituted with sterile water for injection.[16]

Drug Compatibility and Stability

The preparation of IV drugs is accompanied by the risks of incompatibility and instability. Incompatibility is defined as an undesirable reaction that occurs between the drug and the solution, container, or another drug. The three types of incompatibilities associated with IV drugs are physical, chemical, and therapeutic. Stability, on the other hand, refers to the length of time the drug retains its original properties and characteristics.[15]

Drug Incompatibilities

A physical incompatibility refers to a visible reaction, such as a color change, haze, turbidity, precipitate, or gas formation, occurring within the drug.[16] The largest number of physical incompatibilities involve precipitate formation, such as that seen when diazepam is added to dextrose 5% in water.

Chemical incompatibility involves the chemical degradation of the drug and is the result of hydrolysis, reduction, oxidation, or decomposition. It differs from physical incompatibility in that the reaction may not be visible.[16] Such a reaction may occur when penicillin is added to a very acidic or alkaline solution.

Therapeutic incompatibility occurs within the patient and is the result of the overlapping effects of two drugs administered concurrently.[16] Although the effects may not be evident until the patient's response to the drug therapy has been evaluated, knowledge of potential incompatibilities may prevent their occurrence. Specific examples of therapeutic incompatibility were previously discussed as part of the evaluation of drug interactions.

Drug Stability

One of the most important factors in drug stability is the degree of hydrogen ion concentration, or pH, of the solution. Most drugs are stable over a narrow range of pH values. This means that they are unstable in either very acidic (pH below 4) or alkaline (pH above 8) solutions. To maintain the desired pH, drug manufacturers often add buffers to the drug. However, the buffers are usually too weak to counteract alterations in pH when the drug is added to a highly acidic or alkaline solution.[15] The concept of stability is best characterized by penicillin. This drug is most stable in a slightly acidic environment (pH 6.5) but deteriorates if added to a very acidic or alkaline solution. Additional factors that affect drug stability are listed in Table 11–2.

Modes of IV Drug Administration

The mode of IV drug administration depends on the drug used, the patient's condition, and the desired effects of the drug. Generally, it is specified by the physician or other qualified provider. Each of the four primary modes of administration has specific advantages and disadvantages.

Continuous Infusion

Continuous infusion refers to the admixture of the drug in a large volume of solution that is infused continuously over a period of several hours to several days. The solution container is connected to an administration set and the drug (in solution) is infused into the venous access device. Based on the potency of the drug, an electronic infusion control device may be used to deliver the drug accurately at the prescribed rate of flow.

Continuous infusion is used when the drug must be highly diluted, constant plasma concentrations of the drug must be maintained, or large volumes of fluids and electrolytes must be replaced. Examples are infusions of nitroprusside or potassium chloride. Disadvantages associated with continuous infusion are possible fluid overload and potential incompatibilities between the infusion and other IV drugs administered through the same venous access device.

Intermittent Infusion

For an intermittent infusion, the drug is added to a small volume of fluid (25 to 250 ml) and infused over 15 to 90 minutes at intervals. Advantages of the intermittent mode are the ability of the drug to produce peak blood concentrations at periodic intervals, decreased risk of fluid overload, and greater convenience for the patient. However, there are disadvantages. The increased concentration of the drug in the intermittent solution may cause venous irritation, the drug may be less effective than if administered by continuous infusion, and additional equipment is required to administer the drug. IV antibiotics are generally administered using this mode.

Intermittent infusions may be administered in various ways. One of the most common methods is for the drug to be given as a piggyback infusion through the established pathway of the primary solution (Fig. 11–1). Although the primary infusion is interrupted during the piggyback infusion, the drug from the intermittent infusion container comes in contact with the primary solution below the piggyback injection port. Hence, if this method is used, the drug and the primary solution should be compatible.

A second method is simultaneous infusion. With this method, the drug is administered as a secondary infusion concurrently with the primary infusion (Fig. 11–2). Rather than connecting the intermittent infusion at the piggyback port, it is attached to the lower secondary port. One of the major disadvantages of this method is the tendency for blood to back up into the tubing once the secondary infusion has been completed, possibly occluding the venous access device. This does not occur with the piggyback method because hydrostatic pressure closes the back check valve (contained in the piggyback port) once the intermittent infusion is completed. Although drug incompatibility is a possibility with both methods, it is a greater risk with a simultaneous infusion.

Table 11–2		

Factors That Affect Drug Stability

Factor	Effect	Example
Number of additives	The greater the number of drugs contained in the admixture, the greater the chance of one of the drugs becoming unstable.	Multiple additives in TPN solution
Dilution	Limited amounts of a drug are stable in the solution, whereas large doses may be unstable.	Only limited amounts of heparin and hydrocortisone are stable in amphotericin solution
Time	The length of time the drug is in solution may affect stability.	Ampicillin only stable for 4 hours when added to D5W
Light	Some drugs are sensitive to light and exposure may result in degradation of the drug.	Exposure of levarterenol may result in degradation of drug
Temperature	Lower temperatures usually extend the stability of the drug.	Cephalothin only stable for 6 hours at room temperature but up to 48 hours when refrigerated
Order of additives	The order in which drugs are added to a solution affect compatibility and stability.	Addition of lipids to TPN solution
Container	The composition of the container may affect the stability of the drug.	Potency of insulin reduced by at least 20% when added to a plastic container

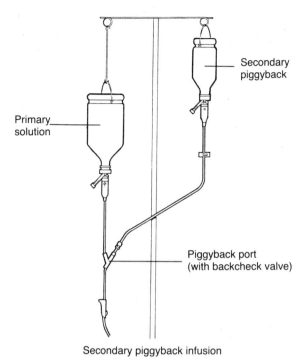

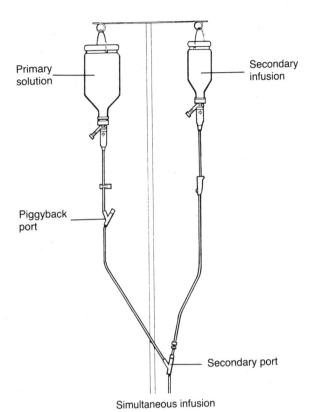

Secondary piggyback infusion

Figure 11–1. Secondary piggyback. (Redrawn with permission from Baptist Memorial Hospital. I.V. Procedure Manual. Memphis, TN: Baptist Memorial Hospital, 1991.)

Simultaneous infusion

Figure 11–2. Simultaneous infusion. (Redrawn with permission from Baptist Memorial Hospital. I.V. Procedure Manual. Memphis, TN: Baptist Memorial Hospital, 1991.)

A third method is the use of a volume control set. Although it was originally designed to control the fluid volume delivered to the patient, a drug may be added to a small amount of solution in the volume control set and infused at the desired rate (Fig. 11–3). This method is associated with many of the disadvantages previously discussed. However, it is still used in some pediatric settings, because it limits the amount of fluid volume the child receives.

The fourth method for administering intermittent infusions is directly into the venous access device. The device must be one that is intended for intermittent administration, such as a peripheral heparin lock or a long-term, centrally placed catheter. The drug is added to a minibag or minibottle and infused intermittently. Between doses, the drug container and tubing are eliminated. This method is generally preferred because it decreases the risk of fluid overload and affords greater freedom of movement for the ambulatory patient. However, failure to remove the empty drug container and tubing promptly and flush the venous access device may result in occlusion of the venous access device.

Technologic developments have produced alternatives for the administration of intermittent doses. One manufacturer has introduced a system whereby the drug is supplied in a powdered form that is attached between the primary solution and the infusion set. Once the drug vial is connected, the solution flows from the primary container through the drug vial and to the patient. Although the use of this system eliminates the costs associated with the preparation and administration of the traditional piggyback, it is only applicable to situations in which the drug and primary solution are compatible.

A second innovation has been the introduction of intermittent doses of drugs that are activated at the time of use.

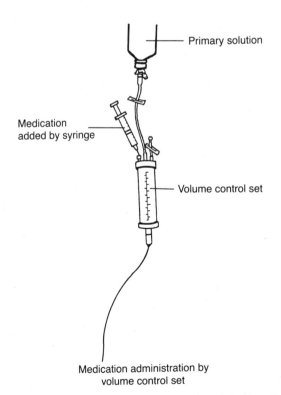

Medication administration by volume control set

Figure 11–3. Volume control set. (Redrawn with permission from Baptist Memorial Hospital. I.V. Procedure Manual. Memphis, TN: Baptist Memorial Hospital, 1991.)

Rather than preparing and refrigerating the drug prior to administration, the pharmacy simply dispenses the drug vial attached to a small container of solution. Immediately prior to administration of the drug, the nurse activates the system by removing the barrier between the drug and the solution. Although this has proven to be a cost-effective system, errors have been reported because of failure to remove the barrier and activate the system.

The third major innovation is the result of the space program and is based on elastomeric technology. The system consists of an elastomeric drug container that is stretched over a specially designed insert to establish a set delivery rate. Once the pharmacist fills the system with the drug, it may be infused at the preset rate by opening the slide clamp on the tubing attached to the container. An advantage of this system is that neither gravity nor electronic assistance is required for precise delivery of the drug.[18] However, not all drugs may be administered with an elastomeric container and, because of the expense, it is usually reserved for the home setting.

Direct Injection

Direct injection, also known as IV push or bolus, is the administration of a drug directly into the venous access device or through the proximal injection port on a continuous infusion. The purpose is to achieve rapid serum concentrations, but this may be accompanied by a greater risk of adverse effects. Instead of regulating the rate of administration by the infusion rate, direct injection only requires the time it takes to push the plunger on the syringe. Many drugs have maximum rates at which they may be administered, so the rate of the injection must be timed and the drug injected in increments. Because the drug may be incompatible with the infusing solution or heparin may be present in the intermittent device, the vascular access device should be flushed with normal saline before and after injecting the drug.

Direct injections may require that the drug be drawn into a syringe prior to administration, or that it be available in a prefilled syringe. A needle 1 inch or shorter should be used to administer the medication, because longer needles may puncture the IV tubing or the vascular access device. Another alternative is the use of a ''needle-less'' system, which also prevents inadvertent puncture of the tubing or device.

Patient-Controlled Analgesia

A fourth mode of administration is patient-controlled analgesia (PCA), which promotes patient comfort through the self-administration of analgesic agents. With this method, an electronic pump (PCA pump) is programmed to administer a small bolus of the drug when activated by the patient. The bolus amount and the time between doses (lockout interval) are predetermined by the physician and programmed into the pump by the nurse. Technologic advances have added features to the pump, permitting both continuous infusion and patient-controlled doses.

DRUG CLASSIFICATIONS

Drug reference books generally list medications alphabetically, even when a classification system is used. Such a

system aids the nurse in clinical practice, but it is not conducive to learning. To assist the nurse in understanding the wide array of IV drugs addressed in this chapter, a prototype approach is used. The drugs are divided into different categories and the drug most representative of each classification is examined in detail. Additional drugs related to the prototype, including antidotes, are then discussed in terms of their differences and similarities or their relationship to the prototype.

Drug dosages vary widely, even among the prototype and its related drugs. To include dosing information on all the drugs discussed would require more pages than are allotted for this chapter. Therefore, drug dosing is only discussed when pertinent to understanding administration of the drugs and their potential side effects. Specific information on dosing schedules for each drug is available in the *American Hospital Formulary Service Drug Information* and *Drug Facts and Comparisons*.[17, 19] These were the primary references consulted for specific drug information, although additional references may be cited to explain the various drug classifications.

Antibiotics

Antibiotics are used to treat infection and represent the largest category of frequently used intravenous medications. Basically, antibiotics may be categorized as either bactericidal or bacteriostatic. Bactericidal agents can destroy the organism by lysis of the cell wall or by prevention of its intact formation. Bacteriostatic agents inhibit growth of the organism by inhibiting protein synthesis. Although bacteriostatics may eliminate the organism in high concentrations, their effectiveness usually depends on the patient's immune system to eradicate the organism once its growth has been inhibited. Theoretically, the bacteriostatic agent inhibits bacterial growth, making administration of a bactericidal agent ineffective because its primary action is against growing cells. Actually, both types of agents may be used in combination to produce a synergistic effect.[6]

The primary contraindication for antibiotics is a known sensitivity to the drug. A patient with a history of hypersensitivity reactions to a certain antibiotic should be considered allergic to all antibiotics within the same group. For example, a patient who has a known sensitivity to penicillin is also considered to be allergic to aminopenicillins. In addition, there is evidence of a cross-sensitivity among some antibiotics, such as penicillins and cephalosporins. Therefore, cephalosporins are used cautiously in patients who are sensitive to penicillin.

One of the major disadvantages of antibiotics is that their prolonged use may result in a bacterial or fungal superinfection. A superinfection occurs when the normal flora of the body is altered by the use of an antibiotic, allowing the proliferation of selected bacteria or fungi that are resistant to the antibiotic.

Penicillins

The penicillins include both natural and semisynthetic antibiotics produced or derived by the fermentation of certain strains of the fungus Penicillium. Because of their relatively low cost, low toxicity, and clinical efficacy in the treatment of many infections, penicillins are still some of the most important antibiotics.

NATURAL PENICILLINS

The mechanism of action of the natural penicillins is bactericidal. These agents disrupt the synthesis of the bacterial cell wall, making the organism osmotically unstable. Instability of the cell wall causes it to lyse, and the organism is destroyed. Because the cell walls of gram-positive bacteria are relatively permeable to most penicillins, these drugs are generally effective against such organisms. However, gram-negative bacteria have an outer membrane around the cell wall that decreases accessibility to the natural penicillins.

Prototype: Penicillin G Potassium. Penicillin G is indicated for the treatment of severe infections caused by some gram-positive and anaerobic organisms. Because it exerts specific antibiotic action against these organisms and is relatively nontoxic to the host, penicillin G is generally considered the drug of choice for streptococcal, pneumococcal, and spirochetal infections. Specifically, penicillin is indicated in the treatment of meningitis, pericarditis, endocarditis, septicemia, and severe pneumonia.

Penicillin G may be administered as a continuous or intermittent infusion, and has a relatively wide margin of safety. Adverse reactions are rare and are usually limited to hypersensitivity reactions. Although the manifestations of a hypersensitivity reaction may only be fever, chills, or eosinophilia, these reactions can be divided into four basic types.

The first type are the dermatologic reactions, which are the most common type of hypersensitivity reaction. Symptoms include urticarial, erythematous, or maculopapular rash accompanied by pruritus. These reactions are delayed in that they do not occur until 48 hours or more following the administration of penicillin G.

The second type are serum sickness-like reactions. This type of reaction is usually evident 6 to 10 days after the initiation of therapy and is characterized by fever, malaise, urticaria, arthralgia, myalgia, lymphadenopathy, and splenomegaly. Although the reaction may be severe, it is usually short-lived and disappears within days or weeks of discontinuing the drug.

The third type of reaction includes hematologic reactions, such as hemolytic anemia, agranulocytosis, and leukopenia. Typically, this type of reaction is associated with large doses of penicillin G. A positive direct antiglobulin (Coombs') test occurs in up to 3% of patients receiving large doses, and a small number of these patients develop hemolytic anemia during or following penicillin therapy. Once the drug is discontinued, the hemoglobin concentration and reticulocyte count return to pretherapy levels, although the Coombs' test may not revert to negative for 3 months or longer.

The fourth and most serious type of hypersensitivity reaction is anaphylaxis. Although anaphylaxis has only been reported in fewer than 0.05% of patients receiving penicillin, it has been fatal in 5 to 10% of reported cases. Anaphylactic reactions to penicillin typically occur within 30 minutes of administration of the drug and are characterized by laryngeal edema, bronchospasm, stridor, cyanosis, and circulatory collapse. Treatment includes immediate discontinuation of the drug and emergency measures such as maintenance of a patent airway and the administration of epinephrine, oxygen therapy, and corticosteroids.

Penicillin interacts with several other antibiotics. Aminoglycosides are physically and chemically incompatible with penicillin and are inactivated if administered in the same IV container or administration set. Bacteriostatic antibiotics, such as chloramphenicol and erythromycin, may reduce the bactericidal action of penicillin, so concurrent use of these drugs is not recommended except in select situations.

Related Drug. Penicillin G is commercially available as a potassium or sodium salt. Both are readily soluble in water and are considered to be aqueous, crystalline penicillins, but penicillin G potassium is usually preferred. The administration of both penicillins requires special consideration because each 1 million units of penicillin G potassium contains 1.7 mEq of potassium and each 1 million units of penicillin G sodium contains 2 mEq of sodium.

PENICILLINASE-RESISTANT PENICILLINS

The critical component of the natural penicillins is the β-lactam ring incorporated into the penicillin molecule. Some strains of bacteria produce an enzyme known as penicillinase, which destroys the ring. Thus, the organism is considered to be penicillin-resistant. To overcome this resistance, the penicillinase-resistant penicillins have been developed. These antibiotics are used exclusively to treat penicillinase-resistant organisms such as Staphylococcus aureus and S. epidermidis. Their mechanism of action, contraindications, and precautions are similar to those of the natural penicillins.

Prototype: Methicillin Sodium. Methicillin sodium (Staphcillin) is mainly indicated for the treatment of infections caused by penicillinase-producing staphylococci. It is also used preoperatively to reduce the incidence of staphylococcal infections associated with certain surgical procedures. Although methicillin may be administered as a direct injection, it is more commonly given as an intermittent infusion.

Some bacteria have been labeled as ''methicillin-resistant,'' but this term is misleading. Certain strains of staphylococci are resistant to all penicillinase-resistant penicillins, not just methicillin. These resistant strains are prevalent in both the hospital and community and are being reported with increasing frequency.

The side effects of methicillin are similar to those associated with the use of penicillin G. Specifically, methicillin may cause transient asymptomatic elevations of serum alkaline phosphatase, alanine aminotransferase, and aspartate aminotransferase levels. In rare instances, transient neutropenia, leukopenia, granulocytopenia, and thrombocytopenia have been reported. Generally, these hematologic effects are not evident until more than 10 days after the initiation of therapy and resolve within 2 to 7 days once the drug is discontinued. There is also a 15 to 20% incidence of acute interstitial nephritis with the use of methicillin.

Related Drugs. Two additional penicillinase-resistant penicillins are nafcillin sodium (Unipen) and oxacillin sodium (Prostaphlin). Both drugs are similar to methicillin, but nafcillin is more likely to cause phlebitis than other penicillinase-resistant penicillins. However, nafcillin may be prescribed more frequently than methicillin, because it is less likely to cause acute interstitial nephritis.

Aminopenicillins

Aminopenicillins have a free amino group added to the penicillin nucleus, which increases their bactericidal effectiveness against gram-negative bacteria. However, they are inactivated by penicillinase-producing organisms.

Prototype: Ampicillin Sodium. Ampicillin sodium (Omnipen-N) is highly effective in the treatment of severe infections caused by Salmonella, Shigella, Proteus mirabilis, and Escherichia coli. Although ampicillin may be administered by direct injection, it is generally administered as an intermittent infusion. Concentrated doses of ampicillin are stable for 4 hours in 5% dextrose in water and 5% dextrose in 0.45% sodium chloride, but potency is extended to 8 hours when added to isotonic sodium chloride without dextrose. When the drug is further diluted in a minibag or minibottle, stability may be extended up to 48 hours.

Adverse reactions to ampicillin are similar to those of penicillin G. It may also produce a distinct, nonimmunologic reaction characterized by a generalized erythematous, maculopapular rash similar to measles. The rash typically occurs 3 to 14 days following the initiation of therapy and generally disappears despite the continuation of therapy. It is more common in patients with mononucleosis and is not indicative of a hypersensitivity to penicillin. Hematologic effects such as neutropenia, agranulocytosis, and thrombocytopenia have also been reported, but these are usually reversible once the drug is discontinued.

Because of the probability of patients with infectious mononucleosis developing rash during therapy, ampicillin is generally not prescribed to those with this disease. In addition, the potential for ampicillin rash is increased for patients receiving allopurinol and ampicillin concomitantly.

Related Drug. Ampicillin sodium-sulbactam sodium (Unasyn) is a combination of ampicillin with sulbactam that prevents inactivation of the drug by penicillinase-producing organisms. It is primarily indicated in the treatment of intraabdominal and gynecologic infections.

EXTENDED-SPECTRUM PENICILLINS

Because of structural differences in the side chains of the extended-spectrum antibiotics, they have a wider spectrum of activity than the other penicillins. Specifically, the extended-spectrum penicillins are effective against gram-negative organisms, including Pseudomonas. Like the natural penicillins, the extended-spectrum penicillins are ineffective against penicillinase-producing organisms.

Prototype: Ticarcillin Disodium. Ticarcillin disodium (Ticar) is bactericidal for several gram-negative, gram-positive, and anaerobic organisms. Specifically, it is indicated for bacterial septicemia and infections of the respiratory, genital, and urinary tracts.

Ticarcillin may be administered by direct injection, intermittent infusion, or continuous infusion. However, administration should not exceed the recommended rates. Too rapid infusion of ticarcillin and higher than normal doses have

resulted in seizures. Other side effects of ticarcillin are similar to those of penicillin G and include dermatologic and hematologic reactions, thrombophlebitis, and anaphylaxis.

Drug interactions associated with ticarcillin are similar to those of the other penicillins. There may also be an increased risk of bleeding in patients who are receiving anticoagulants.

Related Drugs. Other extended-spectrum penicillins include mezlocillin sodium (Mezlin), piperacillin sodium (Pipracil), and ticarcillin disodium-clavulanate potassium (Timentin). Because of their cost, these drugs are usually reserved for patients with infections resistant to ticarcillin.

Cephalosporins

Cephalosporins are bactericidal antibiotics that share a close structural similarity with the penicillins. Because of this, they have similar mechanisms of action, side effects, and contraindications. Cephalosporins are classified by their spectrum of activity, or "generation."

FIRST-GENERATION CEPHALOSPORINS

First-generation cephalosporins are active against susceptible gram-positive bacteria, such as Staphylococcus aureus and S. epidermidis, and some gram-negative organisms. Because of their low cost, they are the preferred drugs for most gram-positive infections.

Prototype: Cefazolin Sodium. Cefazolin sodium (Kefzol) is effective in the treatment of serious infections of the respiratory tract, genitourinary tract, cardiovascular system, and soft tissue. It may be administered as a direct injection or as an intermittent infusion. Because the primary route of elimination for cefazolin is the kidneys, renal impairment requires a reduced dosage.

Although cefazolin is considered relatively nontoxic, allergic reactions have been reported in up to 5% of patients receiving the drug. These reactions are similar to those associated with penicillin G and range from a mild rash to anaphylaxis. Nephrotoxicity has been reported, but it is rare and more likely to occur in geriatric patients or in those with renal impairment.

There are few reported drug interactions involving cefazolin. However, the concurrent use of nephrotoxic drugs such as aminoglycosides and cefazolin may increase the risk of renal toxicity.

Related Drugs. Other first-generation cephalosporins are cephradine (Velosef), cephalothin sodium (Keflin), and cephapirin (Cefadyl). Of these agents, cephalothin has the greatest risk of nephrotoxicity and venous irritation.

SECOND-GENERATION CEPHALOSPORINS

The second-generation cephalosporins have greater gram-negative activity than the first-generation drugs, but are less effective against gram-positive organisms. Their mechanism of action, side effects, contraindications, and precautions are similar to those of cefazolin.

Prototype: Cefoxitin Sodium. Cefoxitin sodium (Mefoxin) is indicated for the treatment of serious infections of the respiratory and genitourinary tracts, gynecologic infections, and septicemia. The increased activity of cefoxitin against anaerobic bacteria also increases its usefulness in intra-abdominal infections. Because it is excreted by the kidneys, a reduced dosage of cefoxitin is required in those with renal impairment.

Related Drugs. Additional second-generation cephalosporins are cefamandole nafate (Mandol), cefonicid sodium (Monocid), ceforanide (Precef), cefotetan disodium (Cefotan), and cefuroxime sodium (Kefurox). The most significant of these drugs is cefamandole, which may increase bleeding tendencies because of the elimination of intestinal bacteria that normally synthesize vitamin K or the inhibition of clotting factor synthesis independent of vitamin K.

THIRD-GENERATION CEPHALOSPORINS

Third-generation cephalosporins have increased activity against gram-negative organisms, including Pseudomonas, but are less effective against gram-positive organisms. An important characteristic of this category of drugs is their ability to cross the blood-brain barrier when the meninges are inflamed. The third-generation cephalosporins share many of the characteristics of the first and second generations.

Prototype: Cefotaxime Sodium. Cefotaxime sodium (Claforan) is indicated for the treatment of bacteremia, septicemia, meningitis, and serious infections of the respiratory and genitourinary tracts. It is usually administered by intermittent infusion, but may also be given by direct injection.

Related Drugs. Related third-generation drugs include cefoperazone sodium (Cefobid), ceftazidime (Fortaz), ceftizoxime sodium (Cefizox), ceftriaxone sodium (Rocephin), and moxalactam disodium (Moxam). Ceftriaxone is generally preferred for home care, because it only requires a single daily dose.

Aminoglycosides

Aminoglycosides are bactericidal antibiotics that are effective against several gram-negative organisms. Their name is derived from the amino sugars contained within their chemical structure.

Prototype: Gentamicin Sulfate. Gentamicin sulfate (Garamycin) is well distributed throughout all body fluids, achieves peak plasma concentrations within 30 minutes to 2 hours of administration, and maintains serum levels for up to 12 hours. It is frequently administered concurrently with penicillin because the two drugs have synergistic bactericidal effects. Specifically, gentamicin is effective in the treatment of serious infections of the respiratory, urinary, and gastrointestinal tracts, septicemia, and infections of the skin and soft tissue.

The most significant side effects associated with gentamicin are ototoxicity (associated with high peak plasma levels) and nephrotoxicity (associated with high trough levels). It has been suggested that this is the result of accumulation of the drug intracellularly in the inner ear and kidneys. Otic effects are manifested by vestibular symptoms, such as dizziness, nystagmus, vertigo, and ataxia, or auditory symptoms, such as tinnitus and hearing impairment. Nephrotoxicity is

evidenced by increased BUN and serum creatinine levels and decreased creatinine clearance and urine specific gravity. Both ototoxicity and nephrotoxicity are more likely to occur in geriatric patients, patients with renal impairment, patients receiving high doses or extended therapy, and patients receiving other ototoxic or nephrotoxic drugs. However, symptoms are usually reversible once the drug is discontinued.

Gentamicin may produce dose-related and self-limiting neuromuscular blockade. Symptoms range from general muscular weakness to seizures and a myasthenia gravis-like syndrome. Gentamicin may also provoke hypersensitivity reactions such as rash, urticaria, stomatitis, pruritus, fever, and eosinophilia.

There is a narrow margin between therapeutic and toxic levels of gentamicin. A therapeutic level of 4 to 8 μg/ml should be maintained and serum concentrations monitored to avoid peak levels greater than 12 μg/ml and trough levels above 2 μg/ml. Monitoring of gentamicin serum levels requires that the trough sample be drawn 30 minutes prior to a scheduled dose, the dose be administered as scheduled, and the peak sample be drawn 30 minutes following completion of the scheduled dose.

Related Drugs. Aminoglycosides similar to gentamicin include amikacin sulfate (Amikin), kanamycin sulfate (Kantrex), netilmicin sulfate (Netromycin), and tobramycin sulfate (Nebcin). These drugs are usually reserved for the treatment of gentamicin-resistant infections.

Tetracyclines

Tetracyclines were the first broad-spectrum antibiotics developed. They are considered bacteriostatic but may have bactericidal activity in high concentrations. Although IV tetracycline is no longer available commercially, there are other tetracycline antibiotics that may be administered intravenously.

Prototype: Doxycycline Hyclate. Doxycycline hyclate (Vibramycin) is indicated for infections caused by susceptible organisms such as rickettsiae and viruses, and as a substitute when penicillin therapy is contraindicated. Doxycycline is usually administered by intermittent infusion in 100 to 200 ml of fluid over 1 to 4 hours.

The most common side effects of doxycycline are dose-related effects on the gastrointestinal tract. Manifestations include nausea, vomiting, diarrhea, and anorexia. Other adverse effects include hypersensitivity reactions and blood dyscrasias. In addition, the administration of doxycycline may cause venous irritation and thrombophlebitis, requiring that the IV site be rotated more frequently than every 48 hours. Photosensitivity reactions may occur, resulting in exaggerated sunburn on areas of the body exposed to the sun. Although it is not a significant risk for hospitalized patients, home patients should be alerted to this potential reaction.

Doxycycline is potentiated by alcohol and hepatotoxic drugs, but is inhibited by cimetidine and alkalizing agents. In addition, doxycycline potentiates the effects of anticoagulants and digoxin.

Related Drug. A related tetracycline is minocycline hydrochloride (Minocin). It is similar to doxycycline in its mechanism of action, side effects, and precautions. However, minocycline is less likely to cause venous irritation.

Erythromycins

Like the tetracyclines, the erythromycins are generally bacteriostatic but may have bactericidal activity when administered in high concentrations. The only erythromycin administered intravenously is erythromycin lactobionate.

Prototype: Erythromycin Lactobionate. Erythromycin lactobionate (Erythrocin) is primarily indicated for staphylococcal, pneumococcal, and streptococcal infections and in the treatment of legionnaires' disease. It may also be used as an alternative in the presence of a penicillin allergy. Although erythromycin may be administered as a continuous infusion, it is generally given as an intermittent infusion in 100 to 250 ml of fluid over 20 to 60 minutes. The infusion time may be extended if the patient experiences venous discomfort during administration.

Erythromycin is relatively free from serious side effects. However, the patient must be monitored for hearing loss secondary to IV erythromycin. The most common complaint is localized venous irritation during administration, which may be minimized by slowing of the infusion rate, further dilution of the medication, and frequent site rotations. Mild allergic reactions such as urticaria and rash have also been reported.

Because erythromycin is unstable if the pH is lower than 5.5, 1 ml sodium bicarbonate (e.g., Neut) may be added to acidic solutions, such as dextrose 5% in water, to increase the stability of erythromycin. When erythromycin is in solution for only a short period, as with an intermittent infusion that is activated at the time of usage, such buffering is considered unnecessary.

Increased serum levels of cyclosporine, digoxin, methylprednisolone, theophylline, and warfarin may occur with the administration of erythromycin. Therefore, if serum levels of these drugs are tested, the results must be interpreted accordingly.

Chloramphenicol

Chloramphenicol is a bacteriostatic antibiotic that may be bactericidal when used in high concentrations. Although different forms of the drug are available for oral and topical administration, only the sodium succinate salt of chloramphenicol may be administered intravenously.

Prototype: Chloramphenicol Sodium Succinate. Chloramphenicol sodium succinate (Chloromycetin) is reserved for serious infections caused by susceptible organisms such as Haemophilus influenzae, Rickettsia spp., and Salmonella typhi. Frequently, it is used in conjunction with penicillin G for the treatment of anaerobic infections of the central nervous system. Regardless of the indication, the preferred method of administration is by intermittent infusion.

Although chloramphenicol is associated with fewer minor side effects than other antibiotics, it is more likely to cause serious and potentially fatal adverse reactions. Most notable are its hematologic effects, and chloramphenicol may cause two types of bone marrow depression. The first is irreversible, not dose-related, and results in aplastic anemia and a mortality rate that exceeds 50%, but it is relatively rare. The second and more common type is dose-related and typically reversible once the drug is discontinued. Symptoms include

reticulocytopenia, anemia, leukopenia, and thrombocytopenia. Because of the possibility of hematologic effects, a serum level should not exceed 5 to 20 μg/ml, and laboratory values should be carefully monitored.

Chloramphenicol potentiates chlorpropamide, phenytoin, cyclophosphamide, oral anticoagulants, and hypoglycemic drugs. It inhibits iron dextran but is inhibited by rifampin. When administered concurrently with penicillin, chloramphenicol extends its own half-life while inhibiting the action of penicillin.

Miscellaneous Antibiotics

Some antibiotics do not belong to a specific classification. Because they share common properties with all antibiotics, only their unique characteristics are discussed here.

Aztreonam. Aztreonam (Azactam) is the first drug in a new class of antibiotics known as monobactams. Although monobactams differ structurally from β-lactams, such as penicillins and cephalosporins, cross-sensitivity between the two classes of drugs may exist. However, because the probability of cross-sensitivity is not as great and does not typically result in a serious, life-threatening allergic reaction, aztreonam may still be indicated in the presence of a β-lactam allergy.

Ciprofloxacin. Ciprofloxacin (Cipro) belongs to a class of antibiotics known as fluorquinolones. These antibiotics contain a fluorine molecule, which increases the drug's potency against gram-negative and gram-positive organisms, and piperazine, which is responsible for antipseudomonal activity. Because ciprofloxacin is associated with venous irritation, it should be administered over at least 60 minutes. Other adverse side effects include convulsions and hypersensitivity reactions.

Clindamycin Phosphate. Clindamycin phosphate (Cleocin) is a bacteriostatic antibiotic that is effective against anaerobic and aerobic organisms. It is chemically unrelated to penicillin, so it is useful in penicillin-sensitive patients. Side effects associated with clindamycin are diarrhea, pseudomembranous colitis, and a generalized rash. Because hypotension and cardiopulmonary arrest have been reported following too rapid administration of the drug, it is recommended that clindamycin be administered by intermittent infusion over a minimum of 10 minutes.

Imipenem-Cilastatin Sodium. Imipenem-cilastatin sodium (Primaxin) is a β-lactam antibiotic that has been structurally altered to increase its antibacterial activity. Because of its wide spectrum of activity, imipenem-cilastatin is effective in the treatment of polymicrobial bacterial infections, including Pseudomonas and many β-lactamase–producing strains of bacteria.

Vancomycin Hydrochloride. Vancomycin hydrochloride (Vancocin) is a bactericidal antibiotic. It is considered the drug of choice for methicillin-resistant staphylococcal infections and for staphylococcal infections in patients who are allergic to penicillin. The two most serious side effects of vancomycin are ototoxicity and nephrotoxicity. In addition, rapid administration results in hypotension and a transient reddish blotching caused by histamine release. This reaction can be avoided if vancomycin is administered over a minimum of 60 minutes.

Other Anti-Infective Agents

Because antibiotics are primarily effective against bacterial organisms, other agents are required to treat infections caused by fungi, viruses, and protozoa. Categories of drugs discussed in this section include antifungal agents, antiviral agents, and antiprotozoal drugs. Although sulfonamide combination products have antibacterial activity, they have been included in this section because of their unique properties.

Antifungal Agents

Systemic fungal infections, although rare, are difficult to treat, and are more common in immunosuppressed patients. Such infections may be treated with antifungal agents that act by binding to sterols in the membrane of the fungal cell. Once the drug binds to the cell membrane, the cell no longer has a protective barrier, the cellular constituents are lost, and the cell destroyed. Because bacteria do not contain sterols in their cell membranes, antifungal agents are not active against these organisms.

Prototype: Amphotericin B. Amphotericin B (Fungizone) is considered the drug of choice for treating progressive and potentially fatal infections such as aspergillosis, blastomycosis, candidiasis, coccidiomycosis, cryptococcus, and histoplasmosis. Because the drug is only effective against susceptible organisms, diagnosis of the organism must be confirmed by histologic studies before initiating treatment.

Prior to the initiation of amphotericin therapy, a test dose is administered to assess the patient's ability to tolerate the drug. Typically, 0.25 mg/kg of amphotericin in 5% dextrose is infused over 4 to 6 hours and the patient's pulse, respirations, temperature, and blood pressure are monitored every 30 minutes. The daily dose may be gradually increased up to a daily dose of 1 mg/kg, or up to 1.5 mg/kg administered on alternative days. Because the maximum daily dose is 1.5 mg/kg, most fungal infections require months of therapy to achieve the total cumulative dose of 2 to 4 g.

Common dose-related side effects of amphotericin include headache, chills, fever, malaise, anorexia, nausea, and vomiting. Antipyretics, antihistamines, and antiemetics may provide symptomatic relief when administered prior to or during therapy, and hydrocortisone may be added to the infusion to decrease the severity of febrile reactions. Another expected reaction to amphotericin is thrombophlebitis at the injection site, but the incidence may be decreased by the addition of 1200 to 1600 units of heparin to the infusion.

The selective binding of amphotericin to sterols accounts for the toxicity of the drug. Some body cells, such as kidney cells, contain sterols that bind to the drug, making the cell subject to alterations in cellular permeability. Some degree of nephrotoxicity occurs in more than 80% of patients receiving amphotericin and may be manifested by elevated blood urea nitrogen and creatinine levels, hypokalemia, and hypomagnesemia. To decrease these nephrotoxic effects mannitol, 12.5 g, or normal saline may be administered intravenously immediately prior to and following each dose of amphotericin.

Amphotericin may also bind with sterols in the cellular membrane of erythrocytes. Consequently, a reversible, normocytic, normochromic anemia occurs in most patients receiving amphotericin. Cardiovascular toxicities such as hypotension, ventricular fibrillation, and cardiac arrest are rare, but may occur with rapid infusion of the drug.

Precautions regarding the administration of amphotericin may include infusing the drug over a minimum of 4 hours to reduce the incidence of side effects and monitoring the injection site for signs of phlebitis. However, more rapid infusion rates are now recommended if the patient's renal function is normal. Throughout therapy, the patient's serum electrolyte levels and renal function require monitoring, and the patient should be assessed for symptoms of electrolyte imbalance.

Amphotericin interacts with a number of drugs. For example, it produces additive nephrotoxic effects when administered with aminoglycosides and it enhances potassium depletion when given with corticosteroids, diuretics, and cardiac glycosides.

Related Drugs. Miconazole (Monistat) is an antifungal agent that works by altering the cell membrane and interfering with intracellular enzymes. Because miconazole is less toxic, it may be an alternative for patients who cannot tolerate amphotericin. However, phlebitis and pruritus are common side effects and rapid administration may result in tachycardia or cardiac arrest.

Another alternative to amphotericin is fluconazole (Diflucan), which is indicated for the treatment of serious systemic candidal infections and cryptococcal meningitis. Although adverse reactions may occur in patients receiving fluconazole, such reactions are more common in HIV-infected patients. Nausea and vomiting, headache, and abdominal pain are among the adverse reactions that have been reported. Serious hepatic reactions and exfoliative skin disorders may also occur, but are less likely in HIV-infected patients.

Antiviral Agents

Treatment for viral diseases is generally less effective than for bacterial infections. Because agents capable of killing the virus can also kill the host cells, antiviral therapy is limited to inhibition of the viral replication process. In addition, viral infections often progress without clinical signs or symptoms early in the course of illness, when the drugs might be most effective.

Prototype: Acyclovir Sodium. Acyclovir (Zovirax), indicated in the treatment of herpes simplex, varicella zoster, Epstein-Barr virus, and cytomegalovirus infections, is one of the most common and useful antiviral agents. The activation of acyclovir by an enzyme produced by the virus causes the drug to inhibit DNA production within the virus, thus preventing viral replication.

Because of the risk of renal tubular damage with rapid administration of acyclovir, each dose is administered over at least 1 hour. Acyclovir crystals may occlude the renal tubules; therefore, adequate hydration and urine output must be maintained prior to and during the infusion. The more common side effects associated with acyclovir are headache and thrombophlebitis.

Other Antiviral Agents. Other antiviral agents include ganciclovir sodium (Cytovene), vidarabine (Vira-A), and zidovudine (AZT). Ganciclovir is structurally and pharmacologically related to acyclovir and is indicated in the treatment of cytomegalovirus in immunosuppressed patients, particularly those infected with HIV. Because of its mutagenic potential, guidelines for handling cytotoxic agents must be followed when preparing and administering ganciclovir. Viradabine, on the other hand, is used specifically for the treatment of herpes simplex encephalitis. One of the newest antiviral agents is zidovudine, which is primarily used to decrease the severity of symptoms in patients with HIV and a confirmed history of Pneumocystis carinii pneumonia. The most serious side effects of zidovudine are hematologic effects, nausea, and headache.

Antiprotozoal Drugs

The two drugs identified for their antiprotozoal activity, metronidazole and pentamidine, also have additional properties that make them effective against certain other organisms.

Prototype: Metronidazole. Metronidazole (Flagyl) is a bactericidal agent that is effective against protozoa and specific anaerobic bacteria. Indications include serious intra-abdominal, gynecologic, and lower respiratory tract infections, Crohn's disease, and antibiotic-related pseudomembranous colitis. Although metronidazole may be given as a continuous infusion, it is typically administered as an intermittent infusion over a minimum of 1 hour.

The most common side effects of metronidazole are nausea, anorexia, headache, and an unpleasant metallic taste. Peripheral neuropathy, characterized by tingling, numbness, or paresthesia of the extremity, has been reported but is reversible once the drug is discontinued. If alcohol is ingested while receiving metronidazole, disulfiram-like reactions, such as flushing, headache, nausea, sweating, and abdominal cramps, may occur.

Related Drug. Another antiprotozoal agent is pentamidine isethionate (Pentam). It is specifically indicated in the treatment of Pneumocystis carinii pneumonia if the patient does not respond to trimethoprim-sulfamethoxazole. Severe hypotensive reactions may occur, particularly if pentamidine is administered over less than 60 minutes. Other adverse reactions include hypoglycemia and diabetogenic effects.

Sulfonamide Combination Products

Sulfonamides are broad-spectrum antimicrobial agents that have been used for more than 50 years. Although their general use has declined with the introduction of penicillins and cephalosporins, they remain an inexpensive and effective antibacterial therapy. Sulfonamides are usually bacteriostatic in action and act by depriving the bacteria of folate products required for DNA synthesis. This inhibits the growth and reproduction of the microorganism. Body cells, unlike bacterial cells, do not synthesize their own folic acid and are unaffected by the drugs.

Sulfonamides are associated with numerous adverse reactions that involve nearly every body system. Because sulfonamide combination products contain a sulfonamide in addition to another drug, all precautions applicable to sulfonamides apply to the combination products.

Prototype: Trimethoprim-sulfamethoxazole. Trimethoprim-sulfamethoxazole (Bactrim, Septra) is a combination of sulfamethoxazole and trimethoprim in a fixed 5:1 ratio. Because of its bactericidal properties, it is indicated in the treatment of severe urinary tract infections, Pneumocystis carinii pneumonia, and shigellosis.

Because it contains a sulfonamide, trimethoprim-sulfamethoxazole is associated with three major types of side effects. First are hypersensitivity reactions, which range from rash to anaphylaxis. These reactions tend to be more common in HIV-infected patients receiving trimethoprim-sulfamethoxazole. Second, sulfonamides may crystallize in the renal tubules, causing renal damage. The risk is reduced by maintaining adequate hydration and urinary output or by reducing the dosage. Third, sulfonamides may have a toxic effect on the bone marrow, resulting in aplastic anemia, thrombocytopenia, and agranulocytosis. Overall, the most common side effects of trimethoprim-sulfamethoxazole are nausea, vomiting, and rash.

Sulfonamides bind to the plasma proteins, either displacing or being displaced by other protein-bound drugs. They potentiate the effects of warfarin and phenytoin, but are inhibited by alkalinizing agents and thiopental. In addition, sulfonamides can be cross-sensitized with other drugs containing a sulfa structure, such as thiazide diuretics and oral hypoglycemics.

Central Nervous System Drugs

The central nervous system (CNS) is biologically complex and susceptible to interference by many pharmacologic agents. Because the CNS controls multiple physiologic functions, drugs that act centrally may have secondary effects on other body systems. There are many ways of classifying CNS drugs, but one of the most useful is according to their mechanism of action.

Analgesics

Analgesics are administered to relieve pain. Narcotic agonist analgesics may cause stupor or insensibility, also known as narcosis. These drugs are often referred to as opiate agonists because they are chemically related to morphine, which is derived from the opium poppy. Another category of analgesics is the mixed narcotic agonist-antagonists. When these drugs are administered to a patient who has received no other narcotic, they produce a morphine-like analgesia and respiratory depression. However, if mixed narcotic agonist-antagonists are administered to a patient who has received a narcotic, they partly antagonize the analgesia and respiratory depression.[6]

NARCOTIC ANALGESICS

Although the narcotic analgesics vary in potency, they share several common properties. Narcotic analgesics act as agonists on specific opiate receptors, share the major side effect of respiratory depression, and cause drowsiness. Repeated administration may produce tolerance to the drug or the phenomenon of cross-tolerance. Cross-tolerance means that, once a tolerance to the action of one narcotic develops, the patient may also be tolerant to the action of other narcotics.

Prototype: Morphine Sulfate. The prototype of all narcotic analgesics is morphine sulfate. By binding to the opiate receptors, morphine relieves severe pain and inhibits the perception of pain. It may also alter the patient's mood, producing a feeling of euphoria. The primary indications for morphine are severe pain and apprehension associated with coronary occlusion or pulmonary edema, chronic pain associated with malignancies, and postoperative pain.

Although morphine may be administered by direct injection or continuous infusion, it may also be administered as patient-controlled analgesia (PCA). Using a PCA pump, the patient may self-administer frequent, small doses based on the patient's requirements for pain relief and the program prescribed for the PCA device.

The major side effect of morphine is respiratory depression. Patients with impaired respiratory function or those receiving morphine by rapid injection are at greatest risk. Other severe adverse effects of morphine include tachycardia, hypotension, myocardial depression, pinpoint pupils, excitation, and coma. Minor side effects such as nausea, vomiting, and constipation are more common.

The contraindications for morphine are based on its pharmacologic effects. Because morphine may produce respiratory depression, it is generally contraindicated in patients with poor pulmonary function, such as those with emphysema and asthma, and in the presence of closed head injuries. Morphine also produces spasmogenic effects on the smooth muscle of the gastrointestinal and genitourinary tracts. Therefore, it is contraindicated for benign prostatic hypertrophy, biliary tract surgery, and diarrhea caused by poisoning.

Morphine is potentiated by several drugs, so that a reduced dosage of both drugs may be indicated. Specific drug categories include phenothiazines, monoamine oxidase (MAO) inhibitors, neuromuscular blockers, and adrenergic blocking agents. Central nervous system depressants, such as alcohol, barbiturates, hypnotics, and sedatives, also potentiate the effects of morphine. Cimetidine, in particular, may prolong or intensify the effects of morphine, causing disorientation, respiratory depression, apnea, and seizures, but these reactions are generally not associated with cimetidine alternatives.

Related Drugs. The other narcotic analgesics are related to morphine but differ in terms of analgesic potency. Hydromorphone hydrochloride (Dilaudid) is approximately five to ten times as potent as morphine, whereas meperidine hydrochloride (Demerol) has an analgesic potency equivalent to 20% of morphine and a shorter duration of action.

Antagonist. Naloxone (Narcan) is a narcotic antagonist that blocks the opiate receptors, thus inhibiting or reversing the narcotic effects. Narcan is specifically used to counteract opiate-induced respiratory depression and narcotic overdose. The usual dosage is 0.4 to 2.0 mg, administered as a direct injection. Potential adverse reactions include nausea, vomiting, hypotension or hypertension, tachycardia, and fibrillation.

MIXED OPIATE AGONIST-ANTAGONISTS

Mixed opiate agonist-antagonists behave as agonists when administered to a patient who has not previously received a narcotic analgesic. In this manner, the drugs interact with the receptors and alter the function of the cells to produce effects similar to those of the narcotic analgesics. However, when mixed opiate agonist-antagonists are administered to a patient who is receiving a narcotic analgesic, they produce an antagonistic effect and inhibit the response to the narcotic analgesic. Mixed narcotic agonist-antagonists are also called opiate partial agonists because their actions are similar to those of opiate agonists, but only under specific conditions.

Prototype: Buprenorphine Hydrochloride. The prototype of the mixed opiate agonist-antagonists is buprenorphine hydrochloride (Buprenex). When administered as a narcotic agonist, buprenorphine is 30 times more potent than morphine. It is therefore indicated for the relief of moderate to severe pain, especially in patients with a hypersensitivity to narcotic analgesics. Although buprenorphine produces an antagonistic effect approximately three times greater than that of naloxone, it is rarely used clinically to reverse the effects of opiates.

The major side effect associated with buprenorphine is excessive sedation. Other effects on the nervous system include dizziness, vertigo, headache, confusion, euphoria, and insomnia. Nausea, vomiting, hypotension or hypertension, tachycardia or bradycardia, and respiratory depression have also been reported following buprenorphine administration.

Buprenorphine may potentiate the effects of CNS depressants, such as tranquilizers and sedatives. The concomitant administration of IV buprenorphine and oral diazepam has resulted in respiratory and cardiovascular collapse.

Related Drugs. Two related mixed narcotic agonist-antagonists are nalbuphine hydrochloride (Nubain) and pentazocine lactate (Talwin). The mechanism of action, indications, and side effects of both drugs are similar to those of buprenorphine. However, the respiratory depression associated with nalbuphine is not increased with increasing doses, as occurs with buprenorphine.

Sedatives, Hypnotics, and Anxiolytics

There are several CNS depressants that cause drowsiness (sedatives), induce sleep (hypnotics), or relieve anxiety (anxiolytics). These drugs may be chemically classified as barbiturates, which produce CNS depression ranging from sedation to anesthesia, benzodiazepines, which relieve anxiety without causing ataxia or sleep, and miscellaneous CNS agents, which produce antiemetic as well as sedative or anxiolytic effects.

BARBITURATES

Barbiturates comprise the traditional group of CNS depressants. They can produce varying levels of CNS depression ranging from mild sedation and hypnosis to coma and death. Generally, barbiturates share the same pharmacologic effects, side effects, contraindications, and drug interactions.

Prototype: Phenobarbital Sodium. Phenobarbital sodium (Luminal) may be used as a sedative because of its slow onset of action and its prolonged effect. However, it may produce a hypnotic effect at higher doses. Intravenous phenobarbital is primarily used as an anticonvulsant in pediatric patients. It inhibits abnormal electrical activity in the brain without producing marked sedation and is therefore indicated in the management of tonic-clonic (grand mal) and partial seizures.

Phenobarbital is administered by direct injection; too rapid administration of phenobarbital may cause respiratory depression, apnea, laryngospasm, and hypotension. The most common side effects of phenobarbital are excessive sedation and ataxia, but facial edema, fever, and thrombocytopenic purpura may occur. In addition, phenobarbital may cause pain or thrombophlebitis at the injection site.

Phenobarbital is contraindicated in patients who have a history of porphyria, which is characterized by excessive formation of porphyrins in the liver. Barbiturates such as phenobarbital stimulate porphyrin synthesis, which causes dermatologic reactions and peripheral nerve damage.

Phenobarbital may potentiate the effects of other CNS depressants and the adverse effects of antidepressants. Because phenobarbital stimulates the hepatic metabolizing enzymes, it increases the metabolism of corticosteriods and digitoxin so that increased dosages of these drugs may be required. It also inhibits the effectiveness of doxycycline, propranolol, oral anticoagulants, and theophylline.

Related Drugs. Other barbiturates that may be administered intravenously are amobarbital sodium (Amytal), pentobarbital sodium (Nembutal), secobarbital sodium (Seconal), and thiopental sodium (Pentothal). These drugs differ primarily in their onset and duration of action. Thiopental is an ultrashort-acting barbiturate used primarily for its anesthetic effects. Pentobarbital and secobarbital are short-acting barbiturates used for preanesthetic sedation. Amobarbital has a longer duration of action than pentobarbital and secobarbital and is used to control seizures caused by eclampsia, poisoning, meningitis, or tetanus.

BENZODIAZEPINES

Benzodiazepines differ from barbiturates chemically but share many of the same indications. Often, benzodiazepines are preferred to barbiturates because they have a greater margin of safety and are less likely to interact with other drugs and to cause physical dependence. Benzodiazepines have four basic actions—they reduce anxiety, produce sedation, relax muscle spasticity, and act as anticonvulsants.

Prototype: Diazepam. Diazepam (Valium) depresses the autonomic, central, and peripheral nervous systems. For this reason, intravenous diazepam is indicated for the management of acute alcohol withdrawal, the emergency treatment of status epilepticus or recurrent seizures, the treatment of skeletal muscle spasm, and the relief of apprehension prior to electric cardioversion, endoscopy, or surgery.

Because of several reports of precipitation or absorption of the drug into plastic tubing, the preferred method of diazepam injection is by direct injection into the vein. When direct IV injection is not feasible, diazepam should be injected into the IV tubing as close to the vein site as possible. If this alternative method is used, the IV cannula should be flushed with normal saline prior to and following the administration

of diazepam. The manufacturers state that diazepam may form a precipitate when mixed with other solutions, including sodium chloride, so the possibility of precipitate formation still exists when flushing the cannula. Nonetheless, most clinicians agree that this risk of precipitation is lower than if diazepam came into contact with other medications in the IV line.

The most common adverse reactions to diazepam are the results of CNS depression and are similar to the side effects associated with barbiturates. They include drowsiness, ataxia, confusion, syncope, and vertigo. Anticholinergic side effects, or "atropine-like" reactions, may also occur and result in blurred vision, mydriasis, and dry mouth. Other adverse reactions such as apnea, hypotension, bradycardia, or cardiac arrest are rare, and are generally associated with rapid administration of the drug.

Because of the possibility of anticholinergic effects, diazepam is contraindicated in patients with acute narrow-angle glaucoma. It is also contraindicated for patients with acute alcohol intoxication in whom the vital signs are depressed and for patients with known hypersensitivity to the benzodiazepines.

Diazepam is potentiated by other drugs that produce similar CNS depression and cimetidine. In addition, diazepam potentiates the effects of narcotics, barbiturates, antihistamines, and phenothiazines. When diazepam is administered concurrently with levodopa, the antiparkinsonian effects of levodopa may be inhibited.

Related Drugs. The three other benzodiazepines that are most commonly administered by the IV route are chlordiazepoxide hydrochloride (Librium), lorazepam (Ativan), and midazolam hydrochloride (Versed). Chlordiazepoxide is primarily used for acute or severe agitation and acute alcoholism withdrawal, and lorazepam is used as a preanesthetic medication for adult patients. Midazolam is a short-acting benzodiazepine that has been effective in producing conscious sedation for endoscopic and cardiovascular procedures in healthy adults younger than 60 years of age. Because hypoxia and/or cardiac arrest may occur following midazolam, administration of the drug should be limited to settings in which respiratory and cardiac function may be continuously monitored.

Antagonist. Flumazenil (Mazicon) is a benzodiazepine receptor antagonist indicated for the reversal of the sedative effects of benzodiazepines. The duration and degree of reversal correspond with the dose of flumazenil administered and the resultant plasma concentration. The usual initial dosage is 0.2 mg administered by direct injection over 15 minutes; additional doses may be administered at 60-minute intervals. The onset of action is usually evident within 1 to 2 minutes after the injection is completed. Adverse effects include cutaneous vasodilation, dizziness, visual disturbances, cardiac arrhythmias, bradycardia or tachycardia, rigors, and pain at the injection site.

Miscellaneous CNS Agents

Two other CNS drugs are frequently administered intravenously. Rather than reviewing their drug classifications, only information specific to these drugs is discussed here.

Droperidol. Droperidol (Inapsine) is classified as a tranquilizer. The primary indications of this drug are for preoperative sedation and for reducing the incidence of nausea and vomiting during surgical and diagnostic procedures. Because of the cardiovascular side effects associated with droperidol, it is generally reserved for use under the direction of an anesthesiologist.

Promethazine Hydrochloride. Promethazine hydrochloride (Phenergan) is a phenothiazine derivative with potent sedative properties. Specifically, promethazine produces antihistamine, antiemetic, antimotion sickness, and anticholinergic effects, and is frequently used as an adjunct for pain control in terminal cancer patients. The most frequent side effects of the administration of promethazine are venous irritation and phlebitis, suggesting that the peripheral IV site be rotated frequently or a central venous catheter be used.

Anticonvulsants

Epilepsy is a neurologic disorder characterized by a recurrent pattern of abnormal neuron discharges within the brain. The result is a sudden loss of consciousness, inappropriate behavior, and/or involuntary body movements. Basically, seizures may be classified as partial, with electroencephalogram (EEG) changes confined to one area of the brain, or generalized, involving the symmetric distribution of abnormal brain discharges. Status epilepticus results when several generalized seizures with convulsions occur successively without intervals of restored consciousness or normal muscle activity. Although anticonvulsants suppress the start or reduce the spread of seizures, they do not treat the underlying cause of the seizures. Therefore, the type of seizure, not the underlying cause, determines the drug of choice.[12]

Many of the drugs previously discussed have anticonvulsant properties. Phenobarbital is indicated for the treatment of generalized and partial seizures, and diazepam is the drug of choice for status epilepticus. Two additional categories of drugs, hydantoins and magnesium sulfate, are also indicated in the management of seizure activity.

HYDANTOINS

Hydantoins are used for the treatment of tonic-clonic and complex partial seizures. Their principal feature is the ability to control seizures without causing the sedation.

Prototype: Phenytoin Sodium. Phenytoin sodium (Dilantin) is a hydantoin derivative. Although it is used primarily for its anticonvulsant features, it also has antiarrhythmic properties similar to those of procainamide. The primary indications for phenytoin are the control of clonic-tonic and psychomotor seizures.

The preferred method for the administration of phenytoin is by direct IV injection at a rate not exceeding 50 mg/min. Because phenytoin precipitates if the pH is altered, the IV tubing and cannula must be cleared by flushing with normal saline before and after administration. This prevents phenytoin from mixing with other drugs. Solutions of 0.9% sodium chloride can be used to infuse phenytoin in concentrations of 100 mg in 25 to 50 ml of diluent. Higher concentrations have also been administered, but the maximum amount of diluent is 100 ml. When this alternate mode of administration is used, the drug infusion must be prepared immediately prior to use, administered within 1 hour, and infused above the filter.

When phenytoin is administered as an anticonvulsant, the most common side effects involve the central nervous system. Sluggishness, ataxia, nystagmus, confusion, slurred speech, dizziness, nervousness, and fatigue may occur. Gingival hyperplasia and excessive growth of the gums may also occur with extended therapy. Because of its antiarrhythmic properties, phenytoin is associated with adverse cardiovascular effects. Hypotension may occur with too rapid administration of the drug, whereas phenytoin toxicity may result in cardiovascular collapse. In addition, status epilepticus may result from abrupt withdrawal of the drug.

There is a narrow therapeutic margin associated with phenytoin. Acceptable plasma levels range from 5 to 20 μg/ml, and signs of toxicity occur once plasma levels exceed 20 μg. Symptoms of toxicity include nystagmus, ataxia, dysarthria, tremors, slurred speech, and nausea and vomiting.

The major contraindication for phenytoin is a hypersensitivity to hydantoins. Because of its effects on cardiac electrical activity, phenytoin should not be administered to patients with sinus bradycardia, sinoatrial block, second- or third-degree heart block, or Stokes-Adams syndrome.

Phenytoin interacts with several other drugs to increase or decrease their effectiveness. Phenytoin is potentiated by anticoagulants, antidepressants, cimetidine, and phenothiazines, but it potentiates CNS depressants and muscle relaxants. Barbiturates and theophylline inhibit phenytoin, whereas phenytoin inhibits corticosteroids and digitalis. In addition, the concomitant administration of phenytoin and sympathomimetic antihypertensive drugs such as dopamine may result in severe hypotension and bradycardia.

MAGNESIUM SULFATE

Magnesium sulfate is a CNS depressant that exhibits anticonvulsant properties when administered parenterally. As such, magnesium sulfate is indicated for the prevention and control of seizures associated with severe pre-eclampsia or eclampsia. The onset of action is usually immediate and lasts for approximately 30 minutes. Other indications for the drug include the treatment of hypomagnesemia and as an additive in total parenteral nutrition (TPN) solutions.

The primary adverse reaction associated with magnesium sulfate is magnesium intoxication. Symptoms of hypermagnesemia begin at serum magnesium concentrations of 4 mEq/liter and include the absence of the knee jerk reflex, hypotension with signs of tetany, hyperthermia, circulatory collapse, and depression of CNS and cardiac function. Because it is considered a CNS depressant, high doses of magnesium sulfate may potentiate the effects of other CNS depressants.

Cardiovascular Drugs

Drugs that alter cardiovascular (CV) function have a variety of actions. They can affect cardiac strength and rhythm, counteract hypotension, control hypertension, and improve blood flow. Because a comprehensive discussion of these agents is beyond our scope here, the focus is on the major categories of cardiovascular agents. The sympathetic nervous system plays a major role in cardiovascular function, and drugs acting on the CNS are discussed as part of CV drugs. Table 11–3 summarizes the cardiovascular drugs typically used in cardiac resuscitation.

Drugs Acting Through Adrenergic Receptors

Adrenergic receptors on the target cells within the sympathetic nervous system mediate the response of the neurotransmitters (norepinephrine and epinephrine). Drugs that elicit biologic responses similar to those produced by activation of the sympathetic nervous system are known as sympathomimetics; drugs that inhibit the effects of sympathetic stimulation are called sympatholytics. Because sympathomimetics mimic the sympathetic nervous system and provoke a response in the adrenergic receptors, they are also known as adrenergic agonists. In contrast, sympatholytics block the sympathetic nervous system and inhibit the adrenergic response, so they are referred to as adrenergic blockers.[12]

Cardiovascular drugs that elicit or inhibit the adrenergic response are also classified according to the subtype of adrenergic receptor site stimulated. There are four major subtypes of adrenergic receptors: α_1, α_2, β_1, and β_2. α_1-adrenergic receptors mediate the typical sympathetic responses such as mydriasis and vasoconstriction, whereas α_2-adrenergic receptors provide a negative feedback to inhibit release of norepinephrine. β_1-adrenergic receptors mediate cardiac stimulation, but β_2-adrenergic receptors mediate noncardiac responses, such as bronchodilation and vasodilation. Cardiovascular drugs that stimulate (or inhibit) both α- and β-adrenergic receptors are considered totally nonselective; the drugs are highly selective if they stimulate (or inhibit) only one subtype of α- or β-adrenergic receptor.

α-β–ADRENERGIC AGONISTS

The α-β–adrenergic agonists act on both the α- and β-adrenergic receptors. Because these drugs are nonselective,

they imitate almost all actions of the sympathetic nervous system.

Prototype: Epinephrine Hydrochloride. Epinephrine hydrochloride (Adrenalin) is the least selective adrenergic agonist and is identical to the epinephrine synthesized within the body. It acts on the cardiovascular system by strengthening the force of cardiac contraction, increasing the contraction rate, and usually increasing cardiac output. Epinephrine elevates the systolic blood pressure and decreases the diastolic blood pressure, resulting in a widened pulse pressure. Because of its actions, epinephrine is considered the drug of choice for anaphylactic shock and is used in cardiac resuscitation. It is also the antidote of choice for histamine overdose and allergic reactions. The usual dosage for cardiac resuscitation is 0.5 to 1.0 mg of a 1:10,000 solution by direct injection; this may be repeated every 5 minutes, as required.

Because epinephrine stimulates both the α- and β-adrenergic receptors, it may produce side effects in any patient receiving the drug. These are often transitory and include anxiety, dizziness, dyspnea, pallor, and palpitations. More serious side effects such as cerebrovascular hemorrhage, fibrillation, severe headache, hypotension, pulmonary edema, and tachycardia are associated with overdose or too rapid injection of the drug.

Epinephrine interacts with many drugs. It is potentiated by anesthetics and antihistamines, but antagonized by adrenergic blockers. Epinephrine may be used alternately with isoproterenol, but the two drugs should not be used together because they are both cardiac stimulants.

Related Drug. Norepinephrine bitartrate (Levophed) is pharmacologically equivalent to the sympathetic neurotransmitter norepinephrine. It is an agonist for the α- and β_1-adrenergic receptors but has almost no effect on β_2-adrenergic receptors. Because it is more selective, the actions of norepinephrine are more limited than those of epinephrine. Norepinephrine is primarily used as a vasopressor agent to raise the blood pressure in acute hypotensive states. Because it is a potent vasoconstrictor, severe tissue necrosis can result from extravasation of this drug into the surrounding tissue.

α-ADRENERGIC AGONISTS

The α-adrenergic agonists mimic the action of naturally occurring norepinephrine on the α-adrenergic receptors, but may also stimulate β-adrenergic receptors of the heart (β_1-adrenergic receptors). The primary effects of these drugs are vasoconstriction and cardiac stimulation.

Prototype: Metaraminol Bitartrate. Metaraminol bitartrate (Aramine) produces vasoconstriction, which results in elevation of the systolic and diastolic blood pressures. It also strengthens cardiac contractility and increases coronary, cerebral, and renal blood flow. Because of these actions, metaraminol is indicated for acute hypotensive states.

Metaraminol is less potent than norepinephrine, but it has similar side effects and precautions. In addition, metaraminol may cause increased arterial pressure, resulting in bradycardia. Although metaraminol may be administered by direct injection in emergency situations at the rate of 5 mg over 1 minute, it is usually administered as a continuous infusion by means of an electronic infusion device. During the infusion,

Table 11–3

Drugs Used in Cardiac Resuscitation

Drug	Indications	Nursing Considerations
Lidocaine (L)	Ventricular dysrhythmia	Bolus may be repeated every 5 minutes until dysrhythmia suppressed; excessive doses may cause seizures; may cause hypotension initially
Epinephrine (E)	Asystole; to elevate perfusion pressure	Inactivated by $NaHCO_3$ Isoproterenol may lead to vasoconstriction and reflex bradycardia
Atropine (A)	Sinus bradycardia; high-degree AV block	Repeated until heart rate is 60 bpm, or higher
Dopamine (D)	Shock syndrome	Incompatible in alkaline solutions or with other drugs
	Hemodynamic imbalances	Titrate to BP

the patient's blood pressure should be monitored every 5 minutes until the desired effect is achieved, and every 15 minutes thereafter. As with norepinephrine, infiltration of metaraminol may result in tissue necrosis and sloughing.

Related Drug. Methoxamine hydrochloride (Vasoxyl) is a potent vasopressor, but it does not produce undesired cardiac or CNS stimulation. Intravenous administration is limited to emergencies in which the systolic blood pressure is lower than 60 mm Hg.

β-ADRENERGIC AGONISTS

Drugs that act only on the β-adrenergic receptors are used primarily to stimulate the heart or dilate the bronchi. When the mechanism of action is limited to only the β_1-adrenergic receptors, the primary effect is cardiac stimulation. If the drugs act on the β_2-adrenergic receptors, bronchodilation and vasodilation result.

Prototype: Dopamine Hydrochloride. Dopamine hydrochloride (Intropin) is a selective β_1-adrenergic agonist that is indicated for the correction of hemodynamic imbalances. It produces a positive inotropic effect by stimulating cardiac contractile force and is sometimes classified as an inotropic agent. Because dopamine increases cardiac output, blood pressure, and urine output, it is administered as an adjunct in the treatment of shock. The patient's response must be carefully monitored based on these effects, and the administration rate adjusted accordingly.

Dopamine is administered by continuous infusion using an electronic infusion device. The usual initial dosage is 2 to 5 μg/kg body weight. The dosage is then gradually increased by 5 to 10 μg/kg/min in 10- to 30-minute increments and titrated based on the patient's response to treatment. The blood pressure should be monitored every 2 minutes until the patient has been stabilized at the desired level, and then every 5 minutes thereafter. As with norepinephrine, there is a risk of tissue necrosis if the drug infiltrates into surrounding tissue.

The side effects of dopamine are associated with its cardiac effects. Bradycardia, tachycardia, hypertension, hypotension, vasoconstriction, and a widened QRS complex may occur. Other side effects include nausea, vomiting, headache, and dyspnea. The rate of infusion should be immediately decreased and the physician notified if there is a disproportionate rise in diastolic blood pressure, an increasing degree of tachycardia, and/or a decreased urinary output.

Related Drugs. Dobutamine hydrochloride (Dobutrex) is a selective β_1-adrenergic agonist that stimulates cardiac contractile force (positive inotropic effect), with less alteration in heart rate than dopamine. Following stabilization of the patient in the hospital setting, dobutamine can be continued in the home environment under closely supervised conditions.

Isoproterenol hydrochloride (Isuprel) differs from dopamine in that it stimulates both β_1- and β_2-adrenergic receptors to produce cardiac and bronchial effects. The primary indications for isoproterenol are the treatment of atrioventricular (AV) heart block, cardiac standstill, and bronchospasm.

β-ADRENERGIC BLOCKERS

β-Adrenergic blockers bind with the β-adrenergic receptors to prevent the action of the naturally occurring β-adrenergic receptor agonists (norepinephrine and epinephrine). Most β blockers are nonselective in that they do not differentiate between β_1- and β_2-adrenergic receptors. In contrast, cardioselective β blockers produce their antiarrhythmic and antihypertensive effects by only inhibiting the β_1-adrenergic receptors. Because the cardioselective blockers have no effect on the β_2-adrenergic receptors that mediate bronchial dilation, they are generally safer for patients who have accompanying respiratory disease.

Prototype: Propranolol Hydrochloride. Propranolol hydrochloride (Inderal) is a nonselective β-adrenergic blocker that acts on both β_1- and β_2-adrenergic receptors. Because it produces antiarrhythmic effects, propranolol is indicated in the management of life-threatening cardiac arrhythmias such as paroxysmal atrial tachycardia, atrial flutter, and atrial fibrillation. Cardiac function and blood pressure should be continuously monitored during administration.

Because of the nonselective β blocking, propranolol may cause cardiovascular, respiratory, and/or metabolic side effects, especially in patients with severe cardiac disease, respiratory disease, or diabetes mellitus. Other side effects include syncope, vertigo, visual disturbances, and paresthesia of the hands.

Related Drugs. Esmolol hydrochloride (Brevibloc) is a fast-acting nonselective β blocker indicated for the treatment of acute episodes of supraventricular or sinus tachycardia and atrial flutter or fibrillation. In contrast, metoprolol tartrate (Lopressor) is a cardioselective β blocker. Although the exact mechanism of action is unknown, metoprolol has been effective in reducing cardiac mortality in patients with suspected or diagnosed myocardial infarction.

α-ADRENERGIC BLOCKERS

The α-adrenergic blockers prevent the naturally occurring α-adrenergic receptor agonists (epinephrine and norepinephrine) from binding to the α-adrenergic receptor sites.

Labetalol Hydrochloride. Because of its effects on the α receptors, labetalol hydrochloride (Normodyne) reduces peripheral vascular resistance, resulting in decreased blood pressure. It also blocks the β-adrenergic receptors to produce propranolol-like depression of cardiac contractility. As a result of these α- and β-adrenergic effects, labetalol is indicated for the management of blood pressure in patients with severe hypertension.

Phentolamine Mesylate. Phentolamine mesylate (Regitine) blocks the α-adrenergic receptors and antagonizes responses to epinephrine and norepinephrine. Because of its ability to reduce blood pressure, phentolamine is primarily indicated for the treatment of hypertensive episodes associated with pheochromocytoma. It may also be added to solutions of norepinephrine or dopamine to prevent dermal necrosis in the event of extravasation of the solution, or may be administered subcutaneously into the tissue if extravasation does occur.

Drugs Affecting Cardiac Strength and Rhythm

When the heart loses its ability to contract with normal strength, drugs are administered to strengthen the cardiac contraction. Such drugs include the β-adrenergic receptor agonists (see earlier), cardiac glycosides, and miscellaneous inotropic agents. In contrast, alterations in cardiac rate and/or rhythm require the administration of antiarrhythmics.

CARDIAC GLYCOSIDES

Cardiac glycosides act directly on the myocardium to increase cardiac contractility and alter electrical impulse generation and conduction. This results in a slower, stronger contraction, with increased cardiac output.

Prototype: Digoxin. Digoxin (Lanoxin) is indicated in the treatment of congestive heart failure, atrial fibrillation and flutter, paroxysmal tachycardia, and cardiogenic shock. Effects begin within 5 to 30 minutes of administration and last up to 3 days.

Digoxin has a narrow margin of safety. Dosages must be individualized because a therapeutic dose for one patient may be toxic to another. Whereas the first signs of toxicity may be detected on electrocardiogram (ECG) monitoring, the most common clinical symptoms are nausea, vomiting, and anorexia. Patients may also experience blurred vision, disturbed color vision, headache, confusion, and diarrhea.

Many drugs interact with digoxin:

1. Drugs that alter serum electrolyte levels, such as potassium-sparing diuretics, can affect the intensity of the response to digoxin.
2. Autonomic agents can alter the effects of digoxin on cardiac conductivity.
3. Drugs that affect the metabolism or excretion of digoxin, such as phenytoin, quinidine, or verapamil, may require adjustment of the digoxin dosage to maintain therapeutic effects.

Antidote. Digoxin immune Fab (Digibind) contains anti-digoxin antibodies that bind to the digoxin molecules, rendering them unable to exert their toxic effects. Because it is obtained from sheep serum, digoxin immune Fab is potentially allergenic.

MISCELLANEOUS INOTROPIC AGENTS

Other inotropic agents enhance the strength of cardiac contraction but differ from cardiac glycosides and β-adrenergic receptor agonists in their mechanism of action.

Prototype: Amrinone Lactate. Amrinone lactate (Inocor) produces both inotropic and vasodilator effects. It is mainly indicated for the short-term management of congestive heart failure (CHF) in patients who have been unresponsive to conventional therapies.

ANTIARRHYTHMICS

Cardiac arrhythmias, sometimes referred to as dysrhythmias, occur when there is a deviation from the normal sinus rhythm. Under normal circumstances, there are changes in cardiac electrical activity that occur in a constant sequence. The normal heartbeat originates in the sinoatrial (SA) node at a rate of 60 to 80 beats per minute (bpm). If the heart rate is greater than 100 bpm, it is classified as a tachycardia; rates lower than 60 bpm are classified as bradycardias. If the impulse originates in the SA node and only the rate is altered, the arrhythmia may be classified as a sinus tachycardia or sinus bradycardia.

Impulses are transmitted from the SA node to the atrial muscle, causing the atria to contract. On ECG monitoring, this electrical activity is reflected by the P wave. The impulse is then passed from the atria to the ventricles through the AV node. Because the atria must complete their contractions before the ventricles are activated, there is a brief delay, demonstrated by the PR interval on the ECG. From the AV node, impulses pass through the bundle of His, bundle branches, and Purkinje fibers to activate the ventricles. This phase is the QRS complex on the ECG.

If the impulse is not delivered to the ventricles from the AV node, the ventricles attempt to beat at their own rate. Such a condition is known as heart block, and it may be partial or complete. The degree of partial heart block is classified in a manner that reflects the number of atrial contractions for each ventricular contraction. In complete heart block, no impulses pass from the atria to the ventricles.

With the normal heartbeat, there is a spontaneous depolarization of the SA node and a sequential conduction of the impulse along specific pathways within the heart. In abnormal conditions, however, a region of the heart other than the SA node may initiate its own impulse. Such an ectopic impulse causes the heartbeat to become unsynchronized, resulting in a serious arrhythmia.

To maintain the normal heartbeat, the myocardial cells have four unique properties. First, the cells have the ability to initiate their own activity by spontaneous depolarization, known as automaticity. Second, the cells depolarize at a regular rate, called rhythmicity. Third, the cells have the ability to transmit impulses at an appropriate rate, known as conduction. Last, the cells have refractoriness, meaning that they are resistant to further stimulation during repolarization.

Cardiac arrhythmias are usually classified according to their site of origin. If there is abnormal conduction above the ventricles, they are categorized as supraventricular arrhythmias. Examples of such arrhythmias are sinus bradycardia and atrial fibrillation or flutter. Sometimes arrhythmias originating in the atria, such as atrial fibrillation or flutter, are further classified as atrial arrhythmias. When there is abnormal conduction in the ventricles, they are referred to as ventricular arrhythmias. Premature ventricular contractions (PVCs) and ventricular tachycardia are examples of ventricular arrhythmias.

Antiarrhythmics are administered to prevent or stop an irregular heart rate or rhythm. Because there is no "universal" antiarrhythmic, no single prototype can be identified. For our purposes here, the antiarrhythmics are grouped according to their mechanism of action and the most common drugs for each group are discussed. Because of the cardiac effects of these drugs, IV administration requires continuous ECG and blood pressure monitoring.

Group A. Some antiarrhythmics decrease the transport of sodium through the cardiac tissue and slow conduction through the AV node. This prolongs the refractory period and decreases the automaticity of the heart. Therefore, these drugs are indicated for the treatment of supraventricular arrhythmias, such as atrial fibrillation and flutter. Examples of such drugs are quinidine gluconate and procainamide hydrochloride (Pronestyl).

Quinidine Gluconate. Quinidine is indicated for the management of atrial fibrillation and flutter. It has also been used to treat Wolff-Parkinson-White syndrome, which is characterized by supraventricular tachycardia. Because quinidine acts by decreasing AV node conduction, adverse effects include AV block, decreased cardiac output, and cardiac standstill. Other adverse reactions include acute hypotension, diaphoresis, tinnitus, and visual disturbances. In rare instances, ventricular tachycardia and fibrillation have occurred.

Procainamide Hydrochloride. Procainamide hydrochloride (Pronestyl) is similar to quinidine but has a more rapid onset of action and is less likely to cause hypotension or cardiac depression. Procainamide acts by slowing the heart rate and conduction, decreasing myocardial irritability, and prolonging the refractory period, and is indicated for the emergency treatment of ventricular and supraventricular arrhythmias. Side effects of procainamide are usually dose-related and are similar to those associated with quinidine.

Group B. This group of antiarrhythmics decreases the refractory period, especially in the Purkinje fibers and the ventricular myocardium. By acting preferentially on areas of the myocardium in which impulse conduction rates and automaticity are abnormal, these drugs promote uniform conduction rates throughout the heart. As a result, ventricular excitability is reduced without a reduction in the force of the ventricular contractions. The best-known example of this group is lidocaine (Xylocaine). Phenytoin, an anticonvulsant, also belongs in this group.

Lidocaine Hydrochloride. Lidocaine hydrochloride (Xylocaine) is the drug of choice for the treatment of ventricular arrhythmias and ventricular tachycardias, especially following a myocardial infarction. The usual bolus dose is 50 to 100 mg administered at a rate not exceeding 25 mg/min. Once the bolus dose is administered, a continuous infusion of 1 to 4 mg/min is initiated to maintain a therapeutic serum level between 1.5 and 5 μg/ml. Greater than recommended doses and too rapid administration rates are likely to cause excessive cardiac depression and CNS stimulation.

Lidocaine has a relatively low margin of safety. Serum levels above 6 μg/ml are usually toxic and may suppress AV transmission, resulting in partial or complete heart block. In addition, high serum levels may produce adverse CNS effects. Sedation and drowsiness are associated with therapeutic blood levels, but higher levels may cause unconsciousness, generalized convulsions, and respiratory arrest. However, more common side effects (even at therapeutic blood levels) include apprehension, blurred vision, lightheadedness, tinnitus, and numbness.

Lidocaine is potentiated by β-adrenergic blockers and phenytoin. The concomitant administration of these drugs with lidocaine may result in cardiac depression and an increased likelihood of excessive CNS effects.

Phenytoin Sodium. Phenytoin sodium (Dilantin) is chemically unrelated to lidocaine, but the two drugs are similar in their antiarrhythmic actions. As discussed earlier, phenytoin is an effective anticonvulsant. However, it is also indicated for the treatment of digitalis-induced arrhythmias because it normalizes AV conduction and suppresses ectopic pacemakers. Adverse reactions and side effects of phenytoin are similar to those of lidocaine. Too rapid administration and/or toxic serum levels may result in severe depression of cardiac contractility, severe hypotension, and excessive CNS effects.

Group C. Antiarrhythmic effects are also produced by the β-adrenergic receptor blockers. As discussed earlier, β-adrenergic blockers inhibit the cardiac response from sympathetic nerve stimulation. They slow the heart rate by inhibiting AV conduction, reduce the force of cardiac contractility, and decrease arterial pressure and cardiac output. β-Adrenergic blockers are particularly effective in the management of arrhythmias caused by excessive sympathetic cardiac stimulation or sympathomimetic drugs. Propranolol hydrochloride (Inderal) and esmolol hydrochloride (Brevibloc) are β-adrenergic blockers used for the management of arrhythmias involving increased sympathetic cardiac stimulation.

Group D. Antiarrhythmics in this group prolong the duration of the action potential, increasing the cellular refractory period and producing an antifibrillatory effect. Although the drugs are chemically unrelated, they share the ability to suppress ventricular tachycardia and prevent ventricular fibrillation. An example of this group of antiarrhythmics is bretylium tosylate (Bretylol).

Bretylium Tosylate. Bretylium tosylate (Bretylol) increases the refractory period without increasing the heart rate and is effective in the treatment of life-threatening ventricular arrhythmias. Because it increases the ventricular fibrillation threshold, bretylium is indicated for the prophylaxis and treatment of ventricular fibrillation. Therefore, bretylium is sometimes classified as an antifibrillatory agent.

The administration of bretylium is associated with adverse effects. However, reactions associated with initial doses differ from those related to subsequent administration. With initial administration, the patient may experience hypertension, tachycardia, or worsening of the dysrhythmia. Because bretylium blocks the release of norepinephrine from the sympathetic nerves, its subsequent administration is often associated with postural hypotension. Other adverse effects include syncope, transient hypertension, substernal pressure, and bradycardia.

Group E. The calcium channel blockers slow electrical impulse conduction rates and increase the cellular refractory period by blocking the influx of calcium into the cells. This action reduces conduction of the impulse through the SA and AV nodes, prolongs the refractory period in the AV node, and reduces ventricular rates. A common calcium channel blocker is verapamil hydrochloride (Isoptin).

Verapamil Hydrochloride. Verapamil hydrochloride (Isoptin) is effective in the treatment of supraventricular tachyarrhythmias and temporary management of a rapid ventricular rate in atrial flutter or fibrillation. Verapamil acts by decreasing the myocardial contractility, afterload, arterial pressure, vascular tone, and oxygen demand within 5 minutes of administration. Potential side effects include dizziness, headache, abdominal discomfort, bradycardia or tachycardia, hypotension, and PVCs.

When administering verapamil, potential drug interactions must be considered. Because digoxin is potentiated by verapamil, lower doses of digoxin may be required. The concomitant administration of verapamil and β-adrenergic drugs must be avoided, because both drugs depress myocardial contractility and conduction through the AV node. Excessive hypotension may result from the administration of antihypertensive drugs and verapamil.

Group F. Atropine sulfate is a drug that is not usually classified as an antiarrhythmic, but it has antiarrhythmic effects. It is an anticholinergic drug that blocks the action of acetylcholine (ACh) on the SA node. Because ACh slows the heart rate, atropine blocks the action and restores the heart rate to a more normal level. Therefore, atropine is indicated in the treatment of sinus bradycardia, syncope associated with Stokes-Adams syndrome, and AV block with profound bradycardia.

Antihypertensives

The treatment of hypertension involves the use of drugs in a logical sequence. This generally accepted plan, known as the ''stepped-care'' approach, is presented in Table 11–4. The approach begins with the lowest effective dose of a single drug. If the drug fails to control the hypertension, small doses of additional drugs are used rather than markedly increasing the dosage of the initial drug. Step I drugs are frequently continued in the subsequent steps, and some step II drugs may be indicated for step I therapy when diuretics or β-adrenergic blockers are inappropriate for a particular patient. (The β-adrenergic blockers were reviewed earlier and thiazide diuretics are presented later with agents for electrolyte and water balance.)

For the management of essential hypertension, these drugs are usually administered orally. Intravenous administration is typically reserved for subacute or acute hypertensive emergencies. Discussion of antihypertensive agents in this section focuses on drugs used for the treatment of severe and abrupt increases of blood pressure, and is limited to those not previously discussed.

Methyldopate Hydrochloride. Methyldopate hydrochloride (Aldomet) is a centrally acting antihypertensive that depresses sympathetic nervous system activity through an action in the central nervous system. Intravenous methyldopate is indicated for the treatment of hypertensive crises, especially for patients with renal or coronary insufficiency.

The usual dosage of methyldopate is 250 to 500 mg ad-

ministered over 30 to 60 minutes as an intermittent infusion every 6 hours. The patient's blood pressure needs to be carefully monitored throughout the therapy and the dosage withheld if the patient's blood pressure is not within the parameters established by the physician. Potential side effects include dizziness, dry mouth, sedation, postural hypotension or paradoxic hypertension, and apprehension.

Hydralazine Hydrochloride. Hydralazine hydrochloride (Apresoline) is a potent antihypertensive drug that lowers the blood pressure through direct relaxation of the smooth muscle of the arteries and arterioles. For this reason, it is sometimes classified as a vasodilator. The primary uses of Apresoline are for the treatment of severe essential hypertension and to promote vasodilation in cardiovascular shock.

Hydralazine is administered as a direct injection at a rate not exceeding 10 mg/min. The usual dosage is 10 to 40 mg, but the dosage may be increased gradually as required to a maximum dosage of 300 to 400 mg/24 hours.

As with methyldopate, the patient's blood pressure must be carefully monitored. Potential side effects include anxiety, paresthesia, dry mouth, unpleasant taste, tachycardia, palpitations, and postural hypotension. The peripheral vasodilation produced by hydralazine may stimulate the carotid sinus reflex, thus increasing the heart rate and cardiac output.

Nitroprusside Sodium. Nitroprusside sodium (Nipride) is a vasodilator that produces effects similar to those of hydralazine. Because the most common side effects are reflex tachycardia and reduced arterial pressure, nitroprusside may be contraindicated for patients with ischemic heart disease.

Nitroprusside is administered as a continuous infusion by an electronic infusion device. The dose is based on body weight but is usually 3 μg/kg/min. Because nitroprusside is converted to thiocyanate prior to excretion in the urine, cyanide poisoning may occur if the recommended maximum dose of 10 μg/kg/min is exceeded. Other potential side effects include abdominal pain, dyspnea, diaphoresis, palpitations, headache, and muscle twitching.

The potency of nitroprusside can be affected by exposure to light, so the solution container (and sometimes the administration set) should be covered with aluminum foil or an opaque material to protect the drug from light.

Diazoxide. Another potent vasodilator, diazoxide (Hyperstat), acts by relaxing the smooth muscle of the peripheral arterioles. Because the drug is administered as a single dose, its use is preferred when an infusion pump and titration monitoring are not immediately available.

Enalapril Maleate. Enalapril maleate (Vasotec) lowers the blood pressure by interrupting the renin-angiotensin-aldosterone system. It acts by inhibiting the angiotensin-converting enzyme (ACE), which inhibits formation of the vasoconstrictor angiotensin II, and by indirectly reducing the blood levels of aldosterone. As a result, the peripheral arterial resistance is reduced and the blood pressure is lowered. Enalapril is administered as a direct injection over 5 minutes. Adverse reactions include dizziness, dyspnea, parasthesia, and abdominal pain.

Hematologic Agents

When a blood vessel wall is injured or severed, the body activates processes to maintain hemostasis. This protective

---

Table 11–4

Stepped-Care Approach to Managing Essential Hypertension

Step	Agent(s) Used
1	Thiazide diuretics; β-adrenergic blockers
2	Centrally acting antihypertensives; peripheral α-adrenergic blockers; catecholamine depleters
3	Direct-acting vasodilators
4	Angiotensin-converting enzyme inhibitors; monoamine oxidase inhibitors; complete peripheral catecholamine depleters

mechanism is accomplished by means of a clotting cascade that is activated through a series of intrinsic and extrinsic factors. Although coagulation is usually the desired reaction, there are several clinical situations in which hemostasis must be inhibited or the coagulation process reversed. Hematologic agents such as anticoagulants and thrombolytics, respectively, are the drugs indicated for such situations.

Anticoagulants

Anticoagulants interfere with the coagulation pathways to prevent clot formation. They are effective in decreasing the risk of clot formation and preventing the enlargement or fragmentation of blood clots, but anticoagulants cannot dissolve existing clots.

Prototype: Heparin Sodium. The prototype for parenteral anticoagulants is heparin sodium. Low doses of heparin inhibit the conversion of prothrombin to thrombin, and larger doses inactivate thrombin and prevent the conversion of fibrinogen to fibrin. Heparin therapy is indicated for the prophylaxis and treatment of venous thrombosis and pulmonary emboli, the diagnosis and treatment of disseminated intravascular coagulation (DIC), and the prevention of coagulation during arterial and cardiac surgery, hemodialysis, and blood transfusions.

To achieve a constant degree of anticoagulation, the preferred mode of intravenous administration of heparin is by continuous infusion. However, heparin may be administered by intermittent injection with the dosage adjusted according to coagulation times. The most common laboratory test for monitoring heparin action is the activated partial thromboplastin time (APTT). A baseline APTT is measured prior to initiation of heparin therapy. Because heparin prolongs the APTT in a dose-dependent manner, the therapeutic range for the APTT during heparin therapy is 1.5 to 2 times the control value.

As a result of the pharmacologic action of heparin, the major adverse effects are bleeding and hemorrhage. The frequency and severity of these effects may be minimized with careful monitoring of the APTT during therapy. Whereas bleeding may occur at any site, the most common locations are the gastrointestinal and urinary tracts and mucosal surfaces, such as the nasal passages and gums. Epistaxis, hematuria, and/or tarry stools may be the first signs of overdosage.

A more infrequent adverse reaction to heparin is thrombocytopenia. The patient's platelet count must be closely monitored, because a paradoxic reaction resulting in platelet aggregation, or white clot syndrome, may occur. Other side effects related to heparin therapy are rare but include hypersensitivity reactions, alopecia, and osteoporosis.

Heparin is contraindicated in the presence of active bleeding, blood dyscrasias, history of bleeding disorder, or known hypersensitivity to the drug. In disease states in which there is a risk of hemorrhage, such as arterial sclerosis, aneurysm, hemophilia, and ulcerative colitis, heparin should be used with extreme caution. If heparin is administered with thrombolytic agents and platelet-activated drugs, the risk of hemorrhage may be increased.

Heparin interacts with a number of drugs. Antihistamines, barbiturates, digitalis, phenothiazines, and tetracyclines may chemically neutralize heparin, reducing its anticoagulant action. Conversely, heparin may be potentiated by chloramphenicol, dextran, ibuprofen, indomethacin, and penicillin.

Heparin may also be used to maintain the patency of venous access devices designed for intermittent use. The usual concentration of the heparin flush is 10 or 100 units of heparin/1 ml normal saline. The amount of solution depends on the device to be flushed but should be enough to reach the tip of the cannula or implanted port. The intervals between flushes are determined by the type of device and the frequency of use. Generally, a heparin flush is administered immediately following each IV medication and/or every 8 to 24 hours. Because heparin is incompatible with several other medications, the SASH technique should be used to instill the heparin flush. With this technique, the device is flushed with 0.9% sodium chloride (S), the medication is administered (A), the device is again flushed with 0.9% sodium chloride (S), and a heparin flush is administered (H).

Antidote. In the event of heparin overdose, protamine sulfate is administered to neutralize the heparin's anticoagulant activity. Protamine molecules that have positive electrostatic charges combine with the negatively charged heparin molecules to form the protamine-heparin complex, which has no anticoagulant activity. The dosage of protamine is determined by the heparin dosage, and approximately 100 units of heparin are neutralized by 1 mg of protamine. Because blood concentrations of heparin decrease rapidly following administration, the dosage of protamine required also decreases as time elapses.

Side effects associated with the rapid administration of protamine include acute hypotension, bradycardia, dyspnea, transient flushing, and pulmonary hypertension. These effects are minimized when protamine is administered slowly and the total dosage for any 10-minute period does not exceed 50 mg. Hypersensitivity reactions are rare but have been reported in persons allergic to fish.

Thrombolytic Agents

In contrast to anticoagulants that prevent the formation of clots or thrombi, thrombolytic agents promote thrombolysis. When a thrombosis or embolism obstructs blood flow in organs such as the heart, lungs, or brain, thrombolytic agents act by dissolving the obstruction and preventing ischemic tissue damage in the organ involved.

Prototype: Streptokinase. The prototype of the thrombolytic agents is streptokinase (Streptase). Streptokinase, a nonenzymatic protein, works in a complex manner to combine with plasminogen found in the thrombi and convert it to plasmin. The plasmin in turn degrades fibrinogen and fibrin clots. Specific indications for streptokinase include lysis of coronary artery thrombosis, acute massive pulmonary embolism, and deep vein and arterial thrombosis. Streptokinase has also been used to clear totally or partially occluded arteriovenous cannulas.

Because streptokinase prolongs the normal coagulation process, particularly the thrombin time, the major side effect is hemorrhage. The administration of streptokinase is intended to lyse thrombi, and this may result in bleeding at injection sites. Geriatric women, especially those with diabetes mellitus, are at particular risk for bleeding complications during streptokinase therapy. Other adverse reactions include febrile and sensitivity reactions, ranging from urticaria to anaphylaxis. When the drug is used to lyse coronary artery thrombi, a reperfusion-induced arrhythmia may result. Phlebitis at the infusion site for streptokinase may occur; this can be managed by further dilution of the drug.

Major contraindications for streptokinase are active internal bleeding, intracranial or intraspinal surgery, a recent cerebral vascular accident, severe uncontrolled hypertension, intracranial neoplasm, or a history of hypersensitivity to the drug. Streptokinase is also contraindicated following recent major surgery and for patients with subacute bacterial endocarditis. Because of the risk of hemorrhage, streptokinase should not be administered concurrently with anticoagulants or platelet-active drugs.

Related Drugs. There are three other thrombolytic agents that are similar to streptokinase. Anistreplase (Eminase), made from streptokinase and human plasminogen, exhibits an action similar to that of streptokinase. Alteplase (Activase) is a biosynthetic form of the enzyme human tissue-type plasminogen activator (tPA). Because alteplase only binds to the fibrin in the thrombus, it may be associated with a decreased risk of hemorrhage. Both anistreplase and alteplase are used to lyse thrombi obstructing coronary arteries in the management of acute myocardial infarction.

Urokinase (Abbokinase) is mainly used to restore the patency of occluded venous access devices. As part of the procedure, 5000 IU of urokinase are instilled into the occluded catheter and the catheter is clamped for 30 minutes. At the end of the 30 minutes, the contents are aspirated and the catheter is flushed with 0.9% sodium chloride solution.

Hemostatics

Hemostatics are indicated for the control of unexpected hemorrhagic episodes. Although all the drugs in this category arrest bleeding, each has a specific indication in clotting.

Prototype: Aminocaproic Acid. Aminocaproic acid (Amicar) is indicated in the treatment of excessive bleeding caused by overactivity of the fibrolytic system. It inhibits plasminogen activator substances and increases fibrinogen activity in clot formation. The primary indication for aminocaproic acid is systemic hyperfibrinolysis associated with heart surgery, aplastic anemia, or carcinoma of the lung, prostate, cervix, or stomach. It has also been effective in the treatment of overdosage of thrombolytic agents.

Adverse effects of aminocaproic acid are generally mild and disappear once the drug has been discontinued. They include nausea, cramping, diarrhea, dizziness, tinnitus, nasal stuffiness, headache, and rash. Bradycardia, hypotension, and cardiac arrhythmias are associated with rapid infusion of the drug but may be avoided if aminocaproic acid is administered as recommended.

Aminocaproic acid is contraindicated in those with DIC unless the patient is receiving heparin concomitantly. It is also contraindicated in patients with active intravascular clotting and possible active fibrinolysis, and in patients with cardiac, renal, or hepatic disease.

Related Drugs. The two related hemostatics, antihemophilic factor (factor VIII) and factor IX complex (Konyne 80), differ from aminocaproic acid in that they are used for

the treatment of hemophilia. Antihemophilic factor is indicated in the treatment of a congenital deficiency of factor VIII associated with hemophilia A, whereas factor IX complex is used in the prevention and control of bleeding caused by hemophilia B. Because both drugs are prepared from pooled plasma, they may be contaminated with viral hepatitis or with HIV.

A third hemostatic is desmopressin acetate (DDAVP), which is used for the management of spontaneous or trauma-induced bleeding in patients with hemophilia A. Desmopressin is a synthetic polypeptide that causes a dose-dependent increase in plasma factor VIII and plasminogen activator. Because of the risks associated with antihemophilic factors prepared from pooled plasma, it has been recommended that desmopressin be used whenever possible in patients with mild or moderate hemophilia A.

Agents for Electrolyte and Water Balance

Fluid and electrolyte balance may be disturbed in many medical conditions and require intervention to restore equilibrium. To maintain homeostasis, drugs may be required to correct acid-base imbalances, mobilize fluid for excretion from the body, expand plasma volume, or replace or maintain electrolyte or fluid levels.

Agents Used for Acid-Base Imbalances

To preserve normal physiologic processes, the pH of the body must be maintained within a narrow range. The body works to maintain the pH of the extracellular fluid by means of various homeostatic buffering mechanisms. When these mechanisms fail, acidosis or alkalosis occurs.

ACIDIFYING AGENTS

Metabolic alkalosis may be caused by vomiting, excessive nasogastric suction, steroid administration, and Cushing's syndrome. The cause of the alkalotic condition must be identified and treated, and acidifying agents may be administered to counteract the alkalosis.

Prototype: Ammonium Chloride. Ammonium chloride is indicated for the treatment of hypochloremia and metabolic alkalosis. In metabolic alkalosis, hypochloremia is usually present, resulting in a bicarbonate excess. Once ammonium chloride is administered it dissociates into an ammonium cation and a chloride anion. In the liver, the ammonium ions are converted to urea, freeing the hydrogen and chloride ions. The hydrogen ions then react with the excess bicarbonate to form water and carbon dioxide, which is excreted by the lungs. The chloride ions combine primarily with the sodium bases in the body, thus correcting the hypochloremic state.[12]

The major side effects associated with ammonium chloride are caused by ammonia toxicity. These include bradycardia, disorientation, headache, pallor, sweating, irregular respirations, coma, metabolic acidosis, and calcium deficit resulting in tetany. Venous irritation and phlebitis may also occur following administration of the drug at a rate exceeding 5 ml/min.

ALKALINIZING AGENTS

Acidosis occurs when the serum pH is lower than 7.35. The blood is acidic because of excess carbonic acid, which alters the bicarbonate to carbonic acid ratio. In this situation, alkalinizing agents are administered to buffer the excess acid and help return this ratio to normal.

Prototype: Sodium Bicarbonate. Sodium bicarbonate is indicated for the treatment of metabolic acidosis caused by circulatory insufficiency. It may also be used to treat hyperkalemia, hyponatremia, salicylate or barbiturate poisoning, and bronchospasm associated with status asthmaticus. Calculation of the appropriate dosage is determined by the pH, $PaCO_2$, calculated base deficit, and clinical response. Although dosages may be prepared from solutions of sodium bicarbonate of varying percentages, the rate of administration of the final concentration should never exceed 50 mEq/hour. In addition, the incompatibility of the drug with other drugs necessitates flushing the IV line with 0.9% sodium chloride both before and after the administration of sodium bicarbonate.

There are several side effects associated with sodium bicarbonate. Because of the hypertonicity of the drug, extravasation may result in chemical cellulitis, tissue necrosis, ulceration, and/or sloughing at the injection site. Rapid administration may cause alkalosis, hypokalemia, hypocalcemia, or cardiac dysrhythmias resulting from an intracellular shift of potassium. Excessive doses or doses administered too rapidly have been associated with intracranial hemorrhage or hypernatremia.

Sodium bicarbonate may potentiate or inhibit several other drugs. For example, ephedrine and quinidine are potentiated by sodium bicarbonate, whereas tetracyclines, chlorpropamide, and salicylates are inhibited.

Diuretics

Diuretics increase the amount of water eliminated through the kidneys, thus decreasing the total volume of water in the body. This occurs primarily because of a natriuretic effect whereby diuretics increase the renal excretion of sodium. There are different classifications of diuretics, but the main types administered intravenously are the loop diuretics, thiazide diuretics, and osmotic diuretics.

LOOP DIURETICS

Loop diuretics are so named because their primary site of renal action is in the ascending limb of the loop of Henle in the kidney. They inhibit the active reabsorption of sodium chloride so that it is excreted in the urine, along with body water.

Prototype: Furosemide. The prototype for the loop diuretics is furosemide (Lasix). Because furosemide is extremely potent and has a rapid onset of action, it is indicated in the treatment of edema associated with congestive heart failure. Typically, the onset of action occurs within 5 minutes and the effects last for approximately 2 hours. Other indications for furosemide include patients with end stage renal disease, acute pulmonary edema, or nephrotic syndrome.

Because furosemide acts by inhibiting the reabsorption of water and electrolytes, major side effects are hyponatremia, potassium depletion, and hypovolemia, with resulting hypotension and circulatory collapse. Other side effects include tinnitus and hearing impairment if the drug is administered too rapidly or administered in conjunction with other ototoxic drugs. It is recommended that high doses of furosemide be administered by slow IV infusion rather than direct injection to reduce the ototoxic effects. High doses should be infused at a rate not exceeding 4 mg/min; direct injections of 20 to 40 mg should be administered over 1 to 2 minutes.

The primary contraindications for furosemide are hypotension and anuria. Because it may decrease the plasma volume and produce a hypotensive effect, administration of the drug to a hypotensive patient may provoke an excessive reaction. Furosemide is chemically related to sulfonamide antibiotics and is therefore contraindicated in patients with a known allergy to sulfonamide antibiotics.

Furosemide interacts with a number of other drugs, primarily because of its ability to reduce blood volume indirectly. Examples are the increased risk of nephrotoxicity from cephalosporins, ototoxicity from aminoglycosides, and excessive hypotensive effects with some antihypertensives.

Related Drugs. Two additional loop diuretics, bumetanide (Bumex) and ethacrynic acid (Edecrin), are similar to furosemide except in action. Approximately 1 mg of bumetanide is equal to 40 mg of furosemide. Ethacrynic acid is similar in potency to furosemide and is usually administered as a single dose of 100 mg. Because ethacrynic acid is not chemically related to the sulfonamides, it may be substituted for furosemide in the presence of a known allergy to sulfonamide antibiotics.

THIAZIDE DIURETICS

Thiazide diuretics enhance the excretion of sodium, chloride, and water by interfering with the reabsorption of sodium in the distal convoluted tubule in the kidney. Compared with the loop diuretics, thiazide produces only modest diuresis.

Prototype: Chlorothiazide Sodium. Chlorothiazide sodium (Diuril) is indicated for the management of edema, toxemia of pregnancy, and diabetes insipidus. Volume and electrolyte depletion may result from the administration of this drug, so many of the precautions discussed for the loop diuretics are pertinent to chlorothiazide. As a result of the potency of chlorothiazide, oral administration is preferable to the IV route. However, chlorothiazide is the only nonloop diuretic available for IV use and as such is often used in combination with loop diuretics when loop diuretics alone have failed. The purpose of this combination therapy is to produce a diuretic synergy. Because chlorothiazide is structurally related to the sulfonamides, cross-sensitivity may occur with use of the two drugs.

OSMOTIC DIURETICS

Unlike the loop diuretics and thiazides, osmotic diuretics do not inhibit the reabsorption of ions through the renal tubules. Rather, they work by the mechanism of osmosis.

Prototype: Mannitol. Mannitol (Osmitrol) is a sugar alcohol that induces diuresis by elevating the osmotic pressure in the renal tubules to hinder the reabsorption of water and electrolytes. It is primarily indicated for the prophylaxis of acute renal failure following cardiovascular procedures, severe trauma, and hemolytic transfusion reactions. Mannitol may also be used to reduce intracranial pressure, high intraocular pressure, and generalized edema and ascites.

The major side effects and contraindications for mannitol are the conditions for which loop diuretics and thiazides are indicated. Mannitol may increase blood volume and pressure causing acute heart failure, pulmonary edema, and/or hypertensive crisis. Minor side effects are limited to chills, headache, and dizziness. Because of the osmolarity of the mannitol, thrombophlebitis may occur at the injection site.

Drug interactions with mannitol are rare. However, the therapeutic effect of drugs eliminated by the kidneys may be reduced as a result of the increased diuresis.

Replacement Solutions

Replacement solutions are indicated for specific fluid or electrolyte deficiencies. Because replacement solutions were discussed earlier with parenteral fluids, this section is limited to electrolyte supplements and volume expanders.

ELECTROLYTE SUPPLEMENTS

Electrolyte supplements are usually contained in electrolyte solutions and solutions of total parenteral nutrition. However, there are specific situations in which additional supplements must be administered as a result of an electrolyte deficiency. Because calcium and potassium are the two most common electrolytes administered in this manner, both are discussed as prototypes.

Prototype: Calcium Gluconate. Calcium is a salt that is naturally present in the body. When there is a deficiency of calcium, tetany may ensue and a calcium supplement may be indicated. Other indications for calcium are as an antidote to magnesium intoxication, because an increase in calcium provokes a reciprocal decrease in magnesium, as adjunctive treatment in cardiac resuscitation, and following blood transfusions to maintain the calcium to potassium ratio.

Calcium gluconate may be administered by continuous infusion or by direct injection at a rate of 0.5 ml over 1 minute. Side effects associated with calcium administration include flushing, bradycardia, tingling, and depressed neuromuscular function.

Although calcium gluconate (Kalcinate) is the most common form of calcium salt used, two other forms of calcium salts are available. Calcium gluceptate has a calcium content equal to that of calcium gluconate, whereas calcium chloride is three times as potent.

Prototype: Potassium Chloride. Hypokalemia may be caused by diuretic therapy, digitalis intoxication, vomiting, diarrhea, diabetic acidosis, and metabolic acidosis. In these situations, the administration of potassium may be warranted. However, intravenous administration of potassium is not without risks. Precise measurement of the potassium deficiency is not possible; therefore, too much potassium may be administered, resulting in hyperkalemia.

The intravenous administration of potassium requires that the drug be diluted in an appropriate volume of solution. Under no circumstances should potassium be administered undiluted as an IV injection; such administration results in cardiac arrest. The usual concentration of potassium chloride is 40 mEq/liter, although higher concentrations may be prescribed. As a result of the venous irritation associated with the IV administration of potassium, it is recommended that the maximum peripheral concentration not exceed 80 mEq/liter. If a central venous catheter is used, the concentration may be increased, up to 240 mEq/250 ml. However, continuous cardiac monitoring is recommended for infusions given at a rate greater than 10 mEq of potassium in 1 hour. Other potassium supplements are potassium acetate and potassium phosphate. Potassium acetate is generally preferred for potassium deficiencies in patients with renal tubular acidosis, because hyperchloremia is probably present. Potassium phosphate is indicated for specific intracellular deficiency not caused by alkalosis, because phosphate is the ion usually attached to potassium in the body.

VOLUME EXPANDERS

Volume expanders increase the plasma volume and provide fluid replacement. These drugs produce a colloidal osmotic effect that draws water from the interstitial to the intravascular spaces.

Prototype: Dextran 40. The primary indication for the use of dextran 40 is as an adjunctive therapy in the management of shock caused by hemorrhage, burns, trauma, and surgery. Dextran 40 is a low-molecular-weight polymer of glucose that increases plasma volume by one to two times its own weight. This means that each gram of dextran 40 holds 25 ml of water in the intravascular space.

Although the initial 500 ml of dextran 40 may be administered over 15 to 30 minutes, the remainder of the initial dose and subsequent daily doses should be evenly distributed over 8 to 24 hours. The patient's pulse, blood pressure, central venous pressure (CVP), and urine output should be monitored frequently during the first hour of the infusion and hourly thereafter. Because of the antigenic properties of dextran 40, allergic reactions ranging from mild urticaria to anaphylaxis may occur. Severe anaphylactoid reactions have been reported during the first minutes of the infusion.

Related Drugs. Whereas dextran 40 has a low molecular weight, the colloidal properties of dextran 70 and hetastarch (Hespan) are approximately equal to those of human albumin. However, the indications, precautions, and side effects of dextran 70 and hetastarch are similar to those of dextran 40.

Gastrointestinal Drugs

Common disorders of the gastrointestinal tract are nausea, vomiting, and peptic ulcers. The intravenous medications administered for these disorders are directed at controlling the symptoms rather than eliminating the underlying cause.

Antiemetics

Vomiting is a complex reflex initiated by the vomiting center in the medulla and affecting the smooth muscle of the upper alimentary tract. Intravenous antiemetics act centrally to control or prevent this process. Although the three antiemetics selected for discussion differ in their mechanisms of action and classification, they all control nausea and vomiting.

Prototype: Metoclopramide Hydrochloride. Metoclopramide hydrochloride (Reglan) is a dopamine antagonist that blocks receptors in the vomiting center in the medulla. It is primarily indicated for the prevention of nausea and vomiting associated with cancer chemotherapy. A single dose is administered 30 minutes prior to the administration of the cancer chemotherapy and doses are repeated every 2 hours for two doses and every 3 hours for three doses. Metoclopramide may be administered either as an infusion over 15 minutes or by injection at a rate not exceeding 10 mg over 2 minutes. If it is administered too rapidly, metoclopramide causes intense anxiety, restlessness, and then drowsiness.

Adverse reactions associated with metoclopramide usually involve the CNS and include headache, fatigue, restlessness, insomnia, and fatigue. Extrapyramidal reactions may also occur, especially in children or when high doses are administered, such as those used to prevent chemotherapy-induced emesis. Once the drug is discontinued, the side effects usually disappear.

Metoclopramide interacts with a number of other drugs. It is antagonized by anticholinergics and narcotics, but potentiated by sedatives, hypnotics, and tranquilizers. Because it stimulates motility of the GI tract, metoclopramide may alter the absorption of oral medications and diminish their action.

Other Antiemetics. Two other antiemetics that may be administered by the IV route are diphenhydramine (Benadryl) and prochlorperazine edisylate (Compazine). Diphenhydramine is an antihistamine that is indicated for the control of nausea and vomiting, as well as for the treatment of allergic reactions to blood products and other agents. Prochlorperazine is a phenothiazine derivative with potent antiemetic properties. As with other phenothiazines, the major side effects include orthostatic hypotension and extrapyramidal effects.

Histamine Antagonists

Histamine stimulates gastric acid secretion through the stimulation of the H_2 receptors. Histamine (H_2) antagonists block the receptors and decrease acid secretion.

Prototype: Cimetidine Hydrochloride. Cimetidine (Tagamet) was the first H_2 antagonist introduced. Because it inhibits gastric acid secretion, cimetidine is indicated for the short-term treatment of active duodenal ulcers, active benign gastric ulcers, and hypersecretory conditions. The usual dose is 300 mg every 6 hours administered as a direct injection in 20 ml normal saline or as an intermittent infusion. When the prescribed dose is ineffective, the frequency of administration, not the amount, is increased. Continuous infusions of cimetidine have been recommended, because they produce pH control.

Because of its chemical structure, cimetidine produces more side effects than the other H_2 blockers. With average doses, bradycardia, confusion, dizziness, delirium, hallucinations, diarrhea, muscular pain, and/or rash may occur. The rapid administration or overdosage of cimetidine may cause cardiac dysrhythmia, hypotension, respiratory failure, and/or tachycardia. Therefore, cimetidine should be administered over at least 2 minutes as a direct injection or over 15 minutes as an infusion.

Cimetidine interacts with a number of drugs because it reduces hepatic blood flow and inhibits the drug-metabolizing enzyme system in the liver. Increased plasma concentrations of coumadin, phenytoin, propranolol, lidocaine, metronidazole, and theophylline may occur if any of these drugs is administered concurrently with cimetidine therapy.

Related Drugs. The related H_2 blockers are similar to cimetidine in that they share the same mechanism of action. However, they are more potent, have a longer duration of action, and are associated with a lower incidence of side effects. Ranitidine hydrochloride (Zantac) is twice as potent as cimetidine and its effects last for 6 to 8 hours. Famotidine (Pepcid) has been shown to be up to 20 times as potent as cimetidine and is effective for 10 to 12 hours.

Hormones and Synthetic Substitutes

The endocrine system controls homeostasis through the release of hormones. When there is hypoactivity of an endocrine gland, replacement therapy with a hormone or its synthetic analogue is required.

Corticosteroids

Corticosteroids are hormones that are secreted by the adrenal cortex, or their synthetic analogues. In physiologic doses, they replace deficient endogenous hormones; pharmacologic doses may be used to decrease inflammation.

Prototype: Hydrocortisone Sodium Succinate. Hydrocortisone sodium succinate (Solu-Cortef) is the drug of choice for replacement therapy in patients with adrenocortical insufficiency. Because of its anti-inflammatory effects, hydrocortisone is also indicated for acute hypersensitivity reactions, aspiration pneumonitis, and systemic lupus erythematosus relapse. In the treatment of neoplastic disease, hydrocortisone may be used alone as palliative treatment or in combination with cytotoxic and immunosuppressive drugs.

The adverse effects of hydrocortisone are generally associated with massive doses or long-term therapy. These include hyperglycemia caused by the drug's effects on glucose metabolism, cushingoid symptoms, characterized by a moon face and buffalo hump, and sodium retention, with resultant edema. In addition, hydrocortisone depresses the immune response, increasing the susceptibility to infection. Because the usual signs of inflammation are masked, infections may be widely disseminated before they are recognized.

Hydrocortisone interacts with several drugs. It inhibits anticoagulants but is inhibited by anticonvulsants and barbiturates. Concomitant administration with theophylline may potentiate its pharmacologic effects.

Related Drugs. Two additional corticosteroids are administered for their anti-inflammatory effects. Dexamethasone sodium phosphate (Decadron) is 20 to 30 times as potent as hydrocortisone, whereas methylprednisolone sodium succinate (Solu-Medrol) is 5 times as potent.

Estrogens

Estrogens are potent female hormones capable of producing widespread effects on the body. Although they may be given as replacement therapy, IV administration is generally used for the palliative treatment of cancer.

Prototype: Diethylstilbestrol Diphosphate. Diethylstilbestrol diphosphate (Stilphostrol) is used in the palliative treatment of prostatic or breast carcinoma, particularly in advanced stages of these diseases. Usually, 0.5 g is administered the first day, 1.0 g the second through fifth days, and then 0.25 to 0.5 g once or twice weekly as a maintenance dose. Each daily dose is diluted in 300 ml of solution and infused at a rate of 1 to 2 ml/min for the first 15 minutes. The rate is then increased so that the entire infusion is completed within 1 hour.

Because diethylstilbestrol is a female hormone, feminization in the male and uterine bleeding in postmenopausal women are expected. In addition, sodium and water retention may occur.

Insulin

Insulin acts as a catalyst in carbohydrate metabolism by facilitating the transport of glucose and promoting glucose utilization in the peripheral tissues. It also stimulates protein synthesis and inhibits the release of fatty acids from adipose cells. Although there are a number of forms of insulin available, only regular insulin is administered intravenously.

Prototype: Regular Insulin. Regular insulin is indicated for the emergency management of acute diabetic acidosis and diabetic coma and as an additive in solutions of total parenteral nutrition. The dosage varies greatly based on the condition and response of the patient, but it generally ranges from 2 to 100 units/hr. Insulin may be administered by direct injection or continuous infusion. However, the potency of an insulin infusion may be reduced because of adsorption of the drug onto plastic IV solution containers or tubing. The percentage of adsorption is inversely proportional to the concentration of insulin so that the greater the concentration, the lower the precentage of adsorption.

Regular insulin may also be administered in combination with glucose for the treatment of hyperkalemia. This is done to facilitate a shift of potassium into the cells, thus lowering the plasma potassium level.

Because insulin is a hypoglycemic agent, the most common adverse reaction is hypoglycemia associated with overdosage. Symptoms range from clammy skin, drowsiness, and headache to disorientation, convulsions, and coma. In addition, the hypoglycemic effects of insulin are potentiated by anticoagulants, salicylates, sulfonamides, and tetracyclines.

Antidote. The specific antidote for an insulin overdose is glucagon hydrochloride. Glucagon acts by converting glyco-

gen to glucose in the liver. The action of the drug is prompt, with the patient awakening within 5 to 20 minutes.

Pituitary Agents

The posterior pituitary gland synthesizes and releases two hormones, vasopressin and oxytocin. Vasopressin promotes water retention by the kidney and constriction of the peripheral vasculature, and oxytocin stimulates the myometrium. The synthetic analogues of these hormones produce similar effects.

Vasopressin. Vasopressin (Pitressin) elicits all the antidiuretic responses produced by endogenous vasopressin. The primary indication is the treatment of diabetes insipidus to control the polyuria and dehydration. Vasopressin has also been used as adjunctive therapy in the treatment of acute, massive hemorrhage caused by esophageal varices and peptic ulcer disease. Adverse effects are usually associated with large doses and include increased blood pressure, bradycardia, heart block, and coronary insufficiency. It is recommended that vasopressin be administered as a continuous infusion at a rate of 0.2 to 0.4 units/min; the rate may be progressively increased up to 0.9 units/min.

Oxytocin. Oxytocin (Pitocin) is a synthetic posterior pituitary hormone that produces rhythmic contraction of the uterine muscle. Because of this, oxytocin is used for the induction of labor or the control of postpartum bleeding. It is administered as an infusion with the rate precisely controlled by an electronic infusion device. Initial administration rates for the induction of labor are 1 to 2 mU/min, whereas control of postpartum bleeding requires an initial rate of 10 to 20 mU/min. Once the infusion is initiated, the rate may be increased or decreased in increments, as necessary. Adverse effects for the mother include anaphylaxis, cardiac arrhythmias, uterine rupture, and subarachnoid hemorrhage; bradycardia and death are possible fetal reactions.

Immune Modulators

The immune system protects the body against foreign invaders. By distinguishing the body's own proteins from foreign proteins, it selectively attacks and destroys foreign substances that enter the body. This is known as the immune response. However, there are certain situations in which the immune system may need to be enhanced or suppressed. Drugs that elicit such responses are classified as immune modulators.[1]

Immunostimulants

Immunostimulants enhance the function of the immune system by producing immunity against certain diseases. Those administered intravenously accomplish this by transferring antibodies to the person who lacks endogenous active immunity. The result is a passive immunity against the infection.

Prototype: Immune Globulin IV. When immune globulin IV (Sandoglobulin) is used for patients unable to produce

Table 11–5

Summary of IV Drugs

Category	Type	Prototype	Related Drugs
Antibiotics			
Penicillins	Natural	Penicillin G potassium	Penicillin G sodium
	Penicillinase-resistant	Methicillin sodium (Staphcillin)	Nafcillin sodium (Unipen)
			Oxacillin sodium (Prostaphlin)
	Aminopenicillins	Ampicillin sodium (Omnipen-n)	Ampicillin sodium/sulbactrim sodium (Unasyn)
	Extended-spectrum	Ticarcillin disodium (Ticar)	Mezlocillin sodium (Mezlin)
			Piperacillin sodium (Pipracil)
			Ticarcillin disodium/clavulate potassium (Timentin)
Cephalosporins	First-generation	Cefazolin sodium (Kefzol)	Cephadine (Velosef)
			Cephalothin sodium (Keflin)
			Cephapirin sodium (Cefadyl)
	Second-generation	Cefoxitin sodium (Mefoxin)	Cefamandole naftate (Mandol)
			Cefonicid sodium (Monocid)
			Ceforanide (Precef)
			Cefotetan disodium (Cefotan)
			Cefuroxime sodium (Kefurox)
	Third-generation	Cefotaxime sodium (Claforan)	Cefoperazone sodium (Cefobid)
			Ceftaxidime (Fortaz)
			Ceftizoxime sodium (Cefizox)
			Ceftriaxone sodium (Rocephin)
			Maxalactam disodium (Moxam)
Aminoglycosides		Gentamicin sulfate (Garamycin)	Amikacin sulfate (Amikin)
			Kanamycin sulfate (Kantrex)
			Netilmycin sulfate (Netromycin)
			Tobramycin sulfate (Nebcin)
Tetracyclines		Doxycycline hyclate (Vibramycin)	Minocycline HCl (Minocin)
Erythromycins		Erythromycin lactobionate (Erythrocin)	
Chloramphenicol		Chloramphenicol sodium succinate (Chloromycetin)	
Miscellaneous		Aztreonam (Azactam)	
		Ciprofloxacin (Cipro)	
		Clindamycin Phosphate (Cleocin)	
		Imipenem/Cilastatin sodium (Primaxin)	
		Vancomycin HCl (Vancocin)	
Other anti-infectives			
Antifungals		Amphotericin B (Fungizone)	Miconazole (Monistat)
			Fluconazole (Diflucan)
Antivirals		Acyclovir sodium (Zovirax)	Ganciclovir sodium (Cytovene)
			Vidarabine (Vira-A)
			Zidovudine (AZT)
Antiprotozoals		Metronidazole (Flagyl)	Pentamidine isethionate (Pentam)
Sulfonamide-combination products		Trimethoprim sulfamethoxazole (Bactrim; Septra)	
Central nervous system drugs			
Analgesic	Narcotics	Morphine sulfate	Hydromorphone HCl (Dilaudid)
			Meperidine HCl (Demerol)
			Antagonist: naloxone (Narcan)
	Mixed narcotic agonist-antagonists	Buprenorphine HCl (Buprenex)	Nalbuphine HCl (Nubain)
			Pentazocine lactate (Talwin)
Sedatives, hypnotics, and anxiolytics	Barbiturates	Phenobarbital sodium (Luminal)	Amobarbital sodium (Amytal)
			Pentobarbital sodium (Nembutal)
			Secobarbital sodium (Seconal)
			Thiopental sodium (Pentothal)
	Benzodiazepines	Diazepam (Valium)	Chlordiazepoxide HCl (Librium)
			Lorazepam (Ativan)
			Midazolam HCl (Versed)
			Antagonist: flumazenil (Mazicon)
	Miscellaneous	Droperidol (Inapsine)	
		Promethazine HCl (Phenergan)	
Anticonvulsants	Hydantoins	Phenytoin sodium (Dilantin)	
	Magnesium sulfate		

Table continued on following page

Table 11-5

Summary of IV Drugs *Continued*

Category	Type	Prototype	Related Drugs
Cardiovascular drugs			
Drugs acting through adrenergic receptors	α-β–adrenergic receptors	Epinephrine HCl (Adrenalin)	Norepinephrine bitartrate (Levophed)
	α-adrenergic agonists	Metaraminol bitartrate (Aramine)	Methoxamine HCl (Vasoxyl)
	β-adrenergic agonists	Dopamine HCl (Intropin)	Dobutamine HCl (Dobutrex) Isoproterenol HCl (Isuprel)
	β-adrenergic blockers	Propranolol HCl (Inderal)	Esmolol HCl (Brevibloc) Metoprolol tartrate (Lopressor)
	α-adrenergic blockers	Labetalol HCl (Normodyne) Phentolamine mesylate (Regitine)	
Drugs affecting cardiac strength and rhythm	Cardiac glycosides	Digoxin (Lanoxin)	Antidote: digoxin immune Fab (Digibind)
	Miscellaneous inotropic agents	Amrinone lactate (Inocor)	
	Antiarrhythmics	Group 1	Quinidine gluconate
		Group 2	Procainamide HCl (Pronestyl)
		Group 3	Lidocaine HCl (Xylocaine)
		Group 4	Phenytoin sodium (Dilantin)
		Group 5	β-adrenergic blockers
		Group 6	Bretylium tosylate (Bretylol) Verapamil HCl (Isoptin)
Antihypertensives			Atropine sulfate Methyldopate HCl (Aldomet) Hydralazine HCl (Apresoline) Nitroprusside sodium (Nipride) Diazoxide (Hyperstat) Enalapril maleate (Vasotec)
Hematologic agents			
Anticoagulants		Heparin sodium	Antidote: protamine sulfate
Thrombolytic agents		Streptokinase (Streptase)	Anistreplase (Eminase) Alteplase (Activase) Urokinase (Abbokinase)
Hemostatics		Aminocaproic acid (Amicar)	Antihemophilic factor (Factor VIII) Factor IX complex (Konyne 80) Desmopressin acetate (DDAVP)
Gastrointestinal drugs			
Antiemetics		Metroclopramide HCl (Reglan)	Diphenhydramine (Benadryl) Prochlorperazine edisylate (Compazine)
Histamine (H₂) antagonists		Cimetidine HCl (Tagamet)	Famotidine (Zantac) Ranitidine HCl (Pepcid)
Hormones and synthetic substitutes			
Corticosteroids		Hydrocortisone sodium succinate (Solu-Cortef)	Dexamethasone sodium phosphate (Decadron) Methylprednisone sodium succinate (Solu-medrol)
Estrogens		Diethylstilbestrol diphosphate (Stilphostrol)	
Insulin		Regular insulin	Antidote: glucagon HCl
Pituitary agents		Vasopressin (Pitressin) Oxytocin (Pitocin)	
Agents for electrolyte and water balance			
Agents for acid-base balance	Acidifying agents	Ammonium chloride	
	Alkalating agents	Sodium bicarbonate	
Diuretics	Loop diuretics	Furosemide (Lasix)	Bumetanide (Bumex) Ethacrynate Sodium (Edecrin)
	Thiazide diuretics	Chlorothiazide sodium (Diuril)	
	Osmotic diuretics	Mannitol (Osmitrol)	
Electrolyte supplements	Calcium	Calcium gluconate (Kalcinate)	Calcium chloride Calcium gluceptate
	Potassium	Potassium chloride	Potassium acetate Potassium phosphate
Volume expanders		Dextran 40	Dextran 70 Hetastarch (Hespan)
Immune modulators			
Immunostimulants		Immunoglobulin IV (Sandoglobulin)	
Immunosuppressants		Lymphocyte immune globulin (Atgam) Azthioprine sodium (Imuran) Cyclosporine (Sandimmune)	
Respiratory agents			
Smooth muscle relaxant		Theophylline	Theophylline ethylenediamine (Aminophylline)
Vitamins			
Multivitamin preparations (MVI-12)			
Phytonadione (Aquamephyton)			

adequate amounts of IgG antibodies, it provides immediate antibody levels for up to 3 weeks. Immune globulin is also used for patients with idiopathic thrombocytopenic purpura or for those with bone marrow transplants to increase platelet counts temporarily. Because the drug is obtained from biologic sources, a wide range of allergic reactions is associated with the use of immune globulin.

Immune globulin is administered as a continuous administration. Although the recommended administration rate is determined by the commercial product used, manufacturer recommendations must be followed. Too rapid injection of the drug may result in a hypotensive reaction.

Immunosuppressants

An active immune system is desirable for protection against infections and neoplasms. However, in situations such as organ transplants and autoimmune disorders, the immune response needs to be suppressed. Because immunosuppressants are relatively new drugs, each is discussed separately.

Lymphocyte Immune Globulin. Lymphocyte immune globulin (Atgam) is a leukocyte-selective immunosuppressant used to delay or reduce renal transplant rejection. A total of 21 doses is administered over 4 weeks, with each dose infused over at least 4 hours. Adverse effects are mainly ''flu-like'' symptoms, allergic reactions, thrombophlebitis, and thrombocytopenia.

Azathioprine Sodium. Azathioprine sodium (Imuran) is an immunosuppressant used to prevent the rejection of a renal transplant. Administration is begun within 24 hours of the transplant, and each dose is infused over 30 to 60 minutes. Side effects associated with azathioprine include leukopenia, thrombocytopenia, arthralgia, and nausea and vomiting.

Cyclosporine. Cyclosporine (Sandimmune) is a potent immunosuppressant used to prevent organ rejection in those with heart, kidney, or liver transplants. Within 4 to 12 hours prior to transplantation, cyclosporine is administered as a continuous infusion over 2 to 6 hours. Possible adverse reactions include nephrotoxicity, hepatotoxicity, and hypertension.

Respiratory Smooth Muscle Relaxants

The smooth muscles of the trachea and bronchi are sensitive to various stimuli and may contract, causing a narrowing of the airways. When bronchospasm occurs, the patient experiences wheezing, coughing, dyspnea, and tightness of the chest. In such situations, drugs that relax the smooth muscles of the respiratory tract are indicated.

Prototype: Theophylline. Theophylline may be classified as a bronchodilator because of its ability to open the bronchial passages or as a xanthine derivative because of its chemical structure. It is primarily indicated for the management of bronchial asthma and reversible bronchospasm associated with chronic bronchitis or emphysema.

The initial loading dose of theophylline is usually 4.7 mg/kg lean body weight infused over 20 to 30 minutes. This is immediately followed by a continuous infusion of 0.5 to 0.7 mg/kg/hr for the first 12 hours, and then 0.1 to 0.5 mg/kg/hr for as long as prescribed. Because theophylline has a low therapeutic index, an electronic infusion device is recommended to infuse the solution and maintain a serum level between 10 and 20 μg/ml. Rapid infusion of theophylline or serum levels in excess of 20 μg/ml may produce toxic reactions such as anxiety, convulsions, ventricular fibrillation, and cardiac arrest.

Theophylline interacts with several other drugs. By altering the hepatic clearance of theophylline, cimetidine, propranolol, erythromycin, and ciprofloxacin increase serum theophylline concentrations, whereas rifampin and phenytoin decrease serum theophylline concentrations. In addition, the concomitant administration of theophylline with ephedrine and other sympathomimetics may predispose the patient to the development of cardiac dysrhythmia.

Related Drug. Theophylline ethylenediamine (Aminophylline) contains 79% theophylline and requires a minimum dilution of 25 mg/ml for administration.

Vitamins

Vitamins may be administered in IV solutions to maintain optimal vitamin uptake following surgery, extensive burns, trauma, or severe infections. Examples of such vitamin additives are beta carotene (Aquasol A) for vitamin A, thiamine hydrochloride (Betaline S) for vitamin B_1, pyridoxine hydrochloride (Hexa-Betalin) for vitamin B_6, folic acid (Folvite) as part of the vitamin B complex, ascorbic acid (Cevalin) for vitamin C, and calcitrol (Calcijex) for vitamin D. These vitamins may also be administered as a multivitamin preparation (MVI-12), which contains vitamins A, D, E, and the B complex vitamins.

Phytonadione (Aquamephyton) contains vitamin K_1 and is used to treat an overdose of warfarin. Because vitamin K_1 is essential for the production of prothrombin in the liver, the dosage and effects of phytonadione are determined by the patient's prothrombin levels. It is recommended that the infusion rate of phytonadione not exceed 1 mg/min; higher rates are associated with the risk of anaphylaxis.

Table 11–5 presents a summary of the classifications of IV drugs discussed in this section.

References

1. Gahart BL. Intravenous Medications, 7th ed. St. Louis: C.V. Mosby, 1991.
2. Rachel MM, ed. LPN expanded role in IV therapy. Miss Bd Nurs Newsletter 1991; 6:2.
3. Sesin P, Wiggins MS. New England Deaconess guidelines for the administration of I.V. drugs. NITA 1987; 10:224–234.
4. Gardner C. Spartanburg General Hospital policy book on I.V. therapy administration—part I. NITA 1986; 9:267–288.
5. Intravenous Nurses Society. Intravenous Nursing Standards of Practice. Belmont, MA: Intravenous Nurses Society, 1990.
6. Shlafer M, Marieb EN. The Nurse, Pharmacology, and Drug Therapy. Redwood City, CA: Addison-Wesley, 1989.
7. Clark B, Queener SF, Karb VB. Pharmacological Basis of Nursing Practice, 2nd ed. St. Louis: C.V. Mosby, 1986.
8. Weinstein SM. Use of investigational drugs. NITA 1987; 10:336–347.
9. Gardner C. Risk management of medication errors. NITA 1987; 10:187–196.

10. Otto SE, LaRocca JC. Nursing diagnosis: Challenge for intravenous nursing practice. JIN 1988; 11:245–248.
11. Baker DL. Measuring outcome criteria: The intravenous nursing care plan. JIN 1990; 13:253–258.
12. Karb VB, Queener SF, Freeman JB. Handbook of Drugs for Nursing Practice. St. Louis: C.V. Mosby, 1989.
13. Korth-Bradley JM. A pharmacokinetic primer for intravenous nurses. JIN 1991; 14:16–27.
14. Crudi C, Larkin M. Core Curriculum for Intravenous Nursing. Philadelphia: J. B. Lippincott, 1984.
15. Sager DP, Bomar SK. Intravenous Medications. Philadelphia: J.B. Lippincott, 1980.
16. Plumer AL, Cosentino F. Principles and Practice of Intravenous Therapy, 4th ed. Boston: Little, Brown and Co., 1987.
17. American Society of Hospital Pharmacists. American Hospital Formulary Service Drug Information. Bethesda, MD: American Society of Hospital Pharmacists, 1991.
18. Caremark. Intermate Home Intravenous Therapy. Lincolnshire, IL: Caremark 1989.
19. Kastrup EK, ed. Drug Facts and Comparisons. St. Louis: J. B. Lippincott 1991.

CHAPTER 12

Parenteral Nutrition

Carolyn D. Ford, MSN, CRNI
Cora Vizcarra, RN, BSN, CRNI

Nutrition support is a rapidly growing specialty in nursing practice. The use of parenteral nutrition therapy is important for the prevention and treatment of many disease states in the hospital and home settings. This chapter provides a framework for assessing, planning, implementing, monitoring, and evaluating the nursing care of patients receiving parenteral nutrition.

Parenteral nutrition refers to the provision of partial or total nutrient requirements through the venous system. Depending on the actual solution components, parenteral nutrition can be administered by the central venous route or a peripheral vein. In this chapter, the terms "peripheral parenteral nutrition" (PPN) and "total parenteral nutrition" (TPN) are used to describe the approaches to delivery of parenteral nutrition. TPN refers to the infusion of a parenteral nutrition containing high concentrations of dextrose and amino acids, along with fat, electrolytes, vitamins, and trace elements, delivered through a central venous catheter into a large-diameter vein (usually the superior vena cava, through the subclavian or jugular vein). This type of parenteral nutrition is indicated for patients requiring long-term nutritional support with calorically dense solutions. TPN provides sufficient nutrients to satisfy total nutritional requirements to replenish or maintain nutritional status. PPN refers to a partial nutritional solution that involves the infusion of low-osmolarity dextrose, amino acids, fat, electrolytes, vitamins, and trace elements that may be infused through peripheral vascular access. This form of nutritional therapy may only meet partial nutritional requirements and is therefore used for short-term or supplemental nutrition support.

Technologic advances and the refinement of delivery systems have helped make the administration of TPN an almost routine aspect of patient care in hospitals today.[1] These advances include the use of total nutrient admixtures, parenteral nutrition as a medication delivery system, and cyclic infusion schedules. Nurses must integrate these new technologies into patient care and apply research findings to clinical practice.[2] Dr. Stanley Dudrick, a pioneer in the development of parenteral nutrition support, has called the nurse an invaluable, if not the most important, member of the nutrition support team. "The importance of the nurse as a patient advocate, communicator, and teacher cannot be overemphasized in any aspect of patient care, but it is especially obvious in the management of nutrition problems."[3]

HISTORICAL PERSPECTIVE

Historically, two major limiting factors have hindered the safe administration of nutrient solutions. One was the volume of solution needed to provide adequate calories. The second was the concentration of the solution that was conventionally administered through peripheral veins.[4] A 5 or 10% glucose solution could be tolerated peripherally, but with only 4 kcal/g would not provide sufficient calories in volumes tolerated by the patient. Therefore, a means for delivering higher, more hypertonic concentrations was needed. This was accomplished with the development of methods for accessing the central venous system with a cannula. Rhode and Vars developed a technique of central venous cannulation by cutdown on the jugular vein. Dudrick subsequently used a method of subclavian puncture described by Aubaniac in 1952 that eliminated the need for a cutdown and allowed highly concentrated solutions of glucose and amino acids, ranging from 20 to 70%. Adequate calories could now be provided using concentrated solutions in volumes tolerated by the compromised patient. In the 1960s, Dudrick used beagle puppies to demonstrate that the long-term infusion of intravenous nutrients could sustain and nourish growing animals. Subsequent studies were conducted on patients in "dire medical condition and suffering profound depletion of nutrients."[3]

Nutritional support has undergone tremendous advancement during the last three decades. Three areas continue to undergo rapid changes. First, as a result of increased knowledge and experience, the substrates for total parenteral nutrition (fat emulsions, amino acids, trace elements) continue to be improved. Second, technological advances have led to new and varied delivery systems, including long-term central venous access catheters, specialized administration sets, and programmable infusion devices that allow for the long-term administration of TPN in the home setting. Nursing care of home parenteral nutrition patients may soon be directed electronically through a nationwide network. Third, documentation of the efficacy of nutrition support has increased, along with the use of nutrition support teams. Past and current efforts in parenteral nutrition support have been directed toward treating the disease process or cause of organ failure in the patient. Dudrick has stated that "the future of nutrition support will be in efforts to maintain optimal function of the maximum number of cells in the body cell mass . . . to ensure optimal organ and system function."[5] Nutrition support nursing continues to develop as a specialized role in the nursing profession.

INDICATIONS FOR PARENTERAL NUTRITION

"Parenteral nutrition is administered to promote wound healing and to avoid malnutrition by providing and maintaining essential nutrients required by the body."[6] Protein-calorie malnutrition occurs frequently in the hospitalized patient secondary to an NPO status for diagnostic studies, critical illness, and severe stress. This results in catabolism, which is the breakdown of body tissue and protein to use for energy. TPN should be initiated before significant protein and calorie deficits occur. It is easier to maintain nutritional status than to replace nutritional deficits. Protein catabolism for energy affects organ function throughout the body. Malnutrition in disease contributes to delayed wound healing, increased morbidity and mortality, septic complications, and immunosuppression.[7, 8] It is considered one of the most frequent causes of immunosuppression in the world today.[9]

Goals of Nutritional Therapy

The goals of nutritional therapy depend on the patient's status, as follows:

Goals of Parenteral Nutrition

1. To provide all essential nutrients in adequate amounts to sustain nutritional balance during periods when oral or enteral routes of feedings are not possible or are insufficient to meet the caloric needs of the patient
2. To preserve or restore the body's protein metabolism and prevent the development of protein and/or calorie malnutrition
3. To diminish the rate of weight loss and maintain or increase body weight
4. To promote wound healing
5. To repair nutritional deficits

In addition, there are a number of considerations for parenteral nutrition support:[10–13]

Considerations for Parenteral Nutrition

Patient evaluation for parenteral nutrition is based on various objective parameters:

1. Any patient who is unable to ingest sufficient nutrients through the gastrointestinal (GI) tract is a potential candidate for parenteral nutrition.
2. The least invasive, least expensive means of supporting a patient's nutritional status must be considered.
3. The GI route should always be used, if appropriate. There can be serious adverse effects associated with a totally resting GI tract. Enteral nutrition preserves intestinal mass and structures, as well as hormonal, enzymatic, and immunologic function, better than intravenous nutrition.
4. Generally, nourished patients unable to eat for as long as 7 to 10 days do not require parenteral nutrition. However, the general rule is that whenever 5 to 7 days have passed with insufficient enteral intake, parenteral nutrition should be considered.
5. The indications and disease states for which parenteral nutrition is clearly beneficial are continually being established and reassessed.

Current accepted guidelines for the use of parenteral nutrition support in adult and pediatric patients have been formulated by the American Society of Parenteral and Enteral Nutrition.[14] "Parenteral nutrition support is used to nourish patients who either are already malnourished or have the potential for developing malnutrition and who are not candidates for enteral support."[14] It is generally accepted that a functional gastrointestinal tract should be used as the route for nutrition support, whenever possible. Additionally, specific indications are influenced by specific diseases and conditions. Disease states in which the use of TPN may be indicated as a primary therapy include short-gut syndrome, enterocutaneous fistula, renal failure caused by acute tubular necrosis, hepatic failure (acute decompensation in the face of cirrhosis), and burns.[12] There are other disease states in which TPN may be indicated as supportive therapy or conditions in which the efficacy of parenteral nutrition has not been clearly demonstrated (e.g., inflammatory bowel disease, anorexia nervosa). The use of TPN for cancer support, sepsis, trauma, and general perioperative support may be appropriate in selected situations. Parenteral nutrition is an expensive intervention and can pose additional risk to the patient in the form of metabolic and septic complications, so the benefits of TPN support should outweigh the risks. The decision to use PPN versus TPN is determined by the extent of nutritional depletion, duration of illness, and clinical course prior to the initiation of parenteral nutrition. An algorithm that outlines the selection process for choosing the route of nutrition support in adult patients is presented in Figure 12–1.[14]

Ethical Concerns

Ethical concerns have become increasingly apparent in justifying the withholding and withdrawing of nutrition support. Kaminski has recommended three guidelines in the decision to withdraw nutrition support humanely:[15]

1. Acceptance of the premise that the death of a terminally ill patient is a natural event and not one that should be associated with guilt
2. Acknowledgment of the patient's right to a useful existence
3. Recognition of the patient's right to a trial of hyperalimentation and to continue with it if he or she so chooses

Some believe that there is a distinction between withdrawing and withholding therapy. There is no ethical requirement that a treatment must be continued once started, especially if the treatment is against the patient's wishes. However, it is admittedly more difficult to withdraw a treatment once started, especially if that action results in the patient's death. This concern should not lead to reluctance to begin treatments. Instituting a time-limited trial of the procedure makes it easier to evaluate beneficial effects objectively and thus make a subsequent decision to withdraw or continue treatment.[16]

CONCEPTS OF NUTRITION

There are three major components in the body: water mass, fat mass, and fat-free mass (skin and skeleton, plasma pro-

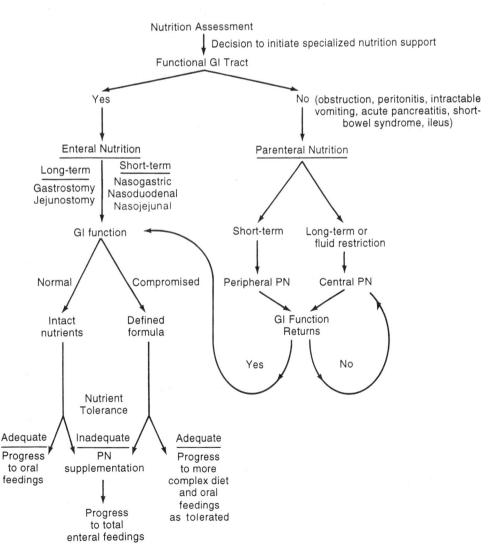

Figure 12–1. Guidelines for the use of parenteral and enteral nutrition in adult and pediatric patients. (From ASPEN. In JPEN [Suppl] 1993; 17:75A.)

Table 12–1

ICD-9-CM Codes for Classification of Malnutrition

ICD-9-CM Code	Description	Criteria*
260	Kwashiorkor	1. >90% of IBW 2. Transferrin <200 mg/dL, or albumin <3.5 g/dL 3. Decreased oral intake >2 weeks 4. Anorexia, nausea, vomiting for more than 2 weeks 5. 3+ for any one physical trait
261	Marasmus	1. <90% of IBW and/or <90% of UBW 2. Transferrin >200 mg/dL, or albumin >3.5 g/dL 3. Weight loss >10% in 6 months 4. Decreased oral intake >2 weeks 5. Anorexia, nausea, vomiting, diarrhea >2 weeks 6. 3+ for any one physical trait
263.8	Hypoalbuminemic malnutrition	1. >90% of IBW 2. Albumin <3.5 g/dL 3. New onset of stress
262, 263.9	Mixed protein-calorie malnutrition	Any combination of the criteria listed for kwashiorkor and marasmus
263, 263.1	Malnutrition of mild to moderate degree	1. 60–90% IBW and/or 60–90% UBW 2. Transferrin of 100–200 mg/dL, or albumin 3.0–3.5 g/dL 3. Weight loss of 5–10% in 6 months 4. Decreased oral intake for 5–14 days 5. Anorexia, nausea, vomiting, diarrhea for 5–14 days 6. 1+ or 2+ for any one physical trait

From Grant JP. Handbook of Parenteral Nutrition, 2nd ed. Philadelphia: W. B. Saunders, 1992:49–73.
*A minimum of three must be present.
IBW = ideal body weight; UBW = usual body weight.

tein, visceral protein, and skeletal muscle).[17] Nutritional balance is achieved when nutrients are provided in sufficient quantities for the maintenance of body function and renewal of these components. This balance depends on three factors:[18]

1. Intake of nutrients (quantity and quality)
2. Relative need for nutrients
3. Ability of the body to use nutrients

Nutritional Deficiency

When nutrient utilization is insufficient to meet the body's requirements, a nutritional deficiency develops. This can be primary, in which there is a deficiency of specific nutrients, or secondary, resulting from impairment of digestion, absorption, or utilization of nutrients. When nutritional deficiency exists, the body's components are used to provide energy for essential metabolic processes. Body stores of carbohydrates, fats, and proteins are metabolized as energy sources. Carbohydrate is stored in the muscle and liver as glycogen (a short-term energy reserve). Adipose tissue is the body's long-term energy reserve of fat. Body protein is divided into somatic and visceral compartments. The somatic compartment refers to muscle protein and the visceral compartment refers to all other body proteins, including solid viscera and secretory proteins. Protein is not stored in excess of the body's needs and, as such, the utilization of protein as an energy source without replacement adversely effects total body function.

Malnutrition

Malnutrition is defined as a nutritional deficit associated with an increased risk of morbidity and mortality.[19] Malnutri-

tion is a result of starvation and added stress of illness. Starvation alters the distribution of carbohydrate, fat, and protein substrates. Brief starvation (24 to 72 hours) rapidly depletes glycogen stores and uses protein to produce glucose (gluconeogenesis) for glucose-dependent tissue, such as the central nervous system. Prolonged starvation (greater than 72 hours) is associated with an increased mobilization of fat as the principal source of energy, reduction in the breakdown of protein, and an increased use of ketones for central nervous tissue fuel. Stress in the form of pain, shock, injury, and sepsis intensifies the metabolic changes seen in brief and prolonged starvation. The hormonal release of catecholamines, glucagon, and cortisol increases the metabolic rate and impairs the body's use of fuel.[20] Fatty acids serve as fuel for cardiac and skeletal muscles, liver, and other tissue. Somatic protein breakdown increases, as does hepatic protein synthesis, to promote the healing process, and results in the wasting of lean body mass.[21]

Three types of malnutrition have been defined and classified by an International Classification of Diseases (ICD) diagnostic code (Table 12–1).[22] The outcome of nutritional assessment determines the category to which an undernourished individual is assigned.

Types of Malnutrition

Marasmus: Protein-Calorie Malnutrition. This condition results from a diet deficient in protein and calories but adequate in water and electrolytes.[23] The individual appears starved, and therefore this type of malnutrition is sometimes referred to as adaptive starvation. This appearance is associated with weight loss, decreased fat, glycogen stores, and muscle mass, but relatively normal visceral protein levels. If starvation continues long enough, the somatic and gut mass are exhausted, compromising visceral protein stores and decreasing cell-mediated immunity. This is usually seen during prolonged starvation, chronic illness, and anorexia, and in the elderly.[17]

Kwashiorkor: Protein Malnutrition. With this type of malnutrition, the caloric intake is adequate or excessive, but the diet consists of almost all carbohydrates, with little or no protein. It is characterized by a ''well-nourished'' or obese appearance, increases in extracellular water, pitting edema, and visceral and somatic protein wasting. The distinction between marasmus and kwashiorkor is significant because the individual with kwashiorkor may appear well nourished, but is clinically at a greater risk for infection and death.[23] It is usually associated with trauma or physiologic stress and the long-term use of routine or standard intravenous infusions.

Mixed Marasmus-Kwashiorkor. Individuals with a mixed marasmus-kwashiorkor malnutrition share some aspects of both conditions. Clinical findings include muscle wasting and visceral protein depletion, decreased fat stores, and immune incompetence. The individual experiences acute catabolism, appears cachectic, and is at an extreme risk of morbidity and mortality.

Effects of Malnutrition

Protein-calorie malnutrition has a great impact on the morbidity and mortality of the patient, especially in the presence of the added stress of illness. The hazards of malnutrition on bodily functions include the following:[20]

Deterioration of Functional Status. Without protein stores in the body, a deficiency of total body protein results first in decreased strength and endurance (loss of muscle mass) and ultimately in decreased cardiac and respiratory muscle function.

Albumin Depletion. Skeletal muscle wasting occurs in a ratio of about 30:1 compared to visceral protein loss. Hypoalbuminemia is accompanied by loss of gastrointestinal function, abnormal distribution of total body water, and delayed wound healing.

Impaired Immune Status. Protein-calorie malnutrition is one of the most common causes of impaired immune function.[9] Both B- and T-cell-mediated immune functions are impaired, causing enhanced susceptibility to infections.

NUTRITIONAL ASSESSMENT

Nutritional assessment is a systematic review of the body systems combined with physical, anthropometric, and biochemical measurements that provide the data necessary to make a statement of nutritional health. The goal of nutritional assessment is to identify high-risk patients and implement the appropriate nutritional therapy.[19] Understanding the components of a nutritional assessment and their relevance to determining and monitoring the patient's nutritional status enable the nurse to provide optimal nursing care and seek appropriate consultation with those in other disciplines involved in nutritional support.

Physical Assessment

Physical examination is an essential part of a standard nutritional assessment. A nurse specially trained in nutritional support is often in the best position to conduct the physical examination, because special emphasis is placed on signs and symptoms relating to nutritional deficiencies. Signs of nutritional deficiencies are observed most commonly in the skin, hair, eyes, and mouth. Less commonly affected are the glands and nervous system. It is important to relate the findings during physical examination to the patient's diet and medical history. Knowledge of specific nutrient functions is also helpful in recognizing nutritional deficiency states. Because physical signs of nutritional deficiencies occur only after significant body nutrition depletion, it is important for the nurse to monitor the patient closely during acute illness for physical signs of nutrient deficiency.

Dietary History

To identify any possible dietary deficiencies, a thorough dietary history can delineate eating patterns, as well as life style and social habits such as alcohol consumption, vitamin usage, and economic problems. Thus, possible overconsumption and underconsumption of nutrients can be identified. The patient's usual and current intake should be assessed by a 24-hour intake report, food records, or food frequency questionnaire. The 24-hour intake report is a simple documentation of what the patient recalls eating for the past 24 hours and is a rough estimation of the patient's usual eating patterns. For patients suspected of having a poor oral consumption, a dietary intake record for a period of 3 to 7 days is valuable. Questionnaires are also available to analyze dietary intake. From these, the dietitian can interpret nutrient intake to define specific nutrient deficiencies.

Anthropometric Measurements

Anthropometrics is the physical measurement of subcutaneous fat and muscle mass (somatic protein stores) in an attempt to estimate the energy stores of the body. The most common anthropometric measurements include weight, height, limb, and trunk circumferences and skin fold thickness at various sites. Anthropometrics can be an unreliable indicator of an individual's nutritional gains because peripheral edema can inflate measurements, repeated measurements can be highly variable as a result of differences in technique used by those collecting data, and benefits from nutritional repletion primarily affect cellular function and cannot be readily detected through increases in somatic mass. The validity of anthropometry is greatly enhanced when the measurements are obtained by skilled, conscientious personnel. Serial measurements over long periods of time (e.g., a month or longer) have the most value in determining nutritional status.[15]

Weight and Height Indices

Body weight is the most used and easily attainable anthropometric measurement. Weight loss is probably the most common variable considered in nutritional assessment. In assessing the importance of weight loss, current body weight is compared with the usual and ideal body weights. Usual weight is the patient's stated weight prior to being ill. The ideal body weight is obtained from standard tables of age, height, and sex, such as the Metropolitan Life Insurance Table. The percentage of usual weight and weight loss are frequently used clinical expressions of weight change. A loss of 10% of the usual weight, or a current weight less than 90% of ideal, is considered to be a risk factor for nutrition-related complications. However, these parameters provide only limited information regarding overall nutritional status. The magnitude of weight loss cannot be necessarily correlated to the severity of malnutrition and, similarly, the lack of significant weight loss does not preclude the existence of malnutrition. The use of body weight and height indices alone in nutritional assessment is not totally reliable. Other factors must be considered, such as body composition and the rate and cause of weight loss. It is important that weight be measured accurately (i.e., same time of day, similar clothing). Serial weight determinations over a long period provide the most reliable and clinically relevant information for nutritional assessment.[15]

Total Body Fat

Skin fold measurements, the mainstay of anthropometric techniques, are used to determine and assess body fat stores by estimating the thickness of subcutaneous adipose tissue at various sites on the body. These include the triceps, biceps, subscapular, abdominal, suprailiac, medial calf, and anterior thigh locations.[15] The use of calipers to assess skin fold thickness as a measure of subcutaneous fat is an easy, non-invasive, and inexpensive test. The most common measurement is the triceps skin fold thickness, which is compared with percentile standards or serial measurements. The actual value of this measurement in nutritional assessment remains questionable for several reasons. First, anthropometric techniques are only indirect measurements of body composition. The validity of these measurements for a given population requires comparison to standard methods of body compositional analysis. Second, normal values and ranges are highly population-specific. Third, the accuracy of a given measurement by one observer and the degree of error among different observers may be large. Last, the assumption that subcutaneous fat is distributed symmetrically around the arm has been challenged by computerized axial tomography analyses. With these limitations in mind, anthropometric measurements of subcutaneous fat must be carefully performed and analyzed.[15]

Alternative methods for determining body composition include the use of radiographic and ultrasound techniques, isotope dilution assays, neutron activation analysis, tetrapolar bioelectrical impedance analysis, and total body electrical conductivity.[22]

Skeletal Muscle Stores

Skeletal muscle represents 60% of the total body protein pool and is the major source of amino acids during times of stress and starvation. The anthropometric evaluation of skeletal muscle mass has been predominantly restricted to the assessment of the upper extremities. Anthropometric measurement of muscle mass is accomplished by using midarm circumference (MAC) and skin fold thickness to calculate midarm muscle circumference (MAMC) and midarm muscle area. The MAC is measured at the same level as the triceps skin fold thickness (TSF). The shape of the arm converts minor discrepancies of the location of the mid-upper arm measurements into major area differences, and this potential for error makes serial comparisons insensitive. For the best overall impression, results should be interpreted in relation to weight percentiles.[22]

Creatinine-Height Index

Creatinine excretion is used as an indirect measurement of body muscle mass. The amount of urinary creatinine excreted is an indicator of muscle mass and total body nitrogen. The creatinine-height index (CHI) is a ratio of 24-hour urine creatinine excretion in a patient compared to the height of matched controls of the same sex, expressed as a percentage. Therefore, an index of 100% indicates a normal muscle mass, provided creatinine excretion is normal. Skeletal muscle depletion is defined by an index of less than 80% of normal. For adequate assessment of the CHI, the patient must be on a meat-free diet, have normal renal function, and be in a steady state of catabolism. Potential errors associated with this technique include the significant individual variation among patients (normal creatinine excretion decreases with age), accuracy of urine collection (small errors can greatly affect results), extrarenal losses, and variable renal clearance.[19, 22]

Laboratory Data Measurements

Routine laboratory tests may be helpful in detecting nutritional status from a biochemical standpoint. There are several laboratory tests that reveal certain aspects of nutritional deficiencies. Determinations of serum total protein, albumin, and transferrin were the first biochemical tests included in nutritional assessment. Serum total protein is of little value as a nutritional index as a result of its lack of specificity, because both nutritional and non-nutritional factors affect the serum total protein. Other visceral proteins with shorter half-lives, such as retinol-binding protein and prealbumin, are significant indicators of nutritional status.[15] The changes in the levels of these proteins should be evaluated together, because they reflect different processes in the body. All visceral protein measurements should be interpreted in the context of the patient's clinical condition, because they are also affected by changing fluid balance, sepsis, medications, and any stressful insult.

Serum Albumin

Albumin is the major protein synthesized by the liver, and has a half-life of 18 days. Approximately 40% of the protein mass is in circulation. This important visceral protein serves to maintain plasma oncotic pressure and functions as a carrier for substances such as metabolites, enzymes, drugs, hormones, and metals in the circulation. The serum albumin concentration is normally between 3.5 and 5.0 g/dL and is considered the best single nutritional test for predicting outcome. However, this long half-life limits its value for detecting acute nutritional changes. An albumin level between 2.8 and 3.2 g/dL represents mild protein depletion, 2.1 to 2.7 g/dL reflects moderate depletion, and less than 2.1 g/dL indicates severe depletion.[22]

Serum Transferrin

Serum transferrin is a beta globulin synthesized predominantly in the liver that transports iron in the plasma. It may prevent bacterial infection by binding iron. Transferrin has a serum half-life of 8 days and is present in the serum at a concentration of 250 to 300 mg/dL.[22] Transferrin can be measured directly by radial immunodiffusion and indirectly by an estimation of the total iron-binding capacity (TIBC) using the following equation: Transferrin = (0.8 TIBC) − 4.3. Levels measured directly are consistently lower than those measured indirectly. The serum levels are affected by nutritional factors and iron metabolism. Levels measured directly that are lower than 100 mg/dL indicate severe depletion.[22] The shorter half-life of transferrin is a theoretic advantage over albumin as a nutritional marker, but clinical studies have not demonstrated any significant difference in their value.[19]

Prealbumin and Retinol-Binding Protein

Prealbumin functions in thyroxine transport and as a carrier for retinol-binding protein. It has a half-life of 2 to 3 days, and is therefore sensitive to acute changes in protein status. However, sudden demands for protein synthesis, as in trauma or acute infection, can result in a rapid fall in protein levels and therefore may not always be clinically useful.[22] Normal serum concentrations range from 15.7 to 29.6 mg/dL. Mild depletion is reflected in levels of 10 to 15 mg/dL, 5 to 9.9 mg/dL reflects moderate depletion, and a level lower than 5 mg/dL indicates severe depletion.[22]

Retinol-binding protein is synthesized by the liver and is normally present in the serum at a concentration of 3 to 5 mEq/dL. Retinol-binding protein functions to transport retinol in the plasma and circulates in a 1:1 molar ratio with prealbumin. It has a half-life of 12 hours. As with prealbumin, this relatively short half-life allows for a more accurate assessment of acute depletion and repletion phases of nutritional change.[14]

Immune Competence

Among many factors influencing the immune response of the body is the nutritional state. Immune competence can be adversely affected by malnutrition, stress, and disease. Studies have shown that cell-mediated immunity is affected earlier and to a greater extent than humoral immunity.[19] Immunologic testing is designed to assess nutritional deficiencies. The most common methods used for the assessment of immunocompetence are the total lymphoctye count (TLC) and delayed cutaneous hypersensitivity, also known as anergy testing.

The TLC is derived from the routine complete blood count with differential. The following formula is used in determining the total lymphocyte count:

$$TLC = \frac{\% \text{ lymph} \times WBC}{100}$$

Usually, a TLC between 1200 and 2000/mm³ indicates mild depletion; a TLC between 800 and 1199/mm³ indicates moderate depletion; and a TLC lower than 800/mm³ indicates severe depletion.[22] The TLC must be interpreted with caution, because many other non-nutritional factors may contribute to decreased lymphocyte counts.

Delayed cutaneous hypersensitivity testing involves the use of a battery of four or more common skin test antigens that are injected intradermally to elicit an inflammatory reaction. A positive skin test occurs within 48 to 72 hours if T lymphocytes are functioning properly. The value of this method as a test of nutritional status or therapy is unclear. Studies have shown that many non-nutritional factors alter delayed cutaneous hypersensitivity and, because of the likelihood of these factors coexisting with malnutrition, this test is not currently used for routine nutritional assessment.[19, 24]

Other Indices

Other parameters are also used to assess overall nutritional status.

Nitrogen Balance

Nitrogen balance is a measure of the daily intake of nitrogen minus the excretion. It is the most common clinical method for assessing protein turnover. The nitrogen intake is determined from calorie-protein intake records by dividing the protein intake by 6.25. The excretion consists of measured urinary nitrogen from a 24-hour urine collection plus a factor for other nitrogen losses through insensible and gastrointestinal losses. Thus, nitrogen balance is determined by this formula: nitrogen balance = nitrogen intake − (total urinary nitrogen − insensible losses − gastrointestinal losses). A positive nitrogen balance indicates an anabolic state with an overall gain in body protein for the day, whereas a negative nitrogen balance indicates a catabolic state with a net loss of protein.

Indirect Calorimetry

Energy balance can be viewed as the difference between energy intake and expenditure. Energy expenditure can be measured using indirect calorimetry or calculated using a predictive formula such as the Harris-Benedict equation. The difficulty with this formula is that it is derived from healthy patients and has limited application in times of illness.[19] Indirect calorimetry is the technique used in the measurement of resting energy expenditure (REE) based on oxygen consumption and carbon dioxide production. The most commonly used instrument for the determination of indirect calorimetry in the clinical setting is the metabolic measurement cart (MMC). Portable systems estimate energy expenditure in nonintubated patients and those requiring ventilatory support. Most metabolic measurement carts have a canopy system for long-term continuous measurements, along with a fully automatic calibration and computerized data system.

The REE in most cases reflects 130% of the daily total energy expenditure.[19]

Multiparameter Indices

In an attempt to improve the sensitivity and specificity of tests for nutritional assessment, a number of mulitparameter indices have been developed. The development of these indices involves comparing outcome results with a large number of nutritional tests and selecting those that combine to form the best predictive model.

The most popular example is the prognostic nutritional index (PNI). The PNI is based on four measures selected by discriminant analysis and a computer-based stepwise regression that are then incorporated into a linear predictive model. The clinically important factors as determined by this analysis include serum albumin concentration, serum transferrin level, triceps skin fold thickness, and delayed hypersensitivity. The PNI model that relates the risk of postoperative morbidity to nutritional status is expressed by the following:[25]

$$PNI\ (\%\ of\ risk) = 158 - 16.6\ (*Alb\ g/dL)$$
$$- 0.78\ (*TSF) - 0.2\ (*TFN,\ mg/dL) - 5.8\ (*DH)$$

A PNI lower than 40% is considered low risk; a PNI of 40 to 49% is intermediate risk, and a PNI greater than 50% is high risk. This index has been validated prospectively in several surgical patients and was found to be a useful tool for identifying patients at high risk of developing nutritionally based complications in the postoperative period.[15]

Measurement of Energy Requirements

Provision of adequate caloric intake depends on accurately measuring or predicting the energy requirements of the patient. Whereas underfeeding could result in further deterioration of nutritional status, overfeeding may result in excessive fat deposition in the liver, deranged liver function, excessive ventilatory requirements, and less effective use of nutrients.[20]

A method of measuring energy requirements that is flexible enough to reflect changes in the clinical state of the patient is the energy balance technique. Energy balance is the difference between energy intake and expenditure. A positive energy balance (food intake exceeds expenditure) results in glycogen and fat synthesis. Negative energy balance results in weight loss as the body uses its own energy stores to meet requirements.[26]

Total daily energy requirements in the healthy individual are divided into three components: resting energy expenditure (REE), the energy expenditure of activity, and specific dynamic activity (SDA). The REE is the amount of energy required to maintain daily metabolic processes. Specific dynamic activity (SDA) is the energy required to process ingested food.[27] The REE includes the basal metabolic rate of the body (BMR), the SDA, and minimal physical activity. The BMR is defined as the "minimum amount of energy required by the body at rest in the fasting state needed to sustain life processes."[18] Factors that affect the BMR are age, sex, size, sleep, and climate.

Energy expenditure can be measured directly or indirectly. Direct measurement is complex and measures the actual heat produced by the body. Indirect measurements of energy expenditure more commonly used today include actual measurement of the rate at which oxygen is consumed and carbon dioxide is produced or estimates of the expenditure using nomograms and equations.

Actual measurements involve noninvasive tests performed by open circuit or closed circuit methods. Both systems require equipment to capture and measure all expired gas accurately. The measured gas exchange reflects actual caloric expenditure under conditions present at the time of the test. Actual measurement of the BMR is performed within 30 minutes of waking with the patient in a supine resting position, after a 12- to 18-hour fast, and in a neutral thermal environment. The REE is measured in a neutral thermal environment with the patient in a resting position for greater than 30 minutes and at least a 2-hour fast. The MMC allows these tests to be done at the patient's bedside. This enables the physician to determine the patient's energy requirements, and adjustments can be made to meet the patient's metabolic capacity. Practical considerations of cost and time have limited the routine use of MMCs for monitoring patients already receiving TPN.

Estimates of energy requirements for weight maintenance in the clinical setting can be made using a formula proposed by Apelgren and Wilmore: REE × 1.25 × stress factor.[27] The REE is calculated by using the Harris-Benedict equation and adding an additional 10% for the SDA of food utilization. A 25% increase (a factor of 1.25) is allowed for physical activity and the stress of hospitalization. An additional 500 kcal/day are added for a weight gain of approximately 1 kg/week. The Harris-Benedict equation and stress factors added to correct for the disease process are given in Table 12–2.

COMPONENTS OF NUTRITION

Fluids

The average healthy adult requires 2 to 3 liters of fluid/day, or approximately 30 ml/kg/day. Fluids are lost through the kidneys, lungs, bowel, and skin. Fluid balance depends

---

*Alb, Serum albumin level; TSF, triceps skin fold; TFN, serum transferrin level; DH, delayed hypersensitivity.

Table 12–2

Harris-Benedict Equation and Stress Factors Used to Correct for the Disease Process

Harris-Benedict Equation*
BMR (male) = 66.5 + (13.75 × W) + (5.0 × H) − (6.8 × A)
BMR (female) = 66.5 + (9.56 × W) + (1.7 × H) − (4.68 × A)

Condition	Stress Factor
Mild starvation	0.85–1.00
Postoperative recovery	1.00–1.05
Cancer	1.10–1.45
Peritonitis	1.05–1.25
Severe infection or multiple trauma	1.30–1.55

*W = weight in kilograms; H = height in centimeters; A = age in years.

on a balance between fluid intake and output, so gains in fluid intake must equal losses in body fluid. Individual fluid requirements vary greatly and can fluctuate on a daily basis. Therefore, accurate patient intake and output records are invaluable to help determine fluid requirements. Most fluid replacement is based on body surface area and has been found to be more constant than when expressed by body weight. Many essential physiologic processes such as heat loss, blood volume, organ size, and respiration rate have a direct relationship to the body surface area. Fluid and electrolyte requirements are also proportional to the body surface area, regardless of age.[28]

Protein

Protein is essential for body growth, maintenance, and repair of tissue. When proteins are digested they are absorbed as amino acids, the basic structural unit of protein. Approximately 22 different amino acids are commonly found in proteins. Nonessential amino acids can be synthesized and are precursors for the synthesis of carbohydrates, fats, and other amino acids. Amino acids that the body cannot make and must be obtained from the diet are called essential amino acids. Essentiality can be the result of a total inability to make the amino acid or, as in young growing children, the inability to make an adequate amount. In either case, additional amino acids must come from the diet, because the body does not store amino acids.[3] Excess amino acids are used as an energy source and excess nitrogen is excreted in the urine as urea.

The metabolism of amino acids occurs primarily in the liver, where it monitors the amino acid uptake and regulates its release. Specific essential amino acids such as phenylalanine, tryptophan, methionine, threonine, and lysine, as well as all the nonessential amino acids, are catabolized in the liver. The liver is also the site for urea synthesis, where nitrogenous wastes must be converted to urea prior to transporting to the kidney for excretion.

Each amino acid has its own distinct metabolic pathway that leads to oxidation, carbon dioxide, water, and urea. Urea contains two amino acid groups, oxygen and one-carbon. Thus, incomplete oxidation results in obtaining less than the energy potentially available from protein. Protein yields approximately 4 kcal/g of available energy. In addition, when some amino acids are split, they yield carbon structures that can produce glucose through gluconeogenesis, in which the carbon structures fit into the glycolytic pathway and are metabolized as if they were carbohydrate to produce energy or resynthesized to form glucose. Other amino acids are ketogenic, in which the carbon structures fit into the lipid metabolic pathways and can form ketone bodies. Ketogenic amino acids cannot contribute to the formation of glucose. Other amino acids have branched chains, meaning that a portion of their carbon structure is glucogenic and a portion is ketogenic. These branched chain amino acids have proven to have an important role in the parenteral feeding of some hypermetabolic states.[3] Table 12–3 presents the classifications of amino acids.

Body proteins are constantly undergoing catabolism and anabolism, and approximately 40% of the body's resting energy expenditure is used for these processes. During

Table 12–3	
Classifications of Amino Acids	
Essential Amino Acids	**Nonessential Amino Acids**
Histidine	Alanine
Isoleucine	Arginine
Leucine	Asparagine
Lysine	Aspartic acid
Methionine	Cysteine*
Phenylalanine	Cystine
Threonine	Glutamic acid
Tryptophan	Glutamine
Valine	Glycine
	Hydroxyproline
	Proline
	Serine
	Tyrosine

*May be essential for premature infants.

growth and in pregnancy, the body is making more protein than it is breaking down. Therefore, the body is in a state of positive nitrogen balance, as described earlier. During other conditions, such as restricted food intake, disease, or trauma, the body might be in negative nitrogen balance. Clinically, the balance between protein synthesis and degradation can be estimated by measuring the nitrogen balance.

Carbohydrates

All carbohydrates are compounds of carbon, hydrogen, and oxygen. Carbohydrates in the diet are classified as complex carbohydrates or simple sugars. The simple sugars are monosaccharides, meaning a one-sugar moiety, or disaccharides, with two-sugar moieties. The major monosaccharides are glucose and fructose and the other two are galactose and mannose. The disaccharides include sucrose, maltose, and lactose.

The metabolism of carbohydrates involves a number of intricate chemical processes that depend on the presence of insulin, glucagon and, to a lesser extent, hormones such as epinephrine and norepinephrine. Carbohydrate metabolism, like all forms of metabolism, has a constructive phase called anabolism and a destructive phase called catabolism. Carbohydrate catabolism is the process whereby the body breaks carbohydrates down into smaller molecules and uses the energy that is released in the process. The three major processes involved in carbohydrate catabolism are glycolysis, the Krebs cycle, and glycogenolysis. The initial process in carbohydrate catabolism is glycolysis, in which sugar is broken down into simpler compounds. This results in a split of the glucose molecule and a partial release of energy. The Krebs cycle completes carbohydrate catabolism, which results in the total breakdown of glucose into carbon dioxide, water, and energy. Whenever the blood glucose level in the body is abnormally low, glycogen stores are converted to glucose by the process called glycogenolysis.

Carbohydrate anabolism is a process whereby catabolic products of carbohydrates, fat, or protein are chemically converted into glycogen and stored principally in the liver. This process, unlike catabolism, does not release energy but, instead, uses the body's energy. There are two major processes involved in carbohydrate anabolism, glycogenesis and glyconeogenesis. Glycogenesis is the process whereby glucose is converted to glycogen. This process is the reverse of glycogenolysis and depends on the release of insulin. Glyconeogenesis is the transformation of fats and proteins into glucose or glycogen for use by cells as fuel. This process occurs when carbohydrates are not available for use as fuel.

Fats

Fats or lipids are organic substances that are relatively insoluble in water but are soluble in organic compounds such as ether, chloroform, and benzene. Lipids are responsible for a wide range of metabolic and structural functions. In parenteral nutrition, they are a major source of metabolic fuel, providing usable energy for a wide range of metabolic processes, and a source of essential fatty acids. Lipids are a particularly efficient form of energy storage because of their high energy content (9 kcal/g) and anhydrous state in stored fat. Structurally, lipids function as a component of cell membranes to pad critical organs and insulate against heat loss. Lipids are precursors of the regulatory compounds, such as the prostaglandins, glucocorticoids, mineralocorticoids, estrogens, androgens, and bile acids. Certain nutrients that are essential to body metabolism, such as vitamins A, D, E, and K, are lipids. The major classes of lipids found in the plasma include triglycerides, phospholipids, cholesterol, and free fatty acids.

The names and classifications of fatty acids are related to the number of carbon atoms and the position and number of double bonds. Those with 6 to 8 carbons are considered short-chain fatty acids; those with 8 to 12 carbons are medium-chain fatty acids, and those with 14 carbons or more are long-chain fatty acids. Each fatty acid can contain one or more double bonds, which determines the degree of saturation. Saturated fats have no double bonds and contain the most hydrogen. Monosaturated fats contain one double bond and polyunsaturated fats contain more than one double bond. Medium- and short-chain fatty acids contain single bonds and are saturated fats.

The two essential fatty acids for humans are linoleic and α-linolenic acids. These fatty acids are necessary for cell membrane structure and stability and are the precursors for prostaglandins.[22] The primary fatty acid in the diet is linoleic acid, a precursor to arachidonic acid. Linoleic is considered essential because the body cannot synthesize it and it must therefore be supplied from an extraneous source, such as diet or parenteral feedings. Arachidonic acid can be synthesized from linoleic acid if there is an adequate supply. The importance of linolenic acid as an essential dietary component is uncertain; only linoleic acid appears to be required in the adult's diet.[22] Essential fatty acid deficiency (EFAD) can occur in as little as 5 days without fat supplementation. The clinical signs and symptoms of essential fatty acid deficiency are as follows:

Dry, thick, desquamating skin
Alopecia
Brittle nails
Increased capillary fragility
Diminished wound healing

Enhanced platelet aggregation caused by decreased prostaglandin synthesis
Thrombocytopenia
Increased susceptibility to infection
Hepatic dysfunction secondary to fatty liver
Growth retardation in infants

Lipids in the diet are emulsified by the action of gastric lipase and bile salts in the small intestine. As with carbohydrate and protein, lipid metabolism is influenced by various hormones (insulin and epinephrine) and vitamins (niacin, riboflavin, and pantothenic acid). Disease states and drugs may alter lipid metabolism by increasing or decreasing fat digestion, absorption, mobilization, and utilization.

Electrolytes

Electrolytes play a critical role in almost all the body's physiologic functions. Disorders of electrolyte homeostasis are associated with many disease states. As a result, in the patient requiring nutritional support, abnormal electrolyte concentrations are encountered that reflect either the primary disease state, its complications, or its treatment. Electrolytes commonly used in a parenteral nutrition formula include sodium, potassium, calcium, magnesium, chloride, and phosphorus. Electrolytes are included in the formula to meet daily requirements and correct deficits. The management of electrolytes for these patients can be one of the most time-consuming aspects of monitoring and managing nutritional support. The key points for minimizing electrolyte complications associated with nutritional support are close monitoring, awareness of pre-existing deficits and factors that predispose a patient to electrolyte imbalance, and the recognition of signs and symptoms of deficiency.

Sodium. Together with chloride and bicarbonate, sodium is the major osmotic force in the extracellular fluid. Sodium is actively involved in the absorption of sugars and amino acids. It is the most abundant cation and contributes to the osmolarity of the extracellular fluid.

Potassium. Potassium is the main intracellular cation. It plays a role in cell metabolism, participating in such processes as protein and glycogen synthesis. Potassium absorption in the ileum is a passive process and depends on the concentration gradient. Potassium loss may be increased by diarrhea and the chronic use of laxatives.

Calcium. Calcium is responsible for the preservation and function of cell membranes, propagation of neuromuscular activity, regulation of endocrine and exocrine secretory functions, blood coagulation cascade, platelet adhesion process, bone metabolism, muscle cell excitation-contraction coupling, and mediation of the electrophysiologic slow channel response in cardiac and smooth muscle tissue. In malnourished patients, serum calcium levels may be low because of decreased levels of albumin, to which half of calcium is bound, whereas ionized calcium levels remain normal.

Magnesium. After potassium, magnesium is the next most abundant intracellular cation. Intracellularly, it is bound to protein and is necessary for a number of vital cellular functions, including membrane and mitochondrial integrity, enzyme activation, such as that of adenosine triphosphate (ATP) and adenylate cyclase, and the synthesis and stability of nuclear DNA. It is also necessary for the control of neuromuscular irritability. Most of the absorption of magnesium takes place in the ileum because of slow transit in that area and the fact that uptake is passive.

Chloride. Chloride is the principal anion of the extracellular fluid. It is essential for the diagnosis and maintenance of appropriate acid-base balance. Along with sodium, chloride contributes to the total osmolarity in the blood and urine and plays a major role in water balance and extracellular fluid volume control. Chloride is generally excreted with sodium.

Phosphorus. Phosphorus is the major intracellular anion. It is the essential element in phospholipid cell membranes, nucleic acids, and phosphoproteins required for mitochondrial function. It regulates the intermediary metabolism of carbohydrates, fats, and proteins, and regulates enzymatic reactions, including glycolysis. Phosphorus is a source of high-energy bonds of ATP; therefore, it is important in muscle contractility, electrolyte transport, and neurologic function.

Essential Trace Minerals

Trace minerals are a subgroup of the trace elements, which constitute less than 0.01% of the total body. Not all these trace elements are minerals, and not all trace minerals have been confirmed as essential nutrients in humans. The trace minerals that have been identified as essential in humans perform a variety of biologic functions, primarily as components of metalloenzymes. As such, they participate in carbohydrate, lipid, and protein metabolism, immune function, cell membrane integrity, oxygen transport, and hormonal activity. The trace minerals for which human deficiency states have been identified are copper, chromium, iodine, iron, manganese, molybdenum, selenium, and zinc. The other trace minerals that are essential to humans, but for which deficiency states have not been recognized, are cobalt, nickel, silicon, and vanadium.

Copper. Copper is a component of cuproenzymes, which primarily participate in oxygen utilization. Copper is involved in energy, cholesterol, and catecholamine metabolism, erythropoiesis, leukopoiesis, skeletal mineralization, phospholipid, elastin, and collagen synthesis, and iron metabolism.

Chromium. Chromium participates in glucose metabolism as a key component of the ''glucose tolerance factor,'' which potentiates the action of insulin.

Iodine. Iodine is required in much smaller quantities and is primarily a constituent of thyroid hormones. These hormones help regulate metabolic activity in the body.

Iron. The principal function of iron is the transport, storage, and utilization of oxygen. Iron deficiency is the most common nutritional deficiency in the US population, largely because of the needs of women and children.

Manganese. Manganese functions in energy metabolism, antioxidant protection, formation of connective tissue, and

synthesis of mucopolysaccharides. It is a soluble cofactor in a number of enzymatic reactions.

Molybdenum. Molybdenum is required as a cofactor of three metalloenzymes—xanthine oxidase, sulfite oxidase, and aldehyde oxidase. It is therefore involved in oxidation reduction reactions.

Selenium. Selenium is a constituent of glutathione peroxidase, which catalyzes the reduction of hydrogen peroxide to water. Therefore, as an antioxidant, it protects the cell membrane and hemoglobin from oxidative damage and hemolysis.

Zinc. Zinc is the most abundant of all the trace elements and is an integral part of many enzymes and enzyme cofactors. Its functions include protein, carbohydrate, and lipid metabolism, membrane stabilization, and RNA conformation.

Vitamins

Vitamins are organic compounds essential to normal tissue growth, maintenance, and function. They are involved in enzymatic processes that are important to energy and macronutrient metabolism. Vitamins function primarily as coenzymes of energy-yielding nutrients, as well as cofactors in the storage and utilization of energy. Based on their chemical properties, vitamins are classified as fat-soluble, capable of being stored in fatty tissues, or water-soluble, which have limited storage. Table 12–4 lists the fat- and water-soluble vitamins. Because vitamins cannot be synthesized by the body, they must be obtained from dietary sources.

Vitamins are essential during nutrition support. Their key role in numerous metabolic processes make their inclusion critical to the appropriate and efficient use of other nutrients. Standard parenteral maintenance doses of all vitamins should be provided as additives to the total parenteral solution on initiation of parenteral nutrition, unless an existing condition requires the limitation or exclusion of selected vitamins.

Fat-Soluble Vitamins

Vitamin A (Retinol). Vitamin A is required for many functions of the body, most prominently the visual process. Retinol is found in the visual pigments of the eye for both dim light vision as well as color vision. In addition, vitamin A is

Table 12–4

Fat- and Water-Soluble Vitamins

Fat-Soluble Vitamins	Water-Soluble Vitamins
Vitamin A (retinol)	Vitamin B_1 (thiamine)
D	B_2 (riboflavin)
E (tocopherol)	Pantothenic acid
K	B_6 (pyroxidine)
	B_{12} (cyanocobalamin)
	Biotin
	C (ascorbic acid)
	Folic acid
	Niacin

required for the synthesis of certain polysaccharides and is essential in the formation of many membranes of the body. Vitamin A is necessary for proper immune function, particularly antigen recognition, and is essential for the integrity of epithelial surfaces.

Vitamin D. Vitamin D is converted to hormones in the body that are directly involved in the regulation of calcium and phosphorus. This regulation includes not only the absorption of calcium but the deposition and release of calcium from the bone and teeth, as well as the entrance of calcium into certain cells or cell nuclei.

Vitamin E (Tocopherol). Vitamin E is an antioxidant that protects other organic compounds from being oxidized. In particular, it prevents the oxidation and destruction of vitamin A and the rancidity reactions of polyunsaturated fatty acids. It prevents the membrane from breaking and the resulting cellular destruction when unsaturated fatty acids are oxidized.

Vitamin K. Vitamin K is involved in blood clotting. It has been shown to be involved in the formation of certain dicarboxylic amino acids that bind calcium. Deficiency of this vitamin is usually manifested by prolonged prothrombin time. Vitamin K is not usually added to commercially available parenteral vitamin preparations, so it is routinely given by separate intramuscular or intravenous injection.

Water-Soluble Vitamins

B Vitamins. Vitamin B_1 (thiamine) is an important vitamin in the oxidation conversion of pyruvic acid and therefore, the Krebs cycle. Thiamine is also part of certain nerve cells and is required for the proper transmission of nerve impulses.

Vitamin B_2 (riboflavin) is necessary for cellular growth and repair. It is also an integral part of several oxidative enzyme systems necessary for electron transport and thus for the efficient production of cellular energy.

Pantothenic acid is a constituent of coenzyme A and is the prosthetic group on an acyl carrier protein. It is necessary for the release of energy from carbohydrates, the breakdown of fatty acids, and steroid hormones.

Vitamin B_6 (pyridoxine) is intimately involved in amino acid metabolism, acting as a cofactor for numerous enzymes. It is essential for the synthesis of heme and glycogen phosphorylase activity.

Vitamin B_{12} (cyanocobalamin) serves as a coenzyme involved in the synthesis of DNA nucleotides and in lipid and amino acid metabolism.

Biotin is required for the normal activity of the numerous enzyme systems involved in carbohydrate, fat, and protein metabolism.

Folate (folic acid) is transformed to numerous compounds (folates), which serve as coenzymes in a variety of one-carbon transfer reactions involved in purine biosynthesis and amino acid metabolism.

Niacin (nicotinic acid) is a component of nicotinamide adenine dinucleotide and nicotinamide adenine dinucleotide phosphate. These coenzymes are involved in many oxidation-reduction reactions occurring in cell respiration, glycolysis, and fat synthesis.

Vitamin C (Ascorbic Acid). Vitamin C is required for normal amino acid metabolism and for the synthesis of collagen, adrenal hormones, vasoactive amines, and carnitine. It is important in cholesterol and folacin metabolism and leukocyte function.

Several food substances possess one or more known biologic activities but have not yet been determined to be essential nutrients. For example, carnitine serves as a carrier molecule for long-chain fatty acid transport across the inner mitochondrial membrane. Under normal conditions a dietary intake of carnitine is unnecessary, but neonates and individuals suffering from different diseases may require exogenous carnitine.

DISEASE STATES AFFECTING NUTRITION

Many disease states have an impact on nutritional status secondary to factors related to the disease process, as well as associated treatments.

Esophageal Dysfunction

Dysfunction of the esophagus disrupts nutrient entry into the digestive process. Disorders affecting adequate propulsion of food to the stomach include the following:

1. Cardiospasm: disorder of esophageal motility with relaxation of the lower esophageal sphincter
2. Chronic central nervous system disorders: myasthenia gravis, Parkinson's disease, amyotrophic lateral sclerosis, Alzheimer's disease
3. Cerebrovascular accidents: cause bilateral or unilateral paralysis, dysphagia
4. Esophageal tumors: affect motility or cause obstruction

Esophageal dysfunction usually does not involve the rest of the GI tract and can be supported with enteral nutritional intervention by nasogastric tube, gastrostomy, or jejunostomy. If the patient presents with severe protein-calorie malnutrition, or requires surgery to correct the dysfunction, parenteral nutrition may be used initially.[29]

Gastric Dysfunction

Dysfunction of the stomach may cause an inability to ingest food orally or to pass on to the small intestine, nausea, and vomiting. Disorders of the stomach affecting nutrition include the following:

1. Delayed gastric emptying: related to mechanical obstruction caused by lesions or tumors blocking the gastric outlet, diabetic gastroparesis in insulin-dependent diabetic patients, or following vagotomy and gastric surgery
2. Rapid gastric emptying: often referred to as the dumping syndrome; may result from gastric resection or vagotomy
3. Peptic ulcer disease: lesions of the gastric mucosa causing bleeding and pain, and often leading to gastric surgery
4. Gastric cancer: causes obstructive lesions

Nutrition support is delivered by the enteral route to the small intestine unless the intestinal tract is involved. Special formulations such as elemental formulas may be used, or parenteral nutrition may be necessary.

Intestinal Dysfunction

Inflammatory Bowel Disease. Inflammatory bowel disease, or IBD, describes two inflammatory intestinal conditions, Crohn's disease and ulcerative colitis, that affect nutrient intake and absorption.[8, 30] Crohn's disease presents as an inflammation of any part of the gastrointestinal tract. The inflammatory process is transmural, often involving the lymph nodes and mesentery. It is characterized by fistulas, abscesses, and bowel wall thickening with stenosis. Symptoms include pain, cramping, diarrhea, fever, nausea, and rectal bleeding.

Ulcerative colitis is primarily limited to the colon and affects the mucosa by producing congestion and edema. Ulcerations eventually produce abscesses. Symptoms include recurrent, bloody diarrhea with pus and mucus, weight loss, weakness, anorexia, nausea, and vomiting.

Malnutrition in patients with IBD is caused by several factors. Decreased oral intake results from the nausea and vomiting associated with the disease process, pain, and cramping, which often increases with oral intake, and side effects of the medications used to treat the disease. Excessive protein losses occur during acute diarrhea. Malabsorption of vitamins and minerals almost always accompanies the disease process. Parenteral nutrition may be used during the course of either type of IBD, although patients with Crohn's disease may benefit more with this intervention.

Pancreatic Disease. The pancreas produces and secretes enzymes and hormones that aid in the digestion of nutrients and maintenance of carbohydrate homeostasis. Pancreatitis may be acute or chronic. The causes of the acute and chronic forms include biliary disease, trauma, postabdominal surgery, hyperlipidemia, and excessive alcohol ingestion. The chronic form is distinguished by its progressive fibrotic nature, whereas the acute form can progress to fulminant necrotizing hemorrhagic disease.[29, 31] The acute phase of pancreatitis manifests with epigastric pain, persistent vomiting, and elevated serum amylase and lipase levels. Malabsorption causes weight loss, diarrhea, and steatorrhea. Almost all patients experience impaired carbohydrate metabolism, fluid and electrolyte imbalance, and hypoalbuminemia.[32] Parenteral nutritional support should be initiated promptly to replace nutritional deficits and provide for the additional requirements imposed by the inflammatory process.[31]

Hepatic Failure. The liver plays a vital role in metabolism and maintenance of homeostasis of the body. Liver failure develops in advanced stages of many diseases and is manifested by hepatic encephalopathy, hemorrhage, coagulopathy, ascites, jaundice, and hepatorenal syndrome.[33] The primary diseases of the liver include hepatitis (inflammation of the liver) and cirrhosis (fibrotic tissue formation). Although hepatitis may resolve with medical treatment, cirrhosis results in irreversible damage.

Metabolic changes include glucose intolerance, alteration in fat metabolism, protein intolerance, and an increase in nitrogen demand as a result of hepatocellular destruction. The combination of protein intolerance and increased nitrogen demand presents an extreme challenge for nutritional management.

Goals of nutritional intervention include providing protein for the regeneration of hepatocytes, restoration of protein homeostasis, and avoidance of complications of infection, ascites, and encephalopathy.[30] Both parenteral and enteral support may be used. Parenteral nutrition may be necessary to maintain adequate nutrition when complications prevent or restrict the use of the GI tract.[22]

Renal Dysfunction

The kidneys maintain fluid and electrolyte balance through glomerular filtration of plasma and tubular reabsorption and secretion of water and metabolites. The entire plasma volume passes through the kidneys about 60 times daily, producing between 1 and 2 liters of urine/day. The normal kidney regulates fluid, sodium, potassium, calcium, and acid-base balance. Renal dysfunction may occur because of decreased blood flow to the kidney or actual damage to the functional parts of the organ.

Acute renal failure (ARF), a sudden cessation of renal function, may occur following surgery, trauma, or burns, and can be caused by hypotension, shock, and/or sepsis. ARF may also be related to adverse reactions to medications; it may resolve itself or necessitate renal dialysis.

Chronic renal failure (CRF), resulting from a gradual, progressive loss of renal function, is related to specific diseases of the kidneys such as chronic glomerulonephritis, pyelonephritis, and polycystic disease. CRF results in constant fluid, electrolyte, and protein imbalance. Routine renal dialysis is usually needed in later stages of CRF. Malnutrition is common in patients with advanced renal failure or those on long-term dialysis. Once dialysis is begun, protein needs increase because of amino acid losses during dialysis.[34]

The goal of nutritional therapy in early renal failure is to improve nutritional status, enhance wound healing and resistance to infection, and preserve remaining renal function. Nutritional intervention for all renal patients focuses on reducing catabolism, maintaining fluid and metabolic balance, and promoting weight gain with an increased sense of well-being.[29] This is accomplished through parenteral or, whenever possible, enteral nutrition.

Cardiovascular Dysfunction

Cardiac dysfunction can impair the perfusion of tissue involved in the digestive process. Valvular heart disease and coronary artery disease, the two major types of heart disease, affect patients differently in terms of nutritional status.

Valvular disease leads to pulmonary blood engorgement, edema, and progressive congestive heart failure. Patients experience fatigue and shortness of breath associated with diminished cardiac reserves. Patient weight may increase because of fluid retention, but other signs of a malnourished state may also be evident. Cardiac cachexia occurs frequently with long-term congestive heart failure, most commonly in patients with chronic valvular disease. Starvation results in the wasting of cardiac muscle, thus depressing cardiac function.[29] The causes of cardiac cachexia are multifactorial but may be related to anorexia, malabsorption, hypermetabolism, and impaired delivery of nutrients and oxygen at the cellular level.

Nutrition support is usually indicated for malnourished patients with valvular disease when surgery is indicated. The route of administration may be enteral or parenteral, and TPN should be continued postoperatively until adequate oral nutrition is possible. The TPN formula for the cardiac patient contains a limited sodium content, and the total fluid volume can be reduced by using a higher dextrose concentration.

Coronary artery disease progresses silently until myocardial damage occurs from decreased cardiac tissue perfusion. Nutritional intervention is usually related to sodium and sometimes fluid restriction, potassium repletion, fat modification, and weight reduction. Severe congestive failure following extensive myocardial damage may result in cardiac cachexia. Parenteral intervention is considered in the event of heart transplantation.

Respiratory Dysfunction

Diseases of the respiratory system interfere with oxygenation of blood and carbon dioxide elimination. Acute episodes in patients with adult respiratory disease syndrome, chronic obstructive pulmonary disease, and pneumonia may require intubation and mechanical ventilation. Ventilator-dependent patients who are malnourished are at higher risk for infection, pulmonary edema, hypophosphatemia, decreased ventilatory drive, respiratory weakness, and atelectasis.[35] Ventilator-dependent patients may be supported nutritionally either by the enteral or parenteral route. Formulas may need to be modified to prevent increased carbon dioxide production caused by high carbohydrate intake. Fat emulsions can be used to increase caloric density without increasing dextrose concentration. Provision of protein in excess of actual needs can stimulate the ventilatory drive and complicate weaning attempts. Providing adequate but not excessive amounts of nutrients increases the success of weaning attempts in these patients.

Cancer

Cancer-associated malnutrition is manifested by weight loss, cachexia, depressed serum protein levels, and impaired immune function. The cause of the cachexia may be related to many factors, including the following: (1) inadequate intake resulting from anorexia or tumor obstruction; (2) side effects of chemotherapy or radiotherapy; (3) catabolic effects of tumors; and (4) abnormal nutrient metabolism.

A meta-analysis of clinical trials of nutritional support in cancer has concluded that generally there is no increase in favorable clinical outcome and an increase in potentially harmful side effects in oncology patients receiving TPN.[36] An exception appears in bone marrow transplant patients in whom early intervention has shown improved response and survival. Other exceptions include patients who have the following conditions: (1) long-term inability for oral intake; (2) cachexia caused by inadequate nutrient intake; (3) ade-

quate clinical supervision to decrease complications; and (4) presence of a tumor expected to respond to chemotherapy or radiotherapy. Enteral intervention may be beneficial by improving the oncology patient's sense of well-being.

Acquired Immunodeficiency Syndrome (AIDS)

Gastrointestinal dysfunction is common in the patient with AIDS and AIDS-related complex (ARC). Gastrointestinal pathology is well documented and can be related to specific causative agents in many of those with gastrointestinal symptoms. These symptoms range from minor to severe weight loss and diarrhea, abdominal pain, malnutrition, and malabsorption.

The irreversible nature of the disease has discouraged the use of aggressive nutritional intervention aside from dietary counselling and the use of oral supplementation. Some institutions have used parenteral nutrition in patients according to the following criteria: (1) greater than 20% weight loss; (2) Cryptosporidium-induced enteropathy unresponsive to chemotherapy; (3) intolerance to enteral nutrition; and (4) partial or complete bowel obstruction.[37] The use of enteral alimentation appears to increase the patient's perception of quality of life, and may decrease the incidence of opportunisitc infections.

Hypercatabolic States

Hypercatabolic states result from trauma, burns, and sepsis. Patients with these conditions require aggressive nutritional support as soon as hemodynamic stability has been achieved. The nature and duration of the hypercatabolic state depend on the severity of injury or stress.

Metabolic changes that occur in the response to stress are neurohormonal and are mediated by the sympathetic nervous system. These changes support central anabolism, peripheral catabolism, and result in negative nitrogen balance.[38] General responses include increased metabolic and catabolic rate, changes in body temperature, increased hormonal secretion affecting carbohydrate, fat, and protein metabolism, hyperglycemia with decreased insulin levels, and fluid and electrolyte imbalance. The stress response has two phases: The initial or ''ebb'' phase, lasting 5 to 7 days, followed by the ''flow'' phase. Nutritional support during the ebb phase is generally contraindicated. Nutritional repletion in the flow phase is used initially to maintain nutritional status and then to promote repletion of muscle and visceral protein. Parenteral nutrition is indicated when the enteral route is nonfunctional or during the hypermetabolic phase prior to resolution of the stress response.

PARENTERAL NUTRITION SOLUTIONS

Conventional intravenous solutions are low in calories—that is, 1 liter of 5% dextrose provides 170 kcal and contains only small amounts of trace minerals or electrolytes. Parenteral nutrition solutions, on the other hand, are complex solutions that provide all the known essential nutrients in quantities that promote weight gain, wound healing, anabolism, and growth.

Components

Parenteral nutrition solutions contain essential nutrients, including protein, carbohydrate, fat, electrolytes, vitamins, trace minerals, and water. The proportions of these ingredients and the total calories provided must be carefully individualized to meet the patient's needs and clinical condition.

Essential Nutrients

PROTEIN

Protein, in the form of crystalline amino acid solutions for parenteral nutrition, is an essential component of every nutrition support regimen. The estimated protein requirement in an individual patient depends on the age, level of activity, nutritional status, renal function, hepatic function, and presence or absence of hypermetabolism. Aside from these quantitative differences, there may also be differences in the requirements for specific amino acids. Certain amino acids perform unique physiologic functions that may have a therapeutic or damaging effect on an individual patient. Thus, the optimal provision of amino acids during parenteral nutrition depends on both the total quantity provided as well as the specific amino acid composition.

Normal protein requirements depend on utilization and losses. Any condition that decreases normal utilization or increases nitrogen losses increases dietary protein requirements. The recommended dietary allowance (RDA) for protein is based on the amount of protein needed to maintain nitrogen equilibrium and the fact that energy needs are met by nonprotein sources. A protein intake of 0.8 g/kg body weight/day is recommended for healthy adults; 2.5 to 3.0 g/kg body weight/day parenterally is recommended for neonates and infants.[39] Infant protein requirements gradually decrease to 1.5 to 2.0 g/kg body weight/day by 12 months. This decline continues until the growth cycle is complete. An adolescent requires approximately 1.0 to 1.5 g/kg body weight/day.[40]

Illness can dramatically influence the body's protein needs. During periods of stress or injury, patients may require as much as 2.0 to 3.5 g/kg body weight/day.[41] Burn patients may require up to 2.5 g/kg body weight/day, and an infected adult may require 1.5 to 2 g/kg body weight/day to achieve a positive nitrogen balance.[42]

Currently available amino acid solutions differ in composition. Based on the specific amino acid profile, standard or specialized solutions are available. Standard amino acid solutions are a balanced profile of essential, semiessential, and nonessential amino acids. Specialized amino acid solutions have a modified amino acid profile to meet age- or disease-specific amino acid requirements. Amino acids also differ in their nitrogen content per gram, electrolyte composition, osmolarity, pH, and available concentration. The most important of these is the electrolyte composition, because electrolytes are also essential components of nutrition and require specific dosage. Amino acid solutions with preadded electro-

lytes usually contain amounts of the most common electrolytes needed to meet an adult's requirements. Therefore, consideration must be given to using amino acids containing only acetate and/or chloride salt forms, especially in patients who have increased or decreased electrolyte requirements, because this allows for individualized electrolyte dosages. Specialized amino acid preparations have been developed for use in specific disorders such as renal and hepatic failure.[1] Disease-specific amino acids are discussed later in this chapter.

An interaction exists between calorie and nitrogen substrates. Increasing the caloric support requires less nitrogen to achieve nitrogen balance, and increasing the nitrogen intake reduces the calories required to achieve nitrogen balance. The optimal calorie-nitrogen ratio in the patient requiring nutritional support remains individualized. The currently used calorie-nitrogen ratio ranges from 100:1 to 200:1. It is logical that patients under severe stress are likely to have a different optimal ratio than the chronically malnourished and those with malignant processes.[15]

CARBOHYDRATES

To ensure that the protein content of parenteral nutrition solutions is used for tissue synthesis rather than a source of energy, nonprotein calories must be administered. Carbohydrates are the body's preferred fuel, as well as its immediate source of energy. One carbohydrate molecule yields 4 kcal of energy/g carbohydrate. The body burns carbohydrates rather than fats or protein, provided the carbohydrate intake is adequate, sufficient insulin is available to allow passage of glucose into the cells, and glycogen is present.

There are no specific minimum requirements for carbohydrates during parenteral nutrition, but it functions as a key component of most parenteral nutrition regimens. The predominant source of nonprotein calories in parenteral solutions is the carbohydrate, dextrose. Dextrose is used almost exclusively in parenteral nutrition solutions as the source of carbohydrate calories. Other sources of parenteral carbohydrate and carbohydrate-like substances, such as fructose, galactose, glycerol, invert sugar, maltose, sorbitol, and xylitol, have also been used. However, with the exception of glycerol, most of these substances are no longer in use because of a high potential for adverse effects.[43]

Dextrose has a low caloric density, providing 3.4 kcal/g, and is available in concentrations ranging from 5 to 70%. Higher concentrations of dextrose are usually used in parenteral nutrition solutions to minimize the volume of dextrose in the overall admixture, thus allowing greater volume for the amino acids, electrolytes, and the micronutrients. Dextrose solutions with concentrations exceeding 5% are increasingly hypertonic. The normal serum osmolarity is approximately 310 mOsm/liter. Parenteral solutions with an osmolarity of up to 900 mOsm/liter may be administered peripherally. However, tolerance of solutions with 900 mOsm/liter or less is highly variable with patient and vein condition. In general, parenteral solutions with a final dextrose concentration greater than 10%, or more than 900 mOsm/liter, should be administered through a central vein.[44]

The optimum dose of dextrose differs for infants, children, and adults. In general, for balanced parenteral nutrition, dextrose is used to provide 40 to 60% of the total caloric intake.

In adults, the optimum dose for maximal suppression of gluconeogenesis and glucose oxidation is 2 to 5 mg/kg/min.[44] This represents a parenteral nutrition regimen that contains 150 to 200 g of dextrose/liter administered centrally at a rate of 1.5 to 2.5 liters/day. Overfeeding by supplying glucose in excess of this rate does not further accentuate nitrogen retention and produces adverse effects such as fatty liver and increased carbon dioxide production, which may aggravate pre-existing respiratory distress. Because of the higher resting energy expenditure and greater energy demands of growth and development in infants and children, their overall energy requirements are greater than those of adults.[45, 46]

Glycerol, a sugar alcohol, is available as an intravenous carbohydrate-like solution used in parenteral nutrition. Glycerol is commercially available as a premixed solution, ProcalAmine, which is ready for infusion after the addition of vitamins and trace minerals. ProcalAmine contains 3% amino acids and 3% glycerol premixed in 1-liter bottles. It has a caloric density of 250 kcal/liter and a solution osmolarity of 735 mOsm/liter, and can therefore be administered by the peripheral route. Because it is a partial nutritional solution, the use of ProcalAmine is limited to patients whose nutritional requirements can be met by the nutrients and electrolytes present.[44]

FATS

Fat, in the form of lipid emulsions, serves two purposes in parenteral nutrition. It is a source of calories and also a source of essential fatty acids to prevent essential fatty acid deficiency. Fat is the most calorically dense substrate available, with more than twice the caloric density of carbohydrate and protein, and provides approximately 9 kcal/g. The currently available fat emulsions provide varying amounts of linoleic and linolenic acids sufficient to prevent or treat essential fatty acid deficiency.

There is no recommended dietary allowance for fat as a nutrient in the diet. In parenteral nutrition, lipid emulsions should be provided in quantities sufficient to prevent essential fatty acid deficiency. Essential fatty acid deficiency can occur in as little as 5 days without fat supplementation. The minimum human requirement needed to prevent essential fatty acid deficiency should represent 2 to 4% of the total caloric intake, or at least 2.4 g linoleic acid/2000 kcal of nutrient intake. Fats are also a source of calories for meeting energy requirements to optimize protein utilization and, when needed, to decrease the carbohydrate load. The optimum dose of lipid for the provision of calories is not known. However, the maximum safe dose is no more than 60% (most patients receive 10 to 40%) of the daily caloric intake, 2.5 g/kg for adults, or 4 g/kg for pediatric patients.[44, 46]

Parenteral lipid emulsions first became commercially available in the United States in 1976. These products are emulsions of soybean oil or a combination of soybean and safflower oils. The other components of these fat emulsions include egg phosphatides, which act as an emulsifier, and glycerol, which adjusts the osmolarity to make the emulsion iso-osmolar. Lipid emulsions are available in two concentrations, 10 and 20%. The total caloric content of 10% lipid emulsion is 1.1 kcal/ml and, for the 20% lipid emulsion, it is 2.0 kcal/ml.

Adverse reactions to intravenous fat emulsions have been reported in a variety of clinical settings, particularly when the cottonseed oil emulsions were still commercially available. These reactions include syndrome of platelet dysfunction, hemolysis, and even death. Since soybean and safflower oil emulsions became available, these adverse reactions have not been reported, although acute reactions such as allergic reactions (including fever, chills, vomiting, and chest or back pain) have been reported. These reactions are associated with a pre-existing allergic reaction to the source of lipid or to the egg used as an emulsifier.

Fat emulsions must be administered with caution to patients with liver disease, compromised pulmonary function, coagulation disorders, or pancreatitis. In infants with elevated bilirubin levels, the administration of lipids may cause increased kernicterus. The serum triglyceride concentration must be measured and monitored and the lipid intake may be adjusted accordingly.

ELECTROLYTES

Electrolytes play a critical role in almost all the body's physiologic functions. Therefore, electrolytes are included in the administration of parenteral nutrition to meet daily requirements and to prevent or correct pre-existing deficits. Electrolytes commonly added to parenteral nutrition formulas include sodium, potassium, calcium, chloride, and phosphorus. Although general guidelines for electrolyte requirements during parenteral nutrition exist for both adults and pediatric patients, meeting individual needs is required to maintain electrolyte balance. An initial assessment of the electrolyte status may indicate whether a patient has an altered electrolyte requirement. Patients with pre-existing conditions, such as long-term diuretic use or patients who have ongoing losses of electrolytes such as with fistulas or diarrhea, can be anticipated to have increased electrolyte requirements. Restricted electrolyte intake may be necessary in patients with severe renal dysfunction, edema, or congestive heart failure.

Electrolytes in parenteral solutions may be added as a single electrolyte product or as a mixture of electrolytes that are commercially available in concentrations designed to meet the standard adult electrolyte requirement. As discussed earlier, several amino acid products contain pre-added electrolytes in amounts close to the adult requirement if 2 liters/day are given. The use of these products in parenteral nutrition is usually limited to stable adult patients whose electrolyte balance can be achieved by the contents of these products. The patient's acid-base status assists in the choice of using a chloride or acetate salt when admixing electrolytes in parenteral solutions.

VITAMINS

Vitamins play an essential role in metabolism and cellular function, and therefore a multiple vitamin preparation is added to each day's parenteral nutrition solution. Pediatric and adult vitamin mixtures that contain both fat-soluble and water-soluble vitamins are available. Most commercially available vitamin products now contain folic acid and vitamin B_{12}. However, adult vitamin formulations do not contain vitamin K, and it must be supplemented weekly either intravenously or intramuscularly. Parenteral vitamin requirements, in general, are significantly lower than dietary vitamin requirements because the parenteral route bypasses digestive and absorptive functions of the gastrointestinal tract. Guidelines for parenteral vitamin intake in adults have been established by the Nutrition Advisory Group of the Department of Foods and Nutrition, American Medical Association.[47] Specific disease states and certain drugs may alter vitamin requirements but may easily be supplemented in the parenteral solutions. Caution must be taken when administering additional fat-soluble vitamins, because overadministration can lead to toxicity.

TRACE ELEMENTS

The efficient use of substrates for energy production and protein synthesis depends on the availability of trace elements for the numerous facilitative functions they perform. To ensure adequate amounts, trace elements are added at the start of parenteral nutrition. The trace elements routinely added to parenteral nutrition solutions are zinc, copper, chromium, and manganese. Assessing trace mineral requirements on an individual patient basis is particularly important in patients who are malnourished and who may have pre-existing specific micronutrient deficiencies, and in neonates who have limited body stores of trace minerals and whose needs are critical for growth. Monitoring of trace element status is based on regular clinical assessment for the presence of the signs and symptoms of deficiency.

Trace elements are inefficiently absorbed through the GI tract from dietary sources, so there are substantial differences between amounts when nutrition is delivered enterally rather than parenterally. The AMA Nutrition Advisory Group has made recommendations for the intravenous administration of chromium, copper, manganese, and zinc.[48] The Subcommittee on Pediatric Parenteral Nutrient Requirements from the Committee on Clinical Practice Issues of the American Society of Clinical Nutrition has also published guidelines for trace element intake in infants and children. There are no formal recommendations for selenium and molybdenum for adults, but clinical practice has suggested inclusion of these trace elements during the parenteral nutrition of select patient groups, including long-term TPN patients and those with pre-existing deficiencies. Recommendations for iron and iodine for adult patients have been made by individual practitioners. Parenteral iron, available as iron dextran, may be administered intravenously, which is the preferred route, or intramuscularly for iron deficiency.

Several products are available to meet guidelines for the daily intake of chromium, copper, manganese, and zinc. Specific products exist for adults, children, and neonates. These products are available as single-component trace elements or as multiple trace element products that also contain selenium, molybdenum, and/or iodine.

WATER

Basic fluid requirements are determined using the formula for hydration therapy, which is 1500 ml/m², and then adjusting for additional losses. For a patient on parenteral nutrition, the range of fluid requirements varies from approximately 35 ml/kg body weight/day for adults, to as much as 150 ml/kg body weight/day for infants, depending on clinical circumstances.

During starvation, injury, and hypermetabolic disease states such as sepsis and burns, fluid requirements may be increased. The standard formula for a catabolic state assumes or estimates a release of about 200 to 300 ml water/day from the intracellular space and oxidation of fat. To ensure adequate fluid replacement or supplementation, calculations must also include measured fluid losses estimated for insensible and third space fluid loss, and an additional 300 to 400 ml of fluid to provide for anabolism.[15] Care must be taken to make appropriate adjustments for patients with congestive heart failure or renal failure, those with excessive fluid and pulmonary edema, and those receiving humidified air.

Other Additives

The compatibility of drugs in parenteral nutrition solutions is often in question and is difficult to answer because of many factors such as the solubility, stability, and pharmacokinetics of drugs. However, a number of drugs have been added to parenteral nutrition solutions without any apparent incompatibility reactions.

INSULIN

Patients with limited capability for producing insulin may require exogenous insulin when dextrose is administered. Hypoglycemia or hyperglycemia frequently result when dextrose infusion is altered. The addition of insulin to the parenteral nutrition solution instead of the traditional subcutaneous administration has been more effective in controlling or preventing hypoglycemia or hyperglycemia, because the insulin dose is changed whenever the rate of infusion is adjusted.[22] Blood sugar levels under 200 mg/dL can be achieved in most patients. If the blood sugar concentration cannot be controlled by exogenous insulin, the amount of dextrose may need to be reduced and additional calories provided from fats.

HEPARIN

Heparin in low doses (1000 to 3000 units/liter) is sometimes added to parenteral nutrition solutions to decrease the potential formation of a fibrin sleeve, which may lead to venous thrombosis. Concerns related to the possibility of heparin-induced thrombocytopenia have decreased this practice.[22] Another pharmacologic effect of heparin is improving the clearance of IV fat emulsion from the bloodstream through the activation of the lipoprotein lipase system.[11]

HISTAMINE 2 RECEPTOR ANTAGONISTS

Histamine 2 (H_2) receptor antagonists inhibit gastric acid secretion and are used during parenteral nutrition to prevent stress ulceration. They are effective in counteracting metabolic alkalosis secondary to nasogastric suctioning and when high acetate content crystalline amino acid solutions are used.[22]

ALBUMIN

Patients receiving parenteral nutrition may require albumin so that the amino acids administered are preferentially used for tissue protein synthesis rather than for albumin synthesis and/or normalizing plasma oncotic pressure. Albumin appears to be physically compatible in parenteral nutrition solutions for 24 hours. Albumin in parenteral nutrition solutions must be carefully monitored and evaluated because of its high cost.

Drug Compatibility Considerations

The complex composition of parenteral nutrition solutions renders them highly susceptible to compatibility and stability problems. The addition of drugs to parenteral nutrition admixtures poses an increased risk of physicochemical incompatibility. Consequently, the clinician should be cautious when considering the addition of any drug in a concentration that varies from published guidelines. The pharmacist must consider the physical and chemical properties of all components of parenteral admixtures and ensure that adequate documentation exists to support the inclusion of various additives, particularly drugs.

In general, only drugs with stable dosage regimens supported by published guidelines and having appropriate therapeutic efficacy when given as a continuous infusion should be considered for inclusion in a parenteral nutrition admixture. Medications frequently added to parenteral nutrition solutions include the following: albumin, aminophylline (stable dose regimen), heparin, hydrochloric acid (in lipid-free TPN), and regular insulin.[49] Most antibiotics are not administered continuously and therefore are not suitable for addition to parenteral nutrition solutions.[50] Although this is a controversial issue, intermittent therapy may be preferred, particularly when high serum concentrations are desirable. In addition, drug therapies in which the dosage fluctuates in relation to the patient's clinical status, such as vasopressor agents, are not practical additions. Such inclusions may reduce drug efficacy, lead to administration errors, or generate significant waste of the parenteral nutrition solution.

The use of parenteral solutions as a vehicle for drug delivery has some advantages, such as consolidation of dosage units and improved pharmacotherapy for certain drugs. It also allows for the conservation of fluids in volume-restricted patients, eliminates multiple entries for drug administration into the vascular access device, and provides the economic benefits of reduced time and material savings to both pharmacy and nursing.[49]

Standard Solutions

Peripheral Parenteral Nutrition

PPN is used most effectively for weight maintenance of nonhypermetabolic patients, as a preliminary mode before central infusion, and as a supplement to enteral feedings. It is associated with fewer hazards and complications related to central venous access. The limitations of peripheral parenteral nutrition are the high tonicity and volume of infusate required to meet caloric demands. Prolonged infusions into small peripheral veins are possible using solutions that are lower than 900 mOsm/liter; consequently, a PPN solution provides fewer calories and less protein per volume. The

availability of fat emulsions has made PPN an attractive means for providing parenteral nutrition. The isotonic, high-calorie lipid emulsions help meet the nutritional needs of many patients by the use of PPN alone. Unfortunately, PPN is usually more difficult to maintain because of frequent episodes of phlebitis in superficial veins and the infiltration of solutions into subcutaneous tissue.

A typical standard solution may contain 50 g dextrose with 35 g amino acids/liter. Final concentrations typically range from 1.75 to 3.5% amino acids and from 5 to 10% dextrose, along with 500 ml of 10 or 20% lipids, electrolytes, trace elements, and vitamins. No greater than a 10% final concentration of dextrose should be infused peripherally.[6]

Total Parenteral Nutrition

TPN formulations vary somewhat, depending on the patient's condition and the institution's preference. An example of a standard formulation is 42.5 g amino acids and 250 g dextrose/liter (500 ml of an 8.5% amino acid solution and 500 ml of 50% dextrose).[49] TPN provides 2000 to 3000 kcal and all other essential nutrients to patients needing 2 to 3 liters of intravenous fluid daily. A standard TPN formula creates a nonprotein calorie to nitrogen ratio of 150:1. Intravenous lipid is usually provided separately twice weekly to prevent essential fatty acid deficiency.

TOTAL NUTRIENT ADMIXTURE

Total nutrient admixture (TNA), trisubstrate system, all-in-one system, and 3-in-1 system are all terms used to describe the combination of dextrose, amino acids, fat emulsion, electrolytes, trace elements, and multivitamins in one container. The addition of the fat emulsion is the unique part of this type of admixture. The components are mixed in one bag with a volume up to 3 liters, and provide a total nutrient supply for a 24-hour period.

There are many advantages associated with the use of TNAs. They may be clinically useful in patients with diabetes or patients with compromised respiratory function by decreasing the amount of calories provided from glucose. The use of a TNA might reduce the risk of microbial contamination because of fewer manipulations of the solution container and tubing. Additionally, there are economic advantages associated with time and material savings for both nursing and pharmacy. TNA systems simplify the administration of parenteral nutrition for the home TPN patient.[51]

A number of considerations are associated with the use of TNAs. Because fat droplets have a mean particle size of 0.4 to 0.5 μ, they clog the standard 0.22-μ filter. However, TNA solutions can be administered through a 1.2-μ particulate filter. The extended use of lipid emulsions imposes limits on the quantity of lipid infused daily secondary to the potential for the development of cholestasis. There is also the potential for fat emulsions that contain long-chain triglycerides to depress the immune system, although further study regarding this phenomenon appears to be warranted.[52] Also, there is a potential for increased waste if this system is used in patients who are clinically unstable, with changing metabolic needs. Catheter occlusion resulting from fat deposits has been reported with long-term use of this therapy. Last, limited data exist on the compatibility and stability of this system with various products and concentrations.

The stability of various amino acid, lipid solutions, and electrolyte and mineral additives is variable and must be considered when preparing a TNA. The most fragile component of a TNA system is the fat emulsion. The destabilization of fat emulsions in the presence of a low pH value or high electrolyte concentration affects the methods used to prepare the TNA.[52] All TNAs need to be visually inspected prior to administration for evidence of deterioration or breaking of the emulsion. When this occurs, there is a change in droplet size and dispersion of the emulsion, and the infusion of undispersed fat aggregates may be toxic. Emulsion stability is influenced by several factors such as pH, electrolyte charge, temperature, and time. The pH and compounding sequence must be taken into consideration by the pharmacist when admixing this system. As with all intravenous admixtures, TNA solutions must be mixed in an aseptic environment, because fat emulsions are an excellent microbial growth medium and should not hang or be at room temperature for longer than 24 hours. Under refrigeration, the physical stability is up to 14 days.

FORMULATIONS FOR INFANTS AND YOUNG CHILDREN

Amino acids such as histidine, tyrosine, cysteine, and taurine, which are nonessential in adults, may be essential for infants and young children. There are special amino acid formulations available to meet these needs.

Disease-Specific Solutions

A number of disease-specific formulas, both parenteral and enteral, have been marketed for patients with renal or hepatic disease, respiratory failure, and stress. These products are briefly discussed here.

Renal Failure

Amino acid formulas high in essential amino acids (EAAs) are formulated with specific indications for patients with renal failure. The essential amino acids are converted to nonessential amino acids in vivo as needed and minimize ureagenesis. The significant clinical advantage of highly essential amino acid products over standard formulations containing both nonessential and essential amino acids in renal failure patients remains controversial. It is believed that nonessential amino acids may be needed to optimize protein synthesis and achieve positive nitrogen balance.[53] Also, during the dialysis process, both essential and nonessential amino acids are removed, and therefore standard amino acid solutions containing both essential and nonessential amino acids are recommended to meet the protein requirements of dialyzed patients.

Hepatic Failure

Patients with hepatic failure have abnormal plasma amino acid profiles characterized by high levels of aromatic amino acids and low levels of branched chain amino acids, which

was theorized as contributing to "false neurotransmitter" synthesis and the development of encephalopathy. Hepatic failure formulas contain little or no aromatic acids and high concentrations of branched chain amino acids. These formulas were developed in an attempt to minimize hepatic encephalopathy in patients with liver failure. However, despite initial promising results using these modified amino acid solutions for hepatic encephalopathy, it has not been clearly demonstrated that the use of a modified amino acid solution is more helpful than the use of standard amino acid infusions in the management of hepatic encephalopathy.[54] As a result, these solutions cannot be routinely recommended.

Stress Formula

Patients become hypercatabolic secondary to the metabolic state created by trauma, sepsis, and burns. Altered protein metabolism is a hallmark of the stressed patient. Protein catabolism with resultant increased nitrogen excretion and altered plasma amino acid concentrations has been observed in both adults and children with sepsis, trauma, and major burn injury. The management of altered protein metabolism in the stressed patient requires both quantitative and qualitative modifications in nutrition support. To offset the increased rate of nitrogen excretion, the protein intake should be increased. Modified amino acid solutions are available and differ from standard amino acid solutions by having an increased content of branched chain amino acids in an otherwise balanced amino acid solution.

Respiratory Insufficiency

The parenteral nutrition formula for a critically ill patient affects the respiratory quotient (RQ) because of the large carbohydrate load. The use of fat emulsions can play an important role as an additional calorie source to reduce the carbohydrate load. The production of CO_2 increases as the amount of infused glucose increases. In a patient with normal ventilatory function, the effect of the infusion on the respiratory quotient (RQ) is not a major consideration when selecting substrates for nutritional support; however, in the patient with compromised ventilation, increasing CO_2 production may precipitate respiratory failure or may delay or prevent weaning from a ventilator. Thus, in patients with respiratory insufficiency, maintenance caloric requirements must be defined more precisely. When a patient is being weaned from a ventilator, the caloric intake is stabilized at maintenance levels. If weaning is hindered by CO_2 retention, the carbohydrate load is reduced to provide about 60 to 70% of the maintenance caloric requirements as glucose and 30 to 40% of requirements as fat emulsion.[55]

ADMINISTRATION OF PARENTERAL NUTRITION

Parenteral nutrition solutions should be compounded in a pharmacy using a laminar flow hood to ensure sterility. The solutions should be used immediately after preparation or refrigerated and removed from 30 to 60 minutes prior to administration. To reduce the risk of bacterial contamination, parenteral nutrition solutions must be infused or discarded within 24 hours after hanging.

Solution Regimens

TPN and PPN Solutions

Initiation. The catheter tip location must be confirmed prior to initiating TPN. Prior to initiating PPN, careful assessment of the peripheral site must be done. Solution labels should always be compared to the physician's order prior to administration. The solution and container should be checked for leaks, cracks, clarity, expiration date and, with TNA solutions, for pink discoloration or separation of oils.

TPN solutions are usually initiated gradually and increased as the patient's fluid and glucose tolerance allows. Changes in rate should be gradual because fluctuations in glucose levels can occur if the infusion is interrupted or irregular in rate. Initial glucose infusions should not exceed 250 g over 24 hours to allow for adequate endogenous insulin secretion. Solution administration may then be advanced to the required nutritional level, increasing by 1000 kcal/day. To avoid potential complications, TPN must be administered at a constant rate and not discontinued abruptly. PPN does not require gradual rate introductions and may be initiated at the desired rate. To maintain a consistent and accurate flow rate, an electronic infusion device should be used.[6]

Discontinuation. PPN solutions can usually be discontinued safely without a tapering regimen. The discontinuation of TPN solutions requires a logical approach. There are several techniques:[20]

1. Transition feeding—initiate oral or enteral feeding while tapering parenteral nutrition concomitantly.
2. Replacement with a peripheral IV—used when a central catheter must be removed suddenly. Dextrose 5 or 10% may be initiated at the same rate of infusion.
3. Tapering technique—tapering the rate over a 2- to 3-day period may be required to reduce the incidence of rebound hypoglycemia if the patient is receiving over 1000 kcal/day. The diagnosis, patient's condition, and length of therapy must be considered to evaluate whether tapering is required for discontinuation. The patient may have complicating conditions that predispose to hypoglycemia following the rapid tapering of TPN, such as concurrent insulin administration or existing renal or hepatic disease. In the unstressed patient, rapid tapering can be accomplished by reducing the rate by 50% over 2 to 4 hours before discontinuing.[56]

Cyclic Regimens. Cyclic administration regimens involve the infusion of TPN on a cyclic basis over 8 to 16 hours rather than the standard continuous infusion over a 24-hour period. Indications and benefits of cyclic infusions are presented in Table 12–5. TPN can be transitioned to cyclic administration once tolerance to 24-hour continuous infusion has been obtained. The switch to cyclic infusion is accomplished by a gradual reduction in the hours of infusion, usually 1 to 2 hours/day. The hourly rate is determined by dividing the total required volume of TPN by the number of hours the TPN is to be infused. Cyclic TPN is usually admin-

Table 12–5
Cyclic Parenteral Nutrition: Benefits and Indications

Benefits
1. Improved quality of life through resumption of normal daily activities; allows the patient freedom from pumps during daytime hours, increased psychologic well-being
2. Allows for increased mobility, which maintains somatic muscle
3. Allows for more physiologic hormonal responses and stimulation of appetite
4. Prevention or treatment of hepatotoxicities induced by continuous TPN; reversal of fatty liver and enzyme level elevations and faster albumin level recovery
5. Prevention or treatment of essential fatty acid deficiency in patients on fat-free TPN; reduced insulin levels during TPN-free periods allows for lipolysis and release of essential linoleic acid

Indications
1. Patients who have been stable on continuous TPN and require long-term parenteral nutrition
2. Patients who are on home TPN
3. Patients who can handle the total infusion volume in a shortened time period
4. Patients who require TPN for only a portion of their nutritional needs
5. Patients who have hepatic steatosis or for prevention of hepatic steatosis

istered at a rate no higher than 200 ml/hour. The ability to tolerate the glucose and fluid volume determines how rapidly the solution can be infused. With the average patient receiving 2 to 3 liters, this usually requires a period of 12 to 16 hours to complete. Patients receiving 2 liters of fluid may tolerate 8-hour infusions. Cyclic infusions are generally infused at night and turned off during daytime hours.[57]

Fat Emulsions

Prior to the administration of fat emulsions, the solution should be inspected for frothiness, separation, or oily appearance. The low osmolarity of fat emulsions permits delivery by peripheral veins. Fat emulsions may be administered through a separate site, or given through a lower Y connector in the existing TPN administration set. Fat emulsions should not be filtered unless infused as part of a TNA, in which case a 1.2-μ filter may be used.

Delivery time for a single container of fat emulsion varies depending on the patient's condition, from 4 to 12 hours, but solutions may hang for up to 24 hours. An initial dose of a fat emulsion should be given slowly to test for possible allergic reactions. To administer a test dose for an adult, a 10% fat emulsion should be infused at a rate of 1 ml/min for the first 15 to 30 minutes, and a 20% fat emulsion should be infused at a rate of 0.5 ml/min for the first 15 to 30 minutes. Symptoms of adverse reactions include nausea, fever, chills, muscle aches, pain in the chest or back, and urticaria.[1] Fat emulsions should be given with caution to patients with hyperlipidemia. A baseline fasting triglyceride level may be obtained and monitored weekly; the weekly serum sample should be drawn 8 hours after infusion.[55]

Vascular Access

Guidelines for vascular access and catheter care are basically the same for parenteral nutrition as for any other infusion. However, it is generally recommended that access devices be dedicated solely to the use of parenteral nutrition to decrease potential contamination. As discussed earlier, peripheral venous access for parenteral nutrition should be limited to lower osmolar solutions and those of shorter duration. Veins large enough to provide adequate dilution should be selected. Central venous access, used for hyperosmolar fluids, generally involves insertion into one of the major veins of the upper neck or chest, with the tip located in the superior vena cava. Tunneled catheters and totally implanted venous ports are generally used for long-term parenteral support, but nontunneled catheters may also be used in certain circumstances.

Perhaps the most critical aspect of the nursing management of TPN patients involves the care of the central venous catheter (CVC) prior to, during, and after insertion. Numerous studies have shown that adherence to strict protocols regarding insertion and care of the CVC reduces complications.[1] The type and frequency of catheter site monitoring is determined by the prescribed therapy, patient condition, age, and practice setting. Observation of catheter access site should be documented every 8 hours in the hospital setting. Peripheral catheter sites should be rotated every 48 hours and immediately for suspected contamination or complication.[6] With CVCs, occlusive gauze or tape dressings should be changed every 48 hours in conjunction with administration set changes or when the integrity of the dressing is compromised.[6] Transparent dressings may also be used and should be changed at established intervals. Strict aseptic technique should be maintained. Consideration should be given to the use of sterile gloves and a mask when changing the dressing.[6]

Equipment

All administration sets used for the delivery of parenteral solutions should be changed immediately using aseptic technique for suspected contamination or when the integrity of the product has been compromised. Peripheral administration sets used for PPN are changed every 48 hours and sets used for TPN are changed every 24 hours.[6] More frequent set changes are required because of the dextrose and protein content of TPN solutions, which provide a greater potential for bacterial growth and contamination. All parenteral nutrition solutions should be filtered with a 0.2-μ filter,[6] or a 1.2-μ filter with TNAs.

Nursing Assessment Parameters

Using the nursing process, the nursing care of the patient receiving nutritional support begins with assessment. Daily physical assessment and observation of the signs and symptoms of a catabolic state provide valuable information.

Signs and Symptoms of a Catabolic State

Increased temperature, pulse, and respirations
Decreased level of consciousness
Poor skin turgor
Lesions of skin and mucous membranes
Dehydration
Changes in bowel activity (number and character of stools)
Decreasing body weight
Tissue edema
Eczema

During the physical assessment, the nurse should focus particularly on the GI tract and, in addition, include the neurologic, cardiopulmonary, and renal systems. Assessment of the GI tract may be difficult if the patient's primary disease has involved this system. The identification of patients at risk for metabolic complications during parenteral nutrition is important and includes the very young, the elderly, those with glucose intolerance, renal dysfunction, neurologic damage or excessive fluid loss such as fistula output or secretions, and patients who are intubated or receiving steroids or diuretics.

The nurse assesses the patient's weight daily at the same time every morning using the same scale and with the same amount of clothing. Weighing is often an unpopular task, but the patient's weight provides a means of assessing whether calorie and fluid needs are being met or exceeded. If the patient continues to lose weight after several days of nutritional support, discussion with the other members of the health team such as the dietitian and pharmacist can be beneficial, particularly if the formula needs to be adjusted.

The nurse should also assess other parameters indicating fluid balance, such as intake and output, vital signs, peripheral or dependent edema, lung sounds, mucous membranes, skin turgor, and jugular vein distention. Nursing actions such as measuring intake and output and vital signs should not be considered routine. These important activities have a meaningful relationship to the metabolic monitoring of the patient receiving nutrition support.

Baseline laboratory values are obtained early in the patient's course of therapy. Daily determinations are necessary to guide the concentration and formulation of the parenteral nutrition solution until the patient is stable. The nurse collaborates with the physician to ensure that tests are ordered and evaluated on a regular basis to assess the objective status of nutrition and endocrine function. Laboratory tests measure total proteins, albumin, blood urea nitrogen, electrolytes, minerals, and vitamins. Additional laboratory tests include the serum magnesium level, CBC, prothrombin time, and liver function tests.

All patients on nutrition support have frequent assessments of blood glucose levels, because hyperglycemia can precipitate osmotic diuresis and hyperosmolar dehydration. Capillary blood sugar tests are often used to monitor glucose levels. Also, urine testing for the presence of glucose and ketones may be done, but the availability of capillary sugar tests has decreased its use. The accuracy of urine testing may be altered by drugs, the freshness of the testing materials and the urine, and/or the patient's renal function. Whenever possible, testing should be done with a double-voided urine specimen. An initial correlation of blood glucose and urine glucose levels may be needed to determine the patient's renal threshold for glucose. Patients with a high renal threshold may require sliding scale insulin coverage, based on frequent blood sampling.[3]

Although parenteral nutrition is viewed by medical personnel as a ''lifesaving'' procedure, often patients are unable to separate the procedure from the disease state as the cause of their hospitalization. The parenteral nutrition is a constant reminder of the disease and the limitation it imposes. These feelings can produce anger until the person resolves the conflict and regains some measure of autonomy. Thus, nurses should not be surprised if patients resent the very procedures that are keeping them alive. It is important to assess negative responses and assist the patient in identifying coping strengths. The information obtained in the assessment is used to assist the patient and family's coping mechanism and to assist the nurse in planning other aspects of care.

Patients receiving parenteral nutrition for long periods may need a great deal of emotional support. Food is normally associated with eating, and not eating can have a major psychologic effect on some people. Initially, patients may have hunger pains and food cravings, but physiologic requirements are being met. Eventually, appetites are suppressed by parenteral nutrition, and the patient needs to be assured that their appetite and bowel activity gradually return to normal when the parenteral feedings are discontinued.

► NURSING DIAGNOSIS

The database from these activities and the original assessment may be used to develop a nursing diagnosis for the patient receiving nutrition support. Individual patient circumstances require additional diagnoses to be formulated, with appropriate nursing interventions. The following is an example of a nursing care plan for a patient receiving parenteral nutrition.

Potential Nursing Diagnosis

The potential nursing diagnosis is alteration in nutrition, less than body requirements.

Goal

The goal is to stabilize weight and gradually increase to 10% of ideal.

Interventions

1. Collaborate with patient to establish a scale of weight outcomes from most desirable to least desirable.
2. Weigh patient daily and record until the desired weight is reached.
3. Administer parenteral nutrition solution as prescribed. Monitor and record intake and output.
4. Collaborate with nutrition support team to monitor and evaluate patient's nutritional status.

Expected Outcomes

1. Weight is stabilized (immediate outcome).
2. Weight gain of 1 lb every 3 weeks is achieved, increasing to 1 lb every 2 weeks (most desirable outcome).

Documentation remains an important nursing function. For a patient receiving nutrition support, the documentation of information regarding their status and response is critical to the success of parenteral nutrition therapy. Because nutrition support is a specialized area, it is best to use preprinted, standardized, nutrition support forms (Fig. 12–2). These forms serve an educational purpose by providing guidelines and limited options for the use of products, laboratory monitoring, and patient care. They can also promote cost-efficient nutrition support by minimizing errors in the ordering, prep-

aration, and administration of parenteral nutrition formulas. The forms may be used to record information pertinent to the patient's clinical progress, nutrition support regimen, fluid intake and output, and laboratory data, facilitating communication and thorough documentation.

Complications

Perhaps the most important complication of nutritional support is the failure to achieve the desired goals of therapy as a result of inadequate monitoring. The general goals of nutritional support are to support the lean body mass and, in turn, support the structure and function of individual organs to prevent specific nutrient deficiencies and, perhaps most important, to do no harm. The nurse plays an important role in the monitoring of patients receiving nutritional support therapy. Data collection, measuring vital signs, recording intake and output, knowledge of the parenteral nutrition prescription, and the ability to observe, interpret, and accurately report changes in the patient's condition and the associated physiologic responses are vital for the successful management and care of the patient receiving nutrition support.

The complications of parenteral nutrition may be divided into three areas—metabolic, technical, and septic. The causes, treatment, prevention, and monitoring of these types of complications are summarized in the following outline:

I. Metabolic
  A. Fluid and electrolyte imbalance
    1. Overhydration
      a. Cause: excessive fluid administration, particularly for renal insufficiency or immediately post-trauma.
      b. Treatment: reduce fluid administration, provide diuretics.
      c. Prevention: initiate parenteral nutrition only after fluid balance is stable, careful intake and output monitoring with calculation of fluid requirements and intake from other sources.
      d. Monitoring: intake and output, daily weights, BUN, hematocrit, and serum sodium level.
    2. Dehydration
      a. Cause: inadequate fluid administration, over-diuresis, excessive unreplaced fluid loss.
      b. Treatment: increase fluid administration.
      c. Prevention and monitoring: same as overhydration.
    3. Hyperkalemia
      a. Cause: renal insufficiency or excessive potassium administration.
      b. Treatment: Reduce potassium or potassium binders provided.
      c. Prevention: careful laboratory monitoring and calculation of potassium needs.
      d. Monitoring: serum potassium level.
    4. Hypokalemia
      a. Cause: inadequate amounts provided; increased losses from diarrhea, fistulas, and burns; increased needs related to anabolism.
      b. Treatment: adjust amount of supplement provided.

TOTAL PARENTERAL NUTRITION (TPN) ORDER FORM

Date _____   Time _____

ATTENTION DOCTORS: Please order electrolyte content in **mEq/24 hours.** Pharmacy will supply a 24 hour amount. Please fill out for any ingredient or rate changes. They will be initiated with the next bag unless otherwise indicated.

Protein Source:
Aminosyn 7% (35 grams/500 ml) _____ mls/24 hours
Aminosyn 10% (50 grams/500ml) _____ mls/24 hours

Carbohydrate Caloric Source:
Dextrose 50% (850 kcal/500ml) _____ mls/24 hours
Dextrose 70% (1190 kcal/500ml) _____ mls/24 hours

Total Volume: _____ mls/24 hours,   Rate: _____ mls/hour

Electrolyte Additions:
Sodium Chloride _____ mEq/24 hours
Potassium Chloride _____ mEq/24 hours
Potassium Phosphate _____ mEq/24 hours
Calcium Gluconate _____ mEq/24 hours
Magnesium Sulfate _____ mEq/24 hours

Multivitamin-12 (10 ml = 1 vial/24 hours) _____ mls/24 hours
Trace Elements (1 ml = 1 vial/24 hours) _____ ml/24 hours
Regular Insulin (Humulin-R, 100 units/ml) _____ Units/24 hours

Fat Emulsion 10 % (550 kcal/500 ml unit)®_____ Unit every _____ day(s)
Fat Emulsion 20% (1,000 kcal/500 ml unit)®_____ Unit every _____ day(s)
Normal Serum Albumin 25% (50ml and 100ml)*

® Each unit will be piggybacked below filter and infused over 4 to 8 hours.

* All albumin shall be infused separately below final filter over no more than 4 hours as recommended by CDC and FDA since it is a blood product.

Refer to I.V. Therapy P/P for standard nursing care of TPN patients (Pol. #10-A,B,C)
☐ Blood glucose fingerstick _____ times per day.
☐ Urine S & A every _____ hours. Report 2+ or over.
☐ Baseline lab if not obtained in last 48 hours including: CBC, Chem Profile-20, Serum Magnesium, Protime & Urinalysis.
☐ Daily lab tests: Blood Sugar, Electrolytes or
☐ Ongoing lab tests including: ☐ Chem. Profile-20 & Serum Magnesium 3x weekly,
        ☐ CBC twice weekly, ☐ Protime weekly.

TO/VO_____ M.D. / _____ R.N./Pharm.D
(Circle one)   (Circle one)

(Addressograph)

Roseville Hospital   333 Sunrise Ave
Roseville, CA
95661

FORM #7183

Figure 12–2. Standard total parenteral nutrition order form. (Courtesy of Roseville Hospital, Roseville, CA.)

c. Prevention and monitoring: same as hyperkalemia.

5. Hypernatremia
   a. Cause: excessive water loss.
   b. Treatment: reduce sodium in infusion and fluid replacement.
   c. Prevention: avoid excessive intake and careful fluid replacement.
   d. Monitoring: serum and urinary sodium levels, intake and output.

6. Hyponatremia
   a. Cause: depletion of fluid through sweating or excessive gastrointestinal losses, excessive diuretic therapy, dilutional states, including congestive heart failure (CHF) and syndrome of inappropriate antidiuretic hormone (SIADH).
   b. Treatment: adjust fluid and sodium intake as condition indicates.
   c. Prevention: provide sodium replacement unless contraindicated by cardiac, renal, or fluid status.
   d. Monitoring: same as hypernatremia.

B. Glucose metabolism
   1. Hyperglycemia
      a. Cause: rapid infusion of concentrated dextrose solution; high-risk conditions include diabetes, sepsis, and steroid medication.
      b. Treatment: provide insulin and/or part of non-protein calories, as lipid.
      c. Prevention: slow initial administration of dextrose, reduce dextrose provided, provide insulin as needed.
      d. Monitoring: frequent blood and urine determinations.
   2. Hypoglycemia
      a. Cause: rapid discontinuation of parenteral nutrition.
      b. Treatment: dextrose administration.
      c. Prevention: taper parenteral nutrition solution; if abrupt discontinuation occurs, hang 10% dextrose to prevent rebound hypoglycemia.
      d. Monitoring: frequent blood or urine glucose determinations, especially during discontinuation.

C. Mineral imbalance
   1. Hyperphosphatemia
      a. Cause: frequently seen in long-term parenteral nutrition with phosphorus-containing solutions; also seen in decreased renal excretion.
      b. Symptoms: paresthesia of the extremities, flaccid paralysis, listlessness, mental confusion, weakness, hypertension, cardiac arrhythmias, prolonged elevated phosphorus levels which may result in tissue calcification.
      c. Treatment: discontinue phosphorus; provide serum calcium repletion.
      d. Prevention: reduce phosphorus as indicated by serum levels.
      e. Monitoring: serum levels once or twice weekly.
   2. Hypophosphatemia

a. Cause: frequently seen in malnutrition; predisposing factors include alcohol abuse, diabetes mellitus, antacid ingestion, and increased phosphorus requirements of anabolism.
      b. Symptoms: may include respiratory distress.
      c. Treatment: administer intravenous phosphate or add phosphate to solution.
      d. Prevention: use phosphorus in parenteral nutrition, 13.6 mmol/day; has been shown to prevent phosphate depletion in most patients.
      e. Monitoring: serum level once or twice weekly, more frequently during replacement.

3. Hypermagnesemia
   a. Cause: excess magnesium administration; inability to excrete magnesium because of renal insufficiency.
   b. Symptoms: sharp drop in blood pressure and respiratory paralysis; cardiac toxicity progressing from increased conduction time, hypotension, and premature ventricular contractions to cardiac arrest as serum levels increase.
   c. Treatment: remove or decrease magnesium in parenteral nutrition; severe cases may require mechanical ventilation, dialysis, correction of fluid deficit, and IV administration of calcium gluconate.
   d. Prevention: restrict as appropriate.
   e. Monitoring: plasma levels may be monitored once or twice weekly, or more frequently as indicated.

4. Hypomagnesemia
   a. Cause: risk factors include alcoholism, diuretic use, gastrointestinal disease, aminoglycoside use, diabetic ketoacidosis, and chemotherapy.
   b. Symptoms: nonspecific symptoms, including gastrointestinal and neurologic changes, possible convulsions, cardiac arrhythmia, or neuromuscular hyperactivity.
   c. Treatment: administer peripheral magnesium or add magnesium.
   d. Prevention: provide magnesium in TPN solution.
   e. Monitoring: measure serum levels of magnesium once or twice weekly during initiation of parenteral nutrition and once a week thereafter; more frequent monitoring may be necessary during hypomagnesemia, repletion, and chemotherapy.

5. Hypercalcemia
   a. Cause: neoplasia, excess vitamin D administration, prolonged immobilization, and stress.
   b. Symptoms: thirst, polyuria, muscle weakness, loss of appetite; nausea, vomiting, constipation, itching.
   c. Treatment: administer isotonic saline, provide inorganic phosphate supplementation, corticosteroids, mithramycin.
   d. Prevention: restrict as appropriate.
   e. Monitoring: plasma calcium levels once or twice weekly.

6. Hypocalcemia
   a. Cause: decreased Vitamin D intake; hypoparathyroidism; reduced calcium intake, increased

gastrointestinal losses, decreased phosphate intake.
b. Symptoms: paresthesia; tetany.
c. Treatment: provide additional amounts of calcium.
d. Prevention: administer approximately 15 mEq calcium daily to achieve calcium balance.
e. Monitoring: plasma calcium levels once or twice weekly; if serum albumin level is depressed, obtain ionized calcium levels.

D. Nutritional
1. Carbohydrate overfeeding
a. Cause: rapid increase of feedings above requirements, particularly in patients with compromised pulmonary or cardiac function.
b. Symptoms: CO_2 retention, cardiac tamponade.
c. Treatment: decrease infusions to an acceptable level.
d. Prevention: carefully calculate nutrient requirements; ensure appropriate distribution of energy substrate.
e. Monitoring: respiratory quotients may be helpful in obtaining the proper energy substrate mix.
2. Protein overfeeding
a. Cause: continued infusion of protein in excess of requirements.
b. Symptoms: elevated blood urea nitrogen levels; excess nitrogen excretion.
c. Treatment: reduce amino acid content.
d. Prevention: carefully calculate protein requirements; provide adequate calories from carbohydrate and/or fat.
e. Monitoring: serum BUN levels once or twice weekly; nitrogen balance weekly.
3. Essential fatty acid deficiency
a. Cause: inadequate fat intake; biochemical signs appear 1–2 weeks on a fat-free regimen.
b. Symptoms: dermatitis, alopecia, alterations in pulmonary, neurologic, and red cell membranes.
c. Treatment: provide lipid emulsion at least twice weekly.
d. Prevention: provide 2 to 4% of caloric needs as linoleic acid, or 8 to 10% of calories from fat; adequate fat intake can be achieved by giving 500 ml of 10% fat emulsion two or three times weekly.
e. Monitoring: physical examination for symptoms.
4. Thiamine deficiency
a. Cause: concentrated glucose infusion without adequate thiamine.
b. Symptoms: elevated blood and urine lactate and pyruvate levels, abnormal electrocardiogram, cardiomegaly, and dyspnea.
c. Treatment: adequate thiamine intake per intravenous RDA.
d. Prevention: provide thiamine daily in parenteral solutions.
e. Monitoring: blood and urine lactate and pyruvate levels several times weekly in patients at risk.

E. Hepatic
1. Fatty liver
a. Cause: presumed to be infusion of carbohydrate in excess of hepatic oxidative capacity; overfeeding of calories and/or fat.
b. Detection: moderate elevation shown in liver function tests.
c. Treatment: reducing the amount of carbohydrate administered; cyclic administration of parenteral nutrition has been suggested, but results are inconclusive; rule out other causes.
d. Prevention: balanced nutrient solutions containing energy from carbohydrate and fat; avoid overfeeding.
e. Monitoring: liver function tests at least once a week.
2. Cholestasis
a. Cause: unknown.
b. Detection: progressive increases in total serum bilirubin; elevated serum alkaline phosphatase.
c. Treatment: reassess needs to prevent overfeeding; usually resolves at discontinuation of parenteral nutrition and resumption of a normal diet; rule out other causes.
d. Prevention: use the gastrointestinal tract if possible.
e. Monitoring: liver function tests at least once a week.

II. Technical
1. Pneumothorax
a. Cause: venous anomalies; inexperience with catheter placement technique.
b. Treatment: a small pneumothorax may resolve untreated; a larger pneumothorax may require chest tube placement.
c. Prevention: experience with catheter placement is necessary; some institutions ensure this by restricting privileges for central line insertion.
d. Monitoring: chest x-ray is performed before the line is used.
2. Air embolism
a. Cause: the central line is interrupted and the patient inspires air while the line is open.
b. Treatment: this complication has a high mortality rate if emergency action is not taken; place patient in reverse Trendelenburg position immediately.
c. Prevention: proper dressing and catheter care techniques; proper training of patient and caregivers.
d. Monitoring: observe for signs of respiratory distress.
3. Catheter embolization
a. Cause: pulling the catheter back through the needle used for insertion.
b. Treatment: surgical removal of the catheter tip.
c. Prevention: remove needle and catheter at the same time.
d. Monitoring: assure catheter is intact when removed; if not, obtain chest x-ray.
4. Venous thrombosis

Table 12–6

Indications for Pediatric TPN

Disorder	Features
Short bowel syndrome	Necrotizing enterocolitis, intestinal atresias, midgut volvulus, complicated meconium ileus
Abdominal wall defects	Gastroschisis, omphalocele, cloacal exstrophy
Inflammatory bowel diseases	Ulcerative colitis, Crohn's disease
Other	Tracheoesophageal fistula, malignancy, trauma, burns, sepsis, hepatic or renal disease, cardiac cachexia, chylothorax

  a. Cause: mechanical trauma to vein; hypotension; infection; solution osmolality; solution precipitates.
  b. Treatment: urokinase, streptokinase, or catheter change.
  c. Prevention: proper selection of catheter material; addition of heparin to PN.
  d. Monitoring: observe corresponding arm for swelling.
 5. Catheter occlusion
  a. Cause: hypotension; failure to flush catheter with heparin; formation of a fibrin sheath.
  b. Treatment: urokinase, streptokinase, catheter change.
  c. Prevention: proper catheter care.
  d. Monitoring: observe for inability to infuse.
III. Septic
 1. Catheter-related sepsis
  a. Cause: improper technique in catheter insertion; infusion of contaminated solution; multiple line violation and manipulation; skin colonization adjacent to catheter site; hematogenous seeding of the catheter by blood-borne organisms from other distant infection.
  b. Symptoms: unexplained fever; red, indurated area; or purulent discharge around the catheter site. A positive catheter tip culture and a positive blood culture to confirm infection.

Table 12–7

Nutrient Requirements

Parameter	Age or Weight	Amount/24 Hours
Fluid	0–10 kg	100 ml/kg
	11–20 kg	1000 + 50 ml/kg over 10 kg
	>20 kg	1500 + 20 ml/kg over 20 kg
Calories	Infants (0–1)	90–120 kcal/kg
	Children (1–7)	75–90 kcal/kg
	Children (7–12)	60–75 kcal/kg
	Adolescents (12–18)	30–60 kcal/kg
Fats		0.5–3.0 g/kg
Protein	Infants	2.5–3.0 g/kg
	Children	1.5–2.0 g/kg

Adapted from Taylor L, O'Neill JA. Total parenteral nutrition in the pediatric patient. Surg Clin North Am 1991; 71:477–492; and from Warner B. Parenteral Nutrition in the Pediatric Patient. In Fischer J (ed): Total Parenteral Nutrition, 2nd ed. Boston: Little, Brown and Co., 1991:299–322.

  c. Treatment: removal of the catheter and replacement at another site and concurrent antibiotic therapy.
  d. Prevention: strict adherence to aseptic technique during line insertion, line manipulation, and catheter care.

PARENTERAL NUTRITION IN THE PEDIATRIC PATIENT

TPN must be modified in pediatric patients to meet their special demands of growth and development. In comparison to adults, children have a higher basal metabolic rate per unit of body weight, an increased evaporative fluid loss compared with adults, and immature kidneys with decreased water clearance.[58, 59] Growth failure in children manifests itself as poor weight gain, below-normal height, and delay of secondary sex characteristics. In the newborn, the ratio of the metabolic rate to body weight is three times that of the adult. Neonates exhibit deficiencies of enzymes essential for the synthesis of certain amino acids (e.g., cystine, taurine, tyrosine, and histidine), so these are considered essential amino acids for this age group. Calcium and phosphorus requirements are greater for normal bone growth. Thus, the tolerance period of starvation by neonate ranges from 1 to 5 days, compared to 7 to 10 days in the older child or adult.[59]

Nutritional assessment of the pediatric patient uses standard growth curves. Calculation of the ratio of weight to height indicates wasting, and calculation of the ratio of height to age indicates stunting of growth. Anthropometric measurements are used as gauges of somatic protein and fat stores. Visceral protein stores are evaluated by determining serum albumin, serum transferrin, prealbumin, and retinol-binding protein levels.[58]

Indications

Pediatric patients requiring parenteral nutrition may fall into two major categories:

- Congenital or acquired anomalies of the gastrointestinal tract
- Intractable diarrhea syndromes

A list of conditions that may require parenteral nutrition is provided in Table 12–6.

Nutritional Requirements

Nutritional requirements for the pediatric patient are presented in Tables 12–7 and 12–8. Fluid requirement calculations should take into account the existing hydration status, body weight or surface area, environmental conditions, temperature, and abnormal losses.

Energy requirements can be estimated by using the pediatric Harris-Benedict Equation (see Table 12–2):[60]

$$\text{BEE (infants)} = 22.10 + 31.05W \text{ (in kg)} + 1.16H \text{ (in cm)}.$$

Energy requirements may also be estimated using standard tables based on body weight and age. Current recommendations for the caloric components in pediatric nutritional sup-

Table 12-8

Nutritional Requirements for the Pediatric Patient

Requirements	Term Infants and Children (dose/day)
Vitamins	
Lipid-soluble	
A (μg)	700
E (mg)	7
K (μg)	200
D (IU)	400
Water-soluble	
Ascorbic acid (mg)	80
Thiamin (mg)	1.2
Riboflavin (mg)	1.4
Pyridoxine (mg)	1.0
Niacin (mg)	17
Pantothenate (mg)	5
Biotin (μg)	20
Folate (μg)	140
Vitamin B_{12}	1.0
Electrolytes and Minerals	Daily Amount
Sodium	2–4 mEq/kg
Potassium	2–3 mEq/kg
Chloride	2–3 mEq/kg
Magnesium	0.25–0.50 mEq/kg
Calcium gluconate	100–500 mg/kg
Phosphorus	1–2 mmol/kg

Adapted from Warner B. Parenteral nutrition in the pediatric patient. In Fischer J (ed): Total Parenteral Nutrition, 2nd ed. Boston: Little, Brown and Co., 1991:299–322.

plementation are that carbohydrates make up 50% of the total calories, protein 15%, and fat 35%.[58] Peripheral parenteral nutrition uses 10 to 12.5% glucose and 2.5% protein. Central parenteral nutrition may use up to 25% glucose and 3.5% protein.

Fats are necessary to prevent essential fatty acid deficiency (EFAD); children require approximately 1 to 2% EFA in their diet. EFAD develops more rapidly in children than in adults, in as little as 1 week using fat-free solutions. The use of lipids may be harmful in the infant with jaundice. Fatty acids displace bilirubin from albumin and produce unbound bilirubin which increases the risk of kernicterus.[61] No more than 60% of nonprotein calories should be from fats to prevent ketonemia. Fats should be administered continuously in infants over a 24-hour period to prevent wide fluctuations in plasma lipid fractions. Therefore, TNA solutions are appropriate for use in the pediatric patient. A positive nitrogen balance usually requires 200 kcal/g nitrogen in children. Carbohydrates must be infused simultaneously with the amino acids to maximize utilization and prevent azotemia.

Vitamins are essential in the pediatric formula. Separate recommendations for adult and pediatric formulations were accepted in 1981 and revised in 1988. Actual requirements for electrolytes and minerals depend on such factors as diuretic administration, electrolyte losses, hydration, and renal function. As stated earlier, a greater need for these minerals exists in early infancy. Trace elements are considered essential in parenteral solution only if parenteral nutrition continues for more than 4 weeks. The exception to this is zinc, whose requirements are determined by infant growth rates. The addition of zinc may be necessary after only 1 to 2 weeks on parenteral nutrition.

Administration

Vascular Access. The basic principles of vascular access and catheter care for adults also apply to pediatric patients. A major responsibility is maintaining asepsis and preventing technical problems with use of the catheter, which is the most common complication requiring interruption of therapy in children.[61]

Monitoring. Monitoring parameters during the initiation of parenteral nutrition include daily weights, strict measurement of intake and output, and daily electrolytes until stabilized (then weekly). Serum glucose measurements may be done every 8 to 12 hours initially in addition to urine glucose measurements. Serum triglyceride and free fatty acid levels are measured weekly. Liver function tests are performed on a biweekly basis. Growth determinations include routine measurements of weight, height, head circumference, and anthropometric measurements for the duration of therapy. Many children require long-term support at home. Parents accept responsibility for routine catheter care and infusion procedures. Infusions are usually cycled over 10 to 12 hours at night to permit normal activities during the day. Some patients have undergone home therapy for over 7 years.[58]

Metabolic Complications. These complications are generally related either to disorders of glucose metabolism or to deficiencies or toxicities of specific components in the solution, as in the adult patient. Hepatobiliary dysfunction is one of the more common complications, second only to technical complications of the catheter. A pattern of cholestasis is seen with conjugated hyperbilirubinemia and elevation of other hepatic enzyme levels.[61] Management includes decreasing protein intake, cycling the infusion, and the addition of even minimal enteral feeding, if possible.

HOME PARENTERAL NUTRITION

Nutrition support was one of the first parenteral therapies to be implemented in the home care environment. A patient with metastatic ovarian cancer was maintained on parenteral nutrition at home for 6 months in 1968. Unfortunately, this patient did not have the benefit of the portable equipment used today, and was therefore essentially confined to the bed at home. During the late 1970s and early 1980s, home care companies expanded to provide both the necessary pharmaceuticals and equipment in addition to specialized clinical personnel. A major drawback to patient satisfaction with this therapy was the cumbersome delivery system. By the late 1980s, ambulatory infusion pumps became available that were lightweight, compact, and featured necessary safety systems and delivery capabilities.

Candidate Identification

Four factors have been identified as key elements in the decision process for successful home parenteral nutrition (HPN).[62] These factors and other influencing variables are listed in Table 12–9. The first factor is patient acceptance of this therapy in the home environment. Without a desire and dedication to make the necessary changes in life style re-

Adapted from Warner B. Parenteral nutrition in the pediatric patient. In Fischer J (ed): Total Parenteral Nutrition, 2nd ed. Boston: Little, Brown and Co., 1991: 299–322.

Table 12-9

Assessment for Home Parenteral Nutrition

Requirement Factors
1. Patient and caregivers desire HPN.
2. Sufficient financial coverage exists to cover supplies, nursing, and pharmaceuticals.
3. Patient and caregiver have sufficient abilities to learn and provide the therapy at home.
4. An appropriate long-term venous access device is in place.

Positive Influential Variables
1. The physician philosophy is positive regarding the advisability of HPN.
2. The prognosis is enhanced, or improved quality of life is expected as a result of HPN.
3. The age and condition of the patient are conducive to the management of HPN.
4. Patient and caregiver expectations of the effect of HPN on the disease process are realistic.

quired by HPN, compliance is negatively influenced, along with therapy outcome. Adaptation to HPN may initially involve depression, alteration in body image, anxiety, and fear. Long-term psychosocial adaptation has been enhanced through close coordination of the health care team and the inclusion of psychologic counseling, when indicated.[63] Patients with chronic illness have shown greater adaptation to HPN than those who had been well and suffered an acute episode requiring this therapy.[64]

Second, the financial impact must be considered. Although less expensive than hospitalization, the cost is considerable. Coverage and limitations of the patient's insurance should be thoroughly understood. Medicare and Medicaid guidelines vary among regional providers, and are changing with the current concerns for health care costs and reforms. Declaration of disability or application for medical assistance may be necessary. Case management strategies may be implemented to assist the patient and family to meet the financial burden.

Third, the patient and caregiver must be intelligent enough to understand and participate in the program at home. They must possess adequate eyesight and dexterity to manipulate the equipment and maintain catheter care. The HPN program is usually more successful if individuals living outside the home are not required to perform daily procedures.[64]

Fourth, there must be adequate long-term IV access for provision of the solution. Peripheral venous access is not suitable for HPN.

Indications

HPN may be required for as little as 1 month to lifelong supplementation. The purpose may be temporary nutrition support during bowel rest, lifelong supplementation to maintain life, or supplementation to improve quality of life for certain incurable disease states.[64] Disease states in which HPN may be indicated include the following:

1. Short bowel syndrome
2. Chronic or pseudo-obstruction
3. Fistulas
4. Chronic radiation enteritis
5. Crohn's disease
6. Congenital bowel defects
7. Carefully selected malignancy patients
8. Disorders of malabsorption including sprue, pancreatitis, cystic fibrosis, bone marrow transplantation
9. Acquired immunodeficiency syndrome

Vascular Access

Venous access must be into a central vein to allow rapid dilution of the HPN solution to prevent phlebitis, pain, and thrombosis. The system should be comfortable for the patient, must not limit mobility, and should be accessible to allow maintenance procedures by the patient, if possible. These systems include subcutaneous venous ports, tunneled catheters, and peripherally inserted central catheters for shorter-term therapy. They may be single, double, or triple lumen, depending on the types of infusions needed.

Dressing procedures vary depending on the condition of the patient (including immunocompetency factors), type of dressing being used, and policies set by the HPN team. Patients with tunneled catheters may be able to eliminate the need for sterile dressing procedures after the exit site is well healed. Because there is no external segment, the implanted ports may be more acceptable to patients who have periods without HPN during remission phases of their disease. The needle usually remains in place for several days when on continuous or cyclic therapy that is limited to several hours daily. Some patients actually prefer to change their needle daily for cyclic regimens. Patient preference and manual dexterity are important when making decisions on the type of catheter to be used.

Administration Considerations

Infusion devices used for HPN range from the larger devices commonly seen in the hospital setting to small, compact, battery-operated devices suitable for the totally ambulatory patient. Devices for the home patient need to have various safety features, including sophisticated alarm systems, variable pressure settings, and tapering features that allow programmed rate changes during the infusion. Tapering programmability allows patients on cyclic therapy to increase and decrease infusion rates automatically within a given time and volume at the beginning and end of their daily infusion. Home parenteral solutions are individualized to meet the patient's caloric needs, but are usually nonspecialized for acute organ failure, as seen in the hospital setting. Fats may be included daily or intermittently, as needed, and are usually admixed with the daily solution as a TNA. The solutions have a stability that allows a week's supply to be delivered and stored in the home refrigerator. Insulin and multivitamins are usually added just prior to hanging the solution by the patient or caregiver.

Continuous infusions are the least desirable in the home care setting, but may be required because of caloric need, glucose fluctuations, or fluid intolerance. Cyclic infusions given over a portion of a 24-hour period allow the patient free time away from the therapy, and foster return to normal life patterns.

Patient and Family Education

The most critical factor in the success of HPN may be the adequacy of preparation of the patient and caregiver. Teaching is begun using an individualized plan prior to discharge from the hospital and is a collaborative effort among the nutrition support team, the nurses caring for the patient, and a nurse from the home care agency. Teaching methods may involve audiovisuals, mannequins, and written procedures. The first phase of teaching is observation of the procedure by the patient and caregiver. In the second phase, the patient or caregiver performs the procedure under nursing supervision. The goal is for the learner to demonstrate proficiency in each phase of the procedure three times before progressing to the third stage of independence. It may take from 1 to 3 weeks before independence is achieved. Each training session should be adequately documented. For an example of a home TPN teaching plan, see Chapter 25, Patient Education.

Patient Monitoring

Home care monitoring begins on the day of discharge. The home care nurse should be in attendance for starting the infusion, evaluating the storage and work areas, and assessing the patient's and caregiver's response to discharge. Reiteration of the procedures is often necessary during the first week at home, and may require frequent visits by the home care agency. Availability of the home care agency for 24 hours is required to handle unexpected problems. Weekly visits continue as the patient becomes stable and more independent.

Clinical self-monitoring is documented in a diary and includes weight, temperature, urine or glucometer testing for glucose levels, and changes in urinary volume. Laboratory monitoring of various blood levels is performed weekly at first, then less frequently as the patient becomes stable.

Complications

No matter which type of system is used, the complications of long-term venous access remain the same. The major complication continues to be catheter-related sepsis. The best treatment is prevention through adequate teaching, reinforcement of technique, and prompt recognition of problems.[64] Although some catheter infections can be successfully treated with antibiotics, catheter sepsis remains the main reason for catheter removal or hospitalization.[65] Catheter occlusion may occur because of improper flushing, resulting in blood clots in the catheter lumen. Thrombolytic agents have been successful in restoring patency to this type of occluded catheter. Catheter occlusion may also occur as a result of medication precipitates. Precipitate occlusions specifically related to TNA solutions have been successfully treated with ethanol.[66] Calcium phosphate crystal precipitate occlusions have been successfully treated with the instillation of 0.1 N hydrochloric acid (HCl).[67] Broken catheters can sometimes be repaired.

Metabolic complications include disorders of glucose metabolism, as in the hospitalized patient. Complications unique to the long-term HPN patient include vitamin and trace element deficiencies. These can be avoided by laboratory testing and adequate supplementation in the TPN solution. A metabolic bone disease has been reported in long-term HPN patients. It is characterized by increased serum calcium levels, excessive losses of calcium and phosphorus in the urine, and low-normal plasma levels of parathyroid hormone. Fundamental abnormalities of bone remodelling have been reported, although fractures were uncommon and bone pain was mild to moderate. The significance of the condition is unclear, as is the cause and treatment.[64]

Generally, HPN has been found to be a safe and efficient method for the continuation of parenteral nutrition outside the hospital setting. Life itself can be prolonged while allowing the patient to return to the home environment.

The administration of parenteral nutrition solutions has become a valuable treatment modality for patients with disease states that result in an impaired ability to ingest or absorb adequate nutrients through the GI tract to satisfy nutritional requirements. However, as demonstrated throughout this chapter, the provision of parenteral nutritional support has become increasingly complex. To ensure delivery in a safe and effective manner, the nurse involved in the administration of parenteral nutrition must demonstrate competency in nutrition assessment parameters, parenteral nutrition solution-related pharmacologic considerations, administration delivery systems and regimens, and patient teaching.

References

1. Worthington PH, Wagner BA. Total parenteral nutrition. Nurs Clin North Am 1989; 24:355–371.
2. Wroblewski B, Young LS. Topics in parenteral nutrition for the 1990s. Focus Crit Care 1991; 18:276, 278–279.
3. Grant J, Kennedy-Caldwell C, eds. Nutritional Support in Nursing. Orlando: Grune & Stratton, 1988.
4. Rombeau JL, Caldwell MD. Clinical Nutrition. Vol II, Total Parenteral Nutrition. Philadelphia: W.B. Saunders, 1986.
5. Dudrick SJ. 1991; Past, present, and future of nutritional support. Surg Clin North Am 1991; 71:439–448.
6. Intravenous Nurses Society. Intravenous Nursing Standards of Practice. Belmont, MA: Intravenous Nurses Society, 1990.
7. Kuhn MM. Nutritional support for the shock patient. Crit Care Nurs Clin North Am 1990; 2:201–220.
8. Tellado JM, Christou NV. Nutrition and immunity. In Fischer JE, (ed). Total Parenteral Nutrition, 2nd ed., Boston: Little, Brown and Co., 1991:127–138.
9. Lehmann S. Immune function and nutrition: The clinical role of the intravenous nurse. JIN 1991; 14:406–420.
10. Bernard MA, Jacobs DO, Robeau JL. Nutritional and Metabolic Support of Hospitalized Patients. Philadelphia: W.B. Saunders, 1986:46–51.
11. Ebbert-Sauer ML. Adult parenteral nutrition. In Koda-Kimble, Young LY (eds). Applied Therapeutics: The Clinical Use of Drugs, 5th ed. Vancouver, WA: Applied Therapeutics, 1992:677–694.
12. Sax HC, Hasselgren PO. Indications. In Fischer JE (ed). Total Parenteral Nutrition, 2nd ed. Boston: Little, Brown and Co., 1991.
13. Fleming RC, Nelson J. Nutritional options. In Kinney JM, Jeejeebhoy KN, Hill GL, Owen OE (eds). Nutrition and Metabolism in Patient Care. Philadelphia: W.B. Saunders, 1985:752–772.
14. ASPEN, Guidelines for the use of parenteral and enteral nutrition in adult and pediatric patients. JPEN (suppl) 1993; 17:1SA–52SA.
15. Kaminski MV, Jr, ed. Hyperalimentation: A Guide for Clinicians. New York: Marcel Dekker, 1985.
16. Knox LS. Ethical issues in nutritional support nursing. Nurs Clin North Am 1989; 24:427–436.
17. Curtis S, Chapman G, Meguid M. Evaluation of nutritional status. Nurs Clin North Am 1989; 24:301–313.
18. Knox LS. Nutritional requirements. In Kennedy-Caldwell C, Guenter P, (eds). Nutrition Support Nursing, 2nd ed. Baltimore: ASPEN, 1988:5–28.

19. Smith LC, Mullen JL. Nutritional assessment and indications for nutritional support. Surg Clin North Am 1991; 71:449–458.
20. Page CP, Hardin TC. Nutritional Assessment and Support: A primer. Baltimore: Williams & Wilkins, 1989.
21. Shikora SA, Blackburn GL. (1991). Nutritional consequences of major gastrointestinal surgery: Patient outcome and starvation. Surg Clin North Am 71 (3), 509-522.
22. Grant JP. Handbook of Parenteral Nutrition, 2nd ed. Philadelphia; W.B. Saunders, 1992; 15–47, 49–73, 171–202, 215–237, 239–274.
23. Gray D, Kaminski M. Protein-calorie malnutrition. In Kaminski M (ed). Hyperalimentation: A Guide for Clinicians. New York: Marcel Dekker, 1985:23–45.
24. Jeejeebhoy KN, Detsky AS, Baker JP. Assessment of nutritional status. JPEN (suppl) 1990; 14:193–196.
25. Luketich JD, Mullen JL, Buzby GP. Preoperative total parenteral nutrition. In Fischer JE (ed). Total Parenteral Nutrition, 2nd ed. Boston: Little, Brown and Co., 1991:217–237.
26. Kennedy-Caldwell C, Guenter P. Nutrition Support Nursing: Core Curriculum, 2nd ed. Baltimore: ASPEN, 1988.
27. Barbul A. Measurements of relevant nutrition data for determining efficacy of nutritional support. Fischer JE (ed). Total Parenteral Nutrition, 2nd ed. Boston: Little, Brown and Co., 1991:153–164.
28. Plumer A. Principles and Practices of Intravenous Therapy, 4th ed. Boston, Little Brown and Co., 1987.
29. Griggs B. Indications for Nutritional Support in the Adult Patient. In Grant J, Kennedy-Caldwell C (eds). Nutritional Support in Nursing. Orlando: Grune & Stratton, 1988:65–89.
30. Hennessy K. Nutritional support and gastrointestinal disease. Nurs Clin North Am 1989; 24:373–382.
31. Latifi R, McIntosh JK, Dudrick SJ. Nutritional management of acute and chronic pancreatitis. Surg Clin North Am 1991; 71:579–596.
32. Englert DA. Nutritional alterations in illness. In Kennedy-Caldwell C, Guenter P (eds). Nutrition Support Nursing, 2nd ed. Baltimore; ASPEN, 1988:217–261.
33. Latifi R, Killam RW, Dudrick SJ. Nutritional support in liver failure. Surg Clin North Am 1991; 71:567–578.
34. Liftman C. Renal function. In Skipper A (ed). Dietitian's Handbook of Enteral and Parenteral Nutrition. Baltimore: ASPEN, 1989:87–102.
35. Spector N. Nutritional support of the ventilator-dependent patient. Nurs Clin North Am 1989; 24:407–414.
36. Lipman T. Clinical trials of nutritional support in cancer. Hematol Oncol Clin North Am 1991; 5:91–102.
37. Crocker K. Gastrointestinal manifestations of the acquired immunodeficiency syndrome. Nurs Clin North Am 1989; 24:395–406.
38. Leupold C. Nutritional alterations in illness: Critical care—stress, trauma, burns, and sepsis. In Kennedy-Caldwell C, Guenter P (eds). Nutritional Support in Nursing, 2nd ed. Baltimore: ASPEN, 1988:413–453.
39. Cochran EB, Phelps SJ, Helms RA. Parenteral nutrition in pediatric patients. Clin Pharm 1988; 7:351–366.
40. Zlotkin SH, Stallings VA, Penchary PB. Total parenteral nutrition in children. Pediatr Clin North Am 1985; 32:381–400.
41. Cerra FB, Siegel JH, Coleman B, et al. Septic autocannibalism: A failure of exogenous nutritional support. Ann Surg 1980; 192:570–574.
42. Baumgartner T. Clinical Guide to Parenteral Micronutrition, 2nd ed.: Fujisawa, USA, 1991:619.
43. Torosian MH, Daley JM. Solutions available. In: Fischer JE, (ed). Total Parenteral Nutrition, 2nd ed. Boston; Little, Brown and Co., 1991:13–23.
44. Dickerson RN, Brown RO, White KG. Parenteral nutrition solutions. In Rombeau JL, Caldwell MD (eds). Clinical Nutrition: Parenteral Nutrition, 2nd ed. Philadelphia; W.B. Saunders, 1993:310–333.
45. Okada A, Imura K. Parenteral nutrition in neonates. In Rombeau JL, Caldwell MD (eds). Clinical Nutrition: Parenteral Nutrition, 2nd ed. Philadelphia; W.B. Saunders, 1993:756–769.
46. Hill ID, Madrozo de la Garza JA, Lebenthal E. Parenteral nutrition in pediatric patients. In Rombeau JL, Caldwell MD (eds). Clinical Nutrition: Parenteral Nutrition, 2nd ed. Philadelphia; W.B. Saunders, 1993:770–789.
47. AMA Department of Food and Nutrition. Multivitamin preparations for parenteral use: A statement by the Nutrition Advisory Group. JPEN 1979; 3:258.
48. AMA Department of Food and Nutrition. Guidelines for essential trace element preparations for parenteral use: A statement by an expert panel. JAMA 1979; 241:2051.
48a. Kerner JA (ed). Manual of Pediatric Nutrition. New York: John Wiley and Sons, 1983:157–173.
49. LaFrance RJ, Miyagawa CI. Pharmaceutical considerations in total parenteral nutrition. In Fischer JE, (ed). Total parenteral nutrition, 2nd ed. Vancouver, WA: Applied Therapeutics, 1988:677–694.
50. Stranz MH, Barfoot KS. Total parenteral nutrition: Compatibility of antibiotic admixtures. JIN 1988; 11:43–48.
51. Driscoll DF. Clinical issues regarding the use of total nutrient admixtures. DICP 1990; 24:296–303.
52. Warshawsky KY. Intravenous fat emulsions. NCP 1992; 7:187–196.
53. Sculer CL, Wolfson M. Nutrition in acute renal failure. In Rombeau JL, Caldwell MD (eds). Clinical Nutrition: Parenteral Nutrition, 2nd ed. Philadelphia; W.B. Saunders, 1993:667–675.
54. O'Keefe SJD. Parenteral nutrition and liver disease. In Rombeau JL, Caldwell MD (eds). Clinical Nutrition: Parenteral Nutrition, 2nd ed. Philadelphia; W.B. Saunders, 1993:676–695.
55. Wilmore DW, Van Woert JH. Enteral and parenteral nutrition in hospital patients. In Rubenstein E, Federman DD (eds). Scientific American Medicine, Vol 4. New York: Scientific American, 1992:1–21.
56. Dickerson D. Question: How fast can I taper TPN in a hospitalized patient? Hosp Pharm 1985; 20:620–621.
57. Bennet KM, Rosen GH. Cyclic total parenteral nutrition. Nutr Clin Prac 1990; 5:163–165.
58. Taylor L, O'Neill JA. Total parenteral nutrition in the pediatric patient. Surg Clin North Am 1991; 71:477–492.
59. Testerman EJ. Current trends in pediatric total parenteral nutrition. JIN 1989; 12:152–162.
60. Pfeifer JA. Pediatric clinical nutrition. In Kennedy-Caldwell C, Guenter P (eds). Nutrition Support Nursing, 2nd ed. Baltimore; ASPEN, 1988:541–575.
61. Warner B. Parenteral nutrition in the pediatric patient. In Fischer J (ed). Total Parenteral Nutrition, 2nd ed. Boston: Little, Brown and Co. 1991:299–322.
62. Lin EM. Nutrition support: Making the difficult decisions. Cancer Nurs 1991; 14:261–269.
63. Englert DA, Lawson M. Ambulatory home nutritional support. In Grant J, Kennedy-Caldwell C (eds). Nutritional Support in Nursing. New York: Grune & Stratton, 1988:281–303.
64. Bower RH. Home parenteral nutrition. In Fischer J (ed). Total Parenteral Nutrition, 2nd ed. Boston: Little, Brown and Co., 1991:367–387.
65. Orr ME. Nutritional support in home care. Nurs Clin North Am 1989; 24:437–445.
66. Pennington CR, Pithie AD. Ethanol lock in the management of catheter occlusion. JPEN 1987; 8:507–508.
67. Breaux CW, Duke D, Georgeson KE, et al. Calcium phosphate crystal occlusion of central venous catheters used for total parenteral nutrition in infants and children: Prevention and treatment. J Pediatr Surg 1987; 22:829–832.

CHAPTER 13 Oncologic Therapy

Mary Ann Doyle, CRNI, MS, OCN

According to statistics generated by the American Cancer Society, cancer is the second leading cause of death in the United States, exceeded only by heart disease. Cancer is a chronic condition that consists of a large group of diseases characterized by uncontrolled growth and spread of abnormal cells. Unlike diabetes, hypertension, or arthritis, cancer is the only chronic disease that can achieve a complete remission. The key is early detection and a treatment that focuses on cure and complete remission, when possible. Disease control and symptom management are the therapeutic goals when cure is not feasible. Treatment modalities include surgery, radiation therapy, chemotherapy and, more recently, immunotherapy, biologic therapy, hyperthermia, and genetic markers. This chapter focuses on intravenous chemotherapy and discusses its side effects and their management, describes the chemotherapeutic agents used, and presents some considerations regarding administration techniques.

ROLE OF THE NURSE

Patient Assessment and History

The professional nurse has always assumed the role of patient advocate. This position has evolved to include increased responsibility and accountability in the management of patient care. Because the oncology patient is different from any other classification of patient, the nurse must be prepared to recognize and respond to the unique differences and complexities in this patient population.

It is advantageous for the nurse to understand the different classifications of cancer, presenting symptoms, and natural course of the disease. This knowledge base assists the nurse in obtaining a patient history. In addition to the usual past medical history, the nurse needs to be particularly alerted to prior organ impairment or any secondary diagnosis that might influence the toxicities, side effects, and treatment modalities. This is especially true when drugs are contraindicated in the presence of specific pre-existing conditions.

Not every patient being assessed by the nurse is newly diagnosed. Depending on the circumstances, the patient may have been at multiple institutions and been heavily pretreated prior to arriving at the current facility. Complete information, including total chemotherapeutic drugs, doses, and any radiation, is necessary to determine the most appropriate treatment at this point in time.[1–5]

A cancer history is involved and is not the sole responsibility of the nurse or clinical nurse specialist, but an understanding of its importance assists with customizing the care plan. It is not enough to know that the patient had surgery for a cancer diagnosis. There are important questions that need to be answered that affect the treatment choices and duration of treatment. For example, it is necessary to know whether all the tumor was resected, the size of the tumor, and whether the margins were clean. Information on how many, if any, nodes were positive and visible signs of metastatic disease at the time of surgery are considered in staging the disease. Tumor that invades surrounding tissue or is wrapped around major organs or blood vessels contributes to the staging, which influences treatment decisions. This staging, at the time of surgery, helps separate patients needing additional treatment from those who achieve a complete remission or cure with surgery alone.[3, 5–9]

Knowing that the patient received radiation therapy is not enough. Many patients can tell you how many treatments they received, but the radiation dose and fraction must be known. Information on the radiation site allows the nurse to inspect the skin for radiation effects and to plan for appropriate intervention. Depending on the time of the last radiation treatment, present symptoms may be related to the radiation. Knowing the radiation field also provides a clue to potential complications related to recent or past chemotherapy-associated recall.[1, 5, 7, 10–12]

Some chemotherapeutic agents have lifetime dose limits. It is necessary to know exactly what drugs and doses the patient has received. Many available treatment modalities have similar side effects. A careful history of the toxicities the patient has experienced in the past and a summary of the management of these symptoms are helpful in determining the best approach to ensure patient comfort with subsequent treatments.

Patients do not always know the details of their disease or treatment. The most accurate way to obtain this information is from the medical record. The medical record belongs to the patient and can be obtained with a release of information from the facility that previously treated the patient.

Physical findings, nutritional status, laboratory and diagnostic imaging studies, and the patient's psychosocial and spiritual state all help define the patient's needs and assist in the decision-making process to determine appropriate intervention.[5, 9, 12]

Education

Right to Information

The patient's right to information includes the option to refuse treatment and an explanation of the ramifications of this decision. The patient needs to know whether there is a realistic chance for cure or whether the focus of therapy is control or palliation. It is sometimes difficult to understand the patient who elects no treatment as an option, but we have an obligation to respect the patient's wishes. Our responsibility as health care providers is to help furnish patients with adequate information to enable them to make informed, intelligent decisions related to their moral, religious, and ethical value system.

The teaching method for the patient depends on his or her readiness to learn, as well as learning styles. Teaching should begin with patient contact and continue throughout the course of the disease. The nurse needs to tailor the education plan to the patient. Some patients require volumes of information, whereas others are overwhelmed with only a few facts. Learning is enhanced when all the senses are used and efforts should be made to supplement verbal information with visual aids. Charts, videos, printed material, and audio tapes are beneficial. Studies have shown that information relayed in the first 10 minutes is usually what is remembered. Retention drops off after that; therefore, it is wise to address the most critical areas first. Academic disciplines have demonstrated that retention improves with repetition. The physician is responsible for providing the patient with information so that the patient may give informed consent, but the nurse is in the unique role of reinforcing and expanding on that knowledge base. Patients should be given written and verbal information. Phone numbers of the primary nurse and physician are reassuring to the patient should any questions or concerns arise. Many institutions tape the teaching sessions so that the patient can replay the instructions. Written information should be easy to read and contain important and pertinent information. The written information should be a quick and easy reference so as to address major concerns. For the patient who requires more detailed information, supplemental reading can be provided. It is essential to find a balance between adequate information and overload. There is a difference in information that is a ''need to know'' versus ''nice to know.''[3, 5, 6, 12-14]

Treatment Objectives

Patient education should include but not be limited to an explanation of the treatment goals and their rationale. The informed patient knows the names of the drugs that are given, the long- and short-term side effects, symptom management, and life style effects. Many institutions give patients written material on the medications ordered. The information should be easy to read, in the appropriate language, describe side effects and any drug and food interactions, and provide other pertinent information. If the patient is receiving multiple medications, especially for a comorbid condition, a pharmacy consult can provide additional and useful recommendations.

Cancer patients have a need and right to function at their maximum level as long as possible and to participate in their usual activities of daily living. It is therefore important that the patient know the treatment plan and schedule. For example, the patient needs to understand that the chemotherapy is to be given daily for 5 consecutive days and then repeated in 21 days versus once a week or whatever schedule the protocol specifies. A calendar or appointment card is helpful in ensuring that the patient understands the importance of timely treatments and coordinates these with personal agendas.

Patients and families should be encouraged to formulate realistic short- and long-term plans around the chemotherapy schedules. A family picnic timed the week before chemotherapy treatment allows the patient recovery time from the previous cycle. Patients should be encouraged to be as active as possible based on their physical capabilities. Rest periods and activities should be planned to maximize patient tolerance and enjoyment.

Because chemotherapy is a new experience for most people, many have a tendency to think that one dose can cure their cancer. Therefore, they need to be psychologically prepared for a long-term commitment to treatment and also need to know the end point. In an adjuvant setting, the end point may be 3 months or as long as 1 year, depending on the histology and initial tumor burden. If the patient has active residual disease, the usual rule of thumb is that chemotherapy is continued for 6 to 12 months after a complete remission has been achieved. Treatment is disease- and stage-specific, as well as patient-specific. Some protocols dictate the total number of cycles of chemotherapy. Whatever the length of treatment, patient education improves patient compliance.

Information about the therapeutic goals and expected outcomes can be encouraging and supportive to the patient and family. A brief explanation of the action of chemotherapy fosters a better understanding of potential side effects (Table 13–1).

The patient has a right to know the potential long- and short-term side effects and appropriate interventions. The patient needs to be able to determine whether the symptoms experienced are a result of the treatments, and thus self-limited, or whether there is a problem that requires medical intervention. For example, the asymptomatic patient should take infection precautions but should not be concerned if the white count is 2.0 mm^3. However, the patient should notify the physician if an oral temperature of 101 F develops, regardless of the white blood count.

Educational information may influence the method of ad-

Table 13–1	
Chemotherapy Toxicities	
Duration	**Action**
Temporary	Affects rapidly dividing cells (e.g., side effects consist of stomatitis, nausea, vomiting, alopecia, tumor lysis syndrome, constipation, diarrhea, dysmenorrhea)
Permanent	Affects organs (e.g., cardiac myopathy, pulmonary fibrosis, sterility)

ministration of the chemotherapy. For example, if the treatments are going to be continued for many months, the patient may consent to a central line rather than have repeated venipunctures. Another option is to have a venous access device surgically implanted. Providing the patient with opportunities to make decisions regarding symptom management, scheduling activities, and personal agendas re-establishes control and brings independence back into the patient's life.

Patients also need to know what kind of monitoring is used to follow their progress. Periodic restaging evaluations are done to determine tumor status and response to therapy. The patient needs to know what tests are included. The testing is patient-specific and depends on tumor type and natural history of the disease. Restaging could include but not be limited to blood work for tumor markers, immune panels, chemistry, and blood counts. Other procedures such as imaging scans, barium enema, MRI, CT scans, mammography, and an intravenous pyelogram (IVP) may also be appropriate. In addition, procedures such as colonoscopy, cystoscopy, spinal tap, bone marrow aspiration, and biopsy are frequently used to follow disease status.

Patients and family members feel more secure knowing that someone is watching and following their progress. Often it is the nurse in conjunction with the doctor who fulfills this role. Frequently, the nurse working in oncology coordinates patient care, develops expertise in recognizing early signs and symptoms of side effects, and activates the appropriate intervention.

The treatment modality that has the worst reputation is chemotherapy. Two of three cancer patients are candidates for chemotherapy at some point in their disease process. Many patients have heard stories about the nightmare side effects of chemotherapy, but it is the most effective treatment presently available for disease status that is not localized. Chemotherapy is also useful when there is concern of a recurrence from microscopic disease. It is estimated that 50 to 70% of all newly diagnosed cancer patients have micrometastasis. Only 30 to 40% of patients can achieve a complete remission with surgery alone. In 1955, Congress directed the National Cancer Institute (NCI) to develop a chemotherapy program to evaluate antineoplastics through clinical trials. NCI initiated a long-range program 3 years later to evaluate 35,000 plants for possible antineoplastic potential. This has resulted in the evolution of our present use of chemotherapy in multiple patient settings.[2, 3, 6, 7, 15–18]

There is a fine line between the dose that is therapeutic and the one that is toxic. Needless to say, chemotherapy should only be given under the supervision of a physician who has experience using antineoplastic drugs. Because of the potential life-threatening toxicities of cancer therapy, it is mandatory that the nursing staff and ancillary systems be available to support and monitor the patient. Clearly, the nursing component plays a major role in patient management, along with pharmacy, laboratory, nutrition, and psychosocial services.

There are many misconceptions about cancer drugs. A lack of accurate information concerning chemotherapy contributes to the fear and anxiety seen in many patients and family members. A common myth is that the side effects of chemotherapy are worse than the disease itself. It is true that chemotherapy has side effects and, at times, life-threatening toxicities, but many of these problems can be prevented, managed, or controlled.

Chemotherapeutic agents can be administered by the oral, subcutaneous, intravenous, intra-arterial, intrathecal, intraperitoneal, intratracheal, intravesicular, and even intralesional routes. The primary focus in this chapter is on the intravenous administration of antineoplastics. However, the practicing oncology nurse must understand the other methods of administration.

Treatment Goals

The treatment goal of chemotherapy is situation-dependent. Chemotherapy can be curative when given as primary treatment. For example, patients with acute lymphocytic leukemia (ALL), Hodgkin's disease, and thyroid and testicular cancer all have the potential for achieving a complete remission with chemotherapy.

The therapeutic goal is also curative when chemotherapy is given in an adjuvant setting for tumors such as primary breast, ovary, or colon cancer. Adjuvant therapy means treatment in addition to primary treatment, which usually consists of surgery or radiation.

Recent years have demonstrated the advantages of neoadjuvant chemotherapy prior to surgery. This type of therapy reduces the tumor size to provide the surgeon with a better chance of achieving complete resection. Neoadjuvant chemotherapy prevents the spread of dislodged cells during surgery. Micrometastasis distal to the resection site can be eradicated with chemotherapy prior to surgery. Neoadjuvant chemotherapy is geared toward improving the potential for a complete resection.

The difference between primary treatment and adjuvant treatment is determined by the amount of disease present. With primary treatment the tumor is macroscopic and there is measurable disease that can be documented by physical examination, x-ray, CT scan, MRI, or blood tests. In the adjuvant setting, the patient is said to be NED (no evaluable disease), and treatment is given to eradicate the microscopic cells known to be present based on historical data.

Chemotherapy can also be given to control the disease when cure is not realistic but the possibility exists to slow down the tumor growth, thereby increasing life expectancy and the quality of life. These situations include patients with advanced stages of breast or prostate cancer and multiple myeloma.

Chemotherapy given for palliation is aimed at comfort. It can decrease pain caused by a tumor by relieving pressure on nerves, decreasing lymphatic congestion, and relieving organ obstruction.

In the 1960s, it was found that, although single-agent chemotherapy is effective, combination chemotherapy demonstrates an increased response. Frei was one of the first to use a combination of drugs to produce and improve tumor response. Combination therapy also reduces the possibility of the tumor developing drug resistance. By using more than one drug, multiple modes of action can be produced. Research has shown that there is a synergistic activity with combination therapy. Drugs that have demonstrated tumor sensitivity with different actions and without overlapping toxicities are a consideration in choosing combination therapy.[1–3, 6, 7, 9, 11, 15–17, 19–24]

There are few absolute rules concerning chemotherapy, but there are some basic considerations. In general, the smaller the tumor burden, the easier the tumor is to treat. Surgical debulking decreases the tumor burden and recruits resting malignant cells to start dividing, therefore increasing the sensitivity to chemotherapy. In most situations, the higher the chemotherapy dose, the better the chance for a tumor response. However, there has to be a balance. It is not desirable to wipe out the patient while eradicating the tumor. Adjustment in supportive measures may need to be considered with dose escalation. Doses of chemotherapeutic agents are altered based on the degree of toxicity the patient experiences. The therapeutic margin is the difference in the dose producing the desired benefit and the dose resulting in unacceptable toxicity. The therapeutic margin of antineoplastics is rather narrow compared with other types of drugs.

The therapeutic index may be improved by several methods. The first is to increase the dose administered to the patient. If the dose-limiting factor is the severity of the toxicity, then better management of the side effects allows higher doses of chemotherapy without compromise to the patient. If the efficacy of the chemotherapeutic agents can be increased, there is a better tumor response with a lower chemotherapy dose. This can be accomplished in some instances through modulation of the cell membrane by the use of such drugs as leucovorin, levamisole, interferon, verapamil, amphotericin B, or by hyperthermia. Perhaps the answer to improved tumor control and cure lies in a combination of all these.[6, 7, 11, 16, 18, 23, 25]

Cell Cycle

To understand chemotherapy, it is necessary to understand the unique biochemical properties of the antineoplastics and their relationship to the cell cycle. Cell division is the same for cancer cells as for normal cells. The initial phase is the resting phase, designated as G0. The cell performs its specific function during this part of the cycle. In other words, renal cells filter the blood and make urine and gastric cells digest food. Many enzymes are needed for DNA synthesis, and are produced in this phase. G0 is frequently referred to as the resting phase of the cell, but it can also be called the postmitotic or presynthetic phase.

When a cell is ready to divide, it enters into the next phase. Synthesis of the proteins for RNA occurs during the G1 phase. This is also the phase with the largest variation of time among the different cells. If a cell is in the G1 phase for prolonged periods, it is sometimes referred to as G0.

Enzymes necessary for the DNA synthesis are activated in the S phase. Usually, the amount of time that the cancer cell is in this phase is different from that of normal cells.

The second gap phase is referred to as G2. At this time the synthesis of DNA stops and RNA and protein synthesis continue as the cell gets ready for mitosis.

Mitosis occurs during the final stage, the M phase, and usually lasts 30 to 90 minutes. This phase is subdivided into four steps. In prophase, the nuclear membrane is broken down and the chromosomes clump. In metaphase, the chromosomes line up in the middle of the cell. During anaphase, the chromosomes segregate into centrioles. In telephase, the final step, there is chromosome replication and cell division, which produces two daughter cells. These then go into the resting phase, G0.[1, 3, 5, 6, 9, 16, 17, 18, 20-24]

There are several terms connected with cellular kinetics

Table 13-2

Cellular Kinetics Terms

Term	Definition
Generation time	Time from midmitosis of parent cell to midmitosis of daughter cell
Doubling time	Time it takes for tumor to double in size
Growth fraction	Percentage of cells actively dividing
Loss fraction	Rate of cell death
Gompertzian growth curve	Indicates that, as tumor size increases, doubling time decreases

(Table 13-2). The generation time of a cell is usually measured by the time it takes the cell to replicate from midmitosis of the parent cell to midmitosis of the daughter cell. The growth fraction refers to the percentage of tumor cells that are actively dividing. This is measured by flow cytometry, and has prognostic significance. The doubling time is the amount of time it takes for the tumor to double in size. A cell divides and replicates and with each division the number of cells doubles, so that one cell becomes two and two cells become four. After 20 doublings the tumor contains 1 million cells and is the size of a pinhead. After 30 doublings the tumor is about 1 cm in size and contains 1 billion cells. As the tumor size increases, the doubling time decreases; this is known as the Gompertzian growth curve. As a tumor expands its growth rate slows because of crowding with other structures, decreased blood supply, and decreased nutrients. The loss fraction is the rate at which the cells die.[1-3, 5-7, 9, 16-18, 20-24, 26]

Chemotherapy Classifications

There are several ways in which chemotherapeutic agents can be classified (Table 13-3). They can be categorized according to their relationship to the cell cycle activity, their pharmacologic or chemical structure, their potential to cause necrosis if extravasated, and their emetic potential.

The cell life cycle classification has two categories, cell cycle-specific drugs and non–cell cycle-specific drugs. Antineoplastics can also be classified according to their chemical structure as antimetabolites, vinca or plant alkaloids, alkylating agents, nitrosoureas, antibiotics, hormones, or miscellaneous agents (drugs that do not fit into the other groups) (Table 13-4).

Antineoplastic agents are most effective while the cell is dividing. Agents that have a specific action on a particular stage of the cell cycle are called cell cycle specific. These

Table 13-3

Chemotherapeutic Agent Classifications

Classification System	Category
Cell cycle	Cell cycle-specific or non–cell cycle-specific
Chemical structures	Antimetabolite, vinca alkaloid, alkylating agent, nitrosoureas, antibiotic, hormone or miscellaneous
Local tissue reaction	Irritant or vesicant

Table 13–4

Mechanisms of Action of Antineoplastic Drugs

Classification	Action
Alkylating agent	Creates molecular bond within nucleic acid, which interferes with duplication and therefore prevents mitosis
Antimetabolite	Mimics essential metabolites, thus disrupting DNA synthesis
Mitotic inhibitor	Acts on microtubular proteins during metaphase, causing inhibition of mitosis
Antibiotic	Disrupts base pairs of DNA, inhibiting DNA and RNA synthesis

drugs are most effective when there are large numbers of cells actively dividing (Table 13–4).

Chemotherapeutic agents that will destroy the cancer cell regardless of the activity of the cell are termed cell cycle nonspecific. These drugs are effective against resting and dividing cells. Their cytotoxic effect takes place during the cell cycle and is expressed when the cell tries to divide or repair itself. The number of cancer cells affected is related to the amount of drug given. This is known as the dose intensity curve.

There is a paradoxical relationship in the rate of cell growth and responsiveness to chemotherapy. Most neoplastic agents modify or interfere with DNA synthesis and therefore are most effective in cells that are preparing for, or are in the process of, cell division. The more aggressive the tumor the greater the chance of a response to chemotherapy. Consequently, the greatest successes with chemotherapy are in the early diagnosed hematologic malignancies, which have a short doubling time; these include leukemia, lymphoma, Hodgkin's disease, and multiple myeloma.

The two major categories of drugs that are cell cycle specific are (1) antimetabolites and (2) vinca alkaloids and plant alkaloids.

Chemotherapeutic agents can also be classified by their potential to cause local tissue reactions. The potential for local toxic effects from drugs ranges from transient local discomfort during administration to severe tissue necrosis, with potential damage to tendons and nerves. There is a lack of uniformity in the literature classifying drugs according to this toxic potential. Many drugs are listed as both a vesicant and an irritant.[1–3, 5–7, 9, 16–18, 20–24]

Chemotherapy Dosing

Chemotherapy doses are calculated using body surface area (BSA) to take into account the various sizes and shapes of individuals so that each patient receives the same amount of drug. Clinical trials have provided a formula (or recipe) to determine the amount of each drug to be used in a particular regimen.

The best way to describe the significance of the BSA is by comparing it to baking a loaf of bread. In the recipe for one loaf, the ingredients are 3 cups of flour, 2 cups of sugar, and 1 egg. If 10 loaves are to be baked, however, the formula (recipe) calls for 30 cups of flour, 20 cups of sugar, and 10 eggs. The total amount of ingredients is different, but the proportion remains the same.

How then do we calculate the body surface area? There is a complex formula using the log of the height and weight, or a nomogram chart can be used. Many pharmaceutical companies have BSA pocket calculators available. Some institutions have computers that are programmed to determine the BSA. In calculating the BSA, first determine the height and weight. Using a nomogram, draw a line connecting the two. The point at which the line crosses the center is the BSA. There is an ongoing debate as to whether the actual body weight or the ideal body weight should be used, because there is a difference in drug metabolism in the presence of fat. Most oncologists round off the BSA. A 10-lb (22-kg) change in weight changes the BSA, and it is therefore necessary to weigh the patient before each course of chemotherapy to determine whether an adjustment in the total dose is necessary to avoid overdosing or underdosing.

The basic formula for determining the chemotherapy dosage is as follows:

$$BSA \times mg/m^2 = total\ dose$$

If Adriamycin is ordered at 50 mg/m^2, 50 mg/m^2 times 1.6 BSA = 80 mg. Therefore, 80 mg is the dose for that treatment. If the patient had a 1.4 m^2 BSA, the formula would not change: 50 mg/m^2 times 1.4 BSA = 70 mg. Both these patients would be receiving the same dose in mg/m^2 but a different total number of milligrams.

This concept is particularly important with drugs that have an accumulated lifetime dose. Lifetime dosing is always calculated in mg/m^2. It is determined by adding the administered mg/m^2 of the drug for each course of chemotherapy that the patient has received. It is necessary to know whether the BSA was determined based on ideal body weight or actual weight.[3, 6, 15–17, 22, 23, 27]

SYMPTOM MANAGEMENT

Nausea and Vomiting

Nausea is one of the most common side effects of chemotherapy. For many patients it is the most distressing symptom that interferes with quality of life. Studies have shown that approximately 85% of all cancer patients receive chemotherapy as part of their treatment plan, and 70% of these patients experience nausea and vomiting. Only 10% of patients state that their nausea is very mild, 70% rate their nausea and vomiting as mild or moderate, 15% note that their nausea and vomiting are severe, 7% complain of very severe nausea and vomiting, and 3% find it intolerable.

Nausea is often regarded as benign and self-limiting but, to the patient experiencing this symptom, it is distressing. Nausea is described as a wave-like sensation in the epigastric area accompanied by tachycardia, weakness, dizziness, feeling hot, sweaty palms, hypersalivation, pallor and, frequently, the desire to vomit. Vomiting is an automatic response to nausea, which results in emptying the stomach through regurgitation.

Patients with a history of motion sickness or morning sickness seem to be more prone to chemotherapy-induced nausea and vomiting. Prior exposure to chemotherapy may stimulate anticipatory nausea and vomiting, and this seems to be more common in younger women. Merely entering the outpatient waiting room or hearing the sound of an IV pole may result in the patient's experiencing nausea.

Not all chemotherapeutic agents cause nausea, and the severity of the symptoms is different for each drug. Chemotherapy can be classified by its emetogenic capacity, which can range from little or no nausea to as high as 90% vomiting. Some chemotherapeutic agents also have delayed nausea and vomiting, which needs to be considered in prescribing antiemetics postdischarge.

Multiple assessment scales have been devised to measure nausea. Because of the subjective element, measurement is not always clear-cut. There are few animal studies dealing with nausea and vomiting, because animals cannot describe how they feel and most animals do not vomit.

Uncontrolled nausea and vomiting not only interfere with the quality of life, but can also cause potential life-threatening complications. Persistent nausea and vomiting result in nutritional deficits, decreased energy, and fluid and electrolyte imbalances.

The ideal pharmacologic intervention would control symptoms without contributing additional side effects. Antihistamines alone or in combination have been helpful in managing nausea. The most common antihistamine used is Benadryl, but many patients prefer Dramamine, Marezine, or Antivert.

Barbiturates can be helpful when there is an anxiety component. Historically, the phenothiazines, including Compazine, Torecan, Phenergan, and Thorazine, have been the most widely used antiemetics. The butyrophenones, Haldol and Inapsine, are strong dopamine antagonists. The cannabinoids, Marinol and THC, have mixed reviews. Many researchers have found that there is a relationship between their effectiveness and prior street drug experience. Steroids have been increasing in popularity for antiemetic control. It is believed that perhaps it is the blocking of prostaglandins that is the mechanism of action in this group of drugs, which includes Decadron and Solu-Medrol. Metoclopramide is a substituted benzamide drug that blocks dopamine stimulation and is a serotonin antagonist in high doses.

Two commonly used benzodiazepines are Valium and Ativan. Both depress the central nervous system, and Ativan minimizes nausea and vomiting by producing amnesia. Zofran is the newest antiemetic available and has markedly improved symptom management. It is a serotonin antagonist that has a minimal effect on dopamine and other neuroreceptors. This results in decreased side effects of sedation, agitation, and extrapyramidal reactions. The major side effect of Zofran is headache. It is available as an oral or intravenous preparation.[1–6, 8–10, 17, 18–22, 28–47]

Many of these drugs are used in combination because of their different actions and side effects. Most of the antiemetics cause sedation, and phenothiazines and metoclopramide can cause extrapyramidal reactions. A slow infusion frequently decreases or avoids these extrapyramidal reactions.

Ordering practices, combinations, dosing, and scheduling antiemetics vary greatly. Because no absolute method results in superior antiemetic control, this is fertile ground for ongoing research.

There are various methods used to administer these drugs. Many are given orally or IV but can also be given subcutaneously (SQ) or intramuscularly (IM). If the patient is unable to take anything orally, the rectal route is also an option.

Drugs such as Ativan have also been given sublingually, with good results.

It is easier to control nausea than vomiting, and it is better to have the patient sleep through chemotherapy than to be awake and nauseated. Patients frequently fear losing control or have an aversion to taking medications, and consequently delay asking for an antiemetic. The nurse has to use judgment and educate the patient who refuses to be medicated with an antiemetic.

Nausea intervention is an area in which the nurse has a lot of latitude and an opportunity for creativeness. It is helpful to obtain a nausea history and institute any intervention that may have been helpful in the past. Many patients find that cold foods or foods served at room temperature taste better and do not have as strong an odor as hot foods. Dry toast or crackers may help to settle the patient's stomach, especially first thing in the morning. Bland foods rather than spicy or strong-flavored foods are tolerated better. Clear liquids such as gelatin, juice, ginger ale or other carbonated beverages, and herb tea provide fluids to prevent dehydration. Sport drinks also furnish limited amounts of electrolytes. Sour or tart foods such as hard candy, dill pickles, or lemons are helpful. Foods that are known to increase nausea such as fried fatty foods or foods with a strong odor should be avoided.

Efforts should be made to control the environment. Soft, relaxing music, low lights, and a quiet atmosphere can be helpful. Some patients respond well to diversional activities such as card games, movies, or crafts. Relaxation tapes, hypnosis, and biofeedback have become more popular, and have good results.

Acupressure in the form of bracelets positioned on the wrist over the acupressure point that controls nausea is a noninvasive, nontoxic intervention. This is particularly helpful for the patient who is only slightly nauseated or who is reluctant to take antiemetics. Acupuncture has also been effective but is still highly regulated by governmental bodies.[48, 49]

The patient should be instructed to eat in a relaxed environment. Strong odors of food and perfume can trigger nausea. Opening covers on the food tray prior to entering the room allows the steam to escape in the hall, avoiding the sudden aroma of food near the patient.

Other nonpharmacologic interventions include having the patient suck on ice chips or a popsicle. Rinsing the mouth frequently with water, mouthwash, baking soda, saline solution, or lemon-flavored or mint-flavored water, helps decrease nausea. Frequent brushing of the teeth is also helpful, especially after an episode of emesis. As nurses, we have the responsibility to fine-tune our interventions continually to facilitate patient comfort.[3, 4, 6, 9, 10, 13, 17, 20–22, 31, 34–37, 45, 50–56]

Myelosuppression

Myelosuppression is the most common dose-limiting factor in chemotherapy administration. All chemotherapeutic agents have some effect on blood counts, but certain agents or a dose escalation can result in severe myelosuppression. Management of this potentially life-threatening side effect is paramount to patient care. Death in the myelosuppressed patient is usually the result of infection or bleeding. Patients need to be instructed in the importance of weekly blood counts so that appropriate intervention can be instituted as soon as possible. Patients also need to be aware that a drop in blood counts, especially WBCs, is expected and wanted. Doses of chemotherapy are escalated until myelosuppression is achieved. When myelosuppression is present, the patient needs to be aware of mechanisms to avoid infection when the WBC is depressed and to institute bleeding precautions in the face of thrombocytopenia. Activities of daily living may need to be adjusted to conserve energy when the hemoglobin and hematocrit values are low.

Patients who are the most likely to develop severe or prolonged myelosuppression are elderly patients with aplastic marrow. Patients who have bone marrow involvement, had prior radiation to the flat bones, or have been heavily pretreated with chemotherapy are particularly prone to hematologic problems. Patients who have diseased marrow with neoplastic infiltrates frequently experience pancytopenias until the marrow has been purged of the malignant cells.

Leukopenia and, more specifically, neutropenia predispose the patient to infection. An absolute granulocyte count, AGC (also referred to as total absolute neutrophil count, TANC, or absolute neutrophil count, ANC), of 1500 to 2000/mm³ puts the patient at a moderate risk for infection. Sometimes patients are placed on prophylactic antibiotics. An AGC lower than 500/mm³ places the patient at a severe risk of infection. These patients should be started on broad-spectrum antibiotics within 12 hours of a drop in the WBC. In the neutropenic patient, an elevated temperature may be the only sign of an infection. Antipyretics should be used with caution in these patients so as not to mask an infection.

Many of the necessary precautions may seem obvious to the health professional but may be foreign to the patient and family. Simple things like washing the hands after using the bathroom and staying away from crowds or other sources of infection can make a difference in the potential complications. The nurse should always be on the alert for sepsis, which in the neutropenic patient is an oncologic emergency.

The use of colony-stimulating factors (CSFs) has had an impact on the management of leukopenia. When used, these biologic agents shorten the nadir and facilitate timely chemotherapy treatments. The most common side effect of CSFs is a flu-like syndrome, which can include muscle and joint aches and sometimes an elevated temperature. Administrating the CSF just prior to retiring for the night and premedicating the patient with Tylenol and/or Benadryl can help reduce these side effects. It is important to determine whether the temperature is produced by an infection or by the biologic preparation.

Normally the platelet count ranges between 150,000 and 400,000/mm³. There is concern for the potential of bleeding when the count is below 100,000/mm³, and necessary precautions need to be taken. Presenting signs of a potential problem include bleeding gums, petechiae, nosebleeds, and multiple bruises. Spontaneous, frank bleeding usually does not occur until the platelet count is below 20,000/mm³. Thrombocytopenia places the patient at risk for CNS bleeding, as well as gastrointestinal bleeding. It has become controversial to transfuse a nonbleeding patient. Some authorities recommend holding transfusions until the patient shows signs of bleeding, whereas others transfuse a patient when the platelet count is below 20,000/mm³.

The patient should be protected from unnecessary bleeding risks. Shaving should be done with an electric razor rather than a blade. Care should be taken to avoid bruising during daily routine. Tampons should be avoided so as not to increase vaginal bleeding. Hazardous activity that may cause injury should be avoided, such as contact sports and working with sharp instruments. Vaginal and anal intercourse may cause bleeding, so other forms of intimacy should be explored during times of thrombocytopenia. Patients should be cautioned against using aspirin, ibuprofen, indomethacin, Coumadin, and quinidine and others that may interfere with clotting.

A differential diagnosis needs to be made in patients experiencing anemia, because many GI tumors bleed. Anemic patients may be asymptomatic or present with headache, dizziness, lightheadedness, shortness of breath, fatigue, pallor, hypothermia, and pale nail beds and conjunctiva. A patient is considered to be anemic if the hemoglobin level is lower than 8 g/dL. Many physicians do not transfuse if the patient is asymptomatic. One unit of RBCs can be expected to raise the hemoglobin level by 1 g/dL. In patients who have chronic anemia and in the absence of acute bleeding as the cause, erythropoietin can be effective in stimulating RBC production.

When fatigue is a factor, patients should be instructed to plan rest periods around activities so that they may enjoy the event. This is also the time to capitalize on assistance offered by friends and family. The patient should prioritize tasks and delegate chores in an effort to conserve energy. It is important that the patient be encouraged to be as active as possible and, at the same time, listen to their body and rest when tired.

Weekly CBCs are needed to adjust the dosage, depending on the nadir. The nadir is the point at which the blood counts are the lowest, and this usually occurs 7 to 14 days after day 1 of chemotherapy. Patients with bone marrow involvement from primary tumor burden or metastatic disease may have prolonged myelosuppression. Cell cycle-specific drugs, as a rule, have a swift nadir, with a rapid recovery. Non–cell cycle-specific drugs have a late nadir, with a delayed recovery. Mitomycin and carmustine frequently cause a second drop in the blood count, and the patient needs to be aware of this possibility.

Blood counts are particularly important just prior to administering chemotherapy, because bone marrow depression is the most significant dose-limiting factor. Chemotherapy may have to be delayed if adequate marrow recovery has not occurred. Subsequent doses of chemotherapy may be reduced if the drop in blood counts has been severe. Chemotherapy affects the stem cells in the bone marrow, which are rapidly dividing, rather than the cells in the circulation, which have already reached maturity. Most protocols require the WBC to be at least 3000/mm³ cells with an absolute granulocyte count of 1500.[2, 3, 5–7, 9, 10, 12–14, 19–21, 23, 34, 45, 53, 57–60]

Anorexia and Taste Alterations

Anorexia, fear of weight loss, and changes in taste pose a problem with adequate nutrition. The psychologic stressors of dealing with a life-threatening illness coupled with nausea, fatigue, and taste alterations from the treatment modalities and disease process itself are responsible for this problem.

Many of the treatments that the patient receives result in taste alterations. Dysgeusia, which is also referred to as taste blindness, is a condition in which the gustatory sense is impaired. This results in familiar foods tasting entirely different and, in some circumstances, unpleasant. Patients receiving cisplatin, Cytoxan, or vincristine frequently complain that nothing tastes right. Some patients experience a bitter or metallic taste. Most patients prefer to have their food served on glass dishes, and many use a plastic fork if they have a metallic taste in their mouth.

There is much that the nurse can do to help the patient and family members deal with this distressing symptom, including the following:

1. Carry out oral hygiene prior to meals.
2. Arrange food attractively.
3. Avoid strong odors.
4. Eat in a pleasant, relaxed environment.
5. Use pleasant odors, such as cloves.
6. Avoid noxious odors, such as fish.
7. Enhance food flavors with herbs, spices, or marinade.
8. Serve cold foods rather than hot foods.
9. Eat frequent, small meals.
10. Administer antiemetics prior to meals.
11. Drink power-packed shakes.
12. Serve food on glass dishes with plastic silverware.

Advise the patient that gum and hard candy, especially the sour types, are beneficial between meals. Instruct patients to brush their teeth frequently to help eliminate the unpleasant taste in their mouth. Sometimes rinsing the mouth with a nonirritating mouthwash makes them feel refreshed. These techniques are especially helpful prior to meals.

The patient and caregiver should be encouraged to experiment with different spices and flavorings. This is particularly important, because the taste buds have changed and need to be stimulated. This is an opportunity to experiment with new and different foods. Most patients find they have an aversion to meats, especially red meats, which usually have a bitter taste. Many foods have an exaggerated sweetness that can increase the patient's nausea. Patients should be made aware that the food is not spoiled, but rather their sense of taste is affected by the chemotherapy. Cold foods or foods served at room temperature are usually better tolerated than hot foods. Cold fruits and cheeses are frequently a better alternative to a hot meal. Many patients can tolerate multiple small meals rather than three large meals. The caregiver needs to be cognizant of the myth that patients must have three hot meals a day; in fact, they may do better with small cold meals that do not overwhelm them. Patients should be encouraged to eat, but never nagged or forced. Antiemetics and radiation to the head and neck cause the patient to experience xerostomia. Hard, dry food can cause discomfort and is difficult to swallow, whereas soft moist foods are more pleasing to the palate.

Depending on the patient's condition and severity of the symptoms, the patient may be a candidate for enteral or parenteral nutrition. Nutritional assessment, including a daily calorie count, indirect calorimetry, weight loss history, and viseral protein stores are factors in establishing criteria for intervention.[2, 6, 9, 10, 13, 20, 21, 34, 45, 51, 55, 57, 61, 62]

Constipation

It is important for individuals to know their particular bowel pattern. What is normal for one person may indicate a problem for another. Constipation is generally considered to be difficulty and discomfort in passing hard, dry stool. The severity of the problem can vary from mild discomfort to an ileus in more than 96 hours. Appropriate intervention should be implemented if 2 days have elapsed since the last bowel movement.

There are many causes for constipation other than chemotherapy. These include but are not limited to anxiety, depression, narcotics, muscle relaxants, hypercalcemia, immobility, dehydration, dietary deficiencies, and tumor involvement resulting in intrinsic or extrinsic compression. Intervention in part depends on the underlying cause which also must be addressed. Patients on narcotics frequently require prophylactic stool softeners, as do those receiving vincristine or vinblastine.

Management of the oncology patient is not the same as for the medical surgical patient. Enemas should be used with caution in the myelosuppressed patient; they can be irritating to the mucous membranes and can cause microscopic tears in the mucous membranes of the bowel. This can result in bleeding in the patient with a low platelet count and can be a source of infection in the neutropenic patient. In the event of an impaction, there may be no other alternative except to administer an enema. Usually, an oil retention enema or a phosphate enema is ordered to hydrate the stool. If an enema is used, care should be taken to be as gentle as possible.

Prophylactic intervention leads to greater patient comfort. Patients at risk for constipation should be instructed to increase their dietary intake of fresh fruits, vegetables, and fiber. Unless contraindicated, the patient should have at least 2 to 3 liters of fluids daily. Cheeses, eggs, refined starches, chocolate, candy, and foods that are known to be constipating should be avoided. Attempts to eat at the same time each day help regulate the patient. Because physical activity and exercise stimulate peristalsis, patients should be encouraged to be as active as tolerable. Patients should be instructed to respond to the urge to defecate immediately and not wait.

There are several oral and rectal preparations on the market today, which in many cases prevent or relieve constipation. Laxatives facilitate the evacuation of feces from the colon. These include stool softeners, cathartics, bulk laxatives, and lubricants. Bulk laxatives keep the stool soft and have been found to be helpful and gentle, and are therefore a good choice for the oncology patient.

Stool softeners cause fluid to shift into the colon, thereby preventing the stool from becoming dry and hard. Laxatives and cathartics stimulate peristalsis and move the waste through the intestinal system. Lubricants such as mineral oil and castor oil lubricate the colon and facilitate evacuation.[3, 5, 9, 10, 13, 19, 20–24, 34, 45, 62]

Diarrhea

Diarrhea is the abnormal passage of five or more loose or watery stools in a 24-hour period. Diarrhea might be accompanied by abdominal cramps and flatus. The GI tract produces up to 8 liters of fluid/day, and the colon reabsorbs the fluid and produces formed or semiformed stool.

Like constipation, there are many causes for diarrhea. Postoperative intestinal resection, inflammatory bowel syndrome, Clostridium difficile and other intestinal infections, malabsorption syndrome, and cancer-related treatments of chemotherapy, radiation, and biologic therapy can cause diarrhea.

The frequency, amount, and consistency of the stool constitute important information for grading the severity of the diarrhea. Patients with grade 3 diarrhea (six loose stools/day) are at risk for dehydration and electrolyte imbalance. Diarrhea has psychosocial ramifications and can be a source of embarrassment for the patient.

Nursing management includes patient teaching on the importance of early intervention as a method to avoid complications related to diarrhea. Patients should be instructed to increase their intake of constipating foods, such as cheese and eggs. Many patients have a lactose intolerance resulting in diarrhea, and consequently need to use caution with dairy products. Buttermilk and yogurt contain Lactobacillus and can usually be tolerated by these patients. Foods high in pectin, bulk, and fiber help slow down peristalsis. Fluid replacement prevents dehydration. Patients should avoid spicy foods, which irritate the GI tract. Fatty or greasy foods stimulate evacuation of the colon. Raw fruits and vegetables, nuts, caffeine, seeds, popcorn, and alcohol should also be avoided.

Nursing interventions also include recording intake and output accurately. The stool should be measured, if possible. The consistency and number of stools should be noted. Three or more stools/day (grade 2 diarrhea) is an indication for intervention. Patients need to have at least 2 liters of fluid/day. Because electrolytes are lost through the diarrhea, an electrolyte solution is recommended. Potassium is one of the major electrolytes lost, and, therefore, fluids and foods high in this mineral should be used. In cases of severe diarrhea, intravenous support is necessary.

Pharmacologic intervention should be started as soon as possible to avoid complications of fluid and electrolyte loss. Several medications available by prescription and over the counter are designed to control diarrhea. Bulk laxatives, in spite of the contradictory sound, have been helpful in controlling diarrhea by adding form to the loose stool.[2, 3, 5, 9–11, 21–23, 33, 34, 45, 62]

Alopecia

This side effect has many psychosocial ramifications and causes a great deal of stress. Alopecia is closely tied to self-image. Many patients experience depression when they start to lose their hair. It is traumatic for the patient to see their hair falling out in large bunches. Patients should be reminded that the hair loss is temporary when associated with chemotherapy. Postradiation alopecia may be permanent in doses exceeding 4000 rad. Many patients find that their hair is easier to manage if it is cut short. Other patients shave their heads when the hair starts to fall out. New growth occurs at a rate of about 0.25 inch/month. Frequently, the new hair is darker or with a reddish tint and curly.

Many patients are concerned that this hair loss will occur immediately, with the first drop of medication, but this is not the case. Not all chemotherapeutic agents cause total alopecia. There is usually some degree of hair thinning, which can vary in severity.

Recommendations for Thinning Hair

1. Wash hair regularly with mild shampoo.
2. Avoid using such appliances as curling irons, hot combs, and blow dryers.
3. Avoid hair styles that place tension on the hair, such as pony tails and braids.
4. Avoid chemicals, such as a permanent or coloring. If you should choose to perm or color your hair, have it done professionally, and tell your hair stylist that you are receiving chemotherapy.

Maximal alopecia usually occurs within 1 or 2 months. Patients therefore have an opportunity to buy a wig, hat, or scarf. When purchasing a wig, the patient needs to compensate for the fit when all the hair is gone. Purchasing a wig prior to balding allows for a closer match of color and style to the natural hair.

Wigs have a tendency to look darker because of the coarse texture; therefore, a wig appears more natural if a shade lighter than the natural hair color is selected. Some women choose to have fun with their wigs and regard alopecia as an opportunity to experiment with a different hair color, style, or length. Most insurance companies cover a prosthesis, but not a wig. However, if you get a prescription for a "cranial prosthesis," the charge is frequently reimbursed. If the insurance company does not pay for the wig, the patient can deduct the cost as a medical expense on their income taxes. Frequently, wigs may be obtained on loan from the local chapter of the American Cancer Society.

Care of the scalp should be the same as for any area of exposed skin. Patients should be instructed to bathe with a gentle soap. Lotion or a moisturizer helps keep the scalp from becoming dry but should not be used during radiation treatments to the head. The skin on the scalp is tender and burns if exposed to bright sun, so it needs to be protected. Scarves, turbans, or hats provide comfort and protection against the sun and heat loss in the winter.

The application of an ice cap or a tourniquet to the head reduces the flow of the chemotherapeutic agent to the skull. Some practitioners believe that this can minimize the hair loss, but this is considered to be an area of controversy. Many oncologists think that these interventions establish a sanctuary for the cancer cells and therefore do not use these methods. The decision for a tourniquet or an ice cap should take into consideration the presence of skin metastasis and/or bone lesions of the skull.[2, 3, 6, 9, 10, 20, 21, 45, 51, 53, 63–66]

Stomatitis and Mucositis

The mucous membranes of the gastrointestinal tract, especially those of the mouth, can become red, irritated, and inflamed. Stomatitis can range from a mild irritation and sensitivity when eating acidic or spicy foods to full-blown sores, with difficulty swallowing. Chemotherapy-related stomatitis usually begins 5 to 7 days post-treatment and lasts about 10 days.

Patients with poor dental hygiene are most likely to develop stomatitis. The following are predisposing factors:

1. Poor oral hygiene
2. Poor nutritional status
3. Head and neck radiation
4. Concurrent steroid therapy
5. High-dose chemotherapy

Patients who are nutritionally compromised or who have undergone head and neck radiation are more prone to develop stomatitis. Steroid use also increases the risk of stomatitis.

There is a considerable amount of nursing research in the area of prevention and palliation of stomatitis. Cryotherapy seems to be helpful in preventing stomatitis. Have the patient suck on ice chips 5 minutes prior to chemotherapy and 30 minutes after to help reduce the mucosal blood flow. A prophylactic mouthwash of allopurinol in patients receiving 5-FU or FUDR and a leucovorin mouthwash in patients receiving methotrexate have been beneficial.

Good oral hygiene is imperative in reducing the amount of bacteria in the mouth and decreasing the potential for infection. A soft toothbrush prevents further irritation to the delicate tissue. When the mouth is particularly tender, it is advisable for patients to remove their dentures or partial plate at night or, if possible, during the day.

Patients find that rinsing with a baking soda or saline solution is soothing to the mucous membranes. Sodium bicarbonate is a mucolytic agent that breaks up mucous secretions. There are many different formulas for a stomatitis cocktail. Most contain Benadryl, an antacid, and a local anesthetic. Sometimes an antifungal such as nystatin is also included. A stomatitis cocktail is generally taken as a swish, swirl, and swallow, and is usually ordered before meals, at bedtime, and as needed. Most commercial mouthwashes contain alcohol, which can burn the delicate mucous membranes, and thus should be avoided.

The patient should be instructed to eat soft foods with a smooth consistency. Usually, cold, wet foods are soothing to the irritated mucous membranes. Special attention should also be given to the lips to prevent cracking and drying. Applying lip balm, aloe vera, or a petroleum-based gel keeps the lips moist and promotes comfort and healing. Care should be taken to provide adequate nutrition and hydration. In cases of severe stomatitis, the patient may need to be hospitalized for fluid support and pain management.[3, 5, 9, 10, 13, 20, 21, 34, 38, 45, 62, 67–74]

Cardiac Toxicity

The side effect that causes the patient the greatest amount of psychologic distress is the cardiotoxicity that can result with the anthracyclines, especially Adriamycin. It is a dilemma for patients to be told that an effective drug for their cancer can damage their heart. Since Adriamycin became commercially available in the 1970s, we have learned a great deal about this drug and its analogues.

Early signs of cardiotoxicity are difficult to detect. An electrocardiogram (ECG) may show a decrease in voltage of the QRS complex or nonspecific ST- or T-wave changes. The anthracyclines can damage the myocytes, which weaken the cardiac muscle. This results in a decreased cardiac output, with progression to congestive heart failure. The patient usually is asymptomatic until signs and symptoms of congestive heart failure appear. Patients complain of shortness of breath, especially on exertion, and a nonproductive cough. The physical examination shows neck vein distention, tachycardia, gallop rhythm, and edema.

Researchers have learned how to monitor for impending cardiopathy with a muga scan or an echocardiogram with an ejection fraction. A drop in the baseline ejection fraction signals a decrease in left ventricular function. In these situations, the risk of cardiac damage and complications must be weighed against a meaningful tumor response. Most physicians obtain a baseline muga scan or an echocardiogram with an ejection fraction and repeat these tests at the halfway point of the total accumulated lifetime dose and at the end of therapy. Frequent ECG monitoring to detect changes in the voltage of the QRS helps identify early signs of impending toxicity. In selected patients, a percutaneous endomyocardial biopsy is indicated to determine the degree of myocyte damage.

Studies have shown that young people who do not have hypertension, arteriosclerotic heart disease (ASHD), or other coronary artery disease tolerate this drug much better. Prior radiation to the mediastinum or left chest wall appears to be a risk factor. The lifetime cumulative dose of Adriamycin is 500 to 550 mg/m². Since the late 1980s, some interesting data have demonstrated a dramatic decrease in cardiac damage when the drug is given by infusion rather than the push method.

Taxol, mitoxantrone, idarubicin, Cytoxan, 5-FU, and FUDR also have the potential of producing cardiac problems. Some studies have shown that cardiac toxicity potential from Adriamycin is increased with Cytoxan. This appears to be particularly true in the bone marrow transplant patient who receives high-dose Cytoxan.[3, 7, 10, 16, 20, 21, 24, 59, 75, 76]

Neurotoxicity

Neurotoxicity can be seen as either central or peripheral. Central nervous system toxicity can be an acute or chronic encephalopathy. Peripheral toxicity causes axonal degeneration or demyelination.

Taxol, cisplatin, carboplatin, and the vinca alkaloids are the agents most likely to cause neurotoxicity. Peripheral toxicity usually does not occur until some time after five or more treatments. The exception to this is taxol, which can produce paresthesia within 5 days of administration. When cisplatin is used concurrently with taxol, the patient has an increased potential for neurotoxicity. Patients usually complain of numbness and tingling of the hands and feet. As the toxicity increases, the patient begins to complain of muscle pain, weakness, and disturbances in depth perception, particularly with ambulation. This can result in safety issues. Patients need to be cautioned about loose rugs, steps, and articles lying on the floor that may cause the patient to trip. Patients need to be careful in handling sharp implements when cooking or shaving. Beverages should not be filled to the top of the glass to avoid spilling.

Because there is a decrease in sensation, the patient needs to exercise caution with temperature changes. Hot water, heating pads, electric blankets, hot stoves, and radiators are more likely to cause burns with decreased perception of temperature. Exposure to cold is also a concern, because these patients are less likely to realize the severity of the temperature. Patients should be adequately dressed for the weather, with special protection for the hands and feet. Double gloves and extra heavy socks help prevent frostbite.

Constipation and paralytic ileus are other concerns in this patient population. Symptoms can be manifested within 2 days, and this is particularly true in patients receiving the vinca alkaloids. Vincristine has good tissue binding capacity, which results in prolonged exposure of the neural tissue. The patient should be observed for abdominal distention and active bowel sounds, and the diet regulated according to patient needs, adding fresh fruits and vegetables, fiber, and fluids. Constipation can be compounded in the patient who is also receiving concurrent narcotics. In this patient population, prophylactic stool softeners can assist in maintaining regularity. Suppositories, oral laxatives, or lubricants may be used. Enemas should be used with caution in the neutropenic patient. Depending on the severity, symptoms of neuropathy usually disappear in a few weeks. If treatment continues, there may not be a return of deep tendon reflexes, and muscle weakness may be a problem for many months. In severe cases, motor function may never return to normal.[3, 7, 10, 13, 16, 20, 21, 77–79]

Renal Toxicity

Renal toxicity is defined as an elevation of the blood urea nitrogen (BUN) and creatinine levels. The chemotherapeutic agents most notorious for causing renal damage are cisplatin, methotrexate, mitomycin C and, to a lesser degree, carboplatin. Caution needs to be taken to protect the patient from this potentially life-threatening complication. Baseline laboratory values of the BUN and creatinine levels need to be obtained prior to administration of these renal toxic agents. A 12- or 24-hour urine creatinine clearance test provides additional information regarding the status of the kidneys.

In the presence of renal compromise, the risk versus benefit ratio must be carefully weighed. Renal toxic chemotherapy that could produce a meaningful tumor response may need to have doses reduced to protect the patient from further renal damage and to compensate for the longer half-life resulting from poor renal function.

Prior to the administration of these nephrotoxic chemotherapeutic agents, vigorous hydration is frequently ordered. Sometimes hypertonic saline is used to maintain high renal flow. Mannitol and Lasix may also be ordered in an effort to flush out the kidneys. Accurate intake and output as well as frequent weights must be recorded. Signs of fluid retention or imbalance should be reported to the physician. Early detection of renal compromise can avert the need for hemodialysis or peritoneal dialysis. This complication is serious and can in some circumstances be considered malpractice.

Methotrexate precipitates in an acid solution, thereby plugging the renal tubules. Raising the urinary pH can be accomplished by administering an alkylating agent to the patient prior to high-dose methotrexate in the form of bicarbonate orally or intravenously. Measurement of the urinary pH is frequently ordered to ensure that the pH is greater than 7. If the pH drops below 7, additional bicarbonate is given.

The risk of hyperuricemia from tumor lysis syndrome is another factor that needs to be considered when administering nephrotoxic drugs. Alkalizing the urine prevents the precipitation of uric acid crystals in the renal tubules, and the administration of allopurinol helps prevent the formation of uric acid crystals. These prophylactic measures usually begin 12 to 24 hours prior to chemotherapy.

The nurse needs to be aware of any concurrent nephrotoxic drugs that the patient may be receiving. Amphotericin, the aminoglycoside antibiotics, and vitamin C all have the potential of potentiating nephrotoxicity.[3, 5, 7, 10, 16, 20, 21, 59, 80–82]

Pulmonary Toxicity

Pulmonary toxicity is damage to the endothelial cells of the lung and results in pneumonitis and interstitial fibrosis, which has been seen in select patients receiving specific chemotherapy agents. Bleomycin in doses exceeding 250 units/m^2 or 400 units total dose and carmustine in total doses of 1500 mg/m^2 predispose the patient to pulmonary toxicity. Toxicity appears to be increased with the concurrent use of Cytoxan. Other antineoplastics known to be responsible for pulmonary toxicity include mitomycin, methotrexate, melphalan, procarbazine, and busulfan.

The patient usually presents with a dry hacking cough and complains of dyspnea, especially on exertion. Auscultation of the lungs reveals fine rales. The chest x-ray is nonspecific or has streaky infiltrates and consolidation. Elderly patients, patients with a smoking history, and patients with a preexisting pulmonary condition appear to be at greater risk for pulmonary toxicity.

A baseline pulmonary function test assists with the early detection of pulmonary toxicity. At the first sign of complications, the offending drug should be stopped. Some studies have shown that the administration of Decadron prior to giving mitomycin C prevents pulmonary toxicity. Steroids have also been useful in the symptomatic relief of pulmonary toxicity.[3, 7, 10, 16, 20, 21, 56, 83, 84]

Gonadal Dysfunction

Cells that are rapidly dividing are most sensitive to chemotherapy. Therefore, functions of the ovaries and testicles are affected by many chemotherapeutic agents. This is particularly true of the alkylating agents.

There is frequently a reduction in the sperm count, resulting in infertility that can be temporary or permanent. It is recommended that the option of sperm banking be presented to the patient prior to the initiation of chemotherapy, especially in younger men. Many men have difficulty achieving an erection while on chemotherapy. This can interfere with a sense of well-being and self-esteem, because the sexual drive remains intact. Currently, there are several devices available to assist men in obtaining and maintaining an erection. In select patients, medications may be ordered to be self-injected into the penis. In patients with persistent problems, a penile implant may be an option. This is especially true in patients who have had hormonal manipulation.

Chemotherapy can suppress ovarian function. Within 6 months of starting chemotherapy, women frequently experience amenorrhea or changes in their menstrual cycle during treatment. Many women have symptoms of a medical menopause, including hot flashes, irritability, insomnia, and vaginal dryness. The use of a water-soluble lubricant relieves some of the symptoms of vaginal dryness. Women who are over 40 frequently do not have return of their menstrual cycle on completion of their chemotherapy. The use of estrogen replacement or estrogen-containing vaginal creams is controversial, especially in hormone-dependent tumors such as breast cancer.

Couples should practice birth control for 1 to 2 years postchemotherapy. The literature has documented healthy live births to couples who have had chemotherapy. There does not seem to be an increase in birth defects, chromosomal abnormalities, or spontaneous miscarriages in couples in whom one person has been exposed to chemotherapy.[2, 3, 7, 10, 16, 20, 21, 64, 85–89]

Extravasation

Frequently, the terms "extravasation" and "infiltration" are used interchangeably. The Intravenous Nurses Society describes an infiltration as an inadvertent administration of a nonvesicant into the surrounding tissue. Extravasation is defined as an inadvertent delivery of a vesicant into the tissues. Vesicants cause blistering, severe tissue damage, and even necrosis if extravasated.[104]

An irritant can cause local sensitivity and should not be confused with an extravasation. Chemotherapeutic agents can be irritants. A vesicant is also an irritant, but in this case the intensity of the irritating action has become so severe that plasma escapes from the extracellular space and blisters are formed. The word extravasation is rooted in the Latin word *vesicare*, which means to blister.

Extravasation can affect multiple areas and its ramifications can significantly impinge on patient outcome. Some consequences of extravasation are as follows:

1. Patient discomfort and physical impairment: débridements, skin grafts, amputation
2. Stress and concern for patient, family, and staff
3. Increased workload for staff
4. Prolonged treatment time for patient
5. Delay in appropriate cancer treatment for patient
6. Increased cost resulting from increased hospitalization, surgery, antidotes, increased staff time, potential liability

When fluid leaks into the tissue, the tissue is compressed because of restriction of the blood flow, which decreases the amount of oxygen to the site and thus lowers the cellular pH. There is a loss of capillary wall integrity, increase in edema and, depending on severity, eventual cell death. It has been suggested that there are more extravasations in children than adults because of their smaller and more restrictive veins, which are more prone to venous constriction.

It is important not to confuse a "flare" with an extravasation. A flare is an erythematous streaking along the vein and patchy local urticaria. A flare usually disappears in 1 to 2 hours and rarely lasts longer than 12 to 24 hours. Flares are generally associated with the infusion of hypotonic solutions. It is important to remember that a flare is not associated with an infiltration or allergic reaction.

There are few absolutes in the treatment of extravasations. Many controversies are clouded by lack of or contradictory scientific information, combined with personal opinion and experience. It is difficult to do controlled studies on extravasations because of ethical issues of using a no-treatment arm of a research protocol. The second issue is the problem of acquiring large numbers of patients to obtain meaningful results. This patient accrual problem is mainly the result of the low incidence of extravasation because of having quality IV therapy nurses. The incidence of extravasation is 0.55%. The standard threshold of anything less than 1% is considered to be acceptable.

The area of the greatest controversy regards the use of steroids and antidotes. A wide variety of drugs have been used in an effort to reduce the trauma of an extravasation and promote healing. Some chemotherapeutic agents have specific antidotes.

Many authorities believe that there is no rationale for using sodium bicarbonate in an Adriamycin extravasation. The theory behind sodium bicarbonate is to alter the pH in an effort to interfere with the bonding of Adriamycin in the cells. A second theory of using bicarbonate is that it cleaves the glycolytic bond in the Adriamycin molecule, leaving an inactive aglycone molecule. There is a question as to whether this course of action has a dilution effect rather than being an actual chemical change. If this is true, then the drug is distributed over a larger area and the injury is increased.

Because some of the chemotherapeutic agents produce free radicals, it has been theorized that DMSO might work by scavenging, thereby creating a beneficial effect. Results are conflicting and, for the most part, studies have been nonreproducible. Propranolol and isoproterenol have been shown to be of some help in mice studies by altering blood flow, but have not been of any significance in humans. Heparin has been tried unsuccessfully with Adriamycin in the hope of precipitating the drug. The use of lidocaine, Mucomyst, Benadryl, and Tagamet made the extravasation worse. There have also been trials using glutathione, L-carnitine, coenzyme Q, triamcidolene, cysteine, WR-2721, and vitamin E, all without any meaningful results.

An oversimplification of the chemistry of an extravasation divides drugs into two categories, those that bind to DNA and those that do not. The drugs that do not bind to DNA cause immediate damage but are quickly metabolized or inactivated. This type of injury is similar to a burn in which the damage is immediate, followed by repair using the normal healing process.

For a small extravasation, conservative treatment is indicated. Large extravasations may lead to contractures, the need for débridement and grafting and, in severe cases, amputation.

The vinca alkaloids do not bind to DNA but inhibit mitosis. Ulceration from these drugs is usually less severe than from the binding drugs. Ulcers from the vinca alkaloids are similar to those from anthracycline but they do not tend to erode to deeper structures, and healing usually occurs in 3 to 5 weeks without surgical intervention.

The instillation of hyaluronidase (Wydase) interdermally or subcutaneously with a 25-gauge needle around the infiltration site is the treatment of choice for a vinca alkaloid extravasation. Wydase is a protein enzyme obtained from testicular tissue and is used to increase the absorption of fluids from hyperdermoclysis. Wydase destroys tissue cement, which helps decrease or prevent injury by allowing for the rapid diffusion of extravasated fluid and rapid reabsorption. The injury is minimized, even though the drug is spread over a larger area.

The second class of drugs are those that bind to DNA and not only cause immediate damage but lodge in the tissue, producing a prolonged effect. Because of this binding effect, the cells lose their ability to heal spontaneously. Electron microscopy demonstrates chronic fibroblast disorganization and a delayed myofibroblastic appearance, which suggests that fibro stem cells are unable to replicate and reproduce.

Drugs that bind to DNA include the alkylating agent nitrogen mustard, which rapidly fixes to tissue and causes immediate injury. The vein irritation can progress over several days to a dark bluish gray color. Applying cold compresses for 6 to 12 hours is recommended, and sodium thiosulfate injected into the infiltration site is the suggested treatment. This compound is used intravenously as an antidote for cyanide poisoning and for prophylaxis of ringworm.

Other chemotherapeutic agents that bind to DNA are in the antibiotic family. Because Adriamycin is one of the most widely used chemotherapeutic agents, it has the largest database of information concerning extravasation. Animal studies have shown a relationship between the Adriamycin concentration and the degree of ulceration. Surgical intervention is recommended, especially with Adriamycin, when the lesion is greater than 2 cm or if there is significant residual pain 1 to 2 weeks postextravasation. There is no benefit in surgical excision if no ulceration has occurred unless there is persistent, severe pain. Once necrosis appears, surgical débridement is necessary. If the lesion is not débrided, it can progress to a thick, leathery eschar surrounded by a 2- to 3-cm rim of red, painful skin. The amount of blood in the insulted tissue determines the degree of ulceration.

The eschar usually does not slough spontaneously, and when it is removed, deep subcutaneous, necrotic tissue is found. Depending on the location, tendons may also be necrotic, resulting in deformities, extensive joint stiffness, neuropathy, and causalgia. A wide excision of the entire necrotic and reddened area of the insult by the residual active drug can salvage deep structures and retain function. It is wiser to sacrifice tendons and accept some degree of functional deficit in exchange for improved wound healing and resolution of pain. Active drug has been isolated from the wound as long as 3 months after an extravasation and up to 5 months post-Adriamycin infiltration. An ulceration containing Adriamycin glows a dull red under ultraviolet light.

Mitomycin ulcers are typically deep and expansive and require a wide excision with split-thickness grafting. Because mitomycin is also an irritant, dilution of the drug can help reduce the degree of irritation.

Extravasation Precautions

These include the following:

1. Educate the patient to report any sensation change. Mon-
itor closely for signs of pain, especially in patients who cannot verbalize discomfort. Be particularly alert for complaints of stinging or burning, which are usually the first sign of an extravasation.
2. Assess the venipuncture site. Check for signs of edema or bleb formation.
3. Look for signs of infiltration, including slowing or cessation of drops or flow from the IV solution, increased resistance when administering the drug, and poor blood return when rechecking needle placement.
4. When in doubt, stop the infusion and restart the IV.
5. Notify the physician of the extravasation.

Extravasation Management

1. If an extravasation is suspected, stop the infusion immediately and evaluate for swelling and blood return. If there is any doubt about the patency of the vein, start a new line.
2. Aspirate before removing the line. Studies have shown that there is a decrease in the size of the lesion with aspiration alone.
3. Apply ice, not heat, for 24 to 48 hours (use heat for vinblastine or vincristine). Different schedules are recommended. Some experts specify 15 minutes qid, whereas others prefer 30 minutes. Ice causes vasoconstriction, decreases local drug uptake, especially with Adriamycin, decreases edema, and slows the metabolic rate of cells. Decreased local blood supply and the cooling effect may decrease local pain. Heat causes vasodilation, facilitates fluid absorption, and may enhance drug absorption, but it also increases metabolic demand of the tissue. Heat and Adriamycin work synergistically, which has an adverse effect on extravasation. Studies have shown that ulcers were four times larger in the presence of hot packs than in the unheated controls. Treatment of extravasations from the vinca alkaloids is the only time when heat is recommended rather than cold.
4. Elevate the extremity. Larson found that, in 115 patients with extravasation of Adriamycin, only 11% experienced ulceration after applying ice and elevating the extremity.
5. Administer the antidote with the needle in place or remove the needle and inject around the infiltration site. Hospitals should have a policy that specifies the administration of a specific antidote.
6. Encourage the patient to resume normal activity with the arm to prevent stiffness and discomfort.
7. Notify the physician and obtain specific orders and/or an antidote.
8. Record the episode. Documentation should include the date and time of extravasation, the needle size, and the type of cannula used. Describe the insertion site and whether it was a new start or an existing IV. The drug sequence is important. Sometimes there is a delayed reaction and it is important to know the order in which the drugs were given. Note the drug administration technique, and whether it was a continuous infusion, a side-arm technique, or a push dose. The amount of extravasation is particularly important with drugs that bind to DNA. Note the intervention that was used. A photograph should be taken at the time of injury and at 24 hours, 48

hours, and 1 week. Have the patient describe the experience and sensation.

9. Describe the appearance of the site. Note whether it is pale, reddened, streaked, or edematous. Document that the physician was notified. In many institutions, a plastic surgeon is called by the primary physician at the time of an Adriamycin extravasation to start immediate planning for management of the injury and early assessment of the surgical potential.

10. Notify the risk manager or other appropriate individuals in the institution.[3, 5, 9, 19–22, 26, 45, 75, 90–110]

CHEMOTHERAPEUTIC AGENTS

Antimetabolites

The antimetabolites have their major activity in the S phase of the cell cycle. They inhibit protein synthesis and deceive cells with erroneous metabolites of a structural analogue. The antimetabolites are antagonistic to folic acid, purine, and pyrimidine by competing for the catalytic site of a necessary enzyme. They are cell cycle-specific. Their major toxicities are hematopoietic and gastrointestinal.[3, 6, 9, 16, 19–23, 68]

Methotrexate

Methotrexate (MTX; Amethopterin; Mexate; Folex) is a folic acid antagonist that interferes with purine and thymidylate synthesis. It is cell cycle-specific in the S phase, and is used in combination with other drugs or as a single agent. Methotrexate has activity against a large number of cancers, including ALL, lymphoma, sarcoma, choriocarcinoma, and breast, lung, head, and neck cancers.

There is a wide dosage range for methotrexate. It can be given as a standard dose of 25 to 50 mg/m^2 every week, every month, or twice a month. High doses of methotrexate range from 1 to 10 g/m^2 as a 12-, 24-, or 48-hour infusion. Methotrexate is also given by the PO, IM, or intrathecal route. Intrathecal doses are usually 10 to 15 mg total, and must be mixed in a preservative-free solution.

Methotrexate can crystallize and precipitate in acidic solution and can cause renal damage in the presence of urine with a low pH. This is particularly true with high-dose methotrexate.

It is recommended that sodium bicarbonate be given PO or IV prior to high-dose methotrexate administration, to neutralize the urine. Depending on the specific regimen, bicarbonate is usually given to keep the urinary pH higher than 7. Because of a 10% potential for renal toxicity, the BUN and creatinine levels should be checked to ensure adequate kidney function prior to the administration of methotrexate. Hydrating fluid is usually given prior to and after methotrexate dosing. The patient needs to be encouraged to increase oral fluids, and the fluid balance should be monitored.

Antiemetics are given prior to methotrexate to control the nausea associated with this drug. Slowing the rate of infusion and using large volumes of fluid to dilute the drug can also be helpful in managing nausea. As with all the antineoplastics that induce nausea and vomiting, improved control can be obtained with prophylactic antiemetic use rather than when symptoms occur.

A methotrexate nadir usually occurs in 5 to 14 days post-treatment. When high doses of methotrexate are administered, leucovorin (folinic acid) is usually given as a rescue 24 to 36 hours after the administration of the drug. Leucovorin is available in oral and intravenous forms. The dosage and frequency of leucovorin are determined by the BUN, creatinine, and serum methotrexate levels. An increase in the BUN and serum creatinine levels decreases the clearance of methotrexate, resulting in elevated serum methotrexate levels and decreased drug clearance. When this occurs, the physician generally increases the leucovorin dose and uses more vigorous hydration. The purpose of the leucovorin is to stop the action of the methotrexate, thereby preventing severe bone marrow toxicity.

Stomatitis and esophagitis occurring on day 5 to 14 can range from mild irritation and tenderness with sensitivity to spicy or acidic foods to full-blown, painful sores. The stomatitis can interfere with eating and swallowing. Some studies have shown that a mouthwash with leucovorin immediately following methotrexate administration is helpful in stomatitis prevention.

An elevation in liver function tests has also been seen, particularly when methotrexate is given on a weekly basis versus every 21 to 28 days. With prolonged use of methotrexate, hepatic fibrosis and occasionally cirrhosis can develop.

Methotrexate can also cause some photosensitivity. The patient's skin has an increased tendency to burn if exposed to bright, intense sunlight. Patients do not have to avoid the sun completely. It is recommended that the patient cover the exposed skin or use a good sunscreen when at risk for sunburn. Radiation recall has been seen with this drug.

Methotrexate given prior to 5-fluorouracil (5-FU) increases 5-FU nucleotide formation. The cytotoxic activity of methotrexate may be inhibited by L-asparaginase, so these drugs should be properly spaced if used concurrently.[6, 10, 13, 16–18, 22, 24, 33, 45, 57, 58, 62, 75, 84]

5-Fluorouracil

Another antimetabolite is 5-fluorouracil and its analogue FUDR (fluorouracil; Adrucil; 5-FU; FUDR; floxuridine; 5-FUDR; 5-fluoro-2-deoxyuridine). These drugs inhibit RNA function through direct incorporation into DNA. Methotrexate, when given first, may increase the biologic effect of 5-FU. Fluorouracil has a short half-life of 10 to 30 minutes, with no detectable drug after 3 hours, but intracellular concentrations persist for many hours. These drugs are used in the treatment of colon, breast, stomach, esophagus, pancreas, prostate, and ovarian cancers.

There are multiple drug regimens using 5-fluorouracil that include drug combinations or 5-FU as a single agent. These drugs can be administered by IV bolus or as a 2-, 12-, or 24-hour continuous infusion. Depending on the specific tumor type and treatment protocol, the patient may receive 1 to 5 days of therapy.

The usual dose-limiting toxicities of 5-fluorouracil and FUDR are stomatitis and diarrhea. Depending on the severity of these side effects, the last dose or two may be withheld. It is important to document not only that the patient has diarrhea but also the number of stools daily. Most institutions use the ECOG (Eastern Cooperative Oncology Group) toxicity scale or a similar grading system. Allopurinol ties up 5-fluorouracil and FUDR and therefore should not be given with these drugs. However, a mouthwash made with allopurinol and administered as a swish, swirl, and spit helps prevent stomatitis, which can occur by day 4.

Leukopenia usually occurs by day 9 to 14 but could occur as late as day 20. Nausea and vomiting are usually not seen with these drugs but, as with all chemotherapy, this is patient-specific. A significant number of patients develop conjunctivitis, and/or hypo- or hyperlacrimal secretion. Liquid tears is helpful to alleviate these symptoms. Like methotrexate, these drugs can cause photosensitivity, so necessary precautions must be instituted.

5-Fluorouracil and FUDR can also cause skin toxicities that result in swelling and/or peeling of the hands and sometimes the feet. This is frequently referred to as foot-and-hand syndrome or plantar-palmar syndrome. The patient can experience a great deal of distress. The local application of creams or lotions and the administration of Benadryl or vitamin B_6 can be helpful. When these drugs are given through a peripheral vein, there can be hyperpigmentation along the vein. It is thought that this may be the result of increased levels of melanin-stimulating hormone. Cutaneous changes usually begin 2 to 3 weeks after the start of chemotherapy and continue for 10 to 12 weeks after the completion of treatment.

5-Fluorouracil is supplied in 500-mg vials, which can be stored at room temperature but should be protected from light. Discoloration does not affect the potency. 5-Fluorouracil precipitates at low temperatures but can be resuspended in a warm water bath with shaking.

FUDR is supplied in 500-mg vials and, when reconstituted with 5 ml of sterile water, is stable for 2 weeks when refrigerated. FUDR can be given without further dilution or mixed with 5% dextrose in water or 0.9% sodium chloride.

There are multiple dosing schedules for these drugs. 5-FU has been prescribed IV in the following dosages:

1. 500 mg/m² every day times 5 days every 21 to 28 days
2. 500 mg/m² every week
3. 1000 mg/m² every week
4. 500 to 1500 mg/m² every day times 5 days over 12 hours, or 24 hours every 3 to 4 weeks
5. 400 mg/m², continuous infusion

Intra-arterial 5-FU dosing also varies extensively:

1. 22.5 mg/kg every day times 5 to 21 days
2. 500 to 800 mg/m² every day times 5 days, continuous infusion
3. 100 mg/m² every day times 14 days, continuous infusion

Traditionally, FUDR was used only as an intra-arterial infusion for tumor involving the liver. New ways of using this drug include IV administration. Currently, leucovorin and levamisole are being studied for use as a modulator with intravenous 5-fluorouracil or FUDR. Responses have been seen in tumors that were previously resistant. IV dosing for FUDR is 500 to 750 mg/m² every day times 5 days. Intra-arterial dosing of FUDR is 100 mg/m² every day times 5 days or 0.3 mg/kg/day continuous infusion times 14 days.[3, 10, 13, 16–18, 22–24, 33, 45, 62, 80]

Ara-C

Ara-C (cytarabine; Cytosar-U; cytosine; arabinoside; arabinosyl cystosine) is derived from the cryptothethyacrypta sponge. Ara-C is a pyrimidine analogue that inhibits DNA polymerase and therefore inhibits DNA synthesis. Ara-C is a cell cycle-specific antimetabolite with its action during the S phase, at which time it is incorporated into the DNA molecule. This drug has a short half-life of only 7 to 20 minutes when standard doses are administered and 3 to 6 hours when high-dose ara-C is given. Ara-C is activated by liver enzymes. The organ of excretion is the kidneys, with 4 to 10% of the drug excreted unchanged. Although most commonly used in the treatment of the hematologic malignancies of leukemia, lymphoma, and Hodgkin's disease, ara-C has demonstrated effectiveness in head and neck cancer.

Freeze-dried ara-C can be mixed with bacteriostatic water with benzyl alcohol and further diluted with normal saline or 5% dextrose in water. Ara-C is stable at room temperature for 48 hours but should be discarded if it becomes hazy. If used for intrathecal administration, it must be mixed with a preservative-free solution. In addition to the intrathecal route, ara-C can be administered by the intravenous and subcutaneous routes.

Intravenous dosing is usually 100 mg/m² as a continuous infusion for 5 to 10 days. Ara-C can also be given as an IV bolus dose or subcutaneous injection of 100 mg/m² every 12 hours for 7 to 21 days. Intrathecal doses are 20 to 30 mg/m² for 4 days or 75 mg/m² every fourth day until the CSF is normal. Doses of 3 g/m² are considered to be high. Ara-C should be administered over 10 to 20 minutes unless the dose is over 1 g, in which case the infusion should be given over at least 2 hours.

Because of the potential of tumor lysis syndrome in patients with hematologic malignancies, uric acid levels must be carefully monitored and appropriate intervention of hydration and allopurinol implemented. About 50% of patients receiving ara-C experience loss of appetite, nausea, and vomiting. A drop in the WBC is expected, with a nadir usually occurring on day 7 to 14, and neutropenia and thrombocytopenia precautions should be instituted. Pancytopenia is not uncommon. A small percentage of patients experience mild and reversible hepatic dysfunction with elevated liver function tests (LFTs). Caution is advised when ordering this drug for patients with hepatic compromise. Mild stomatitis and diarrhea have also been seen.

Neurologic toxicity includes dizziness, lethargy, and somnolence, especially if ara-C is infused too rapidly. Some patients have experienced paraplegia, necrotizing leukoencephalopathy, and cerebellar toxicity, with difficulty in balance. Ara-C administered intrathecally can cause paresthesia.

It is not uncommon for patients to have a flu-like syndrome consisting of muscular aches, bone pain, low-grade temperature, headache, loss of appetite, and diarrhea.

Conjunctivitis is most frequently seen when the patient receives high-dose ara-C, but it can also occur at lower doses. It is believed that the keratitis is the result of the inhibition of DNA synthesis of the corneal epithelium. Treatment for this eye irritation includes Decadron eye drops. Protecting the eyes from bright lights and the application of ice help relieve some of the discomfort.

Ara-C is one of the antineoplastic agents known to cause

cutaneous toxicity. The literature reports that between 3 and 72% of patients receiving ara-C have some degree of skin reaction. This is more frequently seen in patients receiving high doses of ara-C. The patient may experience acral erythema associated with palmar-plantar syndrome or a generalized cutaneous reaction. Symptoms range from swelling and erythema to bullae formation and desquamation. The presenting symptoms are tingling of the hands and feet, which progress to edema and pain. Symptomatic treatment consists of the application of cold, elevation of the affected limb, application of soothing lotions, and the use of systemic and local steroids.[6, 15–17, 22, 24, 45, 59, 77, 78, 111–113]

Vinca and Plant Alkaloids

The vinca alkaloids belong to a broader category of plant alkaloids, which includes the podophyllotoxins and the Taxus family. They are mitotic inhibitors. The vinca alkaloids are derived from the periwinkle plant and have their medicinal benefit based in folklore. Their cytotoxic effects were recognized during studies of antidiabetic drugs. The primary method of action of the vinca alkaloids is binding to microtubular proteins that crystallize the mitotic spindles, resulting in metaphase arrest. They also inhibit RNA and protein synthesis.[3, 6, 9, 16, 17, 20–23, 68, 114]

Vinblastine and Vincristine

Vinblastine (Velban; VLB) and vincristine (Oncovin; VCR) are vinca alkaloids derived from the periwinkle plant and differ only in a side chain on the molecular level. These drugs are cell cycle-specific and affect mitosis. They are active in the treatment of ALL, Hodgkin's disease, lymphoma, rhabdomyosarcoma, neuroblastoma, Wilms' tumor, choriocarcinoma, Kaposi's sarcoma, and testicular and breast carcinoma.

One of the dose-limiting side effects is neurotoxicity, and the first sign is loss of the Achilles tendon reflex. The most common dose-related problem associated with these drugs is severe constipation and, at times, paralytic ileus resulting from neurotoxicity of the smooth muscles of the gastrointestinal tract. Patients prone to constipation may need to increase their fiber and water intake or can take a prophylactic stool softener or stimulant. It is not uncommon to see ascending paresthesia of the fingers and toes after six treatments with vinblastine or 6 mg of vincristine. Nausea and vomiting are rare with these drugs, and many patients do not need antiemetics.

Vincristine is available in 1-, 2-, and 5-mg vials. It should be refrigerated and protected from light. Vinblastine is supplied in 10-mg vials. In solution, it is stable for 30 days when refrigerated. Vincristine is given in doses of 1.4 mg/m², to a maximum dose of 2 mg. Vinblastine is given at doses ranging from 3.7 to 15 mg/m². In patients with a bilirubin level between 1.5 and 3, a 50% reduction of dose is indicated and if the bilirubin is greater than 3 mg/dL, it is recommended that it be reduced by 75%. Both these drugs can be administered by a bolus injection. Because of their short half-life, vinblastine and vincristine are now used as a continuous infusion in an effort to increase the exposure time to the cancer cells. Methotrexate appears to achieve a higher concentration in tumor cells when there is concomitant use of vinblastine and vincristine, but the clinical significance is currently unknown. Seventy percent of vincristine and its metabolites are excreted in the stool and bile.

Bone marrow suppression occurs 5 to 10 days after treatment, with recovery by day 7 to 14. Again, because of their short half-life, these drugs can be administered weekly if blood counts have returned to baseline levels.

It is recommended that a central line be used with the continuous infusion method. Both these drugs are vesicants, which can result in tissue necrosis in case of extravasation. If a peripheral line is used, continuous observation of the insertion site and of the vein integrity is paramount.

Treatment of an extravasation consists of immediately stopping the infusion, aspirating prior to removing the cannula, and installing Wydase around the infiltrated area. The vinca alkaloids are the only drugs for which heat is recommended as treatment for an extravasation.[3, 6, 9, 17, 20, 21, 23, 24, 45, 97, 100, 109]

Etoposide

Etoposide (VP 16; Vepesid) is another plant alkaloid that has a significant place in the treatment of lung, testicular, and ovarian cancers, and hematologic malignancies. It entered clinical trials in 1971. Etoposide is cell cycle-specific, with activity in the G2 and S phases. It is a derivative of podopyllin, which is an alcohol extract of the dried roots of the May apple plant. At high doses, it causes lysis of cells entering mitosis. At lower doses, etoposide inhibits cells from entering prophase. The predominant effect of this drug is inhibition of DNA synthesis.

Bone marrow nadir is seen on day 7 to 14, with recovery by day 21. Patients experience mild to moderate nausea and vomiting, which can be controlled by antiemetics. Alopecia is seen in about 60% of patients, with thinning of the hair in the remainder.

In addition to the previously seen side effects of the plant alkaloids, etoposide can cause severe hypotension if administered too rapidly. It should be administered for longer than 30 minutes, with a usual administration time of 1 to 2 hours.

Etoposide is supplied in 50- and 100-mg vials. The literature recommends that it be diluted to a concentration of 0.2 to 0.4 mg/ml to avoid precipitation. It has a pH of 3 to 4 and can therefore be irritating to the veins. It is not clear whether this drug is a vesicant or irritant, and it is frequently classified as both. In some mouse studies, ulcer formation occurred after large doses of etoposide had extravasated. The phlebitis that occurs is the result of lipophilic diluents, and there can be a decrease in its incidence with an increase in isotonic solution. Burning and pain at the injection site are common. Increasing the diluent and slowing the rate decrease the burning.

Etoposide is given in doses of 100 to 150 mg/m² daily times 3 to 5 days every 3 to 4 weeks. It is synergistic with Cytoxan, BCNU, ara-C, and DDP. It has a half-life of 11 hours and is therefore one of the longer acting drugs. The most common method of administration is the intravenous route; however, it is now also being given orally. The bioavailability of the oral form is 50%, so the equivalent IV dose is doubled. Etoposide is supplied in 100-mg vials and as 50-mg pink capsules.[3, 6, 11, 16–18, 22, 23, 32, 80, 101]

Taxol

One of the newest and most promising chemotherapeutic agents is Taxol (Paclitaxel). This drug received its FDA approval in 1992 and it has shown sensitivity against a variety of tumors. In 1971, Wall and Wani were the first to isolate Taxol. Problems with obtaining and producing the drug as well as difficulties with toxicities caused a slow start. Phase I clinical trials were resumed in 1983 by the National Cancer Institute (NCI). In 1988, the activity of Taxol against ovarian cancer was recognized. In 1991, NCI and Bristol-Meyers Squibb entered into a cooperative research and development agreement (CRADA).

Taxol is in short supply at present and is the subject of controversy with environmentalists. Taxol comes from the bark of the western Pacific yew, which is found in the forests of Oregon, Washington, California, Idaho, and Montana. In Oregon, Washington, and California, there is a court order to delay harvesting of the yew. This tree provides a home for the spotted owl, which is in danger of extinction if the yews are destroyed.

It takes over 825,000 lb of bark to produce enough drug to treat 10,000 patients for 1 year. It takes about 60 lb of bark, or three trees, to provide enough drug for one patient. It is estimated that there are about 50,000 patients who could benefit from taxol each year. The bark is harvested manually using hand tools and light machinery. After the bark is chipped and dried, Taxol is extracted and purified. Since the signing of the CRADA, Bristol-Meyers Squibb has entered into a cooperative agreement with the US Forest Service and Bureau of Land Management, which have allowed increased taxol production.

At present, there is no way of synthesizing the drug or making the drug using recombinant DNA techniques. Taxol has a complex chemical structure, making synthesis difficult. It is hoped that synthetic Taxol will be available by 1997.

Taxol is the first organic compound with a tazane ring. Research is under way to extract the drug from the needles, twigs, and wood of the yew. Work is also being done to devise a way to synthesize taxol from natural products. Rhône-Poulenc-Rohrer is involved with the development of taxoterea, which is related to Taxol. Taxoterea is extracted from the needles of the Pacific yew.

Unlike vincristine, which disassembles microtubules, Taxol's mechanism of action promotes the assembly of cellular microtubules and stabilizes their formation by preventing depolymerization. This results in nonfunctional microtubules. Taxol is metabolized in the liver and excreted by the kidneys.

Research studies are evaluating the efficacy of Taxol for the treatment of breast, ovarian, lung, head, and neck cancers. Major side effects are myelosuppression, with 76% of patients experiencing grade 3 to 4 hematologic toxicity on the ECOG scale. The nadir usually occurs by day 11. Patients with prior radiation experience have a more severe and longer myelosuppression. There is a 33% decrease in Taxol clearance when it is given after DDP, which results in increased myelosuppression. These pharmacokinetic studies indicate that Taxol should be administered prior to giving DDP. Using colony-stimulating factors has aided in preventing the severe drop in blood counts.

Mild peripheral neuropathy in the form of paresthesia is seen in 62% of patients. Only 4% of patients experience severe neuropathy. The incidence of neuropathy is related to dose intensity and the cumulative dose. In patients who have had prior exposure to platinum, there is a 40% incidence of neuropathy.

Also seen are alopecia, mucositis, mild nausea and vomiting, diarrhea, and cardiac arrhythmias in the form of asymptomatic bradycardia. If patients have a severe cardiac condition, they should be monitored during treatment. Mild elevation of LFTs has been seen in about 25% of patients, so caution needs to be taken in those with severe hepatic compromise. Many patients experience myalgias and arthralgias 2 to 3 days after the drug has been administered. The large joints are most commonly affected, with symptoms usually lasting 2 to 4 days.

Taxol is not water-soluble and is therefore dissolved in Cremophor to keep it in solution. This substance is responsible for hypersensitivity reactions, so Taxol should be used with caution in patients with a known Cremophor sensitivity. Mild hypersensitivity reactions occur in about 19% of patients, with symptoms of flushing, rash, and dyspnea. Usually, no intervention is necessary. About 2% of these hypersensitivity reactions are severe, with symptoms of dyspnea, hypotension, and chest pain. Treatment includes the use of bronchodilators, epinephrine, antihistamines, and corticosteroids. Hypersensitivity reactions usually occur in the first 10 to 60 minutes. In some patients, interruption of the drug is the only treatment necessary. Pretreatment prior to the initial Taxol administration and longer infusions have significantly reduced the number and severity of allergic reactions. The administration of Decadron, 20 mg, 12 and 6 hours prior to Taxol; Benadryl, 50 mg, 0.5 to 1 hour prior to Taxol; and cimetidine, 300 mg, or ranitidine, 50 mg, IV 0.5 to 1 hour prior to Taxol has been effective in averting an allergic reaction.

The usual dosing of Taxol is 135 to 250 mg/m^2 every 22 days. If the patient has been heavily pretreated, the starting dose is reduced to 110 mg/m^2. Taxol is stable up to 27 hours after mixing at ambient temperature and lighting. The solution may appear hazy after mixing because of the formulation vehicle. Freezing does not adversely affect this drug. Cremophor can cause DEHP (di-[2-ethylhexyl]phthalate) to leach from polyvinyl chloride infusion bags. To minimize patient exposure to DEHP, Taxol solution should be delivered in glass bottles or polypropylene or polyolefin plastic bags. A polyethylene-lined infusion set should also be used. This drug is usually given as a continuous infusion over 24 hours, and can be divided into two 12-hour bags. Some studies have shown increased tumor response and better tolerance with a 3- to 5-day infusion.[54, 76, 115–124]

Alkylating Agents

Ehrlich, 100 years ago, observed the damaging effects to renal papillae by chemicals that later became known as alkylating agents. The alkylating agents were the first antineoplastic drugs and were developed as a result of government studies of biologic warfare. Alkylating agents produce highly reactive ions that cause cross linking of abnormal protein base pairs and interfere with DNA replication. Most alkylating agents are non–cell cycle-specific but have more activity in the later phase of dividing cells. Clinical resistance to an alkylating agent usually means tumor resistance to the other alkylating drugs.

The major side effects include toxicities to the hematopoietic, gastrointestinal, and reproductive systems. Reversible changes can occur in ovarian and testicular function, resulting in amenorrhea, oligospermia, and azoospermia. Long-term studies of side effects have shown that the alkylating agents can be carcinogenic, but their benefits far outweigh the risks. The major diseases that use alkylating agents for treatment are lymphoma, Hodgkin's disease, breast cancer, and multiple myeloma.[1, 3, 6, 16, 17, 20–23, 68, 120, 125]

Nitrogen Mustard

In 1917, nitrogen mustard (mechlorethamine; mustargen; HN2) was used in chemical warfare, and it was noted that those exposed to the gas developed hematologic toxicity. During World War II, an Allied ship carrying mustard gas was bombed, exposing many sailors to the toxic substance, and many of these men developed leukopenia. The first non-hormonal chemotherapeutic agent was nitrogen mustard, and it is still widely used in the treatment of Hodgkin's disease, non-Hodgkin's lymphoma, chronic lymphocytic leukemia (CLL), bronchogenic carcinoma, and polycythemia vera. Nitrogen mustard is effective in the topical treatment of mycosis fungoides, and has also been used successfully as a sclerosing agent in malignant pleural effusions. It is a cell cycle-specific alkylating drug. Its multiple mechanisms of action result in DNA miscoding, breakage, and failure of the cell to replicate. Nitrogen mustard rapidly binds to tissue and is quickly metabolized.

Nitrogen mustard is unstable and rapidly undergoes chemical transformation and decomposition. Because of these properties, nitrogen mustard should not be mixed until ready to administer. It should be infused over 3 minutes and within 15 minutes of preparation, and be reconstituted with sterile water or normal saline. Given by the intracavitary route, it causes systemic side effects similar to those of IV doses.

Nitrogen mustard is supplied in 10-mg vials and is reconstituted with 10 ml of sterile water to produce a 1 mg/ml solution. The usual doses of nitrogen mustard are 2 to 16 mg/m² if given as a single agent, and 6 mg/m² if used in combination therapy. When used for topical application, the drug is mixed with 60 ml of sterile water. Latex gloves are necessary when applying topical chemotherapy to avoid absorption through the skin. If inadvertent contact with skin occurs, the area should be washed with copious amounts of water followed by a rinse of 2.5% sodium thiosulfate solution.

Nitrogen mustard is a vesicant and can cause severe tissue necrosis and sloughing in the event of an extravasation. A dilute solution of sodium thiosulfate injected into the area helps neutralize the infiltration. The application of ice for 6 to 12 hours post insult helps reduce tissue damage.

The most common side effects seen with nitrogen mustard are nausea and vomiting, which usually start within a half-hour of administration and can last up to 36 hours. Leukopenia is seen, with the nadir in 6 to 14 days, and may last up to 21 days. Bone marrow suppression can be profound when nitrogen mustard is given with radiation therapy. Thinning of the hair without complete alopecia is seen. It is not uncommon for patients on this chemotherapy to develop menstrual irregularities and impaired spermatogenesis.[3, 6, 13, 16–18, 22, 24, 25, 42, 57, 97, 100, 137]

Dacarbazine

Dacarbazine (DTIC-Dome; imidazole; carboxamide) is another alkylating agent that has some antimetabolite activity as a purine precursor. Its major action is non–cell cycle-specific and it inhibits DNA, RNA, and protein synthesis. It is activated in the liver and excreted by the kidneys, and possesses limited ability to cross the blood-brain barrier.

Dacarbazine is active against Hodgkin's disease, melanoma, carcinoid tumors, islet cell tumors, thyroid malignancies, and a variety of sarcomas. It may be administered by IV injection or infusion. The drip method decreases the burning sensation and vasospasm that many patients experience. Sometimes lidocaine is added to the infusion to reduce the pain, and the application of ice above the injection site can also be helpful. Dacarbazine is a vesicant, and an extravasation can cause tissue necrosis.

Dacarbazine is sensitive to heat and light, which may cause the solution to change in color from ivory to pink, an indication of decomposition. It is stable for 72 hours at 4 C.

Dacarbazine is available in 100- and 200-mg vials. The final concentration is 10 mg/ml. The usual dosing is 150 to 200 mg/m²/day times 5 days every 4 weeks, or 800 to 900 mg/m² every 3 to 4 weeks. It can be given push but it is recommended as a half-hour infusion. Its half-life is 40 minutes. Approximately 40% of the drug is found in the urine.

The nadir of dacarbazine is 7 to 14 days. Nausea, vomiting, myelosuppression, and flu-like symptoms are the most common side effects; 90% of patients experience an onset of nausea and vomiting within 1 to 3 hours of administration, which last for up to 12 hours post-treatment. The flu-like syndrome can last for several days, with primary symptoms of fever and myalgias. Many patients complain about a metallic taste, which may interfere with nutritional intake. Skin reactions of pruritus, erythema, and edema have occurred only on sun-exposed skin. The patient needs to exercise precautions by using a good sunscreen when outdoors during the first 2 days postadministration, because photosensitivity can be a problem. Exposure to the sun during those first 48 hours can cause facial flushing, paresthesia, and lightheadedness.[3, 6, 9, 13, 16–18, 20–23, 68]

Cyclophosphamide

Cyclophosphamide (Cytoxan; Endoxan; Neosar; CTX), synthesized in 1958, is one of the most widely used alkylating agents. It is a synthetic agent chemically related to nitrogen mustard. It is effective against carcinomas, sarcomas, hematologic malignancies, and especially testicular, endometrial, breast, and lung cancers. It is non–cell cycle-specific. Cyclophosphamide is activated in the liver by the enzyme phosphamidase into two active metabolites, acrolein and phosphoramide mustard. It has a long half-life of 6 to 8 hours. Allopurinol prolongs the half-life and therefore increases toxicity, including myelosuppression. In the presence of renal compromise, dose reduction can avoid prolonged neutropenia.

The incidence of nausea and vomiting varies with each patient and can be nonexistent to moderate. The degree of nausea and vomiting is related to the dose intensity. Slowing the infusion rate decreases the nausea and vomiting in most patients.

Myelosuppression occurs between days 7 and 14 post-treatment. Cyclophosphamide has been documented to cause hemorrhagic cystitis as a result of chemical irritation from the acrolein metabolites. The kidneys are the major organ of excretion, and the potential for bladder complications can be reduced with an increase in the amount of diluent used and by adequate hydration up to 72 hours after infusion. The patient should be encouraged to increase fluid intake and also instructed to void frequently, especially at bedtime. The urine should be checked for microscopic blood to detect early signs of bleeding. Mesna has also been used to prevent cyclophosphamide-induced hemorrhagic cystitis. In high doses, alopecia results; at lower doses, only 30% of patients experience hair loss.

Cyclophosphamide is available as a powder in 100-, 200-, and 500-mg vials, and in 1- and 2-g vials, reconstituted with 5 ml of sterile water for every 100 mg of cyclophosphamide. The powder does not readily dissolve and vigorous shaking may be necessary. The vial should be carefully inspected for evidence of any undissolved particles. It may be further diluted in 0.9% sodium chloride or 5% dextrose in water. It is usually infused over 20 to 30 minutes, but slowing the infusion helps reduce the nausea and vomiting. The usual dose is 500 to 1500 mg/m^2.

Used in low doses of 50 mg (usually given orally), cyclophosphamide is an immunomodulator, resulting in suppression of the T-suppressor cells. Severe rheumatoid arthritis, Wegener's granulomatosis, nephrotic syndrome, and allograft rejection are nonmalignant conditions that can be treated with cyclophosphamide.[3, 5, 6, 9, 16–18, 20–23, 32, 45, 68]

Ifosfamide

Ifosfamide (IFEX) is chemically related to nitrogen mustard and is a synthetic analogue of cyclophosphamide (Cytoxan). If the tumor develops resistance to a chemotherapeutic agent, there is frequently a resistance to other agents in the same family. One of the major advantages of ifosfamide is that it is not cross-resistant to Cytoxan and, therefore, patients can achieve a tumor response after prior failure with Cytoxan. Like the other alkylating agents, ifosfamide is non–cell cycle-specific. It requires a liver enzyme to activate the active metabolite. This drug has demonstrated efficacy against a wide variety of tumor types. Initial studies were done on testicular primaries, but it is also active against sarcomas, lymphoma, and small cell lung, ovary, and breast cancers.

The usual dosage is 1.2 to 1.6 gm/m^2 daily times 1 to 5 days every 3 to 4 weeks. It is available in 200-mg ampules and 1-g vials. It should not be infused in less than 30 minutes. Ifosfamide can also be administered as a continuous infusion in doses up to 2400 mg/m^2 daily times 5 days, or 3 g/m^2 daily times 2 days, repeated every 14 to 28 days.

Ifosfamide causes moderate myelosuppression, nephrotoxicity, and hepatotoxicity. Alopecia occurs in 83% of patients.

Ifosfamide is excreted in the urine and so there is a high but varying incidence of hemorrhagic cystitis. Studies have shown that 6 to 92% of patients develop hemorrhagic cystitis. Mesna has done much to manage this problem and reduce the incidence of hemorrhagic cystitis to less than 6%. Mesna reacts chemically with the urotoxic metabolite acrolein that is the result of ifosfamide metabolism, and thus it inhibits ifosfamide-induced hemorrhagic cystitis. Ifosfamide has a 7-hour half-life, with most eliminated in 4 hours. Mesna has a 4-hour dosing schedule; it is usually ordered at a dose of 20% of the ifosfamide dose and administered prior to ifosfamide, at 4 and again at 8 hours. If the patient has a continuous infusion of ifosfamide, Mesna is given also as a continuous infusion at 100% of the ifosfamide dose. Mesna is stable in solution with ifosfamide and cyclophosphamide.

Mesna can cause nausea, vomiting, diarrhea, fatigue, headache, and taste alterations. Its use can cause a false-positive test result for urinary ketones, and diabetics may thus need an alternate method of urinary assessment.[3, 5, 6, 9, 16–18, 20–22, 45, 66, 68]

It is important to ensure that the patient is adequately hydrated and voids frequently when receiving ifosfamide. The urine should be monitored for RBCs during and prior to administration. If urinalysis shows more than 10 RBCs per high power field (HPF), ifosfamide should be withheld until the urine is negative.

Cisplatin

Cisplatin (cis-diamminedichloroplatinum; platinum; CDDP; DDP; Platinol) is a heavy metal that forms covalent links and therefore acts like an alkylating agent. It is non–cell cycle-specific and inhibits DNA synthesis. Clinical trials began in 1971.

Cisplatin reacts chemically with aluminum and forms a precipitate, so only stainless steel needles should be used. It has made a significant contribution to the survival of patients with testicular, ovarian, head, and neck cancers, as well as patients with Hodgkin's disease, lymphoma, myeloma, cervical cancer, melanoma, and sarcoma. One of its advantages is that it is not cross resistant with other alkylating agents, and is synergistic with some.

Cisplatin, however, is not without toxicities. Nausea and vomiting can start within 2 hours after administration and can last up to 1 week post-treatment. Working with this drug has provided many opportunities to learn about nausea control. Presently, the antiemetic with the best control is metoclopramide (Reglan) or ondansetron (Zofran) administered pre- and postinfusion of cisplatin. Frequently, Decadron and Benadryl, Ativan, and other antiemetics are used in combination. Ondansetron produces fewer extrapyramidal symptoms than Reglan.

Moderate neutropenia and thrombocytopenia are seen by day 14, with recovery by day 21 to 28. Similar to the vinca alkaloids, cisplatin has the potential for causing peripheral neuropathy. Because of sensory and perceptual alterations, patient education should include safety measures for the prevention of injury. The exact mechanisms of ototoxicity and tinnitus with cisplatin are not known. The hearing loss is often reversible, however, or can be limited.

The most troublesome side effect of cisplatin is related to renal function, but the precise mechanism of tubular necrosis from its use is unknown. The major organ of excretion for cisplatin is the kidney. The kidneys can be protected by using mannitol, Lasix, and vigorous hydration. Fluids should be infused at a rate high enough to maintain a urinary output of at least 100 to 200 ml/hour and should be started 2 hours prior to cisplatin administration and continued for 8 hours after. Cisplatin causes the kidneys to dump magnesium and calcium, so it is important that these electrolytes and renal function be monitored by such parameters as BUN and creatinine levels and creatinine clearance. The problem is amplified in the presence of other nephrotoxic drugs such as the aminoglycosides or vitamin C.

Cisplatin is usually given in doses of 50 to 120 mg/m^2 as a single dose or in divided doses. The infusion rate should not be lower than 1 mg/min, and is frequently given over 8 or 24 hours. Cisplatin should always be diluted in some form of saline, and never in 5% dextrose in water alone.[3, 4, 6, 13, 16–18, 22, 28, 30, 31, 38–40, 58, 77, 124]

Carboplatin

Carboplatin (paraplatin) is an analogue of cisplatin. It is non–cell cycle-specific. Its method of action is to produce interstrands of DNA cross links rather than DNA protein.

Like cisplatin, carboplatin is emetogenic, but to a lesser degree, and symptoms rarely last longer than 24 hours after infusion. Carboplatin has a half-life of 1 to 2 hours and a median nadir of 21 days. Because carboplatin is eliminated by the kidneys, caution needs to be taken with patients who have an elevated creatinine level. Hydration is necessary during carboplatin administration but to a lesser degree than with cisplatin. A dose reduction is indicated in the presence of an elevated serum creatinine level or a creatinine clearance of less than 40 ml/min. Like cisplatin, carboplatin can cause electrolyte loss, especially sodium, potassium, magnesium, and calcium. Therefore, careful monitoring of their levels is necessary. The nurse needs to be alert for an increased potential for nephrotoxicity when other drugs known to cause kidney damage are used simultaneously.

Neuropathy is infrequent, but the risk is increased in patients who have had previous exposure to cisplatin or in those who are over 65 years of age. Although uncommon, there have been reports of anaphylactic reactions occurring within minutes of administration. Because of this, the nurse must be prepared for necessary intervention with epinephrine, corticosteroids, and antihistamines.

Carboplatin is supplied in 50-, 150-, and 450-mg vials. Each vial contains mannitol and can be diluted in normal saline or 5% dextrose in water. Carboplatin mixed in saline must be administered within 6 hours, but it has a longer stability in 5% dextrose in water. The usual dose of carboplatin is 300 to 500 mg/m^2 daily for 3 to 5 days. This drug is usually administered over 30 minutes, but slowing the rate helps reduce the nausea and vomiting associated with its use. There are some situations in which a 24-hour continuous infusion is given. The half-life of carboplatin is 2 hours. The use of aluminum needles causes precipitation and loss of potency, and therefore they should not be used.

Carboplatin is most frequently used in the treatment of ovarian cancer but has also been successful in the treatment of genitourinary, gynecologic, breast, head, neck, lung, and mesothelioma primaries.[3, 6, 13, 16, 17, 22, 24, 58, 79, 80, 89, 126, 127]

Thiotepa

Thiotepa (thiophosphoramide; triethylene) is a stable derivative of mustard gas and was synthesized in 1952. Thio-

tepa is a non–cell cycle-specific drug. Its method of action is to cause cross linking of DNA. Thiotepa is effective against breast and ovarian cancer as well as Hodgkin's disease, and is also widely used in the treatment of superficial bladder cancer. High-dose thiotepa is being used with increasing frequency in bone marrow transplantation for women with breast cancer.

Thiotepa is supplied in 15-mg vials. Reconstitution with 1.5 ml sterile water produces an isotonic solution of 10 mg that is stable for 5 days when refrigerated. However, because thiotepa does not contain a preservative, it should be discarded after 24 hours. The reconstituted drug should be protected from light. The stability of thiotepa is reduced by carbon dioxide, sodium chloride, and humidity. It is unstable in an acid pH and should be kept at a pH of 6 to 7.

Thiotepa can be given by the IV, IM, subcutaneous, intratumor, intraperitoneal, intrapleural, intravesicular, and intrathecal routes. If it is administered intrathecally, it must be mixed with preservative-free sterile water. Intrathecal doses range from 1 to 10 mg/m^2. Systemic doses of thiotepa are 8 mg/m^2 daily for 5 days. Intramuscular or subcutaneous dosing is 30 to 60 mg once a week. Bladder instillation is usually 60 mg in 60 ml of water weekly. Thiotepa is excreted in the urine during the first 8 hours of administration.

Nausea and vomiting are only occasionally seen, and are dose-dependent. Myelosuppression is the dose-limiting toxic effect of this drug. The nadir is 7 to 10 days, but can be as long as 28 days. Both neutropenia and thrombocytopenia are seen, and can be severe. Occasionally, headaches and fevers are reported. There have been isolated incidents of allergic reactions, with symptoms of hives and bronchoconstriction. In animal studies, thiotepa is carcinogenic, mutagenic, and teratogenic.[3, 4, 13, 16–18, 21–23, 30, 111]

Nitrosoureas

The nitrosoureas are lipid-soluble alkylating agents that substitute a hydrocarbon radical for a hydrogen atom. Because of their lipid solubility, they can cross the blood-brain barrier. They inhibit DNA repair and are non–cell cycle-specific. Their major toxicities are hematopoietic and gastrointestinal. Frequently, there is a mild elevation of liver function tests, which usually return to normal within 1 week. The nitrosoureas are the only classification of drugs in which there has never been a reported case of a hypersensitivity reaction.[3, 6, 9, 16, 17, 20–23, 68]

CARMUSTINE

Carmustine (BiCNU; BCNU) is a nitrosourea primarily used in the treatment of brain tumors. Efficacy has also been seen in the treatment of Hodgkin's disease and non-Hodgkin's disease lymphoma, multiple myeloma, and colorectal, gastric, and lung cancers. Carmustine has been used in the bone marrow transplant setting, with mixed results.

Carmustine is non–cell cycle-specific. It carbamoylates cellular proteins and inhibits RNA and DNA synthesis. It is usually not cross resistant to the alkylating agents. Because of its lipid solubility, carmustine is one of the few drugs that crosses the blood-brain barrier, and it is cleared from the plasma in 15 minutes. Its concentration in the cerebrospinal fluid ranges from 15 to 70% of the plasma level. Amphotericin B may modulate the cell and thus increase the cellular uptake of carmustine. It is excreted primarily in the urine within 24 hours, and 10% of the drug is excreted as carbon dioxide. Its half-life is 6 to 70 minutes.

Carmustine is a lyophilized white powder that is dissolved in 3 ml of absolute alcohol and 27 ml of sterile water, and then diluted further. Sodium chloride 0.9% or 5% dextrose in water can be used. The usual dose is 75 to 100 mg/m^2 IV every day for 2 days or 200 mg/m^2 as a single dose. Dividing the dose reduces the side effects. Carmustine is usually repeated every 6 weeks because of its long nadir.

This drug should be infused over at least 30 to 60 minutes. The patient frequently experiences pain and venous spasm on administration. Increasing the amount of diluent, slowing the infusion, and placing ice over the infusion site help decrease these symptoms. A dilute solution of sodium bicarbonate can be used to neutralize a large inadvertent infiltration. Contact with unprotected skin results in temporary hyperpigmentation of the affected area.

Given intra-arterially to the brain, carmustine was found in some studies to increase the tumor response, as compared to IV administration. Placing the catheter above the ophthalmic artery decreases the potential for optic neuritis and atrophy or hemorrhagic glaucoma. The most common side effects include nausea and vomiting for 6 hours, beginning 2 to 4 hours postadministration, and myelosuppression. Myelosuppression is increased when Tagamet is also given. The nadir usually occurs in 4 to 6 weeks, and can be cumulative. Pulmonary fibrosis has been seen after 6 months of therapy, especially with concomitant bleomycin administration or chest radiation, or when the total dose exceeds 1100 to 1200 mg/m^2. A pulmonary function test result of 70% or less of the predicted value can indicate pulmonary toxicity. The facial flushing that is sometimes seen is possibly related to the ethanol used to reconstitute this drug.[3, 6, 7, 13, 16, 17, 24, 33, 56, 83]

STREPTOZOCIN

Streptozocin (Zanosar; streptozoticin) is a nitrosourea and is chemically similar to carmustine. It is sometimes classified as an antibiotic because it is synthetically prepared from the bacteria Streptomyces achromogenes. This is a non–cell cycle-specific drug that inhibits DNA synthesis through cross linking. Streptozocin's major indications are insulinomas, carcinoid tumors, Zollinger-Ellison syndrome, Hodgkin's disease, and colon, liver, and pancreatic carcinomas.

The side effects and administration precautions are the same as for carmustine, and include nausea, vomiting, and myelosuppression. Duodenal ulcers have been seen in certain patients. The most serious dose-limiting adverse side effect is nephrotoxicity, which occurs in 25 to 75% of patients. If the creatinine clearance is below 25 ml/min, a 50% dose reduction is appropriate. Renal dysfunction is demonstrated by proteinuria, decreased glomerular filtration, and elevated BUN and creatinine levels. Urine output and urinalysis should be monitored for impending renal failure. Special attention should be given to patients who are receiving concomitant nephrotoxic drugs. Toxic effects on the beta cells of the pancreas have been seen. This results in a potential for severe hypoglycemia and glucose intolerance.

Streptozocin is soluble in water, normal saline, and alcohol. Its half-life is 40 minutes. There is no intact drug remaining in the plasma after 3 hours. Within 24 hours, 10 to 20% of the drug is excreted in the urine. Streptozocin should be administered as a 1-hour infusion. Slow administration helps decrease the local pain and burning. Ice over the infusion site can also be helpful in reducing pain. Streptozocin is available in 1-g vials. The usual dose is 500 to 1500 mg/m^2 per week, or 500 mg/m^2 per day for 5 consecutive days every 5 to 6 weeks.[3, 6, 7, 13, 16, 17, 24, 33, 56, 58, 81, 83]

Antibiotics

Although the antitumor antibiotics have some anti-infective qualities, their major action is cytotoxic. They interfere with nucleic acid synthesis and inhibit RNA synthesis by intercalation. They react with or bind to DNA and therefore inhibit DNA synthesis. They are non–cell cycle-specific. Their major toxicities are hematopoietic, gastrointestinal, and reproductive. All the antibiotics except bleomycin are vesicants if extravasated.

The largest category of the antibiotics is the anthracyclines, primarily including Adriamycin, dactinomycin, daunorubicin, mitoxantrone, and the newest drug, idarubicin. In addition to myelosuppression, the anthracyclines can cause alopecia, nausea, vomiting, and stomatitis.

If extravasation occurs, there can be severe tissue necrosis. Because Adriamycin is the most widely used vesicant, there is the greatest amount of data available for this drug. With extravasation, the patient usually complains of pain and burning at the site. As with the vinca alkaloids, the infusion needs to be stopped immediately and aspirated with the needle in place. Many antidotes have been recommended for an anthracycline extravasation, with a great deal of controversy surrounding the use of each remedy. The only clear-cut, noncontroversial treatment for an anthracycline extravasation is elevation of the extremity and the application of ice to the affected area. Adriamycin binds to DNA and can therefore continue to cause tissue damage long after the event. The physician needs to be notified immediately. In the case of severe tissue necrosis, plastic surgery with wide excision of the area is necessary.[3, 6, 9, 16, 17, 20–23, 68, 75]

Adriamycin

Adriamycin (doxorubicin) was first found in the soil in India in 1950. Clinical trials started in the 1960s, and Adriamycin has been commercially available since the 1970s.

Adriamycin intercalates between DNA base pairs and inhibits DNA and RNA synthesis. It is one of the most active drugs available for the treatment of breast cancer. It is also used extensively in the treatment of acute leukemia, sarcomas, neuroblastoma, Hodgkin's disease, lymphoma, and bladder, thyroid, lung, and ovarian cancers.

Adriamycin is supplied in 10-, 20-, and 50-mg vials. It may be reconstituted with 0.9% sodium chloride or 5% dextrose in water. Sterile water is not recommended, because a local doxorubicin flare reaction may be increased. Adriamycin has an acid pH with 0.9% sodium chloride and 5% dextrose in water but is stable in a pH range of 3 to 7. Stored at room temperature, Adriamycin is stable for 24 hours, but its stability is doubled when refrigerated. The simultaneous administration of heparin and fluorouracil in the same line with Adriamycin results in precipitation. Amphotericin B may have a cellular modulation effect on tumors and thereby improve the therapeutic index.

Adriamycin has a half-life of 30 hours. It is metabolized by the liver, and 50% of the drug is excreted in the bile. Care needs to be taken when patients have an elevated total bilirubin, and a dose reduction is necessary when this occurs.

Patients should be alerted to the fact that, because Adriamycin is red, it turns the urine red for 1 to 2 days after treatment. This should not be confused with hematuria.

The usual dose of Adriamycin is 50 to 75 mg/m^2 every 21 to 28 days. Newer protocols use lower weekly doses of 20 mg/m^2. To increase the dose intensity, especially when used as a single agent, Adriamycin can be given at a dose of 30 mg/m^2 daily times 3 days every 3 to 4 weeks. Research has shown that the infusion of Adriamycin rather than the push method reduces the cardiotoxicity of this drug. In doses lower than 450 mg/m^2, the risk of cardiac damage is 1 to 2%. Because of the potential of cardiac toxicity, most physicians stop Adriamycin when the cumulative dose reaches 550 mg/m^2. Some studies have shown that the cardiac toxicity potential of Adriamycin is increased with the concurrent administration of Cytoxan and mitomycin.

Nausea and vomiting are common in patients receiving Adriamycin, especially when they are receiving combination chemotherapy. Stomatitis is dose-dependent, usually occurs 5 to 10 days after a treatment, and lasts up to 5 days. Radiation effect is enhanced with Adriamycin, and radiation recall with erythema may occur as late as 1 year post-treatment.

Bone marrow depression can be severe, depending on the dose as well as other concurrent chemotherapy agents. Nadir usually occurs 7 to 14 days after treatment. Alopecia is almost universal with Adriamycin.[3, 6, 13, 15, 16, 18, 19, 22, 57, 62, 75, 80]

Idarubicin

Idarubicin (Idamycin) is a new synthetic anthracycline and is an analogue of daunorubicin. Idarubicin has an inhibitory effect on nucleic acid synthesis and interacts with the enzyme topoisomerase II.

One advantage of the use of idarubicin over the other anthracyclines is an increased rate of cellular uptake, with increased cellular drug concentrations being achieved within a few minutes after injection. Idarubicin is eliminated through the biliary system. An elevation of the total bilirubin increases the drug level and a dose reduction is appropriate in the presence of an elevated bilirubin or creatinine level. Because idarubicin has a long half-life (22 hours, with a mean terminal half-life of 45 hours), it can be detected in the plasma for up to 8 days. Idarubicin is labeled for use in leukemia but has demonstrated efficacy in liver metastasis, especially when administered intra-arterially. Consistent with the other anthracyclines, idarubicin is a vesicant. It can cause severe tissue necrosis in the event of an extravasation and should therefore never be given subcutaneously or as an intramuscular injection.

Side effects include severe myelosuppression, mucositis, nausea, vomiting, alopecia, abdominal cramps, and diarrhea. Hyperuricemia can occur secondary to tumor lysis syndrome. The most distressing side effect is myocardial toxicity, leading to congestive heart failure and cardiac arrhythmias. Patients with prior experience with anthracyclines or a known history of heart disease are more likely to develop cardiac toxicity.

Idarubicin comes in 5- and 10-mg vials. It contains lactose MPH, an orange-red lyophilized powder, which when mixed produces a red color. Usual doses are 12 mg/m^2 daily times 3 days. Patients with hepatic compromise should have the dose reduced to avoid severe toxicity. Idarubicin should be discontinued if LFTs and/or the total bilirubin exceed five times the normal value. It is recommended that idarubicin be infused over 10 to 15 minutes through the side port of a free-flowing IV of 0.9% sodium chloride or 5% dextrose in water. Precipitation occurs when idarubicin is combined with heparin. Prolonged contact with a solution having a pH greater than 7 results in drug degradation. Idarubicin is stable for 168 hours (7 days) when refrigerated and 3 days at room temperature. It can cause skin irritation if improperly handled. In the event of an accidental skin exposure, the affected area should be washed immediately with copious amounts of water and a mild soap.[3, 6, 13, 15–18, 22, 59, 62, 75, 80]

Mitoxantrone

Mitoxantrone (Novantrone; DHAD) is an Adriamycin analogue. Like Adriamycin, it is a non–cell cycle-specific drug and exerts its antitumor effect by intercalation between base pairs, thus interfering with DNA synthesis. It is active against ALL, lymphoma, and breast and ovarian cancers.

Mitoxantrone is supplied as a dark blue concentrated solution, 2 mg/ml, in 20-, 25-, and 30-mg vials. It should be diluted in at least 50 ml isotonic saline or dextrose, and is stable for 2 years. Mitoxantrone can be further diluted and administered as an infusion rather than a bolus over at least 15 to 30 minutes. The usual dose is 10 to 15 mg/m^2 every 3 to 4 weeks, given either as a single dose or divided over 3 to 4 days.

Because mitoxantrone is a vesicant, precautions are necessary to avoid extravasation. Frequently, the first sign of extravasation is a blue streaking in or around the vein. Guidelines for dealing with a mitoxantrone extravasation are the same as for the other anthracyclines.

Mitoxantrone has a short half-life of 21 to 27 minutes, and so it is recommended that it be given as an infusion to increase the exposure time of the tumor cell to the drug. It is metabolized in the liver, and the major organ of excretion is the kidneys. Mitoxantrone is a dark shade of blue and turns the urine varying shades of blue or green, depending on the concentration of the yellow urine. Some patients have a blue tint to the sclera.

Side effects are similar to those of Adriamycin but are less severe. Patients may experience mild nausea and vomiting, which are usually controlled by antiemetics. Only about 13% of patients lose their hair while receiving mitoxantrone. Neutropenia is usually the dose-limiting toxicity seen, with a nadir between 7 and 14 days. Recovery occurs by day 21 to 28. A slight elevation of LFTs has been observed. The overall cardiac toxicity is lower with mitoxantrone than with Adriamycin. There seems to be an increased predisposition to cardiac damage in patients who have had prior exposure to Adriamycin.[3, 6, 13, 16–18, 22, 23, 48, 62]

Mitomycin

Mitomycin (mitomycin C; Mutamycin) is an antibiotic isolated from the broth of Streptomyces caespitosus. It acts as an alkylating agent and inhibits DNA and RNA synthesis. Mitomycin is non–cell cycle-specific. It is a deep blue crystal that is soluble in water. Mitomycin is short-acting, is cleared through the liver and peripheral metabolism, and has a half-life of 15 to 90 minutes.

Mitomycin is available in 5- and 20-mg vials and is reconstituted with 2 ml sterile water/mg. The solution is stable for 14 days under refrigeration and for 7 days at room temperature. Most chemotherapeutic agents are given every 21 to 28 days but mitomycin has a delayed myelosuppression, with a nadir at 4 to 5 weeks. The usual schedule for mitomycin administration is 6 to 8 weeks to allow time to recover from the nadir. Protocols containing mitomycin are generally given every other treatment cycle. Thrombocytopenia develops in 40% of patients with a platelet count of 50,000/mm³ or less. The usual dose is 2 mg/m² daily times 5 days or 10 to 20 mg/m² as a single dose.

Mitomycin is active against gastrointestinal, breast, lung, pancreatic, colon, cervical, and bladder carcinomas. It has been administered topically for carcinoma of the epithelium of the bladder. The bladder should be evacuated using a Foley catheter to avoid local contact dermatitis from urine spillage on the skin.

There is usually only moderate nausea and vomiting associated with mitomycin, with an onset of 1 to 2 hours following administration. The nausea can persist for 2 to 3 days postinfusion. Stomatitis may also occur in about 4% of patients receiving mitomycin. Although alopecia is rare, thinning of the hair is more commonly seen. Mitomycin has the potential for renal toxicity. As evidenced by an increase in the BUN and creatinine levels, these parameters should be checked prior to mitomycin infusion. There is a need to hydrate the patient adequately and maintain accurate intake and output records.

Mitomycin-induced pulmonary toxicity is manifested by dyspnea, a nonproductive cough, or hemoptysis. Bronchospasm has been seen with the concurrent administration of vinblastine. The chest x-ray usually reveals pulmonary infiltrates. Some studies have shown that pulmonary toxicity can be avoided, or at least reduced, with Decadron 10 mg being given prior to mitomycin administration. The treatment of pulmonary toxicity includes supportive care, the use of steroids, and discontinuing the offending drug.

Mitomycin is also a vesicant, so administration precautions are mandatory. Mitomycin ulcers from an extravasation are typically deep and expansive, and sometimes require a wide excision with split-thickness grafting. The package insert recommends the application of ice to the affected area for 24 hours after an extravasation. Because mitomycin is also an irritant, dilution of the drug can help reduce the degree of irritation. Microangiopathic hemolytic anemia and hemolytic uremic syndrome, although rare, can be fatal.[3, 6, 13, 15–18, 23, 56, 62, 83]

Bleomycin

Bleomycin (Blenoxane) is isolated from Streptomyces. Unlike the other antibiotics, it has its major activity during the G2 phase and therefore is a cell cycle-specific drug, but it can also be classified as a non–cell cycle-specific drug. DNA synthesis is impaired and RNA and protein synthesis are inhibited. Bleomycin is eliminated by the kidneys within the first 24 hours postadministration. Its half-life is 2 to 4 hours. Bleomycin is available in 15-unit vials and may be reconstituted with 0.9% sodium chloride, 5% dextrose in water, sterile water, or bacteriostatic water.

Bleomycin has been used extensively in the treatment of testicular carcinoma, lymphomas, and soft tissue sarcomas. It also has activity in treating squamous cell carcinoma of the head, neck, esophagus, vulva, cervix, skin, and lung. Excellent results have been obtained by using bleomycin as a sclerosing agent in malignant pleural effusions.

Bleomycin is primarily excreted in the urine. The usual dose is 10 to 20 units/m² once or twice weekly. It can be given by the IV, IM, subcutaneous, or intra-arterial routes. Some protocols call for bleomycin as a continuous infusion over 24 to 120 hours to capitalize on the biologic effect of the drug.

Bleomycin causes pulmonary fibrosis; this is more commonly seen as interstitial pneumonitis and occurs in about 10% of patients receiving bleomycin. It affects the alveolar type I cells, and elderly patients are more susceptible to pulmonary complications. Lung biopsy reveals the infiltration of eosinophils. Vital capacity and carbon monoxide diffusing capacity tests are used to monitor pulmonary function. A drop of 30% in the pretreatment diffusion capacity is reason to discontinue the use of bleomycin. Dyspnea and fine rales are early signs of toxicity. There is a relationship between the amount of bleomycin a patient receives and pulmonary complications. Bleomycin is usually stopped when a cumulative dose of 220 units/m² or 400 units total dose is reached, whichever is lower. Patients with prior exposure to bleomycin are at risk of developing pulmonary toxicity when receiving a high fraction of inspired oxygen (FIO_2).

About 60% of patients have a febrile response, with temperatures as high as 103 to 105 F. Lymphoma patients with fever-related disease are more likely to experience bleomycin-related temperature elevation. Frequently, the temperature is accompanied by chills, which begin 4 to 10 hours after administration and persist for 48 hours. The severity decreases with successive doses. Tylenol, aspirin, and antihistamines can be helpful in abating hyperpyrexia. In some cases, steroids may be administered.

About 1% of patients have shown a hypersensitivity to bleomycin. The patient should have a test dose consisting of 1 to 5 units administered prior to the first dose of bleomycin. The patient should be monitored every 15 minutes for 1 hour before completing the remaining dose. Resuscitation equipment should be available.

Bleomycin is not associated with bone marrow depression and can be given regardless of the blood counts. Other side effects include an acne-like skin rash and alopecia. There can be some erythema and desquamation over pressure points and over joints, especially the elbows and knees, which may progress to shallow ulcerations. Frequently, there is also hyperpigmentation of the skin and nail beds, with ridging of the nails. Skin care includes cleansing the area with a mild soap. Applying lotion also helps keep the skin moist.

Bleomycin may be administered subcutaneously, intramuscularly, intravenously, or intra-arterially. Burning and pain at the injection site are common. Increasing the diluent and slowing the rate help decrease the burning.[3, 6, 13, 15, 17, 18, 20–22, 56, 69, 83, 84]

Plicamycin

Plicamycin (mithramycin; Mithracin) has cytotoxic potential, but it is used with greater frequency for the control of hypercalcemia associated with advanced neoplasms. It is both cell cycle-specific and non–cell cycle-specific. Plicamycin inhibits bone reabsorption and subsequently lowers serum calcium levels. One-third of patients receiving this drug experience some sort of coagulopathy and careful monitoring of the bleeding profile is necessary. Marked facial flushing after administration is an early sign of hemorrhage.

Plicamycin is supplied in 2.5-mg vials and is reconstituted with sterile water. Within 15 hours, 40% is excreted in the urine. Equivalent blood levels can be achieved in the CSF in 4 to 6 hours. Because of the toxicity of hypocalcemia, clinical trials of its effectiveness as an antineoplastic agent have been limited. In addition to the treatment of hypercalcemia, plicamycin has been used as an antineoplastic agent in the treatment of testicular tumors, glioblastomas, and Paget's disease.

Side effects are dose-related and usually include thrombocytopenia, nausea, vomiting, lethargy, stomatitis, and diarrhea. A slow infusion helps decrease nausea and vomiting but close monitoring of the site is necessary as this drug is very irritating and is a vesicant.

This drug can cause elevation of renal and liver function tests, particularly the lactic dehydrogenase and serum glutamic-oxaloacetic transaminase levels. Because liver damage can result, with hepatic necrosis and coagulopathies, laboratory monitoring is critical.[3, 6, 8, 13, 16–18, 20–23, 45, 58, 59, 62, 95]

Miscellaneous Drugs

Asparaginase

Asparaginase (L-Asparaginase; Elspar) is a high-molecular-weight enzyme derived from Escherichia coli. It hydrolyzes into aspartic acid and thus removes circulating asparagine, halting cancer cell activity. L-Asparagine is a nonessential amino acid that normal cells can synthesize. Malignant cells cannot synthesize L-asparagine, and thus rely on extracellular sources.

Asparaginase is used primarily in the treatment of acute ALL and lymphoma. It crosses the blood-brain barrier. Because asparaginase is a foreign protein it can cause severe allergic reactions, including anaphylactic shock. There are more reported reactions with IV administration than with the intramuscular route. Patients who receive asparaginase as a single agent have a higher incidence of hypersensitivity reactions than with combination therapy. The risk of a hypersensitivity reaction to asparaginase is 5 to 8%, which increases to 33% after the fourth dose, but fewer than 10% of patients have severe reactions. Those with a history of allergies are more likely to have a hypersensitivity reaction. The syndrome consists of a rapid onset of urticaria, chills, fever, flushing, dyspnea, and hypotension. It is therefore recommended that an intradermal test dose be administered, but some experts feel that this has little validity. The nurse should be prepared for the potential of every dose causing a reaction. The appropriate equipment should be available to maintain an adequate airway as well as oxygen, antihistamines, epinephrine, and steroids in case of a reaction. Asparaginase can cause an increase in liver function tests and the glucose level, which requires monitoring during therapy.

The half-life is 8 to 30 hours. Asparaginase is supplied in vials containing 10,000 IU. For IV use, asparaginase is reconstituted with 5 ml water, 0.9% sodium chloride, or 5% dextrose in water. Asparaginase should be infused within 8 hours of reconstitution through a 5-μ filter. Some loss of potency was observed when a 0.22-μ filter was used. Asparaginase should be infused for at least 30 minutes. When asparaginase is to be given IM, it is reconstituted with 2 ml normal saline.

Asparaginase is given at a dosage range of 6000 units/m^2 and can be given IV or IM. It is usually given in combination, and rarely as a single agent.[3, 6, 7, 13, 16–18, 20–23, 58, 62, 80, 101, 111, 128, 129]

CHEMOTHERAPY ADMINISTRATION CONSIDERATIONS

Because of the caustic properties of many of the available chemotherapeutic agents, and their potential for severe complications, much consideration needs to be given to the venous access. The use of scalp vein or flexible, indwelling catheters is preferred to a straight injection from a syringe and needle. The stiff metal needle can be easily dislodged. Small peripheral veins with low blood flow result in higher concentration of drugs than larger veins with rapid flow. It has been suggested that the antecubital fossa be used because it is a large vein and venipuncture is easily accomplished but most recommend avoiding the antecubital fossa. This is such a common site of venipuncture for blood draws that, if there is an extravasation, the local damage is severe.

The recommended peripheral site of administration is the proximal forearm over muscle bulk. The dorsum of the hand is discouraged because of the scant amount of tissue surrounding the area, so there is less tissue for solution absorption. The guiding principle for site selection is to choose an area that offers the best protection to tendons and nerves and results in the least loss of function if an extravasation occurs.

The suggested order of preference for an IV site is the forearm, dorsum of the hand, wrist, with the antecubital fossa as a last resort. The safest way to determine vein integrity is always to use a newly established venipuncture. If a venipuncture is unsuccessful, make a second attempt in the opposite arm. If it is necessary to use the same arm, use the site proximal to the first venipuncture and make sure it is not the same vein. The choice of needle and site depend on the expertise and dexterity of the nurse and the condition of the veins in each patient.

Chemotherapy administration using the sidearm method with a free-flowing IV is preferred over a straight push. This provides the greatest margin of safety and allows for frequent checks on vein integrity.

The longer the IV infusion time, the greater the possibility of needle dislodgement and extravasation. Venous access of central catheter placement through a long line, thoracic subclavian, or implantable port eliminates many but not all the problems of vein selection and extravasation. A central line decreases the chance of phlebitis, and the increased blood flow results in an increased and more rapid dilution of the drug. Central lines contribute their own set of potential difficulties, which primarily include infection and large vein thrombosis.

There is now increased use of electronic pumps for chemotherapy administration. This has added to the safety margin of infusion therapy but certain considerations must still be kept in mind. Most pumps with an occlusion alarm are sensitive to back pressure, and many of these devices exceed limits of 25 lb psi. The pumps with extravasation alarms work on a principle of decreased skin temperature over the tip of the catheter. A cooling blanket, for example, can produce a false alarm, and therefore is not completely reliable.[3, 6, 14, 22, 68, 105, 129–132]

Technique

1. Use a newly established venipuncture. If a venipuncture is unsuccessful, make a second attempt in the opposite arm. If it is necessary to use the same arm, make sure it is not the same vein. One dilemma of a nurse administering chemotherapy is the repeated trauma to the patient's veins from cancer treatment. Over time, the choices of suitable veins dwindle. If the patient is to receive long-term chemotherapy, it may be in the patient's best interest to have a central line inserted.
2. The nurse should challenge the vein with 10 ml normal saline. Some authorities recommend a challenge with methylene blue, 1 mg/ml, to check for patency.
3. Most authorities recommend a 10-minute infusion into a peripheral vein for each drug. When pushing a drug, care should be taken to maintain even pressure so that the force of the administration is lower than the pressure inside the drip chamber.
4. A periodic check of the integrity of the vein serves as an extra safety measure. Most authorities recommend checking the vein after every 2 to 5 ml of administration of the drug that is being pushed.
5. The use of dependent limbs is contraindicated because of the potential of circulatory compromise.
6. Use a site proximal to that used for the previous IV. There have been reports of extravasation distal to the existing IV. Adequate time should be given to ensure healing of the vein to avoid leakage of a chemotherapeutic agent from a previous puncture site.
7. Always observe the site.[3, 6, 14, 22, 68, 105, 129–132]

Biohazard Safety

Safety for the patient, nurse, and ancillary staff should not be overlooked. The standard is never to expose the patient, the nurse, or the environment unnecessarily to potentially hazardous substances. Special care in preparing and administering chemotherapeutic agents eliminates accidental exposure from spills and sprays. Unpowdered latex gloves of 0.007 to 0.009 mm thickness should always be worn when handling chemotherapeutic agents. Research has shown that surgical latex gloves are less permeable to cytotoxic agents than gloves made with polyvinyl chloride, so latex gloves provide superior protection. Some experts recommend double-gloving during chemotherapy preparation and changing the gloves every 30 to 60 minutes. The use of gowns and masks is controversial, because this may have a negative psychologic effect on the patient; therefore, their use is a matter of personal preference. If there is a potential of a splash, eye protection should be worn. In the case of an accidental spray of chemotherapeutic agent in the eye, the eye must be flushed with copious amounts of water. Depending on the agent and the degree of eye irritation, steroid drops may be administered.

A vertical laminar flow hood, class II biologic safety cabinet, is imperative for the preparation of chemotherapeutic agents to avoid aerosol spray in the air and potential exposure to toxic substances. Bottles and bags should be spiked and tubing primed in the chemotherapy preparation area prior to adding the antineoplastic agent. This provides an added safety margin for the nurse when connecting the patient. After the infusion has been completed, the tubing should be flushed with saline to eliminate the potential for an accidental chemotherapy spill while disconnecting the patient. If a chemotherapeutic agent comes in contact with the skin of the patient or staff, the area must be thoroughly cleansed with mild soap and large amounts of water.

Inadvertent chemotherapy spills should be cleaned up immediately. Most institutions have a chemotherapy spill kit that contains a sawdust-type substance or an absorbent, plastic-backed sheet to soak up the solution. Clean spills starting from the outside edges and work toward the center. Limit traffic in the spill area to prevent spread of the contamination. Broken glass should be gathered with a disposable scoop. The involved area should be washed with copious amounts of soap and water at least three times. Protective clothing, including a low-permeability gown or cover-up and safety glasses, face shield, or goggles, should be worn while cleaning a chemotherapy spill and then disposed of properly.

All contaminated material, such as gloves, tubing, and filters, should be discarded in a double thick plastic bag that is leakproof, sealable, and labeled as a biohazard. Sharp instruments, including needles, syringes, and ampules, should be placed in a leakproof, puncture-resistant container and disposed of in accordance with federal, EPA, and OSHA regulations. Individual state regulations may vary and have other specific requirements that must be followed.

Many of the chemotherapeutic drugs are excreted in the urine and stool. Some studies have shown drug levels in the saliva. The nurse needs to exercise caution when handling sputum, emesis, or excreta from patients receiving chemotherapy. Gloves should always be worn when cleaning an incontinent patient or when emptying a Foley catheter or bedpan. The primary caregiver needs to be aware of and use universal precautions when assisting with patient care.[3, 6, 8, 14, 22, 33, 105, 133–141]

The safe administration of antineoplastic agents depends on the skill of those handling chemotherapeutic agents. Clearly, the education and expertise of the intravenous nurse are key components of the oncology team.

Unfortunately, not every cancer patient can be cured, but the nurse can be an active participant in providing quality care and improving the patient's quality of life. Many oncology nurses find caring for the cancer patient professionally challenging, which provides a renewed sense of purpose and a redefined concept of priority in the nurse's own life.

References

1. Bender C. Chemotherapy. In Ziegfeld CR (ed). Core Curriculum for Oncology Nursing. Philadelphia: W. B. Saunders, 1987, 222–235.

2. Dollinger M, Rosenbaum E, Cable G. Everyone's Guide to Cancer Therapy. Kansas City: Somerville House Books, 1991.

3. Groenwald SL, Frogge MH, Goodman MS, Yarbro CH (eds). Cancer Nursing: Principles and Practice, 2nd ed. Boston: Jones & Bartlett, 1990.

4. Goodman M. Management of nausea and vomiting induced by outpatient cisplatin (Platinol) therapy. Semin Oncol Nurs (suppl), 1987; 3:23–35.

5. Ziegfeld CR (ed). Core Curriculum for Oncology Nursing. Philadelphia: W. B. Saunders, 1987.

6. Brown J, Hogan C. Chemotherapy. In Groenwald SL, Frogge MH, Goodman MS, Yarbro CH (eds). Cancer Nursing: Principles and Practice, 2nd ed. Boston: Jones & Bartlett, 1990:231–283.

7. Holleb A, Fink D, Murphy G. American Cancer Society Textbook of Clinical Oncology. Atlanta: American Cancer Society, 1991.

8. Mayer D. Hazards of chemotherapy. Implementing safe handling practices. Cancer (suppl) 1992; 70:988–992.

9. Petersen J. Chemotherapy. In Baird SB (ed). A Cancer Sourcebook for Nurses, 6th ed. Atlanta: American Cancer Society, 1991:73–83.

10. Dodd M. Managing the Side Effects of Chemotherapy and Radiation. New York: Prentice Hall Press, 1991.

11. Hiderley L, Hassey-Dow K. Radiation Oncology. In Baird SB, McCorkle R, Grant M (eds). Cancer Nursing. A Comprehensive Textbook. Philadelphia: W. B. Saunders, 1991:246–265.

12. McNally J, Somerville E, Miaskowski C, Rostad M. Guidelines for Oncology Nursing Practice. Pittsburgh: Oncology Nursing Society, 1991.

13. Burke M, Wilkes G, Ingwersen K. Chemotherapy Care Plans, Designs for Nursing Care. Boston: Jones & Bartlett, 1992.

14. Oncology Nursing Society and American Nurses Association. Standards of Oncology Nursing Practice. Kansas City, KS: American Nurses Association, 1987.

15. Dorr R, Fritz W. Cancer Chemotherapy Handbook. New York: North Holland-Elsevier, 1980.

16. DeVita V, Hellman S, Rosenberg S. Cancer: Principles and Practice of Oncology, 3rd ed. Philadelphia: J. B. Lippincott, 1989.

17. Fischer D, Knobf M. The Cancer Chemotherapy Handbook, 3rd ed. Chicago: Year Book, 1989.

18. Wittes R. Manual of Oncologic Therapeutics. Philadelphia: J. B. Lippincott, 1991.

19. Dorland's Illustrated Medical Dictionary, 24th ed. Philadelphia: W. B. Saunders, 1965.

20. Goodman M. Cancer: Chemotherapy and Care. Evansville, IN: Bristol Laboratories, 1986.

21. Goodman M. Cancer: Chemotherapy and Care, 3rd ed. Princeton, NJ: Bristol-Meyers Squibb, 1992.

22. Knobf M, Fisher D, Welch-McCaffrey D. Cancer Chemotherapy Treatment and Care, 2nd ed. Boston: Year Book, 1984.

23. Perry M. The Chemotherapy Source Book. Baltimore: Williams & Wilkins, 1992.

24. Tenenbaum L. Cancer Chemotherapy: A Reference Guide. Philadelphia: W. B. Saunders, 1989.

25. Williams W, Beutler E, Erslev A, Lichtman M (eds). Hematology. New York: McGraw-Hill, 1990.

26. Dorr R, Alberts D. Temperature dependence of adriamycin, cis-diaminedichloroplatinum, bleomycin, and 1,3-bis(2-chloroethyl)-1-nitrosourea cytotoxicity in vitro. Cancer Res 1983; 43:517.

27. Gelman R, Tormey D, Betensky R, et al. Actual weight in the calculation of surface area: Effects on dose of 11 chemotherapy agents. Cancer Treat Rep 1987; 71:907–911.

28. Angel F. An overview of ondansetron for chemotherapy-induced nausea and emesis. J Oncol Nurs 1993; 16:84–89.

29. Borison H, McCarthy L. Neuropharmacologic mechanisms of emesis. In Laszlo J (ed). Antiemetics and Cancer Chemotherapy. Baltimore: Williams & Wilkins, 1983:6–20.

30. Carr B, Bertrand M, Browning S, et al. A comparison of the antiemetic efficacy of prochlorperazine and metoclopramide for the treatment of cisplatin-induced emesis: A prospective, randomized, double-blind study. J Clin Oncol 1985; 3:1127–1132.

31. Egan A, Taggart J, Bender C. Management of chemotherapy-related nausea and vomiting using a serotonin antagonist. Oncol Nurs Forum 1992; 195:1791–1795.

32. Fraschini G, Ciociiola A, Esparza L, et al. Evaluation of three oral dosages of ondansetron in the prevention of nausea and emesis associated with cyclophosphamide-doxorubicin chemotherapy. J Clin Oncol 1993; 199:1268–1274.

33. Gahart B. Intravenous Medications: A Handbook for Nurses and Other Allied Health Personnel, 7th ed. St. Louis: Mosby Year Book, 1993.

34. Goodman M. Managing side effects of chemotherapy. Semin Oncol Nurs (suppl) 1989; 1:29–52.

35. Grant M. Nausea and vomiting. Nursing management of common problems. Am Cancer Soc 1987; 16–24.

36. Krasnow S. New directions in managing chemotherapy-related emesis. Suppl Oncology 1991; 5:19–24.

37. Kris M, Tyson L, Clark R, Gralla R. Oral ondansetron for the control of delayed emesis after cisplatin—report of a phase II study and a review of completed trials to manage delayed emesis. Cancer (suppl 4) 1992; 15:1012–1016.

38. Kris M, Gralla R, Tyson L, et al. Improved control of cisplatin-induced emesis with high-dose metoclopromide and with combinations of metoclopramide, dexamethasone and diphenhydramine. Cancer 1985; 55:527–534.

39. Morrow G. Chemotherapy-related nausea and vomiting: Etiology and management. CA 1989; 39:2.

40. Morrow G. The effect of susceptibility to motion sickness on the side effects of cancer chemotherapy. Cancer 1985; 55:2766–2770.

41. Weinstein S. Memory Bank for I.V.'s. Baltimore: Williams & Wilkins, 1986.

42. Wickham R. Managing chemotherapy-related nausea and vomiting. The state of the art. Oncol Nurs Forum 1989; 16:563–574.

43. Now patients take control of antiemesis. Am J Nurs 1992; 92:11.

44. Yasko J. Nursing Management of Symptoms Associated with Chemotherapy. Columbus, OH: Adria Laboratories, 1988.

45. Rhodes V. Nausea, vomiting, and retching. Nurs Clin North Am 1990; 25:885–900.

46. Zofran (ondansetron) package insert. Research Triangle Park, NC: Glaxo, Inc., 1991.

47. Dundee J, Ghaly R, Bill K, Chestnutt W. Acupuncture prophylaxis of cancer chemotherapy-induced sickness. J Royal Soc Med 1989; 82:244–245.

48. Dundee J, Ghaly R, Bill K, et al. Effect of stimulation of the P6 point on postoperative nausea and vomiting. Br J Anaesth 1990; 63:612–618.

49. Cotanch P. Relaxation training for control of nausea and vomiting in patients receiving chemotherapy. Cancer Nurs 1983; 6:277.

50. Goldberg R, Tull R. The Psycho-Social Dimensions of Cancer. A Practical Guide for Health-Care Providers. London: Collier Macmillan, 1983.

51. Morrow G, Hickak J. Behavioral treatment of chemotherapy-induced nausea and vomiting. Oncology 1993; 7:83–97.

52. National Cancer Institute. Chemotherapy and You—A Guide to Self-Help During Treatment. Bethesda: US Department of Health and Human Services, 1990.

53. Rogers B. Taxol: A promising new drug of the '90s. Oncol Nurs Forum 1993; 20:1483–1489.

54. Storey P. Medical management of nonchemotherapy-induced nausea and vomiting in advanced cancer patients. Cancer Bull 1991; 43:433–436.

55. Wickham R. Pulmonary toxicity secondary to cancer treatment. Oncol Nurs Forum 1986; 13:69–76.

56. McCorkle M, Hays K. Understanding Chemotherapy, A Guide to Treatment of Leukemia, Lymphoma and Multiple Myeloma for Patients and Their Families. New York: Leukemia Society of America, Program Services Department, 1992.

57. Pagana K, Pagana T. Diagnostic and Laboratory Test Reference. St. Louis: Mosby–Year Book, 1992.

58. Polomano R, Miller S. Understanding and Managing Oncologic Emergencies. Columbus, OH: Adria Laboratories, 1987.

59. Rostad M. Current strategies for managing myelosuppression in patients with cancer. Oncol Nurs Forum 1991; 18:7–15.

60. It's a matter of taste. Tips for overcoming taste loss or alteration. Coping March/April 1993; 42.

61. Ramstack J, Rosenbaum E. Nutrition for the Chemotherapy Patient. Palo Alto, CA: Bull, 1990.

62. Appearing your best. Atlanta: American Cancer Society, 1990.

63. National Cancer Institute. The Breast Cancer Digest. A Guide to Medical Care, Emotional Support, Educational Programs, and Resources. Bethesda, MD: US Department of Health and Human Services, 1984: NIH Publ. 84–1691.

64. Jordan E. Preparing for hair loss. Coping March/April 1993; 44–46.

65. Plan ahead for hair loss. Coping March/April 1992; 34–36.

66. Beck S. A Client's Guide to Oral Care. Cary, IL: Sage Products, 1990.

67. Crudi C, Larkin M. Core Curriculum for Intravenous Nursing. Philadelphia: J. B. Lippincott, 1984.
68. Eilers J. Oral cavity problems experienced in cancer treatment. Nursing management of common problems. Am Cancer Soc Sept. 1987; 9–16.
69. Mahood D, Dose A, Loprinzi C, et al. Inhibition of fluorouracil-induced stomatitis by oral cryotherapy. J Clin Oncol 1991; 9:449–452.
70. McGuire D. Patterns of mucositis and pain in patients receiving preparative chemotherapy and bone marrow transplantation. Oncol Nurs Forum 1993; 20:1493–1502.
71. National Institutes of Health. Consensus Development Conference on Oral Complications of Cancer Therapies: Diagnosis, Prevention, and Treatment. Bethesda, MD: National Institutes of Health, 1989.
72. Naylor G, Terezhalmy G. Oral complications of cancer chemotherapy: Prevention and management. Special Care Dentistry July/August 1988.
73. Poland J. Prevention and treatment of oral complications in the cancer patient. Oncology 1991; 5:45–50.
74. Jones S. Current Concepts in the Use of Doxorubicin Chemotherapy. Milan, Italy: Graficine Milani, 1982.
75. Rowinsky E, McGuire W, Guarnieri T, et al. Cardiac disturbances during the administration of taxol. J Clin Oncol 1991; 9:1704–1712.
76. Kaplan R, Weirnik P. Neurotoxicity of antitumor agents. In Perry MC, Yarbro JW (eds). Toxicity of Chemotherapy. New York: Grune & Stratton, 1984: 365–431.
77. Lundquist D, Holmes W. Documentation of neurotoxicity resulting from high-dose cytosine arabinoside. Oncol Nurs Forum 1993; 20:1409–1418.
78. Whitecare R, Finley R. Paraplatin Administration Guide. Evansville, IN: Bristol-Meyers, 1989.
79. Chemotherapeutic Drug Compatibility: Quick Reference Guide, 2nd ed. Chicago, IL: Abbott LifeCare Omni-Flow, 1992.
80. Lydon J. Nephrotoxicity of cancer treatment. Oncol Nurs Forum March/April, 1986; 13:68–77.
81. Schilsky R. Renal and metabolic toxicities of cancer treatment. In Perry MC, Yarbro JW (eds). Toxicity of Chemotherapy. New York: Grune & Stratton, 1984:317–342.
82. Ginsberg S, Comis R. The pulmonary toxicity of antineoplastic agents. In Perry MC, Yarbro JW (eds). Toxicity of Chemotherapy. New York: Grune & Stratton, 1984:227–268.
83. Jensen J, Goel R, Venner P. The effect of corticosteroid administration of bleomycin lung toxicity. Cancer 1990; 65:1291–1297.
84. Caligiuri M. Leukemia and pregnancy: Treatment and outcome. Adv Oncol 1992; 8:10–17.
85. Donegan W. Cancer and pregnancy. CA 1993; 3:193–214.
86. Shapiro C, Mayer R. Breast cancer during pregnancy. Adv Oncol 1992; 8:25–29.
87. Ward F, Weiss R. Managing lymphoma during pregnancy. Adv Oncol 1992; 8:18–22.
88. Yarbro C, Perry M. The effect of cancer therapy on gonadal function. Semin Oncol Nurs 1985; 1:3–8.
89. Alberts D, Dorr R. Case report: Topical DMSO for mitomycin C-induced skin ulceration. Oncol Nurs Forum 1991; 18:693–695.
90. Beason R. Antineoplastic vesicant extravasation. JIN 1990; 13:111–114.
91. Bleicher J, Haynes W, Massop D, et al. The delineation of adriamycin extravasation using fluorescence microscopy. Plast Reconstr Surg 1984; 74:114–122.
92. Bowers D, Lynch J. Adriamycin extravasation. Plast Reconstr Surg 1978; 61:86–92.
93. Dorr R, Alberts D, Stone A. Cold protection and heat synergism of experimental doxorubicin skin toxicity in the mouse. Cancer Treat Rep 1985; 69:431–437.
94. Dorr R, Alberts A, Salmon S. Cold protection from intradermal doxorubicin ulceration in the mouse. Proc Annu Meet Am Assoc Cancer Res 1983; 24:255.
95. Dorr R. Discussion: What is the appropriate management of tissue extravasation by antitumor agents? Plast Reconstr Surg 1985; 75:403.
96. Larson D. Treatment of tissue extravasation by antitumor agents. Cancer 1982; 49:1796.
97. Larson D. What is the appropriate management of tissue extravasation by anti-tumor agents? Plast Reconstr Surg 1985; 75:397.
98. Larson D. Letter to the editor. Anti-neoplastic drug extravasation. Plast Reconstr Surg 1986; 77:498.
99. Montrose P. Extravasation management. Semin Oncol Nurs 1987; 3:128–132.
100. Oncology Nursing Society. Cancer Chemotherapy Guidelines: Module V. Recommendations for the Management of Vesicant Extravasation, Hypersensitivity and Anaphylaxis. Pittsburgh: Oncology Nursing Society, 1992.
101. Petro J, Graham W, Miller S, et al. Experimental and clinical studies of ulcers induced with adriamycin. Surg Forum 1979; 30:535.
102. Preuss P, Partoft S. Cytostatic Extravasations. Copenhagen: Finsensvej.
103. Reilly J, Neifield J, Rosenberg S. Clinical course and management of accidental adriamycin extravasation. Cancer 1977; 40:2053.
104. Intravenous Nurses Society. Intravenous Nursing Standards of Practice, Revised. Belmont, MA: Intravenous Nurses Society, 1990.
105. Rudolph R, Larson D. Etiology and treatment of chemotherapeutic agent extravasation injuries: A review. J Clin Oncol 1987; 5:1116–1126.
106. Tsavaris N, Komitsopoulou P, Karagiaouris P, et al. Prevention of tissue necrosis due to accidental extravasation of cytostatic drugs by a conservative approach. Cancer Chemother Pharmacol 1992; 30:330–333.
107. Vogelzang N. Adriamycin flare: A skin reaction resembling extravasation. Cancer Treat Rep 1987; 63:2067–2069.
108. Wood L, Gullo S. I.V. vesicants: How to avoid extravasation. Am J Nurs 1993; 42–50.
109. Yucha C, Hastings M, Szeverenyi N. Difference among intravenous extravasation using four common solutions. JIN 1993; 16:277–281.
110. Craig J, Capizzi R. The prevention and treatment of immediate hypersensitivity reaction from cancer chemotherapy. Semin Oncol Nurs 1985; 1:285–291.
111. Richards C, Wujcik D. Cutaneous toxicity associated with high-dose cytosine arabinoside: A literature review. Oncol Nurs Forum 1992; 19:8.
112. Weiss R. Hypersensitivity reactions to cancer chemotherapy. In Perry MC, Yarbro JW (eds). Toxicity of Chemotherapy. New York: Grune & Stratton, 1984; 101–117.
113. Lobert C. Antiemetics in cancer chemotherapy. Cancer Nurs 1992; 15:22–33.
114. Bayha E. Taxol, the race to synthesize the cure. Coping 1992; 17.
115. Chitwood M. The story of taxol. Coping 1993; 26–27.
116. Galassi A. The next generation: New chemotherapy agents for the 1990's. Semin Oncol Nurs 1992; 8:83–94.
117. O'Brien R. Is taxol the cure? Coping 1992; 11.
118. Rowinsky E, Gilbert M, McGuire W, et al. Sequences of taxol and cisplatin: A phase I and pharmacologic study. J Clin Oncol 1991; 9:1692–1703.
119. Rowinsky E, McGuire W, Donehower R. The current status of taxol. Principles and practice. Gynecol Oncol Updates 1993; 1:1–16.
120. Sadilek D. Taxol: A promising new cancer treatment. Oncol Nurs Soc Update 1993; 15:2.
121. Taxol for Injection: Concentrate Administration Guide. Princeton, NJ: Bristol-Meyers Squibb, 1993.
122. Taxol, Background Information. National Cancer Institute. US Department of Health and Human Services, Bethesda, MD: Office of Cancer Communications, 1991.
123. Williams S. Chemotherapeutic management of advanced testicular and ovarian cancer. Issues in Chemotherapy, Vol. 2. New York: Triclinica Communications, 1991.
124. Uhlenhopp M. An overview of the relationship between alkylating agents and therapy-related acute nonlymphocytic leukemia. Cancer Nurs 1992; 15:9–17.
125. Bunn P, Canetta R, Ozols R, Rozencweig M. Carboplatin (JM-8). Current Perspectives and Future Directions. Philadelphia: W. B. Saunders, 1990.
126. Yarbro C. Carboplatin: A clinical review. Semin Oncol Nurs (suppl 1) 1989; 5:63–69.
127. Capizzi R, Holcenberg J. Asparaginase. In Cancer Medicine, 3rd ed. Philadelphia: Lea & Febiger, 1993.
128. Walters P. Chemo: A nurse's guide to action, administration and side effects. RN 1990; 52–67.
129. Huges C. Giving cancer drugs IV. Some guidelines. Am J Nurs 1986; 86:34–38.
130. Oncology Nursing Society. Access Device Guidelines, Recommendations for Nursing Education and Practice. Module I, Catheters. Module II, Implanted Ports and Reservoirs. Module III, Pumps (Infusion Systems). Pittsburgh: Oncology Nursing Society, 1989, 1990.
131. Schulmeister L. Needle dislodgment from implanted venous access devices: Inpatient and outpatient experience. JIN 1989; 12:90–92.
132. American Society of Hospital Pharmacists. Technical assistance bul-

letin on handling cytotoxic drugs in hospitals. Am J Hosp Pharm 1985; 42:131–137.

133. Baldwin D. Management of intravenous hazardous material and hazardous wastes in the work environment. JIN 1992; 15:90–99. March/April, 1992.

134. Dorr R, Griffin-Brown J. Reducing the Risk of Cytoxic Exposure. Evansville, IN: Bristol-Meyers, 1990.

135. Gullo S. Safe handling of antineoplastic drugs: Translating the recommendations into practice. Oncol Nurs Forum 1988; 15:595–601.

136. Laidlaw J, Connor T, Thesis J, et al. Permeability of latex and polyvinyl chloride gloves to 20 antineoplastic drugs. Am J Hosp Pharm 1984; 41:2618–2623.

137. Oncology Nursing Society. Safe Handling of Cytotoxic Drugs: Independent Study Module. Pittsburgh: Oncology Nursing Society, 1989.

138. OSHA. Work-practice guidelines for personnel dealing with cytotoxic (antineoplastic) drugs. Am J Hosp Pharm 1986; 43:1193–1204.

139. Parillo V. Documentation forms for monitoring occupational surveillance of health care workers who handle cytotoxic drugs. Oncol Nurs Forum 1994; 21:115–120.

140. Stevens K. Safe handling of cytotoxic drugs in home chemotherapy. Semin Oncol Nurs (suppl 1) 1989; 5:15–20.

141. Dorr R, Andersen R, Comis N. Working with Cytotoxic Agents: A Compilation of Recent Literature. Evansville, IN: Bristol-Meyers, 1987.

CHAPTER 14 Pain Management

Barbara St. Marie, MA, CRNI

As medical care improves, people will continue to live longer, and with this longevity, an improved quality of life is sought. People are more aware of pain and the significant problems associated with it than in any time in history. "Pain is a more terrible lord of mankind than even death itself."[1] Therefore, it is important that nurses and other health care professionals have up-to-date knowledge of pain and know how to define it and how to intervene. The International Association for the Study of Pain has established three different categories of pain: acute, chronic, and cancer.[2]

Acute pain is caused by such occurrences as traumatic injury, a surgical procedure, or a medical disorder. With acute pain, the patient may show a clinical picture of tachycardia, hypertension, tachypnea, shallow respirations, agitation or restlessness, facial grimace, or splinting. The incidence of acute pain is astounding. Each year over 100 million people have acute pain, 30 million of whom are disabled for 12 days, with a loss of 100 million days of work worth 1 billion dollars.[3]

Chronic pain is persistent, often lasting more than 6 months. However, some practitioners believe that chronic pain may exist before this 6-month period. An individual who has chronic pain may show the same clinical picture as the person suffering from acute pain, or their body may condition all signs of pain with normal heart rate, normal blood pressure, and no facial grimace. It is estimated that back pain alone disables approximately 11.7 million Americans—2.6 million are temporarily disabled and 2.6 million are permanently disabled.[4]

Millions of cancer patients throughout the world experience pain they would rate from moderate to severe. Approximately 30 to 40% of cancer patients in the intermediate stages of cancer and 55 to 90% of terminal cancer patients have pain; 60% of these patients reporting pain express it as of moderate or great severity.[5] Some may achieve pain relief, but only at the expense of losing consciousness before death because of massive doses of narcotics. This tells us we need to do a better job of controlling pain, but there are barriers to effective pain control.

Inadequate knowledge and skills of health care professionals exist in regard to the pharmacology of pain medications, physiology of pain, and techniques of pain control. Attitudes of health care professionals serve as a barrier to effective pain control. Some professionals believe that pain is "normal" or innocuous, whereas others fear addiction.[6, 7] The daily media is filled with information about drug abuse and addiction that feeds the fears of doctors, nurses, and the public about potential drug addiction. Laws and regulations exist that impose penalties designed to prohibit the use of narcotics except in severely limited circumstances. Those concerns and prohibitions can inhibit the use of defined drugs, even though recently acquired information about their use for pain control clearly shows that more effective pain control can be achieved without addiction and patients can maintain awareness of their environment.

State cancer pain initiatives, begun in Wisconsin, are organized efforts to overcome the lack of knowledge and prohibitions of law through physician and nurse education and lobbying efforts with legislators and regulatory authorities. Many of those participating in these initiatives were volunteers who had been close to someone who needlessly suffered cancer pain. The cancer patient's quality of life lies in the balance between the caregiver's fear of professional penalties for the misuse of narcotics, and the lack of understanding of a cancer patient's often increased needs for systemic narcotics.

A landmark study in the *Annals of Internal Medicine* showed that pain is greatly undertreated. This study revealed that physicians underprescribe analgesic agents, nurses administer fewer analgesics than prescribed, patients request fewer analgesic medications than they need, and the prn regimen of administering IM narcotic agents ensures that the patient will experience pain.[8] At first, pain serves the purpose of warning the body that something is wrong, but once it serves that purpose it should be relieved. Pain is harmful to the body if left untreated. There are significant endocrine responses to pain, increases in heart rate and vasoconstriction, and decreased gastrointestinal motility. Pain also causes muscle splinting that can diminish pulmonary function and lead to atelectasis and/or pneumonia. These findings make it even more evident that health care professionals need to take pain control seriously to reduce postoperative complications, reduce the length of the hospital stay, and improve the quality of patients' lives.[7]

DISCIPLINES INVOLVED

The discipline of pain management is rapidly taking form. Physicians from the anesthesiology, neurology, and oncology specialties have chosen to be involved with pain management. Anesthesiology offers a pain fellowship that includes the practice of acute, chronic, and cancer pain management as an adjunct to the practice of traditional pain control in the operating room. The oncologist focuses on cancer pain while focusing on curing patients of their cancer. The neurologist concentrates on the management of pain with a neurologic component, which is usually chronic, nonmalignant pain. The new and rapidly developing discipline of pain management could quickly become obsolete if the supportive foundation of these disciplines were to falter. To prevent this, societies and associations have been organized to advance the art of pain management, provide support for nurses and doctors with educational programs, and promote clinical networking.

Because of the need for improving current pain management systems for acute, chronic, and cancer pain, nursing schools should respond by offering more information on pain management in their curricula. McCaffery and Beebe have offered an excellent contribution to the field of pain management in their text.[9] As more information becomes available about pain pathways, different opiate receptor sites, new medications, and new routes of analgesia administration, we are invited to use our basic knowledge and welcome the advances in pain management. These advances include patient-controlled analgesia, intraspinal narcotics, and local anesthetics. Continuing education regarding advances in pain management warrants high priority.

Knowledge gained through infection control and advances in IV technology have provided the IV nurse with a background that has application in pain management and makes it easier to gain proficiency in pain management. Pain management includes such procedures as piggybacking narcotic infusions and supplying patient-controlled doses of narcotic into maintenance lines. It also involves the delivery of narcotics and local anesthetics into spaces that are not typically used for medication administration, such as epidural and intrathecal spaces. Infusion pumps are becoming ''smarter'' and one must understand computer technology to program these sophisticated pumps correctly.

IV nurses can be valuable members of the health care team concerned with pain management. They have a pre-existing knowledge and expertise that can help resolve problems that occur with pain management. These include an awareness of inappropriate dosages of narcotics, failures of the equipment used to deliver the appropriate medications for pain relief, and complications or adverse reactions that can occur when a patient is subjected to procedures and medications the IV nurse is trained to provide. Special challenges are provided when patients receive these therapies in a variety of settings, such as home, hospital, and outpatient clinics. Knowledge of advances in pain management needs to be acquired by nurses in all settings. As people become more aware that the technology for providing pain relief that was previously unavailable now exists in all health care settings, they will demand it. The IV nurse is positioned to provide pain relief with present technologic skills supplemented by additional training.

PHYSIOLOGY OF PAIN

Matching the clinical indicators with the appropriate pain intervention requires knowledge of the biochemical response to pain, the pain pathway, and opiate receptor sites. Also, correctly interpreting what the patient is communicating about the pain requires a predisposition to hear and believe what is said by the patient.

When there is a cut made on the skin, a chemical is released called a prostaglandin. Prostaglandin is thought to be the precursor to the painful impulse, which allows the impulse to be carried through the afferent or peripheral nerve fibers into the spinal cord. In the spinal cord, the nerve endings release a neurotransmitter called substance P.[11] Substance P allows the pain impulse to be carried through the dorsal horn and ascend to the brain, where the person experiences the painful sensation. Figure 14–1 is a simplified cross section of the dorsal horn; the heavy black lines trace the pain path. Substance P is released at the presynaptic junction and carries the pain impulse forward to the laminae. At the laminae, there is a synapse or firing, which impels the pain impulse through each lamina to the postsynaptic junction. Substance P continues to be released and the pain impulse is transmitted through the spinothalamic tract to the brain—in particular, the thalamus. The pathway continues as the impulse travels to the cerebral cortex, where the pain becomes conscious, and down the descending pathway, where a withdrawal reflex makes the individual pull away from the painful stimuli.[2]

Endogenous Opiates

The body has its own protection from painful impulses, called endogenous opiates.[12] These serve to keep us pain-free through normal daily living. Endogenous opiates include the endorphins and the enkephalins. The endorphins are located in the brain and are mimicked by the systemic administration of narcotics. The enkephalins are located in the spinal cord and are mimicked by the intraspinal administration of narcotics.

Activities that promote the release of endogenous opiates are physical exercise, deep relaxation, sexual activity, crying, and laughter. Situations that decrease the release of endogenous opiates are stress, chronic pain, chemical dependency, and emotional depression.

Opiate Receptors

Understanding opiate receptors helps in understanding how narcotics work to break the painful impulses. Opiate receptors are parts of cells that combine with a particular opiate to create both analgesia and various side effects. There are five known opiate receptor sites, but researchers have gained the most knowledge about three—mu, kappa, and sigma. Each type of opiate receptor has particular characteristics. Table 14–1 lists the opiate receptors and the opiates used to produce analgesia and other effects at these receptors.[2] The most effective opiate receptor for producing superior analgesia is the mu receptor. The kappa receptor is weaker, and is less likely to produce physical dependency. The sigma receptor is very weak and, when combined with narcotics, tends to produce agitation and respiratory stimulation. Little is known thus far about the delta and epsilon receptors. All these opiate receptors are located near the

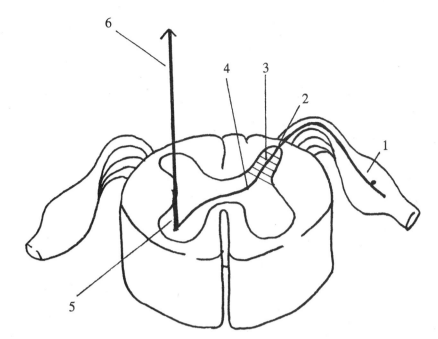

Figure 14–1. Cross section of the spinal cord.

1. Dorsal Root Ganglion
2. Presynaptic Junction
3. Laminae
4. Postsynaptic Junction
5. Contralateral Spinothalamic Tract
6. Brain (Conscious Level)

thalamus in the brain and in the dorsal horn of the spinal cord.[13] Naloxone can reverse any combination of opioids to their respective receptor sites. It has been discovered that there are subsets of the mu receptor, mu-1 and mu-2. Mu-1 is responsible for analgesic effects and mu-2 for side effects. Efforts are now being made to find narcotics that can combine only with mu-1.

Antagonist and Agonist-Antagonist

The advantage of administering narcotics for pain management is that their effects can always be reversed. Early intervention with narcotic side effects allows reversal to take place without the situation becoming an emergency. There

are two types of medications that reverse a narcotic that combines with the mu receptor. A commonly used pure antagonist is naloxone hydrochloride (Narcan). This drug competitively inhibits narcotics at the opiate receptor sites and thus reverses their side effects. However, some reports have indicated that the reversal of the kappa agonist may not be predictable.

An agonist-antagonist can also reverse a narcotic that combines with the mu receptor.[14] Agonist-antagonist narcotics combine at the kappa receptor site, thus producing a lower quality analgesia than a mu agonist. A commonly used agonist-antagonist that combines with the kappa opiate receptor site is nalbuphine hydrochloride (Nubain). Working with agonist-antagonist medications requires understanding when this kappa agonist is administered in relation to a mu agonist.

Table 14–1

Opiate Receptors and the Effects of Opiates

Opiate Receptor	Agonist	Antagonist	Effect of Agonist
Mu	Morphine Meperidine Fentanyl Sufentanil Alfentanil	Naloxone (Narcan) Pentazocine (Talwin) Nalbuphine (Nubain)	Analgesia; decreased respirations; decreased heart rate; physical dependence; euphoria
Kappa	Pentazocine Nalbuphine Butorphanol (Stadol) Buprenorphine (Buprenex)	Naloxone (?)	Analgesia; sedation; decreased respirations; miosis
Sigma	Pentazocine Ketamine	Naloxone	Dysphoria; hypertonia; tachycardia; tachypnea

From St. Marie B. Narcotic infusions: A changing scene. JIN 1991; 14:334–344.

When given alone, nalbuphine hydrochloride produces a mild analgesia. However, if it is given while a mu agonist is in the patient's system, it acts to reverse the mu agonist's analgesia and side effects. For example, a cancer patient who is accustomed to taking oral morphine solution (300 mg/day) is admitted to the hospital for pain control. An order is written for 10 mg IV nalbuphine hydrochloride every 3 to 4 hours prn pain to supplement the oral morphine. Although the thinking behind this nalbuphine hydrochloride order may be that it is preferable because of fewer side effects, it actually acts to reverse the oral morphine, thereby producing severe pain for the patient and, most likely, symptoms of withdrawal.

Pain Nerve Fibers

Specialized nerve endings in the skin and viscera send messages of noxious stimuli, such as mechanical, chemical, or thermal, to the brain. These specialized nerve endings, or receptors, send impulses along specific fiber types, all of which are peripheral nerves. These fiber types are identified as A, B, and C and differ in their rate of impulse conduction and diameter. A fibers are the largest, the most rapid conductors, and myelinated. B fibers are smaller, somewhat slower conductors, and lightly myelinated. C fibers have the smallest diameter, are the slowest conductors, and are unmyelinated. A fibers tend to conduct intense pain but are more receptive to local anesthetics and nonsteroidal anti-inflammatories. B fibers conduct both sympathetic and parasympathetic impulses. C fibers tend to conduct dull pain and are most responsive to narcotics of any route.[2]

Dermatomes constitute the segmental distribution of the spinal nerve sensations and are labeled according to their exit point on the spinal cord. Dermatome charts (Fig. 14–2) are useful for tracking the nerves innervating the area of pain. With a nerve block or the intraspinal route of analgesia, medications can be delivered directly to those nerves that create the origin of an individual's pain.[2]

The IV nurse, with a knowledge of pharmacology, can intervene for those with poorly managed pain by evaluating the current narcotic regimen the patient is receiving. Antagonism between the mu and kappa agonists is easily identified. If a kappa agonist is being used for analgesia and is providing inadequate analgesia, the IV nurse may recommend a mu agonist for superior analgesia. Understanding the function of the A-delta fibers and C fibers in pain conduction can assist the IV nurse in identifying whether the intervention being used for the specific type of pain the patient describes is appropriate.

By understanding the dermatomal distribution of pain when working with epidural infusions of narcotics and local anesthetics, the IV nurse can work with the anesthesiologist to determine the appropriate dermatomal distribution of narcotic and local anesthetic to the painful area. For example, the volume of infusion of lipid-soluble narcotic may need to be increased to widen the spread of analgesia (Fig. 14–2).

PARENTERAL NARCOTICS

The quality of pain management practice depends on the knowledge and expertise of health care professionals. In the

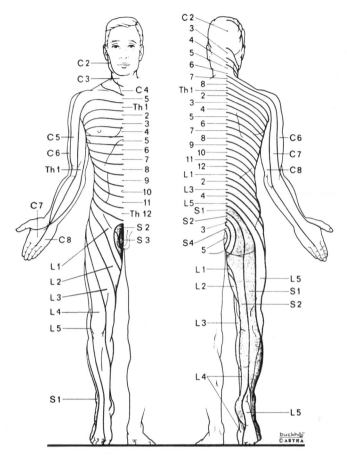

Figure 14–2. Dermatome chart. (Courtesy of Astra Pharmaceuticals.)

ideal health care setting, the professionals are knowledgeable in both conventional methods of pain control and advances in pain control, and are willing to practice quality, up-to-date pain management for their patients.

Parenteral narcotic administration is available to patients in a variety of forms—for example, continuous infusions of narcotics, intermittent doses of narcotics, and combinations of these. Selection of the type of parenteral narcotics for each patient depends on the type of pain indicated by the patient and the availability of the nursing staff for administering it appropriately.

Continuous Infusion. A patient may receive a continuous infusion of narcotics when pain management is desired at a steady state.[15] For example, if the patient states that the pain is rather constant, a continuous infusion of narcotics may be indicated. Before the continuous infusion is given, it is best to administer small doses of narcotic frequently until the proper blood level is achieved to control pain. The continuous infusion is then begun. Continuous infusions of narcotics are appropriately used in trauma, postsurgical, and terminal care settings.[16, 17] The routes of continuous infusion include the intravenous, subcutaneous, and intraspinal (epidural or intrathecal) routes.

Intermittent Doses. Patients may receive intermittent doses of narcotics when they state that the pain is episodic. In these cases, it may be more desirable to treat pain only when experienced, with fast-acting narcotics that are effective for short periods. For example, if the patient has a kidney stone that produces only intermittent yet severe pain, an intermittent dose of narcotic can be effective. Frequent, intermittent doses of narcotics can be administered by the nurse through the oral, sublingual, buccal, rectal, intramuscular, intravenous, subcutaneous, or intraspinal routes. Administering narcotics in larger doses less often can create periods of oversedation in the patient, interrupted by periods of inadequate pain relief (Fig. 14–3).[18] It is more desirable to use small doses of narcotic frequently than large doses of narcotic infrequently.[19] Because the frequent administration of narcotic is time-consuming for the nurse, but is the safest method for administering narcotics, the nurse should consider administering small, frequent doses of narcotics through a patient-controlled analgesia (PCA) delivery system.[20–23]

Combination. A patient may receive a combination of continuous narcotic infusion and intermittent doses of narcotics when it is desirable to produce a steady state of analgesia[24] during painful procedures, increased activity levels, or painful episodes that result from surgery or trauma to organs or tissues.

Routes of Administration

The combination administration of narcotics can occur through the intravenous, subcutaneous, or intraspinal routes. A continuous infusion of narcotics with the patient capability to bolus additional doses is beneficial for cancer pain management. With some infusion pumps, the patient can push the bolus button to administer the dose of narcotic they need, then, after 12 to 24 hours, the nurse can determine how much the patient has used and adjust the hourly rate accordingly. The appropriate assessment of the patient's pain is important here, especially in determining whether the pain is intermittent, constant, or related to activity.[25]

Intravenous Administration

Intravenous narcotics may be administered through central or peripheral venous access. These routes direct narcotics to bind primarily at the opiate receptor sites located in the brain.

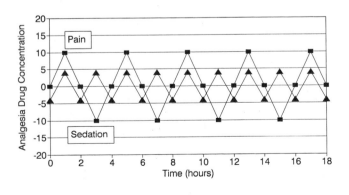

Figure 14–3. Comparison of analgesic levels between IM and PCA narcotics.

Therefore, central nervous system effects, such as sedation or respiratory depression, may easily occur with a patient who is narcotic-naive. Narcotics may be ordered by the physician for intermittent injections administered by the nurse, constant infusion, or PCA. The mechanisms of delivering these narcotics need to be given careful consideration in all settings.

Intermittent injections of narcotics administered by the nurse allow for small doses of narcotics to be given frequently, and require that the nurse be available to the patient for these frequent administrations. Although this may be feasible for nurses attending to patients in critical care settings and postanesthesia care units (PACU), it is not feasible for nurses who work on postsurgical, oncology or medical-surgical floors, where the patient-to-nurse ratio is larger.

A constant infusion is a convenient method for administration and provides the patient with a steady state of analgesia. The problem with this system of narcotic administration is that accumulation may occur, causing the patient to feel oversedated and later to develop respiratory depression. To ascertain the appropriate hourly dose, consideration needs to be given to the patient's age, size, disease process or concurrent diseases, and narcotic tolerance.

The use of PCA allows patients to deliver their own narcotics for pain control. PCA involves low doses of narcotic administered frequently, with the patient's goal being to provide a steady state of analgesia, thus avoiding the peaks and valleys of analgesia, sedation, and pain.[26] PCA delivery of narcotics does not, however, prevent the accumulation of a narcotic and its subsequent side effects. Therefore, patients need to be assessed at regular intervals for respiratory effects and mental status changes. A successful PCA program needs to be safe for the patient while providing adequate pain relief.[27, 28] PCA protocol involves the following: (1) define the type of patient who can use PCA devices and prepare a list of teaching tools; (2) select the appropriate equipment; (3) select the medications and concentrations used; (4) establish consistency of use and dosage; (5) define who can handle the side effects; and (6) provide an appropriate avenue of communication between the patient and nurse to determine the quality of pain relief experienced by the patient. The following types of patients are candidates for PCA:

- Patients who are anticipating pain that is severe yet intermittent, such as those suffering from kidney stones
- Patients who have constant pain that gets worse with activity
- Pediatric patients who can comprehend the technique
- Patients who have the capability to manipulate the dose button
- Patients who are motivated to use this system
- Patients who are not already sedated from other medications

Choosing the proper equipment for PCA administration is imperative. The important features and capabilities of the infusion pump can be listed:[29]

1. The rate of use and doses can be locked in.
2. The narcotics can be locked to the infusion pump to minimize tampering.
3. The pump can deliver a continuous infusion with a bolus capability.

4. The pump measures the amount used by the patient.
5. The pump can be mounted to a pole or be ambulatory.
6. The pump is reliable and durable.
7. The pump is easy to program and easy to learn.
8. The pump is affordable.

Specific patient populations require different parameters for setting the PCA dose and frequency of narcotic delivery. Most narcotics are metabolized in the liver or kidney, so any impairment in these systems may result in the accumulation of narcotic. Precautions such as lowering the drug dose and increasing the time between PCA doses decrease the likelihood of narcotic accumulation. Frequent nursing assessment of the patient's mental status can detect early signs of accumulation so that doses can be adjusted accordingly.

In the elderly population, higher peak effects of narcotic and longer duration of pain relief may be observed after the administration of narcotic.[30] If cognitive impairment is present, this creates barriers to pain management because pain assessment may not be accurate. Pain control for the elderly population must be individualized, making the "routine procedure" of pain management obsolete.

PCA in the substance abuse population is being increasingly used once the cause of pain has been determined (e.g., postoperative pain). The dosage parameters must be increased to achieve analgesia because of the patient's tolerance to opioids.[31] The delivery system for PCA must have specific lock-out intervals and dosage limits within its capability and must be tamper-resistant. By using nonopioid therapies such as transcutaneous electrical nerve stimulation (TENS) units, nonsteroidal anti-inflammatory drugs (NSAIDs), or epidural local anesthetics, the amount of narcotics can be significantly reduced. The nurse must monitor the patient for substance abuse of other narcotics or sedatives during PCA use to prevent the inadvertent potentiation of narcotic, resulting in overdose. Thorough discussion with the patient may determine this potential and/or a toxicology screen can exclude or confirm any suspicions of inaccuracies in the patient's report.

The cooperation of nursing personnel is necessary for a successful PCA program. Infusion devices currently on the market are sometimes difficult to program, lock out, and troubleshoot. When patients sense a nurse's frustration in trying to program the infusion device, their faith in the pain management can waiver. IV nurses can be valuable in selecting the appropriate pain control delivery systems for their facility.

The following questions can be asked when selecting a PCA device:

1. Can the infusion rate be changed easily?
2. Can the infusion pump deliver bolus doses?
3. Can the volume of drug remaining be visually checked?
4. Can it be loaded and started without difficulty?
5. Can the pump hold 12 hours or more of medication?
6. What extra equipment is needed?
7. How much does the drug chamber contain?
8. How much does the pump cost?
9. What potential problems could arise from the use of this pump?

The importance of these questions varies with each setting. By answering these questions, the nurse can select an infusion device that is individualized and appropriate for the facility. Nurses need to have in-service training about the infusion device selected prior to implementation, and should be tested regularly for competency in operating the device.

The Intravenous Nurses Society *Standards of Practice*[32] emphasizes the nurse's vital role in educating the patient. The patient should become familiar with the PCA infusion pump prior to surgery, because the stress of surgery along with amnesic medications received perioperatively may cause the patient to forget any teaching that occurred in the pre-induction area or PACU, or on the surgical floor postoperatively. The concepts used in patient teaching include discussion of the following:

1. How to use patient-controlled analgesia
2. When to push the bolus button
3. When to communicate with the nurse (e.g., pain not controlled with PCA, feeling of sedation)
4. Fear of administering too much medication
5. Fear of addiction to narcotics with PCA therapy
6. Expected outcomes for the patient (e.g., pain rating of 1 or 2, early ambulation)

Efforts in setting up a PCA program are worthwhile. Patients who use PCA are more comfortable. They have control over their own pain management, and can keep their narcotic blood level within therapeutic range so they effectively ambulate and breathe deeply. As Lehman has stated, "PCA is not only suitable to establish and maintain adequate postoperative pain relief but can also yield important information about pain behavior and the patient's pain measurement."[33]

To summarize the use of intravenous narcotics for achieving pain control, the advantages and disadvantages can be considered. In regard to the advantages, it is a route with which most nurses are familiar, there is a rapid onset of action, and it is therefore easier to titrate increasing narcotic requirements with escalating pain. The disadvantages are that vascular access is sometimes difficult to maintain, the accumulation of IV narcotics may not be predictable, and side effects such as somnolence can interfere with the patient's quality of life. Further studies are needed on outcome measures of patient-controlled analgesia, because there are currently conflicting studies as to whether PCA reduces postoperative complications, length of hospital stay, and nursing time.[34, 35]

Subcutaneous Administration

A nurse who readily accepts the role of patient advocate needs to allow the patient the choice of which narcotic administration route is amenable to them. Regardless of the cause of pain, patients can be made aware of the options, including their advantages and disadvantages.

Patients who are intolerant of or unable to take oral or rectal pain medications, or in whom vascular access is not reliable or desired, may want to consider the subcutaneous route of narcotic administration.[36, 37] This is less invasive and less costly than other parenteral narcotic routes. Studies have shown that continuous infusions of subcutaneous narcotics have all the advantages of intravenous narcotic administration, without the need for vascular access. Subcutaneous and intravenous narcotic infusions produce similar blood levels and provide comparable analgesia and side effects.[38–41]

The technique for accessing the subcutaneous tissue is considered a simple procedure. This ease of use makes subcutaneous narcotic infusions desirable for home infusion personnel. The following are needed:

Small-gauge scalp vein needle or cannula
Povidone-iodine swab
Adhesive bandage
Transparent dressing

The skin is prepped with a povidone-iodine swab over the access site desired. Commonly used subcutaneous sites are the subclavicular area, anterior chest wall, and abdomen.[42, 38] The insertion technique used with a small-gauge scalp vein needle involves inserting the needle at an angle under the skin, applying an adhesive bandage over the plastic scalp vein needle wings for stability, and covering the site with a transparent dressing. A Teflon catheter inserted into the subcutaneous tissue is shown in Figure 14–4.

Narcotics used for subcutaneous infusions include morphine sulfate, hydromorphone hydrochloride, levorphanol tartrate, and methadone hydrochloride. Morphine sulfate and hydromorphone hydrochloride are most often used, and no difference has been found between these two narcotics in regard to pain control or side effects.[39] Hydromorphone has a high analgesic potency per milliliter that is five to six times higher than that of morphine. This property minimizes the volume of infusion and is useful in opioid-tolerant patients who require higher hourly dosages for adequate pain relief. The effective elimination half-life of hydromorphone is 2.6 hours. Morphine has a slightly longer effective elimination half-life of 3.1 hours.[40] It has been speculated that higher lipid solubility creates a depot effect and higher water solubility (such as that of morphine) decreases absorption from the subcutaneous compartment into the systemic circulation, resulting in decreased bioavailability, but neither hypothesis has been substantiated through research.[41]

If the patient has a prior history of oral narcotic use, a conversion chart (Table 14–2) can be used to facilitate the initiation of a subcutaneous narcotic infusion.

The following steps can be taken to convert an oral narcotic to the subcutaneous route:

1. Calculate the previous 24-hour oral dose of narcotic required.
2. Convert the oral dose to the subcutaneous dose using Table 14–2.
3. Divide this number by 24 to obtain the hourly subcutaneous infusion and program the pump.

Individual absorption characteristics must be factored in to any route conversions.

Table 14–2

Conversion Chart

Analgesic	Equianalgesic Dose (mg)	
	PO	IM or SC
Morphine sulfate	30.0	10.0
Hydromorphone hydrochloride	7.5	1.5
Levorphanol tartrate	4.0	2.0
Methadone hydrochloride	20.0	10.0

Agency for Health Care Policy and Research. Clinical Practice Guideline. Acute Pain Management: Operative or Medical Procedures and Trauma. Rockville, MD: US Department of Health and Human Services, 1992.

In their study, Moulin and Kreeft showed that plasma concentrations of narcotic subcutaneous and IV infusions are similar at 24 hours, but at 48 hours the plasma concentration of the subcutaneous infusion drops to 78% of an IV infusion.[40] Therefore, adjustments may need to be made during the second day.

Subcutaneous infusions or boluses of narcotics are limited to the absorption of the narcotic at the subcutaneous site. Absorption from injections of subcutaneous or intramuscular narcotic follows comparable time frames.[42] The subcutaneous tissue can tolerate narcotic infusions with less irritation if the infusion rate is lower than 2 ml/hour. Therefore, the preparation of narcotic concentrations is key to the success of subcutaneous infusions for pain control. Local toxicity from chemical irritation of the narcotic is infrequent but more likely to occur with the extremes of higher volume infusions and higher concentrations of narcotic.

Problems associated with subcutaneous infusions are skin irritation at the needle insertion site and subcutaneous scarring.[42] Skin irritation can be resolved with more frequent site changes and less concentrated narcotics. Subcutaneous scarring interferes with the absorption of narcotic, resulting in unpredictable analgesia. Reducing narcotic volume and using more frequent site rotation prevent this from occurring.

IV nurses, with their experience in monitoring vascular access sites and performing vascular site rotations, are in a good position to support the patient receiving subcutaneous infusions. The IV nurse can identify chemical irritation of subcutaneous infusions of narcotics, make recommendations to change the site and concentrate the narcotic infusion, perform the site rotation, secure the subcutaneous needle, and change the dressing.

Transdermal analgesia is an exciting new technology that merits discussion here. Duragesic (Janssen) patches come in various doses of fentanyl citrate gel, such as 25, 50, 75, and 100 μg/hour. Applied to the skin, this patch allows fentanyl to diffuse into the subcutaneous tissue through a rate-controlling membrane. A depot of fentanyl is deposited in the upper skin layers and is carried into the systemic circulation. The patch is applied to the torso area. Prior to placing a transdermal patch, the skin surface needs to be dry and the body hair clipped, not shaved. No soap, oil, or lotions can be used on the skin surface where the patch is to be placed. Areas of abrasion on the skin surface need to be avoided. On the first patch application, the initial concentrations of fentanyl require 12 to 15 hours to peak, and each patch lasts 3 days. Because of the delayed initial peak of narcotic, fast-acting narcotics are needed to provide relief for breakthrough pain

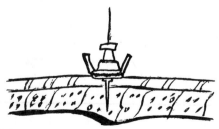

Figure 14–4. Subcutaneous access for narcotic administration. (Courtesy of MiniMed Technologies.)

until adequate plasma concentrations have been reached. With subsequent patches, a more stable plasma level can be maintained.

Nursing Care

Monitoring

Monitoring patients receiving parenteral narcotic medications requires that the nurse document consistently on a flow sheet. The nurse should have knowledge of the pharmacologic implications of the medications along with baseline information about the patient, such as pulse, respirations, blood pressure, known drug allergies, and previous history of narcotic use and amount, before narcotics are given.[32] Flow sheets are useful in the hospital or home setting and should include the ability to monitor the patient for therapeutic response, record untoward side effects, and document nursing intervention. The flow sheet should be part of the medical record. Two samples of flow sheets that can be used in the hospital or home setting are found in Appendix A. State and federal regulations require that controlled substances be discarded appropriately and documented.

Monitoring for respiratory depression is routine to most nurses who administer narcotics. Respiratory depression is usually preceded by signs of changes in mental status, such as confusion or sedation. If the nurse monitors the patient's mental status on a regular basis, such as every hour, the potential problem of respiratory depression can be identified earlier, allowing for changes in the narcotic dose to be reduced or stopped or IV naloxone to be given before the occurrence of respiratory depression.[44] If respiratory rates are counted for the full minute and drop below a predefined limit, such as 8 or 10 respirations/min, or become shallow with poor quality and the patient is difficult to arouse, then the narcotic is stopped and reversal of the narcotic is necessary. Reversal of narcotic overdose can occur with pure antagonist or agonist-antagonist narcotics (if the primary narcotic combines with the mu receptor). IV naloxone can be administered in small increments frequently, such as 0.1 or 0.2 mg every 1 to 2 minutes or with a full ampule (0.4 mg). An abrupt reversal of all analgesia may produce effects in the patients as a result of the sudden onset of severe pain. These include hypertension, tachycardia, rapid respirations, decreased GI motility, and hypercoagulability. By titrating naloxone hydrochloride slowly, the nurse can reverse the side effects, without reversing the analgesia. When reversal takes place, the patient should still be monitored for the return of decreased mental status and respiratory depression because the duration of some narcotics can be longer than the duration of the naloxone, so naloxone may need to be repeated. A low-dose infusion of naloxone might even be considered.

The apnea monitor is a plethysmographic device that detects movements of the thorax, which it records as ventilation rate. It varies in reliability from one patient to another and occasionally can emit loud false alarms that disrupt normal sleep in monitored patients. In many people, normal sleep is characterized by intermittent periodic breathing and short periods of apnea. Patients may develop progressive respiratory depression characterized by rapid, shallow breathing, and this is not detected by plethysmographic apnea monitors.

Significant respiratory depression with infusions of opiates is consistently accompanied by progressive somnolence and obtundation. Therefore, the best monitoring involves hourly nursing checks, with observation of ventilatory patterns and assessment of mental status. During nighttime sleep, patients need only be touched to see that they arouse easily, and the ventilatory rate can be counted without disturbing sleep. Sleep deprivation in patients, related to apnea monitor false alarms, may itself have adverse medical consequences. The use of apnea monitors on cancer patients who are tolerant to the side effects of narcotics may be objected to by the patient as bothersome, and may even be considered punitive by them.

Complications

The nursing management of complications related to the parenteral administration of narcotics requires knowledge and prompt intervention to remedy the situation. Complications include inadequate pain relief and respiratory depression.

INADEQUATE PAIN RELIEF

Nurses often do not know how to respond properly when patients do not receive adequate pain control from their medications. This frustration may reflect a disbelief that the patient has pain or a desire to withhold narcotics from patients because they fear that the patient may become addicted. These conditions frequently occur after a pain control measure sedates the patient so they sleep but, while awake, the patient complains of pain. The nurse needs to realize that patients in pain often do sleep, and that sleep is not a good indicator of a pain-free state. It can be reassuring to the nurse whose patient does not have adequate pain control to realize that there is no perfect method of pain control and that breakthrough pain may occur with any pain control method, but constant attempts to control pain should continue. In general, treating breakthrough pain with small, repetitive doses of IV narcotic is a safe and effective practice that should be used routinely until the medication can be adjusted or the technique of pain management altered. Certain PCA infusion pumps allow the nurse to give these small repetitive doses of IV narcotics to patients without using up the doses the patients can give themselves, or the nurse may choose to bypass the PCA pump to administer IV push narcotic boluses directly. Regardless of the means of administration, one should continually monitor the patient and keep track of the pain medication used (i.e., amount, type, time, and patient response).

RESPIRATORY DEPRESSION

Respiratory depression is a serious complication resulting from overnarcotizing the patient. It may occur with any route of narcotic administration. The important thing to remember is that narcotics that bind with the mu receptor can always be reversed with an antagonist.[45] Respiratory depression is uniformly associated with somnolence or confusion. For this reason, if nurses assess mental status and respirations frequently (e.g., every hour), they can identify and treat the occasional individual who has depression of ventilation. It is important to assess mental status with respiratory rate because some people slow their breathing rate or breathe irregularly during normal sleep or at times of rest during the day. If these patients are awake, alert, and appropriate, it is doubtful that they have clinically significant respiratory depression. However, confusion or somnolence is cause for alarm, even if breathing is not slowed.

Side Effects

Side effects occur with all routes of narcotic administration. These include excessive somnolence or confusion, nausea and vomiting, urinary retention, pruritus, and constipation.

Excessive somnolence or confusion may indicate that significant levels of narcotic are present in the brain, and this is cause for concern. Excessive somnolence may herald impending respiratory depression. The narcotic infusion should be stopped, respiration rate counted for 1 full minute while observing the quality of respirations, and the physician notified. The administration of naloxone may be necessary if the mental status is markedly abnormal and/or if there is poor-quality respiratory status.

Nausea and vomiting may occur from a number of causes unrelated to the use of narcotics, including postsurgical ileus, certain non-narcotic medications, and the effects of general anesthesia. Nausea is often associated with narcotics by any route.[46] Nausea that is narcotic-related tends to occur when patients are ambulatory rather than when they are recumbent, and may be the result of narcotic-enhanced labyrinthine sensitivity to motion.[47] A variety of antiemetics can be used to alleviate nausea or the narcotic can be counteracted by a narcotic antagonist such as nalbuphine or naloxone.

Urinary retention is not a common side effect of systemically administered narcotics. However, when it does occur, it can be treated with medications that contract the bladder, such as bethanechol chloride, if retention is present in the absence of mechanical urinary obstruction. A single bladder catheterization may also reverse the retention problem but may expose the patient to the risk of urinary tract infection.

Pruritus from narcotics given intravenously is a side effect that may be related to a sensitivity or allergy to the drug or its vehicle. Administering an antihistamine is often effective or the narcotic effects can be reversed with an antagonist. Use of another narcotic should be considered.

Narcotics can slow bowel function, resulting in constipation. Bowel sounds need to be monitored, elimination patterns tracked, and stool softeners given when necessary. Managing pain in terminal cancer patients needs to be done simultaneously with managing or preventing constipation. In this population of patients, not only do narcotics reduce GI motility, but so do poorly managed pain, immobility, poor diet, and dehydration. Elimination patterns need to be monitored to facilitate a bowel movement at least every 3 days. A stool softener combined with a peristaltic agent is most likely necessary. If bowel evacuation is delayed for longer than 3 days, the physician should be notified immediately and a more aggressive bowel program defined.

Special Considerations

Adjuvant medications that are not narcotics can be useful in pain control, either by themselves or in combination with narcotics. These drugs include NSAIDs and tricyclic antidepressants. These medications need to be considered in evaluating patients with acute, chronic, or cancer pain.

NSAIDs can be given orally, intramuscularly, or rectally, and are responsible for inhibiting the synthesis of prostaglandin.[16] Because of this prostaglandin-inhibiting activity, studies have shown that the adjuvant use of NSAIDs reduces the amount of narcotics necessary to control pain.[48–53] Careful consideration should be given to the patient before administering NSAIDs. The medical history and physical condition, along with the medications the patient is currently using, need to be identified. For instance, if a patient has a history of renal disease or has an elevated creatinine level, the use of NSAIDs may be contraindicated. If the patient has a coagulopathy or is on anticoagulants, the use of NSAIDs needs to be evaluated carefully.[54, 55] Because certain NSAIDs can be irritating to the stomach, patients with a history of peptic ulcer disease need to be evaluated carefully for this method of pain control.[56] Prostaglandins are responsible for protecting the stomach lining from gastric acids. Patients who have an allergy to aspirin need to be questioned carefully to see whether it is a true allergic reaction. Cross allergies to some NSAIDs occur.

Tricyclic antidepressants are key medications for deafferentation or neuropathic pain. They are beneficial in pain control because of an increase in serotonin in the descending pain pathway, resulting in a release of enkephalin in the spinal cord and a decrease in pain. Because of this function, tricyclic antidepressants are physiologically responsible for terminating nerve-transmitting activity.

Pain management in the home setting involves the transfer of this knowledge to the home health care staff. Home health care nurses need to be familiar with the use of narcotics, NSAIDs, and tricyclic antidepressants for their terminal cancer patients suffering from intractable pain. They need to be able to communicate with the patient to find out their goals for pain management. Educating the patient about various methods and routes of pain control needs to be done to allow the patient to be involved in the decision-making process.[29] The home health care nurse needs to recognize side effects and complications and know how to intervene immediately.

EPIDURAL NARCOTICS

The epidural route can be used for acute[57] and cancer pain management.[58] There are various approaches to the administration of narcotics by the epidural route, and each has its own clinical indication. These include a single bolus injection of narcotic or local anesthetic, a continuous infusion of narcotic with or without local anesthetic, and a continuous infusion of narcotic with a patient-activated bolus. Preservatives in narcotics or local anesthetics used in the epidural or intrathecal spaces need to be avoided to prevent nerve damage.[59, 60] Nurses are better prepared to work with patients receiving epidural or intrathecal analgesic agents through the various methods of administration, if they know the lipid and water solubility properties of the drugs with which they are working.

The lipid and water solubility factors determine the length of time an intraspinal narcotic provides analgesia, how much rostral spread occurs in the cerebral spinal fluid, and the amount of vascular uptake that occurs.[61, 62] Rostral spread is the distribution of the narcotic with the cerebral spinal fluid flow. The amount of rostral spread depends on the fat and water solubility properties of the narcotic. When fat-soluble or lipophilic medications are administered in the epidural space, they quickly diffuse through the dura and arachnoid mater and bind at the spinal cord, where analgesia is achieved. Because these medications bind at the spinal cord, there is limited rostral spread and the analgesia that is achieved is segmental rather than generalized. Because of the lipid solubility factors of certain narcotics, catheters may need to be specifically placed close to the appropriate dermatome for successful analgesia.[63] This allows lipid-soluble medications to be delivered to specific dermatome levels of the nerves that innervate the lesion or incision. An infusion using a lipid-soluble narcotic and local anesthetic can achieve a wider segmental spread of analgesia, with higher rates of infusion.[64] The amount of narcotic administered and the amount of local anesthetic need to be calculated to prevent toxicity from either medication. Conversely, when water-soluble or hydrophilic medications are administered in the epidural space, diffusion across the dura and arachnoid mater is slower and these medications do not bind as quickly along the spinal cord, thereby allowing more drug more time to diffuse rostrally through the spinal fluid.[48] The analgesia created then has a broader segment. The rostral spread of a water-soluble narcotic may produce a delayed respiratory depression when it reaches the respiratory center or medulla.[65] Fentanyl citrate, sufentanil citrate, and hydromorphone hydrochloride are commonly used lipid-soluble narcotics, and morphine sulfate is a commonly used water-soluble narcotic.

Local anesthetic agents are frequently used with epidural narcotics and are instrumental in controlling pain and reducing postoperative complications. Thus, they may reduce the length of a hospital stay.[66–68] Knowledge of the autonomic nervous system is necessary to understand the advantages of adding local anesthetic agents to an epidural narcotic infusion. The autonomic nervous system consists of two systems, the sympathetic and the parasympathetic. Table 14–3 presents a summary of the physiologic responses of each system. With the administration of local anesthetics, the sympathetic system is blocked, thereby reducing postoperative complications such as paralytic ileus,[67, 69] pulmonary complications,[66, 70] and thrombophlebitis.[71] By combining local anesthetics with narcotics in epidural infusions, the amount of narcotics required to control the pain is also reduced.

Contraindications for the epidural or intrathecal routes for analgesic administration include patients with head injuries (i.e., increased intracranial pressure), in whom mental status is difficult to monitor, and those with coagulopathies, infections, and tumor infiltration.[62] Patients who have had back surgery need to be evaluated further by an anesthesiologist before the intraspinal space is accessed.

Mechanisms of Delivery

Single Shot

A single injection of epidural narcotic such as fentanyl or morphine may be used for procedures that produce a short course of postoperative pain.[72] A single injection of epidural morphine may be appropriate for patients having a cesarean section or vaginal hysterectomy, and for some orthopedic surgeries.[73] The advantages of this type of analgesia are that the duration is approximately 12 hours, the analgesia onset is 10 to 15 minutes, and no other type of analgesia may be necessary while the narcotic is in the epidural space. The disadvantage is that respiratory depression may occur in the first 10 minutes from the vascular uptake of the morphine sulfate in the epidural veins or may be delayed 6 to 8 hours because of the rostral spread of the morphine.[74, 75] Therefore, patients who are narcotic-naive need to be monitored for excessive somnolence and respiratory depression for the duration of the medication, up to 12 to 24 hours. Another disadvantage is that if the patient has had a previous, unidentified injection of intraspinal narcotic, an inadvertent administration of additional narcotic by another route may overnarcotize the patient, causing respiratory depression. It is also unpredictable as to when the medication will wear off.[76] When breakthrough pain occurs, narcotic is more safely administered in small doses frequently rather than large doses infrequently, or the breakthrough pain may be handled with an NSAID if the patient passes the screening for their use (see earlier, under Special Considerations). For patients receiving same day surgical procedures, epidural fentanyl provides short-term, postoperative analgesia and normally is eliminated before they go home, creating no danger to narcotic-naive patients who may not be monitored closely at home for delayed respiratory depression.[77, 78]

Continuous Infusion

Epidural narcotic infusions can be administered on a short-term or long-term basis. Indications for a short-term epidural narcotic infusion include patients with pain from surgery, trauma, and acute medical disorders creating severe pain.[79, 80] It may also be indicated for a cancer patient with an acute exacerbation of pain in whom systemic narcotics cloud the sensorium or the systemic administration of analgesic agents is not effective in controlling pain, despite rapid elevations of dosages.

Continuous Infusion with Local Anesthetic Agents

Epidural local anesthetic agents break the pain pathway at the sympathetic chain ganglion outside the spinal cord. By using local anesthetics, narcotic levels are reduced, vascular graft blood flow is improved, the incidence of deep vein thrombosis in the lower extremities is reduced, and there is a

Table 14–3

Physiologic Responses of the Autonomic Nervous System

Parasympathetic System	Sympathetic System
Decreased heart rate	Increased heart rate
Decreased respirations	Increased respirations
Decreased blood pressure	Increased blood pressure
Increased GI function	Decreased GI function
Vasodilation and enhanced vascular return and flow	Vasoconstriction and decreased vascular return and flow

decreased incidence of paralytic ileus.[67, 66, 81] Patients who are predisposed to postoperative complications may be considered for the administration of epidural narcotic with local anesthetic for their postoperative recovery period.

Patient-Controlled Analgesia

Epidural narcotics are safely administered through the patient's control using a lipid-soluble narcotic in the postoperative setting. This allows the patient to administer medications beyond their low infusion rate to accommodate their pain needs with ambulation, incentive spirometry, and coughing. The onset of analgesia is within 2 minutes and the analgesia level is superior to that obtained with the intravenous administration of narcotics.[81–86]

The cancer patient with chronic, intractable pain may be a candidate for epidural narcotic. Allowing for limited PCA in addition to a continuous infusion of narcotic is helpful in controlling the patient's pain. These patients are tolerant to the side effects of narcotic because of their history of pain control using a systemic narcotic. Therefore, the epidural narcotic used may be lipophilic or hydrophilic, with few side effects. In the latter case, the onset of analgesia is within 15 to 30 minutes.

External Catheters

A temporary or permanent epidural catheter may be used externally. A temporary catheter may be appropriate for epidural therapy if it is used for a short period, such as for trauma pain,[49, 87] for postoperative pain management for adults and children,[88] or for cancer pain using a trial epidural catheter system.[89] When an epidural catheter is placed, documentation should include the location of the insertion and the distance the catheter is advanced cephalad. The catheter should be labeled "for epidural use only" to avoid the injection of potentially neurolytic substances. A temporary catheter is commonly used for as little as 3 days to 1 week. Manufacturers do not guarantee a temporary catheter's integrity for long-term use. The long-term use of temporary epidural catheters has been associated with catheter-related problems, such as catheter dislodgment and migration of the catheter.[90–92] The advantage of the temporary epidural catheter is its ease and speed of insertion. The disadvantage of the temporary epidural catheter system (even for temporary, short-term use) is that it cannot be easily secured, and thus falls out readily or begins leaking around the insertion site. Manufacturers have not yet perfected temporary epidural catheter systems and should be challenged to do so.

Permanent epidural catheters are used for long-term therapy for patients with intractable cancer pain[93–96] and for patients with nonmalignant pain, if deemed appropriate.[97, 98] A permanent epidural catheter exits from between the spinous processes and is tunnelled subcutaneously until it exits around the rib, where it can be intermittently accessed or connected to an external catheter.[99] The advantage of the permanent, exteriorized epidural catheter is the length of dwell time.[100] Permanent epidural catheters have been in place and functional for over a year.[101] The disadvantage of the permanent epidural catheter is the chance of infection. Although the incidence of infection is low, the epidural cath-

eter is in an external location, thus creating some risk of infection.[102]

Internal Catheters

The epidural portal system (Fig. 14–5) has the same clinical indications as for the external epidural catheter. There are two main advantages of having an epidural catheter connected subcutaneously to an implanted port. First, dislodgment does not occur as easily because the device is under the skin and second, there are no external components to trail bacteria into the epidural space. The disadvantage of the epidural portal system for patients who have continuous infusions is that the metal needle may be irritating to their skin or become dislodged, but securing it appropriately may alleviate this concern.[103] Obvious labeling needs to ensure epidural use only.

Implantable infusion pump technology (Fig. 14–6) is advancing rapidly.[104–106] One type of implantable infusion pump may be programmed from outside the body by using a laptop computer with a telemetry device that can be placed over the implanted pump, allowing the pump to be programmed accordingly. Another type of implanted infusion pump provides a set rate of infusion of narcotic. When the concentration of the narcotic is changed inside the pump, the dosage the patient receives is changed, and the rate stays the same. These exciting products hold much promise for a number of applications, including long-term pain relief. The advantages of an implantable pump are the following: (1) low risk of infection; (2) the catheter can be placed epidurally or in-

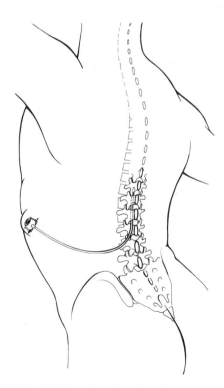

PORT-A-CATH® Implantable Epidural Access System
System Placement
© 1991 Pharmacia Deltec Inc., St. Paul, MN 55112

Figure 14–5. Implantable epidural access system. (Courtesy of Sims Deltec.)

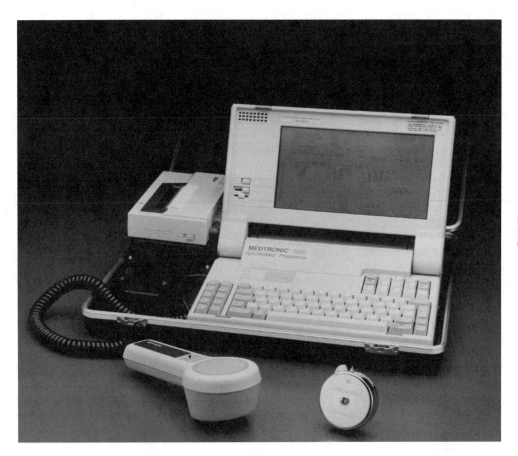

Figure 14–6. Implantable, programmable pump. (Courtesy of Medtronic, Inc.)

trathecally; (3) a reservoir inside the pump holds 10 to 20 ml of fluid so that patients only need to have the pump refilled every 1 to 3 months, depending on the concentration of the medication and the dose the patient requires; and (4) the infusion rates can be changed by computer outside the body or by changing the concentration of the medication inside the pump. The disadvantages are as follows: (1) the initial cost of the equipment and implantation is high (but the longer the pump is used, the more cost-effective it is); (2) the complexity of the technology requires health care professionals who can adapt well to computer technology and internal pump access; (3) there is a needle stick with every fill, which some patients may find uncomfortable without the site being anesthetized with subcutaneous lidocaine; (4) no one knows exactly what problems long-term epidural or intrathecal infusions can cause within the spinal canal because the technology has only been available for a few years; and (5) the life of the pump may be shorter than the patient's life expectancy, requiring surgical replacement of the pump. More research is needed to document outcomes over long periods, and case studies continue to be reported in the literature.[107]

Nursing Care

Monitoring

A flow sheet is used to monitor the patient's response while using epidural technology for pain control. This allows the nurse to track the patient's analgesia and side effects, and enhances the continuity of care provided. Items on the flow sheet may include the patient's mental status, respiratory status, numbness in the lower extremities, signs of infection, bowel function, bladder function, integrity of the epidural system, narcotic dose, and the patient's pain rating.[108–109] Flow sheets can be used in the hospital or in the home setting.[110]

Monitoring mental status while narcotics are being used is a priority. Alteration of mental status is the first indicator that the patient is receiving too much narcotic. Using a level of consciousness scale may be helpful (Table 14–4).

Evaluation of the respiratory status is also necessary (i.e., counting respirations for 1 minute and noting the quality of the respirations). Frequency of mental status checks and hourly respiratory rate checks are the same as when IV narcotics are being infused.[111]

Monitoring for numbness in the lower extremities when local anesthetics are used prevents the patient from an accidental fall.[112] Patient education is important when local anesthetics are infused. The patient should know that when they ambulate for the first time, they must assess for themselves how strong their legs are and whether they can walk. Numbness in the pelvic area does not impede ambulation, but if the local anesthetic used in the epidural infusion is not reduced or eliminated, the numbness gradually goes to the knees and significantly impedes ambulation.[113] This can be prevented by good communication between the nurse and an educated patient.[114]

Infection rarely occurs with short-term epidural infusions, but infections have been documented during long-term infusions of narcotics. Localized infections may occur at the exit

Table 14-4

Consciousness Scale for Monitoring Mental Status
. . . .

Level	Patient Response
I	Alert
II	Sleepy
III	Lethargic
IV	Responds only to maximal stimulation; response to painful stimulus still present
V	Coma

site of the catheter, whether the catheter is permanent or temporary. When this occurs, the catheter should be removed, the tip of the catheter cultured, and the patient placed on antibiotic therapy. Subarachnoid infection appears as a temperature elevation (unless the patient is immunosuppressed), along with severe pain in the back area of insertion. This requires immediate intervention.

Constipation is a problem with narcotics administered by any route. With epidural infusion of narcotics, constipation is less likely because of the tremendous reduction of narcotic that is used.[67] However, bowel sounds and bowel status should continue to be part of the nursing assessment.

Integrity of the epidural system always needs close attention. Research is continuing on the development of epidural systems that do not leak or fall apart but, until these problems are remedied, the nursing assessment needs to include catheter integrity.[92] Signs and symptoms of catheter malfunction include leaking at the distal end of the catheter and leaking at the insertion site.

Home infusion nurses monitor narcotic-tolerant patients receiving epidural infusions for intractable cancer pain by daily contact, either by phone or a home visit, until the patient is stabilized. Monitoring includes mental status evaluation, level of pain relief, side effects, and skin condition around the epidural system.

Site Care

Temporary epidural catheters need to be handled carefully during site care because they are easily dislodged. The dressing change frequency in the hospital or home care setting should follow the Intravenous Nurses Society *Standards of Practice*[32]—which is every 48 hours for gauze dressings—and consideration should be also given to changing transparent dressings every 48 hours.

Dressing Change Technique

1. Wash hands.
2. Secure the temporary catheter close to the exit site with a piece of tape.
3. Remove the old dressing carefully and slowly. Discard appropriately.
4. Apply antimicrobial solution without alcohol in a circular motion, starting at the exit site and working outward.
5. Allow the solution to air-dry.
6. Apply the desired dressing, gauze or transparent, making sure that the catheter is secured well and cannot dislodge accidentally.
7. Document the dressing change, reporting the inspection of the exit site and how the patient tolerated the change.

Permanent external epidural catheters require dressing changes. The frequency of dressing changes is according to the Intravenous Nurses Society *Standards of Practice*,[32] and the technique is the same as with a temporary epidural catheter. Permanent epidural catheters have a Dacron cuff that acts as a protective barrier against bacterial migration along the catheter tract. The Dacron cuff also secures the catheter placement, so securing the catheter during dressing changes is not as great a concern.

Epidural portal systems allow the patient to have the epidural system implanted under the skin.[115] The port requires needle access for the infusion of narcotics or the intermittent injection of narcotics. Skin preparation for needle access includes the use of nonalcohol, antimicrobial solutions applied in a circular motion at the insertion site, working outward. Allow the solution to air-dry, and access the port using sterile technique. The epidural portal system requires access with a noncoring needle. A 90° shaped, noncoring needle may be used for longer infusions of narcotics. The manufacturer requires that these needles be changed weekly. Minimizing irritation of the needle in the port or preventing displacement of the needle can be accomplished by securing the needle adequately.

Site preparation for accessing implantable epidural or intrathecal infusion pumps requires sterile technique, using the same preparations as for an epidural portal system.

Successful epidural pain management in the home setting is totally dependent on the home infusion nurses caring for patients receiving this form of analgesia. Home infusion nurses need to be able to perform all the nursing functions mentioned and to evaluate the patient's response to intervention. Appendix B shows an example of standing orders for permanent epidural catheter management in the home setting. Because pain management incorporates the complexities of a patient and their support systems, the home infusion nurse is challenged to assess the whole individual in addition to the technology being offered to them.[116, 117]

Complications

The nursing management of complications and side effects is important to the safety and efficacy of epidural pain administration.[118, 119] Complications include inadequate pain relief, respiratory depression, infection, and epidural catheter migration.[120] The role of the IV nurse is to educate patients and troubleshoot complications of epidural narcotics, taking appropriate measures to remedy these complications.

INADEQUATE PAIN RELIEF

Patients receiving epidural analgesia must receive effective pain control, whether for acute, chronic, or cancer pain. Therefore, the nurse should treat inadequate pain control seriously. Pain control is no longer viewed as a luxury. Pain can be harmful to the patient by creating a sympathetic response, which delays a postoperative patient's recovery and prevents the cancer patient from having quality of life during their time remaining.

Inadequate pain relief for patients with acute pain may occur for three reasons: (1) epidural catheter migration; (2) insufficient dosages of narcotics and local anesthetics; or (3) an undetermined surgical complication. Inadequate pain relief for cancer patients with intractable pain may occur for three reasons: (1) epidural catheter migration; (2) insufficient dosages of narcotics and local anesthetics; or (3) advancing disease process.

RESPIRATORY DEPRESSION

Respiratory depression that is related to epidural narcotics occurs when the epidural narcotics affect the brain (similar to parenteral narcotics).[121] Respiratory depression from epidural narcotics is managed in the same manner as respiratory depression from intravenous narcotics.[122]

INFECTION

Infections caused by using epidural catheters are rare,[122] but precautions should be instituted to keep the catheter insertion process and exit site sterile. For a patient who is not immunosuppressed, an infection in the epidural space causes temperature elevation, pain in the back where the catheter is placed, drainage at the exit site, and inadequate pain relief. If these symptoms are present, they should be reported to an anesthesiologist and consideration given to removing the catheter immediately. If the infection develops elsewhere in the body, the patient should also be evaluated for removal of the epidural catheter. For cancer pain management, infection may be evident in the epidural space, but the immunosuppressed patient may not exhibit a temperature elevation. Therefore, other signs and symptoms need to be monitored. Infection may exist with symptoms of pain in the back at the catheter site, drainage at the exit site, or inadequate pain control. This can be confirmed by an epiduragram, which is an x-ray of the epidural space following an injection of radiopaque dye through the catheter.

CATHETER MIGRATION

Epidural catheter migration may occur in two different ways.[122, 123] The catheter may migrate through the dura mater into the intrathecal space, creating an overdose of narcotic, or the catheter may migrate into an epidural vein or subcutaneous space, creating inadequate pain relief. Catheter migration with permanent epidural catheter systems is almost unheard of, but catheter migration of a temporary epidural catheter, although not common, has occurred. Catheter migration must be evaluated if pain is suddenly not controlled. Aspiration of the epidural catheter to check for blood return is not a reliable means of evaluating displacement of the catheter into an epidural vein.[124] This is because the epidural veins are pliable and collapse easily with aspiration. A more reliable method of checking catheter placement is by injecting the epidural catheter with a local anesthetic and epinephrine hydrochloride. The patient is monitored for temperature sensation changes around the dermatome area and tachycardia. If tachycardia is present, the epidural catheter is venous, and no further medication should be injected until the anesthesiologist evaluates the catheter. If there is a temperature sensation change, it can be assumed that the epidural catheter is functional. Proper training and the approval of the State Board of Nursing should be obtained before injecting a local anesthetic into the epidural space.

Evaluating epidural catheter migration into the intrathecal space is easier. The epidural catheter easily aspirates 10 ml of cerebrospinal fluid when the catheter is in the intrathecal space. The anesthesiologist should be notified and the patient evaluated for decreased mental status and respiratory depression.

Side Effects

Side effects of epidural narcotics are excessive somnolence and confusion, nausea and vomiting, urinary retention, and pruritus.[122, 123, 125] The use of an antagonist or agonist-antagonist is helpful in handling the side effects of epidural narcotics.[126, 127] If the respiratory rate is low and mental status is changed, and pruritus, urinary retention, and/or nausea occur, a pure antagonist such as naloxone hydrochloride or an agonist-antagonist such as nalbuphine hydrochloride can be used in doses low enough to reverse the side effects without reversing the analgesia. However, some physicians prefer to treat side effects by other means.

The goal in managing the side effects of epidural narcotics is to provide early intervention. The IV therapy department can work collaboratively with the anesthesiology department in establishing protocol so that these side effects can be managed by the nurse at the bedside. The IV nurse, as an educator, can reinforce the use of this protocol to the staff nurse so that relief of these side effects can be provided.

Excessive somnolence or confusion occurs when too much narcotic is being administered. Somnolence improves by decreasing the epidural narcotic infusion, and by administering naloxone hydrochloride in a small dose, such as 0.1 or 0.2 mg IV push. By titrating naloxone hydrochloride to effect, there is a reverse in somnolence without reversing the analgesia.

Nausea and vomiting can be controlled with antiemetics, such as prochlorperazine, droperidol, or scopolamine patch.[128] An antagonist such as naloxone 0.2 mg IV which can be titrated to effect, or an agonist-antagonist such as nalbuphine hydrochloride 5 to 10 mg subcutaneously, can reverse the narcotic enough to reverse the side effects without reversing the analgesia.

Urinary retention may occur 10 to 20 hours after the first injection of intraspinal narcotic. Bethanechol chloride or antagonist drugs can be given for relief. Intraspinal narcotics may prevent the bladder from emptying and therefore cause it to overdistend. This may require catheterization if medical intervention proves inadequate. For postoperative patients, some physicians prefer to maintain the Foley catheter until the epidural catheter is ready to be discontinued.[129]

Pruritus from intraspinal narcotics is not caused by histamine release but by the opiate interacting with the opiate receptor sites in the dorsal horn.[130] It is best treated with an antagonist rather than with diphenhydramine.[131] After an epidural injection, 8.5% of all patients experience pruritus; after an intrathecal injection, 46% experience pruritus.[132, 133]

Table 14–5 compares side effects with various routes of analgesic agents.

Special Considerations

Adjuvant medications, such as NSAIDs and tricyclic antidepressants, can be used with epidural analgesia and with narcotics administered by other routes.

Table 14-5

Comparison of Side Effects of Different Administration Routes*

Side Effect of Analgesic	IV and SC Opiates	Intraspinal Opiates	Intraspinal Local Anesthetics
Respiratory depression	Yes	Yes	No
Nausea	Yes	Yes	No†
Constipation	Yes	No	No
Sedation	Yes	Less frequent	No
Urinary retention	Less frequent	Yes	No
Pruritus	Less frequent	Yes	No
Postural hypotension	Less frequent	No	Yes
Numbness	No	No	Yes

*There are few absolutes in the patient's response while administering narcotic infusions. The reports in this table are based on trends in clinical practice.
†If the hypotension occurs from local anesthetics, nausea may follow.
From St. Marie B. Narcotic infusions: A changing scene. JIN 1991; 14:334–344.

INTRATHECAL NARCOTICS

Intrathecal narcotic infusions may be considered for cancer patients who have a life expectancy of more than a few months, who do not receive adequate pain relief with systemic narcotics, tricyclic antidepressants, or NSAIDs, and who have pain located below the midcervical dermatomes. Intrathecal infusions of narcotics require an implanted infusion pump, not an external pump, because of the risk of infection. Patients have been reported to receive pain relief for 6 months or longer, which merits this therapy for consideration for cancer patients who have side effects from systemic narcotics that interfere with their quality of life.[134]

An implantable infusion pump (see Fig. 14–6) is indicated for long-term intrathecal infusions, similar to epidural infusions.[13, 97] There are differences between the epidural space and the intrathecal space that affect clinical practice. The epidural space contains a vascular system, creating leukocytic activity that decreases the likelihood of an epidural infection. The intrathecal space affords a greater risk for infection and may also cause a spinal headache from a cerebrospinal fluid leak. An intrathecal injection of morphine requires approximately 10 to 12 times less medication than that needed in the epidural space. For example, if 5 mg of morphine is injected into the epidural space to produce analgesia, an equivalent dose of morphine injected into the intrathecal space is 0.2 to 0.5 mg. Parameters for monitoring, site care, and managing complications and side effects are the same as for epidural infusions. Support in the home setting requires knowledge of computer technology to access the implantable pump program through telemetry and refilling the pump.

Intrathecal narcotics given as a single injection are commonly used for postoperative pain management, especially when using preservative-free morphine sulfate. Analgesia from an injection of intrathecal morphine has a rapid onset and may last 18 to 24 hours. This is commonly used for cesarean surgeries, vaginal hysterectomies, and some orthopedic surgeries. The advantages of this type of delivery method are the following: (1) there is no external catheter creating a risk of dislodgment or infection; (2) prolonged analgesia is offered; and (3) it is relatively simple to access. The disadvantages are as follows: (1) the possible presence of pain at high levels as the narcotic wears off, leaving the patient with inadequate pain coverage; (2) risk of respiratory depression;[135] and (3) a greater risk of infection (than epidural) because the cerebrospinal fluid is a good medium for bacteria. Spinal headache may occur, especially in young women. A spinal headache is caused by needle puncture through the dura that does not seal off, and results in cerebrospinal fluid continuing to leak epidurally. The patient could experience a spinal headache for 3 days after the intrathecal injection. Diagnosis of the cause of the headache is confirmed if the patient's headache gets worse when sitting up and improves when lying down. The pain may be located at the back of the head, over the top of the head, or across the forehead. The most effective remedy for spinal headache is a blood patch. This is performed by drawing approximately 10 ml of blood from the patient's arm and injecting the blood epidurally near the level of the original insertion of the intrathecal needle. This blood gels over the dural puncture and prevents cerebrospinal fluid from leaking out of the dural hole, stopping the headache. Patients are instructed to rest and not to exert themselves for a day after placement of the blood patch.

EQUIPMENT USED FOR NARCOTIC INFUSIONS

Knowledge of various types of infusion devices and supportive equipment positions IV nurses within the decision-making process for their respective hospital, home care, outpatient clinic, or long-term facility.

The clinical use of filters with epidural infusions is variable. Bioassay research has confirmed that stability of the medication in cassettes is not a problem.[136] Therefore, 5-μ filters are not necessary, but bacterial studies are not documented. The Intravenous Nurses Society *Standards of Practice*[32] supports using a 0.22-μ filter without surfactant for epidural infusions. This should be considered for home and hospital care.

Medication containers for epidural infusions may include a regular IV bag containing preservative-free medication, or a container that is compatible with an infusion pump. In either case, the containers need to be well marked for epidural use only, so they are not mistaken for an intravenous medication, and vice versa.

Because one purpose of epidural analgesia is to achieve early ambulation, it makes good sense to use ambulatory infusion pumps. There are a variety of ambulatory infusion pumps on the market and careful consideration needs to be given to the selection of a pump.[137] The important features of an infusion pump for administering narcotics have been presented (see earlier: Parenteral Narcotics—Intravenous Administration). The technology is advancing, challenging the intravenous nurse to continue to evaluate new infusion pumps in the marketplace.[138]

NURSING AND PAIN MANAGEMENT

Nurses consider themselves advocates for the patient. Pain management is an aspect of patient care in which patient advocacy is exceedingly important. Nurses who work at the bedside of the patient hear what the patient tells them and know when their patients are experiencing pain. Nurses need to be organized in their approach to pain and can use the nursing process to assist in this organization. Nurses can communicate effectively with other members of the health care team and also need to teach patients how to manage their pain effectively.

It is the responsibility of each nurse caring for a patient to ensure quality pain management. Nurses in various health care settings need to be cognizant of this fact. Interdisciplinary approaches have been successfully implemented throughout the country. Health care professionals from various disciplines such as anesthesiology, neurology, nursing, oncology, and physical therapy have developed pain management strategies, and these team members share the responsibilities of care.

Teams of nurses responsible for pain management have been formed in some hospitals, hospices, and home health agencies.[119] The nursing responsibilities of these teams range from actually administering the pain medications to educating nurses about proper dosing and delivery. A pain team may also serve the purpose of identifying and solving problems associated with pain management.

A pain management medical director is a physician who specializes in pain management. This medical director serves as a resource to those involved in pain management and also acts as liaison and educator of other physicians. The medical director needs to understand and respect the nursing role in pain management, thereby enhancing the care that nurses give to patients in pain.

Assessment of Pain

Pain assessment requires an extensive knowledge of pain and its causes, along with how to use this assessment to manage pain effectively. An in-depth study of pain assessment is beyond the limitations of this treatise, but is essential to conducting clinical pain assessments, as a guide to determine initial pain therapy. A number of resources are available.[139–146]

Assessing the patient's pain is necessary for effective control. There are two types of assessments that are available to assist the clinician involved in pain control: a "brief assessment" and a "comprehensive assessment."

A brief assessment of pain is performed when the patient is in absolute distress and delaying pain management would have harmful effects on the patient. A brief assessment consists of a pain rating according to the patient, timing the pain, the location of the pain, patient's description of the pain, any associated symptoms, what improves the pain or makes it worse, what medications are being used, and identifying any behavioral component. The brief assessment is beneficial for postoperative pain, trauma pain, and acute medical disorders, including acute exacerbations of cancer pain. The goal of a brief assessment is to determine what pathways the pain is taking and to intervene with medications that affect those pathways directly.

A comprehensive assessment of pain is used to formulate a long-term plan for pain management. This approach is useful for cancer pain and for chronic pain from nonmalignant disorders. The following components can be used in assessing chronic pain:

● Overview of pain history
● Sites of pain
● Quality and quantity descriptors, timing
● Exacerbating and relieving factors
● Social evaluation
● Psychologic evaluation

Appendix C presents an example of a pain assessment form. When the parameters of the pain have been determined and systemic narcotics have been administered, it is essential to evaluate the effectiveness of the intervention by asking the following questions:

1. Is pain adequately controlled with systemic narcotics, NSAIDs, and tricyclic antidepressants, where applicable?
2. Are the side effects of the systemic narcotics severe enough to affect the quality of the patient's remaining life adversely?

If the answer to either question is yes, the patient should be evaluated for epidural or intrathecal narcotic administration.[119]

While attempting to control the patient's pain, the nurse should continue to assess parameters to evaluate the effectiveness of these pain interventions. These include vital signs, urinary and bowel function, integument, mental status, pain rating using a pain flow sheet, and coping capability of the patient and family. "The single most reliable indicator of the existence and intensity of acute pain—and any resultant affective discomfort or distress—is the patient's self-report."[147] By looking at the whole picture, the nurse can identify problems that exist earlier and anticipate problems that may surface.

▶ NURSING DIAGNOSIS

Nursing diagnosis "is a clinical judgment about individual . . . responses to actual and potential health problems. . . ."[148] The following nursing diagnoses can be used to assist in the development of a care plan, but are not limited to these.

Anxiety	Characterized by sympathetic stimulation, trembling, voice quivering, facial tension, diaphoresis

Fatigue	Characterized by emotional irritability and decreased performance
Knowledge deficit	Inaccurate follow-through of instruction
Activity intolerance	Related to exertional discomfort
Sleep pattern disturbance	Characterized by irritability, restlessness, disorientation, lethargy, mild, fleeting nystagmus, slight hand tremor, ptosis of eyelid
Altered thought processes	Characterized by cognitive dissonance, inaccurate interpretation of environment, memory deficit

Care Plan

When the particular problem or problems with pain management have been identified, the nursing process continues with planning. Nursing diagnosis acts as a core for nursing care plans by providing a basis for selecting nursing interventions to achieve desired outcomes for which nursing is accountable. Nursing care plans help plan the care of the patient and communicate the plan to the nurse's peers. In developing the care plan, the nurse needs to be informed of what patients want to accomplish in their pain management. For example, cancer patients with intractable pain may express a desire to achieve pain relief while being alert and oriented so they can interact with their loved ones through the rest of their life. Care plans need to address the patient's wishes so that these are communicated and accommodated. This also serves to assist in providing continuity of care, which is so important to a patient in pain. The nursing care plan can be used for postoperative pain, acute medical disorders causing pain, trauma pain, and acute and chronic cancer pain.

Implementation

When the plan has been determined, implementing the plan requires 24-hour cooperation from all nurses in the hospital. In the home setting, this implementation includes assessment of the patient on a daily basis by telephone or visit; after the patient is stabilized, daily contact may not be necessary.

Creating continuity of care for patients in pain cannot be stressed enough. If one or two nurses caring for the patient are not knowledgeable about the level of care given, then the patient is left feeling isolated, helpless, and in pain. There are a variety of methods used to communicate care:

- Educational in-service training with speakers, videotapes, audiotapes, and self-learning packets
- Staff meetings at which pain management is a topic that is discussed regularly
- Verbal "reporting off" on each shift (take the time to emphasize nursing care given for pain control)
- Written documentation in the nursing progress notes for each shift, and documentation on a flow sheet that is left conveniently at the bedside

- Preceptors or nursing instructors may "buddy" with a nurse to facilitate the focus on pain management and serve as a model

Implementation also includes teaching the patient. Teaching patients with all types of pain about their pain management enhances their comfort about the respective pain management intervention. A few key concepts can be applied to any pain control intervention for postoperative, trauma, chronic nonmalignant pain disorders, and cancer pain:

1. Pain rating—explain to the patient they will be asked to rate how much pain they have on a pain scale (define your pain scale). The usual pain scale is 0 to 10, where 0 equals no pain and 10 equals excruciating pain.
2. Tell the patient to let you know whether the pain becomes worse.
3. Explain that side effects may occur and say what they are. Explain the importance of notifying the nurse immediately if side effects are experienced so that they can be treated.
4. Notify the nurse immediately if the medication does not relieve the pain.
5. The patient may be concerned about addiction to narcotics during the postoperative recovery. This fear should be addressed directly. For postoperative pain, you may stress that people do not become addicted if they are taking narcotics directly for pain relief on a short-term basis. For patients who have a long recovery and probably need narcotic pain relief during the painful recovery period, clarify the two different types of addiction, physical dependence and psychologic dependence. Explain that physical dependence can occur when the body is accustomed to receiving narcotics and, if use of the narcotic is abruptly terminated, the patient may go through withdrawal. This is the easiest type of addiction to handle, because the patient is weaned off the narcotic over a short period and the withdrawal is prevented.[149] However, psychologic dependence occurs when the patient craves the narcotic and uses it for reasons other than pain control. Psychologic dependence from postoperative pain management is rare. This type of addiction is more difficult to treat in the usual health care setting, and the patient may need to be referred to a chemical dependency setting. Once patients are educated about these differences, their fears are relieved.

Patient teaching items for patient-controlled analgesia have been discussed (see earlier: Parenteral Narcotics–Intravenous Administration). Patient teaching items for intraspinal narcotics—that is, epidural or intrathecal—are as follows:

1. The infusion pump is preset to deliver medication near the nerve root.
2. If epidural local anesthetic is used, explain to patients that they may experience numbness, but should not be alarmed. They should report it to the nurse, so that adjustments can be made.
3. Physical dependence on an epidural infusion for acute pain has not been documented or noted in clinical practice. The infusion can be stopped abruptly and patients do not go through withdrawal.
4. Patients may ask whether epidural narcotics can take away all their pain. An appropriate response would be

that this technique helps keep their pain at a minimum with less narcotic and fewer side effects. If they *do* have pain, the nurse should be told, and they can be supplemented with additional medication and the epidural dosages adjusted.

Evaluation

Evaluating the patient's response to any pain intervention may be achieved through nurse-patient communication, vital sign monitoring, observation of pupil size, and mental status. If the side effects of narcotics become severe while the patient is still having a lot of pain, a non-narcotic approach should be evaluated for use (e.g., NSAIDs). For example, if a patient has received 12 mg of IV morphine sulfate in a 30-minute period and cannot keep their eyes open, but states they have pain, an injection of ketorolac tromethamine may be helpful to control the pain without producing more sedation.

Monitoring the outcome of all patients on pain intervention validates the need for these advanced pain management interventions to patients, doctors, nurses, and insurance carriers.[150] Any problems in pain intervention can be readily identified and communicated to authorities designated to make recommendations. Improving the quality of pain management means having pain intervention accessible to patients in a timely manner and ensuring that the pain intervention has the desired effect. The goals of effective pain management can be stated as follows:

Goals of Providing Quality Pain Management

- Provide better analgesia with less sedation.
- Improve pulmonary function.
- Decrease the stress response evident in people with pain.
- Produce earlier ambulation.
- Shorten ICU stay.
- Facilitate earlier hospital discharge.

Pain management can be improved through continuous quality improvement. Predetermined clinical indicators can be identified that are related to pain management, such as respiratory depression, breakthrough pain, and somnolence, and these can be monitored quarterly. Other parameters can be determined by using patient satisfaction surveys, and by monitoring costs and charges for pain management interventions. It is through these measures that health care professionals can link cause and effect to intervention and outcome.

In recent years, new therapies have been developed that have increased the effectiveness of pain management. There is reason to hope that patients with intractable cancer, surgical, and trauma pain can benefit even more in the future from more information on how pain can be controlled. The following are advantages of pain service delivery systems:[80, 151]

1. Good communication among physicians and nurses can empower nurses at the bedside to provide effective analgesia to their patients.
2. Effective pain management has been well documented to reduce complications for the patients, thereby decreasing length of hospital stay.
3. Up-to-date approaches to pain management are used efficiently. There have been many new discoveries of pain pathways, opiate receptor sites, NSAIDs, and ways of using old methods of pain management. Pain management is evolving as a specialty in itself. It takes motivated personnel to keep up with the latest information. All these discoveries are there to help patients improve their outcome. Intravenous nurses should seize the knowledge needed to facilitate pain control for their patients. Reading journals that focus on pain management, one might be surprised by what can be done to improve the outcome for patients. Now is the time for intravenous nurses and nurses in other disciplines to open their minds to improved methods of achieving analgesia.

References

1. Schweitzer A. On the Edge of the Primeval Forest. New York: Macmillan, 1931:62.
2. Bonica J. The Management of Pain, 2nd ed, Vol 1. Philadelphia: Lea and Febiger, 1990: 28–35, 40–53, 55, 96–97, 100–101, 104–105, 108–109, 112, 123, 133–139, 146–158, 172.
3. Bonica J. The importance of effective pain control. Acta Anesthesiol Scand (suppl) 1987; 85:1–16.
4. Holbrook TL, Grozier K, Kelsey JL. The Frequency of Occurrence, Impact and Cost of Selected Musculoskeletal Conditions in the United States. Park Ridge, III: American Academy of Orthopaedic Surgeons, 1984.
5. Bonica JJ. Treatment of cancer pain: Current status and future needs. Pain (suppl) 1984; 2:196.
6. Zwarts SJ. The effect of continuous epidural analgesia with sufentanil and bupivacaine during and after thoracic surgery on the plasma cortisol concentration and pain relief. Regl Anaesthesia 1989; 14:183–188.
7. Nimmo WS, Duthie DJ. Pain relief after surgery. Anaesth Intensive Care 1987; 15:68–71.
8. Marks RM, Sacher EJ. Undertreatment of medical inpatients with narcotic analgesic. Ann Intern Med 1973; 78(2):173–181.
9. McCaffery M, Beebe A. Pain: Clinical Manual for Nursing Practice. St. Louis: C.V. Mosby, 1989.
10. Mettler FA. Pain I: What is it? J Med Soc NJ 1964; 61.
11. Sjostrom S, Tamsen D, Hartvig P, et al. Cerebrospinal fluid concentrations of substance P and (met) enkephalin-Arg6-Phe7 during surgery and patient-controlled analgesia. Anesth Analg 1988; 67:976–981.
12. Hughes J. Isolation of an endogenous compound from the brain with pharmacological properties similar to morphine. Brain Res 1975; 88:295–308.
13. Atweh SF, Kuhar MJ. Autoradiographic localization of opiate receptors in rat brain: I. Spinal cord and lower medulla. Brain Res 1977; 124:53–67.
14. Scott DB. Techniques of Regional Anaesthesia. Norwalk, CT: Appleton and Lange, 1989:170–176, 327–332, 337.
15. Hill HF, Mackie AM, Coda BA, et al. Patient-controlled analgesic administration. A comparison of steady-state morphine infusions with bolus doses. Cancer 1991; 67:873–882.
16. Tigerstedt I, Tammisto T, Neuvonen PJ. The efficacy of intravenous indomethacin in prevention of postoperative pain. Acta Anaesthesiol Scand 1991; 35:535–540.
17. Zacharias M, Pfeifer MO, Herbison P. Comparison of two methods of intravenous administration of morphine for postoperative pain relief. Anaesth Intensive Care 1990; 18:205–209.
18. Owen H, Szekely SM, Plummer JL, et al. Variables of patient-controlled analgesia. 1. Bolus size. Anaesthesia 1989; 44:7–10.

19. Holland MS, Gammill BG, Mackey DC. AANA journal course: New technologies in anesthesia: Update for nurse anesthetists—alternatives for postoperative pain management. Am Assoc Nurse Anesthetists J 1990; 58:201–211.
20. Gallion HH, Wermeling DP, Foster TS, et al. Patient-controlled analgesia in gynecologic oncology. Gynecol Oncol 1987; 27:247–253.
21. Lange MP, Dahn MS, Jacob LA. Patient-controlled analgesia versus intermittent analgesia dosing. Heart Lung 1988; 17:495–498.
22. Hadaway LC. Evaluation and use of advanced I.V. technology. Part 2: Patient-controlled analgesia. JIN 1989; 12:184–191.
23. Parker RK, Holtmann B, White PF. Patient-controlled analgesia. Does a concurrent opioid infusion improve pain management after surgery? JAMA 1991; 266:1947–1952.
24. Hansen LA, Noyes MA, Lehman ME. Evaluation of patient-controlled analgesia (PCA) versus PCA plus continuous infusion in postoperative cancer patients. J Pain Symptom Manage 1991; 6:4–14.
25. Citron ML, Johnston-Early A, Boyer M, et al. Patient-controlled analgesia for severe cancer pain. Arch Intern Med 1986; 146:734–736.
26. White PF. Use of patient-controlled analgesia for management of acute pain. JAMA 1988; 259:243–247.
27. McCall LJ, Dierks DR. Pharmacy-managed patient-controlled analgesia service. Am J Hosp Pharm 1990; 47:2706–2710.
28. Mather LE, Owen H. The scientific basis of patient-controlled analgesia. Anaesth Intensive Care 1988; 16:427–436.
29. St. Marie B. Narcotic infusions: A changing scene. JIN 1991; 14:334–344.
30. Kee C. Age-related changes in the renal system: Causes, consequences, and nursing implications. Geriatric Nurs (New York) March/April 1992; 80–83, 89, 93.
31. Agency for Health Care Policy and Research. Clinical practice guideline. Acute Pain Management: Operative or Medical Procedures and Trauma. Rockville, MD: US Department of Health and Human Services, 1992.
32. Intravenous Nurses Society. Revised Intravenous Nursing Standards of Practice. Belmont, MA; Intravenous Nurses, Society, 1990.
33. Lehman K, Ribbert N, Horricks-Haermeyer G. Postoperative patient-controlled analgesia with alfentanil: Analgesic efficacy and minimum effective concentrations. J Pain Symptom Manage 1990; 5:249–258.
34. Albert JM, Talbott TM. Patient-controlled analgesia vs. conventional intramuscular analgesia following colon surgery. Dis Colon Rectum 1988; 31:83–86.
35. Jackson D. A study of pain management: Patient-controlled analgesia versus intramuscular analgesia. JIN 1989; 12:42–51.
36. Bruera E, Legris MA, Kuehn N. Hypodermoclysis for the administration of fluids and narcotic analgesics in patients with advanced cancer. J Pain Symptom Manage 1990; 5:218–220.
37. Bruera E. Palliative care rounds: The use of subcutaneous patient-controlled analgesia. J Pain Symptom Manage 1989; 4:97–100.
38. Storey P, Hill H, St. Louis R. Subcutaneous infusions for control of cancer symptoms. J Pain Symptom Manage 1990; 5:33–41.
39. Bruera E, Bressels C, Michand M, et al. Use of the subcutaneous route for the administration of narcotics in patients with cancer pain. Cancer 1988; 62:407–411.
40. Moulin E, Kreeft J, Murray-Parson N, Bouquillon AI. Comparison of continuous subcutaneous and intravenous hydromorphone infusions for management of cancer pain. Lancet 1991; 337:465–468.
41. IV versus SQ opioid infusions for cancer pain. The American Journal of Home and Palliative Care 1991; 6.
42. Coyle N, Mauskop A, Moggard J, Foley KM. Continuous subcutaneous infusions of opiates in cancer patients with pain. Oncol Nurs Forum 1986; 13:53.
43. Bull P, Mowbray MJ, Markham SJ. Subcutaneous opioids: The painless approach. Anaesthesia 1992; 47:276.
44. Gaukroger PB, Tomkins DP, van der Wait JH. Patient-controlled analgesia in children. Anaesth Intensive Care 1989; 17:264–268.
45. Gueneron JP, Ecoffey CL, Carli P, et al. Effect of naloxone infusion on analgesia and respiratory depression after epidural fentanyl. Anesth Analg 1988; 67:35–38.
46. Robinson SL, Fell D. Nausea and vomiting with use of a patient-controlled analgesia system. Anaesthesia 1991; 46:580–582.
47. Ferris FD, Kerr IG, Sone M, et al. Transdermal scopolamine use in the control of narcotic-induced nausea. J Pain Symptom Manage 1991; 6(6):389–393.
48. Lee VC, Kendrick W, Brown M, et al. Ketorolac given prior to arthroscopic knee surgery decreases postop pain scores and narcotic doses. Anesth Analg 1992; 74:S181.
49. Mackersie RC, Shackford SR, Hoyt DB. Prospective evaluation of epidural and intravenous administration of fentanyl for pain control and restoration of ventilatory function following multiple rib fractures. Anesthesiol Lit Line 1991; 3:3.
50. Gillies GW, Kenny GN, Billingham RE. The morphine sparing effect of ketorolac tromethamine. A study of a new, parenteral non-steroidal anti-inflammatory agent after abdominal surgery. Anaesthesia 1987; 42:727–731.
51. Floy BJ, Royko CG, Fleitman JS. Compatibility of ketorolac tromethamine injection with common infusion fluids and administration set. Am J Hosp Pharm 1990; 47:1097–1100.
52. Peuce RJ, Frogen R, Rembarter D. Intravenous ketorolac tromethamine versus morphine sulfate in the treatment of immediate postoperative pain. Pharmacotherapy 1990; 10:111S–115S.
53. Kenny GN, Gilles GW, Bullingham RE. Parenteral ketorolac: Opiate-sparing effect and lack of cardiorespiratory depression in the perioperative patient. Pharmacotherapy 1990; 10:127S–131S.
54. Reinhart D, Latzen J, Klein K, et al. Effect of ketorolac on coagulation as evaluated by thromboelastograph. Anesth Analg 1992; 74:S248.
55. O'Hara DA. Bleeding diathesis after perioperative ketorolac. Anesth Analg 1992; 74:165–168.
56. Silverstein F. Nonsteroidal anti-inflammatory drugs and peptic ulcer disease: An overview. Postgrad Med 1991; 89:33–60.
57. Haight K. What you should know about epidural analgesia. Nurs 87 1987; 58–59.
58. Lutz LJ, Lamer TJ. Management of postoperative pain: Review of current techniques and methods. Mayo Clin Proc 1990; 65:584–596.
59. Warfield CA, Dohlman LE. Intraspinal narcotics for pain control. Hosp Pract 1984; 148B–148P, 17(9), 1984.
60. DuPen SL. Epidural morphine sulfate: Preservatives or not? Seattle, Swedish Hospital Medical Center, 1987 (reprint).
61. Hicks RJ, Kalff V, Brazenor G, et al. The radionuclide assessment of a system for slow intrathecal infusion of drugs. Clin Nucl Med 1989; 14:275–277.
62. Kreter B. Postoperative epidural anesthesia. Parenterals 1988; 1–3.
63. Chien BB, Burke RG, Hunter DJ. An extensive experience with postoperative pain relief using postoperative fentanyl infusion. Arch Surg 1991; 126:692–695.
64. Sjogren P, Banning AM, Henriksen H. Lumbar epidurography and epidural analgesia in cancer patients. Pain 1989; 36:305–309.
65. Yaksh TL. Spinal opiate analgesia: Characteristics and principles of action. Pain 1981; 11:293–346.
66. Bigler D, Scott NB, Mogensen T, et al. Effects of thoracic paravertebral block with bupivacaine versus combined thoracic epidural block with bupivacaine and morphine on pain and pulmonary function after cholecystectomy. Acta Anaesthesiol Scand 1989; 33:561–564.
67. Thoren T, Sundberg A, Wattwil M, et al. Effects of epidural bupivacaine and epidural morphine on bowel function and pain after hysterectomy. Acta Anaesthesiol Scand 1989; 33:181–185.
68. Gorback MS, Moon RE, Mossey JM. Extubation after transsternal thymectomy for myasthenia gravis: A prospective analysis. South Med J 1991; 84:701–706.
69. Wattwil M, Thoren T, Hennerdal S, et al. Epidural analgesia with bupivacaine reduces postoperative paralytic ileus after hysterectomy. Anesth Analg 1989; 68:353–358.
70. Clyburn PA, Rosen M, Vickers MD. Comparison of the respiratory effects of I.V. infusions of morphine and regional analgesia by extradural block. Br J Anaesth 1990; 64:446–449.
71. Bishop A. The use of epidural analgesia in postoperative vascular surgical patients. J Vasc Nurs 1990; 8:2–5.
72. Sinatra RS, Harvison DM. Comparison of epidurally administered sufentanil, morphine, and sufentanil-morphine combination for postoperative analgesia. Anesth Analg 1991; 72:522–527.
73. Loper KA, Ready LB. Epidural morphine after anterior cruciate ligament repair: A comparison with patient-controlled intravenous morphine. Anesth Analg 1989; 68:350–352.
74. Choi HJ, Little MS, Garber SZ, et al. Pulse oximetry for monitoring during ward analgesia: Epidural morphine versus parenteral narcotics. J Clin Monit 1989; 5:87–89.
75. Shuda MR. Unwanted effects and complications of epidural morphine administration. Parenterals 1987; 5:2–3.
76. Baker MW, Tullos HS, Bryan WJ, et al. The use of epidural morphine in patients undergoing total knee arthroplasty. Arthroplasty 1989; 4:157–161.
77. Hansdottir V, Hednev T, Wrestenborghs R, et al. The CSF and plasma pharmacokinetics of sufentanil after intrathecal administration. Anesthesiology 1991; 74:264–269.

78. Severino FB, McFarlane C, Sinatra RS. Epidural fentanyl does not influence intravenous PCA requirements in the post-caesarean patient. Can J Anaesth 1991; 38:450–453.

79. Lytle SA, Goldsmith DM, Neuendorf TL, et al. Postoperative analgesia with epidural fentanyl. J Am Osteopath Assoc 1991; 91:547–550.

80. Ready LB. Spinal opioids in the management of acute and postoperative pain. J Pain Symptom Manage 1990; 5:138–145.

81. Boudreault D, Brasseur Y, Samii K, et al. Comparison of continuous epidural bupivacaine infusion plus either continuous epidural infusion or patient-controlled epidural injection of fentanyl for postoperative analgesia. Anesth Analg 1991; 73:132–137.

82. Welchew EA, Breen DP. Patient-controlled on-demand epidural fentanyl. A comparison of patient-controlled on-demand fentanyl delivered epidurally or intravenously. Anesthesia 1991; 46:438–441.

83. Owen H, Kenney GN, Toal F, et al. Patient-controlled analgesia. Experience of two new machines. Anaesthesia 1986; 41:1230–1235.

84. Gambling DR, McMorland GH, Yu P, et al. Comparison of patient-controlled epidural analgesia and conventional intermittent ''top-up'' injections during labor. Anesth Analg 1990; 70:256–261.

85. Brownridge P. Treatment options for the relief of pain during childbirth. Drugs 1991; 41:69–80.

86. Marlowe S, Engstrom R, White PF. Epidural patient-controlled analgesia (PCA): An alternative to continuous epidural infusions. Pain 1989; 37:97–101.

87. Ullman DA, Fortune JP, Greenhouse BB, et al. The treatment of patients with multiple rib fractures using continuous thoracic epidural narcotic infusion. Anesthesiol Lit Line 1991; 3:3–4.

88. Haberkern CM, Tyler DC, Krone EJ. Postoperative pain management in children. Mt Sinai J Med 1991; 58:247–256.

89. Dagi TF, Chilton J, Caputy A, et al. Long-term, intermittent percutaneous administration of epidural and intrathecal morphine for pain of malignant origin. Am Surgeon 1986; 52:155–158.

90. Wulf H, Maier C, Striepling E. Pharmacokinetics and protein binding of bupivacaine in postoperative epidural analgesia. Acta Anaesthesiol Scand 1988; 32:530–534.

91. Ali NM, Hanna N, Hoffman JS. Percutaneous epidural catheterization for intractable pain in terminal cancer patients. Gynecol Oncol 1989; 32:22–25.

92. Johnson RG, Miller M, Murphy M. Intraspinal narcotic analgesia. A comparison of two methods of postoperative pain relief. Spine 1989; 14:363–366.

93. Waldman SD. The role of spinal opioids in the management of cancer pain. J Pain Symptom Manage 1990; 5:163–168.

94. DuPen SL, Peterson DG, Bogosian AC, et al. A new permanent exteriorized epidural catheter for narcotic self-administration to control cancer pain. Cancer 1987; 59:986–993.

95. Malone BT, Beye R, Walker J. Management of pain in the terminally ill by administration of epidural narcotic. Cancer 1985; 55:438–440.

96. Yablonski-Peretz T, Klin B, Beilin Y, et al. Continuous epidural narcotic analgesia for intractable pain due to malignancy. J Surg Oncol 1985; 29:8–10.

97. Hassenbusch SJ, Stanton-Hicks MD, Soukop J, et al. Sufentanil citrate and morphine/bupivacaine as alternative agents in chronic epidural infusions for intractable non-cancer pain. Neurosurgery 1991; 29:76–82.

98. Baggerly J. Epidural catheters for pain management: The nurse's role. J Neurosci Nurs 1986; 18:290–295.

99. Malone BT, et al. Management of pain in the terminally ill by administration of epidural narcotics. Cancer 1985; 55:438–440.

100. Williams AR, Beaulaurier KE, Seal DL. Chronic cancer pain management with the Du Pen epidural catheter. Cancer Nurs 1990; 13:176–182.

101. Yue SK, St. Marie B, Henrickson K. Initial clinical experience with the SKY epidural catheter. J Pain Symptom Manage 1991; 6:107–114.

102. Williams A, Molitor RE Jr. Administering and monitoring epidural analgesia. Epidural infusions of opiates and local anesthetic solutions for intractable cancer pain. Oncol Nurs Forum 1988; 15:819.

103. Waldman SD, Feldstein G, Allen M. Troubleshooting intraspinal narcotic delivery systems. Am J Nurs 87(1):63–64.

104. Caballero GA, Ausmen RK, Hemo J. Epidural morphine by continuous infusion with an external pump for pain management in oncology patients. Am Surgeon 1986; 52:8.

105. Yaksh TL, Onofrio BM. Retrospective consideration of the doses of morphine given intrathecally by chronic infusion in 163 patients by 19 physicians. Pain 1987; 31:211–223.

106. Hassenbusch SJ, Pillay PK, Magdinee M. Constant infusion of mor-

phine for intractable cancer pain using an implanted pump. J Neurosurg 1990; 73:405–409.

107. Paice JA. Intrathecal morphine infusion for intractable cancer pain: A new use for implanted pumps. Oncol Nurs Forum 1986; 13(3):41–47.

108. Paice JA. New delivery systems in pain management. Nurs Clin North Am 1987; 22:715–726.

109. McNair ND. Epidural narcotics for postoperative pain: Nursing implications. J Neurosci Nurs 1990; 22:275–279.

110. Sjogren P, Banning AM, Larsen RK. Postural stability during long-term treatment of cancer patients with epidural opioids. Acta Anaesthesiol Scand 1990; 34:410–412.

111. Rosen HF, Calio MM. An epidural analgesia program: Balancing risks and benefits. Crit Care Nurse 1990; 10:32–41.

112. Downing JE, Busch EH, Stedman PM. Epidural morphine delivered by a percutaneous epidural catheter for outpatient treatment of cancer pain. Anesth Analg 1988; 67:1159–1161.

113. Hasenbos MA, Eckhaus MN, Slappendel R, Grelen MJ. Continuous high thoracic epidural administration of bupivacaine with sufentanil or nicomorphine for postoperative pain relief after thoracic surgery. Reg Anesth 1989; 14:212–218.

114. Lubenow TR, Ivankovich AD. Postoperative epidural analgesia. Crit Care Nurs Clin North Am 1991; 3:25–34.

115. Shaves M, Barnhill D, Bosscher J. Indwelling epidural catheters for pain control in gynecologic cancer patients. Obstet Gynecol 1991; 77(4):642–644.

116. Blue CL, Purath J. Home care of the epidural analgesia patient: The nurse's role. Home Healthcare Nurse 1989; 7(4):23–32.

117. St. Marie B, Henrickson K. Intraspinal narcotic infusions for terminal cancer pain. JIN 1988; 11:161–163.

118. Chrubasik J, Magra F. Postoperative epidural opiate pharmacokinetics. Anesth Analg. 1992; 74:S44.

119. Hunter D. Pain control. Relief through teamwork. Nurs Times 1991; 87:35–36,38.

120. Krames ES, Gershow J, Glassberg A, et al. Continuous infusion of spinally administered narcotics for the relief of pain due to malignant disorders. Cancer 1985; 56:696–702.

121. Payne R. Role of epidural and intrathecal narcotics and peptides in the management of cancer pain. Med Clin North Am 1987; 71:313–327.

122. Coombs DW, Mauer CH, Saunders RL, et al. Outcomes and complications of continuous intraspinal narcotic analgesia for cancer pain control. J Clin Oncol 1984; 2(12):1414–1420.

123. Ready LB, Loper KA, Nessly M, et al. Postoperative epidural morphine is safe on surgical wards. Anesthesiology 1991; 75:452–456.

124. Mackie K, Lam AM. The epinephrine-containing test dose during beta-blockade. Anesthesiology 1989; 71:A1146.

125. Rapp SE, Ready LB, Greer BE. Postoperative pain management in gynecology oncology patients utilizing epidural opiate analgesia and patient-controlled analgesia. Gynecol Oncol 1989; 35:341–344.

126. Humphreys HK, Fleming NW. Opioid-induced spasm of the sphincter of Oddi apparently reversed by nalbuphine. Anesth Analg 1992; 74:308–310.

127. Yaksh TL, Noueihed RY, Durant PA. Studies of the pharmacology and pathology of intrathecally administered 4-anilinopiperidine analogues and morphine in the rat and cat. Anesthesiology 1986; 64:54–66.

128. Loper KA, Ready LB, Dorman BH. Prophylactic transdermal scopolamine patches reduce nausea in postoperative patients receiving epidural morphine. Anesth Analg 1989; 68:144–146.

129. Schwartz BR, Gregg RV, Kessler DL, et al. Continuous postoperative epidural analgesia in management of postoperative surgical pain. Urology 1989; 34(6):349–352.

130. Ackerman WE, Guneja MM, Kaczorowski DM. A comparison of the incidence of pruritus following epidural opioid administration in the parturient. Can J Anaesth 1989; 36:388–391.

131. Davies GG, From R. A blinded study using nalbuphine for prevention of pruritus induced by epidural fentanyl. Anesthesiology 1988; 69:763–765.

132. Rosen H. An epidural analgesia program: Balancing risks and benefits. Crit Care Nurse 1990; 10:32–41.

133. Henrikson M, Wild LR. A nursing process approach to epidural analgesia. J Obstet Gynecol Neonatal Nurs 1988; Sept/Oct. 316–320.

134. Penn RD, Paice JA. Chronic intrathecal morphine for intractable pain. J Neurosurg 1987; 67:182–186.

135. Etches RC, Sandler AN, Daley MD. Respiratory depression and spinal opioids. Can J Anaesth 1989; 36:165–185.

136. Allen LV, Stiles MI, Yu-Hsing TU. Stability of fentanyl citrate in

0.9% sodium chloride solutions prefilled in ambulatory infusion reservoirs. 1989; 1572–1574.

137. Kwan JW. Use of infusion devices for epidural or intrathecal administration of spinal opioids. Am J Hosp Pharm 1990; 47(Suppl):S18–S23.

138. White PF. Mishaps with patient-controlled analgesia. Anesthesiology 1987; 66:81–83.

139. Olsson G, Parker G. A model approach to pain assessment. Nurs '87 1987; 17(5):52–58.

140. Portenoy RK. Breakthrough pain: Definition and management. Oncology (Special Suppl) 1989.

141. Howard-Rubin J, McGuire L. Nursing's role in pain management. In Bonica JJ (ed). The Management of Pain, 2nd ed., Vol 1. Philadelphia: Lea and Febiger 1990:1690–1699.

142. Kerns RD, Turk DC, Rudy TE. The West Haven-Yale Multidimensional Pain Inventory (WHYMPI). Pain 1985; 23:345–356.

143. Fishman B, Pasternak S, Wallenstein SL, et al. The memorial pain assessment card: A valid instrument for the evaluation of cancer pain. Cancer 1987; 60:1151–1158.

144. Melzack R. The McGill pain questionnaire: Major properties and scoring methods. Pain 1975; 1:277–299.

145. Daut RL, Clerland CS. Development of the Wisconsin brief pain questionnaire to assess pain in cancer and other diseases. Pain 1983; 17:197–210.

146. Cleeland CS. Measurement and prevalence of pain in cancer. Semin Oncol Nurs 1985; 1:87–92.

147. Agency for Health Care Policy and Research. Clinical Practice Guideline. Acute Pain Management: Operative or Medical Procedures and Trauma. Rockville, MD: US Department of Health and Human Services, 1992.

148. North American Nursing Diagnosis Association. Taxonomy I, Revised—1990 with Official Nursing Diagnoses. St. Louis: North American Nursing Diagnosis Association, 1990; 73–75, 98, 99.

149. American Pain Society. Principles of Analgesic Use in the Treatment of Acute Pain and Chronic Cancer Pain, 2nd ed. Skokie, IL: American Pain Society, 1989:19.

150. Cohen SE, Sibak LL, Brose WG, et al. Analgesia after cesarean delivery: Patient evaluations and costs of five opioid techniques. Reg Anesth 1991; 16:141–149.

151. Macintyre PE, Runciman WB, Webb RK. An acute pain service in an Australian teaching hospital: The first year. Med J Aust 1990; 153:417–421.

NORTH MEMORIAL
MEDICAL CENTER
3300 North Oakdale,
Robbinsdale, MN 55422
(612) 520-5200

CONTROLLED SUBSTANCE
INFUSION
FLOW SHEET

DRUG: _____ **CONCENTRATION:** _____

DATE/TIME DISPENSED: _____ **BY:** _____

RECEIVED BY: _____ **RN** **VOLUME:** _____

Date												
Time												
RES VOL												
CONC. mg/ml (Epidural: Set screen at 0)												
Rate												
Bolus Dose												
Dose Min/Dose Hr												
Dose Given												
Clinician Bolus												
Given 0600-1400-2200 mg or ml												
Other Analgesics (Yes/No)												
LOC *												
Pain Rating **												
Epidural: Qh LOC and Resp. Rate (√)												
Epidural: Numbness (+/-)												
Epidural: Orthostatic Changes (Yes/No)												
Pruritus (+/-)												
Nausea (+/-)												
Dressing/Connection Check (√)												
Nurse's Initials												

INITIALS	SIGNATURE	INITIALS	SIGNATURE	INITIALS	SIGNATURE

LEVEL OF CONSCIOUSNESS KEY (LOC) *

1. Alert, engages in conversation; purposefully travels with eyes, if mute.
2. Lethargic, drowsy, sedate - focuses on personal interchange - but unable to maintain focus.
3. Responds only to maximal stimulation (shaking). Response only a grunt or moan - not a clear sentence.
4. Coma - unable to respond at all.

PAIN RATING (INTENSITY) **

5	Overwhelming
4	Severe
3	Distressing
2	Moderate
1	Mild
0	No Pain

Mix expiration   = 7 days
Hang expiration   = 72 hrs

Mix date/time_____Exp_____
Hang date/time_____Exp_____

Cassette changed or DC'd by _____

Amount Wasted = RES VOL _____

Witness to Wasting of Drug _____

F431 11/92   **Original White = Chart, Yellow = Pharmacy, Pink = Pharmacy**   N21411.dop/bb

APPENDIX 14-A-1

Courtesy of North Memorial Medical Center, Robbinsville, MN.

USE IN ACCORDANCE WITH PROCEDURE AND PROTOCOL
CIRCLE PAIN TREATMENT MODALITY:

1. PO
2. SUBLINGUAL
3. PATIENT CONTROLLED ANALGESIA
4. CONTINUOUS IV OPIOID INFUSION
5. TEMPORARY EPIDURAL INTERMITTENT INJECTION
6. PERMANENT EPIDURAL INTERMITTENT INJECTION

7. IM
8. RECTAL
9. CONTINUOUS SUBCUTANEOUS OPIOID INFUSION
10. INTERMITTENT IV OPIOID INJECTION
11. TEMPORARY EPIDURAL CONTINUOUS INFUSION
12. PERMANENT EPIDURAL CONTINUOUS INFUSION

PAIN SCALE:
0 = none
1 = mild
2
3 = moderate
4
5 = severe

SEDATION SCALE:
3 = Awake and responding
2 = Sleeping, but responds to normal voice
1 = Sleeping, but responds to loud voice or movement
0 = Sedated, doesn't respond

DATE	TIME	MED	BAG OR SYRINGE #	ROUTE #	BOLUS	CONT. RATE or basal	DOSE	PCA DELAY (min)	8 hr total	BP	P/RR	SEDATION	SCALE	PAIN	SKIN ANESTHESIA N=Normal T=Tingling Nb=Numbness A=Absent	SITE	CHECK	Tubing filter &/or SQ needle change	COMMENTS	INITIALS

NURSE INITIALS & SIGNATURE:

ADDRESSOGRAPH:

SWEDISH HOSPITAL MEDICAL CENTER

PAIN MANAGEMENT
NU-1153   Rev. 1/91   FC/SHMC   SN-5885

APPENDIX 14-A-2

Courtesy of Swedish Hospital Medical Center, Seattle, WA.

DATE	TIME	PHYSICIAN'S ORDERS	NOTED BY

PERMANENT EPIDURAL CATHETERS STANDING ORDERS

MD: Please indicate selections with an "X" and fill in all blanks.

Intermittent Injections:
1. Opioid: _____ every _____ hours
   Dilute with _____ ml preservative-free normal saline

Continuous Infusion per Micro Abbott Pump:
1. Opioid: _____
2. Local anesthetic agent and percentage: _____
   Other additive: _____
3. Start infusion at _____ ml/hour
4. ( ) Discontinue intermittent epidural injections previously ordered.

Patient Controlled Epidural Analgesia (PCEA) per Bard pump:
1. PCEA syringe medication same as continuous infusion drug   3. Delay interval _____ minutes
2. PCEA dose _____ ml   4. Basal <u>"OFF"</u>

For inadequate pain relief: (Pain Scale 0 = None, 1 = Mild, 3 = Moderate, 5 = Severe)

    <u>**Intermittent Injections**</u>
        Opioid _____ every _____ hours
        Dilute with _____ ml preservative-free normal saline
        Breakthrough pain relief – Opioid: _____

    <u>**Continuous infusion per Micro Abbott pump**</u>
        If pain level 3:   increase rate to _____ ml/hr.
        If pain level 4:   increase rate to _____ ml/hr.
        If pain level 5:   increase rate to _____ ml/hr.

    <u>**PCEA per Bard pump**</u>   **(Pain level ≥ 3)**
        Increase PCA dose to _____ ml.   Decrease delay interval to _____ minutes
    Call Pain Service STAT (Ext. 2323) (or attending MD) if patient's pain level increases or sustains at a 3 - 5 level.

IV Therapy:
1. IV fluid solution _____ at _____ ml/hr
2. For initiation of local anesthetic agent, patient must have IV access x 48 hrs

Treatment of side effects:
1. For nausea/vomiting:
   ( ) Prochlorperazine (Compazine) 5 - 10 mg IV q 6 hrs prn
   ( ) Lorazepam (Ativan) 0.5 - 1.0 mg IV q 4 hrs prn
   ( ) Metoclopramide (Reglan) 5 - 10 mg IV q 4 hrs prn
   ( ) Other _____
2. Call Pain Service and/or attending MD for the following:
   Sedation level 1 (responds to loud voice or noise) or 0 (no response)   dysphoria
   RR < 8/min   urinary retention
   If BP < _____ or > _____
   Significant increase or sudden onset of numbness or motor weakness
3. If sedation level ≤ 1 <u>**and**</u> RR < 8/min:
   Decrease continuous infusion by 50%.
   Stat oximetry
   Naloxone (Narcan) 0.1 mg IV <u>**slow**</u> push q 5 min x 4; reassess sedation & RR before each dose to determine need for continued dosing. Call Pain Service or attending M.D.
4. If urinary retention: straight cath x 1.
5. Bowel care by nurses

Monitoring:
1. P, RR, BP, sedation, pain, and skin anesthesia (only with local anesthetic agents) q 1 hr x 2, then q 4 hr
2. Postural BP (only with local anesthetic agents) q 8 hr until stable
3. Urinary output q 8 hr – monitor for retention
4. Contact Infusion Therapy instructors at Ext. 6023

☐ _____   _____ , M.D.
          PHONE

☐ Stuart DuPen, M.D.   991-5751   _____

☐ Anna Williams, R.N.   998-6495   _____

A DRUG EQUIVALENT MAY BE DISPENSED UNLESS CHECKED ☐

SIGNATURE IS REQUIRED FOLLOWING ENTRY OF EACH ORDER

SWEDISH MEDICAL CENTER
747 Summit Avenue Seattle, WA 98104-2196

NU-1756   Rev. 9/93   FC/SMC

PHYSICIAN'S ORDERS

APPENDIX 14-B

Courtesy of Swedish Hospital Medical Center, Seattle, WA.

PAIN ASSESSMENT FORM

1. Intensity:

NURSE: _____
PATIENT: _____
DATE: _____

PAIN SCALE

| 0 | 1 | 2 | 3 | 4 | 5 | 6 | 7 | 8 | 9 | 10 |

No
Pain

Worst Pain Imaginable

Pain Rating _____ mm

2. Where is your pain located?   (I = Internal)
    Patient or Nurse mark drawing.   (E = External)

3. How and when did your pain begin?
    Does something trigger your pain?
    _____
    _____

4. How long have you had the pain?
    Is it continuous or intermittent?
    Describe any patterns or changes.
    _____
    _____
    _____

5. Describe in your own words what your pain feels like: _____
    _____
    _____

6. What makes the pain better? _____

7. What makes the pain worse? _____

8. What has helped in the past? _____

9. What has not helped in the past? _____

10. What other symptoms accompany your pain? _____

11. How does your pain affect your: _____
    Sleep? _____
    Appetite? _____
    Physical activity? _____
    Concentration? _____
    Emotions? _____
    Social relationships? _____

12. What do you think is causing your pain now?
    _____

13. Current Analgesic Regimen? _____
    _____

14. Plan/comments _____
    _____
    _____

JPI-DR-019-4A

APPENDIX 14-C

CHAPTER 15 # Types of Intravenous Therapy Equipment

Brenda L. Jensen, BSN, CRNI

The equipment used in health care is changing rapidly to meet the demands of the consumer. In the health care market, the consumer is both the health care provider and the patient. The patient is rarely involved in the decision-making process of equipment acquisition, so the patient's role is more that of a recipient than an actively participating consumer. Because of this unique situation, the nurse makes product decisions for the patient, thereby reinforcing the traditional role of the nurse as the patient advocate. The nurse's role in equipment selection is to ensure the safe, effective delivery of health care to the patient.

A nurse must be aware of the almost unlimited amount of information available from the health care industry. Representatives of the health care industry are aware of medical research in early stages because of their desire to anticipate needs in health care. Research and clinical validation of products can reveal a great deal of information about product capabilities and limitations. These factors make the manufacturer a rich source of information that cumulatively can aid in product selection. The nurse should look at all brands of a specific product to separate salesmanship from product performance before determining the product's acceptability.

Financial accountability is a necessity in health care. The financial profile of any specific population represents a payer mix that should act as a guide to reimbursement expectations. This information is necessary for the formulation of plans to evaluate and procure equipment in a cost-effective manner.

Medical manufacturers pride themselves on the extensive

research and clinical activity used in the design and development of medical products. Many companies have departments of medical professionals who are involved in the evolution of medical products and reimbursement potential. Research and development departments are an invaluable source of information that is often available to the nurse. Not only do manufacturers research the products they develop, but most also submit products for third-party research to validate their own findings. A part of product acquisition is the sharing of research information with the users, nurses, and physicians. The product's capabilities and supporting data are available to anyone who is interested and are frequently catalogued in the institution's purchasing department.

Manufacturers are subject to the laws of supply and demand. If the supply is ample and the demand steady, the cost is usually reasonable. If the demand is high and the supplies are scarce, the cost can be high. Professional networking can help identify substandard products and consequently decrease demand.

In summary, the relationship of industry, health care providers, and the patient is one of mutual dependency. The role of each exists because of the presence of the other two. The public holds industry, medical institutions, and professionals accountable for the safe and effective delivery of health care. Medical products and equipment are the collaborative responsibility of industry and medical professionals.

SOLUTION CONTAINERS

Glass Containers

The first intravenous (IV) infusion container to be mass produced was made of glass. Glass was and is easy to sterilize, and graduations on glass can be easily and accurately read. After 50 years of use, glass remains the container of choice only for solutions that cannot adapt to plastic bags because of incompatibilities with chemicals or properties of plastic. Some plastic-like containers have overcome some of these compatibility issues, and not all researchers even agree that incompatibility presents a risk.

An example of the compatibility problem is IV nitroglycerin. Some studies have shown that nitroglycerin solution adheres to the plastic container, reducing the amount of drug available to be infused into the patient. Accurate administration is therefore difficult to measure. Because the drug dosage is usually adjusted to patient condition, it is not possible to know the actual concentration being delivered.

Another incompatibility issue arises with fat emulsions. This suspension is reported to leach the plasticizer from plastic bags made of polyvinyl chloride (PVC), specifically the plasticizer diethylhexylphthalate (DEHP). This contaminant is suspected of being delivered to the patient along with the fat emulsions. The effects of the plasticizer are very controversial in the literature, therefore, fat emulsions are available only in glass.[1] The admixture of fat emulsions with dextrose for three-in-one total parenteral nutrition is achieved because the solution bags are not made of PVC plastic.

Closed-system glass bottles are sealed with a thick, hard, rubber disk. In the center is a target meant to be easily perforated with the administration tubing spike. The hard rubber disk is covered with an easily removable vacuum seal. Once the seal is removed, the bottle should be used immediately to ensure sterility. The seal must be removed before it is spiked with an administration set and cannot be reapplied or resealed. In a sterile admixture program, solutions can be mixed and a second sterile cover applied for delivery to the patient care area.

Glass bottles must also be vented because of their noncollapsible nature. For the solution to empty from the bottle, air must take its place, which can occur through a venting straw or with vented tubing. If the bottle is made with a venting straw, it runs the length of the bottle to allow air to be pulled in as the solution runs out. The potential for contamination of the solution is increased with the use of a venting straw because no barrier exists between the external sources of contamination and the interior of the bottle.

Most glass bottles are made without venting straws, and vented administration sets are used to relieve the vacuum in the bottle. The tubing spike has a regular channel for the flow of solution and a very small side channel for the introduction of air into the bottle. The infusion set may be made specifically as a vented set or may be considered a universal infusion set, with a capped air channel, requiring the nurse to uncap the air inlet channel when it is used with a glass solution container.

Plastic Containers

The first real commitment to large-scale conversion to plastic IV solution containers came with the need to transport soldiers off the battlefield or from field triage areas with treatment already initiated. The same pressure for plastic came from improved emergency care in regular hospitals. As emergency personnel and treatments evolved and many more treatments were initiated outside the hospital, the need for the safety of plastic over glass became critical for the patient as well as for the health care provider.

The introduction to PVC plastic solution containers met with compatibility concerns, as was discussed earlier. Many concerns have been satisfactorily addressed, and the health care industry has become comfortable with the use of plastic bags as the primary solution container. Solutions that remain a concern with regard to compatibility to plastic are insulin, nitroglycerin, fat emulsions, lorazepam, and others.[2-4] Research on the combination of these drugs and plastic bags and administration sets is ongoing and remains controversial.

Besides compatibility, another concern is that of correctness of the graduations and accuracy in reading the volume remaining in the bag. A study reported by Coles and Fanning in 1987 found that measurements in Viaflex plastic bags were within plus or minus 10% for increments one through nine. However, the first and last graduations were as much as 40% inaccurate.[5]

A word of caution for the use of plastic solution containers is necessary. The bag can be perforated during use. Careful attention should be paid when the bag is spiked because the spike can tear the side of the bag. The tear may result in contamination of the solution or leakage.

Plastic solution containers collapse when they empty, eliminating the need for any kind of venting device either in the bag or on the solution administration set. Because air is not introduced into the bag, very little air can be accidentally infused.

Because of its relatively light and nonbreakable properties, the plastic container is safer and more practical to store, stack, and move from one place to another. Most plastic containers are not sensitive to fluctuations in temperature or changes in environment. Many drugs are provided in prefilled and prefrozen minibags because the bags are able to withstand freezing and thawing.

With the trend toward ambulatory and home care infusions, the plastic solution container has added a significant degree of safety and convenience. The expanding outpatient delivery of IV therapies is possible partly as a result of the development of plastic solution containers.

Semirigid Containers

Semirigid containers were developed to capture the best qualities of both glass and plastic solution containers. Although they do not share the popularity of the plastic bag, they also do not share its shortcomings. The semirigid container holds its shape independent of its contents and is made of rigid plastic. The rigid plastic does not contain plasticizers, reducing drug compatibility issues. The semirigid container is as safe as glass for most drugs that are incompatible with plastic.

The container does not collapse during infusion, so graduations are easily read and reliable. The semirigid container does not perforate during spiking and is difficult to puncture accidentally during admixing.

The semirigid container is lightweight and nonbreakable, making storage, stacking, and transporting safe. The container is, however, more bulky and less flexible. The semirigid container is well-liked in ambulatory and home care infusion situations for its ease of use. However, it does not adapt well to being worn inside pouches or concealed in ambulatory packs.

Besides being too rigid for these ambulatory uses, the semirigid containers must be vented to add air to the infusion system. As is the case with glass, venting straws or vented tubing must be used for solutions to flow correctly. The continuous addition of air to the system contraindicates the use of a semirigid container for many ambulatory situations. The semirigid containers can be cracked if handled roughly or subjected to environmental temperature extremes. This type of container is not well-suited to being frozen.

Other Solution Containers

Syringes can be correctly identified as primary solution infusion containers. The syringe, when used in conjunction with a syringe-loaded electronic infusion pump, acts as a primary container for either intermittent or continuous use. If the pump withdraws or aspirates the contents of the syringe, the tubing must be vented to allow air to displace the solution being extracted. If the pump mechanism is simply compression of the syringe, any tubing may be used with the syringe.

A syringe is easily and accurately readable for volume given or volume remaining. The syringe is nonbreakable, easy to store and transport, and impossible to perforate accidentally. The syringe, in comparison with other solution containers, is inexpensive and is available worldwide. The syringe can be prefilled and prefrozen with an almost unlimited number of solutions and drugs.

The limiting feature of the syringe is the volume it holds. Syringes are seldom seen with volume capabilities of greater than 50 to 60 ml, because syringes of this size are awkward to handle. This is not a limiting feature in neonatal and pediatric applications. In these areas, syringes can be the primary container for all types of infusions, such as crystalloids, blood products, fat emulsions, medications, and parenteral nutrition. In adults, the syringe is most often used for intermittent medications. Continuous infusion via the syringe may be used for small volumes required by such therapies as pain control and nontitrated concentrated medications.

Infusion pump specific containers also fall in the category of solution containers. Most of these are reservoirs made specifically for use with a single, unique infusion device. They are not interchangeable. Efforts to use most of these solution containers in any device other than the one for which they were produced may lead to serious and harmful effects. Some are dedicated not only to a specific infusion system but also to a specific therapy, such as chemotherapy or pain control.

The container systems used for specific devices each have unique limitations, depending on pump functions and therapies delivered. Some of these limitations may be lack of testing for a wider variety of use or problems arising with commonly used drugs in uncommon concentrations or infusion modes.

Venting Rigid Containers

Whether the rigid, nonflexible containers or the collapsible bags are used, the nurse must understand the importance of the free flow of solution. If the container cannot collapse as solution empties, air must be introduced into the container. The most acceptable and current method to introduce air is the use of vented tubing designed to allow air to enter the bottle or rigid container.

The venting mechanism provided by the manufacturer is intended to allow air to enter without solution leaking out the venting device. This concept appears simple but is actually accomplished by an understanding of droplet formation and the physical make-up of the venting outlet. In the absence of this venting device, it is not acceptable for a bottle or rigid container to be vented with a needle through the rubber disk; this method creates a risk of solution contamination and an open entry for infection. This is also an unsafe use of a needle. When a needle is used inappropriately in this way, fluid frequently leaks from the bottle.

Noncollapsible containers require the introduction of air into the bottle to allow the solution to flow correctly. Risk is associated with air being introduced into the solution administration system, and many built-in safeguards exist to counter that risk. These safeguards are addressed throughout this chapter (Fig. 15–1).

Light Sensitivity

Degradation of very specific drugs, such as nitroprusside and Dakin's solution, occurs when the agents have prolonged

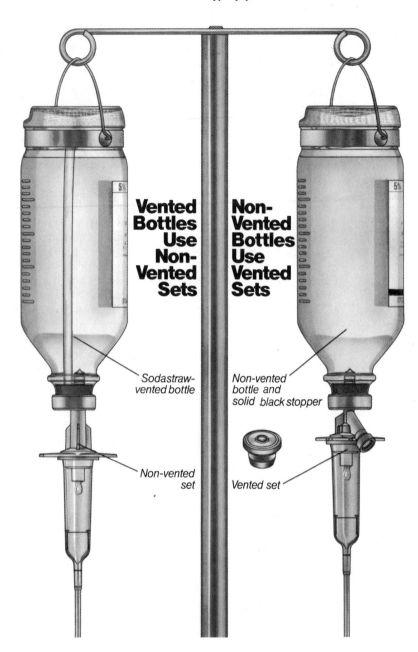

Vented Bottles Use Non-Vented Sets

Non-Vented Bottles Use Vented Sets

Sodastraw-vented bottle

Non-vented bottle and solid black stopper

Non-vented set

Vented set

Figure 15–1. Vented and nonvented bottle tubing. (Courtesy of Baxter Healthcare Corporation.)

exposure to light during infusion. With regard to plastic versus glass, there is apparently no distinct advantage of one material over another. Efforts have been made to provide a container material that addresses this issue, but such development is not economically practical. A simple solution is to protect the solution container from light by placing a dark material over the bag.

Use-Activated Containers

Several complex types of solution containers are available. Use-activated containers are compartmentalized and have premeasured ingredients that form an admixture when mixed. These containers are very helpful for high-use infusions with a relatively short shelf life after admixture. Although they are more expensive than the individually supplied products, use-activated containers offer considerable savings of person-

nel time for admixture. These types of containers play a significant time-saving role in emergency care and enable ease of use in acute situations, such as in ambulances, field use, or transport. Ambulatory and home care settings can also benefit from use-activated containers.

To activate the container, the nurse must deliberately rupture a seal or diaphragm within the container. Usually, this action requires compressing opposing parts or applying pressure to rupture an internal reservoir. The primary disadvantage of the system, however, occurs when this step is not completed appropriately. It is not always apparent when the admixture has not occurred, leaving the primary fluid infusing without the intended medication. The patient is not receiving the medication as intended, although a more severe concern is the belated rupture of the medication reservoir and a potentially harmful concentration of drug being administered. The possibility for administration error does exist with use-activated containers as with all infusion systems.

SOLUTION ADMINISTRATION SETS

Primary Administration Sets

A primary set is typically the main tubing used to carry the infusing solution from the container to the patient. It can be a single entity or it can have many attachments and features. Primary sets can be gravity tubing, infusion pump tubing, or even microbore syringe pump tubing, if the main solution is being infused with the syringe pump.

The primary set can be selected with varying drop size and length, depending on the intended use, the patient's condition, and the rate of infusion. The spike should be designed with a finger guard to aid in spiking the solution container with ease and preventing contamination. The length should be suited to the activity level of the patient and to the bed and equipment arrangement. Primary sets can range from 60 to 110 inches in length.

Any piece of tubing attached to a primary set is considered an add-on device and is generally discouraged. If used with a primary set, add-on devices should have a specific purpose, and their use should be strictly limited. Each add-on device is a potential source of contamination, misuse, and accidental disconnection. Examples of some add-on devices are filters, extension sets, stopcocks, and multiflow adapters.

Primary administration sets should have Luer-Loks to prevent accidental disconnection. The use of needles to access administration set ports should be avoided; needleless or needle protective systems should be used (Fig. 15–2).

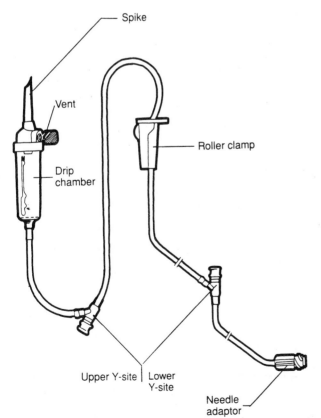

Figure 15–2. Primary administration set. (Courtesy of MiniMed Technologies.)

Secondary Administration Sets

Typically, a secondary set is defined as tubing that attaches to the primary administration set for a specific purpose, which is generally to administer medication. The set may be used intermittently or continuously but must be compatible to the primary infusing solution.

Secondary sets are usually 18 to 70 inches long, but most are around 30 to 36 inches long. Secondary sets can be macrodrop or microdrop, depending on the volume and rate of the secondary solution and the patient's condition. The drip chamber should have a finger guard at the spike for ease of use and for prevention of touch contamination.

Secondary administration sets can be attached to the primary set by use of a blunt, hard plastic cannula to penetrate a soft latex cap that locks in place with Luer-Lok. Another device that may be used is a recessed needle in a rigid cap that penetrates the traditional injection port on the primary set and locks securely. Both the recessed needle and the blunt cannula greatly reduce the risk of accidental disconnection or needle injury.

Vented and Nonvented Sets

Vented solution sets allow air to enter the infusion container to displace the infusing solution. These sets are necessary for use with containers that do not collapse when emptying (glass or semirigid plastic). A vented set is designed with a small air inlet on the spike portion of the tubing. The fit into the container may be tighter than a nonvented spike, requiring more effort to spike the bottle. This characteristic is not considered to be a problem, but the nurse should be aware of it to ensure that the spike is fully inserted into the bottle, preventing accidental dislodgment or impeded flow. Vented sets are available in gravity infusion administration sets as well as in infusion pump sets.

Some manufacturers prefer to offer a universal set that can be vented or nonvented, depending on need. In these sets, a removable cap exists for the air inlet vent. To create a vented set, the capping device is simply removed.

Collapsible plastic containers can physically accommodate a vented spike. If a bag is vented, the infusing solution is displaced by air entering the bag. Air, therefore, is introduced into the infusing system, creating unnecessary risk for the patient.

Nonvented tubing is designed for collapsible plastic containers. No air is admitted into the system; the infusing solution creates a minor vacuum that allows the bag to collapse as it empties. This is an important characteristic when a sterile, closed infusion system is the goal. Nonvented tubing cannot be used with glass or rigid plastic.

Many administration sets are marketed to belong to a specific system or to be used with limited solution containers. It is crucial that these limitations be known to all users. The universal adaptability of administration sets is more common in add-on devices than in primary sets. The best and safest connections and use of primary administration sets are achieved when solution containers of the same manufacturer are used.

Metered Volume Chamber Sets

A metered set contains a small-volume chamber between the primary solution container and the administration set. The metered chamber may or may not be preattached to the administration set. It can easily be obtained as a stand-alone item, which enables the user to use it with various solution sets. It is available with a large variety of preattached tubing. Many pump manufacturers also provide pump sets that have a metered chamber or can adapt to one.

The metered chamber is calibrated in much smaller increments than are other infusion devices. Some may be calibrated precisely, down to 2 ml, but most are very accurate at 5 ml. They are semirigid and may have a ball float at the bottom of the chamber to prevent air from entering the infusion line when the chamber empties.

Metered chamber sets are designed to limit the amount of solution available to the patient, usually for safety, but also as an intermittent infusion routine. The chamber is usually 100 or 150 ml. Some neonatal chambers may be only 10 to 50 ml.

For critical care drugs, titrated drugs, or solutions infusing into severely volume-restricted patients, the use of a controlled volume chamber is crucial. Some pediatric and most neonatal areas require metered volume chamber administration sets on all patients receiving IV infusions with a 1 or 2 hour fill limit of solution to be infused. This limit prevents adverse consequences in the event of uncontrolled intravenous infusions, rates set too high, or tampering mishaps. Metered volume chamber administration sets are equally important in adults receiving critical care drugs, such as aminophylline or lidocaine. The use of the metered set is contraindicated when non-PVC tubing must be used to infuse a specific solution, such as fat emulsions or nitroglycerin.

Another application of the metered chamber is the intermittent infusion of medication. The chamber is filled to a prescribed level to achieve a correct dilution, and the medication is added through an injection port at the top of the chamber. This method is useful when the medication is available in syringe, the medication is admixed immediately before infusion, or the patient's volume is restricted. The primary infusing solution then becomes the diluent. The drawback to this method is that the medication administration rate varies greatly from the primary infusion rate or when the medication is not compatible in solution with the primary fluid (Fig. 15–3).

Drop Factors

The drop factor is the number of drops delivered that equal 1 ml. The drop factor is a specific measurement that is perfected to deliver exact amounts not only for long periods of time but with very little variance in thousands of similar sets manufactured. Each administration set has a predetermined drop factor and can be relied on to deliver solution accurately, plus or minus 10% as an industry standard. The user calculates flow rates based on the number of drops allowed to fall each minute.

Drop factors are manufacturer specific. Each administration set manufacturer has very rigid standards set for its

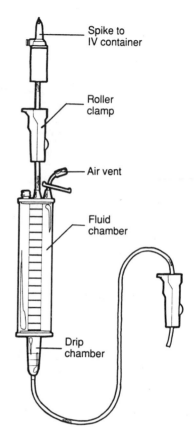

Figure 15–3. Metered volume set. (Courtesy of MiniMed Technologies.)

specific products and unique drop size. Drop sizes may vary from 10, 12, 15, 20, to 60 drops/ml. Drop factors are usually divided into two categories, macrodrop and microdrop.

Macrodrop is also thought of as regular drop size. The 10, 12, 15, and 20 drop/ml sets are macrodrop sets. This common set can be used in any application, although its accuracy decreases as the rate per hour decreases.

Microdrop tubing is the most suitable for infusion rates of less than 100 ml/hour. Microdrop tubing is usually termed pediatric, although it is used as much or more in adults in whom high rates are not necessary. Microdrop sizes are usually 50 to 60 drops/ml.

Microdrop tubing, by restricting the flow even with the control clamp wide open, allows an added safety feature against runaway IV lines or free flow. Both phenomena can still occur, but they are slowed considerably with microdrop tubing. This characteristic makes this tubing especially safe for pediatric, geriatric, or volume-restricted patients.

Electronic infusion pumps sometimes offer administration sets with macrodrop or microdrop options, which should be a consideration if the administration sets are routinely taken from the infusion pumps for use as gravity administration sets. The size of the drop does not factor into the delivery of fluid by an electronic infusion device. These devices measure by fluid displacement or mechanical movement and do not measure drop size or count drops. Any consideration for drop size on infusion pump tubing would be relevant only for use outside the infusion device or as a free-flow protection if the infusion pump does not offer that safeguard.

Primary Y Sets

Primary Y sets are used for rapid infusion or dual administration, usually in critical care, trauma, or surgery patients, and can be found in gravity as well as in infusion pump configurations. Each leg of the Y set is capable of being the primary set. The Y set has two separate spikes, with a separate drip chamber and a short length of tubing with individual clamps. The joining occurs usually 12 to 20 inches below the spikes. At this junction, another drip chamber may be present, but the solutions mix fully at this point. Primary Y tubing cannot be used to infuse incompatible solutions.

Primary Y sets are commonly made with very large bore tubing and clamps that lack the fine-tuning capabilities of general-use tubing, because this tubing is meant to infuse large amounts in acute situations. These sets are not intended for general use and pose a risk if used for general-purpose infusion. The risk of accidental bolus or a runaway IV line is very high because of the design of the tubing.

The primary Y set is ideal, however, for the infusion of blood and some blood products. The infusion leg opposite the portion infusing the unit of blood is commonly used for the administration of 0.9% sodium chloride solution given before and after a unit of blood product is infused. The large inner lumen allows the more viscous blood solution to infuse with ease and decreases trauma to infusing blood cells. Blood can be infused very rapidly with a primary Y set.

A word of caution about the primary Y set: if it is used with a noncollapsible solution container or glass bottle, the air vent will not only fill the bottle, but the air will continue to flow with the infusing fluid from the other side into the patient. Primary Y sets are not provided as vented sets, so this caution applies to bottles with venting straws or a venting apparatus added to the bottle. Any air emboli associated with tubing of this inner lumen size would be significant.

Internal Diameter of Tubing

Internal lumen sizes of solution administration tubings are manufacturer specific. Industry standards refer to a range of inner lumen sizes, and each manufacturer is allowed to market products that are compatible but not uniform. Tubing can be categorized into types based on lumen size, but again, uniformity can not be assumed from all manufacturers. Usually, minuscule differences are acceptable and do not affect performance in situations not calling for such precision. In other instances, these differences can be critical. If performance problems are suspected, the manufacturer of the products should always be consulted to confirm or rule out tubing conflicts. (A tubing conflict means that one piece of tubing interferes with the performance of another.)

Macrobore tubing is commonly used on blood administration sets or primary Y sets for use in trauma or operating room situations. Macrobore means that the tubing inner lumen is larger than standard tubing for the purpose of accomplishing high flow rates; how much larger depends on the manufacturer. Anesthesia sets and some specialty sets are designed specifically with macrobore tubing.

The large inner lumen makes macrobore tubing stiffer and makes accommodating a controlling mechanism, such as a roller clamp, more difficult. The clamp is less reliable for long-term infusion control, making the macrobore set unsuitable for extended use or general care. Macrobore tubing should never be used in electronic infusion pumps that accommodate generic tubing.

Microbore tubing has a smaller-than-standard inner lumen. Because a small tubing is very flimsy, the microbore tubing frequently has a smaller inner lumen but a thicker wall, making it resistant to kinking. Many microbore sets are termed *kink resistant* or *noncompliant* (meaning that it does not bend or stretch). Again, because tubing is manufacturer specific, the qualities of each microbore set should be investigated, not assumed.

Because microbore sets have a narrowed inner lumen, flow is restricted to some degree. Microbore sets can be used as a safeguard against runaway or bolus infusions and offer a very low priming volume, making them a suitable choice in such areas as pediatrics, neonatal units, and volume-restricted adult care areas, such as cardiology or renal units. Microbore tubing is frequently the tubing of choice for syringe pumps, epidural infusion pumps, or ambulatory infusion devices that are designed to deliver small quantities over a long period of time, such as low-dose chemotherapy or pain control medications.

Standard lumen tubing makes up most sets, and almost all infusion therapies can be accomplished with standard-bore administration sets. All standard-bore sets have a common inner lumen size with very little variation from manufacturer to manufacturer. Again, the standard bore sets are within a common range but should never be assumed to be exactly the same.

In-Line Rate-Control Clamps

Roller Clamps. These are found on all standard administration sets and are in-line, which means that they are attached during the manufacturing of the set. The roller clamp allows the tubing to be incrementally occluded by pinching the tubing as the roller clamp is tightened. Most roller clamps are easily regulated with one hand. The clamp is designed to hold its place on the tubing, keeping the infusion rate constant between adjustments. The primary purpose of the roller clamp is to control flow rates of infusion. Standard roller clamps on standard-bore tubing can be as accurate as plus or minus 10%.

The accuracy of standard roller clamps is directly dependent on the number of variables involved in each administration. Patient movement, ambulation, patient transfer, and height of the solution container are just a few of the things that can affect the accuracy of an adjusted roller clamp. Safe rate control with roller clamps requires vigilant observation at frequent intervals by the caregiver to confirm the infusion rates.

Roller clamps should be positioned on the third of the tubing nearest the solution container. This placement is convenient for the nurse, but more importantly, it is out of the way of the patient, to prevent accidental manipulation. The clamp should be repositioned on the tubing at daily intervals because the tubing commonly develops a "memory," making it difficult to regulate. This memory can work in two ways. In the event of "cold creep," the tubing is trying to retain its round shape, pushing the clamp open. The other form of memory is a pinched section of tubing that does not reopen when the clamp is removed. Both of these problems can be avoided by using a set only for the designated number of hours (usually 48) and moving the clamp to an unused portion of tubing when the rate is readjusted.

Some standard sets have a more advanced roller clamp, called a *stationary clamp*, which is positioned on the tubing as an insert. A portion of the PVC tubing is replaced with a small segment of softer silicone tubing. The silicone tubing is not affected by cold creep or memory, therefore, the rate is more easily maintained. These tubings are somewhat more expensive and remain accurate at plus or minus 10%.

Slide and Pinch Clamps. These are provided on some sets but are not regulating clamps. Both are simple, one-handed clamps whose sole purpose is as on-off clamps. Infusions should never be regulated with slide or pinch clamps, because these clamps are not accompanied by accuracy claims. Both of these clamps are capable of creating a serious crimp or crease in the tubing that could be hazardous.

Screw Clamps. These clamps function by turning a screw device to incrementally apply pressure to a point on the tubing, thereby pinching it off. They are easy to adjust with one hand and should be positioned on the upper third of the tubing. Unlike the roller clamp, the screw clamp cannot migrate back, making cold creep impossible. The screw clamp can be moved easily, however, even if it is accidentally bumped. Manufacturers of screw-type clamps do not make claims of substantially greater accuracy than for traditional roller clamps, but most users believe them to be more reliable.

Add-On Manual Flow Control Devices

Add-on manual flow control devices are readily available in many shapes and types. Recent years have seen some exciting new developments in sophisticated flow regulators. These devices are added onto an existing gravity infusion line, either standard or microdrop, at the proximal end near the patient connection. The proximity to the patient is seen as a disadvantage by some clinicians. The pre-existing clamp on the tubing is not used.

These flow regulators generally provide a greater degree of consistency of flow rate than do preattached roller clamps. They are accurate to plus or minus 10% which is the same as for standard tubing with traditional roller clamps. In actual practice, however, some of these clamps have shown that a safety value exists that is not easily quantified. With most add-on controlling devices, significant added protection exists against crimped tubing, cold creep, and drifting of the roller clamp. The add-on controlling devices are not likely to be accidentally reset when bumped or jostled because of patient activity. In addition, added protection from accidental free flow exists.

In recent years, some manufacturers have claimed the ability to compensate for changes in head height, which means changes in patient position or height of solution container in relation to the patient. This feature could be an important asset in the care of ambulatory patients.

An issue that has arisen with some models of add-on regulators is predetermined settings. On these devices, the

nurse sets the dial or indicator to a given number, and the set supposedly delivers at that rate. In actuality, any variable in a patient care setting can alter that rate, such as change in patient position, sharp change in room temperature, or even decreased volume in the solution container. The nurse cannot rely on the numbered setting to indicate the actual flow being delivered. Although the numbered dial may have some advantages of add-on control devices, the number on the indicator may not be what is actually being delivered. Great harm can occur when the caregiver assumes that the delivery rate is the same as the value on the dial indicator and the drop rate is not counted for confirmation.

The use of add-on controlling devices must be determined by close examination of real versus perceived need. The proficiency of the nursing staff, the level of illness being treated, the type of patient population, and the care environment all need to be considered. Add-on regulators significantly add to cost per IV line in any setting and must be changed with the routine tubing changes.

An add-on controlling device is not a substitute for an infusion pump. If patient acuity and drug therapy indicate that an electronic infusion pump is necessary to safely deliver care, an add-on regulator cannot possibly provide any degree of that safety. However, if gravity administration is indicated, some add-on devices may provide an extra measure of safety.

Resealable Latex Y Ports

Most primary IV infusion administration sets are made with one to three injection Y ports located in strategic places along the line. Resealable ports or injection ports are a significant advantage in the administration of many IV therapies. The injection ports are made of dense latex rubber and are secured to a portion of the infusion line where a hard, molded Y exists, with the main infusion line being the other leg of the Y. These rubber caps are tightly secured, frequently with a heat-shrunk band, to prevent any movement or break in the sterility of the infusion line.

The latex rubber port is able to reseal after it is penetrated with a needle, or if it is part of a needleless system, it may reseal after it is punctured with a dull plastic spike. This characteristic makes it possible for the nurse to administer other medications through the existing primary infusion line after confirming compatibility. The latex port should be able to accommodate numerous punctures, although a definitive number does not exist. The port can usually be safely used through the limited life of the infusion line. Caution should be taken if an extraordinary number of punctures occurs. If the latex port is compromised by excessive penetrations, air emboli may occur, and the infusion line is less sterile.

Coring occurs when a large needle or numerous small needles remove a piece of rubber latex from the port during needle penetration. The chance of coring increases with large-gauge needles and some more vulnerable latex materials. Coring may occur after only one puncture or after repeated punctures. The nurse should suspect coring if little resistance is felt when inserting the needle or spike into the latex cap. In these cases, the tubing should be changed immediately.

The latex injection port found on the upper third of the infusion line nearest the solution container is used for IV piggyback administration. It is common practice for the IV piggyback to be attached at this level to infuse either concurrently or sequentially with the main IV solution. The set attached here is referred to as the *secondary set.*

The injection port found nearest the patient is used for IV push medications. This injection port is often 6 to 12 inches from the proximal end of the tubing. This port should never be used for the attachment of a secondary set, because of its close proximity to the patient. One or more other injection ports may be located at various points on the primary administration set. In most cases, the two ports mentioned offer as much flexibility as is ever needed for most administration needs.

Back-Check Valves

Back-check valves or one-way valves are an integral part of many administration sets. These valves allow the fluid to flow in one direction only. Back-check valves work much like a float. When the fluid is passing through the disk, a small float device holds the passage open. If the flow is reversed, the float device closes off the passageway. Another one-way valve appears similar to a flap valve in the fluid path. When fluid is passing correctly, the flap flows open. When the flow is reversed, the flap is forced shut, stopping the flow of fluid. Back-check valves have no other purpose than to direct the flow of fluid.

The most common use of back-check valves is in the administration of IV piggyback medications. The IV piggyback is attached to the injection port on the upper third of the primary administration set. The back-check valve is between this junction and the primary solution container. This configuration prevents the secondary IV piggyback from flowing into the primary infusion container if resistance occurs in the infusion system at the patient end. The primary solution does not flow into the secondary container, because the IV piggyback hangs higher than the primary container.

This same premise applies for back-check valves used in patient-controlled analgesia pump sets. To ensure that the pain medication is flowing from the pump to the patient, the PCA tubing incorporates a back-check valve where the PCA tubing attaches to the primary set. The valve is on the leg of the Y that infuses the primary solution. This configuration prevents the pain medication from flowing upstream into the primary infusion should the IV access device become occluded.

In all cases, the back-check valve prevents the retrograde flow of solution. This measure is necessary in many dual-infusion systems and also inhibits the back flow of blood into the tubing. Back-check valves are standard additions to many infusion systems (Fig. 15–4).

Connections

Manufacturers of IV tubing connections strive to make them universal, which means that male and female fittings for standard devices should make a correct fit when connected. This standard exists for safety and efficiency reasons.

Two basic types of standard connections exist, slip and Luer-Lok. Slip connections are fittings that simply slide into

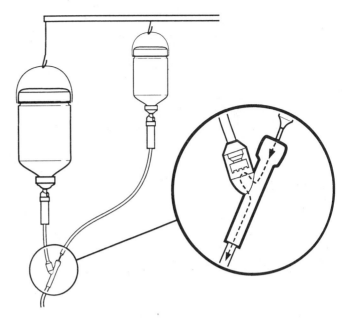

Figure 15–4. Back-check valve or one-way valve. (Courtesy of MiniMed Technologies.)

each other until snug. Many devices are simple slip connections. These are said to be universal but offer no safeguard against accidental disconnection.

Luer-Lok connections screw together two compatible ends. Deliberate twisting motions are required to disconnect a Luer-Lok, making accidental disconnection almost impossible. Most major medical manufacturers offer all infusion tubing and add-on devices with Luer-Lok connections. Luer-Lok connections do not usually add to the cost of the device or tubing, because they are increasingly becoming an industry standard.

Flash Ball

A flash ball is a latex rubber cone located at the patient connection of a primary infusion set. Flash balls were, in the recent past, a standard feature on administration sets. Because of increased understanding in the physiology of IV therapy and improved tubing configurations, flash balls are now seldom seen.

The flash ball is used to inject medication near the patient connection. The newer administration sets have a resealable latex port near the patient connection, making the flash ball unnecessary. The flash ball should never be used to create turbulence in the IV catheter to improve blood flow or restore patency. This action can dislodge microemboli or cause infiltration.

In-Line Hand Pumps

Blood administration sets and some dual-infusion or anesthesia sets are equipped with an in-line hand pump. This device is a clear, chamber-like section of tubing that is usually located on the upper third of the administration set. The chamber is made of soft, pliable plastic, and the inlet into the chamber may be equipped with a one-way valve. The function of the hand pump is to speed the infusion by squeezing the chamber, thereby forcing the fluid to flow more rapidly to the patient.

Adverse affects of inappropriate use of hand pumps include damaged vasculature, severe infiltrations, and loss of the IV site. Other potential problems can be damaged blood cells if blood products are infusing, pulmonary emboli, or speed shock. Because of these affects, hand pumps should be used with caution.

Pressure Bags

A pressure bag for the infusion of gravity drip IV solutions should be reserved for trauma, anesthesiology, surgery, and critical care needs. Pressure bags maintain consistent pressure on the infusing solution to hasten the pace of the infusion. Because this pressure is very difficult to regulate and maintain safely, pressure bags are not routinely used in this manner. Infusion pumps are the method of choice when rapid infusion is necessary.

The most routine use of pressure bags is for the maintenance of pressurized arterial lines. In this case, the pressure bag keeps consistent pressure on an infusing solution of dilute heparin solution or saline but infuses it through a restricted access that maintains the positive flow at a very minimal amount (usually 3 ml/hour). The pressure does not allow any backflow of blood, thereby keeping the arterial catheter patent. Once again, appropriate use is important when pressure bags are used as part of the infusion system.

Nitroglycerin Administration Sets

Continuous IV nitroglycerin infusions are becoming more common in critical care nursing. Nitroglycerin tubing is available in both specific infusion pump sets and gravity administration sets, although because of the critical nature of the drug, nitroglycerin should never be infused by gravity.

Nitroglycerin is somewhat of a challenge in that this drug is considered incompatible with standard PVC tubing. Studies have shown that nitroglycerin adheres to the plastic in the tubing and the plastic solution bag.[6, 7] The percentage of drug lost to bag adherence depends on the exact nature of the plastic, which varies from one manufacturer to another, the length and type of the tubing, and the length of exposure of the nitroglycerin to the plastic. Some investigators have speculated that after prolonged contact, the plastic becomes saturated, stabilizing the amount of nitroglycerin delivered.

This phenomenon of nitroglycerin adhering to PVC tubing prevents the prescribing physician and the nurse administering the infusion from knowing exactly what percentage of nitroglycerin is being delivered. In the clinical setting, the drug is titrated, so the concentration delivered depends on the patient's symptoms, making the actual known concentration given less critical. Not knowing the actual concentration could be problematic if certain interventions are initiated based on the assumption that a predetermined limit of drug infusion has been reached. The saturation point must be reached with each tubing change, potentially creating fluctuations in the drug concentrations delivered. Many clinicians

are uncomfortable dealing with such an unknown factor in conjunction with such a critical drug.

Nitroglycerin sets can be made with non-PVC material, or the inner lumen can be coated with polyethylene or similarly compatible material. Both of these alternatives, together with the use of glass containers, offer a system that does not create an adhering surface for nitroglycerin. Minimal drug loss occurs, making the infusing concentration constant. These nitroglycerin-specific sets are more expensive than standard PVC sets. Actually, the use of specialty sets remains controversial and debated.[8] Safe care can be accomplished with or without the use of nitroglycerin-specific administration sets, as long as the potential risks are understood.

Fat Emulsion–Specific Sets

The infusion of fat emulsions has been an issue of discussion in recent years. The essence of the controversy was that the plasticizer DEHP was found to be leached from the plastic container and tubing into the fat emulsion. The final disposition of the DEHP into the human recipient is the focus of the controversy, and of special concern are neonates and children.

Fat emulsions are provided in glass only. Some researchers feel that the length of time the lipids are in contact with the plastic tubing does not constitute a risk. Regardless, fat emulsions require a vented administration set.[1, 9]

Blood Administration Sets

Blood-specific administration sets are designed to accommodate the viscous properties of blood, allow for rapid transfusion if needed, and provide a dual line for the infusion of normal saline before and after the blood product. Blood-specific sets can be gravity or pump specific and should be used only for their stated purpose. The large-bore tubing and flow regulation clamp in these sets are not intended for routine infusion of crystalloids or medications.

Blood sets usually contain a large screen filter for the removal of coarse fibrin and by-products of stored blood. This filter is usually 170 to 220 μm in size. Add-on filters of smaller pore size, including microaggregate and leukocyte-depletion filters, may be added and are discussed later in this chapter.

Some blood sets incorporate an in-line hand pump to push blood along when rapid infusion is needed. The hand pump should be used with caution, as was discussed earlier.

Blood should be given only through blood-specific sets. Most electronic infusion devices offer blood-specific sets and are safely able to infuse blood without damaging blood cells. Infusion pump manufacturers who do not offer these sets should be consulted before blood is infused through one of their devices. Most blood is infused by gravity through sets specially designed for the safe infusion of blood (Fig. 15–5).

Add-On Devices

The health care market offers an unlimited number of devices that can be attached to any primary IV line. Devices

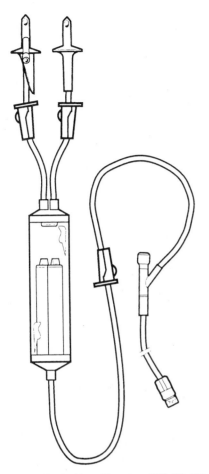

Figure 15–5. Sample blood tubing. (Courtesy of MiniMed Technologies.)

are available for the proximal and the distal connections, as well as for the access ports in between them. The routine use of add-on devices is to be discouraged to reduce the incidence of contamination and of accidental disconnection, as well as to minimize the manipulation of the sterile closed system.[10]

Add-on devices are numerous because they serve many functions. Although their use is to be discouraged, most are added out of necessity and serve a specific purpose. A rule to follow is to constantly justify the use of each item, thus preventing habitual or routine use of add-on devices.

Add-on devices are added to provide length or filtering capability or to increase the overall function of the infusion system. Increased function would be realized with stopcocks, manifolds, multiflow devices, or specialized flow regulators.

Stopcocks

A stopcock is a manually manipulated device used to direct the flow of fluid. The stopcock is generally a three-way or four-way device. For example, one portal on the stopcock is the inlet from the main infusion line, and the second portal directs the fluid to the patient. Turning the stopcock to the third portal allows fluid to flow from a second container to the patient, as well as from the primary container. The fourth portal is an off port, so the first three can be used in any combination of two or three. This device is very useful in

critical care, anesthesia, and trauma settings. The versatility offered by this set accounts for its frequency of use in the marketplace.

The general use of stopcocks is strongly discouraged. Misuse of stopcocks has become a major factor contributing to their unavailability in many health care settings.

The issue of contamination of stopcocks has been addressed in multiple arenas. When the stopcock portals are uncapped, they are vulnerable to touch contamination. The stopcock itself is small and requires handling in such a way that sterility is easily compromised. Frequently, syringes are attached for IV push administration, and the portal is poorly protected after use. Many stopcocks are made without Luer-Lok connections, making accidental disconnection a major issue. If the stopcock is accidentally turned, the infusion may be interrupted or administered incorrectly. The potential for error with stopcocks makes their use worthy of caution.

Extension Sets

Extension sets are used to add length or clamping capability or to restrict flow. To add length, extension sets can be 20, 30, or 60 inches long. Many specially made sets may be any length imaginable. Sets that are made to add clamping capability are usually much shorter, even as short as 2 to 3 inches. Flow restriction from an extension set might be advisable if a standard set is needed for a volume-restricted patient and fluid overload protection cannot be provided by use of an infusion pump. An extension set of microbore tubing would add a measure of safety in this case.

Extension sets should not be added routinely or for convenience unless a clearly defined purpose exists. The potential for contamination exists with any add-on device, especially if excessive length allows tubing to lie on the floor or become entangled. Ensuring that extension sets have Luer-Loks should be a general rule.

Multiflow and Y Connectors

Multiflow adapters and Y connectors allow two or three infusions to be joined into one infusion. These devices are usually designed to connect directly as opposed to requiring a needle. The connecting ends of multiflow adapters and Y connectors should have Luer-Loks. Some are available with color-coded hubs or clamps attached. The versatility of the Y connector or multiflow is enhanced with the addition of pinch or slide clamps on each leg of the device.

The caps provided with many of the multiflow and Y connectors are air vented for easy priming. It is important to remember to prime all infusion legs of the device before their use to prevent small air emboli. Because these caps allow movement of air, they cannot be left in place after the system is primed. The system is not closed and contamination can occur through the cap at this point. If an infusion line is not attached to each leg of the multiflow adaptor, a sterile injection cap must be attached. If the cap provided with the multiflow adaptor or Y connector provides a sterile, air-tight seal, it will need to be removed to accommodate priming and the end should be recapped with a sterile cap. If the multiflow or Y connector does not have capped ends, it is unlikely the device can be used without contamination occurring during set-up.

Catheter Connection Devices

T ports have become a common add-on device. The T port is usually 4 to 6 inches long and is made of standard or microbore tubing with a hard, plastic, T-shaped connector on one end. One side of the T attaches to the IV device, and the other is a resealable latex port. The long leg of the T attaches to standard administration tubing and frequently has a simple slide or pinch clamp attached.

The T connector has gained popularity for several reasons. The clamp allows safe disconnection of the administration tubing without fear of backflow of blood or air emboli. If the IV device is locked off for intermittent use, many patients and practitioners feel more comfortable with the T connector clamped.

If the T connector is to be used on children, care should also be taken to ensure that the slide or pinch clamp is not removable. Some manufacturers make the slide clamp optional and easy to remove. This feature poses a risk to small children, who find the clamps an irresistible item for small fingers and mouths.

J loops and U connectors have the same intended use as T connectors. Both are rigid and hold their shape when attached to the IV site. Their predetermined shape creates a disadvantage at times because the distal end can only be in a specific area, even if the point of connection is in an awkward spot. Their rigid shape is not beneficial in preventing catheter movement with manipulation of the connection (Fig. 15–6).

Latex Injection Caps

Injection ports or caps are small, hard-molded devices with resealable latex rubber caps that are used to cap an IV catheter or female opening on an administration set or an add-on device. This description also implies that it is designed to accommodate needle punctures or, if designed for needleless systems, will reseal after puncture by a specially designed, blunt-tipped spike. Some hard plastic caps solidly occlude an opening and are not included in this discussion, because they serve no purpose except to provide a nonpenetrable cap. All of these devices should be Luer-Loks.

Although these are very small, simple devices, injection ports are worthy of close considerations. One important aspect is their length: injection ports are available in lengths of less than one-half inch to 2 inches. A shorter cap creates less bulk during dressing and less weight during securing, and it allows less dead space during priming, which is an important consideration in neonatal use. Inversely, a short injection port may allow needles to penetrate into the hub of the infusion catheter, potentially puncturing or compromising the catheter or tubing. The use of the needleless design eliminates the need for needles completely in this context.

Coring is a hazard that occurs when large-bore needles or frequent needle punctures remove a plug of rubber from the port, compromising the intact seal provided. Because coring is a risk that is difficult to predict, latex injection caps should be routinely changed in accordance with Intravenous Nurses Society guidelines or institutional protocol. If an extraordinary number of needle penetrations are made daily through an injection port, it is prudent to change the injection port more frequently than scheduled. Again, the hazard of coring

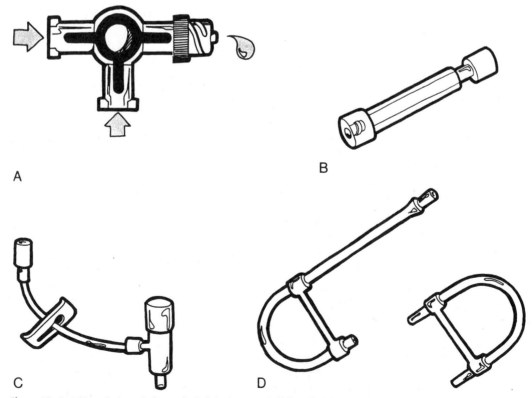

Figure 15–6. Add-on devices. *A.* Stopcock. *B.* Injection cap. *C.* T-Port. *D.* J-Loop. (Courtesy of MiniMed Technologies.)

is greatly diminished and possibly eliminated with the use of a needleless system.

Another hazard of the use of injection ports that is frequently overlooked occurs when blood is withdrawn from the infusion device by use of through-the-cap technique. This means that the injection cap is left in place, and blood is aspirated with a needle or blunt spike through the cap, which is routinely practiced in many places. Adequate flushing after the infusion frequently fails to remove blood cells from under the latex rubber. This blood provides a medium for bacterial invasion into the system. Profuse flushing while the needle or spike is withdrawn is needed to lessen the risk of this occurrence.

INTRAVENOUS FILTERS

Purpose

The Intravenous Nurses Society advocates the use of filters in the *Standards of Practice*, which states that a 0.22-μm filter should be routinely used for the delivery of IV therapy.[7]

Indications for filters include all IV infusions, of both the peripheral and the central route, and intraspinal and intraosseous infusions. Blood filters are advocated for the routine infusion of many blood products. Arterial routes are not filtered, although the introduction of particulates or contaminates in the arterial system has great potential for causing harm. Arterial routes are most often used for monitoring rather than for infusion, and filters negate the clinician's ability to monitor accurately using current technology.

Filters are contraindicated for use with certain medications, which have been shown to be retained on the filter material. Blanket statements cannot be made because filter materials vary greatly. Most adjunct filter tubing is made from PVC, however, and drugs mentioned previously with an incompatibility to the plasticizer in PVC are also contraindicated for use with filters. Filters should also be avoided when administering very small volumes of drugs, because unknown retention by the filter might seriously decrease the volume of medication received by the patient. The Intravenous Nurses Society *Standards of Practice* recommends that filters not be used for doses of less than 5 μg/ml or less than 5 mg over a 24-hour period.

Characteristics

Filters are characterized numerically to differentiate filter pore size. The universal scale of measurement is the micron. Common filters are 5.0, 1.2, 0.45, 0.22 μm retentive filters for use with common IV solutions and medications. Larger filters must be used to filter blood products because they capture large particulates and allow whole human blood cells to pass. Blood filters are discussed separately in this section.

The micron number attached to the filter tells the user that to a degree of certainty, 98% of a given micron size or larger will be retained by the filter. For example, with a 1.2-μm filter, 98% of all the particles in the solution that are greater than 1.2 μm will be retained by the filter.

The function of an infusion filter is multipurpose in today's market, requiring the ability to maintain high flow rates while automatically venting air; retaining bacteria, fungi, particulate matter and endotoxins; tolerating pressures generated by infusion pumps; and acting in a nonbinding fashion to drugs.[11] The particulate matter may include undissolved drug particles, glass, and other debris common in the manufacturing process. The presence of these particles is acceptable in sterile solution to a certain tolerance set by the Food and Drug Administration. These particles do not pose an infectious risk but have been implicated as being at least partially responsible for adverse systemic effects to the body from particle retention in the microvasculature, lungs, spleen, and liver. The byproducts are potential pyrogens, and some clinicians feel that pyrogens present a significant risk to patients.

Another function of the infusion filter is protection from air emboli. The hydrophobic characteristic that allows this effect to occur means that the filter blocks the passage of air and successfully vents this excess air out of the system. All filters currently on the market are air eliminating: air allowed to pass through the infusion line is vented out by the filter. The addition of a surfactant to the filter surface also prevents filters from becoming air locked, which occurs when an air bubble is trapped in a given space in the system, thereby stopping the flow of solution. The air-venting feature is important in both gravity flow situations and in the use of infusion pumps. Modern filters are not position dependent, and the air elimination feature functions well in almost all bedside conditions.

Filters are expected to have high flow capabilities, so in addition to the hydrophobic properties mentioned earlier, the filter also incorporates hydrophilic membranes that are easily wetted and pull the fluid forward, overcoming flow resistance. Most reputable filters can accommodate extremely high flow rates, as much as several liters per hour. The better filters can also continue to allow high flow rates in spite of medications being added or being given via IV push. Filters in past years were problematic during high-flow conditions, but most of these user issues have been satisfactorily addressed.

Pressure tolerance is sometimes a misunderstood feature of the IV filter. Filters used in conjunction with a pressure bag or IV pumps may pose a certain risk if the filter membrane ruptures as a result of excessive pressure. Rupture can also happen if an IV push medication is administered upstream of the filter. If undue pressure causes the filter membrane to rupture, the patient could receive a concentrated infusion of particulate and infectious matter. To prevent this situation from happening, the filter is made with a pounds per square inch (PSI) tolerance in the housing. The housing of the filter is designed to rupture, leaving the filter membrane intact and protecting the downstream flow of solution. When this rupture occurs, the integrity of the infusion system is broken, and solution flows from the filter, necessitating a change in tubing.

Interestingly, most users believe this occurrence of filter breakage to be a malfunctioning filter. This breakage is a patient-protection mechanism that should warn the user to examine activity that precipitated the breakage. If the situation calls for extremely high pressure to be used, such as in trauma cases, then the filter should not be used. If the filter breaks during routine use, the event precipitating the breakage should be carefully examined. Pressure exerted powerfully enough to break the filter could also damage the vasculature or rupture softer internal catheters.

Several philosophies of filter membrane design exist. These designs are the products of much research and medical consumer feedback. The goal of all filters is to give an economical method of providing high-flow sterilizing (0.22-μm) filtration. The *surface area* of a filter refers to the type of filter configuration, and the amount of surface area relates directly to flow capabilities. Filters with increased surface areas are able to achieve higher flow rates.

The depth filter consists of multiple layers of material through which fluid must pass. The pore size is nonuniform; therefore, it captures various-sized particles at different layers. The flow rates provided by the depth filter are usually very good, and particle retention meets all standards. However, these filters do clog when large amounts of particle are retained. A depth filter is not easily discernible from other filters on examination. It usually appears to be a disk with solution passing through from the top or the side to the bottom. Depth filters prime easily and are capable of air elimination.

The membrane filter differs from a depth filter in that the layer of screening material is of uniform pore size. The advantage is more efficient retention of uniform particle size. The disadvantage is that when the particles are retained on one plane, the filter clogs more easily, restricting flow rates. The membrane filter is not visually differentiated from the depth filter in most cases.

The screen filter construction was one of the original concepts and is rarely used. The screen filter has very limited surface area that easily coats with particles, thereby obstructing flow. The screen filter is often problematic to prime, depending on the hydrophilic properties of the screen material.

Hollow fiber filters are designed in the fashion of dialysis filters, to achieve very high flow and very high surface area. The hollow fiber filter housing is cylindrical and is composed of many very fine tubes, each of which is porous and allows the passage of solution through sterilizing membranes. The number of tubes makes high flow rates possible and minimizes clogging over long periods. The hollow fiber filter achieves good air elimination and primes easily.

Configuration

An in-line filter is an infusion filter that is preattached to the primary infusion administration set. The filter is a 0.22-μm filter and is not removable. In-line filters also provide total filtration and give consistency and uniformity of care. Because all solutions cannot be filtered, administration sets that do not contain a filter must also be available, which increases inventory and cost.

Add-on filters can be any micron size, but the 0.22-μm filter is recommended for routine IV infusions. It is critical that the filter be provided in Luer-Lok connections only. The use of the add-on filter allows flexibility in use, product choice, and features desired.

Add-on filters can be added to the proximal or distal end of the administration set, depending on the intended benefit of the filter. If the filter is added to the proximal end of the administration set, it is between the solution container and the tubing spike. The filter at this point ensures sterility and particulate removal from the solution. It also prevents run-dry infusion of air. The filter attached at the distal end of the administration set filters not only the contents of the container but also any contaminants introduced in the system from add-on devices, secondary administrations, or any interruptions to the primary system, including touch contamination. Any air particles would also be safely negated by the filter at the distal position.

Filter sets commonly include an injection port after the filter that is situated between the filter and the patient. This design allows the nurse to give small-volume IV push medications while avoiding the filter.

Blood Filters

The routine use of blood filters is institution specific. The Intravenous Nurses Society *Standards of Practice* states that blood filters are to be used to remove particulate matter during blood administration.[7] The American Association of Blood Banks states that blood must be transfused through a sterile, pyrogen-free transfusion set that has a filter capable of retaining particles that are potentially harmful to the recipient.[12]

Routine IV solution filters and blood filters are not interchangeable. The size of a red blood cell is several hundred times the size of the microorganisms being filtered out of routine IV fluids. Available blood filters are 20, 40, 80, and 170 μm. (IV solution filters are 0.22 μm).

The filter found in-line in some blood administration sets is 170 to 220 μm. A filter of this great pore size removes only coagulated products, micro clots, and debris resulting from collection and storage. The 170-μm filters are a safety net because the particles retained are potentially lethal to the transfused patient. They are visible in the mesh filter after transfusion. Without the large-screen filter, those products are potential emboli to the pulmonary or cerebral circulation.

The 20-, 40-, and 80-μm filters are considered to be microaggregate filters. The 20-μm filter does an excellent job of removing most debris from the transfusion product. Due to the natural presence of a certain amount of debris in all blood products, the 20-μm filter can slow the administration of blood to an undesirable rate. The 40-μm filter allows blood to transfuse easily in the specified period of time, but the filtration is less refined. The 80-μm filter is the filter of choice in many institutions because of its safe level of filtration and high flow rate potential. All three are considered adequate.

Leukocyte-depletion filters are a recent addition to the filter options. These filters are designed to remove leukocytes and leukocyte-mediated viruses, which greatly increases the safety of transfusions to persons with a history of multiple transfusions. They have been shown to improve patient response to blood products in persons requiring frequent, repeated transfusions and to prevent febrile reactions in patients with a history of transfusion reactions. Leukocyte-depletion filters are classified according to efficiency level, not micron size, and remove up to 99.9% of the leukocytes from the red blood cells and platelets.[7]

INTRAVENOUS CATHETERS AND CANNULAS

The original devices used to access the vascular system were hollow feather quills. These were followed by the use of catheters, which are hollow tubes inserted into a body passage. The next generation of products were called cannulas because a cannula has an obturator or something inside the tube that is later removed. Most products routinely used today are actually cannulas. Fortunately, the two terms have become interchangeable. Industry descriptions of the products they provide refer to IV catheters almost exclusively, regardless of the text. For that reason, the term *catheter* here applies to a multitude of access devices.

Peripheral Intravenous Catheters

A peripheral catheter is one that begins and terminates in an extremity (arm, hand, leg, foot, or head). The external jugular access is considered by some to be a peripheral access if the catheter does not extend into the subclavian vein. A peripheral catheter may be any length and includes midline catheters or those that extend 8 to 12 inches from the antecubital insertion site. Intraosseous access is not considered to be a peripheral route.

Catheter Configurations

An incredible evolution of IV access devices has occurred in the past 20 years. A procedure that physicians were once inclined to perform themselves because of its associated risks, IV cannulation is now commonly performed in 80% of all hospitalized patients. The placement of IV catheters is now easier and safer owing to advanced technology and is performed by nurses in all types of health and home care settings.

One of the most basic and time-tested devices is the steel needle with wings. The "butterfly" or scalp vein needle, as it is commonly called, has flexible plastic wings or flaps protruding from either side of the needle hub (Fig. 15–7). Although the needle is steel, the hub is usually plastic and is color-coded for gauge identification. Attached to the hub is a short length of PVC tubing ranging from 3 to 12 inches long. Syringes or IV administration sets attach easily to the connector at the end of the tubing.

The steel needle is biocompatible, and low rates of inflammation or phlebitis have been documented. Because the needle is rigid, blood drawings (aspirations) are usually performed with ease and with little trauma to the vein or blood cells. Users believe that the steel needle is easier to insert than other devices because there are no parts to manipulate. The steel catheter does not flex or yield with resistance and inserts easily with little drag.

The major drawback of the scalp vein needle is the rigid needle that is also its virtue. The steel is unable to move with the patient or soften next to the vein wall. The steel tip easily punctures the vasculature after placement, and the risks increase proportionally to the amount of time the catheter is in place. The steel needle is recommended for use in patients with expected in-dwell times of less than 24 hours. Studies

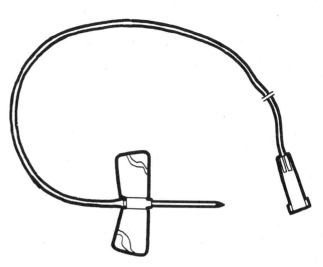

Figure 15–7. Winged steel needle (butterfly or scalp vein). (Courtesy of MiniMed Technologies.)

show excellent phlebitis rates in the use of the steel needle, partly because of its relatively short interval of use.

The most widely used IV device in the Western world today is the over-the-needle catheter. This device is a soft catheter usually made of plastic or plastic-like material with a rigid, color-coded plastic hub. A hollow metal stylet (needle) is preinserted into the catheter; this stylet makes the puncture and guides the catheter as the venipuncture is performed. When the vein is punctured, the flashback appears in a closed chamber behind the catheter hub. The catheter is then threaded off the stylet into the vein, and the stylet is completely removed, leaving the softer, plastic catheter in place (Fig. 15–8). Some of these catheters have preattached PVC tubing that is similar to the scalp vein or butterfly needle, and the stylet is attached to a wire, which enables it to be withdrawn from the tubing completely. This design reduces risk of blood contamination and needle-stick injury.

The through-the-needle catheter with a nonremovable needle for peripheral IV therapy is rarely used today. The steel needle makes the venipuncture, then the softer plastic catheter slides through the needle and into the vein. The sharp needle is pulled back out of the skin, after the vein is cannulated, and is left attached to the apparatus. A protective device covers the needle to prevent catheter shearing or patient trauma.

A new generation of through-the-needle catheters exists that are designed for central and peripheral placement. (The distinction is the proximal tip location of the catheter.) Most of these catheters use a through-the-needle design, but the needles are of steel or plastic that splits or peels away, leaving only a soft catheter exiting the skin. The splittable needle introduced a new generation of access devices.

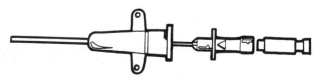

Figure 15–8. Over-the-needle catheter. (Courtesy of MiniMed Technologies.)

Catheter Material

Generically speaking, almost all peripheral IV catheter materials are a variation of plastic. Some of these plastics are simple plastic and have very limited usability. Some are new extrapolations of plastic that come very close to being a new category.

Polytetrafluoroethylene (Teflon) is a plastic-coated catheter material that is less thrombogenic and less inflammatory than simple PVC or polyurethane.[8] Both of these plastics are bioreactive and thrombogenic, but when coated with polytetrafluoroethylene, they become much more compatible to the vasculature.

Vialon is an advancement in IV catheter material; it is a nonhemolytic, hemocompatible polymer that is free of plasticizers. This material is very slick when wetted, and softens after insertion, minimizing vein trauma and clot induction.[13]

Aquavene is an elastomeric hydrogel that undergoes predictable softening and dimension changes after contact with aqueous fluids (blood). The catheter expands at least two gauge sizes after insertion. Manufacturers of this catheter claim it has a lower incidence of complications than those of other common IV catheter materials.

Each year, new and improved materials are introduced, not all of which are discussed here. The most current information comes from trade shows, professional meetings, professional journals, and networking.

Catheter Sizes

The gauge and length of catheters are as varied as their uses. Steel is the material that is most limited. A small steel needle for infusion may be ⅜ inch to 1½ inch long and 27 gauge to 13 gauge.

Plastic catheters have a greater flexibility of length. Typically, the length ranges from ⅝ inch to 2 inches, but can be as long as 12 inches. The catheter sizes range from 27 gauge to 12 gauge, with the most common adult sizes being 22, 20, and 18 gauge.

Catheters that are intended to be threaded 3 to 10 inches are commonly called midarm or midline catheters and may be 16 to 23 gauge to provide the greatest opportunity for use. Some are available in dual-lumen configurations. Peripheral catheters that are designed to terminate in the superior vena cava are discussed appropriately as central catheters. Midline catheters are gaining in popularity, and their insertion technique is much more technical and complex than that of short, peripheral catheters. They are inserted and managed more like long-term peripheral central catheters.

Catheter Design

The thin-walled catheter is constructed of a plastic-type material and is designed with less catheter wall depth. A thin-walled catheter boasts of higher flow rates owing to its larger inner lumen. Thin-walled catheters are supposedly smoother at insertion because there is a more tapered fit to the inner stylet. The thin-walled construction also means the catheter is less able to hold its shape after it is inserted when it is warmed to body temperature. This more flimsy catheter is easy on the vein but collapses with negative pressure, making it more difficult to aspirate blood and less desirable for use as an arterial line catheter.

Thick-walled construction of plastic catheters are the standard design. Users of these catheters claim to be more confident in the insertion process because they feel the vein "give" or "pop" with successful cannulation. A thick-walled catheter may be sturdier in such applications as arterial and jugular puncture. If the arterial line is used to monitor blood pressure, some clinicians feel that the readings have improved accuracy because of the less flexible or noncompliant quality of the thick-walled catheter. Although this finding has not been proved conclusively, it is a popularly held belief.

The stylet inside the plastic catheter must be held stationary during insertion and in a bevel-up position to prevent vein trauma and to receive early flashback. Ideally the nurse must control the stylet assembly, or the catheter must be notched. The notch locks the catheter and stylet in a preset, clinically correct position with the bevel up. This feature is becoming increasingly popular and is a standard feature on many products.

The flashback chamber is a small space at the hub of the stylet. When the stylet punctures the vein during catheter insertion, the increased pressure in the vein is immediately relieved into the catheter stylet with a show of blood in the chamber. The catheters have closed flashback chambers that allow air to escape and blood to fill the chamber.

Some flashback chambers are remarkable feats of engineering and allow blood to travel a micropathway like a maze or an endlessly convoluted path. This capability allows the nurse to see that the blood return is continuing as the catheter is secured. The safest catheters use a flashback chamber that allows the rapid return of blood but prohibits any blood spillage, even with abnormally high flashback pressures. A well-designed flashback chamber minimizes the amount of blood needed to make the flashback apparent.

The addition of wings to the design of IV catheters and scalp vein needles was intended to improve handling and securing. The wings are usually flexible plastic protrusions from the hub of the device and can fit snugly to conform to curves in skin contour. Many nurses feel that a winged catheter allows more flexibility during the securing of the device, without requiring the placement of tape directly over the skin puncture.

Winged catheters also provide more control when the catheter is manipulated. The nurse's fingers never come into contact with the catheter hub during insertion, making the procedure more aseptic. The preference of wings is user dependent. Nonwinged catheters are also very popular, widely used, and accepted. Wings are a feature offered with a variety of products, including catheters with preattached tubing.

Color coding allows for visual recognition of catheter gauge but is not universal or standard in the medical device industry.[14] An inherent danger exists in color coding of IV catheters or any medical product or device because color coding implies that products can be identified without reading the label. For ease of sorting, supplying, or reaching for a product, color codes may be useful. After the product is in hand, the label must be read. Relying on color coding should never substitute for looking at the package label.

X-rays do not penetrate radiopaque materials, making a radiopaque device visible on x-ray. Radiologic visibility issues have been answered with the addition of radiopaque material or striping to most catheters being made today. Although the radiopacity is provided to aid in the identification of a catheter embolus, the incidence of catheter severance is extremely rare. The radiopaque striping is also so small that it may be very difficult to visualize in many cases. Nonetheless, industry has taken steps to provide high-quality peripheral catheters that are radiopaque.

Dual-lumen peripheral IV catheters may also be used and are available in a range of catheter gauges with corresponding lumen sizes. These catheters have a larger total lumen size, necessitating cannulation of a larger vessel to accommodate the dual lumina. Two totally separate infusion channels exist, making it possible to infuse two solutions that are normally not infused together. Because two infusions may be occurring simultaneously, it is also necessary to have as much hemodilution as possible to protect the vessel. Some investigators recommend the antecubital fossa as the site of choice, although this vessel is not the only one that is able to accommodate a dual-lumen catheter.

Simultaneous infusions of known incompatible solutions or medications are controversial because of the proximity of the outlets to each other and the limited hemodilution achievable in any peripheral vessel. A recent study suggests that with the exception of undiluted medications given at bolus injection rates, drug interaction apparently does not occur.[15, 16]

Catheters Designed for Safety

Although the goal of all manufacturers is to design products that perform well and make treatment less problematic for the patient, new emphasis is on safety in the work environment. The care giver also needs protection from harm in the administration of routine and emergent care. Members of the medical industry are providing an array of products that safeguard personnel.

One recently developed product is a self-sheathing stylet that is recessed into a rigid chamber at the hub of the catheter, then safely disposed of at the end of the procedure. Another design puts the stylet at the end of a flexible wire, making accidental needle sticks unlikely. A newly designed scalp vein set allows the steel needle to recess into the hub and wing assembly. Many recent designs are moving away from traditional stylet assemblies in an effort to provide safety. While these products gain in popularity, most nurses continue to select products based on patient comfort and safety, which means that nurses will move to safer IV catheters if the product is equal in quality to the traditional catheters.

Central Venous Catheters

A central venous catheter is commonly called a central line, the line being the device threaded into the central vasculature. The central line has evolved from being an emergent access or long-term access to one that is commonplace in all aspects of health care. Central lines are commonly seen at home, in non–acute care facilities, and the entire range of hospital units.

The medical industry in conjunction with health care professionals and the actual device users (the patients) have worked together to make many central lines safe and functional in many settings and uses. Home health nurses are becoming increasingly adept at delivering therapies via central access at home, greatly enhancing the move from the hospital to outpatient and home settings. Although many central lines are still considered emergent or trauma lines, many more are general or long-term care products.

Even though central lines are becoming commonplace and are easily managed, their insertion and use deserve a great deal of respect.[17] All centrally located catheters should be confirmed for tip location by x-ray, and some long-dwelling catheters should be placed in the operating room only. It is also a significant advantage to the patient if the managing physician has thorough knowledge of the benefits and limitations of the product chosen for insertion.

Percutaneously Inserted Devices

A central line that is inserted by direct skin puncture into the vein is percutaneous, which means that a steel needle (which may be through the needle or over the needle) punctures the skin and is advanced until the vein is entered. The vessel is then cannulated with the central venous catheter. Catheters inserted in this method are usually used for a short time because they are not inserted by the tunneling method and because this method uses the stiffer plastic catheters for easy and accurate insertion outside of the operating room environment. Examples of these catheters are single-, dual-, triple-, and quadruple-lumen subclavian and jugular catheters.

Another percutaneously inserted device is the peripherally inserted central catheter. This is a long-term catheter but does have the advantage of being tunneled. Most of these catheters are designed to stay in place for weeks to months because of their biocompatible composition.

Tunneled Catheters

Tunneling is the method of placement for silicone, cuffed catheters; it allows long dwell times and permits self-care. The placement of silicone catheters is crucial to their usefulness and to patient acceptance. The catheter ideally exits low on the patient's chest so that the patient is able to participate easily in self-care and so that it can be placed discretely under clothing. Types of tunneled catheters include Hickman, Broviac, Raaf, and Groshong catheters, and they may have single or multiple (up to four) lumens.

A very small incision is made at a point near the subclavian vein and is called the entrance site. From this point to a predetermined point lower on the chest where the catheter will exit, a small, pencil-like device called a tunneler is passed. The catheter is drawn through the subcutaneous layer as the tunneler is removed. The tunnel may be 2 to 12 inches long for placement on the chest. If the catheter has a nontraditional entrance and exit site, the tunnel may be even longer. For example, a catheter with a femoral entry site could exit between the breasts.

Placement is determined by the terminal end of the catheter in the central circulation. Catheters able to be trimmed at the terminal end are placed in this manner. Catheters unable to be trimmed owing to uniqueness of design at the terminal end (e.g., valve-tip or staggered lumen ends) must be inserted in reverse. The catheter is placed in the central vessel, and the hub ends (minus the large connectors) are threaded through the skin with the tunneling device from the entrance site to the exit site. Any trimming to make the catheter shorter occurs at the hub end before the Luer connecters are attached (Fig. 15–9).

Catheter Characteristics and Properties

In the evaluation of IV access devices, some qualities are necessary, and others are optional. In determining which catheter is best suited to a particular situation, the nurse should define the problem or need and then select the product that best satisfies that need. Approaching product selection in the reverse manner produces costly mistakes.

Radiopacity

All IV access devices should be radiopaque. For central catheters, the radiopacity helps determine catheter tip placement and location of catheter emboli in the event of catheter shearing or breakage. Although catheter embolism is rare, it does occur, and being able to locate the catheter determines the decision to treat. The degree of radiopacity varies between manufacturers.

Thrombogenicity

Thrombogenicity means the rate of thrombus occurrence related to each catheter material. New catheter materials are researched fully to determine thrombogenicity. All catheters are thrombogenic; the difference is the degree of thrombus occurrence. This degree is based on the time elapsed under normal circumstances until thrombogenic matter accumulates on the catheter and the type of accumulation. Thrombogenicity can be altered by coating the basic catheter material.

Biocompatibility

Biocompatibility, or bio-inertness, is a characteristic that is the goal of most catheter material research. *Bio-inert* means that the tissues of the body do not react to the material

as a foreign substance. Therefore, inflammation and irritation do not occur as a reaction to the material used. Silicone is the most bio-inert material currently used in catheter construction. Because silicone is not without design and performance problems, its uses are limited.

Central Catheter Cuffs

A cuff is a material about 1 cm wide and less than ⅛ cm deep that encircles a catheter. The cuff can be made of various materials, such as nylon or Dacron, although the texture of the cuff before insertion is roughened like Velcro. The cuff, positioned in the subcutaneous tunnel, promotes the growth of a connective tissue seal and enhances catheter stability. The tissue ingrowth reduces the risk of infection by inhibiting bacterial migration along the catheter track. Because the cuff is firmly adhered to the tissue to achieve anchoring, the catheter is designed to pull loose from the cuff when sharp tension is applied. This feature prevents tissue tearing if the catheter is accidentally pulled. After the catheter is removed, the cuff can be left behind or surgically removed using local anesthesia.

Another form of cuff is used to discourage bacterial growth and migration of microorganisms up the catheter to the bloodstream. These cuffs can be used on short- or long-term catheters made of either plastic or silicone. These cuffs, made of silver-impregnated collagen matrix, have been shown to be effective against the organisms most commonly associated with catheter-related infections.[18, 19] Cuffs are no longer used solely for long-term silicone catheters. Silver-impregnated and Dacron cuffs are applied to acute care central lines to increase dwell time.

Chemical Bonding

Chemically bonded catheters are becoming more prevalent, and the types of materials bonded to the catheters are changing rapidly. Initially, the bonding product of choice was heparin. Manufacturers introduced heparin-bonded catheters for two reasons. With heparin bonding, less expensive plastic can be used, making the catheter much more biocompatible at reduced cost. Secondly, the heparin bond reduces the thrombogenicity of the product. The distinct disadvantage

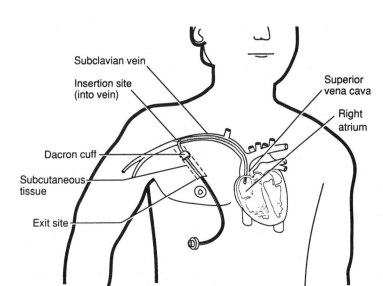

Figure 15–9. Schematic of tunneling technique. (Courtesy of MiniMed Technologies.)

of the heparin-bonded catheter is that it is unsuitable for use in patients who have heparin antibodies, heparin sensitivity, or coagulation disorders of unknown cause.

A newer bonding concept is antiseptic bonding. A recent study with polyurethane catheters bonded with sulfadiazine silver and chlorhexidine showed that these patients demonstrated a two-fold lower likelihood of colonization and a four-fold lower likelihood of catheter-related blood stream infections than patients in a control group with noncoated polyurethane catheters. No evidence of the bonding material was found in the blood stream by use of highly sensitive assays.[20]

Another bonding concept uses surfactant and antibiotics. In a trial study, catheters were coated with penicillins and cephalosporins and had an almost seven-fold reduction in the incidence of infection. No complications or side effects were associated with the antibiotic-bonded catheters.[21]

Safety-Tipped Catheters

A concern about all central catheters is potential damage to the inner lining of the vessel or the myocardium from the chronic rubbing of the central catheter tip. A properly positioned catheter in long-term use should be the suspected cause of this complication. Because of this complication, few central vascular catheters are placed in the right atrium; the superior vena cava is considered the position of choice.

The safety tip on some products anticipates the rubbing caused by the rush of blood with each beat of the heart. The tip is a very soft material, usually silicone, thereby greatly enhancing the safety of the catheters.

Suturability

A standard feature on most central catheters is the presence of a cuff or wing for suturing. The cuff or wing may be stationary, making placement more difficult in some cases. In some catheters, the cuff or wing is attached to the catheter after placement, allowing the physician more flexibility in catheter positioning. If the cuff or wing is not preattached, care must be taken not to damage the catheter during application and suturing. Catheters that do not provide a wing for suturing leave a wide margin for catheter damage and skin stress because the catheter must be sewn directly onto the skin. The presence or absence of the suture wing does not affect the overall performance of the catheter, but it is a feature that affects ease of use and patient comfort.

Clampability

The type of material used to construct the catheter determines whether or not the catheter can be clamped. Silicone is easily damaged and can be clamped only with soft, smooth, "toothless" clamps. Even plastic catheters can be damaged when clamped too aggressively. Catheters with preattached clamps have an extension of the catheter lumen that is made of PVC tubing to allow safe clamping. Several makers of both silicone and polyurethane central lines attach these extensions to ensure product safety and to satisfy the need to clamp. The clamps on the catheters are nonregulating clamps and are suitable for on and off purposes only.

Repairability

Most plastic central vessel catheters are not designed to be repaired. Silicone does not tolerate high pressures and ruptures easily during pressure injections. Because of its elasticity, it can be pressure fitted over a repair coupling to make the catheter whole again. The main criterion for success is to have enough catheter left externally to repair. Usually, tears or ruptures can be trimmed off and a new connecting hub applied. This characteristic of silicone adds to its list of benefits for use in home or extended care settings.

Introducers

The use of an introducer or dilator or the incorporation of a guide wire can be of tremendous benefit in percutaneous central catheter insertion. An introducer is used to cannulate a vessel and to allow nontraumatic cannulation.[22] Introducers are designed to be left in place or removed. Introducers left in place must be specifically designed for use after insertion. The use of an insertion guide wire and introducer is more complex than are traditional through-the-needle or over-the-needle insertions. The risks associated with introducers are greater, although the types of catheters that require introducers and guide wires have advantages that well outweigh the risks.

In some instances, the introducer is deliberately left in place and may incorporate an added infusion port. This feature is most common with the insertion of a Swan-Ganz catheter. In these introducers, the opening that permits insertion of the catheter may have a rubber disk through which the catheter is inserted. This rubber seal holds tight around the catheter, preventing the introduction of air or bacteria. In the absence of the sealing disk, air and bacteria are prevented from entering the port only by the snug fit of the catheter inside the introducer.

An added infusion port appears as a side "pigtail" and exits at the internal tip of the catheter. This side port gives an extra infusion lumen but is not integral to the function of the introducer. The side port does not have a separate lumen but allows flow around the catheter inside the introducer.

The introducer must not be thought of as a central line. The introducer by design is shorter and stiffer than a typical central line, and its intended purpose it not that of an infusion device. When the catheter is removed from the introducer, the introducer should also be removed. The act of removing the catheter may dislodge the introducer, and after the rubber seal has been held in an open position embracing the catheter, it may not seal satisfactorily after the catheter is removed. Its short length and more rigid material may be harmful to the vasculature at the point at which the infusate enters the blood stream. Because not all introducers have the rubber seal, the open port must be capped. Although a cap can be obtained to fit the open end of the introducer in some cases, it is not a universal cap because that port is quite large. Having an injection cap specific to the introducer, yet compatible with other IV catheters, creates additional risk to the patient.

Types of Central Line Devices

IMPLANTED RESERVOIRS

Implanted reservoirs are also commonly called *implanted ports*. These devices are different from the long-term catheters mentioned earlier in that they are totally under the surface of the skin, thereby alleviating the need for daily care. Use of the implanted device requires accessing with a noncoring needle. The use of the term *port* does not imply a specific brand, because many brand names incorporate the word "port." Implanted ports may be single or dual lumen, with a dual port having two totally separate ports and a single catheter with two lumens. The description of implanted catheters here does not specifically include intraosseous accesses, although their use is very similar; however, the intraosseous access port terminates in the bone marrow, whereas those addressed in this section are central vein catheters. Implanted catheters are best suited for long-term intermittent needs. If the implanted port must be used daily for extended periods of time, it may not be the access device of choice.

The implantation procedure is surgical and requires a knowledgeable physician. The incision is made on the chest in a site below the clavicle. At the incision, the subclavian or internal jugular vein is cannulated with the silicone catheter via a splittable introducer. The catheter is trimmed to fit and is attached, or if it is preattached, it is trimmed before it is inserted through the introducer. The reservoir is sutured in place in a small pocket located superficially above the breast tissue. The incision is sutured or suture-taped, leaving no external apparatus.

The implanted ports have a strong, well-made reservoir that is attached to a soft silicone catheter. The catheter is trimmed to fit so as not to extend into the right atrium, and the terminal end may have staggered lumen openings or may be valve tipped.

Ports currently marketed are made of plastic, titanium, steel, silicone rubber and various combinations. The use of steel is becoming less frequent because of its interference in diagnosis (using electromagnetic imaging procedures) and its weight.[23] Titanium has the advantages of metal without the interference problems and is very lightweight. Silicone is rarely used alone but is used in conjunction with hard rubber or plastic. Plastic comes in many types and properties, and when coated with high-quality silicone material, it can be a satisfactory port material. A major difference or preference in port material has not been shown among those on the market.

The reservoir can be many sizes, although most are less than 1 inch in height and are no bigger in diameter than a quarter. Ports must be easily palpable to be accessed and are available in different sizes for children and adults. Smaller ports are called low-profile ports, which are no more than ½-inch high and ½-inch in diameter and have a very low priming volume. If the arm is used for placement, a port designed specifically for that area should be used. The base of the port must have suture holes or must be able to be sutured through the material, such as latex or rubberized plastic. The reservoir itself should be designed to allow thorough and complete flushing without any dead space or corners that will provide a space for build-up of sludge, a blood product residue that impairs use of the catheter. The outlet to the catheter should also be located at the base of the port and should be of lumen size that correlates to the catheter (Fig. 15–10).

The latex rubber septum that accommodates the injection needle deserves note. The septum is critical to the success of the device. The septum is denser and thicker in an implanted

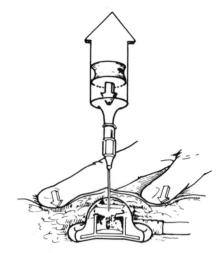

Figure 15–10. Cross section of implanted port. (Courtesy of Bard Access Systems.)

reservoir than in routine injection caps because it not only allows the needle to enter but it is also the only means of stabilizing the needle. The septum must hold the needle tightly upright to prevent damage to the septum, which would render the device unusable, and to prevent tearing or coring of the skin.

The septum is the point of injection and must be palpable. Some implanted ports recess the septum for ease in identification, whereas others have a domed configuration. Experience has not shown remarkable superiority of one design over another. The tissue over the septum commonly becomes calloused or scarred, with a loss of sensitivity resulting from the chronic presence of the device and the needle sticks associated with its use. Experience has shown that ports with softly molded angles cause minimal skin breakdown.

The septum must be protected because it is the key to the device. If traditional needles are used to penetrate the septum, coring and leakage occur after a few punctures, rendering the device useless. Noncoring needles are used exclusively to prevent this complication.

A noncoring needle is one that has the penetration effect of a knife so that when the needle is removed, the septum closes cleanly behind it. The bevel opens on the side of the needle instead of on the end. These needles are very effective and allow the port to be accessed more than 1000 times. Use of smaller-gauge noncoring needles adds to the longevity of the septum (Fig. 15–11).

The silicone catheter attaches to the implanted port at the base. It may be preattached or attached during the insertion

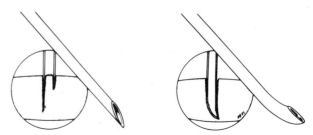

Figure 15–11. Huber tipped needle. (Courtesy of Bard Access Systems.)

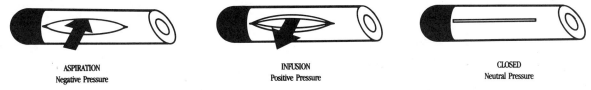

ASPIRATION
Negative Pressure

INFUSION
Positive Pressure

CLOSED
Neutral Pressure

Figure 15–12. Valve-tipped catheter. The three-way Groshong valve opens inward for aspiration, opens outward for infusion, and remains closed when not in use. (Courtesy of Bard Access Systems.)

procedure. The fluid path must make a 90° angle at this point. When the implanted device is evaluated, the outlet of the port into the catheter must be thoroughly examined. Some manufacturers have silicone catheters that are designed to accommodate high flow rates and blood infusions, but the outlet coupling is far smaller than the catheter itself and impairs flow. Implanted catheters with this design frequently have occlusion and low-flow problems.

SILICONE TUNNELED CATHETERS

The most traditional silicone catheter is the tunneled catheter, the most popular of which is the Hickman. Tunneled catheters are between 20 and 30 inches long and have an internal lumen diameter of 22 to 17 gauge. The thickness of the silicone wall varies by manufacturer. A thin silicone wall may be more supple in the vasculature but is prone to rupture and easily pinches off if it is placed near the clavicle and rib cross point. A thicker-walled catheter is less likely to rupture or pinch, but if it is constructed so that the thickness of the wall narrows the lumen, the catheter is sluggish, clots easily, and resists high flow rates. Quality silicone catheters have a tougher, thinner wall that does not impede flow or increase risk of rupture.

Tunneled catheters have a small cuff of slightly abrasive material located on the catheter at a point that would normally be in the subcutaneous tissue. This cuff is usually no more than 1 cm wide and acts to initiate the formation of a scar band, which has a two-fold purpose. The scar band eliminates the need for the catheter to be sutured in place. If sutures are routinely placed during insertion, they are removed 5 to 7 days after insertion. The scar is well developed after 7 to 14 days, and the catheter is usually secure by this time, making accidental dislodgment less likely.

The second vital role of the cuff is to terminate epithelialization of the tunnel. In simplified terms, the bio-inert properties of silicone allow the skin at the exit site to attempt to fully heal, uninterrupted by the presence of the catheter. The epithelium begins to repair, and because it cannot cover the catheter, it follows the catheter up the tunnel. The cuff and scar band stop the epithelialization at that point, making an intact tunnel to the cuff. This well-healed and protected tunnel prevents bacterial migration up the catheter any farther than the cuff, and most bacteria are held harmless, in contact with the epithelialized surface of the tunnel.

Silicone catheters can be dual, single, or triple lumen. Careful consideration of patient need before placement is important because the silicone catheter can stay in place for an indefinite period of time. Additional lumens may be convenient during the initial phase of treatment but are an added care responsibility over a long period. If the life span of the catheter is many months to years, an unused lumen may represent an unnecessary risk to the patient.

The Broviac catheter is a smaller-lumen tunneled catheter. Tunneled catheters made for children are designed with the cuff located with regard to smaller anatomy. Large-lumen catheters are available for children if desired.

When the catheter has multiple lumens, the exterior design of the catheter should be round to best ensure that no leakage occurs when the catheter enters the vein wall. Irregular shapes are difficult for the vasculature to seal around or to use with an introducer, necessitating a cut-down procedure to cannulate the vein.

The inner tip of the silicone catheter has traditionally been a blunt cut, which allows the inserting physician to trim the catheter to the appropriate length before insertion. The Groshong catheter has a closed end with a slit valve located on the side of the catheter near the tip and should not be trimmed at the terminal end.[24] Some versions of the valve tip have two slit valves, one above the other, to ensure catheter function if one valve fails. With infusion, the valve flows open, and with aspiration, the valve opening flows inward. With no pressure exerted in either direction, the valve lies closed, preventing blood flow into the catheter or air flow into the system. The catheter hub can be open to air without adverse affect if the valve is functioning properly. Because blood does not normally flux into the catheter, patency is easily maintained without heparin. A weekly saline flush is recommended (Fig. 15–12).

Many variations exist in the design of silicone catheters. Listing all of them is not possible, and distinguishing one from another is difficult. However, a basic understanding of construction and function is necessary for working with these catheters.

PLASTIC CATHETERS

Plastic is the most widely used material in catheter construction. Many kinds of plastic exist, each with its own indications and associated problems. The cross-mixing of types of plastics makes it difficult to rate them or to make general statements about performance.

PVC is a familiar type of plastic, but it is not the plastic of choice for internal dwelling catheters. PVC is relatively rigid and has been criticized for possible vascular erosion resulting from trauma of the inner vessel from constant rubbing. PVC catheters are radiographic and are easy to insert, but they are not well tolerated by body tissue. PVC can be coated to improve biocompatibility.

Polyurethane is more commonly used in catheter construction because it is less thrombogenic and softens considerably when it is warmed in the blood stream. Increased pliability equates to increased patient safety. Polyurethane is marginally radiopaque, so many manufacturers have embedded radiopaque beads or striping to aid in visualization.

Polyethylene is a polymer that is also used in central catheter construction. This material is available in heparin-coated and non–heparin-coated design. Polyethylene has been implicated in a higher incidence and size of radiologic thrombi than have silicone elastomere catheters.[25]

Elastomeric hydrogel, Aquavene, is used in central catheters. This unique material lengthens, expands, and softens when wetted and warmed after insertion. The material should not be in contact with moisture before it is inserted.

Alternative Access Devices

Swan-Ganz Catheters

The Swan-Ganz catheter is a hemodynamic monitoring catheter that has limited availability (very few manufacturers) and widespread use but limited indications. Its lumens are function specific, and the catheter is primarily used in critical care nursing. The lumens of a Swan-Ganz catheter are for the attachment of data-monitoring devices that determine core temperature, cardiac output, and hemodynamic analysis. The catheter itself is longer than three feet and is used in fully monitored intensive care units and specialty care areas.

Dialysis Catheters

Dialysis catheters can be used not only to administer dialysis but also for routine and intermittent medications in some practice settings. Dialysis catheters are available in both short-term plastic as well as silicone materials for long-term needs. Short-term catheters are used less and less because dialysis is usually not a short-term treatment.

Dialysis catheters have a much larger lumen (usually 13 to 16 gauge) than those of regular central lines and are shorter and less flexible. They have traditionally been more rigid than other lines to allow high blood volumes and rates. These high flow rates are more than infusion volume but an aspiration volume as the blood is circulated out of the body as well as into the body. A catheter that becomes soft enough to collapse with the great flow dynamics would be disastrous to the dialysis process.

The plastic dialysis catheters are problematic in that they are difficult to secure and to dress because of their rigidity. Their large size makes them more painful to the patient during movement. The site bleeds easily, making it difficult to keep the dressing clean and dry. Plastic dialysis catheters do not have a long dwell time.

The newer silicone-type dialysis catheters are softer and more comfortable to the patient. Because they are not as obtrusive as older silicone catheters they are easier to secure and dress, and bleeding at the site is more easily controlled. These catheters may have a cuff to encourage epithelialization of the entrance wound.[26, 27] The connecting hubs are color coded to facilitate the identification of lumens. These silicone products may stay in place for months.

Older dialysis catheters are rarely considered for routine use of infusions and are strictly reserved for dialysis, primarily because of the many problems associated with these rigid plastic catheters. The softer silicone products are more user friendly and have significantly fewer complications. These characteristics increase their versatility, making them much more adaptable to numerous uses, including routine and intermittent infusions.

Shunts

Although many shunts can be put into the human body for a wide variety of reasons, only the artificial venous shunt is discussed here as a vascular access device.

Modern shunts are made of Gor-Tex or silicone material. A shunt bridges two vessels, an artery and a vein. The shunt is usually placed in the forearm between the radial artery and the brachial or cephalic vein. It is accessed with a large-bore dialysis needle and is used for routine hemodialysis.

Newer shunts are able to withstand many needle sticks and are used routinely in some places for IV infusion purposes other than dialysis. Only knowledgeable persons should access a shunt. If it is inadvertently damaged, surgical replacement is necessary.

Arterial Catheters

Catheters that are introduced into the arterial circulation can be used for two purposes: monitoring or organ-specific infusions. When the purpose is monitoring, the arterial catheter provides an access for blood sampling (including blood gases) and blood pressure monitoring, usually at the radial artery located at the wrist.

The catheter must be able to sustain its shape and be long enough to cannulate the artery, which is normally deeper than a peripheral vein. Some of the newer catheter materials are designed to be softer and more pliable after insertion, making them less desirable for arterial cannulation. When properly placed, the arterial catheter may have to bend as it descends to the artery. If the catheter kinks at the bend or collapses on itself with negative pressure, it does not function well as an arterial catheter. As was mentioned earlier, thick-walled catheters are preferred by many anesthesiologists for use as arterial catheters because of their sturdy design. Most peripheral catheters can be used as arterial catheters, and some have superior performance for monitoring as well as for blood sampling for arterial blood gases and general testing. Arterial catheters are routinely used to monitor blood pressure when they are attached to the appropriate nondistensible tubing and transducer set-up.

Peripherally placed arterial catheters are not used for solution infusion. Medication at this point, even in benign volumes and concentrations, can cause tissue damage due to close proximity to the capillary bed or terminal point of circulation. Hemodilution is not sufficient to prevent tissue saturation of drug and resulting cellular hypoxia.

Arterial catheters placed for infusion are organ specific, with the most common being the hepatic artery catheter. These therapies are for specialized infusions, such as chemotherapy to a particular diseased organ. Some are attached to an implanted pump or reservoir that is accessible with a special needle. The care and use of these catheters are the responsibility of specially trained clinicians and physicians.

Intraspinal Catheters

Intraspinal means located within the spinal space; technically speaking, this area can include the epidural and the intrathecal spaces. The intraspinal space has been accessed for many years for many forms of medical treatment, injections, diagnostic tests, and infusions. In the past 10 years, developments in anesthesia have made the intraspinal space more accessible, medically functional, and respected.[28]

The catheters used for intraspinal infusion are 22 to 26 gauge and are approximately 10 to 30 inches long. They are made of biocompatible formulas of polyurethane or silicone-like polymers. They can extend several inches into the epidural space, especially if the catheter is intended to be in place long term. Intraspinal catheters can exit directly from the spinal puncture site or can be threaded subcutaneously to a remote site, similarly to a tunneled catheter.

The catheters are threaded through an introducer apparatus once successful spinal puncture has been performed. If the catheter is intended for a one-time infusion, it is lightly secured until the procedure is over. The rigid needle is not left in place for any length of time. If the catheter is to be left in place for extended periods, it is threaded farther into the epidural space and is taped securely.

Another catheter that introduces infusate into the spinal fluid is the Ommaya reservoir (Fig. 15–13). This is a very specific therapy reservoir that attaches to catheters and terminates in the cerebral ventricular space. The solution infused is usually morphine sulfate without preservative and in concentrated form. This drug bathes the neurons of the brain and spine directly to achieve maximum pain control. This is also called intraventricular therapy.

Needles

A needle is a sterile steel or aluminum tube through which fluids flow. It can be as small as a coarse hair or large enough to drink through. When used to infuse, the needle must be inserted into a fluid space, fluid path, or compartment that can accommodate the introduction of solution.

Hypodermic needles are those that are inserted beneath the skin. IV access can be gained with a hypodermic needle. If a needle is used to perform venipuncture, the vein is easily perforated by the needle's rigid and sharp construction. Hypodermic needles easily penetrate leathery skin and tough vein walls. The disadvantage of these needles is that after penetrating the first wall of the vein, they frequently also penetrate the opposite wall.

Venous perforation and infiltration are common with hypodermic needle venipuncture. This method of venipuncture is reserved for blood drawing and one-time IV push medications. If the needle is to remain in the vein more than momentarily, an IV catheter is the device of choice. The scalp

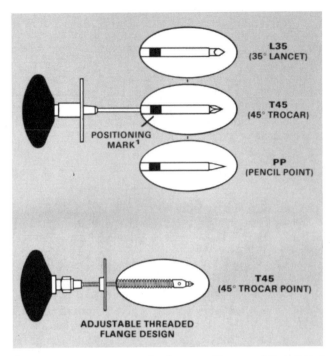

Figure 15–14. Intraosseous needle placement. (Courtesy of Cook Critical Care.)

vein set does not fall into the category of hypodermic needles, although both are made of metal. The scalp vein needle's design greatly increases its dwell time as well as patient safety.

Subcutaneous needles are inserted into the fatty tissue below the skin. This area has minimal pain sensors but good absorption rates, making medications and fluid infused into this compartment effective therapy.

Needles used to access this space can be regular hypodermic needles of less than 1 inch in length. The needle is inserted at a 10 to 20° angle, depending on the patient's fatty tissue depth. Specially designed subcutaneous needles also exist that appear to have a flat disk at the hub for the purpose of leaving the needle in place for a period of time. The needles are ⅜ to ⅞ inch long and are inserted directly into the skin with the disk resting on the skin. These needles are comfortable for the patient and do not easily dislodge. This treatment is called *hypodermoclysis.*

Intraosseous Needles

Intraosseous needles, those inserted into the bone, are categorized with steel needles. The marrow space of the human bone, especially in children, is capable of providing infusion space for almost all IV therapies and carries fluid directly to the vascular system.

An intraosseous needle is "bone chilling" in appearance. The tip end of an intraosseous needle is solidly protected by an obturator, is very sharp, and may have circular screwing threads to aid in bone penetration. The hub end has a large, solid handle that fits into the palm so that pressure can be exerted. The needle recommended for children is an 18 gauge, and 15- to 16-gauge needles are used for adults. The long bones of the leg or iliac crest are usually the point of insertion (Fig. 15–14). Intraosseous administration is thought of as a pediatric procedure, but it can be used in adults. The

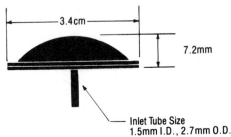

Figure 15–13. Ommaya reservoir. (Courtesy of American V. Mueller.)

complications are bone breakage, infiltration, or bone infection and cellulitis. This technology is special and is reserved for problems that are unable to be resolved by routine means.[29]

The use of an implanted technique in which the bone is cannulated and a reservoir sits on the bone under the skin to allow an intermittent access to the bone has been developed. This method allows administration of chemotherapy directly into the bone in certain patients.

DRESSING MATERIALS

IV dressings run the entire spectrum from simple adhesive bandages to sterile, specialized, semipermeable membranes. Several types of acceptable dressing materials exist, and each has a specific use. Some controversy exists as to whether ointments should be incorporated under dressings, whether dressing changes require gloves, and what the intervals of change should be. These questions are access specific and must be answered in the context of the equipment used, the patient receiving the therapy, the treatment delivered, and the practice setting. Making generalizations about appropriateness of dressing care is not possible.

Gauze

Cotton and cotton blends with synthetics are used to make gauze sponges. Typically, finer-quality sponges have very little lint or are lint-free. Lint-free means that small flecks of cotton do not adhere to the tissue when the gauze is removed. The presence of lint is implicated in problem dressings that stick to soft tissue or granulating areas.

Gauze that has a higher cotton or all-cotton content may be more absorbent than synthetic blended gauze. If the intent of the dressing is to cushion or pad an area, blended gauze can be an excellent choice because the cotton blends also feel very soft to touch. If the function is to absorb, the all-cotton gauze may be superior to the blend.

Appealing aspects of simple gauze are its absorptive quality and clean appearance. The gauze dressing is less costly than other dressings, is easy to apply, and is readily available in almost all health care environments.

The disadvantages of gauze are few but significant. After a gauze dressing is applied, it prevents visualization of the IV site. Once the dressing is lifted to observe the condition of the catheter and the site, a new dressing must be applied. Gauze cannot prevent the migration of bacteria onto the IV site, which occurs when moisture is encountered in normal daily use (including perspiration). It has not been proved that colonization of contaminates occurs at a higher rate with gauze than with other dressings.

Transparent Dressings

Transparent dressings are also called *semipermeable membrane dressings*. They are designed to allow the passage of moisture through the dressing away from the skin surface. The rate of this moisture release varies greatly among products. Even with the best of the semipermeable membranes, the adherence of the dressing is severely tested by wound drainage and perspiration.

Semipermeable dressings are considered to be occlusive. Moisture, and therefore microorganisms, cannot permeate the dressing, a characteristic that makes it an effective shield against contamination. They are able to achieve satisfactory adherence most of the time, minimizing the tape necessary to secure the dressing and the IV device.

Transparent dressings are provided in individually wrapped sterile packaging. Each brand has specific methods of application. This array of application techniques has kept users from accepting these dressings as standardized and contributes to waste and misuse because each dressing technique must be learned. With all transparent dressing brands, the nurse must be vigilant against contamination when handling because the dressing will remain in place for a period of time. There is sufficient time for colonization to occur if the dressing technique is difficult, poorly designed, or contributes to easy contamination.

Antimicrobial Barrier Materials

An innovative dressing is the antimicrobial patch applied under a dressing or used by itself. This patch releases chlorhexidine gluconate incrementally over several days. Chlorhexidine has been proved to reduce gram-positive and gram-negative colonization significantly.[30, 31] The patches are smaller than a regular dressing and have a precut radial slit to allow the catheter to exit at the center. The patches are absorptive, nontoxic, and nonirritating.

The indications for routine use of these patches are institution specific, but they are especially useful in patients with high infection risk. Children with short-gut syndrome, immunosuppressed patients, or patients with recurring line failures may benefit from the use of these patches on any invasive line, such as chest tubes, orthopedic pins, or drains.

INTRAVENOUS INFUSION DEVICES

So many options are available for the infusion of IV fluids other than by gravity that even a clinician with a great deal of IV experience and daily association with infusion pumps would have to make a focused effort to keep abreast of all of them. To simplify the process, infusion devices are discussed in categories of similarities. Specific pumps are not addressed or evaluated in this discussion, and merits or drawbacks about these devices are discussed generally rather than specifically.

The proliferation of infusion devices is directly related to massive cost-cutting efforts after many profitable years in the health care industry. The devices continue to pour forth from research and development labs, but the focus now is cost restraint, economical delivery of care, and administration of safe infusion therapy in many nontraditional settings as delivered by nontraditional care givers.

An infusion device is one that controls the rate or monitors the flow of solution or medication. Some of these devices are very basic, whereas others are very sophisticated pieces of technology. Two kinds of infusion devices exist, mechanical and electronic. Mechanical devices have no outside power

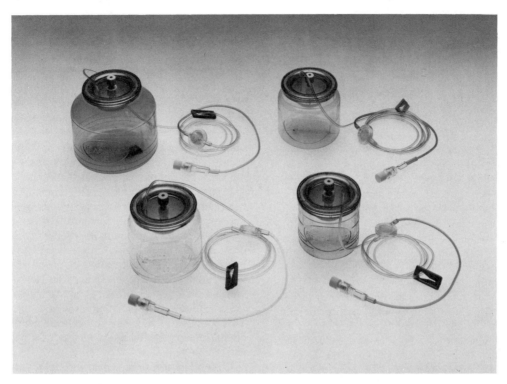

Figure 15–15. Elastomere balloon construction. (Courtesy of McGraw, Inc.)

Mechanical Infusion Devices

Mechanical devices are simple and compact, although not necessarily cost effective. Two types of mechanical devices exist, the balloon and the simple spring. Although neither of these two mechanisms are new, they are new to infusion technology in their current form, and both are very interesting devices.

Elastomere Balloons

Elastomere balloons are made of a soft, rubberized material capable of being inflated to a predetermined volume, with a solution of relatively small volume and a very specific infusion time limit. The balloon is safely encapsulated inside a rigid, transparent container. The container shape is manufacturer specific, some are disk shaped, round, or cylindrical. There is a tamper-proof port for injecting the medication into the balloon, which prevents accidental opening and contamination. There is an outlet port with preattached tubing or a hub to which tubing that is kink resistant can be attached. The tubing must be Luer-Lok with minimal priming volume.

These balloon devices are used primarily for the delivery of antibiotics. Other therapies can be delivered, but intermittent, small-volume parenteral therapies are ideal. Volume-replacement therapy requires larger volumes of solutions. The typical volume for these devices is 50 to 100 ml, but elastomere balloons are available in sizes up to 250 ml. Elastomere balloon devices are not reusable.

The balloons are capable of delivering their preset volume in intervals ranging from 30 minutes to several days. The rate of infusion is not dependent on any characteristic of the balloon. The role of the balloon is to exert constant pressure. The balloon deflates at a rate determined by the diameter of the restricting outlet located in the preattached tubing or in the neck of the container, where the tubing exits from the balloon. The restricting outlet is a very simple and ingenious method of ensuring safe rate control. The outlet is much like a glass capillary with a microscopic tunnel. The size of the tunnel controls the passage of solution. There are no parts to malfunction and no dials to set in error (Fig. 15–15).

The elastomere balloons have been tested extensively for drug compatibility and stability. Not only are most drugs compatible, but many can be premixed and frozen or refrigerated for long periods of time, thawed, and infused with safety.

The PCA elastomere balloon is constructed like the others and functions in the same manner, but the controlling mechanism is unique. A restricting orifice exists in the neck of the rigid container. The patient control option occurs in a push-button regulator on the tubing leading to the patient. The push button holds a dose of prescribed analgesia, which the patient administers to himself or herself when the need arises. The restricting orifice refills the tiny reservoir under the push button at a rate safe enough to prevent an overdose of analgesia. The dose is determined by the dilution of analgesia.

Factors to consider in the evaluation of elastomere balloon devices are few but significant. The devices are so simple that not many aspects create controversy; their simplicity is their best attribute.

One issue of concern is placement of the restricting capillary orifice. When the restricting orifice is placed in the neck of the rigid container, it is relatively safe from interference or breakage. The very fine tube in the center of the orifice may become occluded by particulate matter in the infusate. When this situation occurs, no corrective action can be taken, and the device must be discarded. The restricting orifice at this point also makes priming the tubing very slow.

The restricting orifice placed at the patient connection point makes this glass-like orifice more vulnerable to breakage. The manufacturer does not have a history of problems related to this feature, because the restricting orifice is very small and is well encased in the hard plastic connection device. The tubing is much quicker to prime because no restriction exists between the orifice and the elastomere balloon. There is also a 0.22-μm in-line filter in the kink-resistant tubing. Particulate matter is retained at this point, keeping the orifice free from occlusion.

Cost is also noteworthy. The elastomere balloon is considered to be an ambulatory home infusion device because most hospitals find it more economical to use traditional methods of small-volume infusions, given the large number of small-volume parenteral therapies administered. Ambulatory care settings must demonstrate a defined need to obtain reimbursement for these devices from some providers, especially government payers. Reimbursement is an issue that can be addressed only by each health care provider.

Spring-Coil Piston Syringes

The volume of the spring coil piston syringe ranges from 30 to 60 ml and has a spring with which to power the plunger of the syringe in the absence of manual pressure. The device is incapable of being sensitive to change or interference, such as increased resistance from infiltration. Like the balloon device mentioned earlier, the spring coil piston syringe has limited applications, and the device can be used only once.

The syringe piston is equipped with a spring and is filled by withdrawing the piston and overextending the spring. As the spring attempts to regain its shape, it forces the piston back down, expelling the contents. The orifice at the outlet of the syringe has a restricting tube that allows the syringe to empty at a preset rate. The spring syringes are more bulky than the elastomere balloons, and care must be taken not to interfere with the piston as it collapses. Volume is restricted to the size of the syringe, so many medications are unable to be administered with this system.

The syringe has no incompatibilities associated with its use, which makes it ideal for the infusion of problematic drugs. Its volumes are easy to read, and the technology is familiar to all members of the health care team. Syringes can be prefilled and frozen with success.

Spring Coil Container

The spring coil container is a combination of the spring coil and a collapsible, flattened disk. Unlike the spring syringe devices, the spring coil container may be a multiuse, small-volume administration device. The overextended spring is in an enclosed space between two disks and seeks to collapse, pulling the top and bottom together and forcing the contents out of the restricting orifice. This shape can accommodate many therapies and volumes. Its round, flat shape makes it easy to carry in a sweater pocket while it is discreetly infusing.

Electronic Infusion Devices

Controllers

A significant portion of IV infusion pumps are not actually pumps at all. IV pumps are devices that push with pressure until certain parameters are reached. Reference to *pumps* indicates positive-pressure devices, and the term *controllers* indicates infusion-assist devices that do not create pressure.

Controllers do not exert positive pressure greater than the head height of the infusion bag, which is usually 2 pounds per square inch (psi). Some controllers can reach a psi of 5, but this pressure is uncommon. The function of the controller then, because no infusion pressure exists, is to monitor the infusion for constant operation, to sound an alarm if flow is interrupted, and to provide even, consistent flow. Controllers are safe because a controller is not capable of contributing to large infiltrations or creating vascular trauma from pressure. This purpose is adequate for general populations with uncomplicated problems and is very safe for neonatal, pediatric, and oncology patients.

Controllers use drop-sensor technology. In some devices, a drop sensor attaches to the drip chamber of the administration set and counts drops as they fall in the drip chamber. Accuracy relies heavily on uniform drop size. The absence of the drops tells the pump no flow is occurring. The pump then sounds an alarm to alert the nurse. Many other features exist on a controller, and these are discussed in conjunction with positive-pressure pumps.

Positive-Pressure Infusion Pumps

A pump pushes with pressure to infuse. This pressure overcomes vascular resistance; tubing compromises, such as excessive length; and normal elements of physics that cause an IV to function improperly, such as low head height of the infusion container, tape applied too tightly, and very slow or very fast infusion rates. The term used to describe the measurement of pressure exerted by an infusion instrument is psi. Ten psi is the average for pumps, although newer pumps are set at psi rates as low as five. Older pumps still in use may pump at dangerous pressures of 16 to 22 psi. Pressures greater than 10 to 12 psi should be used with extreme caution. Unusual applications for high psi exist and are discussed later.

Pumps are important for high volume, high-acuity situations, which include complex therapies. Nurses enjoy the fact that few nuisance alarms occur with positive-pressure devices because it takes more infusion resistance for the alarm to sound. The pump delivers accurately as programmed and has many features to safeguard the patient. Positive-pressure pumps account for most of the infusion devices used at home as well as in the hospital.

Mechanisms of Delivery

Volumetric

Volumetric means that the pump calculates the volume delivered by measuring the volume displaced in a reservoir that is part of the disposable administration set. The pump calculates that every fill and empty cycle of the reservoir delivers a given amount of solution.

The reservoir is manipulated internally by a specific action of the pump. This action may be similar to that of a syringe: the piston withdraws to fill and pushes in to pump ("piston device"). Another action is linear peristaltic: fingers in the pump move in a wavelike manner, pushing the fluid out of the chamber. The most accurate mechanism is a series of microreservoirs that fill and empty in sequence and are measurable in hundredths of a milliliter.

The key to accuracy for volumetric devices is that the reservoir may fill and deliver a volume of several milliliters down to parts of a milliliter. If the delivery increment is very small, the degree of accuracy increases, which means that the fill volume may be five ml of a particular pump reservoir, but the pump delivers in microscopic parts. The pump counts what is delivered to the nearest milliliter of the amount that is emptied out of the reservoir. In the case of micropumps (pediatric), the pump counts the amount emptied out of the reservoir to the nearest tenth of a milliliter.

Volumetric pumps and controllers represent some of the finest equipment available in health care today. Although some pump manufacturers feel that they have progressed beyond volumetric pumps, the functional basis of the pumps is unchanged, and for the most part, it is acceptable.

Drop Sensors

The drop sensors mentioned earlier are also applicable in the discussion of drop counters. In a controller, the purpose of the drop sensor is to confirm the presence or absence of flow. In some drop sensors, the device is specially designed to count the number of drops falling and thus calculate the volume flowing. The drop sensor can be located internally on the controller as the flow passes through a chamber, or, more often, it can be attached to the drip chamber of the administration set.

A problem associated with drop sensors is the change in the microvolume of each drop with solution changes. The variance of drop size equates to flow rate errors. The drop chamber also has to remain completely still to ensure that the counter senses or detects each drop as it falls. This feature can be a problem if the counter detects splashes or fails to catch multiple drops in sudden rate changes.

Syringe Pumps

Piston-driven infusion pumps use the common syringe. Syringe pumps arrived early in the infusion market, but because of limitations in volume, their use has always been therapy specific. Most syringe pumps are used for the administration of antibiotics and small-volume parenteral therapy. The use of syringe pump technology for PCA infusions, together with some significant enhancements, has kept syringe pumps in the forefront of infusion therapy. Numerous syringe pumps are also specific to anesthesia, oncology, and obstetric applications.

Syringe pump volume is limited to the size of syringe used in the device, usually a 60-ml syringe, but it can be as small as 5 ml. The rate is controlled by the drive speed of the piston attached to the syringe plunger. Although wide ranges

in infusion rates exist, some syringe pumps infuse over an hour or less, while others are capable of continuous infusion.

Syringe pumps eliminate the concern of drop size or fluid viscosity. They are also unable to detect no-flow situations, unless significant back pressure is exerted. They are not equipped with air sensors or various other safety and convenience alarms. The tubing usually consists of a single, uninterrupted length of kink-resistant tubing with a notable lack of Y injection ports. Syringe pump tubing can be the primary set or the secondary set, depending on the intended use.

INFUSION PUMPS

Characteristics

The alarms on infusion devices should never be assumed to be part of the basic device, nor should it be assumed that every device is equally endowed with the necessary alarms to make all devices safe. For example, all pumps do not have free-flow alarms but are considered safe by current government regulatory standards. A free-flow alarm or prevention device is considered to be a necessary feature not only by nurses but also by those in risk management. However, an abundance of alarms does not ensure a high-performance pump. Each health care environment must establish the alarms necessary for use, as well as which alarms are "busy" alarms that do not add to the performance of the device or the care delivered. The nurse should always remember that alarms are for the protection of the patient not the care giver.

The features noted in the general discussion of infusion pumps refer to the largest application of the pumps, the hospital bedside. Pumps used in the home may not have the same features as those used in the hospital but are absolutely safe and applicable to the alternative health care setting. For example, the following air-in-line discussion refers to air-in-line alarms that are crucial to patient safety when IV solutions are pumped. Several fine home ambulatory devices are positive-pressure pumps and do not incorporate air-in-line alarms, because the solutions and containers are vacuum filled and closed, thereby eliminating the risk of air. Each individual infusion therapy and the setting must dictate what is necessary and safe. General rules regarding safety assume majority application but are not absolute.

Alarms

AIR-IN-LINE

The air-in-line alarm is a basic, necessary alarm. The air-detector device is located on the pump where the administration set exits the device. The detector can be designed to detect only visible bubbles or microscopic bubbles, commonly called champagne bubbles.

Volumetric pumps are the likeliest to be equipped with air-in-line detectors. Some pumps, such as rotary peristaltic or syringe pumps, are rarely equipped with air-in-line detectors, because of the types of infusions and solution containers used. The piston delivers a finite amount in a closed system, and the rotary pump stops functioning when flow is interrupted, making it unlikely the pump could infuse with only air in the line.

The importance of the air-in-line alarm is not to create anxiety over small particles of air in the line, but to alert the nurse that the integrity of the system may be compromised. Air may be entering the infusion line or may not have been properly removed before the infusion commenced. Microscopic bubbles are more frustrating than visible ones because their origin is harder to determine. The presence of microbubbles can also alert the nurse to such problems as gas released by solutions or incompatibilities. Conversely, microbubbles may be meaningless, having come from vigorous movement of the tubing or solution.

Interestingly, air-in-line alarms exist for the patient's protection, but it has long been established that many of the air bubbles detected and tediously removed are far too small to have a harmful effect. Because of this, some pumps allow the nurse to simply push the air through by advancing the bubble with a microbolus. The pump supposedly quantifies the air bubble and does not advance a bubble that is greater than a certain volume. Another pump uses a waste collection bag for air purged through the pumping mechanism and vents this air into the bag. This self-purging process is automatic.

Air-in-line alarms are a necessity for all positive-pressure pumps and infusion controllers. Although the alarm is sometimes annoying, it serves as a legitimate safety factor in infusion therapy.

OCCLUSION

Occlusion alarms have become standard alarms for infusion pumps and controllers. Controllers may only be able to indicate "no flow." Because no forward pressure is being exerted, resistance cannot be detected in most controllers. Controllers are able to indicate upstream (between the pump and the container) or downstream (between the patient and the pump) occlusion by absence of flow. Some infusion devices have the capability to be either a positive-pressure pump or a controller with a simple programming gesture, making alarm capabilities not as pump specific as they once were.

Infusion pumps, because of their positive-pressure design, are able to detect when solution flow is interrupted above the device and when resistance to flow occurs below the device. Many newer pumps are able to differentiate the message in the alarm and to state "upstream" or "downstream."

An upstream alarm is triggered when the fill stroke is unable to be completed because of even the smallest of vacuums created in the upstream line or fill reservoir. The resistance to fill might be from a completely collapsed and empty plastic solution container or from clamped tubing. The newer pumps detect this problem very early in the fill cycle.

Downstream alarms are older technology but are more refined today. A downstream alarm occurs when the pressure required by the pump to push the solution forward exceeds a certain psi limit. The psi on some model pumps is preset by the manufacturer and is usually only adjustable by biomedical engineering departments. Even then, the range is very limited. On most newer versions of infusion devices, the pressure can be adjusted, even by the nurse at the bedside. The psi can be set to a maximum to infuse in problematic situations, such as positional central lines or long-line catheters, although the maximum is rarely greater than 10 psi.

The pressure can be set as low as 2 to 5 psi for infusion of vesicants or routine fluids through healthy veins. Occlusion alarms with low psi settings are common because the pumps are sensitive to even slight changes in pressure. Nurses often term these low-pressure occlusion alarms *nuisance alarms* because changes as simple as the patient turning from one side to the other can create pressure. For this reason, the average variable-pressure setting is not as low as it could be.

Another variation of the occlusion pressure alarm is the ability of the pumps to register a central venous pressure or to detect infiltration or venous occlusion before it is clinically detectable. These features are discussed more fully in the section on pump enhancements.

INFUSION COMPLETE

An "infusion complete" alarm means that a preset volume limit has been reached. Infusion complete alarms are available only on pumps that allow the user to program a volume to be infused. The infusion pump calculates the volume delivered, and when the volume to be infused is reached, the pump sounds an alarm.

Infusion complete alarms are very helpful in preventing run-drys because the alarm can be set to sound before the solution container is completely infused. This feature is responsible for replacing many drop sensors in the industry because the infusion complete alarm is used to call attention to empty infusion containers.

LOW BATTERY OR LOW POWER

"Low-battery" alarms give the user ample warning of the pump's impending inability to function. A low battery alarm means that the batteries need to be replaced immediately or an external power source needs to be connected. Many battery-operated pumps can be recharged while they are being run on regular household current. Others, less ideally, must be recharged while the pump is not being used. Still others have no capacity for external power and require only a battery replacement.

A low power alarm usually indicates a slightly different power problem. The low-power alarm is meant to indicate that the power received from an alternating current is not adequate to support the pump or is causing the pump to pull from battery power even though it is connected to an external power source. This alarm is designed to alert the user that insufficient power is endangering the accurate flow or proper operation of the device. This situation could occur in a home during an interrupted power supply (e.g., brown-out in peak usage times or poor power supply in rural areas). This problem can occur in hospitals when all outlets are not fully supplied during peak demands or when emergency generators are inadequate.

As a protective measure, when low-battery and low-power alarms are continued over a preset number of minutes, the pumps are usually designed to convert to a "keep vein open" (KVO) rate. The actual time frame is manufacturer specific and can range from a few minutes to several hours, depending on the pump. The preset KVO can be 0.1 to 5.0 ml and continues until the battery power is exhausted. The pump may simply cease to function or may sound an alarm one last time. When this occurs, the programmed infusion information and volumes counted may also be lost.

In almost every infusion device, the safety of the patient is well protected by adequate alarms. The pumps also hold the programmed information and maintain the set rate until lack of power triggers the KVO rate. The devices are designed not to drift or to slowly fluctuate downward. The programs or settings are usually safely maintained until all the power is exhausted.

NONFUNCTIONAL

The "nonfunctional" alarm may be worded in many ways. It may be a series of scrambled letters or numbers on a display screen, a light that is completely alien to any other known alarm, or a sound unlike any other alarm sound. A nonfunctional alarm means the pump is outside of its operating parameters and that the problem cannot be resolved. Pumps may go into a nonfunctional status spontaneously or because of improper use or programming.

Regardless of the reason, a pump that indicates malfunction or nonfunction or resists corrective action should be disconnected from the patient immediately. The pump should not be used again unless it is thoroughly checked by a biomedical engineering specialist or the manufacturer.

NOT INFUSING

The "not infusing" alarm indicates to the pump programmer that all of the pump infusion parameters have not been set. For a busy care giver, this alarm is frustrating because it usually occurs after the nurse has left the patient's bedside or when the home health nurse is ready to leave the house. The frustration is tempered with gratitude because the not infusing alarm ensures that the programming is complete and the pump is operational.

Most devices require a deliberate act for operation to begin. This feature prevents some tampering or setting changes from happening accidentally. The pump must be programmed or changed and then told to "start." Without the start command, the pump does not begin infusing or making the designated changes. Instead, it sounds the not infusing alarm.

PARAMETERS

"Parameter" alarms are those that tell the user or programmer that not all of the settings have been completed. These alarms are manufacturer specific. They include set rate, set volume to be infused, secondary rate, and secondary volume. These alarms are instrumental in helping the user to program the pump correctly and in safeguarding against misuse.

TUBING

"Tubing" alarms are provided to ensure proper use of the device. They are capable of preventing the wrong tubing from being used or the correct tubing from being loaded into the pump incorrectly. The tubing alarm can also instruct or remind the user to load the tubing into the pump initially.

DOOR

"Door" alarms indicate that the door that secures the tubing is not closed or is closed incorrectly. In most pumps, the door plays an integral part in the correct pumping mechanism. If the door is not in place properly, the pump can deliver in error. In other cases, the door is part of the free-flow protection mechanism, and incorrect placement of the door jeopardizes this feature. Hence, the door alarm is necessary.

FREE FLOW

"Free-flow" alarms, although not on every infusion device, are lifesaving if the administration set is able to be gravity primed. More simply stated, if the tubing has no restrictive valves or reservoirs that require the motion of the pump to propel the solution, it can be gravity primed. This feature is seen by many users to be a significant advantage because it also means that if necessary, the tubing can be removed from the pump and used as a gravity administration set. The danger in this process is that when the set is removed from the pump, it must be clamped and regulated immediately to prevent free flow, which is the unobstructed, wide-open flow of solution to the patient. This situation has created fatal and many near-fatal situations.

To prevent errors, most pumps have a free-flow alarm that detects the rapid infusion of fluid caused when the pumping or controlling mechanism is partially disengaged. The alarm also sounds if a tubing clamping device is circumvented.

Many newer gravity-primed sets are designed with clamps that lock into place when the tubing is removed from the pump, thereby preventing free flow. The tubing is fully usable as gravity tubing when the user disengages the clamps. Disengaging the clamp requires a deliberate act and cannot occur accidentally.

Additional Safety Features

A wide range of safety features exists: many of these features are taken for granted until their presence is compromised. An excellent example is the actual pump housing. The housing should be sealed to prevent solution from entering the internal mechanisms of the pump. Although the housing is not important to most users, persons in biomedical engineering have witnessed the amazing efforts of infusion devices to function while mired in dextrose solutions. The seal of the housing includes the face, where the indicators and control knobs are located. To achieve a more effective seal, more devices use the touch pad technology with liquid crystal display.

The seal cannot be perfect, however. Somewhere on the housing, a vent must be present to allow gasses from within the pump to escape. Although these gasses are very minuscule in volume, gaseous build-up can cause the pump housing to rupture. The gasses are a natural product of battery storage and pump operation, including the heat generated from use. The vent needed is usually not readily visible, is extremely small, and must be free to ventilate the device.

Automatic KVO features are not available on all devices but are considered to be highly desirable. An automatic KVO feature ensures that instead of a device shutting down when an alarm sounds, such as low battery or infusion complete, the pump goes into a KVO rate. The KVO rate is pump specific but usually ranges from 0.1 to 5.0 ml/hour.

Size is considered to be a safety feature in the current climate of health care delivery. In past years, pumps were all basically the same size, and size was not an issue. This is no longer true, because pumps are available in sizes small enough to fit into a shirt pocket or as large as a medium-sized television. In the context of safety, smaller pumps pose less hazard to the care giver and to the patient in terms of transport and ambulation. Size can cause significant problems in terms of excess weight, bulk, and cumbersome management.

Size can be considered inversely as well. When pumps are miniaturized, certain features, such as the back-up battery, the air-in-line alarm, or the free-flow features, may be compromised. Smaller is not always better or safer; in fact, smaller may have a very high price tag in terms of safety features.

A tamper-proof feature requires that a deliberate series of steps be taken to affect the action of the pump. For both hospital and nonhospital settings, tamper-proof devices are often desired. These steps may not be complex; in fact, they may only include the step of starting the pump after the pump is reprogrammed or initiated. Tamper proof may also include such steps as lock-out programs, which requires the nurse to enter a sequence of numbers to access the programming capabilities of the pump.

Tamper-proof pumps sound like a safe idea but must be tailored to fit the situation. A tamper-proof feature could prove hazardous if it is used in conjunction with life-threatening medications because the time required to override the tamper-proof feature could hinder quick action. All pumps should provide some degree of tamper-proof consideration, especially those used for geriatric and pediatric populations.

Another safety feature is the inability to bypass alarms. Most devices feature an alarm silence button, which is usually self-terminating in less than 5 minutes. This means the alarm can be silenced for only 5 minutes or less. This feature prevents the safety features from being overlooked or deliberately ignored. Repeated attempts to foul a safety feature can result in the pump going into a nonfunctional mode, completely refusing to operate.

Electrical safety is a concern with any equipment connected to an alternating current outlet. Ensure that electrical cords are equipped with grounded plugs and require a grounded outlet. Many devices even call attention to their power source if it is in any way inadequate. When any device is used, both care giver and patient must absolutely be protected from electrical hazard.

ACCURACY

The industry standard for accuracy of an electronic IV infusion pump is plus or minus 5%. This standard has been fluctuating wildly with the introduction of therapy-specific pumps and the wide display of alternative care setting devices. Some claims have been made that accuracy is not an issue for the home infusion of small-volume parenteral therapy. This claim has been answered with concern that the absence of medical support in the home should underscore the need for tightened accuracy for home devices.

Most devices do not have problems, and their error rate is well below 5%. New technology in which micromeasures of solution can be dispensed makes accuracy easier to achieve. In a device that delivers each milliliter in 1/100 increments, accuracy is minutely measurable.

PRESSURE CAPABILITIES

Pressure terminology includes the terms *fixed* and *variable*. With fixed infusion pressure, the pump is set internally to infuse up to a certain psi but not more. "Occlusion limit" alarms sound at that point. Some fixed-pressure pumps can be internally altered by the manufacturer or by biomedical engineering departments. Pumps with altered psi ratings set at greater than the original equipment should be marked with signage on the outside to inform all users and should be restricted to certain applications such as hyperbaric units or dialysis.

Variable-pressure pumps allow the user to use judgment about the psi needed to safely deliver therapy. A variable-pressure pump can be adjusted by the nurse with a simple programming designation or through a lock-out sequence that limits access to a few persons. Variable-pressure devices have a conservative upper limit, usually around 10 psi, and a lower limit that makes the pump function more like a controller, with a two psi setting. A psi setting of four to eight is common.

Pressure greater than 12 to 14 psi is rarely necessary; however, in some instances, pressures of up to 22 psi are appropriate. Greater than normal pressures are needed when the infusion pumps are used in conjunction with specialized high-volume, high-pressure treatments, such as hemodialysis, cardiothoracic surgeries, and arterial occlusion procedures. In each of these cases, which require close medical supervision and specialized nursing personnel, pressures are used for purposes other than simple infusion of fluid. These procedures all accomplish another objective but use infusion technology to aid in the accomplishment.

Another arena for very high pressure is the hyperbaric chamber. Pressures required for the chamber must exceed the greatly exaggerated atmospheric pressure of the therapy delivered. The infusion pump is ideally outside the chamber or room because its pumping capabilities function cannot be guaranteed under high pressure. An extension piece allows the pump to reach the patient through a sealed portal. Although the process is extremely interesting, it presents challenges. A psi of greater than 16 and up to 22 is necessary.

The psi rating on infusion pumps is a safety factor for the patient. Nurses commonly increase the psi limit to decrease alarms, thereby allowing pressure to reach a higher limit before detecting an occlusion or infiltration. A very fine line exists between a nuisance alarm and a safety feature.

Standard Programming Capabilities

RATE

Rate is the amount of time over which a specific volume of fluid infuses. For example a 1000-ml volume infusing over 6 hours will be infused at a rate of 2.7 ml/minute or 166 ml/hour. With very rare exceptions, infusion pumps deliver in increments of milliliters per hour. Therapy-specific pumps, such as those used to administer anesthesia, can be programmed in milligrams per hour.

The most common rate parameters for regular infusion pumps are one to 999.0 ml/hour. With regular infusion pumps, the increment of measure is 1 ml. The rate parameters for microinfusion pumps are 0.1 to 99.9 ml/hour, with the increment in tenths of a milliliter. These numbers, as always, are generalities, and some pumps offer a variation or a combination of these settings.

Many newer pumps are capable of setting rates that satisfy both needs. These usually offer parameters of 0.1 ml in tenth of milliliter increments up to 99.9 ml, and then in 1-ml increments up to 999.0 ml. Many users are excited to have this option because it eliminates the need for both a pediatric and an adult pump. The simplification of infusion sets and distribution of pumps are two reasons this combination pump option is widely accepted.

Implementation of a combination pump should be weighed heavily against the possible danger involved. If the pump cannot be programmed to limit the rate in certain situations, potential for error exists. This danger exists in a health care setting that does not have a designated number of pumps with a preset rate limit for use in pediatric applications. Pumps allowed to freely roam between adult and child care eventually may be programmed on a child by a nurse assuming the decimal to be in place when it is not. This nurse may set a rate of 440 instead of 44.0. Although the reverse mistake can be made on an adult, the consequences are rarely as devastating.

Better-quality pumps that offer combination rates do not allow the rate to be set above 99.9 without a deliberate act to enter the adult or regular pump parameters. Some must even be set into one mode or the other, blocking programming until the designation has been made. Another safety feature prevents the volume to be infused from being programmed above 99.9 ml when the rate includes a decimal.

VOLUME TO BE INFUSED

The volume to be infused is usually the amount of solution hanging in the solution container, but it could be an amount less than that if the nurse intends to only infuse a portion of a container. The pump is designed to sound an alarm when the volume to be infused is reached according to the volume measured by the pump.

Like the rate, the volume to be infused on a regular adult pump is usually between 1.0 and 999.0 ml, measured in 1-ml increments. In a microinfusion pump, the volume to be infused can be programmed at 0.1 to 99.9 ml in increments of one-tenth of a milliliter.

As was stated earlier, with combination pumps that can be regular or microinfusion devices, the potential for error is present unless the pump has built-in safeguards. These safeguards include a deliberate action to limit the threshold to 99.9 ml.

VOLUME INFUSED

The volume infused is a common measurement that the infusion pump provides rather than being a programmable capability. This measurement is the amount the pump has supposedly delivered since the pump was last set to zero.

The volume infused measurement can be used to tell how much of a given solution has infused if the number was returned to zero when the new solution was hung. The nurse can use the volume infused total to show how much solution has infused during a shift by returning the counter to zero at the beginning of each shift. This counter can be extremely valuable to a home health nurse who can monitor the infusion only periodically during the day or over several days. The volume infused measurement is a standard feature on most devices.

Optional Programming Capabilities

TAPERING OR RAMPING

Tapering or *ramping* are terms used to describe the progressive increase or decrease of the infusion rate. Some solutions, specifically those with high dextrose concentrations, such as total parenteral nutrition, are tapered when they are cycled, discontinued, or initiated. Once the pump is programmed to the patient's needs, it begins infusing at a low rate, usually one quarter to one third the final rate. Then, at 1- or 2-hour intervals, the rate increases to half, then to three quarters of the final rate, until the actual full rate is achieved. The hourly increment is individualized, as is the rate increase. Many patients accustomed to the cycle of total parenteral nutrition may taper or ramp in a one- or two-step process over only an hour or two. Tapering is also used in reverse for a patient coming off of total parenteral nutrition. Again, patients accustomed to the process can taper or ramp down more quickly.

Tapering and ramping are not new ideas, and the fact that pumps will do this automatically is gaining popularity. The pump can use its own program to mathematically calculate the ramping rate once the duration of infusion and total volume to be infused is given. These preprogrammed ramping schedules are satisfactory for most applications. The pumps are also able to accommodate individualized schedules.

TIMED INFUSION

Timed infusion refers to the presence of an internal 24-hour clock within the device. With timed infusion, the device must have a sufficient internal back-up battery to maintain the clock accurately at all times.

Timed infusion is used for ramping and tapering, for automatic piggybacking, and for intermittent dosing. The use of a timed infusion feature can greatly simplify many IV regimens both inside and outside the hospital setting, and this feature is becoming increasingly available. It is an exciting feature on a full-sized device that is connected to a standard power source. A smaller ambulatory pump with this feature must be checked frequently to ensure that the internal power source is not depleting to the point of interfering with the internal clock.

Other Infusion Device Considerations

POTENTIAL MISCELLANEOUS ENHANCEMENTS

Although these enhancements are titled miscellaneous, they make the total infusion device package. If the infusion device has most of the aforementioned characteristics, the enhancements described in this section complete the potential of the device. These enhancements enable the acquisition of an infusion device to be based on intended use.

Preprogrammed Drug Compatibility. With this feature, information is available to the user on the display screen. The pharmacist or nurse preprograms drug compatibilities into the infusion pump. When infusions are initiated, the drug dosing is also programmed into the device along with the prescribed concentration. The pump is then able to alert the user to compatibility problems.

Retrievable Historical Data. This feature is available to the nurse on the display screen; it is available on pain control pumps, chemotherapy pumps, and other common devices. Upon request, the pump displays how much solution has infused in a given period (even over days); gives a record of rate changes; and tallies patient requests for pain medications, intermittent doses delivered, and alarm situations sensed by the pump. The value of this information is user specific.

Infiltration or Thrombus Detection. This feature is accomplished by pumps designed to detect very accurately the pressure needed to infuse. The feature is a technical sophistication of variable occlusion pressure capability. The pump displays the infusion pressure on the display screen. If the user monitors the pressure and notes an incremental increase over time, this information may cue the nurse to be aware of the increased likelihood of infiltration or inflammation. An increase in pressure alone is not an indication to remove an IV from the current site; however, combined with careful observation, the pressure-monitoring capability can play a part in early detection of problems.

Central Venous Pressure Monitor. This feature is a side-line enhancement of positive-pressure devices that is able to accurately measure vascular flow resistance. In the same manner that infiltration is detected in the aforementioned description, central venous pressure is measured by infusion pumps attached to central catheters. The internal pump sensor, which monitors for occlusion, does not differentiate between kinked tubing below the pump and vascular resistance. Ideally, the pressure detected by an uncompromised infusion system is the central venous pressure. The value of this enhancement should be carefully weighed to determine if care interventions would be initiated based on the readings of the infusion pump.

Positive-Pressure Fill Stroke. This feature is important in applications in which no tolerance exists for the intermittent loss of positive pressure or intermittent negative pressure. This feature is very important in arterial pumping, neonatal infusion, or infusion of sensitively maintained, titrated medications. The fill stroke occurs when the pump momentum is temporarily interrupted while the pump reservoir refills. If during the refill phase, the pressure in the infusion line is reduced or allowed to "backstroke," even a fraction of a milliliter, blood is drawn into the catheter. If the line is a tiny catheter threaded into an umbilical vessel, the catheter and the infusion are compromised. If the fill stroke stops the consistent forward pressure of medication, blood pressure

may fluctuate, cardiac indicators may vary, and hemodynamic status may be compromised.

Modular Self-Diagnosing Capabilities. These features have made infusion pumps much easier to maintain and repair. The self-diagnosing feature means that in a clinical engineering department, tests can be performed that allow the pump to isolate and communicate mechanical or potential infusion problems. The mechanisms within the device are modular, and repairs can be made to a specific compartment without affecting the remaining parts. Personnel from bioengineering departments are able to quickly repair and return to service pumps that have function problems.

In addition, pumps can be upgraded or enhanced by replacing a specific part that is designed to be integrated into the device for improved function or capability. With technology changing so rapidly, infusion pumps are able to keep pace with changing needs if upgrading involves the addition of a new piece of software for an existing pump.

Printer Read-out. A printer read-out of the activity of the pump is available from several manufacturers. The printer may be centrally located and electrically connected to the infusion device. The printer can be moved from pump to pump, and the information is passed to the printer much like information is down-loaded into a computer. In other pumps, their own printers are individualized, and they print on self-contained paper much like the narrow strips generated by a cash register.

The printer is able to print all of the activity of the pump over a certain time frame. In the case of PCA, this activity might include milligrams and milliliters infused, patient requests, and infusion limits programmed into the pump. Other pumps print out drugs infused, total volumes, alarms experienced, and interruptions in use. The possibilities are many. Printers are somewhat new to the field and are gaining in popularity.

Nurse Call Systems. These systems are being attached to infusion pumps. With these systems, the patient bedside call light can be activated if the pump sounds an alarm. This system can also relay to a central pump diagnostic station. The pump diagnosis screen may be at the nurses' station, where the nurse can problem solve before going to the bedside, often saving a trip and valuable time. The screen at the nurses' station is scored, giving each bedside pump a portion of the screen. The section lighting up corresponds to a specific bedside and a specific device. The screen also indicates the type of alarm sounding.

Remote Site Programming. This programming is accomplished by use of computer technology, which allows communication with the pump by telephone modem. The pump can literally be hundreds of miles from the base unit or can be down the hall. The base unit is at the pharmacy or home health agency. The pump's activities are all able to be monitored from the base unit, making it possible for the care giver to monitor the pump without being present. The pump's infusion settings can be changed by the base unit, so after the remote monitoring occurs, adjustments are made.

These developments may sound like science fiction to some, but they have already proved to be cost effective and efficient in some areas. Trusting in computer technology is the key to accepting this type of technology. The object is not to manipulate care or to monitor the patient without being present. Rather, the goal is to be able to keep a watchful eye on the infusion more frequently and more accurately than nursing time allows. Nursing assessment is not being circumvented but supported.

Syringe Use for Secondary Infusion. This feature is becoming a practical alternative to small-volume piggybacks or tedious IV push medications. The syringe is attached directly to the pump administration set and is vented, allowing the solution to flow from the syringe without requiring pressure to be exerted on the syringe piston.

This option is available with the primary solution in the syringe or with the syringe attached to the primary set, becoming the secondary infusion container. Both options can offer considerable cost savings if this capability eliminates the need for syringe pumps in addition to regular pumps. The largest cost savings are realized by the use of inexpensive syringes in place of more expensive, small-volume plastic bags.

Adjustable Occlusion Pressures. This feature is found on some popular infusion devices. With these pumps, the user can program the pump at the bedside to sound an alarm at high or low occlusion pressures. This feature is probably used as a convenience item by most nurses because its clinical potential is not fully appreciated. Adjusting the pressure upward may silence a persistent occlusion alarm that may need attention.

The real value of the adjustable occlusion pressure is to ensure patient safety during infusion. The oncology nurse may want to use very low occlusion pressures to warn of vesicant extravasations with peripheral chemotherapy. The pediatric nurse may want to use a very low pressure to warn of infiltration while infusing through a scalp vein but may choose a higher occlusion pressure for a central line infusion on an active, inconsolable 2-year-old. Critical care nurses may use high infusion pressure for sensitive medications through a central catheter but may infuse the same drugs at the same rate through peripheral IV lines at a much lower pressure.

Opaque Infusions. These infusions have not always been easily administered. Pumps that rely on certain air-in-line detectors are unable to infuse opaque solutions. Opaque solutions are blood, fat emulsions, and some heavily darkened solutions, such as iron dextran. The air-in-line detectors were bypassed in these cases in the past, which was an unsafe practice.

Newer pumps accommodate opaque solutions easily. The technology of air detection has moved from optic sensors, which are unable to distinguish between solutions of various clarity, to the use of ultrasonography. Ultrasound does not rely upon clarity of solutions, allowing the accurate administration of opaque solutions.

Secondary Rate Settings. These settings are achieved in the same manner as secondary infusions by gravity administration. The secondary container is hung at a higher level than is the primary infusion, so the secondary automatically infuses first. The pump settings are designed to program two consecutive rates. The secondary rate and the secondary volume are intended to run the secondary solution. After the secondary volume is reached, the pump switches back to the primary rate and resumes counting the primary volume. The pump is unable to tell which solution is infusing because it counts volume infused only. The nurse is still responsible to hang the solutions at the correct height to ensure that the pump infuses correctly.

Bar Coding. Bar coding is as useful in infusion management as it is in the grocery store. Amazing new microtechnology has made it possible for the pharmacist to generate the prescription for infusion into a bar code label. An appropriately equipped infusion device reads the bar code with a scanner on the side of the infusion pump, and the pump is programmed. The nurse can check that the parameters in the pump are correct by reviewing the display screen. With this technology, the incidence of human error is significantly reduced.

A pump with this capability allows the nurse to override the system, should unplanned interventions be necessary. This device is more ideal in home infusion practice because it eliminates any accidental program changes or tampering. This pump is a futuristic device, but it is currently being used successfully and represents some of the changes that will soon be commonplace in infusion therapy.

Types

Ambulatory Infusion Pumps

Ambulatory infusion pumps are those devices that are small enough to be easily carried, thereby allowing the patient full ambulation. These devices were developed with the patient's home in mind. Ambulatory devices allow the patient the freedom to return to work, to school, or to a more normal life pattern. Ambulatory devices are capable of delivering most infusion therapy delivered by larger hospital pumps, including the infusion of traditional critical care drugs and blood products.

Ambulatory devices range in size and weight, from small enough to fit into the palm of the hand to large enough to require a backpack. Most of these pumps weigh less than 6 pounds. The solution container is often more cumbersome than the actual pump. Ambulatory pumps have pump-specific tubing made to accommodate only the therapies for which each device is designed. The reduction of programming options is one factor that enables the manufacturer to miniaturize the pump.

Ambulatory pumps have the advantage of being small but have limitations that prevent the small size from being incorporated into the hospital setting. The main inhibiting factor is the power supply. Ambulatory pumps function on a battery system that requires frequent recharging and battery replacement. The lack of a significant major power source built into the pump may limit the in-hospital use of these pumps. Most hospital uses are so rigorous that the ambulatory pump's battery life is too frequently depleted. Ambulatory devices usually infuse at much lower rates or intermittently, requiring significantly less power. Hospitals using battery powered infusion pumps report significant battery replacement costs.

Ambulatory pumps have many features that have improved the quality of life for persons who require infusions outside the hospital. One pump cannot perform all the infusion therapies, but at least one pump exists for every therapy imaginable. Another example is a pump able to be synchronized with the patient's biorhythms, giving medications when needed instead of on a schedule. Another pump is able to deliver several different dose sizes at several different intervals to replicate the secretion of hormones. Several medications may be given sequentially by an internal clock, thereby freeing the patient or care giver from all interventions except reloading of the device. These pumps retain memory of programs, use informational display screens, and have the safety alarms necessary to make their use trouble-free.

Patient-Controlled Analgesia Pumps

The concept of PCA is not new, but the technology to provide this type of pain control is advancing rapidly. PCA pumps are available as ambulatory, semiportable, or full-sized devices. The smallest pumps use microprocessors to achieve miniaturization. The pumps can be programmed in milliliters or milligrams. The programming options are somewhat standardized, although accessory features vary with each pump.

The mechanisms most used are volumetric and syringe-type. The volumetric pumps move the medication through the pump by a fill-and-empty cycle of very small increments. The syringe pump forces down on the syringe piston, collapsing the syringe at a preset rate.

The distinguishing feature of a PCA device is the ability of the pump to deliver doses on demand, which occurs when the patient or family pushes a button on a cord similar to a nurse call light. The pump responds by delivering or denying the dose, recording the request, and perhaps making a small sound to assure the patient that the request was received. Whether or not the dose is delivered is determined by preset parameters in the pump.

Infusion options of a PCA pump can be categorized into three types: basal, continuous, and demand. All three afford some type of pain control with varying degrees of patient interaction. The nurse and physician must understand the terminology of the therapy offered so that PCA pumps can be used to the maximum potential.

The continuous mode of therapy is designed for the patient who needs maximum pain relief without the option of demand dosing. Continuous pain infusions usually do not fluctuate from hour to hour and should completely relieve pain or achieve a constant affect. This mode is used for epidural narcotic infusions, for neonatal infusions, for pain control administration to persons unable to use the demand feature, or for any application requiring a constant rate.

The basal mode differs from the continuous mode in that a basal rate can be accompanied by intermittent doses requested by the patient. The basal dose is designed to achieve pain relief with minimal medication, but not necessarily to achieve a pain-free state, allowing the patient to be alert and active without sedation.

The demand dose is delivered by intermittent infusion when a button attached to the pump is pushed. The demand dose can be used alone or supplemented by the basal rate. Demand doses are limited by a physician-designated maximum amount. The PCA pump must be programmed with parameters to prevent over-medication of the patient. Demand doses are prescribed with the amount per dose, the interval between doses, and the total hourly limit of medication.

PCA pumps are also capable of dispensing a bolus dose. The initial bolus dose is also called a *loading dose* by practitioners. When bolused initially or after a short lapse in medication, the patient may benefit from a one-time dose of medication that is significantly higher than a demand dose to achieve immediate pain relief. After the bolus dose is delivered, the basal or demand doses create the sustained effect of pain control. The bolus dose is not calculated into the hourly limit of medication and cannot be accidentally delivered.

PCA devices may offer a lock-out feature that is designed for patient safety. Lock-out differs from tamper resistance in that tamper-proof pumps require the nurse to repeat a series of simple steps known to any user to change pump settings. Lock-out means that a key or a combination of numbers must be used to gain access to the pump controls. Because PCA pumps normally house a container of narcotic medication, the lock-out capability prevents tampering with the narcotic and the pump settings. In the hospital setting, the PCA device is commonly locked to the IV pole for added security. Narcotic accountability is more defined with the PCA device because the drug is in one reservoir, and all deliveries are automated and recorded on the pump memory.

PCA pumps are built with extensive memory capability, which includes the pump programming, any interventions by the patient or the nurse, and the times of the interventions. The memory is critical for the pump's effective use in pain management. The frequency of patient requests, the tolerated time intervals, and the number of bolus injections are a few of the assessments needed to monitor pain tolerance or change in pain intensity. The programming and memory are able to be viewed on a display screen.

Ambulatory PCA pumps may have the same limitations of use as regular ambulatory devices. They are not built to withstand the rigors of hospital environments unless they are used by a small specialty group. The number of different staff, patient transfers, pump distribution factors, pump accountability, and potential interactions make ambulatory PCA devices more prone to breakdown and malfunction in a hospital environment.

Multichannel and Dual-Channel Pumps

The changing hospital environment dictates infusion pump needs, and rising acuity has resulted in the development of multichannel and dual-channel infusion pumps, which could consist of two devices with an attached housing or several infusion channels within a single device. The best effect is achieved when multiple infusion channels can be regulated independently of each other, in a device that stays within the size and shape configurations of a single pump. Depending on the design, this goal can be achieved with two or more incoming solution lines, each regulated independently and leaving the pump in a single infusing line to the patient. Another design allows each incoming independent line to leave separately and, therefore, multiple lines to infuse to the patient.

Many dual-channel and multichannel pumps are on the market. Some require little adaptation because they appear to be two single-channel devices fused side by side. Others are a two–pump mechanism assembly, with a common control and programming panel. These types of dual-channel pumps use one administration set for each channel, and if one channel is idle, there is no tubing used. Multichannel pumps that require manifold-type sets that set up all channels whether used or not save significant dollars if all the channels are in use. If one or more channels are idle, the sets are no longer cost effective. Each channel must be programmed independently, or the pump is not really dual channel or multichannel.

Intermittent, automatic IV piggyback capability does not fit the description of dual channel unless the IV piggyback is regulated by an internal clock that turns the infusion off and on per a schedule. This feature makes a dual-channel pump invaluable. If the IV piggyback feature is based on head height to deliver a single dose, it does not have dual-channel capability.

Multichannel pumps have three or four channels. Programming a multichannel pump can be complex, and the potential for confusion rises sharply. The need for a three- or four-channel pump should be clearly defined before this complex technology is routinely used. These pumps offer an exciting capacity for infusion, but they are not routinely used in general care.

Cost Considerations in Infusion Pump Technology

The continued theme of defining the patient's need applies to infusion pump technology more than to any other type of IV equipment. If the need is a consistent low acuity patient situation and the pump is a convenience item, a great investment in the latest technology will probably never pay off. On the other hand, older technology with few capabilities may create a significant risk to certain patient populations. The acuity and technology needs are by no means confined to the hospital setting.

Any health care institution must also understand and appreciate the reimbursement capability of the clientele served. Insurance and government payers are involved in decisions regarding appropriate care. If more advanced technology is not reimbursed accordingly, other alternatives should be sought so as to increase fiscal accountability. Responsible care involves assessing and delivering affordable care. Infusion devices too sophisticated for the intended purpose confuse and complicate care unnecessarily. A safe rule of thumb is to use the least difficult equipment and the least amount of supplies necessary to safely and effectively provide the care.

The financial investment in infusion device procurement is significant. This equipment is expensive, and the disposable tubing costs will far outweigh the price of the devices in just a few months. The entire picture should be analyzed, including any changes that will be made when a new system is implemented. These costs should be calculated over the entire length of a contract period because costs are often more significant during the start-up period.

Institutions are able to use one of several finance options when reusable equipment such as infusion pumps are being considered. When equipment is rented, the title to the property stays with the original owner (the agency from which the institution is getting the equipment). In a rental agreement, the upkeep and repair are the responsibility of the owner. There is also more flexibility in obtaining additional

devices or upgrading to newer technology with the same device. The rental agreements usually cover disposable supplies as well.

Leasing of equipment is similar to renting, but in a lease, it is possible to own the devices at the end of the agreement, or to terminate the lease with an intent to buy. In many lease agreements, repair and upkeep are the responsibility of the user institution, and disposable supplies are part of the agreement. Lease options are almost unlimited. In a lease agreement, the receiving institution has temporary ownership.

Purchase options result in transfer of ownership, equipment warrantees, repair contracts, and institutional upkeep. The cost of the disposable supplies is usually less when purchasing the pumps, which sometimes results in the total cost over several years being much less than with rent or lease agreements. The manufacturer has made the profit initially, theoretically making the long-term investment less costly to the buyer. The technology with a purchase agreement is static unless the purchase contract stipulates periodic updating of equipment.

Infusion Pumps in Various Settings

Acute Care

The acute care setting can be a traditional hospital setting or a short-term treatment or surgery center, where the expectations of infusion devices are well defined. The diversity of need is great in the hospital, requiring infusion devices to withstand the rigors of the environment. The number of different users that come in contact with a pump during its use in a hospital include the nurse, the physician, and the persons involved in transporting, cleaning, and storing the device.

Infusion devices in a hospital must be able to satisfy the IV therapy requirements of the patient moving through the system, from the intensive care unit, to surgery, to general care. The device must be user friendly to be used by many nurses and health care professionals without excessive, time-consuming effort being necessary to understand the operation. Constantly changing staff and multiple disciplines should be able to work with the technology easily.

Infusion devices that have specific functions may not be cost effective for hospitals. The cost of tubing, additional accessory items, education, biomedical engineering effort related to parts and service, and many other related costs make lack of equipment standardization expensive. Potential user error is a nonquantifiable cost that could outweigh all other considerations.

Alternative Care

Alternative care settings represent many different types of health care. Active treatment is offered in many settings once reserved for diagnosis or long-term care. Chemotherapy, blood products, and antibiotics are now commonly given in nursing homes, physician's clinics, or outpatient treatment centers. These therapies are given safely when adequate medical support is present, and the equipment selected for use is intended for such a setting.

The infusion devices selected may be therapy specific for safety and convenience. A therapy-specific pump is most likely to have programming features that prompt the user to provide complete information needed to infuse a specific treatment correctly. This information is especially necessary if the treatment being delivered is not administered frequently.

Reimbursement is often a challenge for alternate care settings; some infusion devices have a more reimbursable status than others. Before any equipment is acquired the reimbursement status of the clientele served and the anticipated need should be thoroughly explored so that the profit potential can be maximized.

Home Care

The fastest growing environment for the delivery of health care is the home. The specialized therapies and equipment variations needed to serve patients receiving home health care has generated an evolution in the infusion equipment market, that affects all health care settings.

Instruments used at home must offer the best safety features because the care giver in most situations is the patient. Priming, set-up, and trouble shooting should be easy, uncomplicated, and directed by the pump. Certain parameters of particular treatments may even be locked-out, with the patient unable to do more than start and stop the infusion. Such strategies are popular in pain control or ramping of parenteral nutrition.

Home care infusion devices are designed to allow the patient maximum portability and freedom with minimum interference and inconvenience. Small, quiet, lightweight infusion pumps, with pouches to enclose the infusion container, are available for almost all therapies.

As with alternative care settings, infusion pump use is challenged frequently in home care. Knowledge of the patient's reimbursement status simplifies selection of the appropriate infusion device. If an infusion device is necessary for safe administration of IV medications or solutions in the home, lack of payment should not prevent the use of the equipment. The physician and the payer should collaborate with the health care provider to ensure the safe treatment of the patient in the home.

References

1. Olin BR, ed. Intravenous fat emulsion. In Drug Facts and Comparisons. St. Louis: J. B. Lippincott, 1989:40a–b.
2. Olin BR, ed. Intravenous nitroglycerin. In Drug Facts and Comparisons. St. Louis: J. B. Lippincott, 1991:143a–f.
3. Trissel LA. Handbook on Injectable Drugs, 6th ed. American Society of Hospital Pharmacists, Bethesda, MD, 1988:456.
4. Hancock B, Black C. Effect of a polyethylene-lined administration set on the availability of diazepam injection. Am J Hosp Pharm 1985; 42:335–339.
5. Coles D, Fanning J. Accuracy of Viaflex container graduation marks. NITA 1987; 14:422–424.
6. Little LA, Hatheway GJ. Problems with administration devices for commercially available nitroglycerin injection (letter). Am J Hosp Pharm 1982; 17:400.
7. Nix DE. Intravenous nitroglycerin delivery: Dynamics and cost considerations. Hosp Pharm 1985; 20:230–232.
8. Altavela JL, Haas CE, Nowak DR, et al. Comparison of Polyethylene and Polyvinyl Chloride Sets for the Administration of Intravenous Nitroglycerin to Treat Ischemic Heart Disease (abstract). Presented at the American College of Clinical Pharmacists Annual Meeting, Reno, Nevada, 1993.
9. Badr MZ, Handler JA, Whittaker M, et al. Interactions between plasticizers and fatty acid metabolism in the perfused rat liver and in vivo. Biochem Pharmacol 1990; 39:715–721.
10. Intravenous Nurses Society. Intravenous Nursing Standards of Practice. Belmont, MA: J.B. Lippincott, 1990.
11. Weinstein SM. Plumer's Principles and Practices of Intravenous Therapy, 5th ed. Philadelphia: J. B. Lippincott, 1993.
12. Widmann FK, ed. Standards for Blood Banks and Transfusion Services, 14th ed. Arlington, VA: American Association of Blood Banks, 1991: 39.
13. Deseret Medical. Vialon (product literature). Sandy, UT: Deseret Medical, 1988.
14. Deseret Medical. I.V. Catheter Color Code Conversion Chart (product literature). Sandy, UT: Deseret Medical.
15. Chapolini R. Incompatible Drug Infusion Through the Arrow Two-Lumen Catheter: An In-Vitro Analysis (product literature). Reading, PA: Arrow International, 1987.
16. Collins JL, Lutz RJ. In vitro study of simultaneous infusion of incompatible drugs in multilumen catheters. Heart Lung 1991; 20:271–277.
17. Camp-Sorrell D. Advanced central venous access: Selection, catheters, devices, and nursing management. JIN 1990; 13:361–370.
18. Hickman R. The Etiopathogenesis and Prevention of Catheter-Related Infection in Long Term Central Venous Catheters (product literature). Davol, Cranston, RI, 1988.
19. Maki DG, Cobb L, Garman JK, et al. An attachable silver-impregnated cuff for prevention of infection with central venous catheters: A prospective randomized multicenter trial. Am J Med 1988; 85:307–314.
20. Maki DG, Wheeler SJ, Stolz SM, et al. Clinical Trial of a Novel Antiseptic-Coated Central Venous Catheter (product literature). Reading, PA: Arrow International, 1991.
21. Kamal GD, Pfaller MA, Rempe LE, et al. Reduced intravascular catheter infection by antibiotic bonding. JAMA 1991; 265:2364–2368.
22. Arrow International. The Arrow-Flex Percutaneous Sheath Introducer System with Cath-Gard (product literature). Reading, PA: Arrow International, 1985.
23. Camp-Sorrell D. Magnetic resonance imaging and the implantable port. Oncol Nurs Forum 1990; 17:197–199.
24. C. R. Bard. Groshong Catheters: Minimizing Heparin Use With the Three-Way Groshong Valve (product literature). Cranston, RI: C. R. Bard.
25. Linder LE, Curelaru I, Gustavsson B, et al. Material thrombogenicity in central venous catheterization: A comparison between soft antebrachial catheters of silicone elastomer and polyurethane. JPEN Parenter Enteral Nutr 1984; 8:399–406.
26. Moss AH, McLaughlin MM, Lempert KD, et al. Use of a silicone catheter with a Dacron cuff for dialysis short-term vascular access. Am J Kidney Dis 1988; 12:492–498.
27. Schwab SJ, Buller GL, McCann RL, et al. Prospective evaluation of a Dacron cuffed hemodialysis catheter for prolonged use. Am J Kidney Dis 1988; 11:166–169.
28. Cornwell CM. The Ommaya reservoir: Implications for pediatric oncology. Pediatr Nurs 1990; 16:249–251.
29. Wheeler C. Pediatric intraosseous infusion: An old technique in modern health care technology. JIN 1989; 12:371–376.
30. Maki DG, Ringer M, Alvarado CJ. Prospective randomized trial of povidone-iodine, alcohol, chlorhexidine for prevention of infection associated with central venous and arterial catheters. Lancet 1991; 338:339–343.
31. Shapiro JM, Bond EL, Garman JK. Use of chlorhexidine dressing to reduce microbial colonization of epidural catheters. Anesthesiology 1990; 73:625–631.

CHAPTER 16

Intravenous Therapy Equipment: Preparation, Maintenance, and Problem Solving

Brenda L. Jensen, BSN, CRNI
Dawn G. Frederick, BSN, CRNI

Intravenous (IV) therapy devices and equipment are well represented in the medical marketplace. They can be classified into three types: durable medical goods, reusable products, and disposable products. This chapter deals with product preparation before use, handling of products after use, and care and maintenance required between uses. The aspects of product care vary greatly between the three types.

Durable medical goods are defined as equipment that is used for long periods of time, is cleaned between patient uses, and may be considered to be property or capital equipment. Examples of durable medical equipment are IV poles, infusion pumps, wheelchairs, and walkers.

Reusable products are those that are used for limited periods of time and are cleaned and disinfected between use. A reusable item must be specifically designated as reusable, to prevent extended use not intended by the manufacturer. Few items are able to be reused in IV therapy because IV devices are usually sterile, one-time use products.

Disposable products are those that can be used only once. Their use is limited to one patient and one occurrence before being discarded. Most IV products are disposable, including solution containers, administration sets, IV catheters, and dressing supplies.

This chapter underscores the need for users to be aware of all aspects of devices and products used to administer IV treatments. The care giver has a duty to protect patients from electrical hazards of equipment not checked properly and from mechanical malfunction of devices not used according to manufacturer specifications or used with knowledge of previous malfunction. The user must protect the patient from misuse of equipment by poorly informed care providers, or from equipment used in applications not intended by the maker. The care provider must also protect patients from infectious hazard due to poorly cleaned equipment, reuse of disposable products, or procedures performed with poor technique.

The safety of the nurse and other care givers is of great importance in the development, use, and maintenance of infusion products and equipment. Down to the smallest detail, ease of use and nurse protection have been priorities for manufacturers for many decades. The addition of finger guards to administration sets at the top of the drip chamber to make spiking containers easier and safer is an example of a very small change that represents the safety consciousness of industry.

Employee protection is the responsibility of the institution and of each health care worker. This does not mean that excessive funds must be spent on every device that facilitates product safety; it does mean that product purchases must be made with patient and employee safety in mind. The employee has a right to be protected from electrical hazard by proper grounding of electronic devices and by routine safety checks. Mechanical hazard can be avoided by proper inspection of equipment and thorough, updated education regarding use and upkeep of equipment. For any device brought into an institution, in-service training should be held not only for the user but also for the persons responsible for the upkeep and maintenance of the equipment.

Prevention of chemical hazards requires that employees be well informed regarding the use and risks associated with hazardous chemicals. Employee protection includes the provision of proper receptacles for the disposal of hazardous wastes and accessory supplies needed to use hazardous materials properly, such as gloves, aprons, and protective eye wear.

Protection from infectious hazards has a new urgency since the rapid spread of acquired immune deficiency syndrome and associated diseases. IV therapy has always been considered to be an area of nursing care that represents high infectious risk. However, a thorough understanding of the products and procedures used can reduce the risk factors. Infectious risks can be minimized further with the introduction of some devices developed specifically for infusion safety, but education plays a far greater role.

Protection of employees in the work place includes providing adequate and continuous education. Written information should be available that specifies equipment instructions, procedures, and handling of nonroutine or emergency situations. In-services should be provided when new equipment is introduced and periodically as long as the equipment remains in use. Attendance at educational programs or completion of competencies should be validated in the employee record.

The intended outcome of these extensive efforts is the safe use of medical devices and equipment and, ultimately, the protection of the public. The delivery of health care should not be complicated by the addition of potential harm to the consumer or the health care provider. Prevention of infectious risk to both the employee and the patient is a constant and deliberate focus.

PREPARING EQUIPMENT FOR USE

Ensuring Sterility and Fitness for Use

The nurse is responsible for confirming that equipment is cleaned and safety checked before it is used. Although others perform these functions, the nurse must ensure the usability of equipment. The nurse visually inspects the equipment for breaches in sterility or integrity before using products in any setting.

Materials management and sterile processing departments are responsible for the flow of equipment and supplies from the manufacturer to the user. These two departments share the tasks of product supply and are responsible for making sure that products and equipment arrive ready for use at the patient care area. Ensuring usability in the home setting is the responsibility of the health care provider, regardless of who delivers the products.

Other departments, such as biomedical engineering and infection control, have a sustained purpose of product monitoring and testing. The infection control department usually is involved in monitoring products after an adverse situation has been identified. The biomedical engineering department is directed to maintain a log of electrical safety checks for all equipment and to confirm usability and calibrations at regular intervals, as determined by hospital policy or manufacturer's recommendation. Any devices with a history of problems are evaluated more frequently.

In the home health arena, all of these functions are likewise performed. Equipment rental companies may validate safety and performance, and infection control resources may be regional rather than office specific.

Ensuring Proper Use of Equipment

Before purchase, the intended use of all products should be clearly defined. Products cannot be used for purposes other than that specified by the manufacturer. Manufacturers are not liable for problems resulting from misuse of their products. The Federal Food and Drug Administration (FDA) warns against misuse of products and grants approval of only those products whose documentation clearly states the intended purpose, complete with support studies and data.

Proper use requires education of all users regarding the product. This education should occur when the product is introduced and as often as necessary during sustained use of the product to ensure continued safe practice. Validation of education is mandated by the Joint Commission on Accreditation of Healthcare Organizations (JCAHO). This validation should appear in the employee record or the central education database. Employees in departments responsible for safe handling and cleaning require education as well.

Quality assurance monitors should be developed to measure success in meeting established outcome criteria associated with equipment education. These monitors may include educational in-service attendance on device use and care or time spent viewing an educational program about the product. The monitor may involve spontaneous checks for procedural compliance during use of the product. Variance reports or problem reporting mechanisms also show the presence of an educational need.

Every institution should implement and maintain a device education model. A model defines a series of progressive steps necessary to successfully educate the users of devices. The model should work on the premise that device technology is inadequately addressed in schools of nursing owing to the incredible expense of keeping up with new technology. The model should address the most basic understanding of device function.

One such model is the Abbey-Shepherd device education model, which was developed for the integration of science and mechanical competence into nursing programs and continuing education. This model better equips new nurses to face the onslaught of technology in health care settings. The model represents a logical and complete system for the user to be certain that all critical factors are considered. The model becomes a checklist and can be used to evaluate devices before they are purchased. Use of the model can make it possible to determine what changes to the systems components are required if new technology is introduced into the hospital.[1]

Ensuring Proper Cost Allocation and Reimbursement

Accountability of product use includes the cost of products and reimbursement for their use. Without payment, the system is unable to function. To safeguard the financial integrity of the institution, health care providers are held accountable for the items being charged, and the reimbursement being generated is being scrutinized as never before.

Nurses involved in product selection and education are also responsible for making sure that users understand how to appropriately charge for materials and for confirming patient use of durable equipment. Moving equipment from one patient to another without using an accountability system may put the patient at risk. Tracking and accountability are instrumental in ensuring not only that equipment is appropriately charged but also that it is cleaned and, if necessary, that a safety check is performed between patients.

Correct charging for products and equipment facilitates the reimbursement process. Meticulous care in charging appropriately eliminates suspect charges, which further delay reimbursement. This aspect of nursing care is seldom discussed openly because it is not part of any nursing curriculum; however, it is part of the whole picture that sustains the financial cycle. When products and equipment are introduced into any health care setting, correct patient charging should be taught and validated as well.

CONTROL OF EQUIPMENT

Storage

Medical equipment may be seriously affected by temperature extremes or damaged from excessive dryness or humidity. Although these factors are difficult to control in a warehouse setting, they are important to consider. Generally, disposable products are able to tolerate environmental fluctuations, but they should never be exposed to moisture or allowed to freeze. If stored in areas that are subject to extreme temperature changes, mechanical equipment should be flagged to alert the biomedical engineering department to possible function variations.

Electronic equipment stored away from nursing care areas should be plugged into continuous electric current to prevent depletion of internal batteries, especially under very cold storage situations. If the equipment is battery-powered only, cold storage may damage batteries or may render them useless until they are permitted to return to room temperature.

Cleanliness is critical for storage of medical products. The area should be free of excess dust, lint, rodents, and insects. Mechanical equipment should be covered and protected, and products should be boxed to prevent damage from stacking or crowding.

Equipment and supplies that are stored off-site, requiring movement and transport, are especially vulnerable to damage. Persons responsible for moving equipment should be educated as to the nature of the products entrusted to their care as well as the hazards of damage. If equipment must be transported to the patient care area, proper function and safety should be verified on delivery. In home health care, the verification may be performed by the nurse or by a driver trained in equipment set-up.

Allocation

Allocation of equipment should be delegated to a central resource. In most cases, allocation is a materials management or distribution function that is largely taken for granted. In hospitals, where equipment is stored on the nursing areas and moved from patient to patient as needed, critical elements for equipment upkeep and accountability are often unattended.

Centralized management of equipment is a specialized function of the materials management department, as is charging a daily fee for equipment use. Ideally, it is not the function of the professional nurse. This process is best performed by persons dedicated to the goal of equipment accountability.

There must be physical accountability of equipment at all times, even if the equipment is not returned to a central pool at the end of each use. Logs must be kept that detail safety checks, calibration checks, and validation that proper cleaning occurs between patient uses. Any equipment leaving the system and returning to it must be fully checked by the biomedical engineering department before it is returned to use. Interruption in accountability necessitates that the equipment's function and safety be confirmed.

On discontinuation of therapy, the nurse is responsible for notifying the central equipment pool, or in the case of home health care, the billing office. This action ensures that the patient is not charged needlessly, and that the equipment can be returned to use as soon as it is needed. The nurse must make sure that the persons responsible for cleaning the equipment are aware of its availability.

Disinfection of Durable Medical Equipment

Sterilization and disinfection are not synonymous. *Disinfection* describes a process that eliminates all microorganisms except bacterial spores from an inanimate object. *Sterilization* is the complete elimination or destruction of all forms of microbial life.[2] Sterilization provides the highest level of assurance that an object is void of viable microbes, whereas disinfection reduces the risk of microbial contamination without the same level of assurance.[3]

Sterilization is a process for items intended to be used in a sterile procedure. Mechanical equipment is not sterilized because it is not possible to remove all microorganisms from all parts or to subject mechanical equipment to a sterilization process. Devices or objects that are in constant use in the environment or are considered to be reusable parts of a system are also unable to be sterilized. Items such as IV poles, electric cords, sinks, floors, and walls cannot be sterilized. Items that can be sterilized are drapes, certain instruments, implanted products, catheters, and needles.

Products coming from the manufacturer in sterile packaging do not need to be sterilized before use. In IV therapy, sterilization is used for reusable items, which includes very little because IV products are all provided in sterile prepackaging for immediate use.

Methods used to sterilize products are not legislated or directed by any single source or authority. Methods most used in health care settings are determined by the written policy of each institution and the recommendations from each manufacturer. Chemicals used are registered with the Environmental Protection Agency, which monitors the claims made by manufacturers but does not recommend products used for sterilization or disinfection.

A primary agent for sterilization is ethylene oxide, which is a gas that permeates all surfaces of items easily. This gas must be used with caution to avoid employee exposure during both the sterilization process and the aeration of the product before use. Strict guidelines for the use of ethylene oxide sterilization are available from such organizations as American Operating Room Nurses.

Other methods of sterilization include pressurized steam, which is effective against pathogens and is dangerous if sterilization equipment is not properly maintained or employees are not fully educated on the use of steam sterilization. Dry heat is not used as often as steam.

In addition to the Environmental Protection Agency's monitoring of the use of chemicals and gases for sterilization, the FDA makes recommendations regarding the reuse and sterilization of products. They do not specifically direct the process by stating what method is most suitable for a specific product. Rather, the statements issued by the FDA suggest the best method of sterilizing a type of material; the institution must then decide which materials fit that category.

Statements made by the Centers for Disease Control and Prevention are also worded as recommendations and do not deal with performance of the specific product. The JCAHO states that all sterilization and disinfection procedures must be written, and that policies must be provided that deal with all aspects of decontamination and sterilization.

Disinfection is more applicable to IV therapy equipment than is sterilization. Disinfection shall be established in an institution's policies and procedures, and is applicable to durable medical equipment, which includes IV poles, infusion pumps, teaching models, and nondisposable arm boards. The agent used to disinfect durable equipment should be effective in preventing cross-contamination,[4] which is defined as the movement of pathogens from one source to another.

Common methods of achieving disinfection are germicide use or immersion. Chemicals used for either of these methods should always be considered dangerous. Products disinfected should be allowed to thoroughly dry, and fumes should be avoided. Manufacturers of some chemical disinfection products suggest that the product be aerated for a certain time before reusing.

Other chemicals used include alcohol, which is bactericidal rather than bacteriostatic and is also tuberculocidal, fungicidal, and virucidal but does not destroy spores. Alcohol is used extensively in hospitals, but never as a sterilizing agent. Chlorine is inexpensive, fast acting, and widely used, but it is associated with noxious vapors and corrosive properties. Chlorine compounds are difficult to control because they are relatively unstable and are easily inactivated by organic matter. Other acceptable products are formaldehyde, glutaraldehyde, hydrogen peroxide, iodophors, and phenolics.

Policies regarding the use of chemical disinfectants should include guidelines that protect the employee. Gloves should be worn to protect the hands, the area should be adequately ventilated, and the product should be allowed to dry and aerate before it is reused or is wrapped or packaged. Although this point is seemingly minute, nurses have reported becoming ill from fumes emitted from products in closed areas, even from fumes in face masks from sterile packs.

Durable equipment should be disinfected between each patient use. This means that an infusion pump cannot be moved from one patient to another without validating that thorough disinfection has occurred. In the absence of a centralized equipment pool, knowledgeable personnel on the nursing unit are responsible for such validation; the task should be assigned to a specific person to ensure that this process occurs.

Disinfection should also be performed intermittently during patient use, on a schedule ranging from weekly in the hospital or monthly in the home. The interval is dictated by institution policy and should be delegated to a specific department or individual.

The responsibility of disinfection rests with the professional nurse. Although the actual task can be assigned, the nurse should not initiate the use of any durable medical product without reasonable confirmation that the product does not represent a risk of infection. Items should be tagged or repackaged to clearly indicate fitness for use. It is often not a high-priority task, but it aids in disinfection, a serious aspect of health care delivery.

BIOMEDICAL CONSIDERATIONS

Routine Maintenance

No single authority exists to set standards for equipment validation by biomedical engineering departments. Guidelines are set by manufacturers for periodic checks of equipment function using standardized tests. The JCAHO requires that periodic safety and function tests be performed on all electronic equipment. However, this requirement does not include checking for accuracy. Several other agencies give input into what constitutes acceptable levels of equipment monitoring by biomedical departments.

Institutional policy has priority regarding safety checks of all equipment and frequency of function and programming checks. When new equipment is introduced to an institution, ideally all aspects of its performance are checked, and a baseline is established. After the initial inspection, further performance checks may not be necessary unless a situation arises that indicates a need for testing.

Complete diagnostic tests may be performed on equipment if the hours of use indicate an unreasonably high usage, which the biomedical department might consider to cause undue stress to the equipment, for example, an ambulatory pump that infuses continuously for many months on the same patient. Validation of this device would include performance and electrical safety checks.

The age and service history of a product might trigger extra caution as well. Older devices may have impeccable service histories but should be watched with care because all devices have a predictable life span. However, many infusion pumps from past generations still infuse with the accuracy and reliability of new devices. Older or problematic equipment should be logged and tracked to validate poor performance and extra expense.

In the case of rental infusion equipment, some agencies prefer to monitor performance between each patient use. Because infusion equipment provided by home care is far from the care giver or support systems, equipment malfunction or failure can be inconvenient or even dangerous. To minimize these situations, care of equipment is a full-time effort that requires many more hours and tests than are mandated by regulatory agencies.

All tests and uses of equipment are clearly logged and kept as permanent records, as is mandated by the JCAHO; this regimen should also be a part of institution policy. The maintenance of equipment is a focus of risk management in hospital and home care alike for the safety of the public, the institution, and the employee.

The nurse facilitates problem solving by clearly noting suspected and actual occurrences of malfunction, including questionable product performance. Without clear observation and communication, equipment malfunction may continue undetected.

If equipment is found to be functioning in error or is suspected of operating outside normal parameters, its use should be discontinued immediately. The exact problem should be written down and attached to the device. If the problem is poorly stated, it may not be found in routine examination. For example, if an infusion pump is not delivering at the prescribed rate, a complaint of malfunction to the biomedical engineering department will result in diagnostic tests for operability that may not include long-term infusion accuracy tests. The scope of diagnostic procedures for an infusion pump may need to be altered to isolate the problem identified by the nurse.

It is also helpful if the nurse can describe the situation that precipitated the infusion pump problem. User error should always be suspected initially, an occurrence that is confirmed statistically. A recent review of central venous catheter deaths and injuries reported to the FDA showed that 52% were caused by user technique.[5] Most devices are made with this type of statistic in mind, and a great effort is made to minimize opportunities for misuse.

If user error is confirmed or cannot be determined, it is the responsibility of the nurse or manager and the institution to prevent further error from occurring. Corrective action includes education on use of the product and confirmation that all persons are knowledgeable in problem solving for the device and are aware of situations that might cause the problem to recur.

The nurse should also keep records of product problems. Some institutions provide this record keeping in a centralized location, such as with the IV therapy coordinator, IV team, or the purchasing, materials management, or nursing education department. Isolated incidences rarely receive attention until a central party notices that the complaints and problems represent a trend. Problems with devices should always be considered for inclusion in the medical device reporting program discussed later in this chapter.

Recognition of Malfunction

Statistically, the equipment provided for use in health care is very safe. No allowances are made for critical error acceptability, and the health care industry has tried to design equipment that errs on the side of the patient. This means that if a certain aspect of performance malfunctions, it should decrease danger to the patient rather than increase it. For example, if a microinfusion device for pain medication failed, it would cease to infuse rather than overinfuse. The patient would experience discomfort and inconvenience, but oversedation or death would not result.

Many situations result in permanent injury and death as a result of infusion devices. By law, these situations must be reported to the FDA and the manufacturer. The exact cause of the incident need not be confirmed at the time, but the suspected occurrence must be reported within 10 working days.[6]

Malfunction indicators are built into devices to protect the patient and the care giver. Alarms on infusion devices should never be circumvented. Some devices are still made that allow the alarms to be silenced, a feature that invites certain hazards. All alarms have a specific purpose, and proper use of equipment silences alarms correctly.

Some device problems are not detected by alarms and are discovered by alert care givers. Often, care givers look to confirm that the equipment is functioning without double checking its performance. An example of this type of performance problem is an infusion device set to infuse at a given rate. Each nurse monitors the patient, notes that the pump is infusing, reads the amount infused, and charts the data provided by the pump on the amount infused. Eventually, an observant nurse notices that the solution should have totally infused hours earlier if the pump actually had delivered the amount calculated. In this case, the device operates outside the programmed parameters without causing an alarm. Again, the infusion device must be used as an adjunct to providing safe care, not as a substitution for careful nursing.

Equipment malfunction should always be suspected in situations with negative outcomes. Complications, unexpected deterioration of the patient, or development of a patient crisis should always cue the care giver to check the equipment. If a device or product is even remotely involved in a negative patient outcome, the device should be removed, not altered in any way, taken to the biomedical engineering department, and a full written report made. If the equipment appears to be functioning appropriately but cannot be ruled out as a potential problem, it should be removed as soon as safely possible and checked completely.

The nurse must never allow equipment to substitute for nursing judgment or assessment. If the equipment indicates that the patient is doing well and nursing assessment does not confirm this, the nurse must trust in human skills and actions to take precedence over equipment. Calculating drop factors for infusion pumps is not necessary, but observing the reasonable function parameters is mandatory. If the patient is on a patient-controlled anesthesia device, is pain controlled? If not, is the device functioning? If the patient is somnolent, is the pump delivering medication as programmed? These questions should be answered before the infusion parameters are changed to attain improved patient response.

Equipment failure is statistically less likely to occur than human error. In the example of patient-controlled anesthesia device problems stated earlier, the actual problem would most likely be incorrect programming of the pump or incorrect prescribing of patient-controlled anesthesia variables by the physician.

User-induced malfunctions fall into four categories. These types of problems are the most dangerous, the most challenging to identify, and the most difficult to correct. The first type of malfunction is created when the user bypasses a normal function of the device, such as the air-in-line alarm. New pumps make such bypassing harder to do, but it is possible on any infusion device by a creative nurse, and if the feature is circumvented, the patient is subject to the uninhibited infusion of air. Another example is bypassing the patient lock-out feature on a patient-controlled anesthesia device because the nurse finds it cumbersome, resulting in tampering and possible oversedation of the patient.

The second category is using disposables not approved for use with a specific device. This problem happens with dedicated as well as generic tubing. Infusion devices are tested in controlled situations, and accuracy data are based on use with certain tubing only. Massive overinfusions and underinfusions have been reported when tubings were adapted by the user to function in nonapproved situations.

Another problem in the second category is use of different brands of gravity tubing in pumps designed to use generic gravity administration sets. These pumps are calibrated for use with only one brand of gravity infusion set at a time. Alternating between brands causes great fluctuations in performance. All tubings are not alike, internally or externally, and cannot be used interchangeably without seriously affecting the performance of the device. This is also true of secondary tubing added to pump infusion sets. The infusion device manufacturer must approve of sets used in conjunction with pumps sets, or performance claims may be null and void. Manufacturers are able to condone the mixing of sets if the device is capable of maintaining adequate performance with various sets. However, if the manufacturer is noncommittal, the alternative set should be avoided.

Ignorance or disregard of equipment operation is the third category of user-induced malfunction. All health care providers agree that proper use of equipment depends on understanding of normal operation, yet many nurses assume that all equipment operates alike. Some care givers may not be properly educated in device operation. These care givers are unfamiliar with the equipment and may represent a potential problem. Competency-based learning programs can prevent many errors generated by ignorance.

The fourth category of user-induced problem is the result of equipment used for purposes other than those intended by the manufacturer. Health care journals are full of documented cases of death or injury resulting from unapproved use. A dangerous example is routine infusion pumps and administration sets with Y injection sites attached to epidural drips. The pump may be capable of performing the function correctly, but numerous safety violations are associated with this application. The infusion pump can easily be mistaken for an IV infusion, and the presence of the Y injection sites on the tubing increases the likelihood of accidental infusion.

All of these user-induced problems can be prevented with education, but they continue to plague health care. The health care industry as well as health care professionals must make a concerted effort to address these issues through quality improvement programs designed to identify and correct potential error in the health care setting.

PRODUCT DEFECT REPORTING

Role of the Federal Government

Under the administrative jurisdiction of the United States Department of Health and Human Services, the FDA has monitored health care since 1938. In 1976, the Medical Devices Amendment was enacted to ensure that medical devices are safe and effective for their intended purpose. This is accomplished with the coordinating efforts of the United States Pharmacopeia. The FDA Medical Products Reporting Program (Med Watch) has been developed and put into action. This program is a national effort to encourage product reporting by all health care persons without fear of confrontation. The object of the reporting program is to objectively catalogue problems with medical devices in an effort to safeguard the public from inappropriate or hazardous medical devices.

The Safe Medical Devices Act of 1990 (public law 101-629) specifically states that in the incidence of a device known to have caused or contributed to the death or serious illness or injury of a patient, the facility must notify the FDA within 10 working days.[6] The law further defines the penalties for not reporting, as well as actions to be taken by the

FDA. The FDA notifies the manufacturer that a report has been filed and ensures follow-up by the manufacturer. If the follow-up is deemed inadequate by the FDA, further action is necessary. The FDA fully investigates all device-related deaths that are reported.

The role of the government with regard to medical devices appears to be one of collaboration. Medical manufacturers are allowed to study and report device issues to the FDA, many times without intervention by the government or FDA confirmation of test results. The approval process is considered to be rigorous.

Role of Nongovernmental Agencies

Another organization that monitors and independently tests medical devices and products is Emergency Care Research Institute, located in Plymouth Meeting, PA, which is a nonprofit, tax-exempt institute that has gained recognition worldwide for nonbiased evaluation and data collection regarding products. ECRI publishes volumes of material annually to assist health care agencies in cost-effective and practical approaches for the acquisition of technology. ECRI has an impeccable reputation for representing products in a fair and analytical manner, and endorsement from ECRI is highly prized by medical manufacturers. ECRI provides many excellent publications that are beneficial in the evaluation and selection of products that are available to medical professionals as well as the public.

The Health Industry Manufacturers Association (HIMA), located in Washington, D.C., is also a powerful force in medical device monitoring. Membership in this association includes manufacturers of over 90% of the health care devices on the market today. This group addresses common concerns of quality, education, marketing, and legislation. This group acts as a self-monitoring association to safeguard the public and ensure consistent quality. A major emphasis of this organization is educating the government about how impending legislation will affect health care.

Professional nursing organizations can also be considered among those groups that serve as public safety advocates. The role of such organizations as the Intravenous Nurses Society, the Association of Operating Room Nurses, and the Association of Practitioners in Infection Control is to educate their members to the hazards or potential problems of devices. These organizations offer negative feedback to manufacturers to bring about change if needed, and through professional networking, they are very effective. The endorsement of products by professional organizations is actively sought by manufacturers who value the opinions of the professionals represented.

Role of the Nurse

All other resources combined for product defect input cannot equal the volume and validity that nurses can provide. The nurse is usually represented in all health care settings and is in a position to observe and document the proper or problematic function of devices and products. Most problem products are identified, but not reported, by nurses. In fact, fewer than 5% of all defective products are reported at all.[7]

By being informed and up-to-date on available equipment and technology, the nurse can be a credible source of information. Nursing journals, in-service education, continuing education, and product information updates are widely available and are written specifically for professional nurses. A nurse that stays informed is able to understand new concepts and is quick to recognize potential problems. Nurses must take the initiative to be self-educated in this respect, learning why a product works instead of simply acknowledging its presence.

The FDA's Med Watch is available as a mechanism for nurses. Although anyone can use this program, it is specifically designed for ease of use by nurses. Many nurses are reluctant to report product problems because they are not confident in their ability to recognize situations that are appropriate for reporting.

Med Watch encourages reporting of any device suspected of malfunctioning or of being undependable. Problems might include catheters that break easily, tubing that consistently comes apart with tension, labels that do not include enough information or create confusion, packaging that causes problems when opened, instructions that are incomplete, and user errors that occur at a higher-than-acceptable rate. Products that can be reported include pumps, gloves, transducers, catheters, testing kits, implanted devices, connectors, tubings, and dressings. Death or injury does not have to occur for a report to be initiated; simple observations, if based on intelligent assessment, are all that is necessary.

When reporting a problem, be aware of the whole picture regarding the device. Is the cleaning performed on the nursing unit or in a specialized department? Was the infusion pump delivered to the patient by a rental equipment company or by the home health agency? Professional networking is not necessary before reporting a device, but it can add useful insight into the total scope of the product's uses and reputation. The specialty practice of IV nursing lends itself to this type of collegial communication.

Any device suspected of causing injury or death should be impounded immediately and reported to the FDA within 10 working days. The device should not be cleaned, safety checked, or manipulated in any way. In the case of an infusion pump, all the programming data and history display should be verified by two persons not related to the incident before the pump is turned off. If the pump is battery operated, the battery should not be removed. Legal council should be consulted for further action regarding the device.

When to Report a Problem

Medical devices suspected of being problematic should be reported as soon as the product defect can be defined and user error can be ruled out. It is difficult for manufacturers to be held accountable for problems that can be attributed to the user. Corrective action includes education and competency-based skills testing to verify the ability of the user.

User problems are a common explanation for many device faults. Although many problems arise from care givers' being inadequately prepared to use products, this excuse is acceptable only to a certain point. If the staff must be taught an excessive number of times and they continue to experience problems, perhaps the problem lies with the device and not

the user. The device may be functional and may operate flawlessly, but if the staff cannot use the product efficiently and safely in a reasonable amount of time, then the product may be the source of the problem. The product may be too difficult, too complex, or too time consuming. A product that continues to be difficult to use properly 6 months after acquisition poses user-error risks; this is a reportable product problem.

Any time a problem repeats itself, it should raise a red flag, even if the situation is explainable. Problems may appear to be isolated incidences unless a centralized reporting mechanism exists for every institution, home care agency, or hospital. Many nurses do not realize that other health care givers have experienced the same or similar issues unless a specific forum exists for product issues to be discussed. Most institutions have a committee for material standardization and review. A progressive committee of this type invites product comments by all disciplines to ensure quality and to prevent risk.

Any product-related injury or death of a patient or employee should be immediately reported to the FDA. Suspicion of the product is enough to warrant reporting because careful investigation must begin immediately, and the role of the device must be clarified. Reference to public law 101-629 earlier in this text gives more details regarding reports concerning death or injury.

Active communication with the manufacturer should always be a first step when problems are suspected. The manufacturer must report problems to the FDA and is obligated to investigate all communications that detail problems. Most companies have toll-free numbers for consumer questions and complaints.

The nurse should be realistic about the expected response from the manufacturer. The company is not obligated to detail other reported negative occurrences regarding the product in question. The company will record the complaint or comment and investigate. It is in their own best interest to address and resolve issues before professional publications or nurse networking reveals these product safety issues.

If the product problem is significant and emergent, manufacturers should be notified so that corrective action can be taken immediately. When identifying problems with disposable products, the nurse should keep defective samples—both the FDA and the manufacturer can use the samples to discover the source of the problem. The packaging, including the lot number and any other identifying numbers or markings, should be kept for the manufacturer. All details of the negative occurrence should be written down immediately. Institutional risk management departments should also be appraised of any negative product occurrences. Simple problems, such as misleading packaging or unclear instructions, can be resolved with the manufacturer alone, and the results of the requested change can be almost immediate.

How to Report a Problem

The FDA product problem report is called Med Watch, and it is supplied as preprinted forms that are available to anyone. Institutions may locate forms in nursing administration, clinical engineering, materials management, or purchasing offices. These forms are generated by the government and are simple, one page, straightforward, and concise. They can be reproduced without permission, but the original forms are postage free and can be mailed without an envelope. If assistance is needed in filling out the form, an 800 number is available, or the report can be given verbally (Fig. 16–1).

The report asks the name of the product and a brief description including gauge numbers, lot numbers, or any identifying characteristics. The manufacturer and address are asked, if known, as well as serial numbers and the manufacturer product number. The expiration date and whether or not the device is disposable are also documented.

Reporter information includes the name, facility, and address of the person initiating the problem report. The identity of the reporter can be designated in three ways. The report can be held in strict confidence with no public disclosure. In this case, the reporter's name and address are still important because the investigator may need additional information or follow-up to confirm that the report was received and to offer information regarding the intended course of action.

The reporter may choose to disclose the problem report to the manufacturer only. This option allows the maker to respond to problems and to investigate along with the reporter of the complaint. In most cases, the manufacturer seeks to reassure the user that the complaint has been received and will be addressed. There can be no correction of any problem unless the manufacturer or distributor is fully informed, and the reporter of the problem is the most accurate source of information.

The third identification option is to make the reporter's name available to the manufacturer and to anyone who requests a copy of the report from the FDA. This openness may be intimidating to persons who worry about being confronted. However, the availability of the reporting person lends credibility to the report and makes the free flow of information much easier. Problem identification is often already difficult because of a wide variety of possible contributing factors involved when a problem arises. The availability of the reporter makes quantifying and qualifying problems much easier. Reporter identification is strictly voluntary, and reports that limit the identity of the author are given as much attention as those that do not.

The report asks for a detailed description of the problem as seen by the reporter. Facts are necessary, but suspected flaws or perceived problems can also be included. Sometimes, reports reflect concern that a potential problem may occur. No facts exist in these cases; the report serves only to predict or to warn. User issues are acceptable problems to report, as are specific product function concerns.

It is acceptable to copy the report to the manufacturer; this action will speed the process of response. Ideally, the maker of a product should know of suspected product issues as soon as they occur, which may be some time before the problem is perceived to be widespread enough to warrant a report to the FDA. Nurses should openly communicate with manufacturers to solicit help in education and problem solving. This type of interaction could resolve many issues early in the process. Typically, a nurse who is a care giver assumes that nursing administration communicates with vendors. The irony is that the administrative nurse is rarely the product user or the care giver and therefore has limited hands-on perspective of the problem. Manufacturers respond to the bedside nurse and consider input from the actual care giver

to be of significant value. Problems reported by primary care nurses are a very important contribution and are always welcome by the FDA and the health care industry alike.

All health care institutions have reporting mechanisms as well in the form of variance or incident reports. These are reporting tools for quality improvement and risk management programs, to provide written, ongoing communication regarding real and potential risks in the work environment. Any situation requiring manufacturer or FDA communication should also be processed through quality improvement or risk management programs.

Biomedical engineering departments should be notified first in cases of suspected equipment problems. This department can provide insight into potential risks. The biomedical engineering department may have to impound the device, even if temporarily, to service and test the product before an accurate report can be made. This department is trained to evaluate and anticipate potential and real problems. If the equipment is rented or leased, the original owner or distributor should be notified by the biomedical engineering department.

When a nurse articulates a problem, his or her report, to be considered a credible resource, must be absolutely professional. This means that the report must be free of bias or prejudicial comments. Stating that a product is not as good as that of a competitor is not a problem. The report must provide facts, including dates and times. The report should not stress blame or fault, because these will become evident when the defect is properly identified. The reporter must be interested in corrective action and patient safety more than in assigning fault.

Risk Management

Notification of the risk management department does not always imply that action is needed. The risk management department collects and categorizes information to be assimilated and used if a problem does occur. Allowing this department to collect information and be aware of potential problems allows the institution to better protect itself and the safety of the public.

Legal counsel is notified at the discretion of the risk management department. Usually, legal counsel serves to advise and perhaps correspond with manufacturers regarding situations or events. This action gives more authority to a product complaint issue. Legal counsel is always involved immediately in the case of injury or death.

The risk management department should always be consulted if equipment is to be returned to use after a suspected problem of major impact. The risk management department is able to advise users if problems with the product have been addressed sufficiently to support the continued use or return to use of a device.

SUMMARY

The caregiver must be knowledgeable about the equipment used and must be motivated to initiate change when indicated. The governing institution or agency can provide the access or avenue to action, but it is the responsibility of the

MEDWATCH

THE FDA MEDICAL PRODUCTS REPORTING PROGRAM

For **VOLUNTARY** reporting
by health professionals of adverse
events and product problems

Page ____ of ____

Form Approved: OMB No. 0910-0291 Expires:12/31/94
See OMB statement on reverse

FDA Use Only   H Pad

Triage unit
sequence #

A. Patient information

1. Patient identifier
In confidence

2. Age at time
of event:
or _____
Date
of birth:

3. Sex
☐ female
☐ male

4. Weight
____ lbs
or
____ kgs

B. Adverse event or product problem

1. ☐ **Adverse event** and/or ☐ **Product problem** (e.g., defects/malfunctions)

2. **Outcomes attributed to adverse event**
(check all that apply)

☐ death _____ (mo/day/yr)
☐ life-threatening
☐ hospitalization – initial or prolonged

☐ disability
☐ congenital anomaly
☐ required intervention to prevent
permanent impairment/damage
☐ other: _____

3. **Date of
event**
(mo/day/yr)

4. **Date of
this report**
(mo/day/yr)

5. **Describe event or problem**

6. **Relevant tests/laboratory data, including dates**

7. **Other relevant history, including preexisting medical conditions** (e.g., allergies,
race, pregnancy, smoking and alcohol use, hepatic/renal dysfunction, etc.)

C. Suspect medication(s)

1. **Name** (give labeled strength & mfr/labeler, if known)
#1
#2

2. **Dose, frequency & route used**
#1
#2

3. **Therapy dates** (if unknown, give duration)
from/to (or best estimate)
#1
#2

4. **Diagnosis for use** (indication)
#1
#2

5. **Event abated after use
stopped or dose reduced**
#1 ☐ yes ☐ no ☐ doesn't apply
#2 ☐ yes ☐ no ☐ doesn't apply

6. **Lot #** (if known)
#1
#2

7. **Exp. date** (if known)
#1
#2

8. **Event reappeared after
reintroduction**
#1 ☐ yes ☐ no ☐ doesn't apply
#2 ☐ yes ☐ no ☐ doesn't apply

9. **NDC #** (for product problems only)
_ – _ – _

10. **Concomitant medical products** and therapy dates (exclude treatment of event)

D. Suspect medical device

1. **Brand name**

2. **Type of device**

3. **Manufacturer name & address**

4. **Operator of device**
☐ health professional
☐ lay user/patient
☐ other:
_____

5. **Expiration date**
(mo/day/yr)

6.
model # _____
catalog # _____
serial # _____
lot # _____
other # _____

7. **If implanted, give date**
(mo/day/yr)

8. **If explanted, give date**
(mo/day/yr)

9. **Device available for evaluation?** (Do not send to FDA)
☐ yes ☐ no ☐ returned to manufacturer on _____
(mo/day/yr)

10. **Concomitant medical products** and therapy dates (exclude treatment of event)

E. Reporter (see confidentiality section on back)

1. **Name, address & phone #**

2. **Health professional?**
☐ yes ☐ no

3. **Occupation**

4. **Also reported to**
☐ manufacturer
☐ user facility
☐ distributor

5. If you do NOT want your identity disclosed to
the manufacturer, place an " X " in this box. ☐

FDA

Mail to: MEDWATCH
5600 Fishers Lane
Rockville, MD 20852-9787

or FAX to:
1-800-FDA-0178

FDA Form 3500 (6/93)   Submission of a report does not constitute an admission that medical personnel or the product caused or contributed to the event.

Figure 16–1. MedWatch, Rockville, MD: medical products reporting program.

person providing patient care to initiate the process. The nurse is a patient advocate who strives for the patients' total well-being, a goal that should include not only the care provided but also awareness of the equipment used and corrective action to take, should it be necessary.

References

1. Abbey J, Shepherd M. The Abbey-Shepherd Device Education Model. Nursing and Technology: Moving into the Twenty-first Century Conference Proceedings, 1989:41–53.
2. Rutala WA. APIC guideline for selection and use of disinfectants. Am J Infect Control. 1990; 18(2):100.
3. American Operating Room Nurses. Standards and Recommended Practices for Sterilization and Disinfection. Denver, CO, 1990:Section III:17, pg 1.
4. Intravenous Nurses Society. Intravenous Nursing Standards of Practice. Belmont, MA, 1990:25.
5. Scott WL. Medical-device complication reporting. JIN 1990:178–182.
6. Safe Medical Devices Act: Device User Facility Reporting Sections. US Department of Health and Human Services. Public Law 101-629, 1990.
7. Early warning system for reporting medical device problems to FDA, Intravenous Nurses Society: Intravenous Nurses Society Newsline, 1991:12(1):2.

Product selection and evaluation of intravenous (IV) therapy equipment are significant aspects of the specialty practice of IV nursing. With the vast number of products on the market, the choice of the best equipment at the best price is important to the IV nurse, the patient, and the hospital administrator and requires a methodical approach.

The first steps in the product selection process are recognizing the need for equipment, scanning the market, and identifying essential features of the device. Once the product has been selected, a comprehensive evaluation is conducted, each member of the product evaluation committee having a specific role in the process. Communication of the process, verbal and written, must be conveyed to the users of the equipment so that a proper evaluation can be conducted. Lastly, the financial aspects of purchasing or leasing new products must be addressed. Poor-quality products tend to lead to increased usage, patient trauma, and liability; therefore, basing product selection primarily on price may not be cost-efficient. Cost analysis and justification will enable efficient and appropriate decisions to be made in choosing a new product or in demonstrating the need to continue using a current one.

This chapter discusses the process of product selection and evaluation. It aids the IV nurse in making educated and informed selections of IV products so as to ensure safe delivery of IV therapy without compromising patient care.

NURSE'S ROLE IN PRODUCT SELECTION AND EVALUATION

The *Intravenous Nursing Standards of Practice* states, "The nurse shall be cognizant of all new technological advances and shall participate in the evaluation, selection, and implementation of these products in the clinical setting."[1] The level of education and experience of the nurse should be considered before a product currently in use is replaced or a new product is used by the nurse. The educational background of the registered nurse, coupled with his or her clinical orientation, affords a greater depth of understanding with respect to the scientific principles on which the application of the product is founded. Depending on the policies and procedures of the facility, the professional status of the practitioner may determine who is using the equipment. For instance, a licensed practical nurse may not be allowed to regulate IV infusions via an infusion pump but can operate an infusion controller. If the nursing population is largely made up of licensed practical nurses, the most appropriate choice for that institution would be to purchase controllers.[2]

The practitioner must know how to operate the equipment to ensure that safe IV therapy is delivered to the patient and operator error is minimized. Reading the product literature, familiarizing oneself with the product, and observing precautions are necessary measures to guarantee safe, efficient operation. The staff must be educated on the use and operation of the product, and references should be available and supervision provided should additional assistance be required.

Educational programs should include the reasons for the product evaluation because staff cooperation and understanding can greatly enhance the effectiveness of the evaluation. During the evaluation, the nurse should be aware of the process of reporting a product defect or malfunction, such as documenting the problem, using another product or returning to the former one until the problem is addressed, and contacting the company representative. By taking an active role in the process, the practitioner develops a sense of accomplishment as his or her suggestions and recommendations are applied to clinical practice.[3]

PRODUCT SELECTION PROCESS

Identifying the Need for a Product Change

To begin the product selection process, the need for changing equipment or purchasing a new product must be determined. The rationale for change should fall into one of the following categories: cost considerations, safety considerations, or product effectiveness.

In a time when cost containment and fiscal constraints are critical issues, the prices of products need to be carefully compared. Lower prices may not be equated with higher quality. Therefore, purchasing a less costly item may not be cost-effective, if owing to poor performance, more of the product has to be used. Also, the cost of a custom-made product must be evaluated because the price may be too extravagant to warrant change to that product.

Some products have associated equipment needs. The tubing of an infusion control device may need to be a dedicated set, whereas extension tubings and latex injection ports may be necessary to complete a catheter insertion component. In the case of IV start kits, buying each specific item in it separately may be less expensive than having the kit assembled. When the cost of a device is calculated, the extra amount of the added equipment needs to be included to reflect the true cost of the product.

In addition to the price of the product, consideration needs to be given to the support rendered by the manufacturers. Manufacturers' proposals and competitive bidding should be compared to procure the most appropriate and cost-effective deal for the institution.

When IV products are selected, the issue of patient safety must be addressed. As stated in the *Intravenous Nursing Standards of Practice,* ''the intravenous nurse . . . should interact with other members of the health care team to provide safe, quality intravenous therapy.''[1] As technology has advanced, many innovative products have become available and medications are being administered in more concentrated and potent forms. Therefore, when products are selected and evaluated, specific safety features of the product should be considered. For instance, when infusion control devices are evaluated, features that reduce the risk of accidental free flow and alarms that detect a malfunction, air, or an upstream occlusion should be available on the device. A lock-out mechanism may be necessary to make the device tamper proof. When administration devices are evaluated, needle-stick protection may be investigated. The safety features should include capture of the stylette after catheter insertion and should make accidental or intentional defeat of the safety component difficult. Instituting catheters with protected needle features can reduce the risk of accidental needle sticks to the patient and the practitioner. Potential liability is reduced when safe products are used.

The impact of product effectiveness needs to be addressed when considering a product change. It is important to know if the product will consistently produce the desired results, including a review of maintenance records and product features. The advancements in current technology, the ease of use of the product, and the range of uses also need to be evaluated.

Improving the quality of a product, as well as improving technique, has resulted from advancements in technology. Infusion control devices have become more sophisticated to accommodate the administration of potent medications and therefore are more valuable in the acute care settings. Conversely, some infusion control devices have been designed simply enough that the patient can be taught to use them and are an asset in the home care setting. New catheter materials have been developed whereby insertion is less painful to the patient. Acquiring high-quality products also decreases the risk of IV complications.[4]

Improved technique can be demonstrated by the use of transparent semipermeable membrane dressings. If these dressings, as opposed to gauze dressings, are applied on an IV site, the area can be visualized and inspected without removal of the dressing.[4]

The ease of product use should be investigated. The level of education of the practitioner may be an issue when a new product is introduced. If an institution does not always have the same staff, less complicated equipment may be warranted, so that orientation to it is clear and the chance of making errors is decreased. For patients in the home care setting, the complexity of the machine may be an issue because the patient will need to be taught how to use it competently and safely and should possess knowledge for trouble-shooting if a problem should occur.

The range of uses of the product depends on several factors, including the needs of the patient, the anticipated uses for the product, the patient population the product is to be used on, and the clinical settings in which the product will be used.

The needs of the patient must be considered when new products are deemed necessary. This requirement is apparent in the home care setting. For example, patients who do not have electricity in their home will require a battery-operated infusion device to administer their therapy. Also, for patients who wish to maintain their normal activities, the size of their ambulatory pump is a major concern.

The anticipated uses for the product need to be defined. For instance, when infusion control devices are evaluated, the types of medications to be administered should be considered. Specific features may be required to infuse such therapies as narcotics, chemotherapy, and total parenteral nutrition. IV catheters, whether being used for short- or long-term therapy, vary as to product design and materials. Many types of peripheral, central, and peripherally inserted central catheters may be selected.

The patient population the product is to be used on also must be considered. An infusion pump used in the hospital may be a more sophisticated machine than one that a patient uses in the home. For instance, in the acute care setting medications may need to be titrated into a tenth of a milliliter. Patients requiring the administration of epidural anesthesia, vasoconstrictors, or chemotherapy may need specific equipment that would closely monitor their delivery. In the case of the home care patient requiring cyclic total parenteral nutrition during the night, the infusion device would need a titrating feature that would accommodate that task. Also, patients with implantable ports usually require infusion devices to deliver their treatments. Therefore, the nurse should be aware of the clinical conditions of the patient that may warrant specific products to deliver the appropriate treatments.

The clinical setting in which the product will be used should be considered. If an infusion pump is to be used primarily in an intensive care unit, the size of the machine (i.e., can several pumps be attached safely to one IV pole?) and the ability to titrate medications may be major considerations. The size of a pump would also be a concern for a home care patient who is trying to maintain his or her normal activities; a compact machine that can be carried easily would be preferred. In the case of the patient receiving long-term antibiotic therapy at home, a peripherally inserted central catheter instead of a short peripheral catheter may be the most appropriate method for medication delivery. The peripherally inserted central catheter may remain in place indefinitely, whereas the peripheral catheter would have to be changed every 48 hours or sooner if complications such as phlebitis or infiltration occur. Scheduled follow-up visits by the home care nurse could be planned, to perform dressing changes and evaluate the condition of the peripherally inserted central catheter, as opposed to frequent calls to replace the peripheral catheter.

Timing a Product Change

Incident reports may provide vital information about the need to change a product. If a pattern has evolved that demonstrates errors involving the accuracy of a particular machine or a defect in a product, change is warranted to ensure safe IV delivery.

It is important to review the areas that will affect product selection to ensure that product selection is representative of what the institution needs. It can then be determined whether the proposed product is a necessity or a luxury. For example, an infusion control device should have alarms that detect air, occlusion, and malfunction, but a feature for titration may not be necessary if that mode is seldom used.

Researching for Product Selection

Once the need to change a product has been established, the next step is to research the market of the particular item. There are several ways to obtain information on available products, including conducting a literature review, attending trade shows, and interviewing facilities currently using the product.

Conducting a literature review provides material about the products that are currently available. Articles on IV therapy, nursing and pharmacy journals, and marketing brochures provide useful information on the equipment.[5] The Emergency Care Research Institute, an independent organization that evaluates medical equipment, publishes journals that feature comparative evaluations and ratings of the products, and it reports hazards and problems of medical devices.[6]

Attending trade shows is another method of obtaining product information. At these exhibits, many products can be viewed in one place. The shows offer the opportunity to visualize the product and allow for hands-on use of the device and dialogue with the company representatives. Manufacturing representatives are willing to demonstrate their products, which enables cursory evaluations to be conducted. Time can be conserved later during the institution's actual product evaluation by eliminating equipment that would be inappropriate for the facility.

In addition, interviewing other facilities regarding their experiences with the products used in their institutions can provide useful information about the equipment, including the advantages and disadvantages of the product. Researching the market of available products aids in educated product selection.

Identifying Needed Product Features

Before a product is changed or a new product selected, written criteria should be developed that includes the necessary features of the product. To ensure that all aspects of a product are considered, the most important as well as the least important features should be included in the criteria.[4] Input from all departments that use the product should be considered when the guidelines are developed. This material will be used to narrow the field for the final hands-on evaluation. In addition, this information will be incorporated into a preliminary evaluation form for product selection. Numer-

ous products on the market can be evaluated. Table 17–1 identifies the characteristics that would be assessed in five different products: catheters, infusion control devices, transparent semipermeable membrane dressings, administration sets, and needleless systems.

Preliminary Evaluation Form for Product Selection

Once the product guidelines are established, an evaluation form must be created. The evaluation form may be designed by the IV team, the product evaluation committee, or a task force that is specifically addressing a particular product. This evaluation form is helpful for the preliminary product selection. The form completed in conjunction with the established guidelines enables objective ratings and product comparisons to be accomplished. As many products as possible should be evaluated during this initial phase. This process helps narrow the field for the actual hands-on evaluations because it is not feasible financially or temporally to evaluate all the devices on the market.

To ease the product selection, the entries on the form should coincide with the product guidelines. Spaces for the product name, manufacturer, person evaluating the product, dates of evaluation, and comments should be included.[4] Figure 17–1 and Table 17–2 illustrate the preliminary product evaluation form and guidelines for its use.

Completing the Evaluation Form (Fig. 17–1)

1. Identify the type of product that is to be evaluated, e.g., peripheral catheter or infusion device, on "Product" line.
2. Complete "Evaluation Date" and "Evaluator" entries.
3. Insert product name, or model number, or both, under "Manufacturer" column.
4. Rate each feature of the product according to the scale on the evaluation form.
5. Add scores for each product to determine the "Total Rating."
6. Add "Comments."

Compiling ratings from the evaluation forms: Once a total rating is determined for each product, the committee can narrow the field to a few for the final hands-on evaluation. The products with the highest scores are chosen to be evaluated. The "Comments" section must be taken into consideration because negative comments may override a high score.

CONDUCTING A PRODUCT EVALUATION

Product Evaluation Committee

A product evaluation committee facilitates the making of informed choices regarding product selection and evaluation. This group should be broad based and multidisciplinary; rep-

Table 17-1

Product Guidelines

Features	Considerations
Catheters	
Packaging	Is the package easy to open? Is sterility maintained after the package is opened? Can package be easily stored?
Handling	Is it easy to hold? Do features make it awkward to handle?
Length	What lengths are available?
Gauge	What gauge sizes are available?
Lumens	Is it available with multiple lumens?
Radiopacity	Is it radiopaque?
Ease of insertion	Does the needle penetrate the skin easily or with resistance? Does the needle appear dull?
Catheter advancement	Does it advance easily? Is sterility maintained when catheter is advanced?
Catheter flexibility	Is it too flexible or too rigid?
Blood return	Is blood return visible? Are features available to prevent blood contamination?
Needleless feature	Does it have a feature to capture the stylette after insertion?
Catheter stabilization	Can it be easily secured to prevent movement? Can a dressing be applied that does not interfere with assessment of the insertion site?
Infusion control devices	
Alarm	What alarms are included: air, occlusion, door open, malfunction, low battery, infusion complete?
Battery life	How long will the pump operate on battery power? What types of batteries are needed?
Rate range	What is the rate range? Are tenths of milliliter increments available?
Accuracy	What is the percentage of the margin of error?
PSI	What is the maximum PSI exerted?
Size of machine	Can it fit easily on an IV pole? Can several pumps fit safely on one IV pole?
Titration	Does it have the ability to titrate infusions?
Types of infusates	Can all types of infusates, including opaque TPN solutions, be infused?
Easy to read	Are commands and buttons easy to read? Are panel lights available to illuminate in a dark room?
Directions on machine	Are permanent directions on the pump for quick reference? Are they easy to understand?
Free-flow protection	Do safeguards against free flow of infusates exist?
Tamper-proof characteristics	Does a lock-out mechanism to prevent unauthorized tampering exist?
Piggyback mode	Is piggyback mode available? If available, is it necessary to have?
Associated equipment	Does pump need dedicated infusion sets?
Transparent semipermeable membrane dressings	
Ease of application	Is it easy to apply? Is sterility maintained when applying? Is a one-handed or two-handed method needed for application?
Adhesive quality	Does the dressing adhere adequately to the skin? Is it difficult to remove?
Water resistance	Is it water resistant?
Air permeability	Is it air permeable?
Administration sets	
Injection ports	How many injection ports are available?
Clamps	How many clamps are available? What types of clamps are on the tubing?
Drop size	What drop sizes are available?
Filters	Is an in-line filter available on the tubing? Can a filter be added to the tubing?
Length	What lengths are available?
Luer-Lok design	Is a Luer-Lok feature available?
Types of infusates	Can all types of infusates infuse through the tubing or are other types of sets required?
Compatibility with existing equipment	Can the tubings be used with existing products or devices?
Needleless systems	
Packaging	Is the packaging easy to open? Is sterility maintained after opening? Will storage be a problem?
Number of components	How many components are necessary to complete the system?
Ease of use	Is it easy to handle? Are there features that make it awkward to handle?
Compatibility with existing equipment	Can it be used with existing equipment?
Latex injection port	Is it self-sealing? How many repeated insertions can be made into it?
Types of infusates	Can all types of infusates be delivered via this system?
Injury prevention	Does it automatically guard itself? Is it rendered useless after a single use?
Safety feature	Is the safety feature difficult to defeat accidentally? Is it difficult to defeat intentionally? Does it remain in effect after disposal?
Patient comfort	Is patient comfort compromised; i.e., are more insertion attempts necessary or is needle penetration painful? Is taping and/or securing device to the patient difficult?
Infection control	Does the device increase the risk of infection? Does it prevent changing of needles, which may be necessary to maintain sterile technique? To obtain access, does the system have to be opened to the air?

IV = intravenous; psi = pounds per square inch; TPN = total parenteral nutrition.

resentatives from departments that will be affected directly or indirectly by the use of the product should be included. This committee may be involved in the preliminary selection process, in ongoing product evaluations, and as end-reviewers for product decisions. The product evaluation committee deliberates the products' merits to either support or deny support for purchase and assess the products' range of uses within the facility.[3] The committee should be composed of representatives from the IV therapy, nursing, medical, infection control, pharmacy, materials management, purchasing, and biomedical engineering departments. Each person has specific concerns relative to his or her discipline. In some situations, one committee member may need to represent more than one discipline. For instance, in a small home care company, the pharmacist may also be the purchasing agent and the materials management director. Subcommittees or task force groups may also be formed to evaluate a product specifically related to IV therapy.

Product Selection Process

1. Identify the need to purchase or change to a new product. Is the product being changed to improve cost-effectiveness, safety, or efficiency?
2. Research the market for the product by conducting a literature review, attending trade shows, and interviewing facilities currently using the product.
3. Develop product guidelines by including the most as well as the least important features desired.
4. Complete the preliminary product evaluation form by rating the product using the corresponding guidelines.
5. To narrow the field for the hands-on evaluations, compile the results from the evaluation forms and make the product selections.

Representatives from the IV therapy department are integral members of the evaluation committee. Their clinical expertise will be beneficial to the process, and they can identify favorable and unfavorable features of a product. In addition, they review products for appropriate and safe clinical use. Because the IV nurses are probably the clinicians most involved with the hands-on evaluation, one of them should be the committee chairperson who leads the process. They are also used as resources by others during this evaluation process, and their comments are invaluable when the final product is selected. If IV nurses are not available in an institution, networking professionally and seeking specialty organizational input from the Intravenous Nurses Society would be beneficial in obtaining useful product information.

The committee should be represented by members of the nursing department. Depending on the product to be tested, the staff nurses may be involved in the actual hands-on evaluation of the device. The evaluators must be aware of the importance of completing the evaluation forms and conveying any comments about the product to the designated person on the committee.

Suggestions from physicians are beneficial because they may identify advantages and disadvantages of the product from a different viewpoint. Physicians may also be involved in the hands-on evaluation process.

Pharmacists should also be on the evaluation committee. They have knowledge to share regarding medication administration and infusion capabilities, including parameters to safeguard the patient. They can also provide input on the appropriate distribution of products within the facilities, in particular, infusion control devices.

Input regarding the efficacy and safety of a product from the infection control department may be important to the evaluation process. For instance, when needleless systems are evaluated, individuals from this department may assist the IV nurses in monitoring the nosocomial infection rates related to a specific product. The department may also be helpful when interpreting data from a manufacturer's clinical trials and scientific studies.

A representative from the biomedical engineering department (also referred to as the medical or clinical engineering department) should be included on the committee. Representatives from this department perform accuracy and pressure tests, and they take devices apart to evaluate the quality of design and workmanship.[5] They also have information on the approximate repair and replacement time and cost of a product. In addition, they can warn of any design flaws, possible power inadequacies or incompatibilities with like equipment already in use.

PRELIMINARY PRODUCT EVALUATION REVIEW FORM

Product _____   Evaluation Date _____

Evaluator _____

RATING: 4 = highly satisfactory; 3 = more than satisfactory;
2 = satisfactory; 1 = less than satisfactory;
0 = not acceptable

Guidelines	Manufacturer				
Alarms					
Battery life					
Rate range					
Accuracy					
PSI					
Size of machine					
Titration					
Types of infusates					
Easy to read					
Directions on machine					
Free-flow protection					
Tamper-proof					
Piggyback mode					
Associated equipment needs					
Total					

Comments:

Figure 17–1. Example of a preliminary product evaluation form.

Table 17-2

Infusion Pump Evaluation Guidelines*

Features	Considerations
Alarms	What alarms are included: air, occlusion, door open, malfunction, low battery, infusion complete?
Battery life	How long will the pump operate on battery power?
Rate range	What is the rate range? Are tenths of milliliter increments available?
Accuracy	What is the percentage of margin of error?
PSI	What is the maximum psi exerted?
Size of machine	Can it fit easily on an IV pole? Can several pumps fit safely on one IV pole?
Titration	Does it have the ability to titrate solutions?
Types of infusates	Can all types of infusates, including opaque TPN solutions, be infused?
Easy to read	Are commands and buttons easy to read? Are panel lights available to illuminate in a dark room?
Directions on machine	Are permanent directions on the pump for quick reference? Are they easy to understand?
Free-flow protection	Are there safeguards against free-flow of infusates?
Tamper-proof characteristics	Is there a lock-out mechanism to prevent unauthorized tampering?
Piggyback mode	Is this mode available?
Associated equipment needs	Does the pump need dedicated infusion sets?

*Use these guidelines when completing the corresponding preliminary product evaluation form.

IV = intravenous; psi = pounds per square inch; TPN = total parenteral nutrition.

Materials management representatives are needed to determine a product's storage requirements. The overall size of product packaging has an impact on the amount that can be put in the IV nurses' baskets or carts, as well as department storage units. The materials management department is responsible for storing products that are in easily accessible places in a manner that ensures sterility when needed. They can also address issues that may limit product distribution and can raise awareness of similar products in stock that may be confused with the product in question.

Input from the purchasing department is imperative. These individuals have information on the prices of the products and their shipping costs, as well as on buying groups and contract negotiations that encourage competitive bidding. Their goal is to purchase products at low costs without sacrificing quality. With many facilities facing increasing economic pressures, the price of a product may dictate the decision on whether or not to purchase it. Elaborating on patient safety issues may demonstrate the need to buy a more costly product. In addition, this department is able to perform comparisons of costs. For example, the cost of an infusion pump may be low, but the price of the dedicated tubing required

for its operation may be higher than that of regular tubing. If a custom-designed product is desired, comparisons with other products need to be performed. This department also has insight into reimbursement issues of equipment and products.

Other departments may be affected by a product change, including radiology, anesthesiology, and the emergency and operating departments.[4] Inquiries should be made to see what impact the change may have on different units, and a member from these departments may want to be on the committee.

With all members working as a team, a wise choice can be made on the product selection. Each representative of the committee has valuable information to contribute. The product evaluation committee's goal is to choose safe, cost-efficient products that are appropriate for the facility's needs without compromising patient care.

Product Selection Committee

IV Therapy
Nursing
Medical (physicians)
Infection Control
Biomedical Engineering
Pharmacy
Materials Management
Purchasing

Evaluation Process

The preliminary selection process needs to precede the final evaluation procedure. The IV team or the product evaluation committee rates the products using the established guidelines for that product. Literature reviews, product demonstrations, and manufacturer recommendations aid in completing the preliminary selection process. When the field is narrowed, the products chosen should be those that are appropriate for the institution. Once all the products have been rated by the product evaluation committee, the number to be evaluated by the staff is determined. Usually, no more than two to three products are selected for the actual hands-on evaluation.

Once the number of products to be evaluated has been determined, the actual evaluation process must be delineated. Certain factors about the process need to be addressed, including the length of time for the evaluation, the number of products to be evaluated, the location of the evaluation, and the staff involved with the hands-on process.

The length of time for the product evaluation varies, depending on the device. Weeks or months may be needed to complete an effective evaluation. For instance, time would be the main focus in the evaluation of electronic infusion devices. Familiarizing the staff with the correct operation of the product could take 1 to 2 weeks.[3] Therefore, 2 to 4 weeks per machine may be necessary for all evaluators to have the opportunity to assess the products. Some evaluators may like a product because it is new, and others will dislike it for the same reason. The length of the evaluation should be sufficient to diminish the novelty effect. When a product is used many times each day, it will seem older quicker than one that is used once a day or once a week.[7]

The number of items that will be rated must also be determined. For example, when catheters are tested, insertion of a predetermined number may be the deciding factor for their evaluation.

The location of the evaluation must be determined. In a large institution, several units may be selected to be involved with the study, whereas in a small hospital, the evaluation may be conducted throughout the hospital. Advantages associated with choosing select units within a facility include less in-servicing time to a limited number of staff and concentration on hospital units that frequently use the product and that have a diverse patient population. Units in which central and peripheral catheters are used, multiple types of IV medications are administered, and blood components are transfused can aid the evaluation process because of the varied therapies that are delivered. Data are generated quicker if the department selected uses the product frequently. On the other hand, disadvantages exist to limiting the evaluation to a small number of departments. When a patient is transferred to a unit that is not evaluating the product, the chance of incorrect use of the product and errors in operation can occur if the staff is unfamiliar with the device. Comprehensive information regarding the product may not be obtained when the entire facility is not represented in the evaluation.

The next step is to communicate the evaluation procedure to those involved. An explanation of the importance of the process is essential. When the evaluators understand the purpose of the evaluation, they are more likely to cooperate with the process.

User Education

The next step that needs to be taken before the actual hands-on evaluation occurs is the in-servicing of all evaluators. In-service sessions should be scheduled with the company representative after it is determined when the product will be available, when the evaluation will start, and when it will be completed. The IV nurses and all other evaluators need to know how to use the product correctly, so time should be allowed for hands-on practice. To lessen the chance of details about the product operation being forgotten, the in-services should be conducted as close to the evaluation start date as possible.[4] Written instructions, operating manuals, and videotapes should be readily available as resource materials.

Evaluation Form

The evaluation form is an essential tool for product evaluation. Data can be obtained in various ways. One method is to have the evaluators rank the products on a scale ranging from 0 to 5, from ''highly satisfactory'' to ''not acceptable,'' or from ''strongly agree'' to ''strongly disagree'' with regard to the product's performance. Another way is to ask closed-ended and/or open-ended questions. Closed-ended questions only require ''yes'' and ''no'' answers and may ask the evaluator to compare products. Conversely, open-ended

questions allow the evaluators to respond with subjective comments. An effective procedure is to combine both types of questions on the evaluation form. Closed-ended questions take less time to answer, but additional information can be obtained from responses to the open-ended questions.[7]

The evaluation form can be generic or specific to the product. Whichever form is employed, it should be clear and concise. Figure 17–2 is an example of a generic evaluation form that can be used for any product. If a detailed evaluation is needed for a particular product, specific information is solicited. Figure 17–3 is an evaluation form specific to infusion pumps.

It is imperative that the evaluators understand the importance of returning their completed forms after they have had sufficient time to evaluate the device. The frequency of responses needs to be determined: the evaluators may respond each time they use a product, or they may give their opinions after the products have been in use for a specified period of time. A designated area may be assigned where the forms can be dropped off, or a specific person may have the responsibility for collecting them. Comments, both positive and negative, need to be documented, so that at the conclusion of the process all the information can be compiled for comparison. Equipment problems and complaints need to be reported. An evaluation may need to be terminated before the completion date if extensive difficulties are encountered.

Manufacturer Support

When a product is evaluated, another area that needs to be considered is manufacturer support. During the evaluation process, the availability of the manufacturer and the responsiveness of the company when problems occur should be assessed.

During the trial, the accessibility and receptiveness of the company representative to provide adequate service should be observed. Handouts and teaching material should be available as references. The quality of the in-service training to the staff by the representative needs to be noted. In addition, the follow-up the manufacturer furnishes when addressing requests of the staff or difficulties with the product should be observed. When serious problems occur, it is important to note the response of the representative as well as that of the company's management. These characteristics are indicators of the quality of service the company provides.[4]

Cost Considerations

The *Intravenous Nursing Standards of Practice* states that ''responsibility is required for the financial aspects of IV patient care in order to manage costs while rendering quality care.''[1] Reaching responsible financial decisions regarding new products can be accomplished by the IV nurse's taking an active role in selecting products used in IV therapy.

The cost of the product needs to be justified, and consideration also has to be given to associated equipment needs. The cost of custom-made items needs to be assessed, because they may prove to be extravagant. With custom-made products, the prototype should be retained until the actual item is obtained. If problems arise, a comparison of the item with

GENERAL PRODUCT EVALUATION
REVIEW FORM

Department conducting evaluation _____

Evaluation period to last _____ Days from _____ to _____

	Existing Product	Proposed Product
Description		
Manufacturer		
Model		

Your comments are important to help conduct a thorough product evaluation; please complete this questionnaire and forward to your supervisor.

	YES	NO
1. Have you been in-serviced on the proper use of the product?	____	____
2. Does the product open from its packaging with ease?	____	____
3. If the product is sterile, does it permit sterile transfer from packaging to use site?	____	____
4. Does this product contain all the components necessary for the procedure to be performed?	____	____
If no, which additional items are required?	____	____

_____

5. Does this product contain unnecessary components (resulting in excessive costs) for the procedure to be performed?   ____ ____

If yes, which ones? _____

6. Which characteristics of this product are inferior to those of the existing product?_____

_____

Which characteristics of this product are superior to those of the existing product?_____

_____

7. Do you recommend this product for use in the hospital?   ____ ____

_____   _____   _____
         (Name)   (Date)   (Ext.)

Comments:

Figure 17–2. Example of a generic product evaluation form.

the prototype may be warranted.[4] The written evaluations are effective in rationally proving the quality of the product.

When the field has been narrowed to a few products, a cost analysis should be conducted. The cost of the product, including associated equipment requirements, must be compared. To encourage competitive bidding, hospital negotiators should carefully compare manufacturers' proposals.[2] The cost of the evaluation also needs to be considered; the evaluation price can be reduced by having the manufacturer provide the products, as opposed to the institution's purchasing them for the evaluation process.

At this stage, the purchasing department takes a more active role. New equipment can be obtained in many ways: the institution may purchase the products, rent them, or lease them. Renting or leasing a product may be more advantageous than purchasing it because when the lease agreement expires, an updated version of the product may be obtained. Payment options may include volume discounts, selected option programs, or maintenance contracts with purchase of the product. Group purchasing arrangements may be available to reduce costs.[2] Depending on the product, bidding may be divided in various areas, thereby allowing several manufacturers to bid on an individual item rather than a whole group of products. With new technology constantly improving products, it may be advantageous to limit the length of time of a contract so that newer products can be obtained if necessary within a timely manner.

Product Selection

When the product trials are completed, a final selection can be made. The product evaluation committee or specific

PRODUCT EVALUATION FORM FOR INFUSION DEVICES

Product _____ Evaluation date _____

Manufacturer _____ Evaluator _____

Complete this form by rating each statement and adding any comments. Return to the Product Evaluation Committee representative.

RATING: 4 = highly satisfactory; 3 = more than satisfactory; 2 = satisfactory;
1 = less than satisfactory; 0 = not acceptable

1. The alarms were easy to identify and troubleshoot.   _____

2. The pump was accurate and reliable.   _____

3. The pump could be easily positioned at the bedside or on an IV pole. The weight of the machine did not hinder patient ambulation or transport.   _____

4. The command panel was easy to read.   _____

5. The pump was easy to prime and load.   _____

6. The pump was easy to operate.   _____

7. The directions on the pump were easy to understand.   _____

8. The lock-out mechanism provided additional patient safety.   _____

9. The featured safeguards prevent accidental free-flow of infusates.   _____

10. The in-service education for operation was adequate.   _____

11. Approximately how many times did you use the pump?   _____

Comments:

Figure 17–3. Example of a product evaluation form for infusion devices.

task force tallies the results from the completed evaluation forms and compiles the comments of the evaluations. The advantages and disadvantages of the products are compared. At this point, if the products are comparable, an enhanced feature may be the determining factor when the final decision is made.[4] Also, whether the institution plans to standardize the product within the facility widely influences the selection; it may not be practical to use the same device throughout an entire facility. The manufacturer may be able to offer a product mix to satisfy all the needs of the facility.[2]

Several factors should be addressed when the final product selection is made, including product performance, cost, overall evaluation results, and company representative performance. Product performance must be acceptable and must meet the criteria that were established. From the financial standpoint, the least expensive product may not be a high-quality or efficient device; therefore, cost should not be the only consideration. To justify purchasing an expensive or superior product, features that reduce or eliminate complications may be in its favor. For example, needle safety devices would decrease the risk of needle-stick injuries and the associated complications. Comments from the overall evaluation results must be considered because problems with the product or the service by the company may be discovered. Finally, the responsiveness of the company representative must be assessed with regard to the effectiveness of the in-service training, the frequency of follow-up calls, and the response to problems.[2]

Communication of the Product Selection

Once the product evaluation committee has selected the final product, communication of the decision must be conveyed throughout the institution. Memorandums should be distributed to all units stating which product will be used and when implementation of the device will begin. Policies and procedures will need to be developed for use of the product. The IV nurse should be involved when the procedures and guidelines for use of the new IV-related product are established. Nursing procedure committees, staff education departments, and nursing management may also be involved in this procedure.

The new product may be introduced immediately throughout the entire facility or on a gradual basis, depending on the size of the institution. Smaller institutions may immediately implement the product hospital wide, whereas larger hospitals may find it more effective to in-service the staff unit by unit.

In-service sessions will have to be scheduled. The duration of the in-services will depend on the complexity and sophistication of the product and the skill and training of the staff. Support of the staff during the evaluation and implementation processes must be taken into consideration because the sessions may be time consuming until the staff can familiarize themselves with the product. Round-the-clock in-service sessions with the manufacturer may be necessary for one product, whereas viewing of a videotape may be sufficient instruction for another.[3] For example, operation of an electronic infusion device will probably require in-depth instruction, whereas directions to correctly apply a transparent semipermeable membrane dressing may be demonstrated adequately on a videotape.

Evaluation Process

1. Determine the length of time for the evaluation.
2. Identify the location for the evaluation, i.e., several departments or facility-wide testing.
3. Convey to the evaluators the importance of completing the product evaluation forms.
4. Schedule in-service sessions for proper product operation as close to the evaluation start date as possible.
5. Compile evaluation results and make the final decision for product selection.
6. Communicate throughout the facility which product was chosen.
7. Because this process is ongoing, evaluate new products, as well as the currently used ones, to ensure that the most appropriate product is being used in patient care.

POSTEVALUATION EDUCATION

Once a product has been selected, postevaluation education and problem solving are necessary. Written procedures for proper operation should be available. Resource material and personnel should be readily accessible to the staff using the product. The knowledge and clinical expertise of the IV nurses make them excellent resources. Until the staff is comfortable using the device, extra time is involved in learning the proper operation of the product. If staff appear to have difficulty using the product, additional in-service programs conducted by the company representative may be needed to ensure proper use of the device.

When a product malfunctions or a defect in the device is noted, the serial and lot numbers of the item should be documented. This information aids the vendor in locating a problem that may have developed within the manufacturing process. Incident reports should also be filed. Trends may be illustrated about the product's performance that would require immediate attention from the manufacturer. According to the Safe Medical Device Act of 1990, product defects and failures must also be reported to the Food and Drug Administration.

To ensure quality IV care, evaluation of products must be ongoing. Practitioners may like the product initially but as time progresses may not use it. Reasons for this failure need to be identified. Perhaps more in-service education is needed for the product's intended use, or perhaps the device is faulty or there is an inadequate supply to meet the facility's needs.

Currently used products within an institution should be evaluated, as should products new to the market. This continuous investigation guarantees that the best device is being used in patient care.

CONCLUSION

The IV nurse plays an important role in the process of product selection and evaluation. Educated choices need to be made when products are selected that will enable safe, efficient delivery of IV therapy to the patient. A systematic approach eases this process. Written evaluations aid in demonstrating objective rationales for particular product selection. The process may show that a product can improve technique, patient safety, and product quality and that it is cost efficient, or it may conclude that the product being used is the best one for the patient and the institution. Evaluation of currently used products needs to be ongoing so that the best product is used to deliver high-quality patient care. Active involvement in the product selection and evaluation process by the IV nurse enhances commitment and provides personal satisfaction and a sense of accomplishment as suggestions and recommendations are applied to clinical practice.

References

1. Intravenous Nurses Society. Revised Intravenous Nursing Standards of Practice. JIN (suppl) 1990.
2. Ritter HTM. Evaluating and selecting general-purpose infusion pumps. JIN 1990; 13(3):156–161.
3. Stahler-Wilson JE, Worman FR. A products nurse specialist: The compleat clinical shopper. Nurs Manage 1991; 22(11):36–38.
4. Coggin S. Evaluating and selecting I.V. equipment. NITA 1987; 10(1):52–60.
5. Donnelly EB, Witte KW, Eck TA, LaPlume G. Interdisciplinary Committee on Infusion-Control Devices: Evaluating new products. Am J Hosp Pharm 1988; 45(3):601–604.
6. Lorenz B. Are you using the right IV pump? RN 1990; 53(5):31–37.
7. Monahan RS, Donius M. Product evaluation: Research for practice. Geriatr Nurs 1991; 12(6):305–308.

Selected References

Donnelly EB, Witte KW, Eck TA, LaPlume G. Interdisciplinary Committee on Infusion-Control Devices: Containing related-products costs. Am J Hosp Pharm 1988; 45(3):595–600.

Donnelly EB, Witte KW, Eck TA, LaPlume G. Interdisciplinary Committee on Infusion-Control Devices: Managing product use. Am J Hosp Pharm 1988; 45(3):589–594.

Heenan A. A review of infusion pumps. Nurs Times 1989; 85(41):76–77, 80.

Millam DA. Controlling the flow: Electronic infusion devices. Nursing 1990; 20(8):65–66, 68.

Munz N. Evaluating needleless IV tubing. Am J Nur 1993; 93(2):74–75.

Satwicz MJ, et al. Nursing and product selection = Quality care. Nurs Manage 1991; 22(11):30–31.

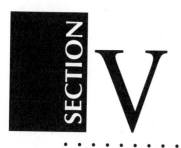

SECTION V

NURSING CARE

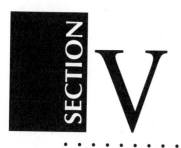

CHAPTER 18 Patient Assessment

Rose Anne Lonsway, CRNI, MA
Maxine Acevedo, CRNI, MPA

Knowledge and recognition of potential problems associated with a fluid or electrolyte imbalance are critical to patient care. This chapter describes basic patient assessment as it relates to fluid volume and electrolyte dynamics. Patient history and clinical assessment as well as correct interpretation of laboratory data are all valuable components of this process.

PATIENT HISTORY

To understand how the body is responding to its internal environment, a description of the patient's fluid and electrolyte status must be obtained from the patient. It is very difficult to determine the absolute amount of total body water and the relationship between that amount and other mechanisms within the body. The more accurate the history obtained from the patient, the more sensitive the monitoring process will be for specific alterations.

Information from past medical and family history should be included in the patient history. For example, the patient may have a familial history of diabetes, even though the patient does not exhibit signs or symptoms of diabetes. As the course of the patient's treatment unfolds, latent diabetes may manifest itself. If this information is obtained from a comprehensive patient history, a nurse can be watchful for signs and symptoms indicating the beginning of diabetic changes in the patient's electrolyte status.

The patient's medical history indicates if he or she is at risk for, or has a history of, fluid and electrolyte alterations and how the alteration and course of treatment were tolerated. Even though the information may not currently be clinically significant, it may be applied to future treatment.

Current Status

When performing a review of systems in conjunction with a physical assessment, one should listen carefully to the patient's description of the chief complaint. If the patient has suffered an injury, the type and degree of injury should be ascertained because many injuries could affect the patient's fluid and electrolyte balance (Table 18–1).

Is the patient suffering from any illness that may have an effect on fluid and electrolyte balance? For example, in congestive heart failure, the patient is at risk for fluid volume excess. Metabolic aberrations, such as diabetes mellitus, can put the patient at risk for metabolic acidosis and fluid volume deficits. Episodes of acute pancreatitis can result in calcium deficits. Conditions such as emphysema cause a respiratory acidosis that results from the patient's inability to exchange carbon dioxide. Some tumors interfere with the utilization or uptake of calcium, leading to calcium excesses.

Many effects are insidious and require careful history taking and careful monitoring to prevent the occurrence of further problems. Prolonged immobilization of a patient may cause a calcium excess that results from loss of calcium from the bone into the extracellular fluid. A patient who drinks excessive amounts of plain water may wash out electrolytes, causing potassium deficits, sodium deficits, or metabolic alkalosis if the condition is not corrected.

Table 18-1

Fluid and Electrolyte Imbalances Associated with Selected Diseases or Conditions

Disease or Condition	Potential Imbalance
Crushing injuries	Potassium excess
	Plasma to interstitial fluid shift
Head injury	Sodium deficit
SIADH	Sodium deficit
Congestive heart failure	Fluid volume excess
Acute pancreatitis	Calcium deficit
	Magnesium deficit
	Hypovolemia
Selected tumors	Calcium excess
Diabetes	Metabolic acidosis
	Fluid volume deficit
Emphysema	Respiratory acidosis
Diuretic therapy	Potassium excess
	Potassium deficit
Prolonged immobilization	Calcium excess
Cirrhosis (hepatic)	Fluid volume excess
	Sodium deficit

SIADH = syndrome of inappropriate antidiuretic hormone.

Medications

A thorough medication history should be obtained because any medications or therapeutic regimens, such as steroids or total parenteral nutrition, have the potential to disrupt fluid or electrolyte balance. Potassium-depleting diuretics cause this problem. Conversely, potassium-sparing diuretics may cause the opposite problems anticipated with the use of diuretics, that of potassium excess. Overuse of laxatives may result in potassium deficits.

Intake and Output

Has the patient suffered a large loss of body fluids from vomiting, diarrhea, or lack of intake? Has the patient suffered dietary alterations or medically imposed dietary restrictions? Questions should be asked of the patient to try to elicit any discrepancies in intake and output. Is the patient producing copious amounts of urine, or is the patient drinking large amounts of plain water? Has the patient experienced any draining wounds or high-output fistulas that would cause a discrepancy between intake and output? The answers to these questions must be examined very carefully when the history is analyzed and must be kept in mind as the clinical assessment is begun.

CLINICAL ASSESSMENT

The clinical assessment of a patient includes an initial intake assessment as well as ongoing assessments to monitor a patient's progress and response to therapy. A systems approach is recommended to assess for fluid and electrolyte balances related to intravenous therapy.

Body Weight

An accurate body weight is one of the initial clinical assessment parameters. Body weight and changes in it accurately reflect fluid loss or fluid gain. It is sometimes easier to obtain an accurate weight or to accurately determine change in weight rather than to depend on an accurate intake and output record. Rapid changes in the patient's body weight can reflect problems with the fluid balance status. One way to approximate the amount of gain or loss of fluid is to compare the equivalent between kilograms and liters of fluid. One kilogram, or 2.2 lb of body weight, is thought to be approximately equivalent to the gain or loss of one liter of fluid. Expressed in pounds, 500 ml of fluid would be equivalent to a gain or loss of 1 lb.

This gain or loss is usually a rapid one. It is usually compared with what is called the "dry weight" of an individual. Even under conditions of starvation, a person will lose no more than 1/3 to 1/2 lb of dry weight a day. Obtaining daily weight assessments is a very important parameter in monitoring for rapid weight gain or loss. If total fluid intake is less than total fluid output, the loss or gain may be categorized as mild, moderate, or severe (Table 18–2).

Third spacing occurs when a patient has a fluid volume deficit of the extracellular space. Body weight is basically unchanged, however, because the loss of fluid is from the extracellular space to other body compartments.

For accurate weights to be obtained, the patient should be weighed at the same time every day, preferably in the morning before breakfast and after voiding. The same scale should be used for each weighing, and the patient should wear the same- or similar-weight clothing.

Intake and Output

Intake and output is a clinical parameter that is used on a daily basis but unfortunately is not always as accurate as hoped. Intake and output can be recorded as a result of nursing judgment and a nursing order; a physician's order is not necessary. The intake and output should approximate one another, maintaining a balance between all sources in and all sources out in any 24-hour period.

The nurse should ask several questions in the course of monitoring and evaluating the patient.

1. How much is the patient drinking? Is it at least 1500 ml of fluid per day if the patient is allowed oral intake?
2. How much is the patient urinating?
3. What does the urine look like? Is it dilute without odor, or is it very concentrated and highly odoriferous?
4. What is the texture of the skin? Is it dry? Is it loose? Is it overly moist or firm?
5. Does the patient have a fever?
6. Is the patient perspiring excessively?

Table 18-2

Rapid Fluid Gain or Loss in the Adult

Category	Fluid Volume Excess (%)	Fluid Volume Deficit (%)
Mild	2	2
Moderate	5	5
Severe	≥8	≥8

7. Is the patient experiencing excessive drainage anywhere, including nasogastric tubes, fistulas, or any portal from which the patient could lose fluids? It is important to include those amounts in the daily intake and output record.

There are many ways to ensure accurate recording of intake and output. First, the importance of the patient's record should be stressed to the clinical staff and to the patient and family so that all may assist in recording all intake and output. If the patient is undergoing parenteral fluid replacement, it is important to remember that intravenous fluid containers may have an overfill of up to 10%. This means that a liter container of fluid may actually contain 1100 ml of fluid rather than the 1000 ml printed on the container by the manufacturer. Whenever possible, intake and output amounts should be measured rather than guessed. In addition, *all* input, such as ice chips (a 200-ml glass of ice chips could equal approximately 100 ml of water) must be recorded.

Output is often referred to as either sensible or insensible loss. Sensible loss is that output that is measurable, whereas insensible loss is output that is difficult to measure, such as perspiration. Water loss by perspiration should be estimated with labels such as excessive, moderate, or mild. The amount of insensible loss in an adult is considered to be 500 to 1000 ml/day.[1] Estimations of fluid from incontinence of stool or urine, wound exudate, and irrigating solutions for bladder or wounds are all important parameters to include in intake and output records. Insensible loss is also increased if respirations are increased to more than 20 per minute.[2] Eight-hour intake and output totals and 24-hour intake and output totals should be reviewed in any patient who is in a delicate state of fluid balance or in imbalance.

Urine Volume and Concentration

During the process of clinical assessment, a nurse needs to be mindful of several things to understand urine volume and concentration and to use that knowledge. Naturally, an accurate intake and output record is extremely important.

Normal urine output averages about 1 ml/kg body weight/hour, or approximately 1500 ml in a 24-hour period in a healthy adult. The urine output can be as small as 1000 ml or as great as 2000 ml in a 24-hour period, which is an average of approximately 40–80 ml/hour in a healthy adult. Children have lesser amounts of urine volume, based on their age and weight. When the body is under stress, urine output may be less than normal because of increased aldosterone and antidiuretic hormone secretion. In stress periods, this may lead to an average of 30–50 ml per hour.

Low or high urine volumes may indicate a fluid imbalance. Urine osmolality and specific gravity give further information on this issue. Urine osmolality is the measure of the number of particles per unit of water. The average normal value is 500–800 mOsm/liter. Again, this value depends on the amount of antidiuretic hormone that is in the blood stream and the rate that solutes are excreted through the kidneys. Urine osmolality more accurately reflects changes in urine content than specific gravity does. The urine osmolality depends on the state of hydration. On average, urine osmolality should be approximately 1.5 times that of the serum osmolality.

Urine specific gravity averages from 1.002 to 1.030. The range of urine specific gravity is a measure of the amount of solutes in the urine and gives a picture of the patient's state of hydration. Urine specific gravity increases with any condition that causes hypoperfusion in the kidneys. Hypoperfusion may lead to oliguria, shock, or severe dehydration. The urine specific gravity decreases when the renal tubules are no longer able to reabsorb water and concentrate urine. This phenomenon would occur, for example, during the early stages of pyelonephritis.

It is also wise to look at urine pH, which may range from 4.5 to 8.0, with an average of 6.0. Urine pH increases in metabolic and respiratory alkalosis and decreases in the presence of uric acid stones or metabolic and respiratory acidosis.

It is important to understand and discriminate between the differences in water diuresis and solute diuresis. A low urinary specific gravity, a low urinary osmolality, and a normal or elevated serum sodium level can indicate either a lack of antidiuretic hormone or the inability of the renal tubules to respond properly. These findings indicate water diuresis.

Solute diuresis occurs when impaired tubular absorption of a solute occurs. Symptoms of solute diuresis are a high urinary specific gravity, a high urinary osmolality, and a normal or low serum sodium level. Solute diuresis may occur in such states as diabetes mellitus or the correction of bladder obstruction.

Water diuresis and solute diuresis usually occur in conjunction with polyuria. The interplay and responsiveness to feedback systems between filtration, reabsorption, and secretion determine the volume and composition of urine released from the body. Diluting and concentrating mechanisms of the nephrons maintain fluid volume in the presence of normal renal blood flow. Dilution results from the kidney's reabsorption of solute, but not the accompanying water. Concentration of urine is the result of reabsorption of water without solute.

Based on this information, it is apparent that the amount of solute and the amount of waste product in the urine can influence volume. In other words, urine volume would be increased in conditions that cause high levels of solute in the urine. The amount of circulating volume in the extracellular space also affects urine volume. Hypovolemia can result in decreased urinary output. Hypervolemia can cause increased urinary output in the presence of normal renal function.

The color of urine normally ranges from pale yellow to deep amber, depending on the degree of urine concentration. Some color changes can occur because of medications or types of food ingested.

Vital Signs

The measurement of vital signs gives important information on the patient's fluid and electrolyte imbalance.

Blood Pressure. Changes in blood pressure may be associated with fluid volume status. Postural hypotension may indicate a fluid volume deficit. Electrolyte alterations may cause fluctuations in blood pressure as well. For example, magnesium deficits may cause hypertension, as may extracellular fluid volume excesses. Sodium excess may cause hypotension and postural hypotension. Potassium alterations may cause hypotension. Good baseline blood pressure measurements and accurate blood pressure monitoring assist in early recognition of, as well as the monitoring of, fluid and electrolyte status.

Respirations. Respirations should be assessed for their depth, rate, and effectiveness because respiration is affected by various alterations. Potassium alterations may cause weakness, or possibly paralysis, of respiratory muscles. Fluid volume excess affects respirations because of the increased effort required to move air in and out of the lungs. Respiration is also altered, as a compensatory mechanism, in the presence of acid-base balance deficiencies. Moist rales in the absence of cardiopulmonary disease indicate fluid volume excess.[3]

Pulse. The quality and rate of the pulse indicate how the patient is tolerating extracellular fluid. Examination of hand veins can provide a way of evaluating plasma volume. When the hand is elevated, the veins will empty in 3 to 5 seconds, and when it is lowered, they will fill in the same amount of time. Filling that takes longer than 3 to 5 seconds may indicate sodium depletion and extracellular dehydration.[4] Slow emptying of the peripheral veins indicates overhydration and excessive blood volume.[3]

Temperature. Body temperature may increase or decrease in response to fluid and electrolyte imbalances. The skin temperature and the core body temperature should be noted when fluid and electrolyte status are assessed. Changes in skin temperature are discussed later in this chapter.

Core body temperature may be decreased in the presence of fluid deficit, or it may become elevated in response to electrolyte imbalances. For example, hypernatremia may cause an elevation of body temperature.

Temperature elevations increase the fluid requirements of the body. A temperature between 101 F and 103 F increases the 24-hour fluid requirement by at least 500 ml, and a temperature above 103 F increases it by a minimum of 1000 ml. Because of increased fluid requirements with fever or temperature elevation, if extra fluid requirements are not met, additional fluid and electrolyte imbalances may occur.

Hemodynamic Monitoring

Fluid volume alterations may be detected through the use of various hemodynamic monitoring techniques. Central venous pressure (CVP) gives information on the status of intravascular volume. The CVP may be measured with a water manometer or with an electronic transducer. Normal CVP values are 8 to 10 cm of water.

The CVP measurement reflects right atrial pressure or the filling of the right side of the heart, known as *preload*; this measurement can be used as a guide to volume replacement. When fluid challenges are performed, the way in which the right atrial pressure responds provides important information regarding the patient's fluid and cardiovascular status.

The CVP can be estimated during the physical examination. With a patient in a supine position, the jugular veins are visually examined for distention. The jugular vein should be distended in this position because it is then at the same level as the right atrium. The patient can then be slowly raised to

a sitting position. When the patient comes to the sitting position, the upper portion of the jugular vein will collapse, but a bulge may be seen where blood vessel distention is still occurring within the vessel.

The distance between the bulge or point of distention and the right atrium is then a measure of central venous pressure. When a person is in a fully upright position, the sternal notch is approximately 5 cm above the right atrium. Measurable distention of the jugular vein above the sternal notch in centimeters is then added to the 5 cm: the resulting value is the CVP. If the jugular veins are not visualized above the clavicle, it is assumed that the CVP is less than 5 cm of water. (Normal CVP values are 8 to 10 cm of water.)

CVP adequately reflects right atrial pressure only in a person with a normal cardiac status. When myocardial dysfunction exists, especially in the presence of right-sided heart failure, the jugular venous pressure is elevated, regardless of the patient's extracellular volume.

Various pressures within the cardiac and pulmonary systems can be measured by use of a Swan-Ganz catheter. Single pressure measurements may be useful, but an advantage of intravenous pressure monitoring is the ability to evaluate pressures over time. The CVP or the pulmonary artery catheter can provide a means to monitor a patient's response to therapy for the correction of volume depletion, as well as determining the volume status of the patient.[5]

Tissue Turgor

The assessment of tissue turgor assists the nurse in evaluating the amount of fluid available to the tissues. Tissue turgor is tested by grasping the skin between the fingers in a pinching action, then releasing the tissue and observing the "tented" skin. If a person is in fluid volume deficit, the skin that has been pinched remains in the pinched or tented position for an extended period of time (usually longer than 3 seconds).

Tissue turgor describes the elasticity available to the skin, which depends, in part, on the presence of interstitial fluid. Tissue turgor is an age-related phenomenon; the geriatric patient commonly has poor skin turgor because the skin loses elasticity with age. Turgor may also be tested over the sternum, the forehead, or the inner aspect of the thighs. Using the skin over the sternum gives the best indication of skin turgor. The tongue can also give information on fluid balance. A person with normal hydration status has one longitudinal furrow. In a dehydrated patient, additional furrows are present, and the tongue may actually appear smaller. Tongue turgor is generally not affected by age, as is skin turgor.

Thirst

The sensation of thirst is a normal function of the body that encourages the system to ingest sufficient amounts of water needed for metabolism. If a person has suffered water losses, the thirst mechanism encourages him or her to attempt to ingest more water. If the thirst mechanism fails for some reason, a patient may be at risk for developing hypernatremia as a result of lack of circulating fluid.

The thirst mechanism is affected only if the patient is conscious or has water available. The use of antianxiety agents, sedatives, or hypnotics can lead to confusion and disorientation, causing a patient to forget to drink fluid.[3] Psychogenic alterations can also encourage the patient to drink copious amounts of water, thereby leading to water intoxication and placing the patient in danger of fluid volume overload. People expressing a sense of thirst may often complain of a dry mouth; however, a dry mouth may also result from a person using excessive mouth breathing. Oral dryness resulting from mouth breathing can be differentiated from dryness resulting from fluid volume deficit by an examination of the membrane inside the cheek and gum. When this area is dry, the dry mouth results from fluid volume deficit.

Appearance of the Skin

Assessment of the skin may provide clues to the patient's fluid status. These changes are related to the amount of fluid in the interstitium. For example, in extracellular fluid volume deficits, the skin and mucous membranes are dry. Skin appears cold and clammy and possibly cyanotic if the patient is progressing to shock. Conversely, in intracellular fluid volume deficits, the skin may be warm and flushed. The skin may feel cool and clammy in acute pancreatitis, whereas in respiratory acidosis, it may appear warm and flushed.

Edema

Edema is the retention of excessive fluid in the interstitial space. Edema may be classified as *pitting* or *dependent*. Systemic symptoms seen in edema are weight gain, high blood pressure, and dyspnea. Pitting edema is generally not seen until there has been a weight gain of 10% of body weight or retention of 5 to 10 lb of excess fluid. Pitting edema is identified by pressing into the tissue with the fingers. If an indentation from the fingers remains, pitting edema is present. It is best to test the ankles or feet of an ambulatory person or the sacral area of a bedridden person. A more accurate means of determining edema is by daily measurement with a measuring tape. Pitting is classified from a +1 to a +4, with 4 being the most severe.

Dependent edema is generally related to gravity. Fluid accumulates in any portion of the body that is dependent. If a person is ambulatory, dependent edema may be seen mostly in the feet and ankles, or possibly in the buttocks if the patient has been sitting for a long period of time. The sacral area of the patient on bed rest should be evaluated for dependent edema.

Some edema is refractory, meaning that it persists after appropriate therapy, such as diuretics or salt-restricted diets, has been implemented. Persons with refractory edema may have persistent weight gain and are usually hypertensive. Edema usually results from an increase in the total body sodium content. Circulatory overload may cause edema and is generally associated with heart failure, which could result from sodium and water retention, or renal failure, resulting from sodium and water retention.

Edema may also be associated with overly aggressive infusion of hypertonic intravenous solutions. The cause of this edema is generally thought to be a rise in plasma hydrostatic pressure, which forces fluid into the interstitial spaces. Edema may also occur when low plasma protein is present, resulting in decreased plasma oncotic pressure. A decrease in plasma protein occurs in kidney disease, when there is a loss of protein, cirrhosis, serous drainage, or hemorrhage. Edema may also be associated with interference in venous return or obstruction of the lymphatic system.

It is important to remember that edema may manifest itself in various ways, not just in dependent areas of the body. The patient's history may reveal such symptoms as swollen feet, the feeling of a tightness in the lower legs, or puffiness of the face or fingers. Rings may fit too tightly. A patient may complain of a rapid weight gain. If the lungs or heart are involved, a patient may speak of dyspnea on exertion or at night. Obtaining daily weights can be beneficial in identifying and monitoring the edematous state and its treatment.

Tearing and Salivation

Tearing and salivation are most useful in assessing fluid balance in an infant or child. If a child is suffering from a fluid volume deficit of moderate proportions, tearing and salivation will not occur.

Behavioral and Sensory Changes

Behavioral changes may occur in relation to fluid and electrolyte imbalance. If a patient is suffering from a fluid deficit, he or she may be apprehensive and restless. Coma may occur in severe cases. Fluid volume excess may cause hyperirritability, disorientation, and mental disturbances. Metabolic acidosis may cause apathy, disorientation, delirium, or stupor. Metabolic alkalosis may cause belligerence, irritability, disorientation, or lethargy. Potassium deficit may cause changes in speech, lethargy, apathy, irritability, and mental confusion. Calcium excess may cause lethargy, exhaustion, mental confusion, a loss of interest in surroundings, and irritability. Magnesium deficiency may cause hallucinations, illusions, extreme confusion, or aggressive behavior. As seen by these examples, it is important to have a baseline understanding of a patient's normal behavior and reaction to his or her surroundings so that subtle changes in behavior can be recognized.

LABORATORY DATA

Obtaining and evaluating a patient's laboratory data is an important adjunct to the physical and clinical assessment. Laboratory data most useful in evaluating fluid and electrolyte status are the blood urea nitrogen, serum creatinine, hematocrit, hemoglobin, serum osmolality, and serum electrolyte values (sodium, potassium, chloride, calcium, magnesium, phosphate, and bicarbonate), as well as arterial blood gases (pH, PaO_2, $PaCO_2$, bicarbonate, and base excess). Table 18–3 provides normal values for the above-mentioned tests, as well as other parameters that are useful in evaluating patients with other problems related to intravenous therapy.

Table 18–3

Selected Laboratory Values

Parameter		Parameter	
Blood chemistry/electrolytes	**Normal values**	**Blood chemistry/electrolytes** (Continued)	**Normal values** (Continued)
Blood urea nitrogen (BUN)	10–20 mg/dL		
Serum creatinine	0.7–1.5 mg/dL	Magnesium	1.3–2.1 mEq/liter or 1.8–3.0 mg/dL
Creatinine clearance	Male: 110–150 ml/min	Chloride	97–110 mEq/liter
	Female: 105–132 ml/min	Carbon dioxide	24–30 mmol/liter
BUN:creatinine ratio	10:1	Phosphate	Adults: 2.5–4.5 mg/dL (1.8–2.6 mEq/liter)
Hematocrit	Male: 44–52%		Children: 4.0–7.0 mg/dL (2.3–4.1 mEq/liter)
	Female: 39–47%	Zinc	77–137 μg/dL (by atomic absorption)
Hemoglobin	Male: 13.5–18.0 g/dL	Lithium	0.8 mEq/liter (therapeutic level 8–12 hours after
	Female: 12.0–16.0 g/dL		administration)
Red blood cells	Male: 4600–6000/mm³		
	Female: 4200–5400/mm³	Serum proteins	
Mean corpuscular volume	80–95 mm³	Total	6.0–8.00 g/dL
Mean corpuscular hemoglobin	26–34 pg	Albumin	3.5–5.5 g/dL
Mean corpuscular hemoglobin	32–36%	Globulin	1.5–3.0 g/dL
concentration		Lactate (arterial blood)	4.5–14.4 mg/dL
Complete blood count		Serum ketones	Often >50 mg/dL in diabetic ketoacidosis
Total leukocytes	4500–11,000/mm³		Usually under 20 mg/dL in salicylate intoxication
Myelocytes	0	Serum salicylates	Therapeutic range: 20–25 mg/dL
Band neutrophils	150–400/mm³ (3–5%)		Toxic range: >30 mg/dL
Segmented neutrophils	3000–5800/mm³ (54–62%)	Anion gap	12–15 mEq/liter
Lymphocytes	1500–3000/mm³ (25–33%)	Aspartate aminotransferase (AST)	7–40 mμ/ml (30 C)
Monocytes	300–500/mm³ (3–7%)	Alanine aminotransferase (ALT)	5/35 mμ/ml (37 C)
Eosinophils	50–250/mm³ (1–3%)	Alkaline phosphatase	20–90 mμ/ml (30 C)
Basophils	15–50/mm³ (0–0.75%)	Serum bilirubin	
Platelets	150,000–300,000/mm³	Total	0.3–1.1 mg/dL
Reticulocytes	0.5–1.5%	Direct	0.1–0.4 mg/dL
Red cell volume	Male: 20–36 ml/kg	Indirect	0.2–0.7 mg/dL (total minus direct)
	Female: 19–31 ml/kg	Lactate dehydrogenase [LOW]	100–190 mμ/ml
Plasma volume	Male: 25–43 ml/kg	Urine chemistry/electrolytes*	
	Female: 28–45 ml/kg	Sodium	80–180 mEq/24 hours (varies with Na⁺ intake)
Clotting time	8–18 minutes	Potassium	40–80 mEq/24 hours (varies with dietary
Prothrombin time	11–15 seconds		intake)
Iron	60–90 μg/dL	Chloride	100–250 mEq/24 hours
Total iron-binding capacity	250–420 μg/dL	Calcium	100–150 mg/24 hours (if on average diet)
(TIBC)			Varies with dietary intake
Serum transferrin	>200 mg/dl (measured directly)	Osmolality	Typical urine is 500–800 (mOsm/liter [extreme
	(0.8 TIBC) −4.3 estimated from TIBC)		range is 50–1400 mOsm/liter])
Partial thromboplastin time	Standard: 68–82 seconds		Usually about 1½–3 times greater than serum
	Activated: 32–46 seconds		osmolality
Fibrinogen	160–415 mg/dL	Specific gravity (SG)	1.002–1.030 (most random samples have an SG of
Serum osmolality	280–295 mOsm/kg		1.012–1.025)
Serum amylase	25–125 mμ/ml	pH	4.5–8.0
Serum glucose	70–110 mg/dL	Arterial blood gases	
Serum electrolytes		pH	7.35–7.45
Sodium	135–145 mEq/liter	PaO₂	80–100 mm Hg
Potassium	3.5–5.0 mEq/liter	PaCO₂	38–42 mm Hg
Calcium	Total: 8.9–10.3 mg/dL or 4.6–5.1 mEq/liter	Bicarbonate	22–26 mEq/liter
	Ionized: 4.6–5.1 mg/dL	Base excess	−2 to +2

*Measurement of electrolytes may be of limited value because of recent administration of diuretics and/or lack of knowledge of dietary intake.

These values may vary among facilities. ''Normal'' values must be referenced with the laboratory performing the tests.

SUMMARY

It is imperative that nurses be competent in assessing for fluid volume and electrolyte imbalances. By using the systems approach for clinical assessment and the information obtained from the patient's medical history, one can more accurately determine a patient's current fluid and electrolyte status. The more accurate the assessment, the better the potential outcome for the patient.

References

1. Metheny NM. Fluid and Electrolyte Balances: Nursing Considerations, 2nd ed. Philadelphia: J. B. Lippincott, 1992.
2. Metheny NM. Why worry about I.V. fluids? Am J Nurs 1990; 90(6):50–55.
3. Phillips LD. Manual of I.V. Therapeutics. Philadelphia: F. A. Davis, 1993.
4. Metheny NM. Quick Reference to Fluid Balance. Philadelphia: J. B. Lippincott, 1989.
5. Kokko J, Tannen R. Fluids and Electrolytes. Philadelphia: W. B. Saunders, 1986.

Selected Reading

American Association of Blood Banks. Technical Manual, 11th ed. Arlington, VA: American Association of Blood Banks, 1993:649–651.

Black J, Matassarin-Jacobs E. Luckman and Sorensen's Medical Surgical Nursing: A Psychophysiologic Approach, 4th ed. Philadelphia: W. B. Saunders, 1993.

Griffin J. Hematology and Immunology: Concepts for Nursing. Norwalk, CT: Appleton-Century-Crofts, 1986.

Horne M, Heitz U, Swearington P. Fluid, Electrolyte and Acid-Base Balance: A Case Study Approach. St. Louis: Mosby–Year Book, 1991.

Smith E, Kinsey M. Fluids and Electrolytes: A Conceptual Approach, 2nd ed. New York: Churchill Livingstone, 1991.

Tennebaum L. Cancer Chemotherapy: A Reference Guide. Philadelphia: W. B. Saunders, 1989.

CHAPTER 19

Intravenous Therapy Calculations

Gloria Pelletier, CRNI

A physician is responsible for ordering patient medications, but the nurse must ensure that the medication is ordered in a safe and accurate manner. This chapter primarily focuses on methods that can be used for various calculations so that the ordered medication can be administered correctly.

The responsibility for the preparation of intravenous medications often rests with the nurse. This is especially true in those institutions that have limited pharmacy coverage and in others that function without the benefit of a comprehensive pharmacy intravenous admixture program.

Even when a health care institution has a comprehensive intravenous admixture program, it is important for the nurse to remember that, although another professional prepared the medication, whoever administers any drug must verify that the correct drug is administered to the correct patient at the correct dose, rate, route, and time.

Nurses tend to have difficulty with calculations. This may be attributed to the increased demands that have been placed on them. Current technology requires the nurse to keep abreast of the many facets of nursing mandated by our profession and health care systems. As a result, nurses have become dependent on calculations completed by others without confirmation of their accuracy.

This chapter intends to help facilitate the various calculation processes associated with intravenous medication administration. It is hoped that this review can help the reader recall knowledge previously acquired.

MEASUREMENTS: METRIC SYSTEM

The metric system is universally accepted by the medical profession. It provides the most accurate means for calculating the dosage of crucial drugs. The effects of a drug administered directly into the vascular system may be immediate. The precise measurements attainable by using the metric system makes it preferable over the use of the apothecaries and household measuring systems.

Abbreviations

The units of the metric system are based on measurements of weight, volume, and length. For intravenous drug calcu-

lations, the four most frequently used weights are the kilogram (kg), gram (g), milligram (mg), and microgram (μg). As listed, the kilogram is the largest and the microgram the smallest weight. The liter (L) and milliliter (ml) are units of volume. To reduce confusion, liter is usually abbreviated as the upper case letter, because the lower case letter (l) could be mistaken for the number one. Milliliter and cubic centimeter (cc) are identical measurements (1 ml = 1 cc), but milliliter is preferred. Although units of length such as millimeter (mm) and centimeter (cm) are used, they are seldom required for intravenous dose calculations (Table 19–1).

Conversions

The metric system uses decimals for calculating fractional amounts. A larger unit can be converted to the next smaller unit by moving the decimal point three places to the right.

Example 1: A kilogram is larger than a gram, so move the decimal point three places to the right.

$$1 \text{ kilogram} = 1.000. \text{ grams}$$
$$1 \text{ milligram} = 1.000. \text{ micrograms}$$
$$1 \text{ liter} = 1.000. \text{ milliliters}$$

A smaller unit can be converted to the next larger unit by moving the decimal point three places to the left.

Example 2: A gram is smaller than a kilogram, so move the decimal point three places to the left.*

$$1 \text{ gram} = 0.001. \text{ kilograms}$$
$$1 \text{ microgram} = 0.001. \text{ milligrams}$$
$$1 \text{ milliliter} = 0.001. \text{ liters}$$

An alternate method for converting a larger unit to the next smaller unit is to multiply by 1000. To convert a smaller unit to a larger unit, divide by 1000 (Table 19–2).

CALCULATIONS

Drug Dosage Determinations

In determining dosages, most nurses are familiar with the ratio-proportion or formula method. Each method is reviewed here but it is not necessary to learn both. Readers should use their preferred method.

Ratio-Proportion Method. To use this method effectively, it must be remembered that a ratio is a comparison between two related items, and a proportion is the equality of two ratios.

---

*A zero should always be placed to the left of the decimal point when the number is less than 1. This is a precautionary measure to prevent dosage calculation errors.

Table 19-1

Metric System Abbreviations

Weight	Volume	Length
Kilogram = kg	Liter = L	Centimeter = cm
Gram = g	Milliliter = ml	Millimeter = mm
Milligram = mg	Cubic centimeter = cc	
Microgram = μg		

When setting up a ratio, place the information that is known on the left of the equal sign (=). The known information (on the drug label) is the strength of the drug on hand (H) and volume of the drug on hand (V). The ratio for the dose desired is the relationship of the dose ordered (D) and the amount to give (G), and this is placed on the right of the equal sign (=):

$$H:V = D:G$$

Thus, the strength on hand (H) is related (:) to the volume (V) as (=) the dose ordered (D) is related (:) to the amount to give (G).

For an answer to be correct, the product of the means must equal the product of the extremes. The extremes are always the two outside numbers, as in the following example.

The means are the two inside numbers.

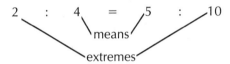

Multiply the extremes together (2 × 10 = 20). Multiply the means together (4 × 5 = 20). Thus, the product of the means equals the product of the extremes.

When one of the numbers in the proportion is unknown, identify it with an X, which represents the unknown number. Using the same example as above, the 10 is replaced with an X:

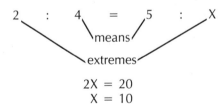

$$2X = 20$$
$$X = 10$$

Table 19-2

Metric Conversion Factors

		Weight		
1 kilogram	×	1000	=	1000 grams
1 gram	×	1000	=	1000 milligrams
1 milligram	×	1000	=	1000 micrograms
1 microgram	÷	1000	=	0.001 milligram
1 milligram	÷	1000	=	0.001 gram
1 gram	÷	1000	=	0.001 kilogram
		Volume		
1 liter	×	1000	=	1000 milliliters
1 milliliter	÷	1000	=	0.001 liter

To prove the answer is correct, replace the X with 10 and repeat the calculation process. If the product of the means equals the product of the extremes, the answer is correct.

Never assume that your initial answer is correct without completing the second equation for proof. When administering drugs into the vascular system, it is imperative that the correct dose be administered.

Formula Method. The terminology applied to the ratio-proportion method remains the same for the formula method. The equation then becomes:

$$\frac{\text{Dose ordered (D)}}{\text{Strength on hand (H)}} \times \text{volume (V)} = \text{amount to give (G)}$$

In the ratio-proportion method, the example was presented as

$$2:4 = 5:X$$

In the formula method, the example becomes

$$\frac{5}{2} \times 4 = \frac{20}{2} = 20 \div 2 = 10$$

The answer remains as 10.

Example 1: A vial contains clindamycin phosphate, 600 mg/4 ml. What volume must be given to administer 300 mg?

Ratio-Proportion Method

$$H \text{ (mg)}:V \text{ (ml)} = D \text{ (mg)}:G \text{ (ml)}$$
$$600:4 = 300:X$$
$$600X = 1200$$
$$X = 2 \text{ ml of clindamycin phosphate}$$

Proof:

$$600:4 = 300:2$$
$$1200 = 1200$$

The product of the means equals the product of the extremes.

Formula Method

$$\frac{D}{H} \times V = G$$

$$\frac{\text{Dose ordered}}{\text{Dose on hand}} \times \text{volume} = \text{amount to give}$$

$$\frac{300 \text{ mg}}{600 \text{ mg}} \times 4 \text{ ml} = \frac{1200}{600} = 1200 \div 600$$
$$= 2 \text{ ml of clindamycin phosphate}$$

Example 2: A 10-ml vial contains calcium gluconate, 0.45 mEq/ml. What volume must be given to administer 2.25 mEq?

Ratio-Proportion Method

$$H \text{ (mEq)}:V \text{ (ml)} = D \text{ (mEq)}:G \text{ (ml)}$$
$$0.45:1 = 2.25:X$$
$$0.45X = 2.25$$
$$X = 5 \text{ ml of calcium gluconate}$$

Proof:

$$0.45:1 = 2.25:5$$
$$2.25 = 2.25$$

The product of the means equals the product of the extremes.

Formula Method

$$\frac{D}{H} \times V = G$$

$$\frac{\text{Dose ordered}}{\text{Dose on hand}} \times \text{volume} = \text{amount to give}$$

$$\frac{2.25 \text{ mEq}}{0.45 \text{ mEq}} \times 1 \text{ ml} = \frac{2.25}{0.45} = 2.25 \div 0.45$$
$$= 5 \text{ ml of calcium gluconate}$$

Example 3: A vial contains cefuroxime sodium, 1.5 g/ml. What volume must be given to administer 750 mg? The dose on hand and dose ordered are not identical units of measure. Through use of the metric conversion factors (Table 19–2), grams can be converted to milligrams:

$$1.5 \text{ g} \times 1000 = 1500 \text{ mg}$$

Ratio-Proportion Method

$$H \text{ (mg)}:V \text{ (ml)} = D \text{ (mg)}:G \text{ (ml)}$$
$$1500:1 = 750:X$$
$$1500X = 750$$
$$X = 0.5 \text{ ml of cefuroxime sodium}$$

Formula Method

$$\frac{D}{H} \times V = G$$

$$\frac{\text{Dose ordered}}{\text{Dose on hand}} \times \text{volume} = \text{amount to give}$$

$$\frac{750}{1500} \times 1 = \frac{750}{1500} = 750 \div 1500$$
$$= 0.5 \text{ ml of cefuroxime sodium}$$

Percent Solutions

The majority of solutions administered intravenously are in the form of a percent solution. These solutions are administered routinely with little consideration of their composition until the nurse is required to calculate and prepare a solution that is not routinely available.

It should be understood that a percent solution is a measure of parts per hundred. This means that 1 g of a drug in 100 ml of solution is a 1% solution. A 100-ml solution containing 10 g of a drug is a 10% solution. To make 1000 ml of a 10% solution, 100 g of a drug is necessary. This can be determined through either the ratio-proportion or formula method.

Ratio-Proportion Method

$$g:ml = g:ml$$
$$10:100 = X:1000$$
$$100X = 10,000$$
$$X = 100 \text{ g of drug required for a 10\% solution}$$

Formula Method

$$\frac{10}{100} \times 1000 = \frac{10,000}{100} = 10,000 \div 100$$
$$= 100 \text{ g of drug required for a 10\% solution}$$

Earlier, in the Drug Dosage Determinations section, the examples determined the amount of drug to give. When applying these methods to percent calculations, the amount of drug to be added to the solution must be determined.

Example 1: The time is 2:00 AM and the pharmacy is not open. A 1000-ml solution of 10% dextrose and 5% amino acids in a flexible container is inadvertently punctured. Available is 50% dextrose in water, 7% amino acids, sterile water for injection, and a 1000-ml empty evacuated container. Prepare the 1000-ml solution of 10% dextrose and 5% amino acids.

Step 1: Determine the amount of 7% amino acids needed.

Ratio-Proportion Method

$$\%:ml = \%:ml$$
$$7:1000 = 5:X$$
$$7X = 5000$$
$$X = 714 \text{ ml of 7\% amino acids needed}$$

Formula Method

$$\frac{5}{7} \times 1000 = \frac{5000}{7} = 5000 \div 7$$
$$= 714 \text{ ml of 7\% amino acids needed}$$

Step 2: Determine the amount of 50% dextrose in water needed.

Ratio-Proportion Method

$$\%:ml = \%:ml$$
$$50:1000 = 10:X$$
$$50X = 10,000$$
$$X = 200 \text{ ml of 50\% dextrose in water needed}$$

Formula Method

$$\frac{10}{50} \times 1,000 = \frac{10,000}{50} = 10,000 \div 50$$
$$= 200 \text{ ml of 50\% dextrose in water needed}$$

$$\begin{array}{rl} 714 & \text{ml of 7\% amino acids} \\ + \ 200 & \text{ml of 50\% dextrose in water} \\ \hline 914 & \text{ml} \end{array}$$

A total volume of 1000 ml is needed.

$$\begin{array}{rl} 1000 & \text{ml} \\ - \ 914 & \text{ml} \\ \hline 86 & \text{ml of water for injection is needed} \end{array}$$

The combination of these three solutions in the empty evacuated container makes the 1000 ml of 10% dextrose and 5% amino acids solution.

An alternative and perhaps more difficult way to solve this problem is through the use of grams. As previously indicated, grams and percentages are interchangeable. Let us see whether this hypothesis is correct.

Step 1: A 7% amino acid solution contains 7 g/100 ml.

$$g{:}ml = g{:}ml$$
$$7{:}100 = X{:}1000$$
$$100X = 7000$$
$$X = 70 \text{ g in } 1000 \text{ ml}$$

Needed: 5% amino acid solution

$$g{:}ml = g{:}ml$$
$$5{:}100 = X{:}1000$$
$$100X = 5000$$
$$X = 50 \text{ g in } 1000 \text{ ml}$$

We now know that there are 70 g in 1000 ml of 7% amino acids, and that 50 g are needed.

$$g{:}ml = g{:}ml$$
$$70{:}1{,}000 = 50{:}X$$
$$70X = 50{,}000$$
$$X = 714 \text{ ml of 7% amino acids needed}$$

Step 2: 50% dextrose in water contains 50 g/100 ml.

$$g{:}ml = g{:}ml$$
$$50{:}100 = X{:}1000$$
$$100X = 50{,}000$$
$$X = 500 \text{ g in } 1000 \text{ ml}$$

Needed: 10% dextrose in water

$$g{:}ml = g{:}ml$$
$$10{:}100 = X{:}1000$$
$$100X = 10{,}000$$
$$X = 100 \text{ g}$$

We now know that there are 500 g in 1000 ml of 50% dextrose in water, and that 100 g are needed.

$$g{:}ml = g{:}ml$$
$$500{:}1{,}000 = 100{:}X$$
$$500X = 100{,}000$$
$$X = 200 \text{ ml}$$

$$\begin{array}{rl}
714 & \text{ml of 7% amino acids} \\
+ \ 200 & \text{ml of 50% dextrose in water} \\
\hline
914 & \text{ml, which is identical to the previous,} \\
& \text{less complicated calculation process}
\end{array}$$

Example 2: A 10-ml vial contains 10% calcium chloride. What volume must be given to administer 700 mg? Recall that a 10% solution contains 10 g of drug in 100 ml, and that grams and percentages are interchangeable.

Ratio-Proportion Method

$$g{:}ml = g{:}ml$$
$$10{:}100 = X{:}10$$
$$100X = 100$$
$$X = 1 \text{ g of calcium chloride in } 10 \text{ ml}$$

Formula Method

$$\frac{10 \text{ g}}{100 \text{ ml}} \times 10 \text{ ml} = \frac{100}{100}$$
$$= 1 \text{ g of calcium chloride in } 10 \text{ ml}$$

Grams and milligrams are not identical units of measure, so convert the gram to milligrams (Table 19–2).
$$1 \text{ g} \times 1000 = 1000 \text{ mg}$$

Ratio-Proportion Method

$$mg{:}ml = mg{:}ml$$
$$1000{:}10 = 700{:}X$$
$$1000X = 7000$$
$$X = 7 \text{ ml of 10% calcium chloride,}$$
$$\text{which is equal to } 700 \text{ mg}$$

Formula Method

$$\frac{700 \text{ mg}}{1000 \text{ mg}} \times 10 \text{ ml} = \frac{7000}{1000} = 7000 \div 1000$$
$$= 7 \text{ ml of calcium chloride}$$

Example 3: A 30-ml vial contains 23.4% sodium chloride. What volume must be added to 500 ml of 10% dextrose in water to make a 10% dextrose in 0.225% sodium chloride solution?

Ratio-Proportion Method

$$\%{:}ml = \%{:}ml$$
$$23.4{:}500 = 0.225{:}X$$
$$23.4X = 112.5$$
$$X = 4.8 \text{ ml (rounded to nearest}$$
$$0.1 \text{ ml of 23.4% sodium chloride)}$$

Formula Method

$$\frac{0.225\%}{23.4\%} \times 500 \text{ ml} = \frac{112.5}{23.4} = 112.5 \div 23.4 = 4.8 \text{ ml}$$
$$\text{(rounded to nearest 0.1 ml of 23.4% sodium chloride)}$$

Units

A unit may be defined as a measurement of specific drugs. The number of units in a specific drug is based on the strength of that drug. A unit is not interchangeable with any other measurement, but dosages can be calculated through use of the methods discussed earlier.

An abbreviation for unit is U. Accuracy is crucial when administering a drug based on unit strength, and it is imperative that the ordered dose not be exceeded. The abbreviation of U may erroneously be interpreted as a zero, so it is recommended that the term ''unit'' always be written out.

Insulin was formerly available as 40 units/ml and 80 units/ml. To standardize the concentration and reduce the potential for dosage error, production of these preparations is on the decline.

The following examples of insulin calculations refer to 100 units/ml, which is the concentration most commonly used. Some institutions have eliminated use of the 100-unit syringe for the administration of 100 units/ml insulin. They believe that the availability of 100 units/ml insulin reduces the absolute need for use of an insulin syringe. An identical level of accuracy can be obtained with the 1-ml tuberculin

(TB) syringe. The number of insulin units required is always equal to an equivalent number of hundredths of a milliliter. Although the syringe adopted by the institution should prevail, profound attention and caution by the nurse are required when the 1-ml TB syringe is used for the administration of 100 units/ml insulin. On one side of the syringe is the 1-ml scale. The calibration is broken down to tenths and hundredths of a milliliter. Next to the 1-ml scale is a section not identified but recognized as a minim scale. There is absolutely no reason for the use of minims in drug calculations. Personnel using the TB syringe must use extreme caution so that the minim scale is not used when preparing drugs.

Profound attention is mandatory. *Do not* relate tenths of milliliters with units. For example, when drawing up 8 units of insulin, there is a tendency to draw up 0.8 ml, which equals 80 units rather than 8 units.

Example 1: How much 100 units/ml insulin is needed to administer 40 units? (When using a 100-unit syringe, draw up insulin to the 40-unit calibration mark.)

When using a TB syringe, one of the following methods can help in preparing the correct dose.

Ratio-Proportion Method

units:ml = units:ml
100:1 = 40:X
100X = 40
X = 0.4 ml of 100 units/ml needed to give 40 units

Formula Method

$$\frac{40 \text{ units}}{100 \text{ units}} \times 1 \text{ ml} = \frac{40}{100} = 40 \div 100$$
$$= 0.4 \text{ ml of } 100 \text{ units/ml needed to give } 40 \text{ units}$$

Example 2: A heparin solution contains 25,000 units in 500 ml of 5% dextrose in water. The administration rate is 16 ml/hour. What is the hourly heparin dose?

Ratio-Proportion Method

units:ml = units:ml
25,000:500 = X:16
500X = 400,000
X = 800 units/hour

Formula Method

$$\frac{16 \text{ ml}}{500 \text{ ml}} \times 25,000 \text{ units} = \frac{400,000}{500}$$
$$= 400,000 \div 500 = 800 \text{ units/hour}$$

Example 3: A vial of penicillin G potassium contains 200,000 units/ml. What volume must be added to a solution to administer 4,000,000 units?

Ratio-Proportion Method

units:ml = units:ml
200,000:1 = 4,000,000:X
200,000X = 4,000,000
X = 20 ml of drug are needed

Formula Method

$$\frac{4,000,000 \text{ units}}{200,000 \text{ units}} \times 1 \text{ ml} = \frac{4,000,000}{200,000} = 4,000,000 \div 200,000$$
$$= 20 \text{ ml of drug are needed}$$

Milliequivalents

A milliequivalent (mEq) is not interchangeable with any other measurement, but dosages can be calculated through the use of the methods discussed earlier.

Example 1: A vial of calcium gluconate contains 0.45 mEq of calcium/ml. How much must be added to a solution for a dose of 9 mEq?

Ratio-Proportion Method

mEq:ml = mEq:ml
0.45:1 = 9:X
0.45X = 9
X = 20 ml of drug are needed

Formula Method

$$\frac{9 \text{ mEq}}{0.45 \text{ mEq}} \times 1 \text{ ml} = \frac{9}{0.45} = 9 \div 0.45$$
$$= 20 \text{ ml of drug are needed}$$

Example 2: A 500-ml solution contains 40 mEq of potassium acetate. The rate ordered is 50 ml/hour. How much potassium is being administered hourly?

Ratio-Proportion Method

mEq:ml = mEq:ml
40:500 = X:50
500X = 2000
X = 4 mEq/hour

Formula Method

$$\frac{50 \text{ mEq}}{500 \text{ mEq}} \times 40 \text{ ml} = \frac{2000}{500} = 2000 \div 500$$
$$= 4 \text{ mEq/hour}$$

Example 3: A 50-ml vial of sodium bicarbonate contains 44.6 mEq. What volume must be given to administer 25 mEq?

Ratio-Proportion Method

mEq:ml = mEq:ml
44.6:50 = 25:X
44.6X = 1250
X = 28 ml need to be given

Formula Method

$$\frac{25 \text{ mEq}}{44.6 \text{ mEq}} \times 50 \text{ ml} = \frac{1250}{44.6} = 1250 \div 44.6$$
$$= 28 \text{ ml need to be given}$$

Body Surface Area

Use of the body surface area (BSA) parameter is one of the most accurate methods for calculating adult drug dosages. This method is frequently used to determine dosages for antineoplastic agents.

To determine the BSA, the height and weight of the patient must be known and a nomogram chart must be available. The West nomogram (Figure 19–1), most applicable for determining the BSA in children, is also appropriate for use with adults. This nomogram is one of several available for this purpose.

Nomogram Procedure

1. Find the patient's height in the column labeled height.
2. Find the patient's weight in the column labeled weight.
3. Using a ruler or straight edge, draw a straight line between these two values.
4. In the BSA column, note where the line intersects. This value represents the BSA in square meters (m^2).

Example 1: What is the BSA for a patient who weighs 130 lb and is 60 in tall?

Drawing a line between 68 in and 130 lb on the West nomogram indicates that the BSA is 1.7 m^2.

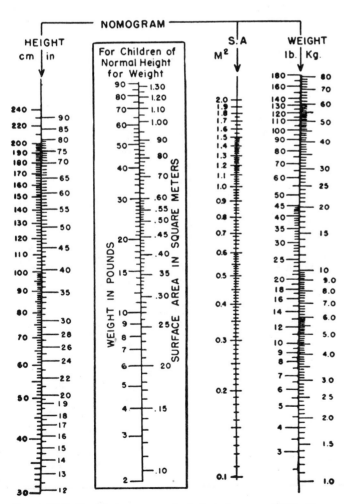

Figure 19–1. The West nomogram for body surface area (BSA). (From Behrman RE, Vaughan VC. Nelson Textbook of Pediatrics, 14th ed. Philadelphia: WB Saunders, 1992.)

Example 2: Applying the 1.7 m^2 answer above, what dose should be prepared for a patient who requires doxorubicin hydrochloride (Adriamycin), 70 mg/m^2?

$$70 \text{ mg} \times 1.7 \text{ m}^2 = 119 \text{ mg of doxorubicin hydrochloride}$$

Body Weight

There are many drugs whose dose is calculated according to the weight of a person in kilograms. The use of kilograms instead of pounds provides more precise dosage administration. The need for accuracy when preparing drugs in the form of units was discussed. Drugs based on kilograms of body weight require the same respect. An error in dosage calculations can result in irreversible consequences.

Universally, it is acceptable to consider that

$$1 \text{ kilogram (kg)} = 2.2 \text{ pounds (lb)}$$

Divide by 2.2 to convert body weight in pounds to kilograms. For example,

$$88 \text{ lb} \div 2.2 = 40 \text{ kg}$$

To prove the answer, multiply the kilograms by the 2.2 figure. The answer is in pounds:

$$40 \text{ kg} \times 2.2 = 88 \text{ lb}$$

If you forget whether to multiply or divide when determining the kilogram weight, remember that you are looking for a smaller number to work with, so that the number of kilograms is always smaller than the pound weight. Note that a gain or loss in body weight may require dosage adjustments when additional doses are ordered.

Example 1: An aminophylline dose of 6 mg/kg has been ordered for a patient who weighs 198 lbs. How much aminophylline should be administered?

Step 1: Convert pounds to kilograms.

$$198 \text{ lb} \div 2.2 = 90 \text{ kg}$$

Proof:

$$90 \text{ kg} \times 2.2 = 198 \text{ lb}$$

Step 2: Determine the ordered dose to be administered.

Ratio-Proportion Method

mg:kg = mg:kg
6:1 = X:90
1X = 540
X = 540 mg of aminophylline

Formula Method

$$\frac{6 \text{ mg}}{1 \text{ mg}} \times 90 \text{ kg} = \frac{540}{1} = 540 \text{ mg of aminophylline}$$

Example 2: An acyclovir sodium (Zovirax) dose of 15 mg/kg in three divided doses has been ordered for a 132-lb patient. How much acyclovir should be administered with each dose?

Step 1: Convert pounds to kilograms.

$$132 \text{ lb} \div 2.2 = 60 \text{ kg}$$

Proof:

$$60 \text{ kg} \times 2.2 = 132 \text{ lb}$$

Step 2: Determine the total dose ordered.

Ratio-Proportion Method

$$\begin{aligned} mg:kg &= mg:kg \\ 15:1 &= X:60 \\ 1X &= 900 \\ X &= 900 \text{ mg of acyclovir} \end{aligned}$$

Formula Method

$$\frac{15 \text{ mg}}{1 \text{ mg}} \times 60 \text{ kg} = \frac{900}{1} = 900 \text{ mg of acyclovir}$$

Step 3: Determine the amount in each dose to be administered.

$$900 \text{ mg} \div 3 = 300 \text{ mg}$$

Acyclovir sodium (Zovirax) 300 mg should be administered times three doses, for a total dose of 900 mg.

Example 3: An infusion of lidocaine hydrochloride (Xylocaine), 1 g in 500 ml of 5% dextrose in water at a rate of 20 µg/kg/min, has been ordered. The patient weighs 154 lb. Determine the rate in ml/min.

Step 1: Convert pounds to kilograms.

$$154 \text{ lb} \div 2.2 = 70 \text{ kg}$$

Step 2: Determine the ordered dose/min.

$$20 \text{ µg} \times 70 \text{ kg} = 1400 \text{ µg/min}$$

Step 3: Determine the number of micrograms in solution.

$$1 \text{ g} \times 1000 = 1000 \text{ mg}$$

$$1 \text{ mg} \times 1000 = 1{,}000{,}000 \text{ µg}$$

Step 4: Determine the ml/min dose.

Ratio-Proportion Method

$$\begin{aligned} \mu g:ml &= \mu g:ml \\ 1{,}000{,}000:500 &= 1{,}400:X \\ 1{,}000{,}000X &= 700{,}000 \\ X &= 0.7 \text{ ml/min can deliver } 20 \text{ µg/kg/min} \end{aligned}$$

Formula Method

$$\frac{1400 \text{ µg}}{1{,}000{,}000 \text{ µg}} \times 500 \text{ ml} = \frac{700{,}000}{1{,}000{,}000}$$

$$= 700{,}000 \div 1{,}000{,}000 = 0.7 \text{ ml/min can deliver } 20 \text{ µg/min}$$

Pediatric Dosage Formulas

The formulas reviewed here are not considered to be absolutely accurate for dosage determination. Dosing for the child and, in particular, the neonate also requires the evaluation of other parameters, such as clinical and laboratory values. The BSA and body weight formulas are commonly used. The remaining formulas in this section are of limited value. They are described as a reference for the reader.

The therapeutic range for neonates and children may be small and a calculation error could prove fatal. Remember to be careful when rounding off dose calculations. The following should be considered when rounding off weight or volume doses:

Weight

Less than 1 mg: round to two decimal places.

1 to 10 mg: round to one decimal place.

More than 10 mg: round to a whole number.

Volume

Less than 1 ml: round to two decimal places.

More than 1 ml: round to one decimal place.

Body Surface Area

As discussed earlier, the use of BSA is one of the most accurate methods for calculating drug dosage. There are two ways to determine a pediatric BSA:

1. If the child is considered to be of normal height and weight, refer to the section on the right of the West nomogram (see Fig. 19–1). The figure opposite the weight in pounds represents the BSA in m^2.
2. Use the actual height and weight of the child. Determine the BSA from the nomogram procedure given earlier. The BSA method is used when a dose in m^2 is ordered.

Alternatively, a pediatric dose based on an accepted adult BSA of 1.73 and the recommended adult dose can be determined. The formula is

$$\frac{\text{BSA of child } (m^2) \times \text{recommended adult dose}}{\text{BSA of adult } (1.73 \text{ m}^2)}$$

$$= \text{pediatric dose}$$

Example 1: A child weighs 22.7 kg and the height is 50 in. What is the BSA? Drawing a line between 22.7 kg and 50 in on the West nomogram indicates that the BSA is 0.9 m^2.

Example 2: A child of normal height weighs 10 kg. What is the BSA?

1. Convert 10 kg to pounds: 10 kg × 2.2 = 22 lb.
2. In accordance with the section on the right of the West nomogram (see Fig. 19–1), the BSA is 0.465 m^2.

Example 3: What is the dose for a child with a BSA of 0.7 m² if the recommended adult dose is 750 mg?

$$\frac{\text{BSA of child (m}^2) \times \text{recommended adult dose}}{\text{BSA of adult (1.73 m}^2)} = \text{pediatric dose}$$

$$\frac{0.7 \text{ m}^2 \times 750 \text{ mg}}{1.73 \text{ m}^2} = \frac{525}{1.73} = 525 \div 1.73$$
$$= 303 \text{ mg (rounded to nearest mg)}$$

Body Weight

Calculations based on body weight or BSA are the most common methods used for pediatric drug dosing. Body weight calculations appear simple, because all that is required is to convert the weight in pounds to kilograms and then multiply by the ordered dose per kilogram. Because it is one of the most frequently used methods, there is an increased potential for error. Many people use calculators or mental recall to obtain the answer. Most important, especially with pediatric dosing, is the need to verify the answers on paper.

Remember that 1 kg = 2.2 lb. Divide by 2.2 to convert body weight in pounds to kilograms.

For example,

$$22 \text{ lb} \div 2.2 = 10 \text{ kg}$$

To prove your answer, multiply the kilograms by the 2.2 figure. The answer is in pounds.

Example 1: A physician has ordered 10 mg/kg of phenytoin (Dilantin) to be administered at a rate of 0.5 mg/kg/min. The child weighs 35 lb. Determine the total dose ordered, dose per minute, and administration time.

Step 1: Convert pounds to kilograms.

$$35 \text{ lb} \div 2.2 = 15.9 \text{ kg}$$

Step 2: Determine the total dose.

$$10 \text{ mg} \times 15.9 \text{ kg} = 159 \text{ mg}$$

Step 3: Determine the dose per minute.

Ratio-Proportion Method

$$\text{mg/kg} = \text{mg/kg}$$
$$0.5{:}1 = X{:}15.9$$
$$1X = 7.95$$
$$X = 7.95 \text{ mg/min}$$

Step 4: Determine the administration time.

$$\text{mg/min} = \text{mg/min}$$
$$7.95{:}1 = 159{:}X$$
$$7.95X = 159$$
$$X = 20 \text{ minutes}$$

Formula Method

(Steps 1 and 2 remain the same.)

Step 3: Determine the dose per minute.

$$\frac{\text{Dose ordered}}{\text{per kg}} \times \text{total kg} = \text{dose/min}$$

$$\frac{0.5}{1} \times 15.9 = 7.95 \text{ mg/min}$$

Step 4: Determine the administration time.

$$\frac{\text{Min}}{\text{Dose/min}} \times \text{total dose} = \text{administration time}$$

$$\frac{1}{7.95} \times 159 = \frac{159}{7.95} = 159 \div 7.95 = 20 \text{ minutes}$$

Example 2: Tobramycin sulfate (Nebcin), 4 mg/kg, has been ordered in two divided doses for a neonate who weighs 2.86 lbs. How much should be given with each dose?

Step 1: Convert pounds to kilograms.

$$2.86 \text{ lb} \div 2.2 = 1.3 \text{ kg}$$

Step 2: Determine the total dose.

$$4 \text{ mg} \times 1.3 \text{ kg} = 5.2 \text{ mg}$$

Step 3: Determine the amount to be given with each dose.

$$5.2 \text{ mg} \div 2 \text{ doses} = 2.6 \text{ mg/dose}$$

The ratio-proportion or formula method can also be used.

Ratio-Proportion Method

$$\text{mg:dose} = \text{mg:dose}$$
$$5.2{:}2 = X{:}1$$
$$2X = 5.2$$
$$X = 2.6 \text{ mg/dose}$$

Formula Method

$$\frac{\text{Dose ordered}}{\text{Number of doses}} \times \text{each dose} = \text{mg/dose}$$

$$\frac{5.2}{2} \times 1 = \frac{5.2}{2X} = 5.2 \div 2 = 2.6 \text{ mg/dose}$$

Bastedo's Rule

Bastedo's rule determines the child's dose based on the child's age + 3 divided by 30, and on the average adult dose.

$$\frac{\text{Age (years)} + 3}{30} \times \text{average adult dose} = \text{child's dose}$$

Clark's Rule

Clark's rule determines the child's dose based on the child's weight in relation to the average adult body weight and dose.

$$\frac{\text{Weight (lb)}}{\text{Average adult weight (150 lb)}} \times \text{average adult dose}$$
$$= \text{child's dose}$$

Cowling's Rule

Cowling's rule determines the child's dose based on the child's age and the average adult dose, divided by 24.

$$\frac{\text{Age (years) on next birthday}}{24} \times \text{average adult dose}$$
$$= \text{child's dose}$$

Dilling's Rule

Dilling's rule determines the child's dose based on the child's age and average adult dose, divided by 20.

$$\frac{\text{Age (years)}}{20} \times \text{average adult dose}$$
$$= \text{child's dose}$$

Fried's Rule

Fried's rule determines the infant's dose based on the infant's age in relation to the average adult body weight and dose. This rule is effective only for infants younger than 1 year.

$$\frac{\text{Age (in months)}}{\text{Average adult weight (150 lb)}} \times \text{average adult dose}$$
$$= \text{infant's dose}$$

Young's Rule

Young's rule determines the child's dose based on the child's age and average adult dose, divided by the child's age + 12.

$$\frac{\text{Age (in years)}}{\text{Age (in years)} + 12} \times \text{average adult dose} = \text{child's dose}$$

ADMINISTRATION OF IV SOLUTIONS

Flow Rate Determination

To administer an intravenous solution accurately, the flow rate must be regulated carefully. Flow rates may be ordered in the form of an infusion over a period of hours, milliliters per hour or minute, or number of drops per minute. The responsibility for administering the solution rests on the nurse. Sets available in the institution must be evaluated and the one most appropriate for administering the solution selected. Criteria for set selection include knowledge of the flow rate required and capability of the set to deliver this rate.

When determining drops per minute the drop rate must be rounded to a whole number, because it is impossible to deliver a part or fraction of a drop. The milliliters per hour rate also needs to be rounded to a whole number when solutions are to be administered by gravity. (Specific electronic infusion devices are available that permit the administration of solutions in fractions of milliliters.)

Milliliters per Hour

Several formulas provide the information necessary for the delivery of a precise flow rate.

Three-Step Method. This method is a comprehensive flow rate calculation because it determines the rate in milliliters per hour and milliliters per minute, and also the number of drops per minute for solution administration.

Example: A physician has ordered 3000 ml of solution to be administered over a 24-hour period.

Step 1: Determine the flow rate per hour.

Formula Method

Total volume ÷ administration time = milliliters per hour

3000 ml ÷ 24 hours = 125 ml/hour

Step 2: Determine the rate per minute.

Formula Method

Milliliters per hour ÷ minutes per hour (60)
= milliliters per minute

125 ml ÷ 60 min = 2.08 ml/min

Step 3: The administration set drop factor is 15 drops (gtt)/ml. Determine the number of drops per minute.

Formula Method

Milliliters per minute × drop factor = drops per minute

2.08 ml × 15 gtt = 31.2 gtt/min (rounded to 31 gtt/min)

An infusion at this rate administers the 3000 ml over a period of 24 hours.

Ratio-Proportion Method

The same example as in the three-step method can be used to determine whether the answer is identical to that obtained with the ratio-proportion method. The example stated that a physician has ordered 3000 ml of solution to be administered over a 24-hour period.

Step 1: Determine the rate per hour.

Ratio-Proportion Method

$$
\begin{aligned}
\text{ml:hours} &= \text{ml:hours} \\
3000{:}24 &= X{:}1 \\
24X &= 3000 \\
X &= 125 \text{ ml/hour}
\end{aligned}
$$

(Determining the drops per minute is identical to the three-step method, so the calculation can continue.)

Step 2: Determine the rate per minute. Hours and minutes are not interchangeable, so convert the hour to minutes (60).

$$ml:min = ml:min$$
$$125:60 = X:1$$
$$60X = 125$$
$$X = 2.08 \text{ ml/min}$$

Step 3: The administration set drop factor is 15 gtt/min. Determine the number of drops per minute.

$$gtt:ml = gtt:ml$$
$$15:1 = X:2.08$$
$$1X = 31.2 \text{ gtt/min (rounded to 31 gtt/min)}$$

Formula Method

For the benefit of those who prefer the formula method, the same example is presented. It was given that a physician ordered 3000 ml of solution to be administered over a 24-hour period.

Step 1: Determine the rate per hour.

$$\frac{3000 \text{ ml}}{24 \text{ hours}} \times X \text{ hours}$$

$$\frac{3000}{24} = 3000 \div 24 = 125 \text{ ml/hour}$$

Step 2: Determine the rate per minute. Hours and minutes are not interchangeable, so convert the hour to minutes (60).

$$\frac{125 \text{ ml}}{60 \text{ min}} = X \text{ min}$$

$$\frac{125}{60} = 125 \div 60 = 2.08 \text{ ml/min}$$

Step 3: The administration set drop factor is 15 gtt/min. Determine the number of drops per minute.

$$\frac{15 \text{ gtt}}{1 \text{ ml}} \times 2.08 \text{ ml/min} = \frac{31.2}{1}$$
$$= 31.2 \text{ gtt/min (rounded to 31 gtt/min)}$$

Milliliters per Minute

Using the ratio-proportion and formula methods, calculations for a rate per minute in milliliters can be presented.

Example: A 10-ml vial (800 mg) of quinidine gluconate has been added to 40 ml of 5% dextrose in water. A rate of 16 mg/min is ordered. What is the milliliter per minute rate? The total volume of the solution is 50 ml (10 ml of drug + 40 ml of solution).

Ratio-Proportion Method

$$mg:ml = mg:ml$$
$$800:50 = 16:X$$
$$800X = 800 \text{ ml}$$
$$X = 1 \text{ ml/min can deliver 16 mg/min}$$

Formula Method

$$\frac{\text{Dose ordered (D)}}{\text{Strength on hand (H)}} \times \text{volume (V)} = \text{amount to give (G)}$$

$$\frac{16 \text{ mg}}{800 \text{ mg}} \times 50 \text{ ml} = \frac{800}{800}$$
$$= 1 \text{ ml/min can deliver 16 mg/min}$$

Drops per Minute

To regulate a solution accurately by the gravity method, the number of drops per minute for the infusion is required. Several methods can be used to determine the infusion rate. (Some electronic infusion devices also require that the drops per minute be programmed. Others require programming in milliliters per hour.)

The drip chamber inlet determines how many drops per minute the set can deliver. The larger the inlet, the fewer drops are required to equal 1 ml. The smaller the inlet, the more drops are required to equal 1 ml. The drop factor is usually determined by the set brand and can be found on the outer packaging. Administration drop factors to be reviewed include the following:

$$10 \text{ gtt} = 1 \text{ ml}$$
$$15 \text{ gtt} = 1 \text{ ml}$$
$$20 \text{ gtt} = 1 \text{ ml}$$
$$60 \text{ gtt} = 1 \text{ ml}$$

Excluding the 60 gtt/ml factor, all of these sets are known as macrodrop sets. The 60 gtt/ml set is known as a microdrop set and is frequently indicated for use in pediatrics and for adult infusions of solutions at rates lower than 60 ml/hour.

Method 1: This is the longest method presented because it requires that the ml/min be known before the gtt/min can be determined.

Step 1: Determine the milliliters per minute.

$$ml/hour \div 60 \text{ min/hour} = ml/min$$

Step 2: Determine the drops per minute.

$$ml/min \times \text{drop factor} = gtt/min$$

Examples: The flow rate is 90 ml/hour. What is the rate in drops per minute?

$$90 \text{ ml/hour} \div 60 \text{ min/hour} = 1.5 \text{ ml/min}$$

$$1.5 \text{ ml/min} \times 10 \text{ (drop factor)} = 15 \text{ gtt/min}$$
$$1.5 \text{ ml/min} \times 15 \text{ (drop factor)} = 23 \text{ gtt/min}$$
$$1.5 \text{ ml/min} \times 20 \text{ (drop factor)} = 30 \text{ gtt/min}$$
$$1.5 \text{ ml/min} \times 60 \text{ (drop factor)} = 90 \text{ gtt/min}$$

Method 2

$$\frac{\text{Drop factor}}{\text{Time}} \times \text{volume} = \text{flow rate}$$

The drop factor is determined by the brand or type of set to be used. The time is always 60, because there are 60 minutes in 1 hour. The volume is the amount to be infused in 1 hour. The flow rate is the infusion rate in drops per minute.

Examples

$$\frac{10 \text{ gtt/ml set}}{60 \text{ min/hour}} \times 125 \text{ ml/hour} = \frac{1250}{60}$$
$$= 1250 \div 60 = 21 \text{ gtt/min}$$

$$\frac{15 \text{ gtt/ml set}}{60 \text{ min/hour}} \times 125 \text{ ml/hour} = \frac{1875}{60}$$
$$= 1875 \div 60 = 31 \text{ gtt/min}$$

$$\frac{20 \text{ gtt/ml set}}{60 \text{ min/hour}} \times 125 \text{ ml/hour} = \frac{2500}{60}$$
$$= 2500 \div 60 = 42 \text{ gtt/min}$$

$$\frac{60 \text{ gtt/ml set}}{60 \text{ min/hour}} \times 125 \text{ ml/hour} = \frac{7500}{60}$$
$$= 7500 \div 60 = 125 \text{ gtt/min}$$

A macrodrop set is recommended for infusions over 60 ml per hour.

Method 3: This is a simple way to determine drops per minute. The milliliter per hour rate is simply divided by a specific number associated with the drop factor.

As an example, a drop factor of 15 gtt/ml means that 1 ml contains 15 drops. Mentally, associate the "15" with minutes rather than drops. There are 60 minutes in 1 hour. Divide 60 minutes by 15 "minutes" and the answer is 4. Once the milliliters per hour are known, divide this rate by 4 to obtain the drops per minute.

In the list that follows, all one needs to remember is the specific number related to the brand of administration set.

Drop Factor	Specific Number
10 gtt/ml	6
15 gtt/ml	4
20 gtt/ml	3
60 gtt/ml	1

Examples: The flow rate is 120 ml/hour. What is the rate in gtt/min?

The drop factor is 10 gtt/ml; the specific number is 6.

$$120 \div 6 = 20 \text{ gtt/min}$$

The drop factor is 15 gtt/ml; the specific number is 4.

$$120 \div 4 = 30 \text{ gtt/min}$$

The drop factor is 20 gtt/ml; the specific number is 3.

$$120 \div 3 = 40 \text{ gtt/min}$$

The drop factor is 60 gtt/ml; the specific number is 1.

$$120 \div 1 = 120 \text{ gtt/min}$$

The drop factor can also determine the milliliters per minute a solution is infusing.

Examples: A solution is being infused at a rate of 21 gtt/min. What is the ml/min rate?

The drop factor is 10 gtt/ml.

$$\frac{21}{10} = 21 \div 10 = 2.1 \text{ ml/min}$$

The drop factor is 15 gtt/ml.

$$\frac{21}{15} = 21 \div 15 = 1.4 \text{ ml/min}$$

The drop factor is 20 gtt/ml.

$$\frac{21}{20} = 21 \div 20 = 1.05 \text{ ml/min}$$

The drop factor is 60 gtt/ml.

$$\frac{21}{60} = 21 \div 60 = 0.35 \text{ ml/min}$$

Method 4: Manufacturers of solutions and administration sets provide, at no cost, specific slide rules to assist in determining drops per minute and milliliters per hour infusion rates. These devices may be obtained from the manufacturer's representative who services your facility.

Total Volume Based on Milliliters per Hour

For accurate documentation, the ability to calculate the total amount of solution a patient has received is required. This total may also need to be determined as part of the patient assessment process.

Example 1: A 1000-ml solution container has been infusing at a rate of 50 ml/hour. At the start of your shift, 150 ml have been infused. What amount of solution should be documented as IV input for your 8-hour shift?

Formula Method

Milliliters per hour × hours infused
$$= \text{amount of fluid infused}$$

50 ml × 8 hours = 400 ml infused on the 8-hour shift

Example 2: A 500-ml solution was ordered to be infused at a rate of 40 ml/hour. The rate was increased to 75 ml/hour after 3 hours. Two hours later, it was decreased to 60 ml/hour for 3 hours. What volume did the patient receive during the 8-hour period?

ml/hour × hours = fluid infused

40 ml/hour × 3 hours = 120 ml infused
75 ml/hour × 2 hours = 150 ml infused
60 ml/hour × 3 hours = 180 ml infused
450 ml infused during the 8-hour period

Length of Administration and Flow Rate

The hours for administration are based on milliliters per hour. On occasion, it may be necessary to determine the hours required for an infusion. The calculation can be completed through the use of simple arithmetic.

Formula Method

Volume to be infused (ml) ÷ ml/hour

= number of hours

Example: A physician orders that a patient receive 1000 ml of solution at a rate of 80 ml/hour, and then be discharged. Seven hours later, the patient requests an approximate discharge time. How much longer must the patient receive the infusion?

80 ml/hour × 7 hours = 560 ml infused

$$\begin{array}{rl} 1000\ ml & \text{total solution to be infused} \\ -\ 560\ ml & \text{infused} \\ \hline 440\ ml & \text{remains to be infused} \end{array}$$

Volume to be infused ÷ ml/hour = number of hours

440 ml ÷ 80 ml/hour

= 5.5 hours to infusion completion

The ratio-proportion or formula methods are also appropriate for calculating this example.

Previously discussed were formulas for converting milliliters per hour to drops per minute. The conversion of drops per minute to milliliters per hour can also be determined.

Formula Method

$$\frac{\text{Drops/min}}{\text{Drop factor}} \times 60\ \text{min/hour} = \text{ml/hour rate}$$

Example: An administration set with a drop factor of 15 gtt/ml is infusing a solution at a rate of 25 gtt/min. What is the hourly rate?

Example: An administration set with a drop factor of 15 gtt/ml is infusing a solution at a rate of 25 gtt/min. What is the hourly rate?

$$\frac{\text{gtt/min}}{\text{Drop factor}} \times 60\ \text{min/hour} = \text{ml/hour rate}$$

$$\frac{25}{15} \times 60 = 1500 \div 15 = 100\ \text{ml/hour rate}$$

Solution Container Overfill

The infusion of a medication through an administration set is known as drip administration. The infusion may take place over a period of minutes or hours. The infusion of a small volume (usually 100 ml or less) over a short period of time and/or at specific intervals is known as an intermittent infusion. An infusion of a large volume (usually over 100 ml) over a period of hours is known as a continuous infusion.

When an infusion is not completed within the calculated time frame, blame is usually placed on factors such as the administration set, roller clamp, or container head pressure. The most important factor, which is usually overlooked, is container overfill.

The exact amount of solution in a manufacturer's container is unknown. When a solution is ordered at a specific rate, it must be assumed that the total volume, including

additives, is as listed either on the manufacturer's or institution's admixture label. The most accurate solution container volumes are those compounded by the institution using an empty container. The volume listed on the admixture label, although perhaps not absolute, is the most accurate listing.

Intravenous solutions compounded by a manufacturer may contain an overfill. As presented in Table 19–3, the "Target" indicates the proposed amount to be inserted into a specific solution container. The "Acceptable Range" represents the minimum and maximum amounts of solution permitted for a specific container. Some of these solutions, such as the 150-ml glass container, may contain a 33% overfill.

Because the exact amount of solution in a container is unknown, institution policy should indicate the preferred method for the infusion rate. In policy development, consideration should be given to the following:

- Whether it is the intent of the physician that the patient receives fluids at the rate ordered
- Whether the physician is aware of solution container overfills
- The importance, if any, of infusions being completed over a specific number of hours
- Drug classifications and requirements for a consistent infusion rate

If policy determines that the ordered rate be divided by the stated container volume, the infusion time for each container should be fairly constant.

As an example (see Table 19–3), a 1000-ml plastic container of 5% dextrose in water to which 1 g of aminophylline has been added could actually contain 1130 ml:

$$\begin{array}{rl} 1090\ ml & \text{5\% dextrose in water} \\ \underline{40\ ml} & \text{aminophylline, 1 g} \\ 1130\ ml & \text{total} \end{array}$$

The ordered infusion rate is 75 ml/hour.

Depending on institution policy, if the infusion is administered at a rate exactly as ordered, it may take up to 15 hours for completion:

1130 ml ÷ 75 ml/hour = 15 hours of infusion time

Alternatively, if the infusion rate is to be based on a 1000-ml container, rate adjustments may be required. This method requires the nurse to determine the amount of solution remaining to be infused after a period of time. Based on the

Table 19–3

IV Solution Container Volumes

Label	Target (ml)	Acceptable Range (ml)
5-ml syringe	5.5	5.3– 5.8
10-ml syringe	10.8	10.3– 11.3
20-ml syringe	21.6	20.5– 22.5
150-ml glass	175	150 – 200
250-ml glass	275	250 – 300
500-ml glass	535	500 – 570
1000-ml glass	1035	1000 –1070
250-ml plastic	280	250 – 310
500-ml plastic	545	500 – 565
1000-ml plastic	1065	1000 –1090

container calibrations, the volume remaining is divided by the hours of infusion time remaining and the rate is adjusted:

$$
\begin{array}{ll}
1130\ ml & \text{total infusion over 13 hours} \\
-150\ ml & \text{75 ml/hour} \times \text{2 hours} \\
\hline
980\ ml & \text{remains to be infused 2 hours} \\
& \text{after initiation}
\end{array}
$$

$$980\ ml \div 11\ hours = 89\ ml/hour$$

An increase in rate from 75 ml/hour to 89 ml/hour at that time should result in infusion completion over 13 hours.

The author recommends that the reader select a preferred method (ratio-proportion versus formula) for specific calculations. The consistent use of a particular method results in ease of use, decreased time required, and increased accuracy of dose determinations.

Caution should be observed when devices such as calculators are used. Such devices are not infallible. Errors can be attributed to decreased battery power and to human mistakes. The slightest calculation error could be detrimental to a patient. Nurses should not rely solely on the results obtained from these devices. Calculations should be completed on paper and then, if necessary, a calculator used for answer comparison.

As stated at the beginning of this chapter, the information presented should assist in the recall of knowledge previously acquired. The application of this knowledge ensures that the dose of medication ordered is calculated accurately.

Bibliography

American Society of Hospital Pharmacists. AHFS Drug Information 94. Bethesda: American Society of Hospital Pharmacists, 1994.

Aurigemma A, Bohny B. Dosage Calculation: Method and Workbook, 3rd ed. New York: National League for Nursing, 1987.

Medici GA. Drug Dosage Calculations, 2nd ed. Norwalk, CT: Appleton and Lange, 1988.

Norville MAF. Drug Dosages and Solutions: A Workbook. Norwalk, CT: Appleton and Lange, 1988.

Wilson BA, Shannon MT. A Unified Approach to Dosage Calculation. Norwalk, CT: Appleton and Lange, 1991.

CHAPTER 20 | Obtaining Vascular Access

Roxanne Perucca, BSN, CRNI

When nurses first began to administer intravenous (IV) therapy, the sole requisite was the ability to perform a venipuncture skillfully. Today, with the technologic development of IV catheters, the use of multiple delivery systems, and the administration of highly specialized therapies, the nurse must be knowledgeable and clinically proficient to administer IV therapy safely and competently. The nurse must be committed to ensuring the delivery of safe, high-quality IV care.

Before IV therapy can be initiated, consideration must be given to the nursing process. A holistic approach is used to assess the patient's health care status, to develop and implement nursing interventions, and to evaluate patient outcomes. A nursing history is obtained to facilitate the development of a description of the whole patient. The following questions may be asked during a nursing history interview: Has the patient had previous experience with IV placement? What was the patient's outcome? What are the ramifications for the present IV interventions? What are the patient's perceptions and expectations of the prescribed therapy? The nursing history provides patients with an opportunity to express their concerns and fears related to IV therapy and to be active participants in their care.

The collection of information during the nursing history interview provides the nurse with an opportunity to assess the patient. An assessment is an ongoing observation that requires nursing judgment regarding the appropriateness of therapy and the achievement of desired patient outcomes.[1] An assessment of a patient is performed, during which consideration is given to subjective and objective information. Subjective data are contained in the patient's clinical record, including the patient's medical history and progress notes.

Examples of information that might be documented in the patient's history include previous surgeries of an upper extremity that would contraindicate future catheter placement, previous complications associated with vascular access placement, or history of IV drug abuse. The progress notes might provide information about the patient's coping mechanisms regarding IV treatment, the family support system, or the patient's compliance regarding health care.

Objective information consists of the nurse's observations and the overall status of the patient. Laboratory data, such as an abnormal red or white blood cell count, decreased platelet count, or altered coagulation factors, require nursing consideration and judgment. The condition of the skin, the fitness of the veins, and the patient's mental status are evaluated.[2] Nursing observations of torn, thin, or bruised skin require that special consideration be given to catheter insertion techniques and the application of dressings. A hypotensive, diaphoretic patient with labored respirations requires nursing interventions and decisions regarding the type and size of the IV device to be inserted. Nursing judgments are required before the placement of an IV catheter. The patient who is confused, combative, or physically restrained necessitates decisions about ensuring safety. The nurse must decide how the IV catheter can be protected to prevent the patient from pulling it out, and how to protect the patient from harm if an infiltration occurs.

The information acquired in the patient assessment requires nursing judgments based on knowledge, experience, and observations. The needs and problems of the patient are identified and prioritized into nursing diagnoses. Frequently encountered problems in the administration of IV therapy include the potential for infection, anxiety, and impairment of skin integrity.[3] A nursing care plan is developed and implemented to organize and provide goal direction to the patient's nursing care. The nursing care plan and goals must be documented and communicated to the patient and other members of the health care team. The IV nurse must plan and provide the necessary specialized interventions. The patient's outcomes are assessed by an ongoing evaluation process.

Positive patient outcomes result from the use of the nursing process and from the delivery of IV care according to established policies and procedures. Policies and procedures describe acceptable nursing interventions and actions to promote the delivery of safe, high-quality IV care. The development and implementation of IV policies and procedures should be based on established professional standards of practice. The Intravenous Nurses Society has established professional standards in the publication *Intravenous Nursing Standards of Practice.*[1]

PREPARATION OF PATIENT AND EQUIPMENT

Verification of Prescribed Therapy

The initiation of IV therapy requires a physician's order, which must be written in the patient's medical record. The order must be complete and must consist of the name of the specific solution or medication to be used; the dosage; the volume to be infused; and the rate, frequency, and route of administration. The nurse must assess and ensure that the order is appropriate for the patient. If the order is incomplete, illegible, unclear, or inappropriate, the physician should be contacted for clarification.

Compatibility Check

After the order has been verified, the nurse assesses the order and its implications for the patient. Particular attention is given to identifying allergies to medications, iodine, or tape. The current status of the patient is evaluated, and the outcome goal for the patient is reviewed.

When multiple solutions or medications are to be infused, consideration must be given to compatibility potentials. More than one infusion site may be required if the medications to be infused are incompatible. A pharmacist or pharmaceutical compatibility reference guide should be consulted to determine compatibilities.

If the compatibility of the solution or medications is not known, the IV system must be flushed with a compatible solution. The IV tubing or device can be flushed by using a syringe of 0.9% sodium chloride, or by establishing a 0.9% sodium chloride or 5% dextrose and water administration system that is used before and after the administration of incompatible medications. Some facilities have established flushing policies that take into consideration the number of medications to be administered per day. For example, if two or fewer medications are administered per day, then the IV line is flushed by using the sodium chloride syringe method. If more than two medications are to be administered per day, then a separate administration system to flush the IV line must be established.

Equipment Check

After the orders have been verified and the type of infusion system to be used has been determined, the nurse gathers the equipment. The collected solution container is verified against the physician's order regarding type of solution, volume, and whether medications are to be added. The container is checked for leaks, and the expiration date is verified. The solution is observed for clarity and particulate matter. If any questions exist regarding the IV solution, it must be returned to the dispensing department.

Initiating the Intravenous Set-Up

The following procedure may be used to begin a solution container and an IV administration tubing set:

1. Verify physician's order.
2. Gather administration set, electronic infusion device if needed, and labels.
3. Wash hands.
4. Remove container outer wrap and discard, if applicable.
5. Observe container and fluid. Check for particulate matter, cloudiness, and leaks.
6. Close roller clamp on tubing.
7. Remove protective cap from solution container.
8. Remove protective cap from administration tubing. Caution must be taken to avoid touch contamination of the tubing. If it is accidently contaminated, a new tubing must be obtained.
9. Insert administration set spike into container.
10. Hang container on IV pole.
11. Squeeze chamber to at least ⅓ to ½ full.
12. Open clamp slightly and allow tubing to fill slowly.
13. Invert medication ports and tap to clear air. If an electronic infusion device is used, purge air from tubing according to manufacturer's recommendations.
14. Close roller clamp.
15. Write date and time initiated on time strip, and tape it to solution container.
16. Document in patient's medical record the type and amount of solution, the flow rate, and medication that is added, if any.

If the IV device is to be inserted for intermittent therapy, a 2-ml syringe of 0.9% sodium chloride and an injection cap must be collected. The remaining venipuncture equipment is gathered. Start kits are advantageous because they can contain all the necessary insertion equipment except the cannula. Often, when equipment is gathered individually, an item may not be available; therefore, it is eliminated while the procedure is performed. Many start kits are available that provide any combination of the following venipuncture equipment; 70% isopropyl alcohol, antimicrobial solution, antimicrobial ointment, sterile gauze, transparent dressing, tape, tourniquet, and label. The required venipuncture equipment to be gathered is determined by the institution's policies and procedures for IV cannula insertion.

Patient Identification and Orientation

Before the IV device is inserted, patient identification must be confirmed. The patient should be asked to state his or her name. The nurse should verbally repeat the patient's name to ensure accuracy and correct patient identification. Patient identification should then be confirmed by an identification band. The patient's given name should be verified with the medical record and the physician's order sheet.

After the patient has been properly identified, the nurse identifies himself or herself to the patient. Next, the nurse assesses the psychological preparedness of the patient while explaining the following: the purpose of therapy, the possible duration of therapy, the method of administration, the insertion procedure, the expected side effects, the care and maintenance of the device, and any limitations or restrictions in mobility.

It is essential for the nurse to establish trust. The patient should be approached in a calm and reassuring manner. Encouraging the patient to ask questions provides information that helps to alleviate fear and anxiety. When answering a patient's questions, the nurse must be honest and forthright. The nurse should always convey self-assurance and appear confident.

Occasionally, despite appropriate patient teaching and reassurance, the patient remains uncooperative. These situations require careful nursing assessment and judgment. The patient has the right to refuse treatment. When the patient refuses to cooperate with the ordered medical intervention, the rationale for therapy should be re-explained and the patient's physician notified. Possible alternative routes of medication administration should be assessed with the physician and the patient. The nurse's actions and the physician's orders are recorded in the patient's medical record.

VASCULAR ASSESSMENT

After the patient has been properly identified, the nurse should provide privacy for the patient by pulling the curtain around the patient's bed, asking visitors to step outside the room, and closing the door to the patient's room. In addition, adequate lighting of the environment is essential for performing accurate venous assessments and IV insertions. If the lighting in the patient's room is inadequate, the patient may be transported to a treatment room that has adequate lighting.

The nurse then ensures that the patient is in a comfortable position. The patient should be able to extend and stabilize his or her arm on a firm, flat surface. Sometimes, it is helpful to place a pillow or roll a blanket or towel under the extended arm. Attention must also be given to the comfort of the nurse. The height of the bed can be adjusted, if necessary, to prevent unneccessary bending.

After ensuring privacy and comfort, the nurse's hands must be washed before the vascular assessment is performed. Before the venous access of the patient is evaluated, the nurse needs to consider the following rationale for the prescribed therapy: Will the prescribed therapy be long or short term? What clinical procedures are to be performed? What extremity or location does the patient prefer? Which arm is dominant? Prior consideration of these factors often determines the success of the infusion, which ultimately results in preserving the patient's veins. To determine which arm should be selected, the nurse performs an overall assessment of the patient's upper extremities. Any injury or absence of sensation to the arm restricts the use of the extremity for venipuncture.

An arteriovenous fistula or graft is inserted usually for dialysis only and requires special consideration for cannula placement. An extremity with an arteriovenous fistula or graft should not be used for routine peripheral IV insertions. The cannulation of grafts and arteriovenous fistulas should be established within institutional policies and procedures.

The placement of a cannula into the affected extremity of a patient who has undergone a cerebral vascular accident should be avoided because of the extremity's decreased or absent neurologic sensation. If the IV device infiltrates or develops phlebitis, the patient would be unable to detect these problems. Often, because of decreased mobility, the affected extremity has limited venous access potential.

The affected arm of a patient who has undergone a mas-

tectomy should be avoided. According to the *Intravenous Nursing Standards of Practice,* a physician's order is required for cannula placement in the arm of a patient who has undergone a mastectomy. Before these veins are accessed, the nurse should evaluate the patient for the presence of lymphedema and ascertain when the surgical procedure was performed. If permission for cannulation is given by the physician, the patient's arm must be closely monitored for any increase in swelling.

The application of a tourniquet promotes venous distention. The tourniquet should be applied snugly enough to impede the venous, but not the arterial, flow. To prevent the spread of nosocomial infections, tourniquets are for single-patient use. The tourniquet is applied around the upper forearm to promote dilation of the veins. A blood pressure cuff may also be used to distend veins. The cuff should be inflated and the pressure released to just below the diastolic pressure. When a patient has extremely fragile veins, the tourniquet must be applied very loosely. Sometimes, nurses elect not to apply a tourniquet if a patient bruises easily.

After the tourniquet has been applied, the veins must be given time to fill. Other methods that may be used to promote venous distention are lowering the extremity below the level of the heart and having patients open and close their fist. Lightly tapping the vein promotes venous distention; however, caution must be taken when using this method. If a vein is tapped too hard, a hematoma may occur. When these methods fail to promote venous distention, warm, moist compresses may be applied to the extremity for 10 to 15 minutes before insertion. The application of warm, moist compresses increases blood flow to the area, which promotes venous filling. Several commercial products are available that may assist in identifying the location of veins.

Veins that are tender, phlebitic, sclerotic, or located in a previously infiltrated area are unacceptable for venipuncture. If damaged veins are used for venipuncture, greater injury to the skin tissue and vascular system will occur. Also, if previous phlebitic or infiltrated areas are used for cannulation, accurate site assessments cannot be performed.

Cannulation of the lower extremities in adults should be avoided because of the increased risk of thrombophlebitis and pulmonary embolism.[4] The cannulation of lower-extremity veins is acceptable in children until they are of walking age. If a cannula is inserted in the lower extremity of an adult patient, it should be changed as soon as a central line or an appropriate site in an upper extremity can be established. Institutional policy should address the authorization and approval process for cannulation of a lower extremity.[1]

Palpation of the vein is an important assessment tool that is used to evaluate the condition of a vessel. By always using the same finger to palpate veins, one develops a sensitivity for assessing veins. Usually, the index finger and the third forefinger of the nondominant hand have the most sensitivity for palpating veins. A sclerosed vein can be identified by a hard, cordlike feeling. Successful venipuncture requires a healthy vein that feels soft and bouncy as one palpates over and across the vessel. Valves can be detected by a hard lump or knotlike feeling. Resilient veins, which are easily depressed, are required for venipuncture. Palpation helps determine if the vein is located in the superficial fascia or deep tissues. Stroking the vessel downward and observing the venous refill is helpful in determining the condition of the vein. Performing venipuncture in areas where valves are palpated or where two veins bifurcate should be avoided. The insertion site should be proximal to a valve or a bifurcation (Fig. 20–1).

Palpation also assists in differentiating arteries and veins. The selected vein must not pulsate; aberrant arteries pulsate and are located superficially in an unusual location. Frequently, aberrant arteries occur bilaterally on the hand or wrist, and usually on a thin, emaciated person. An aberrant artery should not be used for peripheral cannula insertion.

PERIPHERAL INTRAVENOUS ADMINISTRATION

Site Selection

The most distal site on the extremity should be selected for peripheral IV insertion. Peripheral IV therapy can be maintained longer by starting at the lowest point on the arm and working upward with future IV insertions. Sites located below previous insertion sites, as well as phlebitic, infiltrated, or bruised areas, should be avoided. Areas of flexion, such as the wrist or antecubital fossa, are also not recommended. The antecubital veins should be preserved for as long as possible and are not to be used for routine IV therapy. A cannula inserted in the antecubital fossa veins is at greater risk for the occurrence of mechanical phlebitis and infiltration. The metacarpal, cephalic, basilic, and median veins are recommended for venipuncture because of their size and location.

Site Preparation

Health care personnel must wash their hands before and immediately after all clinical procedures. Soap and water washing is adequate for peripheral cannula insertions. However, if long-term IV catheters are being inserted, antiseptic hand-washing solutions should be used.

Universal precautions must be used for cannula placement. Gloves are worn to prevent contact with blood and to provide protection for the patient and the health care worker. When splashing of blood is likely to occur, for example, with the use of a breakaway needle, protective eyewear must be used.

If the patient is unusually dirty, the selected extremity should be washed with soap and water before the insertion site is prepared. Acceptable antimicrobial solutions are 1 to 2% tincture of iodine, iodophors (povidone-iodine), 70% isopropyl alcohol, or chlorhexidine. Unacceptable antimicrobial solutions are aqueous benzalkonium-like solutions and hexachlorophene.[1]

Preparation for peripheral IV insertion begins with the alcohol preparation. The application of 70% isopropyl alcohol removes fatty acids from the skin.[5] The isopropyl alcohol should be applied with friction, working from the insertion site outward. The prepared area should be 2 to 3 inches in diameter. After the isopropyl alcohol is allowed to air dry, the povidone-iodine is applied in a circular motion, working outward from the insertion site (Fig. 20–2). For the antimicrobial solution to be effective, it should be allowed to air dry for a minimum of 30 seconds. Fanning, blowing, and blotting of the prepared area are contraindicated.

If a patient is allergic to iodine, the site should be cleansed with 70% isopropyl alcohol. Apply the alcohol with friction for a minimum of 30 seconds and cleanse the area until the final applicator is visually clean. Applicators are intended for single-patient, one-time use only.

If hair removal is necessary, it should be clipped with scissors. Shaving can be harmful to the skin because it can cause microabrasions, which can harbor bacteria. Depilatories are not recommended because of allergic reactions, which can cause skin eruptions. Surgical clippers with disposable clipper heads are acceptable for removing excess hair. To prevent cross contamination, the clipper heads should be changed after each patient use.

The routine use of 1% lidocaine hydrochloride (Xylocaine) for cannula insertion is not recommended. The use of lidocaine for cannula insertion is a controversial practice. Some clinicians believe that lidocaine use before catheter insertion increases patient comfort and decreases anxiety. However, its use increases the risks for a potential allergic reaction, anaphylaxis, possible inadvertent injection of the drug into

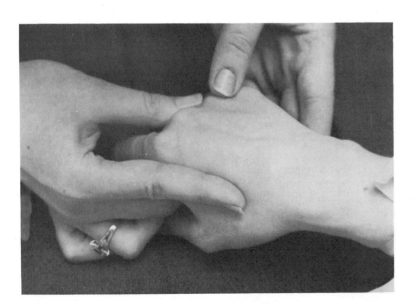

Figure 20–1. Vein assessment

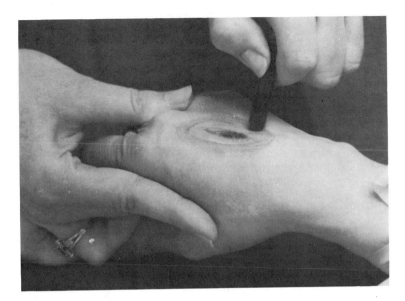

Figure 20–2. Prepping solution is applied in a circular motion, working outward from the insertion site.

the vascular system, and obliteration of the vein.[1] One alternate method is intradermal injection of 0.9% sodium chloride to the side of the vein before the cannula is inserted; this method produces an anesthetic effect without increasing any risks to the patient.[6, 7] A second alternate method is the application of a dermal analgesic cream to produce anesthesia. A disadvantage to using an analgesic transdermal cream is that it must be applied for 60 minutes before the venipuncture procedure. The use of a transdermal cream is contraindicated in patients who have a known allergy or sensitivity to local anesthetics of the amide type. When a clinician has expertise in the insertion of IV devices, local anesthesia is rarely necessary.

Cannula Selection

Cannulas or over-the-needle catheter type devices are the most commonly used peripheral IV devices. Some dual-lumen peripheral cannula devices are available for multiple infusions. The plastic cannula was first introduced in 1945.[8] As the dwell time of cannulas has lengthened, the prevalence of sepsis and phlebitis has increased. Catheter composition has evolved from polyvinylchloride and polytetrafluoroethylene (Teflon) to various polyurethane and elastomeric hydrogel materials. Much controversy exists over the advantages and disadvantages of the available cannula materials. Further advances in polymer technology seek to develop a catheter material that further decreases thrombogenicity.[9] To promote patient safety, IV cannulas are radiopaque.

The smallest gauge and the shortest length of cannula that will accommodate the prescribed therapy should be selected (Table 20–1). This plan causes less trauma to the vessel, promotes proper hemodilution of the infusate, and allows adequate blood flow around the catheter walls. All of these factors lengthen cannula dwell time.

The duration of therapy determines which IV device to insert. Stainless steel winged needles are intended for short-term duration, usually 1 to 4 hours. Winged stainless steel needles are frequently used to administer a single dose of medication. A winged set with a flexible catheter is also available for intermittent or general infusion therapy. The device is available open ended with a Y adapter or with an injection cap already in place.

Midline catheters are over-the-needle devices. The catheter is flexible and is introduced in an antecubital vein with the tip extending into the upper arm of an adult. Some of these catheters are composed of a special catheter material that expands in size and length after insertion. The use of midline catheters is not fully established but may be indicated when patients require frequent restarts of their peripheral IV cannulas, depending on the type of therapy they are receiving. Midline catheters should be inserted by persons who have clinical expertise in IV insertion or are supervised by someone who is skilled in such insertion.

If venous access will be needed for weeks, multiple venipunctures can be prevented by the insertion of a peripherally inserted central catheter (PICC). These catheters may be inserted by nurses who have advanced IV therapy skills and specialized education pertaining to the insertion of PICCs.

Veins can be preserved by initiating therapy on the distal area of the upper extremity. Subsequent cannulation should be performed proximal to previously cannulated sites. The condition of the patient influences cannula selection. In emergency situations, larger catheter access is necessary to accommodate the rapid infusion of fluids. Cannulas inserted in emergency situations should be restarted as soon as the patient has stabilized but within 24 hours of the emergency. These cannulas are restarted because one cannot ensure that the site was adequately prepared or that aseptic technique was maintained during insertion.

Table 20–1	
Recommendations for Cannula Selection	
Cannula Size	**Clinical Applications**
14–18 gauge	Trauma, surgery, blood
20 gauge	Continuous, intermittent infusions, blood
22 gauge	Intermittent or general infusions, children and elderly patients
24 gauge	Fragile veins for intermittent or general infusions

The diameter of the vein and the therapy to be delivered determine the size of the cannula inserted. A smaller-gauge catheter allows greater blood flow around the catheter, which promotes less irritation to the vessel wall. Small veins should not be used for vesicants or irritants. If a large-gauge cannula is required, then a larger vein should be selected.

Increased osmolality of the solution increases venous irritation. Hyperosmotic solutions of greater than 320 mOsm must be administered through veins with a large blood volume to dilute the IV solution and to reduce vein wall irritation. Examples of hyperosmotic solutions are 5% dextrose in Ringer's lactate solution (524 mOsm), and 5% dextrose in 0.45% sodium chloride (406 mOsm).[10]

Fluids with a greater viscosity, such as packed red cells, require a larger cannula. An 18- or 20-gauge catheter has a larger inner lumen, which permits the flow of viscous components. A smaller-gauge cannula may be used in children.

Cannula Placement

Before the venipuncture is performed, the cannula bevel is inspected for product integrity. The patient is informed of the venipuncture. Skin stabilization is an important element of successful venipunctures. Veins are stabilized by applying traction to the side of the insertion site with the nondominant hand. The application of traction prevents veins from rolling. Traction may be applied to the forearm by the palm of the nondominant hand, which is holding the whole forearm while the index finger and the thumb pull the skin away from the insertion site. For patients with poor muscular tone, it may be helpful to apply three-way traction. Using this method requires that a second person apply traction, pulling the skin upward, while the inserter applies traction downward.

With the bevel up, the cannula is held at a 10- to 30-degree angle, as it enters through the skin. The angle used to enter the skin varies slightly with cannulas from different manufacturers (Fig. 20–3). The depth of the vein in the subcutaneous tissue also determines the angle used to enter the skin. A vein located superficially requires a smaller can-

nula angle. However, a vein located deeper in the subcutaneous tissue requires a greater cannula angle. Venipuncture can be accomplished by a direct or an indirect approach into the vein. Using the direct method, the cannula enters the skin directly into the vein. An advantage of the direct method is that the vein is entered immediately. The disadvantage of this method is that with small, fragile veins, direct insertion can cause the vein to bruise more easily or can pierce the other side of the vein wall. With the indirect method, the cannula is inserted thru the skin, the vein is relocated, and the cannula is then advanced into the vein. An advantage of this method is that a small tunnel space exists between the area of entry through the skin and the vein. This method approaches the vein more easily with a gentle entry into the vessel. When small, fragile veins are cannulated by the indirect method, bruising is less likely to occur.

After the skin has been penetrated, the angle of the needle is decreased to prevent puncturing the posterior wall of the vein. The flashback chamber is checked for a blood return. With small-gauge catheters or hypotensive patients, a slow or minimal blood return may be obtained. If blood return is obtained the cannula should be advanced an additional 1/16 inch before stylet removal is begun.[11] The cannula is advanced gently into the vein. The catheter can be threaded into the vein by use of a one-handed or a two-handed technique. With the one-handed technique, the same hand that performs the venipuncture also withdraws the stylet while advancing the catheter into the vein. This technique allows for skin traction to be maintained while the catheter is advanced. It is also an advantage with the uncooperative patient because the skin traction is maintained as well as the hold on the patient. In the two-handed technique, one hand performs the venipuncture and the opposite hand grasps the catheter hub while withdrawing the stylet and advancing the catheter with the dominant hand. This method requires the release of skin traction while the stylet is pulled back.

Once the cannula is totally advanced into the vein, the tourniquet is removed. If any bruising occurs while the venipuncture is performed, the tourniquet is immediately removed to prevent a hematoma from forming. A stylet must not be reinserted into a catheter. If this situation occurs, the catheter wall can be punctured or severed, possibly resulting

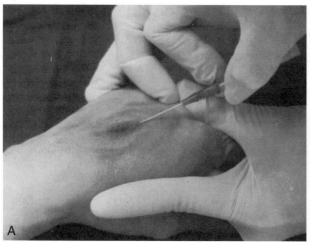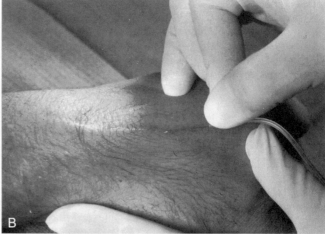

Figure 20–3. *A,* The cannula is held at a 10- to 30-degree angle as it enters the skin. *B,* After the skin has been penetrated, the angle of the needle is decreased as the cannula is advanced into the vein.

in catheter fragmentation and catheter embolism. Sometimes the stylet is removed from the cannula, and the solution in a syringe or administration set is used to advance the catheter into the vein. If any difficulty is encountered in advancing the cannula, or if the cannula cannot be advanced in its entirety, the insertion should be discontinued, and a new attempt at cannulation should be made.

If a venipuncture is unsuccessful, a new catheter must be used with each attempt. Once a catheter has been used, it is contaminated. As the cannula enters through the skin, it acquires any microorganisms that are contaminating the skin. Also, once a cannula has been used to puncture the skin, catheter tip fraying is likely to occur. No more than two attempts at cannulation are recommended. If a nurse has made two unsuccessful insertion attempts, the nurse with the most advanced IV skills should evaluate the patient's venous access. Further insertion attempts should be made only if the venous access is deemed to be adequate. Multiple unsuccessful attempts limit future vascular access and cause unnecessary trauma to the patient. When the patient has limited venous access and the veins cannot be successfully cannulated, the patient's physician should be notified. If the patient has limited venous access, another type of vascular access device needs to be established or other alternative routes for medication administration need to be evaluated.

Cannula stabilization and care are discussed in detail in Chapter 21. Patient preparation before the insertion of any vascular access IV device includes an explanation of the type of catheter, the placement procedure, the rationale, the common complications, and the expected outcome. The patient is encouraged to ask questions. The nurse can reduce the patient's anxiety by encouraging him or her to be an active participant in the placement process; active participation communicates that the patient's concerns are important and that the nurse is interested in the whole person and not just in the technical performance of the procedure. The patient should also be encouraged to report any discomfort experienced during or after the insertion procedure.

The following is a suggested procedure for the insertion of a peripheral intravenous cannula.

Peripheral Intravenous Line Insertion

1. Gather equipment.
2. Wash hands using antiseptic soap.
3. Ascertain the presence of allergies.
4. Explain procedure and rationale for therapy to patient.
5. Set up equipment.
6. Apply tourniquet.
7. Assess veins, keeping in mind the rationale for therapy and the duration of therapy.
8. Apply alcohol with friction in circular motion for a minimum of 30 seconds. Allow to air dry.
9. If antimicrobial preparation is used, apply in circular motion. Allow to air dry for a minimum of 30 seconds.
10. Apply gloves.
11. Perform venipuncture while stabilizing skin with the nondominant hand.
12. Enter skin at a 10- to 30-degree angle. Decrease angle when skin has been penetrated. When blood is obtained in flashback chamber, advance catheter $1/16$ inch, then slightly pull stylet back, advancing catheter gently into vessel.

13. Remove tourniquet.
14. Remove stylet and connect IV administration set. Begin infusing fluids slowly. Observe insertion site for any signs of swelling. If catheter is inserted for intermittent therapy, attach injection cap or needleless device and flush slowly with 2 ml of 0.9% sodium chloride solution.
15. Stabilize cannula with chevron taping, if necessary.
16. Apply dressing.
17. Write date, time, gauge, and length of catheter and name of nurse inserting catheter on the dressing label.
18. Document insertion in medical record.

Midline Catheter Insertion

Midline catheters are to be inserted by nurses who are experienced and have excellent IV insertion skills. Controversy exists about the necessity of a physician's order for the insertion of a midline device. Some agencies require a physician's order because of the increased dwell time of the catheter; other agencies do not require a physician's order, because the catheter is not entering the central venous system. Each institution should have a written policy regarding the necessity of obtaining a physician's order before the insertion of a midline device.

Although the actual procedure varies slightly with different midline devices, the following is a sample procedure for the insertion of a midline catheter:

1. Gather supplies and equipment.
2. Assist the patient to a comfortable supine position.
3. Fully extend the patient's arm, which should be supported by a towel roll.
4. Abduct the arm at a 45-degree angle.
5. Prepare the work area.
6. Position protective covering under the patient's arm.
7. Place tourniquet on the mid-upper arm for final vein assessment.
8. Clip hair 8 to 10 inches from around the antecubital fossa.
9. Apply sterile gloves.
10. Cleanse insertion area three times with 70% isopropyl alcohol swab sticks starting at the insertion site; apply in a circular motion, working outward to an area 4 to 5 inches in diameter.
11. Repeat cleansing with povidone-iodine swab sticks. Allow to air dry.
12. Remove and discard gloves.
13. Apply tourniquet.
14. Don second pair of sterile gloves.
15. Drape arm with a fenestrated drape or sterile towels, leaving an opening for the venipuncture.
16. Venipuncture site should be two to three fingerbreadths above the bend of the arm or one fingerbreadth below the bend of the arm.
17. Perform venipuncture.
18. Insert catheter according to the manufacturer's recommendations.
19. Slowly continue to advance the catheter to the desired initial length.
    Caution: If resistance is met during advancement, stop immediately. Techniques that can be used if resistance is

met include moving the arm at a different angle, rotating the wrist, or having the patient open and close his or her fist. If resistance continues to be met, catheter insertion must be discontinued.

20. Attach IV tubing or injection cap. Begin infusing fluids slowly while observing upper arm for any indications of swelling. If catheter is to be used for intermittent therapy, slowly flush with 0.9% sodium chloride solution, followed by heparinized saline solution.
21. Apply sterile occlusive dressing.
22. Some midline catheter manufacturers recommend the patient leave the arm immobilized for 30 minutes, which allows the catheter material to soften and minimizes venous irritation.

Cannula Securement

Peripheral cannulas may be secured using various taping methods. Minimizing cannula movement helps to prevent mechanical irritation to the lining of the vein. Transparent and gauze dressings are frequently used dressing materials. Transparent dressings are popular because they allow direct visualization of the insertion site. If gauze dressings are used, all the edges must be taped to occlude air flow.

ARTERIAL ADMINISTRATION

Site Selection

The placement of an arterial cannula may be indicated for drawing samples for arterial blood gas determinations, for obtaining continuous and accurate arterial pressure readings, and for assessing the cardiovascular effects of vasoactive drugs.[12] The vessel should be assessed for the presence of a pulse. The radial and brachial arteries are recommended insertion sites because these locations promote ease of insertion and reduce the risk of infection. Occasionally, the femoral artery may be used. In the radial and brachial areas it is much easier to keep an occlusive dressing intact than in the femoral area. When the radial or brachial artery is used, the Allen test should be performed to assess the collateral circulation to the hand (see Chapter 23).

Site Preparation

Arterial site preparation follows the same cannula site preparation procedure as that for a peripheral site, except that it is a sterile procedure. Arterial cannula insertion requires the application of a mask, sterile gloves, and a face shield when splashing of blood could occur.

Cannula Selection

Cannula selection for indwelling continuous arterial access requires the use of a radiopaque catheter in the smallest gauge and shortest length possible. Stainless steel needles may be used for intermittent arterial blood sampling. Cannu-

las are available that are specifically made for arterial cannulation.

Cannula Placement and Securement

See Chapter 23 for a basic step-by-step procedure for arterial insertion. Arterial catheters may be secured by sterile tape or sutures and covered by a sterile air-occlusive dressing.

CENTRAL VASCULAR ADMINISTRATION

Site Selection

Peripherally Inserted Central Catheters

When the therapy is anticipated to be a few weeks' to several months' duration, the placement of a PICC may be indicated. The administration of long-term antibiotic therapy; total parenteral nutrition; or pain control, vesicant, or irritant medications are some of the clinical situations warranting PICC insertion. Long-term antibiotic therapy is usually defined as lasting from 2 or 3 weeks to several months. PICC placement is also preferable when a patient has pulmonary involvement. One of the risks associated with central line insertion is the inadvertent puncturing of the lung because of the anatomic proximity of the lung to the subclavian vein. When the pleural space is inadvertently punctured, pneumothorax occurs. Because the needle used for PICC insertion cannulates the antecubital vein, the risk of a pneumothorax is eliminated.

The basilic and cephalic antecubital fossa veins are the preferred sites for PICC placement. The basilic vein is the largest and usually the best vein for PICC insertion. The cephalic vein is smaller, and the curvature is greater where it anastomoses with the subclavian vein. Previously damaged, sclerotic veins should not be used for PICC insertion, because the use of such vessels can cause increased injury to the vessel and surrounding tissue. As a result, an increase in the occurrence of complications, such as phlebitis and infection, could result from PICC placement. An extremity affected by a mastectomy, an arteriovenous graft, or a fistula is also not recommended for PICC placement.

Short-Term Percutaneously Inserted Central Venous Catheters

A short-term percutaneous central venous catheter (CVC) is inserted in patients who require vascular access for a few days to several weeks. These catheters are considered to be short-term because no tunneling of the device is involved. For this reason, these catheters may be associated with an increased risk of complications. Occasionally, with proper maintenance and meticulous site care, these catheters may remain in place longer than several weeks.

A percutaneously inserted catheter enters through the skin directly into the vein. The subclavian and internal jugular veins are the commonest locations for placement of a CVC. The preferred vein for most CVCs is the subclavian vein. At jugular insertion sites, an intact sterile dressing is difficult to maintain, and the patient's mobility and comfort are altered. Subclavian insertion is contraindicated in patients who have superior vena cava syndrome, subclavian stenosis, tumor blockage, bilateral neck dissection, upper torso trauma, or a history of central placement problems. In these patients, the femoral vein may be used. The femoral veins are primarily used for short-term vascular access. At femoral insertion sites, an occlusive sterile dressing is difficult to maintain, and the catheter inhibits the patient's mobility and may be associated with an increased risk of infection.

Site Preparation

Central site preparation is a sterile procedure. The insertion of a PICC requires the use of a mask, sterile gloves, a gown, a surgical scrub, and sterile drapes. A mask and sterile gloves are worn by the clinician. Protective eyewear should be worn if a breakaway needle is used. Sterile towels and drapes are used to create a sterile field.

Long-term venous access devices, such as tunneled devices and implantable ports, are usually inserted in specialized surgical facilities. Short-term percutaneously inserted CVCs may be inserted at the patient's bedside, and nurses may be required to perform site preparation before the placement of these devices. The site preparation method for the insertion of a CVC follows the same principals as those detailed earlier for peripheral cannula site preparation, except that it is a sterile procedure. The same antimicrobial solutions recommended for peripheral cannula site preparation (70% isopropyl alcohol, tincture of iodine 1 to 2%, iodophors, and chlorhexidine) are also recommended for CVC site preparation. The intended insertion site, if unusually dirty, is cleansed with soap and water, and any excess hair at the intended insertion site is removed with surgical clippers. Sterile surgical preparation consists of cleansing in a circular motion with 70% isopropyl alcohol from the intended insertion site, working outward. The actual size of the prepared area varies depending on the specific CVC to be inserted, but usually an area of 8 to 10 inches is prepared before the placement of a CVC. Starting at the intended insertion site, working outward, repeat cleansing with povidone-iodine. Some facilities use a povidone-iodine scrub, which is removed with a sterile towel, and then apply povidone-iodine paint. Regardless of the actual preparatory method used, the povidone-iodine solution is allowed to air dry and is not removed. The prepared area is draped with sterile towels, creating a wide sterile field.

Catheter Selection

Some of the types of central vascular access devices available are single-lumen and multilumen PICCs, tunneled catheters, and implantable ports. Central vascular access devices are available in many catheter materials that are designed for short- and long-term therapy. Catheters used for long-term therapy, such as PICCs, tunneled catheters, and implantable ports, are usually composed of a soft material, such as silicone. Short-term catheters are usually composed of polyurethane and may have multiple lumens. Multiple-lumen cathe-

ters allow the simultaneous administration of incompatible medications and fluids. Catheters with multiple lumens may be associated with increased catheter-related infection and sepsis because when multiple lumens are available, the IV system has increased manipulation, which increases the risk for contamination.[13]

Central vascular access devices are inserted either percutaneously or surgically. PICCs and various short-term subclavian and jugular multilumen catheters are inserted percutaneously, and tunneled catheters and implantable ports are inserted surgically. Some of the factors to be considered when a vascular access device is chosen include the diagnosis of the patient, the length of therapy, the maintenance of the device, and the preference of the patient.

The PICC is a long, radiopaque, flexible catheter that is introduced in an antecubital fossa vein with the tip extending into the superior vena cava. Tip placement is confirmed by radiology. The length of the selected catheter should allow for appropriate placement without altering tip integrity. According to the *Intravenous Nursing Standards of Practice,* the desired catheter tip location is in the superior vena cava.[11]

PICC placement requires a physician's order, and in some states, the board of nursing through the Nursing Practice Act forbids nurses from inserting PICCs altogether. The physician's order must be verified and documented in the medical record. An informed consent from the physician must be signed by the patient or legal guardian, but before consent is obtained, the physician or nurse should explain to the patient the rationale for placing a PICC, the insertion procedure, the potential complications, and the maintenance requirements of the catheter.

Short-term percutaneously inserted CVCs are available in many lengths and gauges. Smaller-gauge and shorter-length catheters are used in children and neonates. CVC catheters are available in the following lengths: 15, 20, or 30 cm. An average-sized adult requires a 20-cm catheter for the tip to be properly located in the superior vena cava. Larger adults or left-sided insertions may require a 30-cm catheter for the tip to be in the superior vena cava.[14] Some short-term CVCs are large-bore catheters designed for hemodialysis or for rapid infusion of IV solutions.

A tunneled catheter is a long-term catheter that exits partially through the skin. Tunneled catheters have a Dacron cuff, around which fibrous tissue grows. The cuff and tunnel anchor the catheter and impede the migration of microorganisms through the subcutaneous tract. The insertion of a tunneled catheter is considered to be a surgical procedure. A very small incision is made at the point of entry near the subclavian vein. Next, a subcutaneous tunnel from the subclavian vein is formed between the sternum and the nipple. The lower point is called the "exit site."

After the catheter has been tunneled under the skin, it is inserted into the vein percutaneously or by cutdown. Usually, the catheter is inserted percutaneously by using a breakaway introducer. Placement of the catheter is determined by the specific design of the tunneled catheter. Catheters that can be trimmed at the terminal end are inserted in the manner just described. If the terminal end is closed and not able to be trimmed, it is inserted in reverse. The catheter is inserted in the superior vena cava, and the hub end (the hub connectors are absent) is tunneled subcutaneously through the skin from the entrance site to the exit site. The closed-end tunneled catheter is trimmed at the hub end before the connectors are attached.

An implantable port is a system for IV, intra-arterial, epidural, or intraperitoneal delivery of drugs and fluids. It permits repeated access for the administration of medications by bolus injection or infusion, for the administration of blood products and total parenteral nutrition, and for the withdrawal of blood specimens. The system consists of either a stainless steel or plastic chamber with a silicone septum in the center. A silicone catheter locks onto the portal chamber. The catheter system is surgically implanted into the subcutaneous tissues and is sutured, and the catheter is threaded into the superior vena cava, right atrium, or the appropriate cavity. The procedure is performed by a surgeon in the operating room with the patient under local or general anesthetic. The implantable port can be accessed only with a noncoring needle, which has a specially designed bevel that prevents the rubber diaphragm from being removed with the needle insertion.

The nurse should explain the advantages and disadvantages of the various types of venous access devices. The nurse, patient, and physician should decide which vascular access device would be in the best interest of the patient. Information regarding other vascular access devices, the insertion procedure, the potential complications, and the care and maintenance of each catheter is provided to enable the patient to make an informed decision.

Catheter Placement

Peripherally Inserted Central Catheters

PICCs are to be inserted by nurses who have advanced IV therapy skills, except in those states that prohibit nurses from inserting PICCs by means of the state Nursing Practice Act. The insertion procedure varies slightly depending on the PICC product used. PICC cannula selection can be of several designs. The catheter may be inserted through a breakaway needle or cannula with or without a guidewire. With the breakaway needle design, the catheter is passed through a splittable needle. After the catheter is placed, the needle is split and peeled from around the catheter. With the cannula design, an over-the-needle plastic cannula is used as the introducer for the catheter. The needle is removed, leaving the cannula in place, and the catheter is threaded through the plastic cannula.

Some catheter designs have a guidewire, which adds firmness to the silicone catheter. Guidewires enhance the advancement of the catheter and increase the visibility of the catheter on the radiology film. Guidewires are seldom used with the smaller-gauge PICC catheters or in children, who have smaller vein diameters. The guidewire design requires venous access to be established with a needle. Then, a guidewire is threaded through the needle, the needle is removed, and the catheter is threaded over the guidewire. This technique is commonly referred to as the "Seldinger method."[15]

Although the actual procedure varies with different manufacturer's products, the following procedure is suggested for the insertion of a PICC:

1. Assist patient to dorsal recumbent position.
2. Ascertain patient's allergies.
3. Scrub hands using antiseptic soap for 60 seconds.
4. Don mask.
5. Prepare work area.
6. Position protective covering under patient's arm.
7. Place tourniquet on mid-upper arm for final vein assessment.
8. Measure arm with sterile tape. For PICC placement in the superior vena cava, measure from the antecubital insertion site up the arm to the shoulder and across the shoulder. Continue to the sternal notch and down to the third intercostal space.
9. Select vein and release tourniquet.
10. Clip hair 8 to 10 inches around antecubital fossa.
11. Apply nonpowdered sterile gloves.
12. Cleanse with 70% isopropyl alcohol, starting at insertion site and cleansing outward in a circular motion in an area 8 to 10 inches in diameter. Repeat three to five times.
13. Repeat cleansing with povidone-iodine.
14. Remove and discard gloves.
15. Apply tourniquet snugly.
16. Don second pair of sterile gloves.
17. Drape arm with sterile towels, creating a sterile field.
18. Inject subcutaneously 0.5 ml or less of 1% lidocaine to anesthetize the insertion site.
19. Make venipuncture while applying reverse traction with the other hand to stabilize vein.
20. After venipuncture is obtained, pull back stylet and slowly advance introducer (Fig. 20–4A).
21. Remove stylet (Fig. 20–4B).
22. Slowly advance catheter to prevent damage to the vein (Fig. 20–4C).
23. Release tourniquet.
24. Continue to advance catheter slowly over 5 to 10 minutes.
25. When catheter is advanced midway, have the patient turn his or her head toward the insertion site with the chin placed downward on the clavicle.
26. Remove the introducer (Fig. 20–4D).
27. Slowly advance the remaining catheter to the measured length that was determined before insertion.
28. Gently remove guidewire from catheter.
29. Prime and attach extension tubing and injection cap.
30. Flush with 0.5 ml of 0.9% sodium chloride solution.
31. Aspirate with 0.9% sodium chloride to check for blood return.
32. Assess blood for type of flow, color, consistency, and pulsation.
33. Flush vigorously with remaining sodium chloride, followed by heparinized saline.
34. Tape with Steri-Strips or suture in place.
35. Cover with 4 × 4 gauze and a sterile wrap for 24 hours.
36. Obtain chest x-ray for catheter tip placement. Tip should be in the superior vena cava.
37. Document in medical record.
38. After 24 hours, assess insertion site and upper forearm by performing sterile dressing change. Intermittent warm moist packs may be applied to the upper forearm to prevent the occurrence of phlebitis.

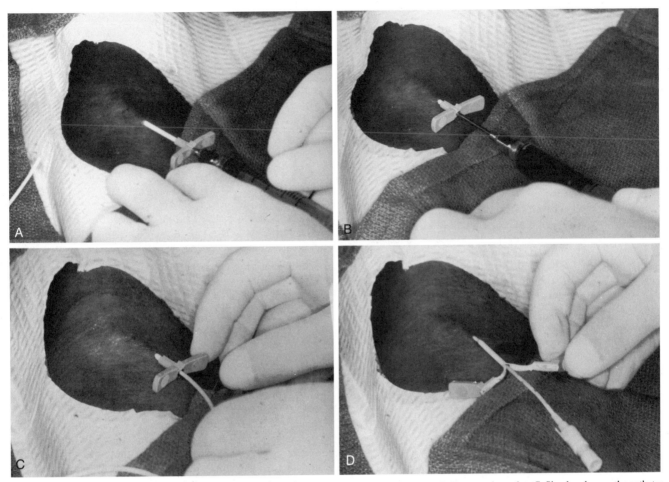

Figure 20–4. *A*, After venipuncture has been obtained, aspirate with a syringe to verify blood return. *B*, Remove the stylet. *C*, Slowly advance the catheter to prevent trauma to the vein intima. *D*, Remove the breakaway introducer before advancing the remaining catheter.

Short-Term Percutaneously Inserted Central Venous Catheters

The insertion of a short-term percutaneously inserted CVC must be performed by a physician. Nurses may assist physicians with the placement of these catheters. Often, nurses are responsible for gathering the supplies, positioning the patient, performing the skin preparation before PICC insertion, and flushing the catheter before and after insertion. Before insertion, signed consent must be obtained from the patient or legal guardian.

The actual procedure varies depending on the physician performing the insertion and with the type of CVC used. The following is a suggested procedure using the Seldinger technique, which is the most commonly used technique.

1. Position patient in the Trendelenburg or supine position, with a rolled towel between the shoulders.
2. Ascertain patient's allergies.
3. Wash hands using antiseptic soap for 60 seconds.
4. Don mask.
5. Prepare work area.
6. Clip hair around intended insertion site area.
7. Position protective covering underneath patient's shoulder and neck.
8. Apply sterile gloves.
9. Cleanse with 70% isopropyl alcohol, starting at insertion site and working outward in circular motion to an area 8 to 10 inches in diameter (actual prepared area may vary in size, according to physician's discretion).
10. Apply povidone-iodine detergent scrub for 2 minutes.
11. Pat dry with sterile towel.
12. Apply povidone-iodine paint for 2 minutes. Allow to air dry.
13. Drape insertion site with sterile towels, creating a wide sterile field. (Note: The remaining procedure is performed by the physician.)
14. Apply second pair of sterile gloves (if the physician performed the sterile surgical preparation).
15. Anesthetize the insertion site with 1% lidocaine.
16. Perform venipuncture into jugular, subclavian, or femoral vein.
17. Remove syringe from needle.
18. Insert spring guidewire through the needle.
19. Remove needle. Sometimes, vein dilator is used.
20. Thread catheter over the guidewire.
21. Suture catheter into place, if necessary.
22. Flush catheter with 0.9% sodium chloride, aspirate for blood return, flush with remaining sodium chloride solution, then flush with heparin.
23. Attach injection caps or needleless device as needed.
24. Apply sterile occlusive dressing over insertion site.

25. Obtain chest x-ray to verify tip placement and to rule out pneumothorax before initiating therapy. The correct catheter tip placement should be in the superior vena cava. If the femoral vein was used for insertion, the correct tip location is the inferior vena cava.
26. Document patient tolerance during insertion and monitoring in the medical record.

Implantable Port Access

Because an implantable port is placed totally under the skin, the nurse must be familiar with the patient's specific type of port. Numerous portal devices are available. Palpation of the portal device assists in determining the type of port, as well as the length of needle to use for accessing. If the port is located in deeper subcutaneous tissue, a longer needle must be used. Many types of noncoring needles are available in different gauges and lengths. A bent or 90-degree, curved, noncoring needle is used for continuous infusion. A straight, noncoring needle may be used for aspirating blood, heparinizing, or injecting a bolus. Patency is always determined by obtaining a blood return before any medication is infused or injected. IV and intra-arterial ports must always be flushed with heparinized saline between uses. If an IV port is not in use, it may be flushed every 4 weeks. An intra-arterial port that remains unaccessed must be flushed every week.

A procedure that may be used to access an implantable port follows:

1. Gather supplies and equipment.
2. Explain procedure to patient.
3. Wash hands thoroughly for 1 minute with antiseptic soap.
4. Palpate site to locate septum.
5. Put on mask and sterile gloves.
6. Cleanse with three swab sticks of 70% isopropyl alcohol, starting with the center of the septum and moving outward in a circular motion. Cover an area that is 4 inches in diameter.
7. Repeat cleansing with povidone-iodine solution. Allow to air dry.
8. Remove and discard gloves.
9. Don second pair of sterile gloves.
10. Locate port by palpation.
11. Immobilize port with index finger and forefingers.
12. Insert needle perpendicular to the septum. Push firmly through the skin and septum until the needle tip contacts the back of the port.
13. Aspirate for blood return to establish patency.
14. Flush with 10 ml of 0.9% sodium chloride solution if medication is going to be administered. Use heparinized saline if the port is not going to be used. To avoid reflux, maintain positive injection pressure while simultaneously withdrawing the needle and syringe from the port.
15. If port is to remain accessed, anchor noncoring needle using sterile tape and sterile 2 × 2 gauze to pad and support needle. To prevent portal erosion and needle dislodgement, secure needle to eliminate any to-and-fro movement.
16. Cover needle and gauze with sterile occlusive dressing.
17. Label dressing with date, time, needle gauge, and length.
18. Document procedure in the medical record.

Blood Sampling

1. After aspirating to establish patency, withdraw 5 ml of blood and discard.
2. Attach sterile syringe and withdraw blood volume.
3. Flush vigorously with 10 ml of 0.9% sodium chloride solution, followed by heparinized saline if port is being used intermittently.

Cannula Securement

PICCs and short-term percutaneously inserted CVCs may be secured by sterile tape or sutures and covered by gauze and a transparent dressing. IV tubing junctions must be secured, preferably with Luer lock connections, clasping devices, or tape. Accidental tubing separations can cause air embolism, hemorrhage, and contamination of the IV system.

Postinsertion Verification

The insertion of IV devices requires verification that the placement is correct. The presence of a blood return does not always provide absolute verification. If the tip of the IV catheter punctures the posterior wall of the vein, leaving the greater part of the cannula in the vessel, a blood return may be obtained, but at the same time the solution could be infiltrating into the tissue. It is important to assess the insertion site for swelling, hardness, coolness, and any patient discomfort. Comparing the infusion site with the same area on the opposite extremity helps to determine if any swelling is present. To ascertain if an infiltration has occurred, a tourniquet can be applied proximally to the insertion site. When a tourniquet is applied, the venous flow is restricted. However, if the infusion continues regardless of the applied venous obstruction, infiltration of the fluid is confirmed. If any questions exist regarding the patency of the device, the site should be discontinued immediately and a new cannula restarted.

Arterial placement can be verified by observing the pulsation of blood into the tubing or a syringe without applying any traction on the syringe. Central venous placement is verified by obtaining a blood return and by radiologic confirmation. If any questions remain regarding CVC placement, fluoroscopic and radiologic examination can confirm catheter placement.

PATIENT DIAGNOSES

With the recent technologic advancements in vascular access devices and infusion equipment and the evolution of nursing research, IV therapy has developed into a highly specialized practice. The nurse must be able to readily identify and define patient care problems and to plan and provide the necessary specialized interventions. The identified problems are referred to as *potential nursing diagnoses*. Frequently encountered problems related to IV administration are fluid volume deficit or excess, nutrition related to an alteration in less than body requirements, impairment of skin, potential for injury in relation to infection, knowledge deficit, anxiety, and noncompliance.

Fluid volume deficit or excess can be prevented by performing an ongoing assessment of the patient and the prescribed therapy and by frequently monitoring the IV infusion. Determining intake and output and monitoring weight and assessing the integrity of the patient's skin can be used to verify that the patient's daily nutritional requirements are being met. The potential for infection and the impairment of skin integrity exist when any IV cannula is placed. Careful site preparation, skillful insertion technique, and meticulous assessment of the insertion site during site care all reduce the occurrence of infections from IV cannulas. A knowledge deficit exists for all patients receiving IV therapy. One of the most important aspects of care is the education of the patient and the family. Teaching begins before the cannula is placed and continues throughout the duration of therapy until the cannula is discontinued. By providing adequate teaching, patient and family anxiety will be reduced and compliance will be increased.

PATIENT OUTCOMES

The nurse continuously evaluates patient outcomes to determine if the nursing interventions are appropriate. Desired outcome statements for the patient receiving IV therapy include the following: maintaining adequate intake of fluid and electrolytes as evidenced by the relief of symptoms of dehydration, exhibiting decreased peripheral edema, identifying factors that increase the potential for injury, verbalizing fears and anxiety related to health care needs, and describing the rationale and procedure for treatment.

Although IV therapy has seen great technologic advancements, from steel needles to a variety of long-dwelling cannulas, from the acute care setting to the home, from continuous to intermittent administration, it is paramount that the nurse provides quality patient care. To ensure the delivery of quality IV care, potential patient problems must be rapidly identified. Nursing care must be goal directed, and appropriate nursing interventions must be provided. The delivery of IV therapy is practiced according to policies and procedures that are based on established professional standards of practice. Patient outcomes are evaluated, and appropriate interventions are reimplemented and communicated to all members of the health care team.

References

1. Intravenous Nurses Society. Intravenous Nursing Standards of Practice. Belmont, MA: Intravenous Nurses Society, 1990.
2. Ryan KA. Standardized care plans for I.V. therapy. JIN 1989;12(2):94–97.
3. Otto S. Nursing diagnosis: Challenges for intravenous practice. JIN 1988;11:(4)245–248.
4. Weinstein SM. Plumer's Principles & Practice of Intravenous Therapy. Philadelphia: J.B. Lippincott, 1993:59.
5. Larson E. Guideline for use of topical antimicrobial agents. Am J Infect Control 1988;16(6):253–266.
6. Milam DA, Warren J. Using a local anesthetic for I.V. insertion: Boon or bane? Nurs Life 1985;5(1):52–53.
7. O'Donnell J. Lidocaine use for placing I.V. cannulas. NITA 1985; 8(1):69–71.
8. Tobin CR. The Teflon intravenous catheter: Incidence of phlebitis and duration of catheter life in the neonatal patient. J Obstet Gynecol Neonatal Nurs 1988; 17:(1)35–41.
9. Gaukroger PB, Roberts JG, Manners TA. Infusion thrombophlebitis: A prospective comparison of 645 Vialon and Teflon cannulae in anaesthetic and postoperative use. Anaesth Intensive Care 1988; 16:265–271.
10. Spencer V. Phlebitis. NITA 1981; 4(3):182–183.
11. Coulter K. Peripheral venipuncture: Site placement and management. Am J Nurs 1991; 1–3.
12. Delaney CW, Lauer ML. Intravenous Therapy: A Guide to Quality Care. Philadelphia: J.B. Lippincott, 1988:234.
13. Bennet JV, Brachman PS. Hospital Infections. 3rd ed. Boston: Little, Brown and Co., 1992:849–898.
14. Baranowski L. Central venous access devices: Current technologies, uses, and management strategies. JIN 1993;16(3):167–194.
15. Goodwin M. The Seldinger method for PICC insertion. JIN 1989; 12(4):238–243.

CHAPTER 21 Intravenous Monitoring and Catheter Care

Roxanne Perucca, BSN, CRNI

The administration of intravenous therapy subjects the patient to numerous risks, such as local or systemic complications. Local complications, such as phlebitis, infiltration, and needle or cannula occlusion, occur more frequently than systemic complications, which include septicemia, circulatory overload, and embolism, and can be life threatening. For this reason, monitoring and catheter care are critical components of intravenous administration. Early detection, thorough monitoring, and meticulous catheter care can prevent many of these complications. Monitoring provides information regarding the patient's response to therapy and the accurate delivery of fluid and medications, and it detects imminent complications. Catheter care is essential in preventing, detecting, and decreasing the occurrence of complications.

The nurse is responsible for observing and assessing the patient's response and providing appropriate nursing interventions. For example, after beginning the infusion of a newly ordered antibiotic, if a nurse observes that the patient is extremely anxious, short of breath, and has hives on the face and chest, the nurse should intervene immediately. Interventions for this situation include stopping the remaining antibiotic from infusing, notifying the patient's physician, and assessing the patient's vital signs. The patient's response to the administration of intravenous fluids or medications must be documented in the medical record and communicated to the other members of the health care team.

MONITORING PERIPHERAL SITES

The parameters to be monitored in the intravenous administration system include the following: the fluid container, the administration tubing, the flow rate, the electronic infusion device, the intravenous site dressing, the vascular access device, and the insertion site. The frequency for monitoring a peripheral intravenous site is determined by the prescribed therapy, the condition and age of the patient, and the practice setting. Intravenous sites should be monitored at 1- to 2-hour intervals.[1] The pediatric, geriatric, or critically ill patient requires more frequent site assessments. A thorough assessment of the insertion site should be performed when the dressing is changed. The patient receiving care in the home should be taught how to assess his or her intravenous access device and insertion site several times daily. If this patient is administering any medications, the insertion site must be assessed before the catheter is flushed or any medication is administered. Frequent follow-up and close supervision must be provided by the home care nurse.

The performance of a systematic and organized assessment of the intravenous administration system begins with the fluid container and progresses down the tubing to the vascular access device and insertion site. The type of solution and medications added are verified against the physician's order, as is the information printed on the fluid container label. The container must be labeled with the date and time that it was hung. Containers can be labeled with times they are hung and flow levels in numerous ways. Several types of flow strips are manufactured that identify the time the container was hung and have interval markings indicating the fluid level at specified times. Sometimes a tape strip is placed on the container that indicates the time when the container is hung and the fluid level. No matter how the hang time of the container is labeled, the label should not be placed over important information printed on the solution container, such as the solution name or the "medication added" label. The fluid container should not be labeled by writing with a pen or a felt tip marker on the plastic surface, because the ink can penetrate the plastic and leak into the intravenous solution.

The next monitoring parameter to note is the amount of solution remaining in the container. The nurse determines how much fluid should remain in the fluid container based on the prescribed flow rate and the indicated time. The appearance of the fluid remaining in the container is noted: the solution should be clear and free from cloudiness and particulate matter.

The correct tubing should be hanging with the fluid container and the electronic infusion device. Solutions contained in glass bottles require vented intravenous tubing. Most electronic infusion devices require that a specific manufacturer's tubing be used. If a solution is being infused by gravity at a very slow infusion rate, microdrop tubing should be used.

The electronic infusion device is evaluated to determine whether it is infusing at the prescribed flow rate. When a gravity administration set is being used, the drops of fluid per minute are counted to determine the flow rate. The flow rate is altered by the following factors. The height of the fluid container should be placed 30 to 36 inches above the patient. Raising the height of the container increases the flow rate. The flow rate can also be altered by any change in the patient's position. If the venipuncture site is located on an extremity near a point of flexion, any time that the patient bends an arm or wrist, the flow rate is altered. Sporadic flow rates result in an inaccurate delivery of fluids and medications and should be avoided.

Armboards may be used when an insertion site is located near an area of flexion. Care must be taken when an extremity is placed on an armboard to ensure that it remains in a functional position. Contractures, unnecessary discomfort, and neural injuries to the extremity can occur if an armboard is applied incorrectly. The armboard may be secured by tape or gauze. If tape is used, it should be back-strapped to avoid placing tape directly on the patient's skin. Tape should never be applied to encircle an extremity, because such a practice impairs circulation to the extremity. If gauze is used to secure an armboard, a window should be left that allows easy observation of the insertion site.

The flow rate is affected by the viscosity of fluids. Fluids that are thick, including blood, lipid emulsions, or colloidal solutions (e.g., albumin or dextran), can have altered flow rates. It may be necessary to administer viscous solutions through a larger-gauge cannula. The temperature of solutions also affects the flow rate. Refrigerated fluid should be brought to room temperature before it is infused. Cool solutions can induce venous spasm, which further slows the flow rate. Solutions cannot be submerged in warm water to hasten warming.

The administration tubing can alter the flow rate if any of the following conditions are present: the tubing is crimped, it is dangling below the bed, a filter is occluded, or, with vented administration sets, the air vent is occluded. When the administration tubing is assessed, it is usually helpful to start the evaluation at the drip chamber and work down the length of the tubing, assessing tubing and piggyback junctions, then continuing down to the cannula-tubing junction site. If the filter or an air vent becomes occluded, a new administration set must be attached.

If the position of an intravenous cannula changes, the flow rate can be altered. If the tip of a cannula lies against the vessel wall or next to a bifurcation in the vein, it can become occluded. Sometimes, this condition can be corrected by backing the cannula out a very small amount, ⅛ of an inch or less. When the cannula is moved back, care must be taken to avoid withdrawing the cannula out of the vessel, or infiltration will occur. The intravenous cannula can become occluded if venous pressure increases. An increase in venous pressure occurs when a blood pressure reading is taken on an extremity that has an intravenous site or when a wrist restraint is placed on or above the intravenous cannula. Blood pressure readings should be taken on an extremity that does not have a vascular access device. Wrist restraints must be loosely applied and should never be placed directly over an intravenous cannula.

A change in the flow rate occurs if an undetected infiltration, phlebitis, or thrombus is present. As the infiltration progresses, the infusion rate decreases, and the electronic infusion device might sound an alarm. If the electronic infusion device infuses fluid using positive pressure, it may not detect an infiltration and continues to infuse the fluid into the subcutaneous tissues. The insertion site must be assessed when any alteration in the flow rate occurs or when the electronic control device sounds an alarm.

The monitoring of the intravenous infusion system continues to assessment of the electronic infusion device. Many electronic infusion devices are available, and health care professionals must be familiar with the intravenous equipment being used for each patient. The nurse oversees the overall mechanical operation and the troubleshooting when an alarm sounds. Equipment should be monitored so that accurate delivery of the prescribed therapy is achieved with minimal deviation. To ensure accurate flow rates, the fluid container should be labeled with the date and time it was hung. Some electronic infusion devices decrease the flow rate when the programmed amount of fluid has been administered. Other electronic control devices decrease the flow rate if the battery becomes low. When the electronic infusion device is assessed, it is helpful to read the display panel and to note the amount of fluid infused to ensure that the machine is operating properly.

If the tubing-cannula junction site has already been assessed, the nurse can proceed to the intravenous site dressing. The dressing is monitored to ensure that it remains dry, closed, and intact. An intact dressing is one in which all edges of the dressing are sealed to the skin. If the dressing is damp or the integrity is compromised, it must be changed immediately. Intravenous dressing changes are discussed in greater detail later in this chapter under "Catheter Care."

The monitoring of the intravenous system proceeds to the assessment of the insertion site. To thoroughly perform an assessment of the intravenous device, the nurse must know the type and length of the intravenous device. Many types of vascular access devices, both peripheral and central, are available in various gauges and lengths. Peripheral intravenous cannulas may be as short as ½ inch and as long as 22 inches when the tip of the catheter is located centrally. The length of the intravenous device determines the area of the patient's arm that requires assessment. If the catheter is 22 inches long, the area of the patient's arm that needs to be assessed begins at the insertion site and follows the catheter tract up the arm, around the shoulder, and down to the third intercostal space. For this reason, the length of the vascular access device must be documented on the insertion site dressing and in the medical record.

The intravenous site must be assessed for pain and tenderness. If a patient experiences pain or discomfort from the peripheral cannula, the site should be discontinued, and a new cannula must be inserted. Pain can be a precursor to phlebitis. Another cause of discomfort is infusion of cool solutions. The tunica media, or the middle layer of the vein, contains nerve fibers. When cool solutions are administered, the veins constrict, and venospasm can occur. For this reason, refrigerated solutions should be allowed to warm to room temperature before they are infused. Solutions can be warmed to room temperature by removing them from the refrigerator 1 hour before they are administered. If the solution cannot be warmed in this way, such as when blood is administered, the infusion should be begun slowly and the solution allowed time to warm before the infusion rate is increased. Application of warm moist packs to the vein promotes vasodilation, relieves venospasm, increase's blood flow, and relieves pain.

The peripheral intravenous site must be assessed for any signs of swelling at or above the venipuncture site. Even though a blood return may be obtained, the intravenous solution can infiltrate into the tissues. If the tip of the intravenous catheter punctures the posterior wall of the vein, leaving the greater part of the cannula in the vessel, a blood return may be obtained, but the solution could be leaking into the tissues. If an infiltration occurs, the insertion site must be changed, and a new cannula must be inserted. The size of the arm with the inserted intravenous device should be compared with that of the opposite extremity. If the arm with the intravenous device is larger or if swelling is observed above the insertion site, the cannula must be discontinued.

Blanching is a white, shiny appearance at the insertion site. It is an indicator of an infiltration, or a fluid leak into the tissue. If any fluid leakage is noted at the insertion site, the intravenous site should be restarted. Leaking sites indicate that the integrity of the skin tissue is compromised. Any intravenous site from which fluid leaks should be evaluated for signs of cellulitis, which manifests as edema, redness, pain, and irritation that is usually noted by weeping skin. Cellulitis is an inflammatory response within the subcutaneous tissue that can be caused by the infiltration or extravasation of irritating medications, the lack of aseptic technique during site preparation or, the use of contaminated equipment or fluid. Any indications of cellulitis should be reported promptly to the patient's physician.

Redness at the insertion site indicates phlebitis, which is an inflammation of the vein. An intravenous site should be discontinued when the first signs of erythema or redness are observed. Some of the other clinical indicators of phlebitis are swelling, induration, tenderness, and palpation of a venous cord. The degree of phlebitis should be measured according to a uniform phlebitis scale, which provides a consistent standard for measuring the degree of the phlebitis. A recommended phlebitis scale is available in the *Intravenous Nursing Standards of Practice.*[2] The accepted phlebitis rate is 5% or less in any given patient population.[2] The degree of phlebitis should be documented in the patient's medical record. The presence of phlebitis may require the application of warm moist compresses or a medical intervention, such as changing medications, doses, dilution, delivery, or vascular access devices.

Suppurative thrombophlebitis occurs when purulent drainage is present at the insertion site. A swab culture of the drainage is obtained, blood cultures are drawn, and the hub and catheter tip are cultured. Removing the cannula does not make the infection disappear. In fact, if any of the infecting organisms are present in the circulatory system, bacteremia or septicemia can result. The first signs of septicemia may appear 2 to 10 days after the cannula is removed.[1] The clinical indicators of sepsis are fever, a positive blood culture, and a positive catheter tip culture.

MONITORING CENTRAL SITES

All the previously mentioned intravenous monitoring parameters apply to the assessment of central sites. The monitoring of central sites starts with the fluid container and progresses down the tubing to the vascular access device. The establishment of monitoring parameters for central intravenous sites depends on the type of vascular access device used. The nurse must be knowledgeable about the various types of vascular access devices that are available. When a central vascular access device is assessed, the nurse must differentiate a tunneled catheter from an implantable one. The various types of vascular access devices, regardless of where or how they are inserted (subclavian, jugular, tunneled, implanted, or peripherally), have similar monitoring parameters.

The catheter tract and insertion site must be evaluated for swelling and the skin around the insertion site assessed for indications of swelling or induration. Swelling around the neck or clavicles is an indicator of superior vena cava syndrome. Obtaining a blood return does not guarantee catheter integrity; the integrity of the catheter and any leakage of solution can be confirmed by fluoroscopy. If the catheter integrity is compromised, the physician should be notified, and medical intervention should be undertaken immediately.

The insertion site, the catheter tunnel and exit site, the portal pocket and the catheter tract are assessed for pain and tenderness. To thoroughly evaluate the catheter tract, the nurse must know the length of the inserted catheter and the location of the catheter tract. The insertion site, the entire length of the catheter tract or tunnel, the sutures, and the portal pocket are assessed for erythema, which is an indicator of inflammation. The size of the erythemic area should be documented in the medical record and communicated to the other members of the health care team for continued assessment. An inflamed portal pocket of an implantable device is usually left unaccessed until the redness and inflammation are resolved. Any painful, reddened, or inflamed insertion site, catheter tract, or portal pocket should be closely monitored. The results of the assessment should be reported to the physician, and medical intervention may be necessary.

The catheter insertion site should be assessed for drainage. If drainage is present, its amount, color, and consistency should be noted. A swab culture of the drainage should be sent to the laboratory, and the physician should be notified immediately. A description of the drainage and the nursing actions that are implemented should be documented in the patient's medical record. A catheter that has purulent drainage is inflamed and possibly infected and needs to be monitored closely. Usually, the catheter is discontinued, and systemic antibiotics are prescribed for the patient. If fever is present, semiquantitative blood cultures should be performed to determine the causative organisms and the source of the infection. The definitive method to determine catheter sepsis is to perform a culture of the catheter tip. The most frequently used method to perform a culture of the catheter tip is the semiquantitative culture. A disadvantage of using this method is that the catheter must be discontinued. After 72 hours of incubation, growth of 15 or more colonies of bacteria confirms that the catheter is infected.[3]

Allowing an infected catheter to remain in place can result in hematogenous seeding of the organism throughout the bloodstream. Hematogenous seeding can result in catheter sepsis if another source or site of infection seeds microorganisms on the intravascular catheter. Many factors affect catheter seeding, such as the patient's clinical status, the length of time the catheter has been in place, and the degree, type, and duration of the causative pathogen. If a fever is present with positive blood cultures, the intravascular catheter must be discontinued immediately.

MONITORING OTHER SPECIALTY SITES

The frequency of monitoring of epidural, intrathecal, ventricular reservoir, and intraosseous sites is determined by the condition and age of the patient, the prescribed therapy, and the practice setting. Flow rate is one of the evaluation parameters for all of these infusion devices.

The catheter insertion site of epidural, intrathecal, ventricular reservoir, and intraosseous infusions should be monitored and assessed for pain, tenderness, inflammation, and swelling. If swelling occurs, the placement of the catheter should be assessed. Epidural catheter placement is determined by aspiration and the absence of spinal fluid. Intrathecal and ventricular reservoir placements are ascertained by aspiration and the presence of spinal fluid. Intraosseous catheter placement is determined by aspiration of bone marrow. (See Chapter 13 for further details on the care and maintenance of epidural and intrathecal catheters, and Chapter 26 for further details on intraosseous infusions.)

CATHETER CARE

Peripheral

Peripheral intravenous catheter care should be performed after an intravenous catheter is inserted and when the dressing is soiled or no longer intact. The guidelines for peripheral site care are established in the *Intravenous Nursing Standards of Practice*.[2] First, the skin-cannula junction should be cleansed with an acceptable antiseptic solution (tincture of iodine, 1 to 2% iodophors, 70% isopropyl alcohol, or chlorhexidine). Then, a small amount of antimicrobial or antibiotic ointment may be applied at the skin-cannula insertion site.[2] An iodophor ointment is effective in killing gram-positive and gram-negative bacteria, including antibiotic-resistant strains, fungi, viruses, protozoa, and yeast. The benefit of applying ointment at the insertion site remains unestablished. Clinical trials regarding the use of ointment have not been conclusive and do not firmly establish decreased infection rates with its use.[4] However, an iodophor ointment should not be applied if the patient is allergic to iodine.

During catheter care, the cannula should be stabilized so that movement of the cannula is minimized. Stabilization of the cannula reduces the risk of phlebitis, infiltration, sepsis, and cannula migration. Various chevron taping methods may be used to stabilize the cannula. When tape is used, it should be applied only to the wings-cannula hub so that the assessment and monitoring of the skin-cannula junction site is not interrupted (Fig. 21–1). Tape should never be placed over the insertion site, but it may be placed on the hub of the cannula.

Many types of dressing materials for intravenous catheters are available. Some of the desired qualities for intravenous dressings are ease of application, viewing capacity, proper adhesion, appropriate size, moisture proof characteristics, permeability, durability, patient comfort, ability to immobilize the catheter, ease of removal, and cost effectiveness. The *Intravenous Nursing Standards of Practice* recommends that a sterile gauze or a transparent semipermeable membrane dressing be aseptically applied over the insertion site.[2] The commonest dressing materials are gauze or a transparent semipermeable membrane, which is a sterile dressing that allows visualization of the insertion site, is water resistant, and is permeable to air. If gauze is used, the entire surface and all edges must be secured with tape to ensure that the dressing is closed and intact. A Band-Aid dressing is not recommended, because it is nonocclusive.

A transparent semipermeable membrane dressing is frequently used on peripheral intravenous cannula sites to enable observation of the insertion site. For peripheral intravenous cannulas, after the dressing has been aseptically applied, a label should be attached to the dressing identifying the date and time, the gauge and length of the cannula, and the name of the nurse who inserted the cannula. If tubing is being attached to the peripheral cannula, the tubing should be looped and the loop taped to the patient's skin. This measure helps stabilize the cannula and keeps the tubing out of the patient's way. Several tubing devices are available that attach to the tubing and the cannula, forming a loop.

Even though the tip of a midline catheter is not in a central vein, the dressing is changed using sterile technique. Most agencies administer catheter care for midline catheters by following the same policies and procedures as those used for central vascular access devices. Central intravenous, subclavian, jugular, and peripherally inserted central catheters; implanted ports; and midline peripheral catheters require sterile dressing changes. Prepackaged dressing kits ensure the availability of all the required supplies and promote continuity in the delivery of care. Sterile central line dressing changes require the use of a mask and sterile gloves.

Central

For central catheters, a combination of dressing materials may be used. Sometimes, gauze is applied under the transparent dressing. The *Intravenous Nursing Standards of Practice* states that when a transparent semipermeable membrane is placed over gauze, it is considered a gauze dressing and must be changed every 48 hours when the administration set is changed.[2] Much controversy exists over the colonization of bacteria and the type of dressing material used.[5-7] Central catheter dressings should be labeled with the date and time of the dressing change and the name of the nurse who changed the dressing.

Jugular cannulated dressings are difficult to maintain in a manner that is intact and occlusive to air. A jugular area insertion site and movement of the neck create a challenge in applying a dressing so that it is comfortable to the patient and remains occlusive. If the jugular insertion site is located near a tracheostomy, moisture repellant is a requirement. With diaphoretic patients, adhesion can be enhanced by the application of a skin sealant around the outer perimeter before and after the dressing is applied. Numerous skin protectants are available in sterile, single-application packages. If the upper layer of the skin is broken or denuded, the application of a skin sealant is contraindicated because of the alcohol content in these preparations. The application of tincture of benzoin is not recommended, because of its drying effect to the skin, which can cause skin irritation.[8]

The frequency of central line dressing changes has not been established. Current practice is that subclavian and jugular dressings should be changed at least every 48 hours.[9] The *Intravenous Nursing Standards of Practice* recommends that gauze dressings on central cannula sites be routinely changed every 48 hours and states that the optimal time interval for changing transparent semipermeable membrane dressings is unknown.[2] However, the *Standards of Practice* recommends that consideration be given to changing these dressings every 48 hours in conjunction with the administration set change.[2] Dressing changes are required if the dressing is damp, soiled, or no longer intact. More frequent dress-

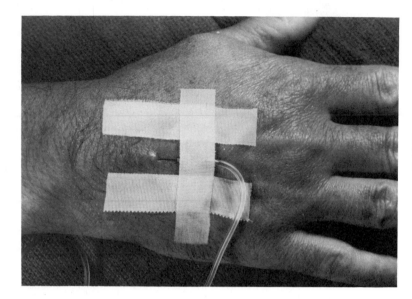

Figure 21–1. Apply chevron tape to the wings and cannula hub only, to allow assessment and monitoring of the insertion site.

ing changes are necessary if visual inspection of the insertion site is required.

The following is an example of a procedure incorporating the recommendations of the *Intravenous Nursing Standards of Practice* for administering site care and changing the dressing on a central venous catheter:

1. Wash hands with antimicrobial soap.
2. Ascertain allergies of patient.
3. Instruct patient to keep head turned away from insertion site.
4. Apply mask.
5. Apply nonsterile gloves.
6. Remove old dressing.
7. Assess insertion site for signs of inflammation, tenderness, or drainage.
8. Apply sterile gloves.
9. Cleanse with 70% isopropyl alcohol, beginning at insertion site and applying outward in a circular pattern. With last swab stick, cleanse catheter and sutures.
10. Repeat with iodophor solution (Fig. 21–2).
11. Allow to air dry.

12. Apply either a transparent or a sterile gauze dressing and tape over the entire gauze dressing, securing all edges.
13. Write date, time, and signature of nurse on label and attach to dressing (Fig. 21–3).
14. Document dressing change and site assessment in medical record.

Dressings on tunneled catheters may be made of gauze or transparent semipermeable membranes with or without gauze. During the first 7 days after insertion, the dressing on a tunneled catheter is changed by use of sterile technique. Dressings on tunneled catheters should be changed at least two to three times weekly and more frequently if the dressing is damp, soiled, or no longer intact. After the exit site has healed, the dressing change procedure for patients with tunneled catheters can be modified. The presence of the Dacron cuff assists in preventing bacteria from migrating along the catheter tract and anchors the catheter in place. When the exit site has healed, and if the patient is not immunocompromised, the dressing can be changed by use of aseptic technique. Thorough hand washing is always required. Some practitioners do not require home patients to use an occlusive

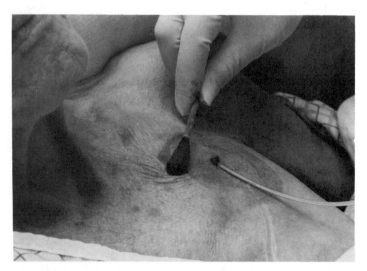

Figure 21–2. Cleanse with iodophor solution, beginning at the insertion site and applying outward in a circular pattern.

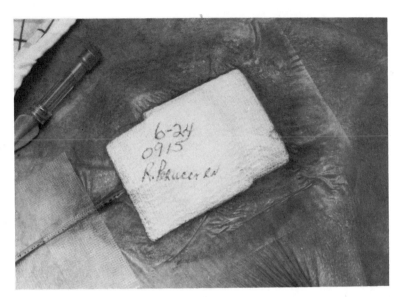

Figure 21–3. After the dressing is changed, label with date, time, and signature of the nurse.

dressing if the exit site has completely healed, usually 3 to 5 weeks after insertion, and if the patient's granulocyte count is above 200/mm³.[10] During periods of hospitalization and as a protection against nosocomial infections, the exit site should be covered by an occlusive dressing. Once the exit site is healed, patients with tunneled catheters are usually allowed to participate in water activities. An occlusive dressing should be applied before swimming and should be changed immediately afterward. The injection cap should also be changed before swimming.

During hospitalization, the current practice is to change a peripherally inserted central catheter dressing using sterile technique every 2 to 7 days, if transparent semipermeable dressings are used. Transparent dressings are preferred because they promote stabilization of the catheter and provide visualization of the insertion site. If the catheter is secured with sterile wound-closure strips, new strips should be applied at each dressing change. The dressing should be changed immediately when it becomes damp or soiled, or if the integrity is compromised. Some patients receiving home care who are not immunocompromised have family members or their caregiver change their peripherally inserted central catheter dressings using clean technique.

When not in use, unaccessed implanted ports do not require any site care except flushing with a heparinized saline solution every 28 days to maintain patency. Because accessing an implanted port is a sterile procedure, sterile gloves and a mask should be used. When the port is accessed, the noncoring needle should be changed at least every 7 days.[2] A sterile occlusive dressing should be placed over the noncoring needle to anchor it and stabilize the needle. Frequently, the noncoring needle is anchored with gauze and a transparent membrane dressing is applied over the needle, which allows the insertion site to be observed. This method of applying a dressing permits edema occurring from the infiltration of the noncoring needle to be detected if the needle becomes dislodged. The dressing must be changed if it becomes damp or soiled or is no longer intact.

Injection Caps and Needleless Systems

Peripheral intravenous cannulas and central intravenous catheters are used frequently for intermittent infusions and injections. Latex injection caps are placed on catheters and cannulas that are used intermittently. All injection caps should have a Luer lock design to decrease the risk of an air embolus. A latex injection cap attached to a peripheral cannula should be changed when a new cannula is inserted or if the integrity of the cap becomes compromised. The integrity of the injection cap depends on the number of needle punctures, the gauge of the needle inserted, and the composition of the latex. The integrity of the injection port should be confirmed before and immediately after each use. If the integrity of the cap is compromised, it should be changed immediately. The optimal period of time for changing latex injection ports on central and peripherally inserted central catheters is unknown. However, the latex injection ports on all central catheters should be changed at least every 7 days.[2] Ideally, the injection cap change should coincide with the dressing change and the flushing of the catheter.

The needleless system is replacing the use of standard injection caps and needles. Blunt-ended plastic insertion devices and reflux valves eliminate latex injection caps that require standard needle access and raise the possibility of accidental needle punctures. Various needleless systems are available. Most needleless devices require minimal change in administration techniques or methods. Needleless devices are changed by following the recommendations outlined for latex injection caps.

Flushes

After an intravenous cannula is used at routine intervals, the patency of the cannula can be maintained by flushing with a heparinized saline solution. A Groshong catheter, which has a two-way slit valve next to a rounded, closed tip, is routinely flushed with 5 ml of 0.9% sodium chloride solution. To maintain catheter patency, the lowest possible concentration of heparin should be used. The strength of heparin used varies from 10 to 1000 U/ml, depending on the patient's condition. The volume of the heparinized saline flush should be equal to twice the internal volume capacity of the catheter.[2] Information on the internal volume of a catheter can be obtained from the manufacturer. Many institutions flush intermittent peripheral cannulas with 0.9% sodium chloride solution only. Most studies that have compared the use of saline versus the use of heparin have specifically addressed their use with peripheral venous access devices.[11, 12]

When a vascular access device is flushed, positive pressure must be maintained on the lumen of the cannula to prevent a reflux of blood into the cannula lumen. Positive pressure is maintained by keeping a forward motion on the syringe plunger as the needle is removed from the injection port. If resistance is met during flushing, no further attempts to flush should be made. Pressure should not be exerted on the catheter in an attempt to restore patency; applying pressure to an occluded catheter can dislodge the clot into the vascular system or can rupture the catheter. The amount and the frequency of the flush should be such that the patient's clotting factors are not altered; if the patient has decreased coagulation factors, a more diluted heparinized saline may be required.

The catheter should be heparinized as soon as the medication is infused or when blood samples have been withdrawn. When blood samples have been withdrawn, the catheter should be flushed with 0.9% sodium chloride to remove the residual red blood cells before the catheter is flushed with the heparinized saline solution. The cannula should also be flushed when continuous fluids are discontinued and when the cannula is left in place for intermittent therapy. If a catheter is capped off and no medication is being administered intravenously, the catheter must be flushed to maintain patency. The frequency of flushing vascular access devices varies from institution to institution. Intravenous catheters may be flushed with a heparinized saline solution every 12 to 24 hours. Implantable venous ports are usually routinely flushed with a heparinized saline solution every 28 days to maintain catheter patency. Because of the closed-valve feature of Groshong catheters, which are not used on a routine basis, they may be flushed weekly with 0.9% sodium chloride solution. To decrease some of the confusion regarding the amount, the frequency, and the concentration of routine flushes, many institutions have established standardized flushing protocols to be used for the various vascular access devices.

BLOOD WITHDRAWAL

Central intravenous catheters are commonly placed in patients who have limited peripheral venous access. Therefore, central venous catheters are commonly used for the drawing of blood specimens. Some institutions require a physician's order permitting these devices to be used for this purpose. Serious consideration must be given when blood specimens for prothrombin time or partial prothrombin time determinations are to be drawn from a heparinized catheter. Erroneous laboratory values have been reported on blood specimens obtained from central catheters. For example, altered aminoglycoside serum concentration results have been reported when the blood was withdrawn from central venous Silastic catheters.[13] In addition, errors in measuring potassium levels have been identified when laboratory specimens have been withdrawn from newly inserted central catheters. These erroneous laboratory values were secondarily attributed to the sensitivity of certain analyzers to the presence of benzalko-

nium salts on newly inserted central catheters.[14] If the laboratory values withdrawn from a central vascular access device are significantly altered in a previously stable patient, the laboratory test should be repeated before any treatment is implemented.

When multiple-lumen catheters are used for the withdrawal of blood specimens, the proximal lumen is the preferred site from which the specimen should be obtained.[10] Before the blood is withdrawn, the nurse's hands must be washed, and gloves must be worn. All infusions being administered through the catheter must be stopped before the blood sample is obtained. Some agencies flush the catheter with 5 to 10 ml of 0.9% sodium chloride to confirm catheter patency and to remove any drug within the catheter lumen before the blood to be discarded is withdrawn. (Approximately 5 to 10 ml of blood is commonly withdrawn and discarded.) Smaller waste volumes are used for neonates and children. An alternative waste method is to flush the catheter with 0.9% sodium chloride and then aspirate or flush back and forth multiple times to clear the catheter prior to withdrawing the laboratory sample. A Vacutainer system or a needle and syringe can be used to withdraw the blood. Occasionally, when central catheters are used to withdraw blood specimens, the blood may be difficult to aspirate. If this occurs, it is sometimes helpful to ask the patient to sit, lie down, or turn from side to side, or to ask the patient to cough. After the blood has been withdrawn, the catheter should be flushed with 10 to 20 ml of 0.9% sodium chloride solution to remove any residual red blood cells. The catheter may then be flushed with a heparinized saline solution as established in the flushing protocol.

Many patients are discharged from the hospital with intravenous catheters. Patients and caregivers are taught to manage the catheters and are provided with professional support from a home care nurse. The frequency of visits to determine compliance depends on the patient's condition and age and the therapy being administered. Compliance visits by the home care nurse should reinforce the need for the patient or caregiver to use aseptic technique while performing dressing changes and administering medications. The nurse should give reinforcement to encourage the reporting of any abnormal findings immediately. Abnormal findings include elevated temperature, inflamed insertion or exit site, unusual catheter discomfort, or equipment or catheter malfunction.

NURSING DIAGNOSES

When nurses are knowledgeable about the array of vascular access devices available, the monitoring parameters associated with each device, and the catheter care requirements, quality patient care is given, and the risks to the patient are minimized. Nurses must be able to quickly identify the wide variety of intravenous devices and to plan and make appropriate nursing interventions to prevent the occurrence of complications. The identification of problems are referred to as *potential nursing diagnoses.* Appropriate nursing diagnoses associated with intravascular devices include alteration in comfort (including acute pain), impairment of skin integrity related to a potential for infection, knowledge deficit in relation to vascular access devices, anxiety, and noncompliance.

The potential for an alteration in comfort, including acute pain, can occur with the insertion of any intravascular device. Patients should be encouraged to promptly report any unusual discomfort related to their intravenous catheter. Whenever an intravenous catheter is in place, the integrity of the skin is impaired, and a potential for infection exists. Many patients who require central intravenous catheters are immunocompromised and are at increased risk for acquiring a nosocomial infection. Many patients are discharged from the hospital with long-term intravenous catheters. Whenever a patient has an intravenous catheter, a knowledge deficit may exist regarding the purpose and the function of the device. Patients and caregivers are often anxious about the management of the intravascular device. After discharge from the hospital, some patients may be noncompliant in administering their medications or maintaining their catheter.

PATIENT OUTCOMES

When the patient's pain is acknowledged, desired patient outcomes regarding an alteration in comfort are achieved. If the intravascular device is a peripheral cannula, the device should be discontinued and a new one restarted. Application of warm moist packs may be required if the pain is associated with phlebitis. If the pain experienced is from a central venous catheter, the insertion site should be frequently monitored and meticulous catheter care should be administered.

Peripheral cannulas should be discontinued immediately if the patient reports discomfort. If phlebitis occurs with a peripheral or central venous cannula, close monitoring and possible treatment with the application of warm moist compresses may be required. It is important that patients verbalize fears and anxiety related to health needs. Compliance is increased when the patient's ability and willingness to learn has been properly assessed. Consideration must be given to the home environment, the availability of the caregiver, and the family's previous intravenous experience and expectations. Much anxiety can be alleviated when the patient and caregiver are instructed on the purpose and the management of the intravenous device. When patients and caregivers are taught the importance of good hand washing,

of administering medications on time, and of assessing the insertion site accurately, they will be more compliant in the care and maintenance of their intravenous catheter. After such instruction, the patient and caregiver should be able to identify factors that decrease the occurrence of potential complications.

The goal of intravenous therapy for all patients receiving intravenous therapy is to complete treatment with minimal or no complications. When nurses deliver intravenous care according to established policies and procedures, which are based on professional nursing standards of practice, the risks associated with an intravascular device are significantly decreased.

References

1. Delaney CW, Lauer ML. Intravenous Therapy: A Guide to Quality Care. Philadelphia: J.B. Lippincott, 1988.
2. Intravenous Nurses Society. Intravenous Nursing Standards of Practice. Belmont, MA: Intravenous Nurses Society, 1990.
3. Bennet JV, Brachman PS. Hospital Infections, 3rd ed. Boston: Little, Brown, & Co., 1992:849–898.
4. Baranowski LB. Central venous access devices: Current technologies, uses, and management strategies. JIN 1993; 16(3):167–194.
5. Aly R, Bayles C, Maibach H. Restriction of bacteria growth under commercial catheter dressings. Am J Infect Control 1988; 16(3):95–100.
6. Conly JM, Grieves K, Peters B. A prospective, randomized study comparing transparent and dry gauze dressings for central venous catheters. J Infect Dis 1989; 159(2):310–319.
7. Farber BF. The multi-lumen catheter: Proposed guidelines for its use. Infect Control Hosp Epidemiol 1990; 9(5):206–208.
8. Bryant RA. Saving the skin from tape injuries. Am J Nurs 1988; 88(2):189–191.
9. Beam TR, et al. Preventing central venous catheter-related complications. Infect Surg 1990; 9(10):1–13.
10. Hadaway LC. Evaluation and use of advanced I.V. technology: Part 1. Central venous access devices. JIN 1989; 12(2):73–82.
11. Fry B. Intermittent flushing protocols: A standardization issue. JIN 1992; 15(3):160–163.
12. Goode CJ, Titler M, Rakel B, et al. A meta-analysis of effects of heparin flush, and saline flush: Quality and cost implications. Nurs Res 1991; 40(6):324–330.
13. Franson TR, Ritch PS, Quebbeman EJ. Aminoglycoside serum concentration sampling via central venous catheters: A potential source of clinical error. J Parenter Enteral Nutr 1987; 11(1):77–79.
14. Johnston JB, Messina M. Erroneous laboratory values obtained from central catheters. JIN 1991; 14:(1)13–15.

CHAPTER 22

Changing and Discontinuing Intravenous Therapy

Roxanne Perucca, BSN, CRNI

The delivery of high-quality intravenous nursing care requires changing solution containers and administration sets, rotating peripheral intravenous cannulas, changing dressings, and performing site assessments.[1] Careful maintenance of the intravenous system, performance of appropriate nursing interventions, and close monitoring minimize the risks to the patient and improve patient outcomes. The nurse administering intravenous therapy must be knowledgeable about the risks involved and must be able to implement measures to prevent their occurrence.

CHANGING THERAPY

A physician's order is necessary to change the fluids or medications being administered intravenously. The physician's order of assessment, planning, and implementation must be clearly written. The nurse uses the nursing process to evaluate the rationale for changing the therapy and intervenes appropriately. Before changing or administering the intravenous fluid or medication, the nurse is responsible for assessing the appropriateness of the prescribed order: the nurse assesses the patient's age and condition as well as the dosage, route, and rate of the intravenous solution or medication to be administered. The nurse must be knowledgeable about the indications, actions, dosage, side effects, and adverse reactions associated with each solution or medication administered.

The nurse is accountable for administering medications and solutions safely and making appropriate nursing interventions. For example, if the nurse questions the prescribed dosage or determines that the patient's condition does not warrant the prescribed medication or solution, the order should not be carried out until it is clarified. If any questions exist regarding the prescribed therapy, the physician should be contacted to clarify the plan of care and to verify the medication order.

The nurse closely monitors the intravenous system and the patient's response to the solution or medication being administered. The type and degree of change in the patient's status determine how promptly the nurse must intervene. Discontinuation of the therapy may be necessary before the physician is notified. For example, if a patient develops hives, hypotension, diaphoresis, and respiratory distress, the nurse must intervene immediately by stopping the medication. These signs and symptoms are indicators of an anaphylactic reaction, and appropriate therapy must be initiated immediately to reverse the complications of reaction.

Solution Containers

Intravenous solution containers may be changed to add a sequential container, to avoid exceeding "hang time" restrictions, or in response to a change in the prescribed therapy. Before a new intravenous fluid container is used, the fluid in the container should be inspected for clarity and for the presence of particulate matter. The solution container should be inspected for cracks, leaks, or punctures, and the expiration date should be verified. If the appearance of the solution is questionable or if the integrity of the container is compromised, the container should be returned to the pharmacy or dispensing department and should be clearly labeled with the reason for the return. If the expiration date has expired or will expire during the infusion, the container should be returned to the originating department or disposed of according to institutional policy.

After a medication has been added to the solution container, or when an administration set has been attached, the solution container must be used or discarded within 24 hours.[1] Once a solution container has been accessed, the potential for bacterial growth is increased; therefore, intravenous solution containers must not hang longer than 24 hours.[2] The solution container should be labeled with the date and time that it was initiated.

Administration Sets

The primary administration set change should coincide with the hanging of a new intravenous solution container or with the changing of the peripheral intravenous cannula. Each entry into the intravenous delivery system increases the risk of contamination. The *Intravenous Nursing Standards of Practice* has established that continuous peripheral and central primary sets and secondary administration sets should be changed every 48 hours. Total parenteral nutrition administration sets and primary intermittent sets should be changed every 24 hours.[1] Primary intermittent sets deliver medication through latex injection caps or needleless system devices. Intermittent devices have a greater risk of touch contamination than continuous devices because of the interruption involved in initiating and discontinuing solutions. Total parenteral nutrition requires the administration set to be changed every 24 hours because of the greater potential for bacterial and fungal contamination with this therapy.[3]

The administration set should be labeled with the date and time that it was initiated and documented according to institutional policy. The tubing should be labeled to communicate to subsequent shifts when the tubing must be changed.

The administration set, dome, and pressure tubing used for hemodynamic and arterial pressure monitoring should be changed every 48 hours.[4] If the integrity of the system has been compromised and contamination has occurred, the system must be changed immediately. The changing of the tubing is done using aseptic technique. Greater detail about the hemodynamic and arterial pressure monitoring system may be found in Chapter 23.

The following procedure can be used to add a solution container to an existing administration set:

1. Close the flow control clamp or shut off the electronic flow device.
2. Remove the protective cap from the new container.
3. Remove the old solution container from the intravenous pole.
4. Remove the spike from the old container and insert it into the new container. Be careful to avoid touch contamination of the administration set spike or the solution port.
5. Hang the new container.
6. Regulate the flow clamp or turn on the electronic flow device.
7. Label the new container with the date and time it was initiated.
8. Discard old container according to facility policy.
9. Document in medical record the type and volume of solution, the date and time initiated, the rate of flow, and the amount infused.

The initiation of a solution container with a new administration set is described in Chapter 19.

Dressing

The intravenous insertion site dressing should be changed simultaneously with the administration set change. Each break into the intravenous system increases the risk of contamination and infection. The procedure to perform peripheral cannula care and to change a central line dressing is detailed in Chapter 20. Peripheral cannula care is performed using aseptic technique. If the catheter is a peripherally inserted central catheter, the dressing should be changed using sterile technique. Changing the intravenous insertion site dressing allows the skin-cannula junction to be observed and evaluated. Peripheral and central gauze dressings should be changed every 48 hours. If a transparent dressing is placed over gauze on a peripheral or central catheter insertion site, it is considered to be a gauze dressing and should be changed every 48 hours.[1]

The frequency of transparent central line dressing changes has not been established. The optimal frequency for transparent semipermeable membrane dressing changes is unknown, but consideration should be given to changing these dressings every 48 hours, when the administration set is changed.[1] Regardless of the established dressing change policy, dressing changes are required if the dressing is damp, soiled, or no longer intact. If visual inspection of the insertion site is required, more frequent dressing changes may be necessary.

Vascular Access Devices

When intravenous therapy is changed, the nurse must assess if the current intravenous device and equipment can be used with the new therapy. For instance, if the patient has been receiving peripheral parenteral nutrition and the order has been changed to total parenteral nutrition, a central venous access device will need to be inserted. When the glucose concentration of a solution exceeds 10%, the solution becomes very irritating to small peripheral veins. Solutions whose glucose concentration exceeds 10%, or whose protein concentration exceeds 5%, or both, must be administered through a central venous access device.[5]

Peripheral Cannulas

The *Intravenous Nursing Standards of Practice* recommends that stainless steel needles and peripheral cannulas be removed every 48 hours.[1] When a peripheral intravenous site rotation policy is strictly followed, venous access can be prolonged, and the complications of phlebitis and infiltration are significantly reduced. For routine peripheral site rotations, the extremities should be alternated whenever possible. Using the opposite extremity allows previous insertion sites time to rest and phlebitic or infiltrated areas time to resolve. If a subsequent insertion site is restarted in the same extremity, it must be located proximal to the previously cannulated site. Inserting a cannula proximal to a previously infiltrated or phlebitic site prevents further damage to the tissues.

Some institutions have policies that allow cannula dwell time to be extended in patients who have limited venous access. In these situations, an order must be obtained from the physician to continue the present site, and the physician's order must be documented in the patient's medical record. Peripheral venous sites that are extended beyond the 48-hour catheter dwell time must be monitored very closely and discontinued at the first indication of tenderness, infiltration, or phlebitis. Documentation by the nurse should include the location and appearance of the insertion site; site care, if administered; and any nursing actions taken to resolve problems associated with the cannula.

Cannulas that have been placed in emergency situations should be replaced as soon as possible because aseptic technique or skin preparation may be compromised when intravenous cannulas are inserted during emergencies. Peripheral cannulas must be removed immediately if phlebitis, an infiltration, or cannula occlusion occurs. If the peripheral cannula appears to be infected, the cannula and insertion site should be cultured when it is removed. Culturing will identify the microorganisms that might be the source of the infection and will determine the medical interventions that follow.

Central Catheters

The optimal time interval for changing central venous catheters is unknown.[1] The Centers for Disease Control and Prevention states that the proper frequency for changing central lines, including those for pressure monitoring, is unknown.[6] As a result, no established practice exists regarding the dwell time of central vascular access devices. Critical care units usually have the most specific policies for the changing of short-term percutaneously inserted central catheters. Some critical care units change multilumen subclavian and jugular catheters over a guidewire using sterile technique every 3 or 4 days, others change lines every 7 to 10 days, and still others leave multilumen central catheters in place until complications develop.[7]

Peripherally inserted central catheters must be removed when an infection or inflammatory process is evident or if the catheter tip is malpositioned. Because of their small diameter and the insertion procedure used for these catheters, veins in the upper extremity may develop mechanical phlebitis several days after the catheter is inserted. Depending on the patient's condition, the inflammation may be treated with the application of warm moist compresses, which usually results in a decrease in the tenderness and the size of the inflamed area. If the inflammation does not decrease within 24 hours of the application of warm moist compresses, or if it does not resolve within 72 hours, the catheter should be removed.

Catheter tip placement should be confirmed intermittently by radiography. Occasionally, the tip of a peripherally inserted central catheter migrates outside of the superior vena cava or the subclavian vein. If this situation occurs, the catheter can no longer be considered a central line. The catheter must be removed if the prescribed therapy requires central access, such as the administration of total parenteral nutrition. A catheter that has been partially withdrawn out of the vein cannot be readvanced, because the external portion of the withdrawn catheter is no longer sterile and introduces microorganisms into the vascular system if it is reintroduced.

Long-term catheters, such as tunneled catheters and implantable ports, are frequently left in place for several years. If complications occur, such as fever or sepsis, the catheter must be considered as a possible source of the infection. Blood cultures can be drawn through the device and compared with peripherally obtained blood cultures. The catheter should be cultured to identify the presence of microorganisms. If the source of infection cannot be identified and the patient remains septic, the long-term catheter must be removed.

It is important to explain to the patient the rationale for the medication being administered, the purpose for changing the intravenous access device, or the reason for changing the dressing over the insertion site. A patient's anxiety and apprehension are decreased when he or she understands the reason for changing the therapy. For example, if a patient receiving intravenous therapy at home understands the importance of maintaining a dry and intact central venous catheter dressing to decrease the risk of infection, compliance will be increased.

Any change in the intravenous therapy solution or medication, the administration set, the cannula, or the insertion site dressing should be documented in the patient's medical record. The date and time of the change and the nurse's name should be charted. When a cannula or a dressing is changed, the condition of the site as well as the reason for changing the site should be documented. With peripheral cannula changes, the cannula type, gauge, and length, and the location of the insertion site must be documented. When patient education is provided on the care of an intravenous catheter, the communication should be documented.

DISCONTINUING THERAPY

The physician's order to discontinue intravenous therapy must be clearly written. The nurse then uses the nursing process of assessment, planning, and implementation to evaluate the rationale for discontinuing the therapy. Intravenous access may be discontinued because it is no longer required by the patient or because the patient decides not to continue treatment. Because of the risk of complications carried by central venous catheters, they are usually removed when they are no longer indicated. A catheter should be removed immediately if its integrity is compromised, for example, if a hole or tear is observed in the catheter wall, because the risk of infection is greatly increased if such a catheter is left in place. If a catheter is removed because it is defective, it should be saved and the problem reported to the manufacturer and the Food and Drug Administration.

Before an intravenous cannula is removed, the procedure should be explained to the patient. The patient should be encouraged to ask questions regarding the process; answering a patient's questions decreases anxiety and alleviates apprehension.

At any time during the therapy, the patient or the legally authorized representative has the right to request that the therapy be discontinued. Any intervention that results in the discontinuation of therapy should be communicated to the physician.

Peripheral Cannulas

Peripheral cannulas should be removed immediately if contamination is suspected, if the patient experiences discomfort, or if phlebitis or an infiltration is detected. The delayed withdrawal of an infiltrated or phlebitic intravenous catheter extends the duration and the severity of the tissue damage. If the insertion site is tender and reddened with a palpable cord, warm moist compresses may be applied for 20 minutes several times a day to alleviate the discomfort associated with phlebitis.[8] If a vesicant medication has been administered and extravasated, the treatment protocol should be initiated before the cannula is removed. The severity of the tissue damage is decreased if the extravasation protocol is implemented immediately.

After the cannula has been removed, the insertion site requires ongoing observation and assessment because postinfusion phlebitis can occur after the cannula has been removed. Usually, postinfusion phlebitis is evident within 48 hours after cannula removal. Some investigators have reported that greater than 40% of catheter-associated phlebitis occurs more than 24 hours after the cannula has been discontinued.[9] Depending on the severity of the phlebitis, nursing interventions may include the application of intermittent warm moist compresses to the phlebitic area. In cases of severe phlebitis, medical intervention may be necessary. The treatment of severe phlebitis may include the administration of systemic antibiotics or lysis of the phlebitic vein.

Peripheral Cannula Removal

1. Verify physician's order.
2. Wash hands with antiseptic soap.
3. Explain cannula removal to the patient.
4. Close the flow clamp.
5. Assess the cannula insertion site for evidence of local complication.

6. Remove the tape and dressing, and stabilize the cannula with one hand. *Do not* use scissors to remove the tape.
7. Put on gloves.
8. Withdraw cannula using a slow steady movement and keeping the hub parallel to the skin.
9. With the extremity elevated, gently apply pressure with a sterile dry gauze to the insertion site until the bleeding stops.
10. Assess cannula integrity and length.
11. Tape a sterile dressing over the insertion site.
12. Document the type, gauge, and length of the cannula removed; the assessment of the insertion site; and the date and time the cannula was removed.

Arterial Catheters

The *Intravenous Nursing Standards of Practice* recommends that peripheral arterial catheters be removed every 96 hours.[1] If the arterial catheter becomes contaminated, occluded, infiltrated, or infected, or if circulatory impairment develops, the catheter should be discontinued immediately. Arterial catheter removal is detailed in Chapter 23.

Central Catheters

Before a central venous access device is removed, the nurse must determine if the intervention is a medical act. In many health care settings, subclavian, jugular, and peripherally inserted central catheters are removed by a registered nurse in accordance with the institution's policies and procedures. The removal of central catheters requires that precautions be taken to minimize the risk of an air embolism. Two such precautions are positioning the patient to a dorsal recumbent position with the head of the bed in a flat position and having the patient perform a Valsalva maneuver while the catheter is being withdrawn. The Valsalva maneuver raises intrathoracic pressure, which impedes air from entering into the vein. A patient may be instructed to perform the Valsalva maneuver by bearing down against a closed glottis after taking a deep breath.[10]

When a peripherally inserted central catheter is removed, precautions should also be taken to prevent an air embolism. When a peripherally inserted central catheter is to be removed, the patient's arm should be abducted. If resistance is encountered as the catheter is withdrawn, the nurse should not remove the catheter. A peripherally inserted central catheter may resist removal because of the occurrence of venous spasm, vasoconstriction, phlebitis, valve inflammation, and thrombophlebitis, or the presence of a fibrin sheath. The application of warm moist compresses may alleviate venous spasm and vasoconstriction, resulting in easier removal of the catheter.[11] Any catheter that is not withdrawn with smooth, gentle pressure should be left in place and covered with a sterile dressing, and the physician should be notified. A catheter embolism can occur if too much withdrawal pressure is applied to a resistant catheter.

A tunneled catheter must be removed by a physician. This procedure may require the dissection of the Dacron cuff from the subcutaneous tissue. After a tunneled catheter is removed, the exit site should be covered with a sterile, dry dressing.

The nurse is then responsible for observing the exit site and making appropriate interventions.

Implanted ports may be surgically removed when the treatment requiring them is no longer necessary. After removal of an implantable port, the insertion site must be assessed for signs of inflammation. Tunneled catheters and implantable ports are often removed as an outpatient procedure; in these cases, the patient must be instructed to monitor the incision site for signs of tenderness, redness, drainage, or an elevated temperature. If any signs of inflammation are observed, the patient should contact his or her physician immediately.

If a catheter has purulent drainage at the insertion site or is considered to be a source of infection, it should be cultured as it is removed. This measure will identify any microorganisms that are present on the catheter surface.

The following procedure may be used for the removal of a central catheter:

Central Catheter Removal

1. Wash hands with antiseptic soap.
2. Assist patient to dorsal recumbent position. Note: the head of the bed must be in a flat position.
3. Close flow clamp.
4. Apply gloves.
5. Remove the tape and dressing.
6. Assess the insertion site.
7. Clip and remove sutures, if present.
8. Instruct the patient to perform the Valsalva maneuver.
9. Remove the catheter with gentle pulling motion (Fig. 22–1).
10. Instruct patient to breathe normally.
11. Apply gentle pressure at the insertion site with sterile, dry gauze until bleeding stops.
12. Cleanse with an antiseptic solution and apply a small amount of antimicrobial ointment at the insertion site.
13. Apply sterile, air-occlusive dressing over the insertion site to prevent a delayed air embolism (Fig. 22–2).
14. Assess the length and integrity of the discontinued catheter and visually inspect the tip for smoothness.
15. Document the date, time, site assessment, patient response, and nursing interventions in the patient's medical record.

After the catheter has been removed, the patient's condition must continue to be monitored. The patient should remain flat and supine for a short time after central catheter removal; this position helps to maintain a positive intrathoracic pressure and allows the tissue tract time to seal. The condition of the insertion site and surrounding tissues should continue to be assessed and documented. The *Intravenous Nursing Standards of Practice* recommends that the insertion site dressing be changed and assessed every 24 hours after central line removal until the site has epithelialized.[1] Catheters that have had a longer dwell time require a longer period of time for the insertion site to close.

▶ NURSING DIAGNOSIS

Maintaining and monitoring the intravenous system are nursing responsibilities. Frequently encountered problems of nursing diagnoses related to changing and discontinuing intravenous therapy are knowledge deficit in relation to intra-

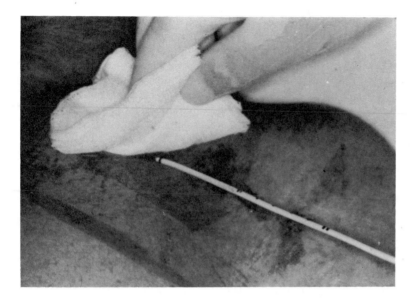

Figure 22–1. Remove catheter with a gentle pulling motion. Apply pressure at the insertion site with sterile gauze until bleeding stops.

vascular devices, potential for injury related to infection, impairment of skin integrity, and noncompliance.

A knowledge deficit exists with all patients who have intravenous devices. It is important for patients to understand that if their peripheral cannula site is tender or painful while their antibiotic is infusing, they should report it to the nurse. Failure of patients to be honest when they are asked about the comfort of their intravenous site results in increased phlebitis and inflammation.

Today, many patients are sent home with long-term central venous catheters. Some of these catheters are inserted during the patient's hospitalization, and the patient and caregiver are instructed regarding catheter care and management before the patient is discharged. In other patients, the catheter is inserted as an outpatient procedure, these patients are discharged immediately with a long-term central venous catheter. Patients must be instructed on the potential for injury and infection related to the maintenance of an intravenous catheter. The signs of inflammation (i.e., redness, tenderness, drainage, and temperature elevation) should be explained to the patient or caregiver. If the patient observes inflammatory indicators, it

is essential that he or she notifies their physician or home care nurse immediately. When patients or caregivers do not understand the risks involved, they may become noncompliant in reporting discomfort.

An impairment in skin integrity results in an increased risk of local or systemic complications. The nurse delivering intravenous care must understand the importance of changing the administration set and solution container according to established professional standards of practice. The nurse must understand the risks involved to the patient when aseptic technique is not used while a peripheral cannula is restarted.

PATIENT OUTCOMES

The delivery of high-quality intravenous care requires that the nurse evaluate patient outcomes on an ongoing basis. The evaluation of patient outcomes determines if the nursing interventions used are appropriate. Desired patient outcomes related to changing and discontinuing treatment are complet-

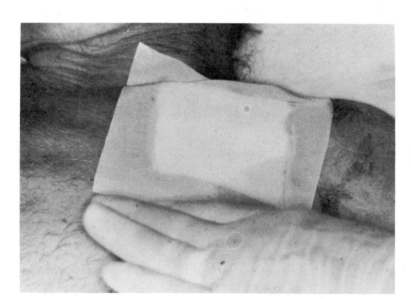

Figure 22–2. Apply a sterile, air-occlusive dressing over the insertion site to prevent a delayed air embolism.

ing therapy with minimal or no complications, identifying factors that decrease the potential for injury, and verbalizing the rationale for treatment.

Rotating cannula sites, changing central line dressings and administration sets, and performing insertion site assessments allow many patients to complete their course of intravenous therapy with minimal or no local complications. When patients receiving intravenous therapy in the home understand the risk factors related to intravenous therapy, they are more compliant in the administration of their catheter care. Compliance is increased when patients understand the rationale for monitoring their insertion site for signs of inflammation.

Nurses must be knowledgeable about the risks involved in intravenous therapy. Today, many patients are immunocompromised and have extended hospitalizations and are critically ill; these patients are at risk for developing local and systemic complications. To prevent the occurrence of complications, the nurse must be committed to the principles and rationale involved in changing and discontinuing intravenous devices and equipment. When the nurse adheres to professional standards of practice, safe, high-quality intravenous nursing care will be delivered.

References

1. Intravenous Nurses Society. Intravenous Nursing Standards of Practice. Belmont, MA: Intravenous Nurses Society, 1990.
2. Delaney CW, Lauer ML. Intravenous Therapy: A Guide to Quality Care. Philadelphia: J. B. Lippincott, 1988:133.
3. Weinstein SM. Plumer's Principles and Practice of Intravenous Therapy, 5th ed. Philadelphia: J. B. Lippincott, 1993:364–374.
4. Bennett JV, Brachman PS. Hospital Infection, 3rd ed. Boston: Little, Brown, and Co., 1992:885.
5. Clinical Skillbuilders. I.V. Therapy. Springhouse, PA: Springhouse Corp., 1990:189–192.
6. Centers for Disease Control Working Group. Guidelines for prevention of intravenous therapy-related infections. Infect Control 1981; 3:62–67.
7. Beam TR, Goodman EL, Farr BM, et al. Preventing central venous catheter-related complication. Infect Surg 1990; 9(10):1–13.
8. Phillips LD. Manual of I.V. therapeutics. Philadelphia: F. A. Davis, 1993:237.
9. Hershey CO, Tomford JW, McLaren CE, et al. Natural history of intravenous catheter-associated phlebitis. Arch Intern Med 1984; 144(7):1373–1375.
10. Thielen JB, Nyquist J. Subclavian catheter removal: Nursing implications to prevent air emboli. JIN 1991; 14(2):114–118.
11. Baronowski L. Central venous access devices. Current technologies, uses, and management strategies. JIN 1993; 16(3):167–194.

Hemodynamic Monitoring

Terri A. Miller, CRNI

• •

• •

Hemodynamics is defined as "the forces involved in the circulation of the blood."[1] The effectiveness of the heart to contract and circulate blood depends on the strength of the heart muscle itself and the pressures surrounding it. These pressures within the surrounding major vessels, heart valves, and lungs are generated by the blood volume with contraction (systole) and relaxation (diastole) of the heart. Hemodynamic monitoring catheters and equipment translate the pressures into graphs and numbers.

Arterial, venous, and balloon flotation or pulmonary artery catheters have been developed to allow measurement of these pressures. Bedside monitoring of these pressure values, or readings, aids the physician in preoperative and postoperative evaluation of cardiac function, fluid volume delivery, and intravenous medication administration for optimum cardiac function.

Nurses are responsible for maintaining many of these invasive monitoring catheters while caring for their patients in a critical care setting. To ensure proper care of the patient, the nurse should have a basic understanding of the pressures within the circulatory system, be familiar with the similarities between catheter systems, recognize normal and abnormal pressure patterns, and respond with appropriate nursing actions.

GENERAL HEMODYNAMIC MONITORING

Arterial and venous pressure waveforms all reflect atrial and ventricular contraction (systole) and relaxation (diastole). Also, the closing of the heart valves may sometimes be seen. The contraction of the heart chamber is an upward, or positive, stroke on the pressure tracing, and the relaxation is the downward, or negative, stroke. Valvular closure, when seen, is also an upstroke, reflecting the increased pressure in the monitored chamber of the heart. Central venous, arterial, and pulmonary artery monitor tracings are represented by a, v, and c waveforms, which refer to atrial, ventricular, and valvular closure pressures in all of the monitoring systems.

Intra-arterial blood pressure, central venous pressure (CVP), pulmonary artery pressure, and pulmonary wedge pressure (PWP) are the basic pressure waveforms monitored in the critical care setting. Pulmonary artery catheters also have the ability to determine cardiac output and mixed venous oxygenation and may have a port for pacing wires.[2]

These types of monitoring require the same basic equipment. A fluid system, a transducer, and a monitor translate the pressures in the vascular system into digital values and visible waveforms, which appear on the bedside monitor. Most critical care units have a central monitor system that is capable of visualizing and storing the information for later printout.

The fluid system needed to translate the patient pressures to the transducer is placed under pressure via a pressure bag at 300 mm Hg. The intravenous solutions used may be heparinized sodium chloride in a concentration of 1 to 4 U of heparin per milliliter of solution. Patients with clotting disorders or low platelet counts may be given only saline flush solutions.

The bag used to pressurize the flush solution may have a pressure gauge attached for proper inflation via a bulb or a handle that automatically reaches proper pressure when it is fully cranked and locked. Either method gives a continuous infusion at 3 to 5 ml/hour when the bag is inflated to 300 mm Hg. The system can also be flushed intermittently via a fast-flush device (Fig. 23–1).

The tubing for this system is stiff and noncompliant and contains stopcocks for calibration to zero and for blood sampling. The length of tubing is kept to a minimum to prevent distortion of the signal; it is generally 3 to 4 feet long (Fig. 23–1).

The fluid system is connected to the transducer, which senses changes in flow, temperature, concentration, pressure, light intensity, and other physiologic variables. Disposable and reusable transducers are available. External, disposable, strain gauge, and pressure transducers are the most widely used. This type has a diaphragm that transfers the pressure it senses to a bedside monitoring system.

Placing the transducer level with the patient's right atrium negates the effect of atmospheric pressure. This plane is known as the phlebostatic axis and is located at the fourth intercostal space, at the mid-axillary line.[2-6] Marking the phlebostatic axis position on the patient's chest ensures the accuracy of each reading (Figs. 23–2 and 23–3).

The patient is placed in a supine position when the transducer is set to zero to facilitate the accuracy of the reading. If the transducer is below the level of the heart, a falsely high pressure can be recorded. When placed too high, the transducer reflects a falsely low reading.[5] Setting the monitor at zero on the scale being utilized will cancel the effect of atmospheric pressure and allow the pressures within the circulatory system to be recorded.

If the patient's head is kept elevated (e.g., because of cerebral injury), the phlebostatic axis should be marked on the patient's chest with an indelible marker, and the degree of elevation should be noted on the Kardex. Some institutions lock the bed in this position to ensure that it is kept elevated to the ordered degree and to ensure the accuracy of hemodynamic readings.

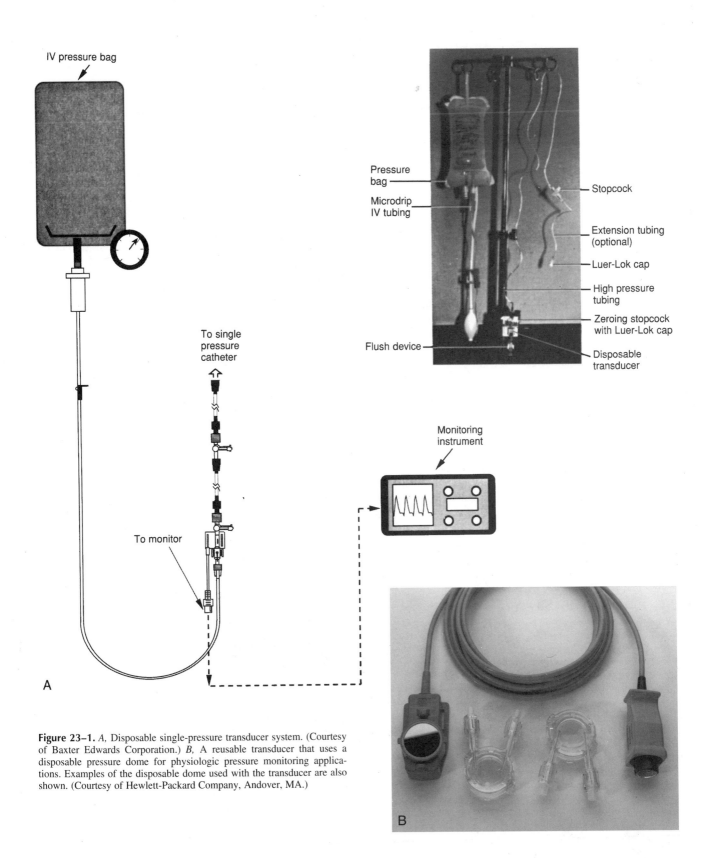

IV pressure bag

To single
pressure
catheter

To monitor

A

Pressure
bag

Microdrip
IV tubing

Flush device

Stopcock

Extension tubing
(optional)

Luer-Lok cap

High pressure
tubing

Zeroing stopcock
with Luer-Lok cap

Disposable
transducer

Monitoring
instrument

B

Figure 23–1. *A,* Disposable single-pressure transducer system. (Courtesy of Baxter Edwards Corporation.) *B,* A reusable transducer that uses a disposable pressure dome for physiologic pressure monitoring applications. Examples of the disposable dome used with the transducer are also shown. (Courtesy of Hewlett-Packard Company, Andover, MA.)

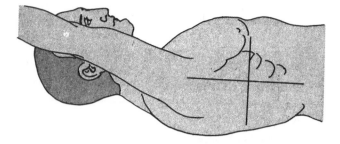

Figure 23–2. Transducer leveling from different positions. (From Boggs RL, Wooldridge-King M [eds]. AACN Procedure Manual for Critical Care, 3rd ed. Philadelphia: W.B. Saunders, 1993:290.)

A cable attached to the transducer carries the signals to the bedside monitor, which is an amplifying device for these signals or pressure readings. Basic monitor functions include digital read-outs, an oscilloscope to display waveforms, indicators for the various pressures being obtained, alarm systems with high and low adjustments, waveform size (gain) control, and controls for setting the machine to zero and for calibrating. Simultaneous monitoring of various pressures is possible with newer monitoring systems.

Inserting a hemodynamic catheter is a sterile procedure. Equipment for insertion may be gathered from unit supplies, or prepackaged insertion kits may be used. Supplies needed include sterile gowns, gloves, masks, hats, drapes, towels, gauze, dressing, local anesthetic, suture equipment, flush solution, and a catheter. A stocked cart containing additional supplies in case of defect or contamination may be taken to the patient's bedside.

Preparation

Placement of a hemodynamic catheter requires obtaining informed consent from the patient or the family, if the patient cannot consent. Ample time should be provided for the patient and family to ask questions; lessening patient apprehension can facilitate insertion. The patient should be told that the nurse will assist with the procedure and will answer questions or will explain the steps as the procedure progresses. After consent is obtained, the system should be prepared (Table 23–1). Then the patient should be prepared to provide a sterile entry area. A 5- to 10-minute scrub with a

povidone-iodine solution or chlorhexidine is performed by the nurse or physician, and a sterile towel is placed over the prepared site. The towel protects the site from accidental contamination and is removed just before the catheter is inserted. The catheter may be inserted into the antecubital area or directly into the central system via the subclavian, internal or external jugular, or femoral vein.

A sterile field is prepared either during preparation of the equipment and fluid system or while the patient is being prepared. In some institutions, the physician prepares the patient while the nurse prepares the equipment and field, or two nurses may prepare the patient and sterile field, then be available to help with the insertion.

When a pulmonary artery catheter is placed, the balloon is checked for leakage before the catheter is inserted. If a multilumen catheter is used, the ports are all preflushed with either 0.9% sodium chloride or a heparinized solution. Other items placed on the sterile field include a local anesthetic, suture equipment, sponges, and dressing equipment. A separate table may be used for sterile gowns, drapes, and towels. The nurse preparing the field dons a gown and gloves and may help the physician don gown and gloves, if necessary.

Insertion

The patient is placed in the Trendelenburg position unless it is contraindicated. This position engorges the jugular and subclavian vessels to ease insertion. The antecubital or femoral insertion does not require the Trendelenburg position. The nurse assisting the physician passes equipment, observes

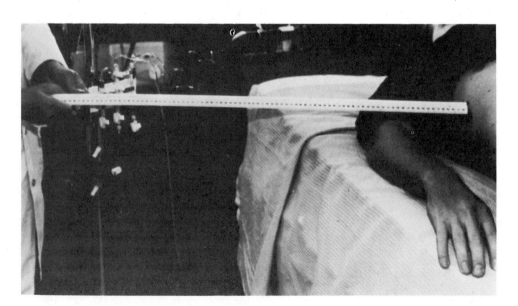

Figure 23–3. Leveling transducer to phlebostatic axis. (From Boggs RL, Wooldridge-King M [eds]. AACN Procedure Manual for Critical Care, 3rd ed. Philadelphia: W.B. Saunders, 1993:292.)

Table 23-1

System Preparation Before Hemodynamic Catheter Insertion

1. Turn on the monitor. Allow it to warm up according to manufacturer's recommendation.
2. Prepare and label the flush solution, spike the bag with microdrop tubing, and prime tubing.
3. Carefully remove the transducer tubing from the package. Tighten all connections and replace the open stopcock caps with dead-end caps.
4. If using a disposable dome, a drop of sterile normal saline may be placed atop the transducer to facilitate transmission before the dome is attached.
5. Attach the transducer system to the monitor.
6. Attach the flush solution and tubing to the stopcock at the transducer.
7. Use the fast-flush device on the transducer tubing to prime it. Inspect tubing for air bubbles and prime again as needed.
8. Place the pressure bag over the flush solution. Wait to inflate the pressure bag until the monitor has been set to zero to avoid contamination or electrical hazard from leakage of fluid. This measure also will decrease pressure on the transducer tubing created by the system being closed to itself and will lessen the chance of diaphragm rupture.
9. Align the transducer to the phlebostatic axis by using a carpenter's level. Mark the spot on the patient's chest with a waterproof marker.
10. If the patient cannot be supine, note the degree of elevation used for leveling the transducer on the flow sheet and Kardex.
11. Inflate the pressure bag. The system can now be calibrated, and a pressure-monitoring range selected.
12. Follow the manufacturer's directions for calibrating and setting the monitor to zero. This may be accomplished by pushing a button and holding it in until the monitor has been set to zero and calibrated, or the monitor will perform its functions automatically after the desired function is selected.

the monitor for cardiac and waveform changes, inflates the balloon if a pulmonary artery catheter is inserted, reassures the patient, and places the sterile dressing over the insertion site. Both bioclusive and traditional silk or gauze dressings may be used to cover the catheter after it is inserted. Dressings are changed using sterile technique every 24 to 48 hours and whenever they are not intact.[6]

Some institutions use a second nurse to attach the transducer tubing to the catheter. This nurse calibrates the bedside monitor, observes the patient's cardiac status, and records all waveform pressures as noted by the physician. This second nurse may obtain additional equipment, if needed, and may provide additional reassurance to the patient during the procedure.

Most monitors are able to run continuously, which is a convenient feature if only one nurse is assisting. These monitors store the digital pressure readings and waveforms so that they can be placed in the chart when the catheter insertion is completed. The type of catheter placed and its location, the person inserting it, and how the patient tolerated the procedure are recorded in the nurses' notes.

Complications occurring with subclavian or jugular vein placement include hematoma, pneumothorax, and hemothorax. Arterial puncture or laceration and nerve damage can occur with both venous and arterial insertions.[2-5] A chest x-ray is performed to verify proper location of the catheter tip after any central line insertion. The x-ray is also used to assess for lung complications if the catheter placement was jugular or subclavian (see Chapter 24 for treatment of insertion complications).

Initiating Therapy

Patient care after hemodynamic line placement focuses on both patient safety and interpretation of hemodynamic values. Many patients may need restraints to prevent catheter or line dislodgement. If restraints are needed, institutional policies regarding their use should be followed.

In most institutions, blood samples for laboratory testing can be drawn by registered nurses and physicians. When heparin is used to maintain line patency, the results of coagulation studies may be altered. Care must be taken to maintain the monitoring system integrity because contamination and accidental blood loss may result if line disconnection occurs. Blood loss from an arterial line can be rapid. The use of a transparent dressing alone or over gauze permits arterial insertion site visualization. High and low alarm limits should always be set to assess significant changes and to prevent accidental line disconnection.

The recording of pressure readings varies according to the severity of the patient's illness and the institutional guidelines. Fifteen- to 30-minute readings are commonly required for unstable patients, whereas readings obtained every 2 hours may be routine after the patient is stabilized. Wedge pressures from a pulmonary artery catheter are not obtained as frequently to prevent vessel trauma and balloon rupture. The pulmonary artery diastolic pressure may be recorded instead of repeated inflation of the balloon. Care and pressure readings may be documented on a flow sheet. Clinically significant changes should always be addressed in the narrative section of the patient's chart.

Discontinuing Therapy

When hemodynamic monitoring is no longer needed, the nurse may receive a physician's order to remove the catheter. The central catheter placed for hemodynamic monitoring is removed using the method noted in Chapter 22. The pulmonary artery catheter balloon must be deflated before it is removed to prevent damage to the cardiac valves. Pressure is applied at the insertion site for 5 to 10 minutes after the device is removed. Arterial lines, or those removed from patients with coagulation abnormalities, should be assessed after 10 to 15 minutes, and pressure should be held longer, if needed. A sterile dressing should be placed on the site after bleeding ceases.

After the line is removed, the condition of all insertion sites should be documented in the nurses' notes. Early recognition of signs of infection, phlebitis, or hematoma facilitates early intervention. Documentation includes when and how the line was removed, the type of dressing applied, and how the patient tolerated the procedure.

TYPES OF HEMODYNAMIC MONITORING

Intra-arterial Monitoring

As the heart contracts, pressure from the blood volume is exerted against the arterial walls. The amount of blood in the

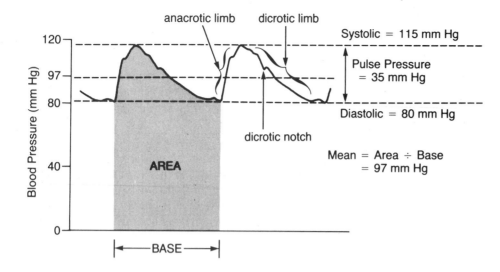

Figure 23–4. Normal arterial waveform. (From Darovic GO. Hemodynamic Monitoring. Philadelphia: W.B. Saunders, 1987:109.)

left ventricle, the elasticity, and the integrity of the arterial system determine the amount of pressure needed for contraction.[2] Intra-arterial monitoring is used to obtain direct measurements of the systolic and diastolic pressures occurring during the cardiac cycle.

The arterial line waveform has three separate components that reflect the cardiac cycle. The upstroke, or positive deflection, occurs at the peak of systole and ranges from 90 to 140 mm Hg. The dicrotic notch occurs with aortic valve closure and reflects the beginning of diastole. The lowest point of the waveform is end-diastole and ranges from 60 to 90 mm Hg (Fig. 23–4).

Most bedside monitors provide mean arterial pressure (MAP) in addition to systolic and diastolic values.

$$MAP = \frac{Systole + 2\,(Diastole)}{3}$$

Factors affecting MAP include the cardiac output and the elasticity of the vessels (systemic vascular resistance). MAP is reflected on the monitor screen by a number that is an average of the systolic and diastolic readings or can be measured alone by use of an anaeroid sphygmomanometer gauge. A normal MAP ranges from 70 to 105 mm Hg. Catheter size and location can cause pressure readings to vary, but the MAP is not affected by these characteristics. MAP is an indicator of organ perfusion.

Intra-arterial monitoring is used with patients who require frequent blood gas samplings, in those receiving vasoactive drugs, in critically ill patients undergoing other invasive monitoring, and in patients who have undergone or will undergo surgical procedures.

Arterial catheter placement is determined by the collateral circulation and the size of the artery to be cannulated. The Allen test or a modified version of it is used to determine adequate collateral circulation. Both arteries on the limb being used for insertion are occluded simultaneously. The limb is raised slightly above the torso while the hand is clenched several times. The pressure on each artery is released separately, and the hand is observed for return of color, which indicates adequate collateral circulation. Slowed return of color is a negative test result, and another site should be selected (Fig. 23–5).[2]

Catheters are usually placed in the radial, brachial, or femoral arteries, and less often, in the dorsalis pedis, axillary,

temporal, and umbilical arteries. The catheter is placed either by direct arterial puncture or by cut-down if the vessel cannot be cannulated. Catheter changes are recommended every 3 to 5 days.

Preparation and Insertion

The system and patient are prepared as previously described. A short length of pressure tubing is added to the sterile tray. This tubing has a stopcock near the proximal end, which will be attached to the catheter after it is inserted. The tubing may be preflushed with a syringe or is flushed just before arterial insertion by connecting the distal end to the transducer tubing. After the pressure tubing is attached to the transducer tubing, it may be held by the nurse who is assisting, or it may be covered with a sterile towel and clamped on the field.

After the catheter is inserted, the system is set to zero and calibrated, the stopcock is opened to the patient, and readings

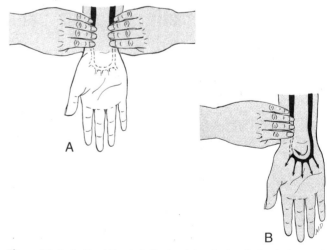

Figure 23–5. In the Allen test, the hand is raised and clenched several times. The radial and ulnar arteries are compressed, and then the hand is lowered. A, When the hand is opened and arteries are still occluded, the client's hand is pale. B, When either the ulnar or the radial artery is released, the entire hand should become pink as a result of collateral circulation. (From Black JM, Matassarin-Jacobs E, eds. Luckmann and Sorensen's Medical Surgical Nursing: A Psychophysiologic Approach, 4th ed. Philadelphia: W.B. Saunders Company, 1993.)

are obtained. The nurse assists the physician either by being scrubbed and handing equipment to the physician or by attaching the monitoring tubing and recording pressure readings. The catheter is usually sutured in place, and a sterile dressing is applied. A pressure dressing is recommended if bleeding from the site occurs.

Types of catheters used for arterial monitoring include a catheter over needle and a catheter over needle with a guidwire. Some catheters are designed solely for arterial use, or a venous access catheter may be used. The length of the catheter chosen depends on which artery is used, the size of patient, and the preference of the inserter.

Complications occurring with arterial line placement include bleeding, infection, arterial spasm, pain, nerve damage, circulatory decrease in the ipsilateral side, thrombus formation, and air embolism. If complications occur, catheter removal is indicated in most cases. Infection is usually treated with systemic antibiotics. Fasciotomy or arterial repair, or both, may be indicated if thrombus formation and occlusion, severe swelling with circulatory decrease, or excessive, uncontrolled bleeding occurs.[2-13]

Nursing Care

Nursing care of the patient with an arterial line includes assessment of the catheter, the system, and the pressure waveform. The site should be observed for redness, tenderness, swelling, or drainage. The involved extremity should be inspected for color, size, warmth, and sensation distal to the insertion site. The dressing should be changed every 24 to 48 hours or if it is loosened or soiled. Documentation on the appropriate form is performed according to institution policy.

The system should be checked for loose connections, proper pressure on the flush solution, dead-end caps on the stopcocks, and proper labeling of the tubing that includes any changes. The flush solution should be changed ever 24 hours and the tubing, every 48 hours. The monitor should be set for the proper range (300 mm Hg), and alarms should be turned on. The high and low alarm limits need to be set according to individual patient blood pressure. Usually, these limits are 10 to 20 mm Hg above and below the patient's pressure or as indicated per physician order when vasoactive medications are administered.

Changes in the waveform may signify a change in the patient's condition or a change within the system. The physical status of the patient should be assessed, and if no changes are noted, the system should be evaluated.

A poorly defined or dampened waveform is softer, rounder, and less clearly defined on the monitor (see Fig. 23–12). A dampened waveform can be caused by air or blood in the tubing, inadequate pressure on the flush solution bag, inaccurate calibration, or a positional catheter. Blood or air can be removed by aspirating and then fast-flushing through a stopcock. The blood or air should always be aspirated before the fast-flush device is used so that a clot or air embolus is not introduced into the patient.

The pressure on the flush solution bag should remain at 300 mm Hg. The system should be recalibrated and set to zero with each shift change, change of the line and solution, or whenever the waveform changes character. The phlebo-static axis should be verified before the system is recalibrated and set to zero.

Observing the blood pressure and reporting changes is a major responsibility of nurses caring for patients with arterial lines. If a significant drop or elevation is noted and the system is intact, a cuff blood pressure should also be obtained. Catheter size and location can cause variations between cuff and arterial pressures of between 5 and 20 mm Hg. Hospital protocol may provide guidelines for assessment of arterial line blood pressure's correlation with cuff pressure.

If the patient is taking medication that affects blood pressure, specific orders for notification of the physician are written. The nurse should always assess the physical status of the patient when interpreting arterial monitoring changes.

Blood samples can be obtained from an arterial line. The system may have a reservoir to draw blood back into (Fig. 23–6), or the syringe method with aspiration may be used. Gloves should be worn when blood is obtained from an arterial line (Table 23–2).

As previously stated, care and observation of the line can be documented on a flow sheet designed for that purpose. Abnormal findings or a change of site should be recorded on the nurse's notes.

Discontinuing Therapy

A minimum of 5 minutes of direct pressure should be applied to an upper extremity artery after the line is removed. Femoral catheters or those in patients with abnormal coagulation study results should have pressure applied to the insertion site at least 15 minutes after catheter removal. In patients receiving coagulation therapy, the therapy may be discontinued for 1 or 2 hours before the line is removed. All bleeding should cease before a pressure dressing is applied. Physicians commonly order bedrest for 6 to 8 hours after removal of a femoral line.[2-5, 8-13]

The site should be checked at each assessment and redressed if bleeding occurs. The nurse should always check under the affected limb for bleeding. Patients should notify the nurse at once if they feel wet, warm, or sticky sensations under the dressing or affected extremity.

Central Venous Pressure Monitoring

CVP is a measure of right heart function, or the pressure of blood in the right atrium or vena cava. The waveform for a CVP tracing reflects the contraction of the atria and the concurrent effect of the ventricles and surrounding major vessels. It consists of a, c, and v ascending, or positive, waves and x and y descending, or negative, waves. Because systolic atrial pressure (a) and diastolic (v) pressure are almost the same, the reading is taken as an average or mean of the two (Fig. 23–7).

Normal parameters may vary, depending on the method used for measurement and on the patient's underlying condition. CVP values are affected by circulating volume, cardiac contractility, and vascular tone. Water manometer pressures range between 4 and 12 cm of water. If a transducer and monitor are used, the pressures are between 0 and 8 mm

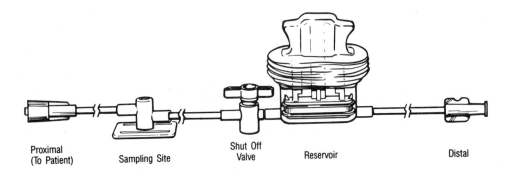

Proximal (To Patient)   Sampling Site   Shut Off Valve   Reservoir   Distal

Figure 23–6. VAMP system for needleless blood withdrawal from hemodynamic lines. (Courtesy of Baxter-Edwards Laboratories.)

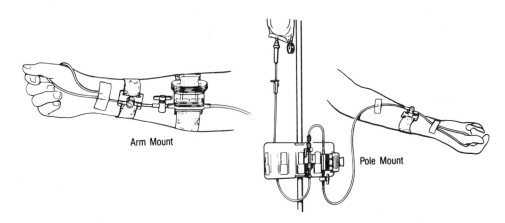

Arm Mount   Pole Mount

Hg. Physician orders direct the frequency of CVP readings and interventions for abnormal values.

The approach for placement of a CVP line varies. Some lines are inserted by the antecubital route, whereas others are inserted via the subclavian or jugular routes. The tip of any device placed for CVP readings should lie in the distal superior vena cava to prevent right atrial irritation, dysrhythmia, and erosion of the catheter through the atrium. Because no valves exist between the right atrium and the superior vena cava, a tip in this location provides accurate reflection of values from the right side of the heart.

Table 23–2

Syringe Method for Obtaining Arterial Blood Samples

1. Obtain necessary supplies, including syringes in the appropriate volume for specimen collection, clean gloves, 4- × 4-inch gauze pads, new stopcock caps.
2. Remove the cap from the stopcock closest to the insertion site, and attach a sterile syringe to the portal.
3. Turn the stopcock off to the solution, and aspirate 3–5 ml of blood into the syringe.
4. Turn the stopcock off to the syringe, remove it, and replace with a second syringe. This syringe may contain heparin if it is needed for the test being performed.
5. Turn the stopcock off to the solution and aspirate the amount of blood needed.
6. Turn the stopcock off to the syringe and remove it. Use the fast-flush device to clear the line of blood distal to the stopcock.
7. Turn the stopcock off to the patient, and flush the portal free of blood. Turn the stopcock off to the portal, and recap with a new, sterile cap.
8. Document the amount of blood withdrawn, the type of laboratory test for which it was drawn, and the return of the initial waveform after flushing the portal free of blood.
9. Recalibrate if needed.

Pressure monitoring setups for CVP readings are identical to those previously noted. The setting used on a monitor when CVPs are read is on the 50 mm Hg scale.

CVP readings can also be obtained by use of a water manometer; this method is most frequently used outside the critical care setting when other hemodynamic tracings are not needed. Water manometers use a fluid column and continuous-drip intravenous solution instead of a pressure line to keep the system patent. Infusion is performed with a three-way stopcock.

When readings are needed, the stopcock is turned off to the solution and is turned on to a fluid chamber. The pressure in the right atrium is reflected in this fluid. When the pressures equalize, the reading is taken from the markings on the fluid chamber (Fig. 23–8).

The distal port of a multilumen catheter is used to measure CVP. The proximal port of a pulmonary artery catheter is used. Infusions through the other ports on both types of catheters may need to be turned off during readings for an accurate pressure to be obtained. However, if infusates cannot be temporarily stopped, this inability is documented to maintain consistency between persons performing the measurement.

Nursing Considerations

Routine care of hemodynamic catheters has previously been described. Dressing, administration, setup of the line, and changes should all be performed and charted according to the *Intravenous Nurses Society Standards of Practice*.

CVP readings indicate changes in the preload (filling pressure in the right ventricle) of the heart. Abnormal readings may result from inadequate or increased preload, decreased

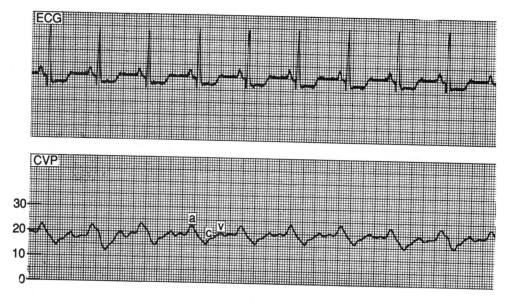

Figure 23–7. Central venous pressure waveform with *a*, *c*, and *v* waves present. The *a* wave usually is seen just after the P wave of the electrocardiogram (ECG). The *c* wave appears at the time of the RST junction on the ECG. The *v* wave is seen in the TP interval. (From Boggs RL, Wooldridge-King M [eds]. AACN Procedure Manual for Critical Care, 3rd ed. Philadelphia: W.B. Saunders, 1993:304.)

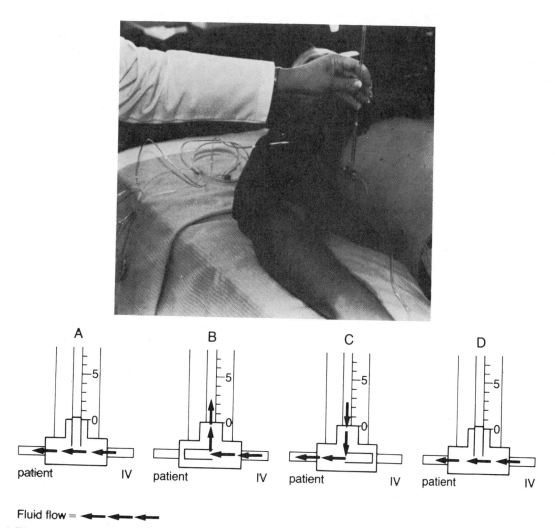

Figure 23–8. *A*, Water manometer placed at phlebostatic axis on patient. (From Boggs RL, Wooldridge-King M [eds]. AACN Procedure Manual for Critical Care, 3rd ed. Philadelphia: W.B. Saunders, 1993:290.) *B*, Proper stopcock positioning sequence in a venous pressure manometer. (From Darovic GO. Hemodynamic Monitoring. Philadelphia: W.B. Saunders, 1987:128.)

contractility, or increased afterload (pressure the left ventricle contracts against). If the waveform is low or dampened, line integrity should be assessed. Abnormal CVP readings are seen in patients with tricuspid stenosis and regurgitation, cardiac tamponade, constrictive pericarditis, pulmonary hypertension, chronic left ventricular failure, and volume overload or depletion.

Complications

Complications occurring with CVP lines are the same as those previously noted. If the antecubital approach is used, the patient may experience mechanical phlebitis after the insertion. Application of warm moist heat is used to treat the phlebitis.[14] If the phlebitis is not resolved in 24 to 36 hours, the catheter is removed.

Pulmonary Artery Catheter Monitoring

Pulmonary artery catheter or balloon flotation catheter pressures reflect left ventricular function. The catheters pass through the right side of the heart into the pulmonary vessels. When the balloon of the catheter is inflated, it wedges in a pulmonary artery (Fig. 23–9). Wedge pressures reflect left ventricular end-diastolic pressure in patients with normally functioning mitral valves. Pulmonary artery pressure can be assessed preoperatively or postoperatively to give the physician more extensive knowledge of the patients' cardiac and circulatory status. Pulmonary artery catheters are also placed in trauma patients and in patients with acute respiratory and cardiac impairment. Pulmonary artery catheters are used only in critical care settings.

Pulmonary artery catheters are multiluminal and can be used to measure CVP, pulmonary artery pressure, PWP, cardiac output, and mixed venous oxygen saturation, as well as for temporary pacing of the heart. The number of lumens within the catheter dictates how many functions it is able to perform (Fig. 23–10).

Normal pulmonary artery pressure ranges from 20 to 30 mm Hg systolic over 8 to 12 mm Hg diastolic. Pulmonary artery pressure reflects pulmonary blood volume and vascular resistance. Systolic pressure represents right ventricular contraction, and diastolic pressure represents resistance to blood flow within the small arterioles and pulmonary capillaries. If no obstructions to blood flow exist, the diastolic pressure reflects the PWP. Normal PWP readings range from 4 to 12 mm Hg.[2–6]

The cardiac output reflects how well the heart is pumping; specifically, cardiac output equals the amount of blood the left ventricle ejects in 1 minute. A specialized computer measures the cardiac output by determining the length of time it takes a predetermined amount of solution to reach the temperature thermistor at the tip of the catheter. The normal cardiac output ranges from 4 to 8 L/minute.[2–6]

The vessels of choice for placement of a pulmonary artery catheter are the subclavian and jugular veins; the femoral and antecubital veins are less frequently used. As the catheter is passed through the heart, pressure readings in the right atrium, right ventricle, and pulmonary artery, as well as PWP, are noted. The waveform on the monitor changes with the passage of the catheter through the heart and reflects the specific location of the tip. Characteristic waveform variations and pressure measurements facilitate passage at the patient's bedside without the need for fluoroscopy (see Fig. 23–9).

Commonly observed waveforms when pulmonary artery catheters with bedside monitoring are used include the pulmonary artery and PWP. The pulmonary artery form has an abrupt upstroke (systole) with a gradual downstroke followed by a dicrotic notch (pulmonic valve closure, designated *c*). The PWP has a and v waves owing to atrial contraction and ventricular systole (Fig. 23–11).

Preparation and Insertion

Along with the routine setup previously described, preparation for pulmonary artery catheter insertion includes check-

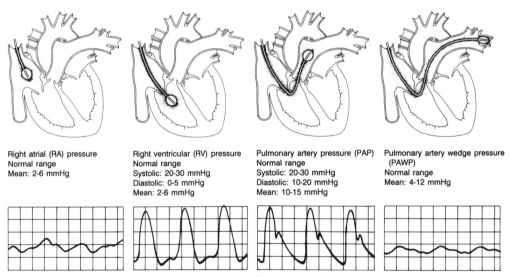

Right atrial (RA) pressure
Normal range
Mean: 2-6 mmHg

Right ventricular (RV) pressure
Normal range
Systolic: 20-30 mmHg
Diastolic: 0-5 mmHg
Mean: 2-6 mmHg

Pulmonary artery pressure (PAP)
Normal range
Systolic: 20-30 mmHg
Diastolic: 10-20 mmHg
Mean: 10-15 mmHg

Pulmonary artery wedge pressure (PAWP)
Normal range
Mean: 4-12 mmHg

Figure 23–9. Flow-directed balloon-tipped catheter as it passes through the right side of the heart, wedging in a distal pulmonary artery with corresponding pressure waveforms and normal values. (From Alspach JG [ed]. AACN Core Curriculum for Critical Care Nursing, 4th ed. Philadelphia: W.B. Saunders, 1991:194.)

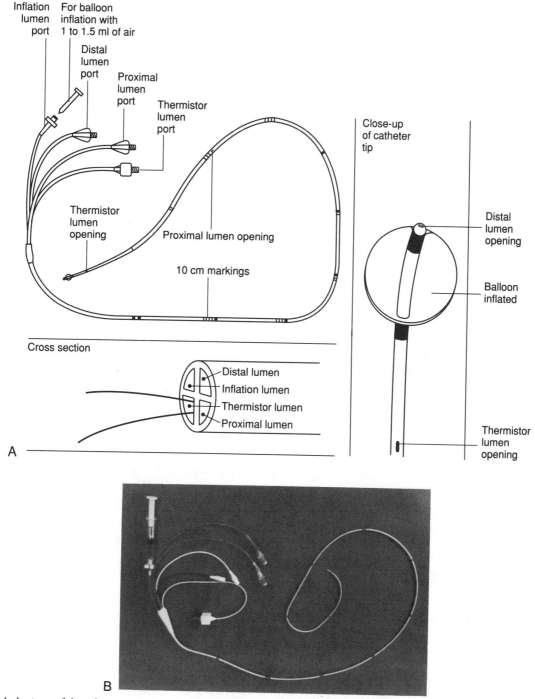

Figure 23–10. *A,* Anatomy of the pulmonary artery (PA) catheter. The standard no. 7 French thermodilution PA catheter is 110 cm in length and contains four lumens. *B,* PA catheter with atrial and ventricular pacing lumens. (From Boggs RL, Wooldridge-King M [eds]. AACN Procedure Manual for Critical Care, 3rd ed. Philadelphia: W.B. Saunders, 1993:315, 376.)

ing the integrity of the balloon. The balloon is inflated and placed in a cup of sterile water or saline to observe for leaks. Care must be taken not to rupture the balloon by overinflation. The balloon port is labeled with the inflation amount (0.8 ml to 1.5 ml). The nurse who prepares the sterile field and scrubs with the physician is responsible for checking the balloon, preflushing the other ports, and attaching the sterile sheath to the catheter.

After the catheter is placed, a routine dressing for central lines is applied. Documentation should include the insertion site location, the length of the catheter inserted to obtain PWP, the initial readings, and the patient's tolerance of the procedure. Subsequent pressure readings can be documented on a flow sheet.

Nursing Considerations

The frequency and type of readings obtained depend on the severity of the patient's condition and the physician's orders. Various medications to help improve or ease preload

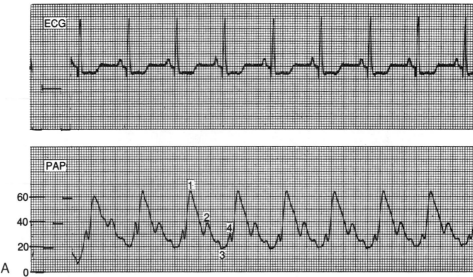

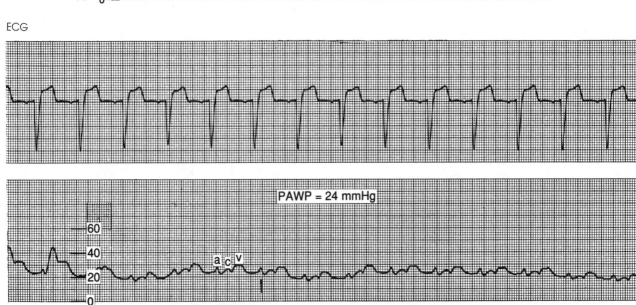

Figure 23–11. *A,* Pulmonary artery (PA) waveform and components: *1* = PA systole, *2* = dicrotic notch, *3* = PA end-diastole, *4* = anacrotic notch of PA valve opening. *B,* Normal PA wedge pressure waveform and components. Note delay in *a, c,* and *v* waves owing to the time it takes for the mechanical events to show a pressure change. This waveform is from a spontaneously breathing patient. The arrow indicates end-expiration, where the height of *a* wave pressure is measured. (From Boggs RL, Wooldridge-King M [eds]. AACN Procedure Manual for Critical Care, 3rd ed. Philadelphia: W.B. Saunders, 1993:316.)

and afterload may be ordered based on pulmonary artery, PWP, or cardiac output readings. The nurse must be sure that each reading is performed accurately to assess trends that indicate need for therapy.

Changes in pressures can be seen in patients with conditions that increase the pulmonary blood flow, including pulmonary hypertension and embolus, mitral stenosis and left ventricular failure, and exacerbation of pulmonary disease (chronic obstructive pulmonary disease). Cardiac tamponade, constrictive pericarditis, or volume overload may also result in elevated pressures. Decreased pressures may indicate hypovolemia or a reduction in afterload, as occurs with vasodilator administration.

Complications

Insertion complications with a pulmonary artery catheter include those noted for any central line insertion, as well as dysrhythmias as the catheter floats through the right side of the heart. The irritation to the endocardium is the mechanical cause of these dysrhythmias. Pulmonary infarction and balloon rupture can also occur.

After the catheter is inserted, the nurse should observe for waveform changes that indicate problems within the system. These changes include dampening or poor waveform, catheter fling, respiratory variations from ventilation, catheter migration into the wedge, and balloon rupture. If the patient's physical status has not changed, the waveform change may result from system problems.

A dampened wave is less defined and more rounded than a normal wave. The upstroke may be slowed and the dicrotic notch absent. The pressure bag should be checked for proper inflation, all connections should be tightened, and any air or blood in line should be removed and the system recalibrated and reset to zero (Fig. 23–12).

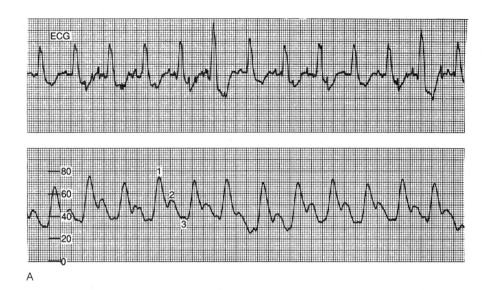

A

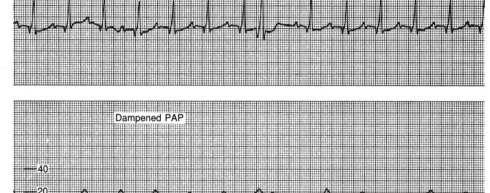

B

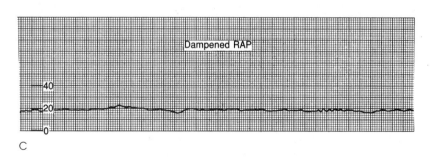

C

Figure 23–12. Effects of dampening on pulmonary artery pressure (PAP) and right atrium pressure (RAP) waveforms. *A,* Normal PAP waveform. (*1* = PA systole, *2* = dicrotic notch, *3* = PA diastole.) *B,* Dampened PAP waveform. *C,* Dampening of RAP waveform. Dampening of the waveform may result from clots at catheter tip, catheter against vessel or heart wall, air in lines, partially closed stopcock, deflated pressure bag, or patient hypotension. (From Boggs RL, and Wooldridge-King M [eds]. AACN Procedure Manual for Critical Care, 3rd ed. Philadelphia: W.B. Saunders, 1993:304.)

If the wave has developed an artifact or is exaggerated, the catheter may have developed "fling" or "whip" owing to the movement at the insertion site as the patient moves. Fling may result from the location of the catheter in the pulmonary artery. The nurse should be sure the patient is lying flat or at the recorded angle of elevation and is still when values are recorded. The physician may need to pull the line back to compensate for the internal location or may need to reposition it entirely if the catheter has coiled in the ventricle.

When the catheter is inserted in a patient with a ventilator or if the patient is receiving mechanical ventilation after the insertion, pulmonary artery pressures may increase owing to positive thoracic pressure. Readings, PA and PWP, should be taken at the end of the respiratory cycle (end-exhalation). To avoid jeopardizing respiratory status, patients are not routinely taken off ventilators to obtain readings.

When the catheter migrates into a smaller branch of the pulmonary artery, it may occlude the artery without balloon inflation. This migration results in a "wedge" waveform on the monitor. If the system is intact and the balloon is deflated, migration is suspected. If the initial length of catheter inserted has been documented, the dressing should be removed and the amount of catheter lying outside the patient checked against the length recorded at insertion. If the catheter is further inside the vein, migration has occurred. Before the physician is called to reposition the catheter, the nurse may attempt to dislodge the wedged catheter. Having the patient cough, suctioning an entubated patient, or turning the patient on either side may cause migration back to a pulmonary artery pattern. If such attempts are unsuccessful, the catheter will need to be pulled back until a pulmonary artery pattern appears on the screen. The balloon is then inflated, and a PWP is obtained. The physician may need to resuture the catheter, or it can be more securely taped.

Balloon rupture can occur if the balloon is overinflated or is frequently inflated. The amount of air needed for PWP to be obtained (0.8 ml to 1.5 ml) should be noted with the initial insertion, and no more than this should be used each time. Using the full balloon capacity may not be necessary to obtain a wedge. After the reading is obtained, the syringe is then removed from the port for deflation. If blood is noted in the balloon port or if a wedge pattern cannot be obtained after the system has been thoroughly checked, rupture is suspected. The port should be locked off and taped over to prevent it from being used. The catheter may be replaced, or the pulmonary artery diastolic reading may be used in place of a wedge reading.

Any complications should be documented in the narrative section of the patient's chart. Routine pressure readings and care may be noted on a flow sheet. Documentation of removal of the catheter includes the deflation of the balloon, the position of the patient (Trendelenburg), the amount of time pressure applied to site, the type of dressing applied, and how the patient tolerated the procedure.

▶ NURSING DIAGNOSIS

The nursing diagnosis for patients with hemodynamic lines may include reduction of anxiety, recognition and treatment of any insertion complications, potential for bleeding, infection, monitoring problems, and potential problems during or after catheter removal.[13]

The expected patient outcomes will be a less anxious patient and family, complication-free insertion, and absence of or prompt recognition and treatment of any bleeding, infection, mechanical problems, or problems occurring with removal.[13]

OTHER TYPES OF MONITORING

Some catheters enhance cardiac perfusion and measure left atrial pressures, cerebral pressures, and other vital organ pressures. These catheters are considered hemodynamic devices more advanced than those routinely used by all critical

care units. Many critical care references describe these types of hemodynamic monitoring devices in detail.[2-6]

CONCLUSION

Hemodynamic monitoring is a more advanced nursing practice that requires basic critical care assessment skills and an understanding of basic cardiovascular physiology. Nurses in a critical care setting are familiar with the different types of hemodynamic monitoring catheters. The ability to interpret the waveform and its values in conjunction with physical assessment of the patient enables prompt interventions to be performed. When basic knowledge and practice of good infection control techniques with regard to intravenous therapy are also used, good patient care is ensured.

References

1. The Random House Dictionary of the English Language, 2nd ed. Unabridged.
2. Daily EK, Schroeder JS. Techniques in Bedside Hemodynamic Monitoring, 4th ed. St. Louis: C. V. Mosby, 1990.
3. DeAngelis R. Diagnostic studies. In Alspach J (ed). Core Curriculum for Critical Care Nursing, 4th ed. Philadelphia: W. B. Saunders, 1991:191–200.
4. Kadota LT. Hemodynamic monitoring. In Clochesy JM, Breu C, Cardin S. Critical Care Nursing. Philadelphia: W. B. Saunders, 1993:155–178.
5. Lough M. Introduction to hemodynamic monitoring. Nurs Clin North Am 1987:22(1):89–110.
6. Yang SS, Bentivoglio LG, Maranhão V. From Cardiac Catheterization Data to Hemodynamic Parameters, 3rd ed. Philadelphia: F. A. Davis, 1988.
7. Intravenous Nurses Society. Revised Intravenous Nursing Standards of Practice. Philadelphia: J. B. Lippincott, 1990.
8. Rountree WD. Removal of pulmonary artery catheters by registered nurses: A study in safety and complications. Focus Crit Care 1991; 18(4):313–314, 316–318.
9. Masters S. Complications of pulmonary artery catheters. Crit Care Nurse 1989; 9(9):82–91.
10. Biga CD, Bethel SA. Hemodynamic monitoring in postanesthesia care units. Crit Care Nurs Clin North Am 1991; 3(1):83–93.
11. Covey M, McLane C, Smith N. Infection related to intravascular pressure monitoring: Effects of flush and tubing changes. Am J Infect Control 1988;16(5):206–213.
12. Crow S, Conrad SA, Chaney-Rowell C. Microbial contamination of arterial infusions used for hemodynamic monitoring: A randomized trial of contamination with sampling through conventional stopcocks versus a novel closed system. Infect Control Hosp Epidemiol 1989; 10(12):557–561.
13. Hazinski M. Hemodynamic monitoring. In Johanson BC, Dungca CU, Hoffmeister D (eds), Standards for critical care (2nd ed.). St Louis: C. V. Mosby, 1985:191–201.
14. Hadaway LC. Evaluation and use of advanced IV technology: Part 1. Central venous access devices. J Intravenous Nurs 1989; 12(2):73–82.

Maxine Perdue, BSN, CRNI

Up to 80 to 90% of all hospitalized patients in the United States receive some form of intravenous therapy. Other patients receive some form of intravenous therapy in the alternative care setting, such as the physician's office, the ambulatory clinic, and the home. Although most intravenous therapy is administered without problems, complications do occur and range from minor to very serious. Some of the more serious complications can result in death if immediate medical intervention is not provided.

The potential for complications is always present in the patient receiving intravenous therapy. Complications increase hospital stays and length of therapy, increase nursing responsibilities, and can put the patient at risk for other medical problems. Furthermore, the patient experiences additional discomfort, and overall expenses are increased.

Fortunately, most of these complications are preventable. A thorough knowledge and understanding of the risks involved with intravenous therapy and the use of measures to prevent their occurrence can eliminate many of the hazards associated with this treatment. Patient education in the recognition of signs and symptoms for complications and frequent monitoring by the nurse result in early detection and treatment of complications. These measures may prevent further associated complications from occurring and may promote prompt healing of problems associated with existing complications.

LOCAL VERSUS SYSTEMIC COMPLICATIONS

Complications associated with intravenous therapy are classified according to their location. Local complications are usually seen at or near the site or occur as a result of mechanical failure. These complications are more common than systemic complications and are not usually serious. Immediate recognition of associated signs and symptoms coupled with nursing intervention can prevent more serious complications from occurring.

Systemic complications are those occurring within the vascular system, usually remote from the intravenous site. Although these complications are rarely seen, they are usually very serious and can be life threatening without appropriate medical intervention. Some local complications can lead to more serious systemic complications. For example, throm-

bophlebitis can develop into a pulmonary embolism if the thrombus becomes detached and free-floating in the vascular system. Systemic complications are more difficult to treat than local complications; preventing systemic complications is far easier than treating them.

Local Complications

Local complications result from mechanical problems associated with the infusion system or result from trauma to the intima of the vein (Table 24–1). Mechanical problems can result in depriving the patient of urgently needed fluids, or medications, or both, if vein access is lost. Trauma to the intima of the vein can lead to extensive edema, which can also deprive the patient of needed fluids and medications; to necrosis of surrounding tissue, resulting in a need for skin grafting; thrombophlebitis, with the subsequent danger of embolism; and sepsis, if an infection at the site is not detected early or goes untreated. Individuals performing intravenous procedures must use techniques to prevent trauma to the vein intima and must frequently monitor the system to detect both mechanical difficulties and signs of potential complications. The frequency of monitoring should be stated in established policies and procedures, and compliance should be monitored under the institution's quality improvement program.

Mechanical Complications

Mechanical complications are related to a failure of the intravenous system to adequately deliver therapy at the prescribed rate. They are usually resolved by correction of the identified problem. If a mechanical problem is suspected, five major areas should be evaluated (Table 24–2).

INTRAVENOUS SITE

The site should be checked for swelling at, above, and below the insertion of the cannula. By observing for potential problems associated with the site, one can immediately rule out site-related problems.

CANNULA

Proper placement of the cannula should be verified. A cannula tip that lies against a bifurcation or a valve or a

Table 24–1
Local Complications of Intravenous Therapy

Mechanical failure	Thrombophlebitis
Infiltration	Fragmented or broken catheter
Extravasation	Ecchymosis or hematoma
Phlebitis	Site infection
Postinfusion phlebitis	Venous or arterial spasm
Thrombosis	

419

Table 24–2

Steps in the Evaluation of Mechanical Complications
· ·

Check the site.	Check the tubing.
Check the cannula.	Check the involved extremity.
Check the solution container.	

cannula that is kinked or bent can slow or stop the infusion. Frequently, pulling back slightly on the cannula can eliminate this problem. Bent cannulas should be discontinued and replaced to prevent possible cannula breakage and subsequent catheter emboli. Taping the cannula to prevent in-and-out motion can help prevent bending or kinking of a cannula.

Placement of a cannula in a flexion area can also affect the infusion rate. If not obvious, one can easily check for a positional rate by having the patient flex and extend the extremity. If the flow rate slows or increases, the cannula is positional. If venous status is limited and the cannula cannot be changed, the application of an armboard should be considered. Sites in flexion areas should be avoided, if possible, because they can lead to further complications.

Infrequently, a cannula may leak at the point at which it attaches to the hub, or the cannula may be obstructed as a result of the manufacturing process. If either of these situations occurs, the cannula should be removed. The package and the cannula should be saved and returned to the manufacturer so that the cannula can be checked for defects. The lot number should be noted, and the cannula should be placed in a puncture-resistant container that meets the standards of the Occupational Safety and Health Administration (OSHA).[1] Other cannulas from the same lot should be monitored for defects. Partially or completely obstructed cannulas, regardless of cause, should be removed; these cannulas should not be flushed, since a clot may be dislodged, and the resulting embolus could cause a more serious complication.

SOLUTION CONTAINER

The solution container should be assessed. An empty container or a lack of adequate gravity flow can lead to an inaccurate flow rate or to no flow rate at all. This problem is easily corrected by hanging another bag or by adjusting the height of the intravenous pole.

The solution container should be checked for a patent air vent. Intravenous solution bags do not need to be vented; however, bottles that are nonvented require that a vented adapter or vented tubing be used. A vacuum cannot be created within a bottle, and solution will not flow from a bottle unless it is replaced with air. Using a needle to vent a bottle is inappropriate.

Another concern is the bag entry port; if it is obstructed, solution cannot pass. The outlet port seal must be completely penetrated by the administration spike for solutions to flow freely.

Refrigerated solutions should be removed from the refrigerator and allowed to reach room temperature before they are administered. The administration of cold solutions can produce venospasms with vasoconstriction and subsequent slowing of the infusion rate.

TUBING

Tubing that is pinched, crimped, or kinked prevents the delivery of an accurate flow rate. Tubing may need to be taped or retaped to prevent this problem from occurring. Filters can also become blocked by particulates and can slow the infusion rate, particularly with the administration of certain medications, such as tetracycline. The filter should be changed when this problem occurs.

PATIENT

The involved extremity should be checked for constrictive clothing, identification bracelet, jewelry, and restraints. Anything placed above an intravenous site that constricts the arm may act as a tourniquet and may slow the rate or stop the infusion.

Infiltration

Infiltration is the inadvertent administration of a nonvesicant solution or medication into surrounding tissues as a result of dislodgement of a cannula.[2] It can usually be recognized by increasing edema at or near the venipuncture site (Fig. 24–1).

The first symptom recognized by many patients is the feeling of skin tightness at the venipuncture site that makes flexing or extending the involved extremity difficult. If a large amount of fluid is trapped in the subcutaneous tissue, the skin may appear taut or stretched. As more fluid gathers in the tissues, blanching and coolness of the skin may occur, the infusion may slow or stop, and the patient may experience tenderness or discomfort at the site. The amount of discomfort experienced by the patient is also determined by the type of solution or medication being infused. Whereas isotonic solutions generally do not produce much discomfort when an infiltration occurs, solutions with an acidic or alkaline pH or those that are slightly more hypertonic are more irritating and usually cause discomfort.[3]

Unless obvious, an infiltration may go undetected owing to dependent edema or the administration of fluid at a very slow rate. The intravenous site must be monitored frequently to prevent this problem from occurring.

PATIENT ASSESSMENT

A complete assessment of the patient, the intravenous site, the involved extremity, and the infusion system may be necessary to determine the presence of an infiltration. The site around the tip of the cannula and the extremity should be inspected for swelling, blanching, stretched skin, firm tissues, and/or coolness. Comparison of the site with the same area on the opposite extremity may also be helpful. If both extremities appear edematous, the patient's medical status should be evaluated. Patients with hemodynamic problems, congestive heart failure, toxic conditions, compromised kidney function, hypothermia, and vascular insufficiency are particularly prone to vascular edema. The immobilized patient or the patient with muscular weakness or paralysis of an extremity may experience edema of the extremity that is totally unrelated to a problem at the intravenous site.[3]

If an assessment of the involved extremity and the pa-

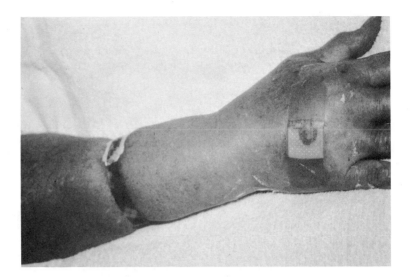

Figure 24–1. Infiltration: the inadvertent administration of a nonvesicant solution, or medication or both, into surrounding tissues. (Courtesy of Johnson and Johnson Medical, Inc., Vascular Access, Arlington, TX.)

tient's medical status are inconclusive, the application of pressure on the vein about 2 inches above the insertion site (must be above the tip of the cannula) with a finger or tourniquet will decrease or stop the infusion rate if the cannula is in the vein. If an infiltration is present, the rate will remain unchanged. If the infusion continues despite the venous obstruction, an infiltration has occurred.

Checking for a blood return, or backflow of blood, is not a reliable method for determining the absence of an infiltration. A blood return may not be present when small veins are used, because they may not permit blood flow around the cannula; one may think the infusion has infiltrated when it has not. Additionally, the use of veins that have had previous punctures or veins that are very fragile may seep fluid at a site above or below the vein cannula entry point; a blood return may be present, yet an infiltration is occurring. The movement of a cannula, such as in-and-out motions, can cause the skin and the vein entry site to enlarge, allowing fluid to seep at the vein entry site, causing an infiltration.

NURSING INTERVENTIONS

To prevent or minimize infiltration-associated problems (Table 24–3), it is imperative that once an infiltration has been identified, the cannula be discontinued. The type of solution being infused should also be considered. If the solution is isotonic and has a normal pH, the patient may not feel much discomfort unless a large amount of fluid has infiltrated. In these cases, warm compresses, such as warm, moist towels or chemical packs, may help alleviate the discomfort and help absorb the infiltration by increasing circulation to the affected area. Sloughing can occur from the application of warm compresses to an area infiltrated with certain medications, such as potassium chloride. In these instances, the application of cold compresses is preferred.[3] Established policies and procedures should dictate the use of compresses. The involved extremity should be elevated to improve circulation and to help in the absorption of infiltrated fluid.

If weeping of the tissues occurs because of an extensive infiltration or loose thin tissue, as is often present in the elderly, the application of a sterile dressing to the affected area may be necessary. It is usually better to leave these areas open because the application of a dressing means the use of gauze and possibly tape, which can increase tissue damage. If a dressing is used, it should be loosely applied and should be nonconstricting.[4] Extreme care should be given to prevent infection. The physician should be notified and measures should be carried out as ordered. If an infusion is needed, a cannula is placed in the opposite extremity or in a site above and away from the previous site.

PREVENTIVE MEASURES

Not all infiltrations can be prevented, but adherence to certain measures can aid in their prevention and minimize their severity. Flexion areas should be avoided if possible. The cannula should be taped securely, and the site should be protected from excessive movement or pressure by use of an armboard, or restraints, or both. Restraints must be applied with extreme caution and within the guidelines established by the Joint Commission on Accreditation of Healthcare Organizations[5] (JCAHO) and by the Food and Drug Administration (FDA).[6] They should be well padded and applied so that they do not cause nerve damage, constrict circulation, or cause pressure areas, and they should be removed at frequent intervals and nurse-assisted range of motion exercises performed. Inadequate or improper use of armboards or restraints can cause very serious complications; policies and procedures should be established to guide their use.

Patient education can be a key factor in the prevention and early recognition of signs and symptoms of an infiltration. Patient knowledge about the care of the intravenous site and system can prevent activities that may cause an infiltration from occurring, such as manipulating the cannula, pulling on

Table 24–3

Effects of an Infiltration
. . . .
Deprives the patient of medications and/or solutions at the prescribed rate that is essential for successful therapy.
Limits mobility of an extremity.
Limits availability of veins for therapy.
Causes tissue damage.
Causes unnecessary patient discomfort.

the tubing, picking at the dressing, and using the extremity excessively. If he or she knows what to look for, the patient can also alert the nurse to the early signs of an infiltration, and immediate care can be rendered, thereby preventing the possibility of more serious complications.

Extravasation

Extravasation is the inadvertent administration of a vesicant solution and/or medication into the surrounding tissues.[2] A vesicant solution is a solution or medication that causes the formation of blisters, with subsequent sloughing of tissues occurring from tissue necrosis (Fig. 24–2).[7]

PATIENT ASSESSMENT

It is essential that an extravasation be noted early before extensive fluid is allowed to infiltrate the interstitial tissues. A complete assessment of the patient, the intravenous site, the involved extremity, and the infusion system should be performed at regular intervals. The flow rate should never be increased to determine the infiltration of a vesicant, nor should a blood return be used as a reliable method to determine an infiltration. Fluid can seep into the tissues from a previous puncture site or the vein insertion site, and increase the potential for tissue necrosis (refer to *Infiltration* for the assessment process).

Initial indications that tissue sloughing may occur include pain or burning at the site with progression to erythema and edema. Tissue sloughing is usually apparent within 1 to 4 weeks because of tissue necrosis.[8] Necrosis can involve a small area or a large area, including underlying connective tissues, muscles, tendons, and bone, necessitating surgical intervention.

The severity of damage is directly related to the type, concentration, and volume of fluid infiltrated into the interstitial tissues. The most harmful of the vesicant medications are the antineoplastic agents, with doxorubicin (Adriamycin) causing the most severe tissue necrosis.[3] Other medications that act as vesicants and cause tissue necrosis include dopamine hydrochloride (Dopastat, Intropin), norepinephrine (levarterenol bitartrate, Levophed), potassium chloride in high doses, amphotericin B (Fungizone), calcium, and sodium bicarbonate in high concentrations.

NURSING INTERVENTIONS

When an extravasation is suspected, the infusate is discontinued immediately. Treatment protocols established in written policies and procedures are initiated, and a new site is established, preferably in the opposite extremity or in a site above and away from the extravasated site.

Institutional policies vary as to the treatment of the tissues in which an extravasation has occurred. Usually, the cannula is left in place until after any residual medication and blood are aspirated, and an antidote particular to the vesicant is instilled into the tissues.[8, 9] (See Chapter 13 for protocols related to the management of extravasation.) After the cannula is removed, a dry, sterile dressing is applied to the site, and either cold or warm compresses are applied. Cold compresses are usually used for the alkalating and antibiotic vesicants, whereas warm compresses are applied to an extravasation of the vinca alkaloids.[3] The extremity is elevated and observed regularly for erythema, induration, and necrosis. The physician is notified, and tissue damage is evaluated by the physician for the possibility of surgical intervention.

PREVENTIVE MEASURES

Every effort should be made at preventing the potential for an extravasation; such measures include the following:

1. Only qualified registered nurses who have been trained in venipuncture and drug administration skills and who have a knowledge of drugs with vesicant potential should be allowed to administer vesicants. Their training should include how and over what interval these drugs are administered, early signs of extravasation, preventive measures, and associated treatment protocols.
2. The intravenous site and the surrounding area should be checked for patency before, during, and after the administration of a vesicant. Infusion of 5 to 10 ml of saline before the administration of a vesicant can help determine vein patency.
3. Institutional policies should specify the role of the nurse

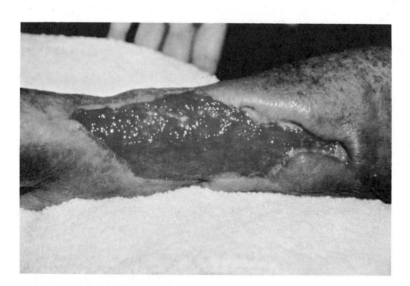

Figure 24–2. Tissue sloughing associated with extravasation, the inadvertent administration of a vesicant solution or medication, or both, into surrounding tissues. (Courtesy of Johnson and Johnson Medical, Inc., Vascular Access, Arlington, TX.)

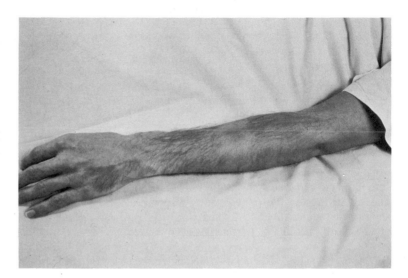

Figure 24-3. Phlebitis: inflammation of the vein characterized by pain and tenderness along the course of the vein. (Courtesy of Johnson and Johnson Medical, Inc., Vascular Access, Arlington, TX.)

during the administration of vesicants. Some policies state that a nurse must be in constant attendance during the infusion of a vesicant, whereas others state that the patient and the site should be monitored at specified intervals during the infusion. Also, some institutions require that two licensed nurses verify vein patency before the administration of a vesicant.[4] The degree to which the patient and site are observed may depend on the location of the patient at the time the vesicant is administered.

4. When a vesicant is administered directly into a vein with a syringe, the plunger of the syringe is pulled back every 3 to 4 ml to note blood return. Although a good blood return does not guarantee that an extravasation has not occurred, any change in blood return could indicate the need to investigate the possibility of an extravasation.

5. A vesicant should be administered through a side port of a free-flowing infusion because the vesicant is usually concentrated and the severity of tissue damage is related to the amount and concentration of the vesicant. A free-flowing infusion indicates a patent line.

6. Cannulas should be properly taped to prevent an in-and-out motion, which can enlarge the vein entry site and create an opportunity for the vesicant to seep into interstitial tissues, resulting in an extravasation.

7. Vesicants should not be administered in areas of flexion.

8. The hands should be avoided as intravenous sites for vesicant administration because of the close network of tendons and nerves that would be destroyed if an extravasation occurs.

9. Gravity and heat (which maximize vasodilatation) should be used to distend small fragile veins, especially those that have been used repeatedly for the administration of cancer cytotoxic agents. Venipuncture should be performed without a tourniquet or with a loosely tied tourniquet to decrease the potential for an extravasation in these patients.[9]

10. Sites should be protected from excessive movement with the use of armboards, or restraints, or both, when indicated. The use of restraints should be outlined in written policies and procedures.

11. If a cannula has been in place longer than 24 hours,

consideration should be given to changing the site, preferably to the opposite extremity, before a vesicant is administered.

12. Consideration should be given to the placement of a central venous access system. Some institutions administer vesicants only through central venous catheters, even when good peripheral veins are available. The use of a central venous catheter should not provide false assurance that an extravasation cannot occur; extravasation has been documented to result from catheter rupture, catheter leakage, backtracking of an infusate along a fibrin sheath, separation of the port, and dislodgement of the port needle.

Knowledge of the vesicant potential of infusions and medications and identification of associated risk factors are essential to the safe administration of these infusates. The nurse must know if the patient has a history of multiple venipunctures, where they were located, and how long ago the sites were used. Vesicants have been known to seep into the tissues at the vein entry site of a previous infusion.

The patient should be educated in the care of the infusion, including the recognition of potential problems, what to do if a problem occurs, and the dangers associated with extravasation. A well-educated patient can be a vital asset in preventing an extravasation and in minimizing the effects of an existing extravasation.

Phlebitis

Phlebitis, a condition in which inflammation of the intima of the vein occurs, is a commonly reported complication of intravenous therapy. It is characterized by pain and tenderness along the course of the vein, erythema, and inflammatory swelling with a feeling of warmth at the site. Note the erythema along the vein line in Figure 24-3.

Factors that substantially increase the risk for infusion phlebitis include the following:

- Improper cannula material, length, and gauge
- Lack of skill of individual inserting the cannula
- Incorrect anatomic site of cannulation
- Prolonged duration of cannulation
- Infrequent dressing changes

- Properties and character of the infusate
- Host factors, such as age and presence of disease

Phlebitis is classified according to the causative factors and can be chemical, mechanical, or bacterial. Phlebitis should be rated according to a uniform scale. The scale recommended by the *Intravenous Nursing Standards of Practice* is given in Table 24–4.

CHEMICAL PHLEBITIS

Chemical phlebitis is associated with a response of the vein intima to certain chemicals infused into or placed within the vascular system. An inflammatory response can be created by the administration of solutions and/or medications, or as a result of the cannula materials used for access (Table 24–5).

Normal blood pH is 7.35 to 7.45 and is slightly alkaline.[7, 10] The normal pH for solutions is 7.0, which is neutral. The ph for alkaline, or basic, solutions ranges from 7 to 14; that for acid solutions ranges from 7 to 0.[7] The *United States Pharmacopeia's* specifications for the pH of dextrose solutions range from 3.5 to 6.5. Acidity is necessary to prevent carmelization of the dextrose during autoclaving and to preserve the stability of the solution during storage. Some manufacturers also include an additive in the solution to increase its pH. However, this additive may alter the solution's compatibility status when other medications are added to it.[10]

Solutions or medications with a high pH or osmolality predispose the vein intima to irritation. The more acidic an intravenous solution, the greater the risk of phlebitis. Glucose-containing admixtures, which are acidic; amino acids; and lipid emulsions used in parenteral nutrition are all far more phlebitogenic than is normal saline. Moreover, additives, such as potassium chloride, and various intravenously administered medications, such as vancomycin hydrochloride (Vancocin, Vancor), amphotericin B, most β-lactam antibiotics, benzodiazepines (diazepam [Valium, Zetran] and midazolam [Versed]), and many chemotherapeutic agents, can produce severe venous inflammation.

Also, the addition of certain medications can alter the pH of a solution. For instance, the addition of vitamin C to intravenous fluids further decreases the pH, whereas the addition of sodium heparin increases the pH, rarely causing phlebitis.

Osmolality refers to the measure of solute concentration and, depending on the solute present, can irritate the vein intima and predispose the patient to phlebitis. Parenteral solutions are classified according to the tonicity of the solution in relation to normal blood plasma. The osmolality of blood plasma is 290 mOsm/liter. Solutions that approximate 290 mOsm/liter are considered isotonic. Those with an osmolality significantly higher than 290 mOsm are considered hypertonic, whereas those with an osmolality significantly lower than 290 mOsm are hypotonic.[3] (See Table 24–6 for the osmolalities of the most commonly used intravenous solutions.) The tonicity of solutions infused into the circulation has an effect not only on the patient's physical status but also on the vein intima. The vein intima can be traumatized by the administration of hyperosmolar fluids (solutions having an osmolality higher than 300 mOsm/liter), especially if they are administered at a rapid rate or through a small vessel. Isotonic solutions may become hyperosmolar when they are mixed with certain medications, such as electrolytes, antibiotics, and nutrients, especially when certain medications are added to solutions less than 100 ml.[3]

Improper mixture or dilution of medications can result in incompatibilities and the possibility of a precipitate formation, thus increasing the risk of phlebitis. When medications are mixed without regard to pH or compatibility, the effect of the drug may be altered. Interactions can occur with no apparent change, but rendering one or both of the medications or solutions ineffective or causing a physical change in which crystals are formed and a precipitate is observable.

The infusion rate can be a major factor in the development of phlebitis. A slow rate is thought to cause less venous irritation than a rapid rate. Rapid infusion rates irritate the vessel walls by providing a larger concentration of medications and solutions. Slower rates provide longer absorption times, with hemodilution of smaller amounts of solutions or medications.

Table 24–5

Factors Contributing to Chemical Phlebitis
. . . .

Administration of irritating medications or solutions
Administration of medications improperly mixed or diluted
Administration of medications or solutions at a rapid rate
Administration of particulate matter
Cannula material or structure
Cannula dwell time

Table 24–4

Assessing the Severity of Phlebitis
. . . .

Severity	Assessment Findings
1+	Pain at site Erythema and/or edema No streak No palpable cord
2+	Pain at site Erythema and/or edema Streak formation No palpable cord
3+	Pain at site Erythema and/or edema Streak formation Palpable cord

From Intravenous Nurses Society. Intravenous nursing standards of practice. JIN ISSN 0896-5846, 1990; S26–S80.

Table 24–6

pH and Osmolality of Common Intravenous Solutions
. . . .

Solution	pH	Osmolality
5% dextrose in water	3–5	252 mOsm/liter
5% dextrose in water with 0.33 sodium chloride	4	365 mOsm/liter
5% dextrose in water with 0.45 sodium chloride	4	406 mOsm/liter
5% dextrose in water with Ringer's lactate solution	5	524 mOsm/liter
Ringer's lactate solution	6.5	274 mOsm/liter

Particulate matter within intravenous solutions or medications may also contribute to the formation of phlebitis. Particulates are formed when medication particles are not fully dissolved during the mixing process. When infused, they irritate the vein intima, causing inflammation. When intravenous medications are prepared for administration, the use of a 1- to 5-μm particulate matter filter eliminates this problem. The use of a particulate matter filter does not eliminate the need for a 0.2-μm bacteria retentive filter, which is recommended for routine use for the delivery of intravenous therapy.[11]

The use of catheters for intravenous therapy can predispose the patient to phlebitis. Although several different materials are used in the manufacture of catheters, none is absolutely foolproof for the prevention of phlebitis. Catheters made of silicone elastomer and polyurethane have a smoother microsurface, are thermoplastic, are more hydrophilic, become more flexible than polytetrafluoroethylene (Teflon) at body temperature, and induce less venous irritation. In studies performed by Maki and Ringer,[12] peripheral intravenous catheters made of PEU-Vialon were shown to be much safer for use than those made of polyvinylchloride or polyethylene and were substantially less phlebitogenic than catheters made of FEP-polytetrafluoroethylene. Maki and Ringer also showed that the incidence of phlebitis increased progressively with the increasing period of cannulation. Their studies revealed the risk to be 30% by day 2, and 39 to 40% by day 3.[12]

The basic principles of aseptic technique and measures for the prevention of chemical phlebitis must be carried out. Many of the problems associated with chemical phlebitis can be eliminated by implementation of the following:

1. Use of filters
2. Use of recommended solutions or diluents when mixing medications
3. Dilution of known irritating medications to the greatest extent possible
4. Administration of intravenous push medications through a port of a compatible free-flowing infusion
5. Administration of medications or solutions at the minimal rate recommended
6. Rotation of peripheral sites at recommended intervals
7. Use of large veins for the administration of hypertonic or acidic solutions to provide greater hemodilution
8. Use of the smallest-gauge cannula that will adequately deliver the ordered therapy

The pharmacist should always be consulted if any questions exist about the mixing of medications or solutions and should be made aware of frequent occurrences of phlebitis associated with certain drugs. Sometimes, the addition of a buffering agent can aid in the prevention of a chemical phlebitis.

MECHANICAL PHLEBITIS

Mechanical phlebitis is associated with the placement of a cannula. Cannulas placed in flexion areas often result in the development of mechanical phlebitis. As the extremity is moved, the cannula irritates the vein intima, causing injury and resultant phlebitis. A large cannula placed in a vein that has a smaller lumen than the cannula irritates the intima of the vein, causing inflammation and phlebitis. Cannulas that are poorly taped have a tendency to move in and out of the vein, allowing the cannula tip to irritate the vein intima and resulting in phlebitis. Extensive, unrestrictive movement of an extremity can also result in unwarranted movement of the cannula within the vein.

The experience of the person inserting an intravenous cannula clearly influences the risk for phlebitis. In comparative trials, the availability of an intravenous therapy team of highly experienced nurses who insert intravenous catheters and provide close surveillance of infusions resulted in a two-fold lower rate of infusion-related phlebitis and an even greater reduction in catheter-related sepsis.[12]

BACTERIAL PHLEBITIS

Bacterial phlebitis is an inflammation of the intima of the vein that is associated with a bacterial infection and is the less frequently seen type of phlebitis. It can, however, be more serious and can predispose the patient to the systemic complication of septicemia. Contributing factors include those described in Table 24–7.

Hand washing is the single most important procedure for preventing nosocomial infections.[13, 14] The hands should be washed before therapy is initiated and after the procedure has been completed. Universal precautions dictate that health care providers are required to wear gloves when performing venipunctures.[1] Even when gloves are provided in the immediate area, the hands should be washed before the gloves are donned; otherwise, contaminants are easily carried into the area and then deposited on the gloves.

All equipment should be checked for expiration date, package integrity, particulate matter, cloudiness, or any signs indicating the presence of contaminants. Bags should be squeezed to reveal punctures, and bottles should be held up to the light and rotated to reveal very fine cracks.

Aseptic technique is essential in the preparation of an insertion site. Appropriate cleansing of the insertion site reduces the potential for infection by minimizing microorganisms on the skin. If the skin is very dirty, it should be washed first with soap and water before an antimicrobial solution is applied. Shaving is not recommended, because a potential exists for causing microabrasions, which can allow microorganisms to enter the vascular system.[11] Antimicrobial solutions that can be used in the preparation of the skin for venipuncture include tincture of iodine, 1 to 2%; iodophor, isopropyl alcohol, 70%; or chlorhexidine. The solution should be applied in a circular motion, starting at the intended site for puncture and working outward to prevent contaminants from being carried from an uncleansed area to

Table 24–7

Factors Contributing to Bacterial Phlebitis

Poor hand washing techniques
Failure to check equipment for compromised integrity
Poor aseptic technique in preparation of the site or system
Poor cannula insertion techniques
Poorly taped cannula
Extended cannula dwell time
Infrequent site observation with failure to notice early signs of phlebitis

a cleansed area. The preparatory solution should be allowed to completely air dry; blotting of excess solution should not be allowed.[11]

Aseptic technique should be maintained during the insertion of the cannula. Sterility of the cannula should not be violated by laying the cannula on the skin during insertion or by touching the cannula with the fingers. Only one cannula is used for each venipuncture attempt because cannulas that have penetrated the skin for venipuncture are considered contaminated. Sterile tape to prevent unwarranted movement of the cannula and a sterile dressing are applied over the cannula site. The cannula is then taped to prevent in-and-out movement of the cannula.

Maintenance care of the system includes measures to prevent bacteria from entering the system. Routine site care should consist of changing the dressing at established intervals according to the *Intravenous Nursing Standards of Practice*. Both types of dressings should be changed immediately if the integrity of the dressing is compromised. Site care should be routinely given and should consist of cleansing the skin-cannula junction with the application of an effective antiseptic solution (e.g., tincture of iodine, 1 to 2%; iodophors, isopropyl alcohol, 70%; or chlorhexidine), and application of a sterile dressing.[11] Consideration should be given to wearing sterile gloves and a mask when care is administered to a central venous catheter or to the immunocompromised patient.[11]

PATIENT ASSESSMENT

The best treatment for phlebitis, whether chemical, mechanical, or bacterial, is prevention. The site is checked frequently and is changed at the first sign of tenderness, redness, or inflammation. The skin is palpated at the tip of the cannula by use of slight pressure to check for tenderness, and the skin is observed for warmth, edema, and vein induration.

NURSING INTERVENTIONS

If an infection is suspected, the cannula should be removed and cultured using established policies and procedures. The surrounding skin should be cleansed with 70% isopropyl alcohol and allowed to air dry. If purulent drainage is present, a culture of the drainage should be taken before the skin is cleansed. The recommended method of culturing is the semiquantitative technique.[11, 15, 16] Consideration should be given to obtaining blood cultures to determine proliferation of cannula-related infections. The cannula should be relocated to the opposite extremity, if possible, or to a vein into which the phlebitic vein does not empty. The application of warm, moist compresses promotes healing and patient comfort.

Postinfusion Phlebitis

Postinfusion phlebitis, another commonly reported complication of intravenous therapy, is associated with inflammation of the vein that usually becomes evident within 48 to 96 hours of cannula removal. Factors that contribute to the development of postinfusion phlebitis include:

- Cannula insertion technique
- Condition of the patient
- Condition of the vein being used
- Type, compatibility, and pH of solutions or medications being infused
- Ineffective filtration
- Gauge, size, length, and material of cannula
- Cannula dwell time

PATIENT ASSESSMENT

The patient is assessed for postinfusion phlebitis by monitoring of the intravenous site for signs of inflammation after the intravenous cannula has been removed. The site is observed for erythema, edema, and drainage. The site is palpated for warmth and for vein induration. The degree of postinfusion phlebitis should be measured according to the uniform scale used to measure phlebitis (see Table 24–4).

NURSING INTERVENTIONS

Generally, hot or cold compresses are applied, as described earlier, to the infusion site once a postinfusion phlebitis is detected. Depending on the degree of postinfusion phlebitis, medical intervention may be required.

PREVENTIVE MEASURES

Measures to prevent postinfusion phlebitis are the same as those designed to prevent phlebitis and include those outlined in Table 24–8.

Thrombosis

A thrombosis is the formation of a blood clot within a blood vessel. It is caused by any injury that breaks the integrity of the endothelial cells of the venous wall and usually occurs at the point at which the cannula touches the intima of the vein. Platelets adhere to the injured wall, and a thrombus is formed. Contributing factors include those listed in Table 24–9.

Table 24–8

Measures for Preventing Postinfusion Phlebitis
. . . .
Performance of venipuncture by skilled professional
Use of aseptic techniques when using or manipulating venous system
Checking compatibility of solutions and medications before mixing and administering
Use of filters when preparing medications and solutions
Use of final filtration when administering medications and solutions
Addition of a buffer to known irritating medications and to hypertonic solutions
Use of a cannula that is smaller than the vein to promote hemodilution of infusions
Use of large veins for the administration of hypertonic or acidic solution to promote hemodilution
Rotation of infusion sites as outlined in the *Intravenous Nursing Standards of Practice*.[11]
Changing solution containers every 24 hours
Changing latex injection peripheral ports on intermittent devices at the time of cannula change and when the integrity of the port has been compromised

Table 24–9

Factors Contributing to the Formation of Thrombosis
. . . .

Venipuncture by an unskilled professional
Multiple venipuncture attempts
Use of a cannula that is larger than the vein lumen
Poor circulation with venous stasis
Administration of medications incompatible with solutions
Administration of solutions or medications with high pH or tonicity
Ineffective filtration
Use of catheter materials that are thrombogenic

PATIENT ASSESSMENT

When an infusion slows or stops, the causative factors should be assessed. Mechanical and other problems should be ruled out. The possibility of a thrombus should be considered because the formation of a thrombus narrows the lumen of the vein, allowing less fluid to be infused. Usually, a thrombus goes undetected until either the infusion stops or the extremity becomes swollen owing to circulatory involvement. The area becomes very tender, and redness appears. The degree of circulatory involvement in the involved extremity should be assessed because a thrombosis can cause the loss of use of a limb because of tissue damage resulting from the lack of circulation.

The patient should also be assessed for the possibility of a systemic infection or a pulmonary embolism. Thrombi form an excellent trap for bacteria, whether stationary, carried by the blood stream from an infectious process located somewhere else in the body, or introduced through a subcutaneous orifice. Although a thrombus is usually well attached, it may, in rare circumstances, become unattached.

NURSING INTERVENTIONS

If thrombosis occurs, the infusion should be discontinued immediately, and the site should be relocated to the opposite extremity. Cold compresses should be applied to the site initially to decrease the flow of blood and increase platelet adherence to the clot that has already formed. The physician should be notified, and the site should be assessed to determine whether surgical intervention is needed; vein ligation may be necessary if the degree of circulatory impairment is sufficient to cause extensive tissue damage. The site should be monitored until symptoms completely resolve.

PREVENTIVE MEASURES

To prevent these injuries from occurring, atraumatic venipunctures by skilled professionals are necessary. Cannulation of the lower extremities in adults should be avoided because these veins are very small and allow pooling of blood with subsequent damage to the vein intima and clot formation. The selection of the appropriate venipuncture device is also very important; use of the smallest and shortest device possible to deliver the prescribed therapy decreases the potential of injury to the endothelial lining. Veins over flexion areas should be avoided, and cannulas should be anchored securely with tape to avoid in-and-out movements. Consideration should be given to the placement of central venous catheters when venous access is poor.

Thrombophlebitis

Thrombophlebitis is a condition denoting a two-fold injury: the presence of a thrombus and the occurrence of inflammation. Usually, the first symptom noted is inflammation along the vein line that is characterized by erythema. Edema, pain at the site and along the vein line, and a feeling of warmth usually follow. The vein becomes hard and tortuous as the vein thromboses. As this occurs, marked erythema, increased edema, marked pain along the vein, and aching of the extremity occur.

Any irritation to the intima of the vein can predispose the vein to inflammation and clot formation as platelets adhere to the traumatized wall of the vein. The incidence and degree of inflammation increase with the duration of the infusion. Other causative factors have been previously discussed under "Phlebitis" and "Thrombus."

PATIENT ASSESSMENT

The intravenous site and vein line should be observed at frequent intervals for signs and symptoms consistent with thrombophlebitis. The vein should be palpated for induration and tenderness. The patient should be questioned about the presence of pain at the site, along the vein line, and in the involved extremity. The patient should also be observed for chills and fever, and the laboratory values should be evaluated for an elevated white blood count (WBC).

If the condition goes untreated, the vein becomes sclerosed and is unavailable for future therapy. Although the inherent danger of an embolism always exists when a thrombus forms, these thrombi are generally well attached to the vein wall and do not migrate. The risk of septicemia or bacterial endocarditis is greater, particularly if the inflammation is the result of sepsis.

The degree of phlebitis should be measured according to the recommended scale (see Table 24–4). Thrombophlebitis is usually rated a 3 on this scale owing to the presence of a palpable cord.

NURSING INTERVENTIONS

When thrombophlebitis occurs, the infusion should be discontinued immediately, and the physician should be notified. If an infection is suspected, the cannula should be cultured using a semiquantitative technique.[11, 15, 16] The skin surrounding the cannula should be cleansed with 70% isopropyl alcohol and allowed to air dry before the cannula is removed for culture. When a purulent drainage is present, the culture of the drainage should be taken before the skin is cleansed.[11]

If infusion therapy is still necessary, a new cannula with new tubing and solution container should be placed in the opposite extremity, if possible. If using the opposite extremity is impossible, a separate vein that does not form a tributary of the traumatized vein should be used.

Cold compresses should be applied to the site initially to decrease the flow of blood and increase platelet adherence to the clot already formed. Then, warm compresses should be applied. The extremity should be elevated, and the patient should be cautioned that rubbing or massaging the area can cause an embolus. The extremity and the patient are monitored for the development of further complications.

PREVENTIVE MEASURES

Thrombophlebitis can lead to serious systemic complications, and measures should be taken to prevent their occurrence. These measures should include those outlined earlier under "Phlebitis" and "Thrombus."

Ecchymosis and Hematoma

Ecchymosis is a term used to denote the infiltration of blood into the tissues, whereas *hematoma* usually refers to uncontrolled bleeding at a venipuncture site, usually creating a hard, painful lump. Figure 24–4 illustrates ecchymosis with hematoma formation. Ecchymosis and hematomas are commonly associated with venipunctures that are performed by unskilled professionals or in patients who have a tendency to bruise easily. Patients receiving anticoagulants and long-term steroid therapy are particularly susceptible to bleeding from vein trauma. Ecchymosis and hematomas frequently occur when multiple entries are made into a vein, or when attempts are made into poorly visible veins or those that cannot be palpated.

The presence of both ecchymosis and hematomas limits veins for future use and produces damage to tissues. If a hematoma is severe, it may limit the use of an extremity.

PATIENT ASSESSMENT

The intravenous site and the area around the site should be observed for swelling during cannulation. Ecchymosis may or may not be noted immediately, owing to tissue turgor and

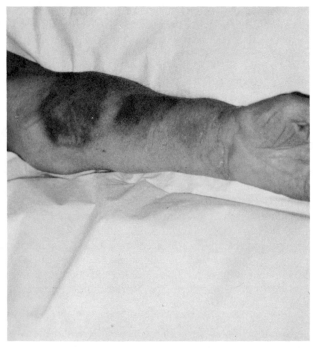

Figure 24–4. Ecchymosis with hematoma. The infiltration of blood into the tissues with uncontrolled bleeding can create a hematoma. (Courtesy of Johnson and Johnson Medical, Inc., Vascular Access, Arlington, TX.)

the amount of blood escaping into the tissues. Ecchymosis occurs first, and if bleeding is allowed to continue, a hematoma is formed. If sufficient bleeding is present, it is noted at the moment the cannula pierces the vein as blood escapes into the tissues. Discoloration may be immediate or slow, depending on the amount of subcutaneous tissue between the vein and the skin exterior.

NURSING INTERVENTIONS

If ecchymosis occurs during venipuncture, the cannula should be removed, and light pressure should be applied. If heavy pressure is applied, fragile veins within the area may rupture and increase bleeding. These areas usually feel sore, are unsightly, and take 1 to 2 weeks to disappear.[3]

If a hematoma is noted during a venipuncture attempt, the cannula is removed immediately, direct pressure is applied to the area, catheter integrity is assessed, and the extremity is elevated until the bleeding has stopped. A dry, sterile dressing is applied to the site and the area is monitored for signs of breakthrough bleeding. Ice may be applied to the area to prevent further enlargement of the hematoma. The extremity is monitored for circulatory, neurologic, and motor function.

PREVENTIVE MEASURES

Ecchymosis cannot always be prevented. Usually, hematomas can be prevented by the performance of venipunctures by highly skilled professionals. Inexperienced individuals should never perform venipunctures on patients with very fragile veins or veins that are not visible or easily palpable.

Hematomas can also result from excessive pressure being applied to a venipuncture site when a cannula is removed. Direct pressure with a dry, sterile dressing should be applied when cannulas are removed. Elevating the extremity while continuing to apply pressure for 1 or 2 minutes helps stop bleeding and prevent hematoma formation. Alcohol pads should not be used, because they inhibit clotting.

Occluded Cannula

Both peripheral and central venous cannulas can become occluded if monitoring or proper maintenance and care are not carried out. Cannulas can become occluded with blood when solution containers run dry and when flush solutions are not administered appropriately. The administration of incompatible solutions or medications can also lead to precipitate formation within the catheter with subsequent occlusion.

PATIENT ASSESSMENT

Usually, the first sign of a partially occluded cannula is the inability to maintain an accurate flow rate. The infusion slows, and, even with readjustment of the infusion rate, the flow cannot be increased. As the occlusion intensifies, the infusion stops. Resistance is met when attempts are made to flush an occluded cannula. Prescribed therapy cannot be administered if the catheter is occluded; in addition, a danger exists of thrombophlebitis or pulmonary embolism.

NURSING INTERVENTION

Cannulas should never be flushed to remove an occlusion. Clearing a cannula occlusion by force releases the occluding substance directly into the vascular system, creating a potential for an embolus. A peripheral cannula should be removed, the cannula should be examined for integrity, and a dry, sterile dressing should be applied to the site. If therapy is to be continued, a new cannula should be placed in another vein. Interventions for occluded central venous catheters are discussed under ''Complications Associated with Central Venous Catheters.''

PREVENTIVE MEASURES

Solution containers should be changed when less than 100 ml of solution remains. The use of time tape to designate the time that the solution will reach certain levels is very helpful in determining when a container will be empty.

Solutions and medications should be evaluated for compatibilities before they are mixed and administered. The pharmacist should be consulted when questions about compatibilities arise.

Policies and procedures should be established for the flushing of cannulas used as intermittent devices. The American Society of Hospital Pharmacists (ASHP) recommends the use of 0.9% sodium chloride to maintain patency of peripheral indwelling cannulas.[17]

Heparinized saline is used for flushing central venous catheters. The lowest possible concentration of heparin should be used. The amount and the frequency of the flush should be such that the patient's clotting factors are not altered. When medications are administered that are incompatible with heparin, the cannula is flushed with saline before and after the administration of the medication.

All cannulas used as intermittent devices are flushed as follows:

- After each administration of a medication
- After the administration of blood or blood products
- After withdrawal of blood
- When converting a continuous infusion to an intermittent device
- Every 8 to 12 hours when the cannula is not in use

The volume for maintaining patency is equal to the volume capacity of the cannula times two, added to the volume of the injection cap and to that of an extension set (if an extension set is used). Positive pressure within the cannula lumen must be maintained during and after the administration of a flush solution to prevent the reflux of blood into the cannula lumen and the formation of an occlusion. One way of maintaining positive pressure is to exert a continual push on the syringe plunger while withdrawing the syringe during the administration of the last 0.2 ml of flush solution. Withdrawing the syringe while continuing to push on the plunger replaces the space occupied by the needle during flush with the flush solution, thereby preventing reflux of blood within the cannula tip.

Infection at the Venipuncture Site

An infection can occur at the venipuncture site in the absence of phlebitis. It is usually a local infection at the cannula-skin entry point.

PATIENT ASSESSMENT

The intravenous site should be assessed for signs of local infection at frequent intervals while in use, at dressing and site changes, and when therapy is discontinued. The cannula-skin entry site should be observed for swelling and inflammation, and the surrounding tissue should be observed for discoloration and purulent drainage. The occurrence of an infection at the site may be apparent before or after the cannula has been removed.

NURSING INTERVENTIONS

If the cannula is in place, it should be removed and cultured to determine if it is the source of the infection. Any drainage from around the site should be cultured, and the skin should be cleansed with 70% isopropyl alcohol before the cannula is removed for culture. A sterile dressing should be applied, and the physician should be notified; usually, an antibiotic ointment with sterile dressing changes is ordered. Systemic antibiotic therapy may be necessary, and occasionally surgical intervention is necessary. The site should be monitored until the infection has resolved.

PREVENTIVE MEASURES

Usually, the causes of an infection at the site are related to a break in aseptic technique either during catheter insertion, during performance of catheter care, or during catheter removal. The use of contaminated equipment or supplies, the use of improper hand washing technique before care is performed, or the patient's picking at the site can predispose the site to an infection.

Aseptic technique must be maintained during cannula insertion, during intravenous therapy, and during catheter removal. An infection at the site provides an excellent opportunity for bacteria to enter the venous system unless early recognition occurs and appropriate interventions are carried out.

Venous or Arterial Spasm

A spasm is a sudden, involuntary contraction of a vein or an artery (vasoconstriction), resulting in temporary cessation of blood flow through a vessel. Stimulation by cold infusates or by mechanical or chemical irritation may produce spasms in arteries and veins.

Because arteries supply circulation to large areas of the body, arterial spasms are far more serious than are venous spasms. Unlike arteries, many veins supply a particular area, and if one becomes injured, blood is supplied to the area by collateral circulation; in these cases, the area's supply of blood may be decreased but not to the extent that it would be in an artery.

PATIENT ASSESSMENT

It is most important to recognize the signs and symptoms of a spasm. Cramping or pain above an infusion site or a feeling of numbness is usually the first symptom experienced by the patient. Patients experiencing arterial spasms may or may not complain of pain initially; they may not feel pain until tissue damage has occurred. When the patient complains of one of these symptoms, the involved extremity should be observed for localized blanching and the absence of a pulse; these signs would indicate an arterial spasm and a loss of blood flow to the area supplied by the artery.

NURSING INTERVENTIONS

If an arterial spasm occurs, it is usually related to the inadvertent puncture of an artery instead of a vein during venipuncture. If this occurs, the cannula should be removed immediately, pressure should be applied to the site over sufficient time to ensure hemostasis, and a dry, sterile dressing should be applied.

If a venous spasm occurs, discontinuing the infusion is not necessary. The infusion rate should be decreased, and if possible, the medication or solution should be further diluted. If a spasm has occurred as a result of the administration of a cold solution, warm compresses should be applied above the site; the heat provides vasodilatation and increases the blood supply, thereby relieving the pain and the spasm.

Some institutional protocols allow the use of 0.25 ml of lidocaine 1% (Xylocaine) to alleviate pain associated with spasms.[9, 10] This medication should be given only with a physician's written order and after an allergy history has been obtained. Established policies and procedures should govern the use of lidocaine for spasms.

PREVENTIVE MEASURES

The occurrence of many spasms can be prevented. The performance of venipuncture by skilled, experienced nurses can decrease the possibility of an inadvertent arterial stick. Venous spasms can also be prevented or minimized by infusing known irritating medications or solutions at slower rates and by diluting them as much as possible. Blood warmers should be used for rapid transfusions of potent cold agglutinins, for exchange transfusions in neonates, and for treatment in patients with hypothermia. Fluid warmers may be used to warm intravenous solutions to prevent or reverse hypothermic conditions. All refrigerated medications and parenteral solutions should be allowed to reach room temperature before they are administered.

Systemic Complications

Systemic complications are those occurring in circulation with the possibility of affecting the entire body. Systemic complications are usually very serious and require immediate interventions (Table 24–10).

Table 24–10

Systemic Complications of Intravenous Therapy

Septicemia	Pulmonary edema
Pulmonary embolism	Speed shock
Air embolism	Allergic reactions
Catheter embolism	

Table 24–11

Risk Factors Associated with Septicemia

Patient susceptibility
  Age
  Alteration in host defense
  Underlying illness
  Presence of other infectious processes
Use of intravenous therapy
  Solution container
  Contaminated equipment
  Stopcocks
  Catheter material and structure
  Experience of professional inserting cannula
  Insertion site
  Hematogenous seeding
  Manipulations of infusion system
  Certain transparent dressings
  Presence of monitoring devices
  Duration of cannulation

Septicemia

Septicemia is a pathologic state or a pyrogenic reaction that is usually accompanied by systemic illness. It occurs when pathogenic bacteria invade the bloodstream.

PATIENT ASSESSMENT

Usually chills, fever, general malaise, and headache are the first symptoms noted when pathogenic bacteria invade the blood stream. As the fever increases, the pulse rate increases, and prostration occurs. These symptoms may be accompanied by flushed face, backache, nausea and vomiting, and hypotension.

Patients receiving intravenous therapy should be monitored for these symptoms, and, if they occur, patients should be evaluated in terms of diagnosis, medications being administered by all routes, and any pending conditions that might be present. If no other cause can be found, the diagnosis of septicemia should be considered. If the condition goes undetected or untreated, symptoms become more severe, and cyanosis, increased respirations, or hyperventilation are noted. As the organisms overcome the system, vascular collapse, shock, and death can occur.

CONTRIBUTING FACTORS

Contributing factors placing the patient at risk for septicemia can be divided into two major categories: those that make the patient susceptible to the infectious process and those that allow microorganisms to enter the system (Table 24–11).

Solution Container. The solution container can be a focal point not only for contamination but also for microbial growth. Solutions can become contaminated during the manufacturing process, storage, and set-up or while they are in use as a result of manipulation or improper handling. The gram-negative organisms, the *Klebsiella, Serratia,* and *Enterobacter* species have been associated with contamination during the manufacturing process, whereas *Enterobacter cloacae, Enterobacter agglomerans,* and *Pseudomonas cepacia* have been associated with sepsis from contaminated infusates while in use.[15, 18] In addition, the composition of the infusate may actually promote the growth of microorganisms. *Klebsiella, Enterobacter, Serratia,* and *P. cepacia* show rapid growth within 24 hours in 5% dextrose in water solutions.[19] Blood products also provide an excellent source for *Klebsiella* microorganisms to grow, and total parenteral nutrition solutions support the growth of *Candida* species.

Other characteristics of the solution that can increase the risk of contamination include the tonicity, the pH, and the presence of particulate matter. Hypertonic solutions containing large amounts of particulates tend to irritate the vascular intima, causing an inflammatory reaction. This situation predisposes the vessel to thrombus formation, which provides a nidus for infection if the area becomes contaminated, either by contiguous infection or by hematogenous seeding.[20]

Solution containers that are allowed to hang longer than 24 hours may also cause septicemia because bacteria proliferate in solutions after 24 hours of use.[15, 20]

Contaminated Equipment. Equipment may become contaminated at the factory, en route from the factory, during storage, or at the time of use. If the integrity of the package is compromised, it should be discarded and new equipment used.

Stopcocks. Studies have shown that three-way stopcocks used as part of the infusion system have frequently been the cause of microorganisms entering the intravenous system.[20] Microorganisms enter the system from the hands of personnel during frequent manipulations of the stopcocks; from syringes that are used either to flush or to draw blood specimens; from residual blood that remains in a port after use, serving as a breeding ground for bacteria; and from failure to keep a sterile cap on the stopcock when it is not in use.

Catheter Material and Structure. The catheter material and structure contribute to the risk of infectious complications associated with the administration of intravenous therapy. Larger catheters come in contact with a greater skin area, produce a larger hole in the skin and vessel, are more difficult to anchor, and are often used for purposes that require more frequent entries into the system. Some studies state that the use of multilumen catheters increases the risk of infections as much as 12.8%[20] because of the increased number of entry sites into the vascular system.[18] Stiffer catheters also increase the risk of infection by provoking thrombogenesis and an inflammatory response that may facilitate colonization.

Microorganisms are able to adhere to some catheter materials more readily than to others. The *Candida* species have been shown to adhere to polyvinylchloride catheters much better than to polytetrafluoroethylene catheters. Differential adherence of microorganisms to catheters of various compositions may influence the microbiology of infection. Although some catheter materials are less thrombogenic than others, most authorities believe that all catheters become encased in a fibrin sheath within several hours of implantation.[18, 20] Whether this sheath represents an asset or a liability is unclear. Some catheter materials appear to promote the adherence of certain pathogenic strains of microorganisms; in these materials, the fibrin sheath may be relatively protective. Conversely, other catheter materials do not promote microbial adherence; in these materials, the fibrin sheath may represent a nidus for infection.

Experience of Practitioner. The technical skill of the person placing the catheter influences the potential for infection. Studies have shown that good insertion techniques actually lower the risks of infection.[18, 20–22]

Insertion Site. Many authorities believe that the primary route by which microorganisms gain access to the vascular system is by entry along the catheter insertion site, whereas others have demonstrated a rather loose association between skin colonization and subsequent development of infection by the same organism, with the exception of *Staphylococcus aureus.* Skin organisms gain access to the transcutaneous tract (the space between the catheter and the subcutaneous tissue) at the time the catheter is inserted.[23] Intravenous cannulas can be contaminated during the time of insertion by microorganisms on the hands of personnel.

When serial cultures were performed, two thirds of all persons carried *S. aureus* on their hands. Washing the hands with soap and water while employing mechanical friction for a least 15 seconds is sufficient to remove most transiently acquired bacteria.[18] If not removed, these organisms can be deposited into the blood stream and can produce bacteremia or fungemia.

Studies have also shown that microbial growth occurs when intravenous sites are not cleaned appropriately and dressings are not changed. These microorganisms also migrate along the tract and enter the blood stream, producing bacteremia or fungemia.[12] Access to the intravascular portion of the catheter by microbial flora residing in and on the skin depends on several factors, such as insertion technique, catheter composition, microbial adherence to the catheter, and catheter movement in the insertion site.

Hematogenous Seeding. Another factor that causes catheter sepsis is hematogenous seeding from a distant foci. Microorganisms are carried from a remote site or from another source of infection, such as a tracheostomy, the urinary tract, or a surgical wound, and actually seed on the intravascular catheter. Most vascular access yeast infections appear to be the result of hematogenous dissemination from another site.[16, 18, 20] This route appears to be less common for the spread of *S. aureus.*[20, 23]

Hematogenous seeding can also occur if a catheter is inserted into a patient who has a high-grade bacteremia or candidemia. Factors that affect catheter seeding include the causative pathogen, the degree and duration of bacteremia, the patient's clinical status, and the length of time the catheter has been in place.

Manipulation of the Delivery System. Frequent manipulations of the cannula or the intravenous system greatly increase the risk of sepsis.[20] Each time the system is entered, the potential exists for microorganisms to enter the intravascular system. The system may be entered for the addition of medications to the solution container, for injections of medications into the tubing, for administration of blood products, for flushing of tubing or cannulas, for manipulation to reposition catheters, and for obtaining blood samples. Because a Swan-Ganz or arterial catheter is manipulated many more times per day than other catheters, it is reasonable to expect the risk of infection to be greater for these devices per day of catheterization.[12]

Transparent Dressings. In early studies performed by Beam and colleagues,[23] a significant relationship was demonstrated between the application of a polyurethane dressing on central venous catheter sites and the development of infection. These investigators reported a build-up of liquid moisture under these dressings, causing an increase in colonization of the site and the risk of catheter-related infection. Other studies have shown that replacing the transparent dressings and cleansing the site with an antiseptic solution every 48 hours result in minimal build-up of flora and no significant increase in the risk of infection.[23] Now, newer transparent dressings are available that have improved moisture permeability, which may actually decrease the potential for infection.

Pressure Monitoring Systems. Research has shown that pressure monitoring systems used in conjunction with arterial catheters have been associated with both epidemic and endemic nosocomial intravascular infections.[24, 25] The common pathway for microorganisms to enter the blood stream, leading to bacteremia, is the fluid column in the tubing between the patient's intravascular catheter and the pressure monitoring apparatus. Microorganisms in a fluid-filled system may move from the pressure monitoring apparatus to the patient or from the patient to the pressure monitoring system.[25] Pressure monitoring systems have also been reported to be contaminated by contaminated infusate,[26] by the use of nonsterile calibrating devices,[27] by ice used to chill syringes,[28] by introduction of microorganisms into the system from contaminated disinfectant used on the domes,[29] and by contamination of the monitoring system related to blind, stagnant columns of fluid between the transducer and infusion system.[25]

Duration of Catheterization. Length of exposure is listed by some authorities as the most important risk factor for vascular access infections.[18, 20] Investigators have concluded that an approximate fourfold range exists in the risk of infection for different types of catheters per day of catheterization. Studies have also shown that arterial catheters have an increased incidence of positive catheter cultures after 2 to 4 days.[23] In general, no catheter should be considered as having a low risk of infection, and because the risk is cumulative, no catheter should be left in place any longer than is absolutely necessary.[18, 20, 23]

NURSING INTERVENTIONS

Early symptoms of septicemia must be evaluated for possible causes. In the absence of other causes, such as the presence of a kidney, respiratory, or wound infection, the solution and the delivery system must be considered. Some authorities feel that fever in a person with a central venous catheter should be attributed to the catheter until proven otherwise.[20] Erythema at the site of insertion is an unreliable sign of sepsis because virtually all catheters under transparent polyurethane dressings show erythema; however, erythema at the site should be monitored because it could indicate an infectious process that could lead to sepsis. In most of these patients, no other signs of infections are present. Vital signs should be monitored, and if sepsis is suspected, the physician should be notified immediately. If a physician's order is required to perform cultures, the physician should be asked for orders to culture the cannula, the infusate, and the patient's blood.

The cannula should be removed and cultured only after the skin around the cannula has been cleansed with 70% isopropyl alcohol and allowed to dry. The recommended method of culture is the semiquantitative technique.[11, 15, 16] The infusate should also be cultured. Consideration should be given to obtaining blood cultures to determine the proliferation of an infusate-related infection.

A new infusion site with new tubing and solution container should be initiated as soon as possible. The patient should be monitored for signs of shock, and emergency measures should be carried out, if necessary. The physician usually orders antibiotics, which should be started as quickly as possible after the cultures are drawn.

Some authorities believe that central venous catheters suspected of being infected should not be routinely removed from patients who have limited sites for central venous access or from those who would be put at risk of mechanical complications or bleeding that results from insertion of a new catheter at a new site. In these patients, quantitative blood cultures are drawn through the catheter and peripherally. Empiric antimicrobial therapy is initiated based on the assessment that a bacteremia is present, and the catheter is removed only if all cultures are positive for infection.[23] Another option is to change the central venous catheter in the same site over a guide wire by use of aseptic technique. The old catheter is cultured, and if the old catheter shows heavy colonization, the new catheter that has just been placed is removed because it has been placed into an infected site. The exception to both options is the presence of *Candida* or any other fungus because candidemia cannot be eradicated in a person with a central line.[23] Policies should be established that give specific guidelines on the procedure that should be followed when sepsis from an intravenous system is suspected.

PREVENTIVE MEASURES

The best treatment for septicemia is prevention. Strict adherence to the guidelines listed in the box below can aid in the prevention of septicemia related to the administration of intravenous therapy.

Numerous studies have also shown that catheter-related infections can be greatly reduced by the insertion of peripheral catheters and the administration of care to both peripheral and central venous catheters by a team approach.[12, 20] This finding was most evident in studies of patients receiving total parenteral nutrition solutions in which infection rates were reduced from 25 to 30% to 3 to 5%.[20] In comparative trials, Maki and Ringer concluded that the availability of a team of nurses who are highly experienced in intravenous therapy and who insert intravenous catheters and provide close surveillance of infusions resulted in a two-fold lower rate of infusion phlebitis and an even greater reduction in catheter-related sepsis.[12]

Guidelines for the Prevention of Septicemia

1. The hands should be washed, rinsed, and dried before initiating an infusion and before handling any part of the intravenous system.
2. All solutions should be checked before administration for clarity, cracks, or leaks and for the presence of a vacuum.

3. The site for cannula placement should be cleansed with an antimicrobial solution applied with friction, working outward from the center to the periphery. Tincture of iodine, 1%–2%; iodophors; isopropyl alcohol, 70%; or chlorhexidine may be used to cleanse the site. If both alcohol and an iodophor are used, the alcohol should be applied first, then the iodophor. The iodophor should not be removed with the alcohol, because its action depends on the release of iodine over a period of time. The preparatory solution should be allowed to dry completely.

4. Excessive hair over the venipuncture site should be clipped.

5. Cannulas should be taped to prevent an in-and-out movement of the cannula, which promotes the transport of cutaneous bacteria into the site and the vascular system.

6. Cannula site care should be administered at the time of dressing change and at the intervals stated in the *Intravenous Nursing Standards of Practice.*[11] The site is observed for signs of redness, swelling, or inflammation. The site is cleansed with an antiseptic solution (e.g., tincture of iodine, 1%–2%; iodophors; isopropyl alcohol, 70%; or chlorhexidine) and an antimicrobial or antibiotic ointment, as indicated by policy, and a sterile dressing is applied. Sterile gloves and a mask are worn during the administration of site care to a central venous catheter.

7. Lines are not broken to allow patients to ambulate or to change gowns.

8. Aseptic technique is used when initiating therapy or manipulating the line. The cannula is not touched at any time during insertion. Cannulas inserted in an emergency are replaced at the earliest opportunity.

9. All solution containers are changed every 24 hours, preferably at the same time the tubing is changed.

10. Peripheral cannulas are changed according to the *Intravenous Nursing Standards of Practice.*[11]

11. Peripheral and central primary and secondary intravenous tubings are changed according to the *Intravenous Nursing Standards of Practice*[11] and immediately if contamination is suspected or if the integrity has been compromised.

12. Connections on central venous catheter hubs and tubings are cleaned with a povidone-iodine solution and allowed to dry before they are disconnected for a tubing change.

13. Primary intermittent administration sets are changed according to the *Intravenous Nursing Standards of Practice.*[11]

14. Luer-Lok connections are used when possible, and other connections are secured with connecting devices to avoid accidental separation.

15. The use of add-on devices is limited to situations in which an absolute need exists because the addition of a device allows an opportunity for bacteria to enter the system. If use of an add-on device is necessary, the device is changed at the same time the administration set is changed.

16. Injection ports are disinfected with an antimicrobial solution (iodine, 1%–2%, iodophor, isopropyl alcohol, 70%; or chlorhexidine) before they are used.

17. Latex injection caps on peripheral lines are changed at the time the cannula is changed or whenever the latex injection port is suspected of being compromised. Latex injection caps on central lines are changed at least every 7 days and when the latex port is suspected of being compromised.

18. Needles are changed on secondary medication sets before subsequent use. If secondary medication sets are disconnected from the primary line, needles are changed.

19. Defective equipment or equipment whose package integrity has been broken is never used.

20. The intravenous site is observed frequently and is changed at the first signs of inflammation. Policies and procedures are written specifying the frequency for site checks.

21. Peripheral arterial cannulas are changed every 96 hours, and pulmonary artery catheters are changed every fourth or fifth day.

22. Plugged or sluggish cannulas are not flushed or irrigated. Not only do they represent a nidus for infection, but an embolus can also be released into the vascular system.

23. Intravenous cannulation of the lower extremities is avoided because of the higher incidence of associated complications.

24. The smallest needle possible is used when an injection port is used. Needles that are 25 to 20 gauge and do not exceed 1 inch in length are recommended.

From Intravenous Nurses Society. Intravenous nursing standards of practice. JIN 1990; ISSN 0896-5846, Journal Supplement S26–S80.

Recent studies have shown that catheter-related infections of central venous catheters can be reduced by the use of an attachable cuff impregnated with silver ions.[23–26] The ions have a very broad spectrum of antimicrobial activity and are effective against both bacteria and fungi that are likely to cause catheter-related infections. The cuff is placed beneath the skin at the insertion site when the catheter is inserted. The cuff inhibits the migration of bacteria along the external surface of the catheter, preventing colonization of the subcutaneous segment and the tip of the catheter. Subcutaneous tissue grows to the cuff, providing a mechanical barrier, and the silver ions provide a chemical barrier against organisms. Studies have shown the use of the cuff to cause a threefold reduction in the incidence of colonization and a fourfold reduction in the incidence of septicemia.[23, 27]

Studies have also shown that the use of catheters molecularly bonded with antimicrobial substances are four times less likely to produce a bacteremia.[28]

Pulmonary Embolism

A pulmonary embolism occurs when a mass of undissolved matter, usually a blood clot, becomes free floating and is carried by venous circulation to the right side of the heart and into the pulmonary artery. The embolus may obstruct the pulmonary artery or its branches that supply the lobes of the lung, thus occluding arterial openings at major bifurcations. If the pulmonary artery is obstructed, the patient will experience cardiac disturbances. If multiple emboli are passed into the pulmonary circulation, the patient will experience pulmonary hypertension and right-sided heart failure.[29, 30]

PATIENT ASSESSMENT

The patient receiving intravenous therapy should be monitored for signs and symptoms of pulmonary embolism. These symptoms include dyspnea, pleuritic pain or discomfort, apprehension, cough, unexplained hemoptysis, sweats, tachypnea, tachycardia, cyanosis, and low-grade fever. If any of these are noted, the chest should be auscultated for a pleural friction rub.[30, 31]

NURSING INTERVENTIONS

If a pulmonary embolism is suspected, the patient should be placed in semi-Fowler's position, and the patient's vital signs should be assessed. The physician should be notified. Medical interventions usually include the administration of oxygen to maintain blood gas levels, a lung scan to verify a pulmonary embolism, a prothrombin time determination to have as a baseline clotting time before anticoagulant therapy is initiated, and a bolus of heparin followed by a heparin infusion.[4, 30]

PREVENTIVE MEASURES

The best treatment for a pulmonary embolism is prevention. Measures to prevent the formation and the release of pulmonary emboli into the vascular system include

1. Use of a filter to remove particulates from solutions or medications being administered.
2. Administration of blood and blood components through a filter designed to retain blood clots and other debris.
3. Avoidance of the use of the lower extremities for venipuncture in the adult patient.
4. Use of measures that prevent injuries to the vein intima. Such measures include the performance of venipunctures by skilled professionals, the use of the smallest cannula possible to deliver the prescribed therapy, the use of large veins when irritating solutions or medications are administered to promote hemodilution, and the use of proper taping techniques to prevent cannula movement.
5. Use of good judgment when intravenous lines are flushed. Positive pressure should never be used to flush a line, because a blood clot can be released into the vascular system. Irrigating lines to improve flow rates is dangerous and should not be practiced.
6. Examination of solution containers for particulate matter before they are used.
7. Clipping of excessive hair and cleansing of the area to remove the potential for hair to be severed and carried into the vascular system with venipuncture.

Air Embolism

An air embolism is caused by the entry of a bolus of air into the vascular system. The embolism is propelled into the heart, creating an intracardiac air lock at the pulmonic valve and preventing the injection of blood from the right side of the heart.

PATIENT ASSESSMENT

When an air embolism occurs, the patient complains of chest pain and shortness of breath and may complain of shoulder or low back pain, depending on the location of the air embolus. The patient appears cyanotic. Assessment reveals hypotension and a weak rapid pulse. On auscultation, a continuous churning sound may be heard over the precordium. The patient may faint or lose consciousness. If signs

and symptoms go unrecognized or untreated, shock or cardiac arrest may result.

NURSING INTERVENTIONS

If an air embolism is suspected, the patient should be placed immediately on the left side in Trendelenburg's position; this measure keeps the air in the pulmonary outflow tract to a minimum by trapping it in the right heart chambers and great veins proximal to the pulmonic valve. If the air embolism results from an open or leaking infusion line, the line should be changed immediately and replaced with new tubing that is filled with solution. The source of air intake must be corrected immediately, or air will continue to be drawn into the system. The physician should be notified, and the patient's vital signs should be monitored. Oxygen is usually administered in these cases.

PREVENTIVE MEASURES

Every effort should be made to prevent the formation of an air embolus. Infusion tubings and extensions on catheters should be clamped when tubings are changed. A negative pressure is created within the vein when the extremity receiving the infusion is elevated above the heart[29]; a negative pressure within the vein increases the potential for air to be drawn into the system. Infusions through central venous catheters are at a greater risk of having air drawn into the system; as intrathoracic pressure is decreased below atmospheric pressure, negative pressure occurs within the central vein, causing a sucking effect that can draw air readily into the vein. To prevent this event from occurring, the patient should lie flat and perform the Valsalva maneuver (forced expiration with the mouth closed) when central lines are inserted or discontinued and when tubings are changed. The use of an air-eliminating filter can prevent air from passing into the vascular system by removing the air as it travels through the filter.

Solution containers should be changed before they are completely empty. Leaking infusion tubings should be changed as soon as they are discovered to eliminate the possibility of air being drawn into the vascular system. Luer-Lok connections should be used to prevent the accidental separation of infusion systems, which can also create a negative pressure in the vascular system and pull air into the system. Infusion sets should be purged of all air before an infusion is initiated, and air should be removed from all syringes before medications are administered.

Patient education on the appropriate care and maintenance of a central venous catheter to prevent an air embolism and in the recognition of signs and symptoms of an air embolism should be initiated immediately after a central venous catheter is placed.

Catheter Embolism

A catheter embolism occurs when a piece of catheter is broken in the vein and enters the circulatory system. This event can occur with a through-the-needle catheter if the catheter is pulled backward and then threaded forward; the needle may pierce or sever the catheter. Catheter embolism can also occur with an over-the-needle catheter if the needle stylet is partially withdrawn, then reinserted into the catheter. In these two instances, the professional inserting the catheter may be aware that the catheter has been severed; however, one does not always have the opportunity to detect an embolism at the time of occurrence, because a defective catheter can break or rupture after placement. Silicone catheters may rupture if a medication or a flush solution is administered with positive pressure. Catheters can also rupture as a result of the pinch-off syndrome created by their anatomic placement between the first rib and the clavicle.

Once the catheter is completely severed or even a small segment is broken, it may be released into circulation and block a major vein, causing loss of circulation, or the catheter embolism may travel to the heart, causing cardiac irritability and cardiac arrest. A catheter may also rupture without releasing a fragment into the circulation, such as could occur with a tunneled catheter; however, the danger of an embolus is always present.

PATIENT ASSESSMENT

An immediate sign that a peripheral cannula has broken is cannula and hub separation or a severed cannula on withdrawal. When a central venous catheter has ruptured, the patient may be asymptomatic, and the rupture may not be discovered until the catheter is used. Central venous catheters should be assessed for patency each time they are used. If the nurse suspects that a catheter has been released into the vascular system, the patient should be observed for cyanosis, hypotension, increased central venous pressure, tachycardia, fainting, and loss of consciousness. The severity of symptoms is totally dependent on the location of the catheter embolism.

NURSING INTERVENTIONS

Immediate intervention to prevent an embolus is necessary if a peripheral catheter is broken. A tourniquet is placed on the patient's arm above the venipuncture site, and bed rest is prescribed for the patient to minimize the rapidity with which the cannula travels in the vascular system. The physician is notified immediately, and the patient is monitored for signs of catheter migration. An emergency cart should be readily available in the event of a cardiac arrest.

If a central venous catheter embolism is suspected, strict bed rest is prescribed, the physician is notified, and the patient is monitored for signs of further distress and treated for shock, if necessary.

Radiographic studies are ordered to determine the exact location of the catheter fragment. In most instances, the catheter fragment can be retrieved with a specially designed snare. The procedure involves the intravenous passage of the snare under fluoroscopic control to remove the catheter fragment. If the fragment cannot be removed successfully, a thoracotomy may be required to remove the embolized catheter.[30]

PREVENTIVE MEASURES

Measures for preventing catheter emboli include those listed in Table 24–12.

Table 24–12

Measures for Preventing Catheter Emboli
. . . .
Cannulas should be inspected for defects before use.
Through-the-needle catheters should never be pulled back through the needle.
Over-the-needle catheters should never be withdrawn and reinserted once they have been partially or fully threaded.
Positive pressure should not be exerted when a flush solution or a medication is administered through a silicone catheter.
Consideration should be given to the use of syringes of no less than 10 ml when medications or flush solutions are administered through silicone catheters.

Pulmonary Edema

Pulmonary edema is a condition that is precipitated by the presence of more fluid volume than the circulatory system can manage. When an excess of fluid volume occurs, there is an increase in venous pressure and the possibility of cardiac dilatation. If the condition is allowed to persist, congestive heart failure, shock, and cardiac arrest can result.[30, 32] Frequently, this condition is precipitated by infusing too much fluid or infusing fluids too fast,[30] which is particularly hazardous to the elderly patient, the pediatric patient, and the patient with renal or cardiac problems.

PATIENT ASSESSMENT

The nurse must be alert to the early signs of pulmonary edema. Early signs include restlessness, slow increase in pulse rate, headache, shortness of breath, cough, and possibly flushing. As more fluid continues to build, the patient becomes hypertensive, becomes severely dyspneic with gurgling respirations, and starts to cough up frothy fluid. The patient should be assessed for venous dilatation, which is indicated by engorged neck veins, pitting edema in dependent areas, elevated pulmonary wedge pressure, and moist rales on auscultation. Some patients also experience puffy eyelids as fluids start to collect within the circulatory system.[30]

NURSING INTERVENTIONS

The occurrence of pulmonary edema creates an emergency situation. The infusion should be slowed immediately to a rate that keeps the vein open, and the patient should be placed in a high Fowler's position. The patient's vital signs and fluid balance should be monitored. The physician should be notified, and oxygen should be administered as ordered. Medical intervention may include (1) the administration of diuretics intravenously to produce rapid diuresis; (2) the administration of an intravenous vasodilator, such as sodium nitroprusside, to decrease afterload; (3) the administration of morphine sulfate to decrease myocardial workload, by decreasing preload through peripheral venous vasodilation, and afterload, by decreasing arterial blood pressure; and (4) phlebotomy to relieve the workload of the heart and to reduce venous pressure.[30]

PREVENTIVE MEASURES

Measures for the prevention of pulmonary edema are detailed in Table 24–13.

Measures for Preventing Pulmonary Edema

Patients are assessed before the initiation of intravenous therapy for a history of problems associated with having previously received intravenous therapy; for a history of cardiac and respiratory problems; and for present status relative to their ability to tolerate fluid volume.
Patients receiving intravenous therapy are monitored closely for tolerance to the administration of solutions and/or medications.
Infusion rates are maintained as ordered unless such rates would compromise the well-being of the patient. Rates are not increased to allow for solutions whose rates have gotten behind.
The infusion rate is slowed if signs or symptoms of fluid overload are observed and the physician is notified for orders to decrease the infusion rate.
Volumetric chambers, infusion control devices, or both, are used when solutions or medications are administered that require accurate measurement and when solutions or medications are administered to the neonate, the pediatric patient, and/or the elderly patient whose condition warrants critical management to prevent fluid overload.

Speed Shock

Speed shock is a systemic reaction that occurs when a substance foreign to the body is rapidly introduced into circulation. This phenomenon usually results from the administration of a bolus medication at a rapid rate or from the rapid administration of an infusion containing a medication. Speed shock should not be confused with pulmonary edema. Pulmonary edema relates to volume whereas speed shock relates to the rapidity with which a medication is administered and can occur even when a small volume of medication is given. Rapid injections of a medication enter the serum in toxic proportions and flood the heart and the brain with medication.

PATIENT ASSESSMENT

When medications are administered, the patient should be observed for dizziness, facial flushing, headache, and symptoms associated with the administration of the medication. It is vital to note these symptoms early because progression is immediate, with the patient experiencing tightness in the chest, hypotension, irregular pulse, and anaphylactic shock.

NURSING INTERVENTIONS

The infusion should be discontinued immediately on recognition of the first symptom, and an intravenous line should be maintained for emergency treatment. The patient should be treated for symptoms of shock, if necessary. The physician should be notified, and the patient should be given additional treatment as needed.

PREVENTIVE MEASURES

Speed shock can be prevented. Individuals administering a medication should have knowledge of the medication being given and should administer the medication at the recommended rate. Gravity flow administration sets should be checked frequently to make sure that they are infusing at the appropriate rate. Solution containers should be time-taped so that the amount that has infused can be readily observed.

Electronic flow control devices or volumetric chambers should be used for patients who are at great risk for developing complications and when critical solutions or medications are administered.

Allergic Reactions

An allergic reaction is a response to a medication or solution to which the patient is sensitive. Reactions may also occur from the passive transfer of sensitivity to the patient from a blood donor, or the patient may be sensitive to substances normally present in the blood, as is seen in transfusion reactions. Reactions may be immediate or delayed. The most common reactions are those seen as a result of the administration of antibiotics and blood products. (Reactions to blood and blood products are discussed in Chapter 10.)

PATIENT ASSESSMENT

Patients receiving intravenous therapy should be monitored for symptoms of allergic reactions. The patient may experience chills and fever with or without urticaria, erythema, and itching. Depending on the internal response to the allergen, the patient could experience shortness of breath with or without wheezing. The patient may also experience angioneurotic edema.

NURSING INTERVENTION

The infusion should be stopped immediately, the tubing and solution container should be changed, and the vein should be kept open for the possibility of anaphylactic shock. The physician should be notified, and interventions should be carried out as ordered. Antihistamines are usually administered to relieve mild symptoms; epinephrine or steroids are administered for more severe reactions. Sometimes, antihistamines are used prophylactically when an allergic reaction is considered likely.

PREVENTIVE MEASURES

Preventive measures include the following:

1. An admission assessment should be performed of the patient's previous drug allergies, sensitivities, or idiosyncrasies. An identification bracelet should be placed on the patient, and the medical record should be flagged so that nurses are aware of all allergies. The pharmacy profile should list all allergies so that all medications can be cross-referenced for allergic reactions.
2. Adequate screening of donor and recipient blood can aid in the prevention of blood reactions. Policies and procedures should specify the procedures for drawing blood samples for crossmatching, for the crossmatching process, for the identification process before the blood is administered, and for the interventions to be carried out if a reaction occurs.

Complications Associated with Central Venous Catheters

Central venous catheters are being used more now than ever before. As more patients are placed on long-term intravenous therapies, receive intravenous therapy within the home, and receive medications or solutions that can produce adverse effects if an infiltration occurs, the frequency of the use of central venous catheters will continue to rise. The difficulty of maintaining vascular access for the length of extended therapies and the complications associated with the use of smaller, more fragile blood vessels have required the use of these catheters. In many clinical settings, central venous catheters are being placed early in the treatment process, long before peripheral access is exhausted.

Modern technology has risen to the occasion, and many different types of central catheters have been developed. The availability of these catheters has led to mass confusion for many health care professionals as to which device is best for the therapy prescribed. Additionally, with each type of device comes different protocols for insertion, care and maintenance, and removal. Health care providers must establish policies and procedures for the use of each catheter.

Each type of central catheter is unique and has special advantages and disadvantages. The use of these catheters is not without risks or complications. The nurse and the patient must be knowledgeable about, and alert to, the complications of the catheter being used. Many complications that relate to central catheters have already been discussed under "Systemic Complications"; however, other complications are specific to central catheters.

Insertion-Related Complications

Complications associated with the placement of central venous catheters are rare, but they can be very serious. Complications related to the subclavian vein approach include pneumothorax, hemothorax, hydrothorax, extravascular position, chylothorax, and brachial plexus injury, whereas the antecubital cephalic vein approach is associated with hematoma and tendon or nerve damage. Complications related to both approaches include arrhythmias; perforation of vein, artery, or heart; venous thrombosis; thrombophlebitis; severed catheter; infection; and catheter malposition.[33]

Pneumothorax

A pneumothorax is a collection of air in the pleural space, the space between the lung and the chest wall.[30, 32] It results from puncture of the pleural covering of the lung during insertion of a central venous catheter, usually as a result of the anatomic proximity of the lung to the subclavian veins. The lung may also be punctured, creating an associated danger of an air embolism from puncture of the vein as well as surgical emphysema.[30]

Signs and symptoms depend on the size of the pneumothorax. The patient may experience a sudden onset of chest pain or shortness of breath while the procedure is being performed, or the patient may be asymptomatic and the pneumothorax may not be discovered until radiographic confirmation of catheter tip placement is made. On auscultation, a crunching sound with heartbeat is heard that results from mediastinal air accumulation. If the pneumothorax is severe, the patient will have marked dyspnea.[30]

If symptoms are noted during catheter insertion, the physician should remove the catheter and insertion needle immediately. The color of the patient's face, the respirations, and the pulse should be monitored, and the patient should be observed for signs of pleural shock and effusion. Oxygen is usually administered, and a chest tube may be inserted. If no respiratory distress occurs and the pneumothorax does not create tension within the chest, the pneumothorax may slowly resolve without evacuation of the air. However, if the size of the pneumothorax increases on repeated chest radiographic studies or if respiratory distress or progressively increasing subcutaneous emphysema occurs, a persistent air leak from the injured lung may be present. The patient should be observed and monitored for these delayed events. If any of these findings are present, the physician should be notified, radiographic studies performed, and the patient prepared for chest tubes.

If the pneumothorax is not diagnosed until radiographic confirmation of catheter tip placement is made, the physician is notified and medical interventions are carried out as ordered.

A pneumothorax cannot always be prevented, because of the anatomic location of the subclavian veins and the lungs; however, some measures can aid in the prevention of a pneumothorax (Table 24–14).

Hemothorax

A hemothorax occurs when blood enters the pleural cavity as a result of trauma or transection of a vein during insertion of a central venous catheter.[30] The patient may experience a sudden onset of chest pain with mild-to-severe dyspnea while the catheter is being inserted or the patient may be asymptomatic, depending on the amount of blood released into the pleural cavity. Frequently, bleeding is slow and constant into the pleural cavity, which can be particularly alarming if a patient has a clotting problem. Delayed symptoms that may occur as blood accumulates within the chest include tachycardia, hypotension, dusky skin color, diaphoresis, and hemoptysis. Percussion may disclose dullness of the affected side of the chest, and auscultation may detect decreased or absent breath sounds over the affected side.[30]

If symptoms of a hemothorax are noted during catheter insertion, the physician should remove the catheter and the insertion needle, and pressure should be applied to the site. If a tunneled catheter is being inserted, pressure should be

---

T a b l e   2 4 – 1 4

Measures That Aid in the Prevention of Injuries Associated with the Insertion of Central Venous Catheters
· ·
Only highly skilled professionals should insert central venous catheters. The insertion of centrally placed catheters is a medical act; nurses who insert peripherally placed central venous catheters should be educated in insertion, management, associated complications, and removal of these lines.
Patients with a centrally placed venous catheter should be placed in Trendelenburg's position with a rolled towel placed along the spine between the clavicles to facilitate placement of the catheter by hyperextending the neck and elevating the clavicles.
The patient should be given a thorough explanation (if he or she is coherent) of the procedure and should be given emotional support during the placement of a central venous catheter. Patients fear what they do not know or understand and often respond unfavorably. Patient understanding elicits cooperation, which facilitates catheter placement.

applied over the vein entry site. The patient's vital signs should be monitored, and symptoms should be treated. Oxygen is usually administered, and a chest tube may be placed if the hemothorax is associated with a pneumothorax.[30] If symptoms occur after the catheter has been inserted, the physician should be notified and medical interventions carried out as necessary.

The risk of hemothorax is decreased by following the same guidelines as those for decreasing the risks of a pneumothorax (see Table 24–14).

Chylothorax

Chylothorax is a condition in which chyle (lymph) enters the pleural cavity as a result of transection of the thoracic duct on the left side where it enters the subclavian vein. Chyle is the milk-like contents of the lacteal and lymphatic vessels of the intestines and consists of the products of digestion and principally absorbed fats. It is carried by the lymphatic vessels to the cisterna chyli and then, by way of the thoracic duct, to the left subclavian vein, where it enters the blood system.[32] Because of the anatomic position of the thoracic duct, the left supraclavicular approach to the subclavian vein is usually avoided.

Symptoms of chylothorax are similar to those of hemothorax. The patient may experience a sudden onset of chest pain with dyspnea as the thoracic duct is transected and lymph fills the pleural cavity. Frequently, chylothorax is noted by the clinician at the time of transection of the thoracic duct because of the withdrawal of a milklike substance into the needle or catheter.

The leaking of a cloudy material from around the catheter site suggests the possibility of a chylous fistula. Any cloudy fluid leaking from around the catheter site should be aseptically collected if possible and checked for glucose content. A low glucose content suggests that the liquid is a body fluid, whereas a high glucose content suggests a lymphatic leak. If a lymphatic leak is found, the physician should be notified for removal of the catheter, and the patient's vital signs should be assessed. Oxygen and chest tubes may be necessary, depending on the amount of lymph emptied into the thoracic cavity.

Hydrothorax

Hydrothorax occurs when intravenous fluids are infused directly into the thoracic cavity as a result of transection of the vein and placement of the catheter into the thorax. Signs and symptoms include chest pain with dyspnea, absence of vesicular breath sounds, and a murmur with a flat sound over the location of the fluid.

Medical interventions include removal of the catheter, aspiration of fluids from the pleural space, and possibly, insertion of chest tubes. The patient is monitored, and interventions are carried out as necessary. Oxygen may be administered, depending on the severity of the hydrothorax.

A hydrothorax can be prevented by obtaining radiographic confirmation of catheter tip placement before the therapy is initiated. Many institutions currently cap central lines as heparin locks or intermittent devices until radiographic confirmation of catheter tip placement is received. This practice prevents fluid from being administered into the thoracic cavity.

Brachial Plexus Injury

The brachial plexus is the network of lower cervical and upper dorsal spinal nerves that supplies the arm, forearm, and hand.[32] Because of the anatomic position of these nerves (Fig. 24–5), they may be injured during the insertion of a central venous catheter. If such an injury occurs, the patient may experience tingling sensations in the fingers, pain shooting down the arm, and/or paralysis.

The physician is notified, and medication is usually administered for pain. Physical therapy is helpful in the treatment of brachial plexus injuries. Treatment is palliative and does not always resolve the injury. Preventive measures include those listed in Table 24–14.

Inadvertent Arterial Puncture

Inadvertent puncture of an artery during insertion of a central venous catheter is usually not a serious problem, unless the carotid artery is punctured. If symptoms are noted at the time of insertion and the artery can be located, pressure should be applied to the artery for at least 5 minutes; pressure must be applied longer if a patient has a bleeding or platelet disorder. Pressure cannot be applied to all arteries; the ability to apply pressure to an artery depends on the location of the artery.

If symptoms are not recognized immediately, the patient can develop a hematoma with signs and symptoms of tracheal compression, or respiratory distress, or both. If a subclavian artery is accidentally catheterized, air or debris that enter the artery may embolize to the brain and result in a central neurologic deficit. Laceration of the subclavian artery can also produce a hemothorax.

Extravascular Malposition

An extravascular position of a central venous catheter exists when the catheter penetrates the vessel, and the tip of the catheter lies outside the vascular system. During the process of threading a catheter, the needle or introducer through which the catheter is passed may slip out of the vein. Hydromediastinum occurs when the catheter tip is placed in the mediastinum and medication is infused into the space where the heart and great vessels are located.[33]

The patient may experience symptoms associated with a pneumothorax if the pleural covering of the lung has been punctured. He or she may experience symptoms of a hemothorax as blood enters the pleural system. If the vein is transected and the catheter tip is placed within the neck or chest area outside the pleural cavity, the patient may not experience any symptoms until the catheter is used. At this time, the patient may experience a hydrothorax as fluid is infused into the chest, or he or she may experience arm or neck swelling as fluid accumulates in the area adjacent to the tip of the catheter.

Radiographic confirmation of catheter tip placement before its use can prevent an extravascular malpositioned catheter from being used and from causing more serious complications.

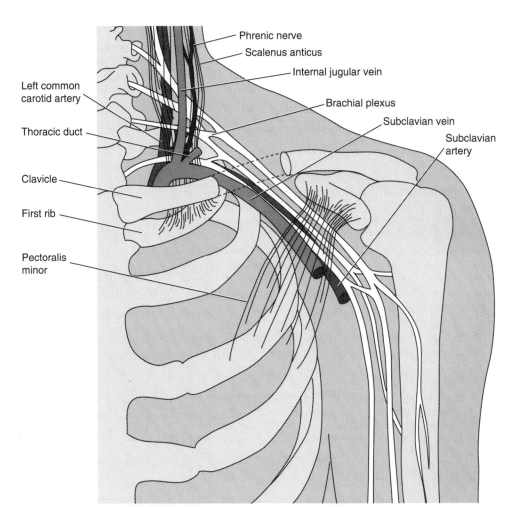

Figure 24–5. The brachial plexus in relation to the central vessels.

Labels on figure:
- Phrenic nerve
- Scalenus anticus
- Internal jugular vein
- Brachial plexus
- Subclavian vein
- Subclavian artery
- Left common carotid artery
- Thoracic duct
- Clavicle
- First rib
- Pectoralis minor

Medical interventions include removal of the catheter and treatment of associated complications. The patient is monitored, and vital signs are assessed. Oxygen and chest tubes may be necessary if a pneumothorax, hemothorax, or hydrothorax has occurred.

Intravascular Malposition

The incidence of malpositioned central venous catheters verified radiographically varies from 5.5 to 29% by the subclavian approach, and 21 to 55% by the antecubital vein approach.[33–36] Most authorities consider the optimal position for the tip of a central venous catheter to be the superior vena cava.[11, 35–38] Central venous catheters are usually misplaced into the internal jugular vein instead of the subclavian vein because of anatomic location of the internal jugular and the subclavian veins. Misplacements have also been documented in the contralateral innominate vein, the azygos vein, the right and left internal thoracic veins, the superior intercostal veins, and the accessory hemizygous veins.[33, 35, 38] The most common misplacement with the subclavian approach is in the internal jugular vein,[33, 38, 39] and the most common malposition of the cephalic vein is the axillary vein.[33]

Signs and symptoms of catheter malposition are frequently noted when the catheter is used. Difficulty with aspiration or infusion through the catheter may be noticed. In addition, the patient may complain of discomfort or pain in the shoulder, neck, or arm. Edema may also be noted in the neck or shoulder area. Infusions through a catheter aberrantly placed in the internal jugular vein have been associated with a benign annoyance called the ''ear gurgling'' sign, which patients frequently describe as the sound of a ''running stream'' rushing past the ear.[33, 34, 38] The infusion of medications through a catheter located in the internal jugular vein has often produced undesirable neurologic effects resulting from retrograde perfusion into the intracranial venous sinuses and the tributary vein.[33]

A malpositioned catheter is not always removed. Studies have indicated that misplaced central venous catheters can be safely and effectively repositioned without subjecting the patient to the potential morbidity associated with repeated percutaneous cannulation.[33] Most misplaced silicone catheters can be repositioned by rapid flushing of the catheter with 20 ml of normal saline at 4 to 5 ml/second. Catheters that loop back into the axillary or peripheral veins in the axilla have a lower rate of being repositioned. The rapid flushing technique is not successful with double- or triple-lumen catheters or with rigid or semirigid single-lumen catheters, because of the inflexibility of the catheters. Catheter rupture has occurred during use of the rapid flush technique because of catheter obstruction; therefore, this technique should be performed only when no resistance to injection occurs and the patient exhibits no signs of venous occlusion.[32]

Repositioning of the patient is very helpful when the catheter is repositioned. Before the catheter is flushed, the patient is placed in Fowler's position if the catheter is misplaced into the internal jugular vein. The patient is placed in an ipsilateral position with the head of the bed slightly elevated if the catheter is in the contralateral vein, and in a position contralaterally to the insertion with the head of the bed slightly raised for a malpositioned catheter in the axillary vein. Catheters with simple looping into the subclavian vein, the innominate vein, or the internal jugular vein can frequently be repositioned in the above positions, which allow gravity and blood flow to reposition the catheter overnight.[33]

With experience, malpositioned catheters with the tip in the subclavian, internal jugular, or innominate veins can be replaced in the appropriate vein by guide wire exchange. Catheters malpositioned beyond the superior vena cava into the right atrium or ventricle can be partially withdrawn, provided the catheter is not a nonflexible catheter with memory that is looped in the great vein. Direct fluoroscopic visualization is the safest and most reliable method of repositioning a central venous catheter. Radiographic techniques are also available to reposition these catheters.

Certain measures can help reduce the misplacement of a central venous catheter. Only well-qualified, highly skilled professionals should place central venous catheters. Measuring the distance from the proposed insertion site to the right atrium can prevent catheter malposition when peripheral central venous catheters are placed. This procedure can be easily performed by measuring the distance from the proposed site on the skin along the presumptive anatomic course of the veins to the right chondrosternal junction, or to one third of the way down the suprasternal notch to the xiphoid process.[33, 39]

Proper positioning of the patient is essential for the appropriate placement of a central venous catheter. For instance, a peripherally placed central catheter inserted through the basilic vein tends to pass along the cephalad wall of the subclavian vein to enter the jugular vein. By turning the patient's head toward the side of insertion to make the angle between the subclavian and the internal jugular vein, this problem can be avoided.[40] Placing a patient in Trendelenburg's position with a rolled towel between the scapulae facilitates the placement of a catheter into the subclavian vein and the threading of it into the superior vena cava by the subclavian approach.

The use of soft catheters, such as those made of a silicone elastomer, further enhance the possibility of placing a central catheter into the appropriate vein. The softer catheter materials enhance the blood's ability to carry the catheter tip and allow the catheter to readily follow the contours of the vein.

Radiographic confirmation of tip placement can frequently prevent complications associated with the use of a malpositioned catheter. However, it can be difficult to determine the correct position of a catheter placed in the left side of the mediastinum because of the close proximity of the internal thoracic vein to the superior vena cava when the area is viewed in a frontal chest radiograph. The location can be confirmed by obtaining a lateral chest radiograph and by injecting a contrast medium.[32, 39]

Pericardial Tamponade

Pericardial tamponade is a condition caused by penetration of the atrium by a centrally placed catheter. Cardiovascular collapse with neck vein distention, a narrow pulse pressure, and hypotension, with or without symptoms of congestive heart failure, suggest that the wall of the atrium has been penetrated. Symptoms are usually delayed because blood or solution must leak into the pericardial space and compress the heart to cause this complication.[31] Symptoms suggestive of this complication require emergency intervention by the physician.

The treatment for pericardial tamponade is aspiration of the pericardial sac from just below the xiphoid process of the sternum. The catheter is removed and replaced only after resuscitative measures are complete.

Preventive measures include performance of central vein cannulation by a highly skilled professional and use of the softer catheters, such as those made from silicone.

Complications Associated with Central Venous Catheters Remaining in the Vascular System

Central venous catheters place the patient at risk of complications during insertion, and the patient continues to be at risk while the catheter remains within the vascular system. Central venous catheters must be monitored, and appropriate care must be administered while these catheters are in place. A lack of monitoring or inappropriate care can place patients with these catheters in life-threatening situations.

Dislodgement and Twiddler's Syndrome

Central venous catheters are usually sutured in at the time of insertion. However, these catheters can still fall out, become dislodged, or be pulled out. Also, ports can become freely movable and migrate from one area to another, or patients may develop the nervous habit of ''twiddling'' with their ports, resulting in displacement of the port.[41]

Although it is fairly obvious when a catheter has been pulled out or when a port moves when accessed, catheter dislodgement may not be so obvious. When an assessment of a central venous catheter is made, the length of the external part of the catheter should be assessed.[42] If the external part appears longer, the catheter tip may no longer be at the position it was on insertion. The exit site and tunnel should be palpated for coiling.[42] In certain catheters, the exposure of a Dacron cuff can also alert the nurse that the catheter has become dislodged. Difficulty with aspiration or infusion through the catheter, leaking of solution from the catheter exit site, edema, a burning sensation, or pain when solution is infused can also indicate a displaced catheter.

Careful observation skills are sometimes necessary to determine the displacement of a central venous catheter. If catheter displacement is suspected, the physician should be notified. Usually, venographic studies are performed to determine catheter tip placement; depending on radiologic findings, the catheter may or may not be repositioned. If the catheter cannot be repositioned, it should be removed, and a new one with new tubing and solution container should be placed. The catheter should be secured with sutures, and the patient should be taught not to manipulate his or her catheter.[42]

If a central venous catheter is pulled out, a sterile occlusive pressure dressing, such as Vaseline gauze or Telfa covered with antibiotic ointment, should be applied,[43] and the physician should be notified. Usually, the dressing can be removed within 24 to 72 hours. The patient should be prepared for reinsertion of the catheter, if necessary.

Preventive measures for central venous catheter dislodgement include[42]

1. Suturing the catheter at the skin exit site
2. Looping and taping the catheter to prevent pull on the catheter at the skin exit site
3. Educating the patient in care of the catheter and the danger of pulling the catheter out
4. Use of an occlusive dressing

Catheter Migration

Migration associated with a central venous catheter refers to movement of the catheter tip from one position to another. When central venous catheters are placed, the catheter tip often migrates into the right atrium or into the internal jugular vein. Migrations have also been documented in the axillary veins.

Spontaneous migration of the catheter tip has been reported frequently.[23, 36] Some investigators have suggested that catheter tip migration may result from forceful flushing of the catheter or from changes in intrathoracic pressure associated with coughing or sneezing.[36] In some instances, migrations have been noted as a result of a disease process. For instance, in patients with congestive heart failure, catheter tip migration has been thought to result from the reduced flow of blood and the dilated vessels associated with the disease process.[33] Also, migrations have resulted from displacement by invading tissue (tumor) or venous thrombosis.

A change in functional capability can be an indication that the catheter tip has migrated. The inability to inject fluids can mean that the catheter tip is no longer at the desired position. Arrhythmias are very indicative of catheter migration into the right atrium or ventricle. The ear gurgling sound[42] described earlier is frequently heard when a catheter migrates into the internal jugular vein. Palpation of the catheter in the internal jugular can affirm migration to the jugular vein.[33]

When catheter migration is suspected, the physician should be notified, and venographic studies should be performed to verify catheter tip location. The nurse should prepare the patient for either repositioning of the catheter under fluoroscopy or removal of the catheter and possible reinsertion of another catheter. All infusions should be discontinued.[42]

Catheter migration cannot always be prevented. Avoiding trauma to the catheter site and placing a catheter near the site of local disease with suturing of the catheter can aid in the prevention of catheter migration.[42]

Fibrin Formation with Occlusion

All catheters inherit the potential for fibrin formation at the tip or along the catheter line where the catheter touches the vessel. Catheter occlusion resulting from a blood clot may result from inadequate heparinization, pump malfunction, break in the catheter system, or hypercoagulability of the patient's blood.[44] Catheters can also become occluded when medications or solutions are not mixed appropriately to avoid incompatibilities. The most common precipitates are calcium, diazepam, and phenytoin.[44]

Signs and symptoms of a partially occluded catheter include

1. Discomfort, pain, or edema in the shoulder, neck, arm, or insertion site[42]
2. Resistance when a solution, flush, or medication is instilled
3. Difficulty infusing a solution
4. Bubbles in tubing (blood is foamy)
5. Leaking of fluid from the insertion site as fluid tracks back along a fibrin trail (fibrin sheath formation)

A catheter is completely occluded when blood cannot be withdrawn from the catheter and complete resistance is met when the catheter is used.

Catheters that are allowed to remain clotted predispose the patient to infection and the possibility of an embolus. When a central venous catheter is thought to be clotted, the nurse must initially assess the entire line and catheter for patency. The solution container, the tubing, and the infusion device must be checked for proper operation.

Catheters suspected of being occluded should be assessed for catheter placement; the catheter could possibly be pinched between the clavicle and the first rib because of its anatomic location, or the outlets (particularly on multilumen catheters) could be lying against the wall of the vessel (one-way obstruction). On aspiration, the wall is sucked into the catheter, blocking blood withdrawal; an infusion, however, forces the tip away from the wall and restores patency. Repositioning the patient may restore the ability to aspirate from a port. The patient should change position, sit up, lie down, raise the arm above the head, and cough in an attempt to open the catheter.

Only attempts using very light pressure and a 10-ml syringe should be made to flush a catheter suspected of being occluded; if the catheter cannot be flushed without resistance or if flow of an infusion cannot be established, an attempt should be made to aspirate the occlusion using a gentle push-pull technique with normal saline. If blood cannot be drawn, solution cannot be infused, or aspiration cannot be performed (two-way obstruction), the cause of the occlusion should be determined. Catheters occluded because of precipitant formation are usually removed. The use of ethanol, hydrochloric acid,[44, 45] or sodium bicarbonate has been advocated for the absorption of precipitates; institutional policies and procedures should dictate the use of these medications.

If an implanted vascular access device appears occluded, the Huber point needle should be removed, and the device should be reaccessed with a new needle. Frequently, the needle may be accidentally pulled out of the septum; the needle should not be pushed back into the portal, because this practice could cause microorganisms to be carried into the system. Once reaccessed, the system should be re-evaluated for patency using normal saline and a gentle push-pull, as previously stated.

If the occlusion results from a blood clot or a fibrin sheath, the catheter should be declotted using a thrombolytic agent designed specifically for lysis of catheter clots. Urokinase (Abbokinase Open-cath) is the preferred drug for declotting central venous catheters because of the decreased risks associated with an allergic reaction.[4] The recommended concentration is 5000 IU/ml. The volume administered should be equal to the volume of the catheter. The physician should be notified and the catheter declotted by established policies and procedures; policies and procedures should specify which catheters can be declotted because all catheters do not expand and cannot support the addition of even a small amount of medication when they are occluded.

Frequently, central line occlusions or fibrin formation at the catheter tip can be prevented. Recommended guidelines include

1. Complying with established policies and procedures for maintenance of patency
2. Maintaining positive pressure when lines are flushed
3. Using infusion pumps when indicated
4. Frequently monitoring intravenous system and catheter for mechanical difficulties (e.g., empty solution container, kinked tubing, malfunctioning infusion control device)
5. Mixing medications with the appropriate diluent and compatible medications or solutions
6. Preventing pull on catheters and tugging on implanted vascular access devices
7. Using low-dose oral anticoagulant therapy, especially with patients who have hypercoagulability problems[42, 44, 46]

Vessel Thrombosis (Catheter-Related Thrombosis)

Vessel thrombosis is the formation of a blood clot in a vessel within the neck, chest, or arms that occurs in the presence of a central venous catheter. The pathophysiology of a vessel thrombosis has been identified as being a triad of thromboses: stasis, vessel wall injury, and hypercoagulability.[46, 47] Stasis can result from the effect of intrapulmonary or mediastinal disease. Vessel wall injury can be attributed to the aggregation of platelets on the catheter surface and mechanical irritation of the vessel intima by the catheter tip. Injury to the vessel wall can also occur at the site of the catheter's entry into the vein, can be related to catheter infection, or can be related to the exposure of the vessel wall to total parenteral nutrition solutions and chemotherapeutic agents. Hypercoagulability is frequently associated with a malignancy; patients with cancer have a tendency for hypercoagulation.[46, 47] Other factors that appear to be associated with thrombosis in tunneled catheters include suboptimal internal catheter tip location and left-sided catheter placement.[47]

Vessel thrombosis should be suspected if the patient complains of chest pain, earache, jaw pain, or edema of the neck, the supraclavicular area, or the extremities. Associated dangers include pulmonary embolism, cerebral anoxia, laryngeal edema, bronchial obstruction, and death.

The physician should be notified immediately if a vessel thrombosis is suspected. Radiographic studies using dye (venography) are usually performed to verify catheter placement. The patient is usually placed on anticoagulant therapy (systemic heparin, coumadin, or both). Depending on the size of the clot and the area of impaired circulation, the clot may have to be lysed; lysis is achieved by imbedding a peripheral catheter into the clot by use of fluoroscopic guidance and administering a kinase infusion.

Vessel thrombosis can be prevented by the use of low-dose anticoagulant (warfarin) therapy for patients at high risk of clotting disorders,[46, 47] the insertion of central venous catheters by highly skilled professionals, and the placement of central venous catheters into the right subclavian vein. A recent Food and Drug Administration task force recommended that "except for pulmonary artery catheters, the catheter tip should not be placed in, or allowed to migrate into the heart. The superior vena cava is considered the recommended (optimal) location for the tip of a central venous catheter, and placement in the right atrium is contraindicated."[47]

Damaged Catheter

Central venous catheters can easily be damaged if appropriate measures are not used when care is provided. The use of scissors at or near the catheter during dressing changes can result in the catheter being cut if extreme caution is not taken to separate the catheter from the dressing. Catheters are made of a nonresealable material, and if penetrated with a needle, pinholes with subsequent leaking will occur. Catheter rupture can also occur when force is exerted, when a syringe smaller than 10 ml is used to flush the catheter, or when the pinch-off syndrome occurs—the catheter is pinched owing to the anatomic location of the subclavian vein and the clavicle; over time the catheter cracks because of repeated pinching and it ruptures.

Central venous catheters should be monitored and assessed for pinholes, cuts, leaks, tears, and ruptures at frequent intervals. An assessment should include observation of the dressing, the catheter, and the area around the catheter. A wet dressing or leaking at the insertion site during an infusion or catheter flushing may indicate catheter damage. Swelling in the chest area may indicate rupture of a catheter and infusion of solution into the chest wall. Tunneled and implanted catheters can usually be palpated to the point at which they enter the subclavian vein; if the catheter has ruptured, swelling may be felt at the point of catheter rupture if the rupture is in the tunneled segment of the catheter.

At the very moment an assessment reveals a damaged catheter, a nonserrated clamp should be applied proximal to the damaged part of the catheter, if possible. The damage should be assessed and the appropriate action taken.

Damaged catheters must be repaired or removed without delay to prevent serious complications. Any opening in the catheter can serve as a portal of entry for bacteria or air into the vascular system. The entrance of bacteria into the system can predispose a debilitated patient to septicemia. Air may also be drawn into the system because of the negative pressure created within the heart, and the patient can suffer an air embolism directly to the heart. Policies and procedures should be established for the repair of a catheter according to the manufacturer's guidelines. If the catheter cannot be repaired, the physician should be notified immediately, and the catheter should be removed.

One of the most serious dangers of an implanted vascular access device is the rupture of the catheter. Implanted vascular access devices are also known for port-catheter separation. Although this phenomenon can cause severe complications if a vesicant is infusing, usually there is less risk of an embolus than there is when the catheter ruptures. If either of

Table 24–15

Guidelines for Preventing Damage to Central Venous Catheters

Use clamps on clamping sleeves provided on silicone catheters. If using a clamp at another area on the catheter becomes necessary, use a flat, toothless clamp only.

Avoid the use of scissors or other sharp objects around the catheter.

Use only small-bore needles (22–25 gauge) with a needle length 1 inch or shorter when accessing latex injection ports on the catheter.

Administer medications without force. Consider the use of 10-ml syringes when administering medications via a silicone catheter.

Educate patient regarding catheter and problems associated with "twiddling" of ports and of playing with external catheters.

these conditions is suspected, the infusion should be discontinued, the patient should be placed on bed rest, and the physician should be notified. Radiographic studies should be performed to verify a rupture or a port-catheter separation, and the patient should be prepared for removal of the port and possible replacement of the catheter. Every effort must be made to prevent damage to central venous catheters (Table 24–15).

Superior Vena Cava Syndrome

Superior vena cava syndrome is a condition caused by a blood clot, fibrin formation, or both, that occludes the superior vena cava. This condition can also be caused by a tumor or enlarged lymph nodes compressing the superior vena cava or by the placement of a central venous catheter.[48, 49] The cause must be established before it is assumed that the condition results from the central venous catheter.

Signs and symptoms include progressive shortness of breath, dyspnea, cough, sensation of skin tightness, unilateral edema, and cyanosis of the face, neck, shoulder, and arms. Extensive edema of the upper body without edema of the lower body parts, often called "short cap edema," may also be noticed. Edema and cyanosis of the mucous membranes of the mouth, pharynx, larynx, thorax, and occasionally the hydropericardium also occur. The jugular, temporal, and arm veins are engorged and distended. Usually, a prominent venous pattern is present over the chest as a result of dilated thoracic vessels. If the condition goes unnoticed and untreated, headache owing to increased intracranial pressure, visual disturbances, and altered mental status occurs. A danger of cerebral anoxia, bronchial obstruction, and death exists.[48, 49]

The physician must be notified immediately when the first symptoms of superior vena cava syndrome are observed. Diagnosis is confirmed by radiographic studies.

Depending on the severity of the symptoms, the ability to initiate an alternate intravenous route, and the type of catheter in place, the catheter may or may not be removed. Anticoagulant therapy is usually prescribed for the patient, and symptoms are treated. The patient should be placed in a semi-Fowler's position, and oxygen should be administered to facilitate breathing. These patients become very anxious and fearful because of the feeling of suffocating, so it is important to provide emotional support. The patient's fluid volume status should be monitored to minimize further edema, and the cardiovascular and neurologic status should be monitored.[48]

Superior vena cava syndrome is rare; however, it can be very serious. The insertion of a central venous catheter by a well-trained, experienced professional can aide in the prevention of superior vena cava syndrome. An inexperienced individual can traumatize the endothelial lining of the vein and actually predispose the vein to clot formation. Anticoagulant therapy has proved to be most effective in the prevention of superior vena cava syndrome. Anticoagulants should be considered, particularly with the use of long-term catheters in patients who are at high risk for the development of clotting problems.[44, 48]

Site Infection

The insertion and use of a central venous catheter predisposes the patient to the possibility of an infection with subsequent septicemia. Septicemia has been discussed under "Systemic Complications." However, the patient may experience an infection at the catheter exit site with or without septicemia.

The catheter exit site should be observed for redness, edema, and drainage, and the patient should be questioned about tenderness or pain around the catheter. Laboratory values, such as white blood cell count, should be monitored. If the patient experiences sudden chills with fever, general malaise, headache, nausea and vomiting, hypotension, and cyanosis, he or she should be immediately treated for sepsis.

The physician should be notified immediately of any symptoms related to an infection of the catheter. The physician may have the catheter removed or may choose to replace it over a guide wire. Blood cultures are usually drawn both peripherally and from the central line. The patient is usually given antibiotic therapy and may be given anticoagulant therapy because the development of a thrombus within the catheter or at the tip can trap bacteria and predispose the patient to sepsis. If the catheter is removed, consideration should be given to culturing the catheter tip, and care is given to the site until healing has occurred. If an implanted vascular access device is in place and has not been accessed, it is not used until the origin of the infection has been determined.

Site infections associated with the use of central venous catheters are preventable. By strict adherence to the guidelines listed in Table 24–16, the chance of an infection is greatly reduced.

Skin Erosion

Infrequently, a patient with an implanted vascular access device may experience a skin tear or an erosion of the skin

Table 24–16

Guidelines for Prevention of Site Infections Associated with Central Venous Catheters

Maintain aseptic technique during the insertion of a central venous catheter.

Wash hands before gloving for insertion of catheter, for changing of dressings, and before manipulation of catheter.

Wear sterile gloves and a mask when performing dressing changes.

Assess all equipment for package integrity and sterility before its use.

Change dressings and provide site care according to the *Intravenous Nursing Standards of Practice*.[11]

Table 24–17

Necessary Knowledge for an Accurate Diagnosis of Complications Associated with Intravenous Therapy
· ·
Anatomy of vascular system
Disease processes related to therapy and associated complications
Various therapies used, including drug classifications
Recommended dose and volume relative to age, height, and weight, or body surface area
Drug and solution properties, actions, side effects, and adverse reactions
Methods of intravenous administration and infusion systems used
Interventions necessary for treatment of complications

over the portal septum, or a patient with a tunneled catheter may experience skin erosion over the catheter. Skin erosions are usually seen in patients who have very poor nutritional status, are very thin, and have experienced a large weight loss. Skin erosions have been seen also as a result of trauma over a tunneled catheter or portal septum. Signs of an erosion include visible skin abrasions or tears over a port or catheter with redness, edema, or both.

The physician is notified of a skin erosion over a port or a catheter. The catheter is usually removed, and, depending on the patient and the therapy being administered, another catheter may be placed.

The possibility of skin erosions over ports or tunneled catheters can be minimized by maintaining a positive nutritional status, by avoiding pressure or trauma to the area surrounding the catheter or port, and by rotating the site each time the port is accessed.

NURSING CONSIDERATIONS

Nurses must be able to accurately diagnose complications associated with the insertion, use, and removal of venous and arterial devices. By use of the nursing process and the holistic approach, the nurse must implement nursing interventions that provide immediate treatment, promote healing, and prevent further complications. The nurse must constantly evaluate the care rendered in terms of patient outcomes to promote quality improvement in the performance of intravenous therapies. In forming an accurate diagnosis of complications associated with intravenous therapy, the nurse should have knowledge in all areas stated in Table 24–17. In addition, the nurse should be able to translate knowledge into practical use when assessing the patient for complications and intervening when necessary.

The clinical diagnosis of complications is related to the nurse's ability to evaluate the patient's signs and symptoms. Using objective, subjective, and cardinal evaluations, the nurse can make an accurate nursing diagnosis. Objective symptoms are those that are visible (e.g., edema, erythema, and blanching). Subjective symptoms are those that have an internal or mental origin; they relate to the patient's perception of what he or she feels (e.g., pain, tingling sensation, or feeling of suffocation). Cardinal symptoms are those symptoms that relate to the physical body (e.g., pulse, temperature, and blood pressure). Additionally, signs and symptoms occur locally or systemically. Complications that occur locally usually appear at the site of the invasion of the body and usually produce visible signs and symptoms. Systemic complications

occur within the body and usually affect the systemic circulation and other bodily processes.

Other tools often used for the evaluation of signs and symptoms include differential evaluations, exclusion evaluations, pathologic evaluations, and roentgenographic evaluations. Differential evaluations can be extremely helpful, such as comparing one arm against another to determine infiltration. Exclusion evaluations are frequently performed when no other reasonable explanation exists for a complication. For example, a patient with a central venous catheter may suddenly develop an elevated temperature, and no other possible explanation exists for the elevated temperature. Sepsis related to the catheter is considered, and interventions for catheter-induced septicemia are initiated.

Pathologic evaluations are used to verify the presence of pathologic organisms; they are usually performed when drainage from a wound or an elevated temperature occurs, suggesting an infectious process. A good example is the

Table 24–18

Outcome Criteria for Peripheral Intravenous Therapy
· ·
Outcome Criteria: The patient will remain free of complications related to the administration of IV therapy.

1. Goal
  Patient will remain free from infection related to IV therapy.
Interventions
  IV site will be inspected for signs of infection at least every 4 hours.
  IV catheter and tubing will be changed every 48 hours.
  IV solution containers will be changed every 24 hours.
  IV catheter will be securely taped to prevent movement of catheter in and out of the vein.
  IV equipment and solution containers will be inspected for contamination before use.
  A final filter will be placed at the distal end of the IV tubing.
2. Goal
  Patient will remain free of chemical phlebitis associated with the administration of medications.
Interventions
  All medications and solutions will be mixed in the pharmacy under a laminar flow hood. Known irritants will be mixed to the fullest extent possible.
  All solutions and medications will be administered at the recommended rate.
  The IV site will be checked every 2 hours for redness and inflammation associated with a chemical phlebitis.
3. Goal
  Patient will remain free of local complications.
Interventions
  IV sites over flexion areas will not be used unless absolutely necessary.
  Catheters will be taped according to policy and procedure to prevent movement of catheter.
  An armboard will be placed if necessary to limit movement of the extremity, using measures to prevent constriction of circulation and pressure on nerves and skin.
4. Goal
  Patient will take part in the care and maintenance of his IV system.
Interventions
  Patient's level of knowledge for learning will be assessed.
  Patient will be taught care of system.

  • Performance of routine activities—bathing, movement in bed, and ambulation.
  • Emergency measures—for pulling out line, loose or wet dressing, kinking of tubing.
  • Signs and symptoms of complications.

IV = intravenous.

Outcome Criteria for Placement of Implanted Vascular Access Device
· ·

Outcome Criteria: The patient will remain free of complications associated with the implantation of a vascular access device.

1. Goal
Patient will remain free from infection associated with placement of implanted vascular access.
Interventions
Site and surrounding area will be checked every 2 hours for swelling, bleeding, and inflammation.
The dressing on the site will be changed daily and as needed.
Dressing changes will be sterile.
The site will be cleansed with alcohol followed by povidone-iodine each time the dressing is changed.
The patient's temperature will be monitored every 4 hours for elevation.
2. Goal
Patient will remain free of associated infections resulting from use of the device.
Interventions
Solution containers will be checked for possible leaks and contamination.
All equipment will be checked for defects and contamination.
Solution containers will be changed every 48 hours.
Intravenous tubing will be changed every 48 hours.
3. Goal
Patient will experience minimal discomfort at insertion site.
Interventions
Patient will be assessed frequently for pain in site area.
Analgesics will be administered as needed.
Relief of pain from analgesics will be evaluated.
Cold compresses will be applied to the site for edema for the first 24 hours after insertion.
Warm compresses will be applied to the site for comfort after the first 24 hours following insertion, unless the site is bleeding.
4. Goal
Patient will receive education relating to care of vascular access device.
Interventions
Patient's ability to learn will be determined.
Patient will develop understanding of how device is used.
Patient will assist in care by taking preventive measures to maintain catheter and dressing.
Patient will be alert to signs and symptoms of complications.

culturing of the catheter site, the catheter, or an infusate, when a vascular infection is suspected. A pathologic evaluation is a very good tool to use because it can verify the disease source. However, it should never be the only tool used, because pathologic reports usually take time, and complications do not wait to be diagnosed—they frequently progress very rapidly once they start. Roentgenographic evaluations can be used to prevent complications (e.g., taking an x-ray to verify placement of a central venous catheter before its use), or they may be used to verify a complication (e.g., verifying a pulmonary embolus). The nurse must be alert to all signs and symptoms and must evaluate each one individually. Early recognition of potential complications can actually prevent further complications and can promote quick healing and restoration of health.

Although observation for and evaluation of signs and symptoms is very important, it is far better to prevent complications from occurring. The ideal situation is delivery of intravenous therapy that is free of complications, thereby promoting positive patient outcomes. Outcomes should be established that deliver high-quality care protecting the pa-

tient and the nurse from risks associated with intravenous therapy.

Outcome criteria can be written generically to cover an entire aspect of intravenous nursing care, or they can be written to cover only one aspect. One example of a care plan that could apply to all patients receiving peripheral intravenous therapy is represented in Table 24–18. In comparison, Table 24–19 is a plan of care outlining outcome criteria for a newly implanted vascular access device. Both care plans expect high-quality performance and positive patient outcomes. Goals have been written to define the expected outcomes and the care necessary to achieve the outcome.

Outcome criteria promote the delivery of high-quality intravenous care by expecting performance at the optimal level. Each model for outcome criteria promotes delivery of care that prevents complications associated with intravenous therapy—a goal that should be strived for by nurses practicing intravenous therapy.

In addition to establishing criteria for patient outcomes, nurses should also monitor patients' outcomes. Statistics should be kept regarding the incidence of complications, interventions, and outcomes. They should be reported to staff, the risk management department, the quality improvement council, and various others involved in the process. They should be used as a tool to recognize areas for improvement.

References

1. Occupational Safety and Health Association (OSHA). Bloodborne pathogens. Federal Register 1991; 56:235(12):61476–61477.
2. Crudi C, Larkin M. Core curriculum for intravenous nursing. NITA 1984; 121–123.
3. Millam DA. Managing complications of I.V. therapy nursing. Nursing '88 1988; 18(3):34–42.
4. IV Therapy Policy and Procedure Manual. Administration of chemotherapeutic medications. High Point Regional Hospital, 1993.
5. Joint Commission on Accreditation of Health Care Perspectives. Joint Commission Perspectives: Interpretations: Limitations on hospital patient movement that constitute restraint. Joint Commission on Accreditation of Health Care Organizations 1992; Sept/Oct:11–12, 15–16.
6. Food and Drug Administration. FDA Safety Alert: Potential hazards with restraint devices. Food and Drug Administration 1992; 7.
7. Tabor CL. Tabor's Cyclopedic Medical Dictionary, 17th ed. Philadelphia: F.A. Davis, 1993:531, 1277.
8. LaRocca JC, Otto SE. Pocket Guide to Intravenous Therapy. St. Louis: C.V. Mosby, 1989:187–190.
9. Dorr RT, Fritz WL. Cancer Chemotherapy Handbook. New York: Elsevier, 1980:191–192.
10. Plumer AL, Cosentino F. Principles and Practices of Intravenous Therapy. Boston: Little, Brown and Co., 1987:269–289, 314–316.
11. Intravenous Nurses Society. Intravenous nursing standards of practice. JIN ISSN 0896-5846, 1990; S26–S80.
12. Maki DG, Ringer M. Risk factors for infusion-related phlebitis with small peripheral catheters. Am Coll Physicians 1991; 114(10):845–854.
13. Garner JS, Favero MS. Guidelines for Handwashing and Hospital Environmental Control. Hospital Infections Program, Atlanta Centers for Disease Control, 1985.
14. Wenzel RP. Prevention and Control of Nosocomial Infections, 2nd ed. Skin cleansing. 1993, Baltimore: Williams & Wilkins, 450–451.
15. Bennett JV, Brachman PS, et al. Hospital Infections, 2nd ed. Boston: Little, Brown, and Co., 1986:561–574.
16. Linares JA, Sitges-Serra A, Garau J, et al. Pathogenesis of catheter sepsis: A prospective study with quantitative and semiquantitative cultures of catheter hub and segments. J Clin Microbiol 1985; 21(3):357–360.
17. American Society of Hospital Pharmacists. ASHP Report: ASHP therapeutic position statement on the institutional use of 0.9% sodium chlo-

ride injection to maintain patency of peripheral indwelling intermittent infusion devices. Am J Hosp Pharm 1994; 51:1572–1574.

18. Henderson DK. Intravascular device-associated infection: Current concepts and controversies. Infect Surg 1988; (6):365–371, 398–399.

19. Conley JM, Grieves K, Peters B. A prospective, randomized study comparing transparent and dry gauze dressings for central venous catheters. J Infect Dis 1989; 159:310–319.

20. Hampton AA, Sherertz RJ. Vascular-access infections in hospitalized patients. Surg Clin North Am 1988; 68(1):57–66.

21. Eisenberg PG, Howard P, Gianino MS. Improved long-term maintenance of central venous catheters with a new dressing technique. JIN 1990; 13(5):279–284.

22. Sitzmann JV, Townsend TR, Siler MC, Barlett JG. Septic and technical complications of central venous catheterization. Ann Surg 1985; 202:768–770.

23. Beam TR, Goodman EL, Maki DG, et al. Preventing central venous catheter-related complications: A roundtable discussion. Infect Surg 1990; 10:1–12.

24. Solomon SL, Alexander H, Eley JW, et al. Nosocomial fungemia in neonates associated with intravascular pressure-monitoring devices. Pediatr Infect Dis 1986; 5:680–685.

25. Maki DG, Hassemer CA. Endemic rate of fluid contamination and related septicemia in arterial pressure monitoring. Am J Med 1981; 70:733–738.

26. Phillips I, Eykyn S, Curtis MA, Snell JJS. Pseudomonas cepacia (multivorans) septicemia in an intensive care unit. Lancet 1972; 1:375–377.

27. Fisher MC, Long SS, Roberts EM, et al. Pseudomonas maltophilia bacteremia in children undergoing open heart surgery. JAMA 1981; 246:1571–1574.

28. Stamm WE, Colella JJ, Anderson RL, et al. Indwelling arterial catheters as a source of nosocomial bacteremia—An outbreak caused by Flavobacterium species. N Engl J Med 1992; 292:1009–1102.

29. Weinstein RA, Emori TG, Anderson RL, Stamm WE. Pressure transducers as a source of bacteremia after open heart surgery. Report of an outbreak and guidelines for prevention. Chest 1976; 69:338–344.

30. Anderson AJ, Kransnow SH, Boyer MW, et al. Hickman catheter clots: A common occurrence despite daily heparin flushing. Cancer Treatment Rep 1987; 71(6):651–653.

31. Maki DG, Cobb L, Garman JK, et al. An attachable silver-impregnated cuff for prevention of infection with central venous catheters: A prospective randomized multicenter trial. Am J Med 1988; 85(9):307–314.

32. Hadaway LC. Evaluation and use of advance i.v. technology: Part 1. central venous access devices. JIN 1989; 12(2):73–81.

33. Flowers RH, Schwenzer KJ, Kopel RF, et al. Efficacy of an attachable subcutaneous cuff for the prevention of intravascular catheter-related infection: A randomized, controlled trial. JAMA 1989; 261(6):878–883.

34. Maki DG, Wheeler SJ, Stolz SM. Study of a novel antiseptic coated central venous catheter. Presented at the Society of Critical Care Medicine Annual Symposium. Washington, D.C., May 1991.

35. Matheny NM. Fluid and Electrolyte Balance, 2nd ed. Philadelphia: J.B. Lippincott, 1992:164–165.

36. McMahon E, Ambrose ML, Deutsch D, et al. Diseases. Springhouse, PA: Springhouse Corp, 1993:625, 627, 635–639, 644–647.

37. Vazquez M, Lazear SE, Larson EL. Critical Care Nursing, 2nd ed. Philadelphia: W.B. Saunders, 1992:229–231.

38. Miller BF, Keane CB. Encyclopedia and Dictionary of Medicine, Nursing, and Allied Health, 4th ed. Philadelphia: W.B. Saunders, 1987:175, 257–258, 406, 568, 982.

39. Lum PS, Soski M. Management of malpositioned central venous catheters. JIN 1989; 12(6):356–365.

40. Conces DJ, Holden RN. Aberrant locations and complications in initial placement of subclavian vein catheters. Arch Surg 1984; 119:293–295.

41. Dunbar RD. Radiologic appearance of compromised thoracic catheters, tubes, and wires. Radiol Clin North Am 1984; 22:699–722.

42. Lang-Jensen T, Nielsen R, Sorensen MD, et al. Primary and secondary displacement of central venous catheters. Acta Anaesthesiol Scand 1980; 24:216–218.

43. Black R. Vein extravasation: A severe complication of IV therapy. Parenterals 1988; 6(4):1–2, 5–8.

44. Dunbar RD, Mitchell R, Lavin M. Aberrant locations of central venous catheters. Lancet 1981; i:711–715.

45. Malatinski J, Kadlic T, Majek M, et al. Misplacement and loop formation of central venous catheters. Acta Anaesthesiol Scand 1976; 20:237–247.

46. Hadaway LC. An overview of vascular access devices inserted via antecubital area. JIN 1990; 13(5):297–305.

47. Wilkes G, Vannicola P, Starck P. Long-term venous access. Am J Nurs 1985; 85(7):793–796.

48. Camp-Sorrell D. Advanced central venous access: Selection, catheters, devices, and nursing management. JIN 1990; 13(6):361–369.

49. Thielen JB, Nyquist J. Subclavian catheter removal, nursing implications to prevent air emboli. JIN 1991; 14(2):114–117.

50. Richardson D, Bruso P. Vascular access devices: Management of common complications. JIN 1993; 16(1):44–48.

51. Shulman RJ, Reed T, Pitre D, Lane L. Use of hydrochloric acid to clear obstructed central venous catheters. JPEN 1988; 12(5):509–510.

52. Bern MM, Lokich JJ, Wallach SR, et al. Very low doses of warfarin can prevent thrombosis in central venous catheters: A randomized prospective trial. Am Coll Physicians 1990; 112:423–428.

53. Brown-Smith JK, Stoner MH, Barley ZA. Tunneled catheter thrombosis: Factors related to incidence. Oncol Nurs Forum 1990; 17(4):543–548.

54. Parish JM, Marschke RF, Dines DE, et al. Etiologic considerations in superior vena cava syndrome. Mayo Clin Proc 1981; 56:407–413.

55. Santiego SM. Superior vena cava syndrome after Swan-Ganz catheterization. Chest 1986; 89(2):319–320.

CHAPTER 25 Patient Education

Rebecca Kochheiser Berry, RN, MS

The current emphasis on health promotion, consumer satisfaction, cost containment, and early discharge challenges the intravenous therapy nurse to devise patient education strategies that provide patients and caregivers with the information and self-care abilities necessary to complete the therapy, prevent complications, and reduce readmissions to the hospital or home care. Patient education is not an optional extra that is "nice to do if you have time," but is mandated by accrediting bodies such as the Joint Commission on Accreditation of Healthcare Organizations.[1, 2] It is also considered a standard of practice by the Intravenous Nurses Society.[3] The benefits of patient education far outweigh the costs and time involved in teaching patients. To meet the educational needs of patients and caregivers, intravenous therapy nurses must understand educational principles, be skilled in the educational process, and be knowledgeable about available resources.

The first step toward understanding the principles and process of patient education is to become familiar with basic terms. The following list defines some of these:

Learner: The person who acquires knowledge, skill, or behavior change as a result of instruction or study.
Learning: An interactive process that creates knowledge or skill and may bring about a change in behavior.
Learning style: The way an individual processes information. Preference for a particular style may change over time. There is no one preferred style of learning; all are of equal value if knowledge is gained by the learner.
Patient education: The process of assisting people to learn and incorporate health-related behaviors into everyday life.[4]
Self-care: Any action or psychologic process undertaken to promote, assess, maintain, or restore one's own health, comfort, or perceived well-being.[5]
Teacher: The person or program that facilitates learning.
Teaching: Communication specifically structured and sequenced to produce learning.[6]

Patients and their families have the right to be informed

about the patient's condition and care. This information enables them to make informed decisions and assume health care responsibilities. Six of the rights listed in the American Hospital Association's *A Patient's Bill of Rights*[7] relate to patient education.

Patients, health care organizations, and society all benefit from patient education. These benefits can be summarized as follows:

I. Patient benefits
  A. Improved patient outcomes, such as
    1. Improved adherence and compliance to therapeutic regimen
    2. Increased patient satisfaction
    3. Enhanced patient self-determination
    4. Enhanced patient recovery following surgery
  B. Increased knowledge
  C. Improved self-care
  D. Decreased anxiety
  E. Reduced disruption in daily functioning
  F. Enhanced self-concept and self-esteem
  G. Increased satisfaction with care
  H. Improved pain control
  I. Improved physical status, when possible
II. Health care agency benefits
  A. Cost savings resulting from
    1. More timely hospital discharges
    2. Reduced losses in agency productivity
    3. More appropriate use of services
    4. Reduced need for acute care
  B. Enhanced patient satisfaction
  C. Reduction in malpractice suits
III. Society benefits
  A. Disease prevention
  B. Increased control of chronic illness
  C. Reduced numbers and lengths of hospital stays
  D. Less absenteeism from school and work
  E. Acquisition of positive health-related behaviors

Nurses also have an opportunity to benefit from patient education through the therapeutic alliances with patients and families that foster both personal and professional satisfaction. How satisfying it is to see patients become so comfortable in their knowledge and skills that they volunteer to become involved in teaching other patients.

Professional standards also address the nurse's responsibility for patient education. The *Intravenous Nursing Standards of Practice*[3] has stated that patients have the right to receive information on all aspects of their care. The patient education standard addresses the responsibility of the intravenous nurse to provide comprehensive patient instruction in both the inpatient facility and the home.

Health professionals and agencies are also mandated by law, accreditation standards, and reimbursement policy to provide patient and family education. The nurse's teaching role and responsibilities are addressed in most state nursing practice acts. The Joint Commission on Accreditation of Healthcare Organizations has addressed patient education re-

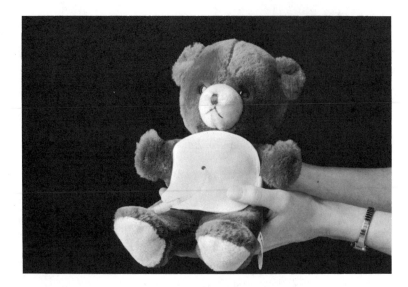

FIGURE 25–1. Pediatric central line training vest on a child's teddy bear for instruction and play. (Courtesy of Caremark, Inc., Northbrook, IL.)

quirements throughout the hospital and home care standards.[1, 2] Landmark legal cases have supported the right of individuals to make an informed choice about their care. For example, in *Cantebury v. Spence* and subsequent cases, it was ruled not permissible to withhold information merely to negate the possibility that the patient will refuse treatment or make a ''wrong'' decision.[8] Nurses can help ensure that the patient's consent is truly an informed consent by educating the patient thoroughly and effectively.

The goals of patient education are to provide instruction to promote health, prevent illness, and cope with illness.

HISTORICAL CONSIDERATIONS

Nurses have been teaching patients for decades. In 1860, Florence Nightingale addressed patient education in her *Notes on Nursing*. In 1918, the National League of Nursing addressed the need to cover preventative and educational factors for visiting nurses in nursing schools' curricula. Historically, the quantity and quality of patient education available in the United States have appeared to be inversely related to the degree of social distancing between health care providers and patients.[9]

The self-care movement that began in the 1960s greatly influenced the practice of educating patients. As the public sought to understand medical practices, the health care system was pressured to respond to the need for patient education. During the 1960s, a group of nurses developed a theory of nursing based on self-care. Within this concept, the patient was empowered through increased knowledge to become an integral part of the decision making process.

As patient education began to be discussed in the literature in the early 1970s, the insurance industry, policy makers, and legislators became interested in the potential contribution of patient education to cost containment. Financial support was also made available for research on patient education. In 1972, *A Patient's Bill of Rights* was developed by the American Hospital Association.[7] In this document, many areas of patient teaching were covered.

Today, patient education is an integral part of the nurse's responsibility in all health care settings. In the hospital, pa-

tient education is necessary to provide the patient, family, and/or caregiver with an understanding of the patient's condition and therapeutic regimen. Such education can be the impetus for reducing patient anxiety during procedures. Nurses are also charged with preparing the patient for early release from the hospital. Early discharge and the increasing number of outpatient procedures change the patient's and caregiver's responsibilities for care. Nurses in alternate health care settings, such as home care and ambulatory clinics, must ensure appropriate patient self-care through effective initial and ongoing patient education.

Early discharges and a shortage of nurses have decreased the amount of time nurses can spend educating patients and caregivers. Preprinted materials and audiovisual media are available for assisting in the patient education process. Guidelines for choosing and evaluating these materials are discussed later in this chapter.

PRINCIPLES OF PATIENT EDUCATION

The intravenous therapy nurse must understand the principles of patient education to teach patients effectively. These principles vary according to the age, condition, and cognitive abilities of the learner.

Pediatric Patients

Patient education does not apply only to the adult patient. Children who receive adequate, age-appropriate instruction are often less anxious and more cooperative during procedures. The challenge of teaching children is gearing the instruction to the child's cognitive level (Fig. 25–1). Table 25–1 provides general guidelines for age-appropriate approaches to pediatric patient education.[10]

Adult Patients

Malcolm A. Knowles, often referred to as the father of adult education, noted that the adult's patterns of learning are

Table 25–1

Pediatric Patient Education Guidelines

Age	General Characteristics of Patient	Patient Education Tips
Infant (0–12 months)	Developing a sense of trust; attached to parent; stranger anxiety; rapid growth and development; sensorimotor phase	Instruct parents; keep parent in infant's line of vision; encourage parents to comfort child
Toddler (12–36 months)	Limited understanding; striving for independence; egocentric; limited language skills; limited concept of time; unable to reason	Instruct parents; allow child to participate during instruction (e.g., hold dressing or open package); give simple explanations; explain procedures in relation to what child sees, hears, tastes, smells, and feels; emphasize aspects of procedures that require cooperation (e.g., lying still); communicate using behaviors; use play—demonstrate with dolls and small replicas of equipment (see Fig. 25–1); limit teaching sessions to 5–10 minutes; prepare child immediately before procedures
Preschool (3–5 years)	Developing sense of initiative; increased language skills; limited concept of time; illness and hospitalization often viewed as punishment; fears bodily harm	Explain procedure in simple terms and in relation to how it affects the child; demonstrate use of and allow child to play with equipment; encourage "playing out" on a doll to clarify misconceptions; use neutral words such as "medicine under the skin" for "shot," "hurt" for "pain," and "tube" for "catheter"; avoid overestimating child's comprehension; encourage child to verbalize; limit each teaching session to 10–15 minutes; state directly that the procedure is not a form of punishment; point out on drawing, child, or doll where procedure is to be performed; explain unfamiliar situations such as noises and lights; involve child in instruction and care (e.g., hold equipment, open packages, tear tape); instruct parents
School age (6–12 years)	Developing a sense of industry; increased language skills; interested in learning; improved concept of time; increased self-control; developing relationships with peers	Explain procedures using correct terminology; explain reasons for procedures using anatomic drawings; explain function and operation of equipment in concrete terms; allow manipulation of and practice with equipment; allow for questions and discussion; limit teaching sessions to 20 minutes; instruct in advance of procedures; suggest ways child can maintain control (e.g., deep breathing, counting, relaxation); include child in decision making (e.g., preferred site for venipuncture); may instruct in small groups or encourage teaching other peers; instruct parents
Adolescent (12–20 years)	Developing a sense of identity; increasing capability for abstract thought and reasoning; conscious of appearance; developing peer relationships and group identity	Involve in all decision making and planning; provide reasons for and benefits of procedures; explain long-term consequences of procedures; encourage questioning regarding fears; discuss how procedures may affect physical appearance and what can be done to minimize it; suggest methods for maintaining control; be cognizant of adolescent's difficulty accepting authority; instruct in groups and encourage peer instruction; teaching session may be as long as 45 minutes

Adapted from Whaley LF, Wong DL. Nursing Care of Infants and Children, 4th ed. St. Louis: C. V. Mosby, 1991.

distinct from those used by the child. He suggested that, because of their extensive backgrounds and greater independence adults bring more to a learning experience, and that educators should serve more as facilitators, with an opportunity to benefit as much as the learner through their exchange. Knowles coined the term "androgogy" to describe the art and science of helping adults learn. Table 25–2 presents practical recommendations for using these principles of adult learning to provide more effective patient education.

As with children, life stages within adulthood are an important consideration when educating the adult. Young adults (ages 20 to 40) and middle adults (ages 40 to 60) should be approached with an empathetic and nonjudgmental attitude. This approach, as well as the application of principles of adult learning, also applies to adults in their later years (over 65 years of age), along with some additional considerations:

- Approach each patient as unique. Do not stereotype because of age.

- Be aware that aging is a multidimensional process in which multiple factors affect functioning.
- Capitalize on the elderly patient's strengths.
- Refrain from using first names unless invited to do so.
- Speak clearly and concisely.
- Avoid patronizing.
- Motivate learning by showing how the acquisition of new skills and knowledge can improve the quality of life.
- Provide large-print reading materials.
- Limit teaching sessions to 20 to 30 minutes.
- Present one idea at a time, with frequent summarization.
- Keep all training sessions well organized and slow-paced.

THE EDUCATIONAL PROCESS

Patient education is a process that includes thoroughly assessing the learner and teacher, developing a teaching plan

Table 25-2

Application of Knowles' Principles of Androgogy

Assumptions	Applications for Adult Patient Education
1. Adults are independent learners.	Allow the adult to control the learning situation as much as possible (e.g., determine time frames, information addressed, and instructional techniques); show respect for the adult's independence.
2. Adults use their life experiences as a learning resource.	Assess the adult's past experiences prior to developing a teaching plan; draw on the adult's past experiences whenever possible throughout the educational process; show respect for the adult by giving credence to past experiences; provide opportunities for the adult to share knowledge and experience with others.
3. Adults' learning is oriented to developmental tasks of their role.	Assess the adult's current developmental stage and life tasks and problems (e.g., parenthood, career building, retirement); increase the adult's motivation to learn by applying the needed information to the adult's current life situation.
4. Adults' time perspective in learning is related to immediacy of application.	Be considerate of the many compelling and conflicting demands on the adult's time and thought processes; focus education on information that the learner views as being needed now.
5. Adults' orientation for learning is problem-centered.	Provide an opportunity for the adult to find answers to questions or problems; focus education on the adult's perceived needs.
6. Adults see themselves as doers.	Provide opportunities for the adult to apply learning through doing (e.g., return demonstration, restating information).
7. Adults resist learning under conditions that are incongruent with their self-concept.	Avoid learning situations that are potentially humiliating or detrimental to the adult's self-concept.

based on assessment results, effectively implementing the teaching plan, and evaluating the results.

Assessment

Effective teaching depends on a complete and accurate assessment of both the learner and teacher. Thorough assessment of the patient (learner) should include needs, level of comprehension, readiness and motivation to learn, maturational level and age, and cultural, social, religious, and economic factors. Sources for assessment information include interviews with the patient, family, and other caregivers, review of the patient's chart, including nursing care plans, discussions with other health care team members involved in the patient's care, patient questionnaire, and observation of the patient.

To be effective, information must not only be received by the learner but also understood. There are various ways of assessing comprehension. ''Grades completed in school'' is not useful information for making assumptions about comprehension levels, because many high school graduates score far below the expected twelfth-grade level of comprehension.[11] Direct methods for assessing comprehension include the Cloze test for reading comprehension, listening tests, and word recognition tests.[11] Indirect methods for assessing learner comprehension include restatement of information

read and, perhaps the least threatening way, patient choice of instructional media.

If the learner is not ready or motivated to learn, no learning occurs. Many factors can affect learner readiness, including level of acceptance of diagnosis, stress, patient comfort, and energy level. Redman has stated that every patient is ready to learn something, but it is up to the teacher to find out what it is.[6] Learner readiness may increase when even the smallest need is met. Instructing the learner about the need for learning specific information may also improve readiness and motivation.

Although often not considered, it is also important to assess the teacher who is providing patient education. Being a nurse does not instantly qualify one as a capable teacher. Four factors to consider when assessing a nurse's ability to teach are energy, attitudes, knowledge, and skill.[12] The potential impact of the nurse's value system on the effectiveness of teaching is also an important consideration.[13] An example of such impact may be when the nurse strongly disagrees with the patient's religious beliefs and thus finds it difficult to spend time with the patient without these differences becoming an issue.

Planning

Another important step in the educational process is developing the teaching plan. The time spent assessing learner needs is wasted unless these needs are included in an individualized patient teaching plan. The teaching plan must be based on patient goals and objectives or outcomes, which are developed as a result of the assessment with the active input, when possible, of the patient (learner). The following illustrates patient assessment prior to developing a teaching plan.

Sample Teaching Plan for Home Infusion of Total Parenteral Nutrition (TPN)

Patient name:	Mr. RY
Patient assessment:	Mr. RY is 53 years old and a high school graduate. He is currently hospitalized and is to be discharged home on cyclic TPN infusion through a Hickman catheter. This is the first time Mr. RY has had a Hickman catheter and, prior to hospitalization, had never heard of it or TPN. He appears anxious to learn so that he can go home and return to work on his farm and spend time with his grandchildren. He has no past medical education but has worked closely with the veterinarians who care for his farm animals and has been trained to give injections to the farm animals. His wife is available to assist him, but

| | he prefers to carry out as much of his care as possible. Mr. RY is a Methodist and is active in the small farm community where he has lived all his life. He is emotionally close to his family, all of whom live in neighboring communities. Mrs. RY has debilitating arthritis in her hands and appears nervous about having any responsibility for her husband's therapy. |
| Learner input: | Mr. RY states that he was never a star student in school and does not read books because it takes too long. He reads the newspaper and farm magazines, and enjoys watching TV. He doesn't enjoy studying and related a "bad" experience he had when studying to become certified in CPR. Mr. RY states that he learns best when he can see things done and can then do them himself. He wants to learn everything he can about his therapy and hopes that he can remember everything and do the procedures correctly. |

Objectives should be written in behavioral terms that can be measured. The teaching plan should include a content outline developed from the objectives, along with preplanned time frames for teaching. The steps in designing the plan include identifying the material to be covered, determining the sequence of the material, and selecting the teaching methods to be used to deliver the material.[13] These steps can be included in a teaching plan, as shown in Appendix I.

Whenever possible, the environment in which teaching takes place should be controlled and planned. A well-organized teaching plan can be ineffective if the environment is not conducive to learning. Environmental considerations include comfortable seating with good visibility, comfortable temperature, limited number of persons in attendance, adequate space for teaching supplies, equipment available for audiovisual materials, and limited distractions or interruptions from television, radio, and other patients.

Various formats and resources are available that are appropriate for patient education. The most effective teaching plan includes varied teaching approaches to ensure that the learning style most appropriate for that particular patient is met, and that more of the patient's senses are involved in the learning process. According to Patterson,[14] individuals remember 10% of what they read, 20% of what they hear, 30% of what they see, 50% of what they hear and see, 80% of what they say, and 90% of what they say and do. Thus, if

the patients' only source of education is a printed booklet, they will remember only 10% of the information read. The patient remembers only 20% of verbal instruction, such as a lecture or audiotape. If the teaching session includes verbal instruction along with a demonstration, 50% of the information is likely to be retained. If the patient is given an opportunity to repeat the instruction, retention increases to 80%. The most effective instructional technique is return demonstration and instruction, when 90% of the information is retained.

Written education materials are frequently used to carry out and enhance patient education. Patient use of written educational materials must be carefully considered based on the patient's level of comprehension. Studies have shown that many printed patient instruction materials developed today are at a comprehension level many grades higher than that of 60% of the US population. To ensure that as many patients as possible comprehend the written instructions given to them, it is recommended that all printed materials be written at a fifth-grade level of comprehension. Techniques for testing the readability of written materials include the SMOG test and the Fry readability formula.[11] The most common characteristics evaluated are the difficulty of vocabulary used and the average sentence length. With the necessary information, these tests can be administered by members of the nursing staff or education department.

Printed patient education materials may be developed by the nurse on an individual basis for each patient, developed generically by the hospital or agency, or acquired from an outside source. Here are some tips for writing patient education materials:

Tips for Writing Patient Education Materials

- Limit information to that which is absolutely necessary to know.
- Use visual messages as much as possible (e.g., Use simple line drawings, when appropriate).
- Break down complex information into small individual parts.
- Use a logical sequence to present information.
- Put the most important points first.
- Use a conversational, informal writing style such as "you will feel" rather than "the patient should feel."
- Use short words (two syllables or less, when possible, or define longer words) and short sentences (less than 15 words).
- Remove all unnecessary words that obscure the main point.
- Use headings to let the reader know what is coming.
- Be consistent with wording (e.g., don't switch from "tube" to "catheter").
- Consider the cultural and language needs of the patient population.
- Test readability using accepted published formulas, such as the SMOG formula or the Fry index of readability.[11]
- Summarize and review at the end of each section.
- Have patients or other laypersons review and provide feedback on the written piece prior to printing.

Many free patient education materials are also available for intravenous nurses from product and service companies. Requests can be sent directly to companies; their address is usually included on the package labelling or can be obtained from the local company sales representative. Appendix II lists sources of free patient education materials.

Patient education materials that are printed by an outside source should be carefully evaluated for teaching applicability. The following are criteria for selecting preprinted patient education materials:

1. Are the facts, pictures, and subject matter accurate and up to date?
2. Is the material at the appropriate comprehension level for the patient population?
3. Are the learning objectives consistent with those of the teaching plan?
4. Is too little or too much information given?
5. Are the language and material as simple as necessary for the intended audience?
6. Do all procedures and directions follow hospital, clinic, or agency policy?
7. Is the information well organized?
8. Is the print clear and large enough to be easily read?
9. Are the illustrations appropriate and adequately labelled?
10. Do the pictures and drawings reflect a patient population with which the patient can identify?

Verbal instructions and demonstrations are the most commonly used approaches to patient education. The advantages of this one-on-one approach are the immediate ability to answer questions, reassess learning needs, and make changes in the teaching plan.

Audiovisual media are being used at an increasing rate. Studies have shown that this approach can be just as effective as the use of written materials and verbal instruction.[15] Audiovisual materials include videotapes, audio tapes, and television programs. Benefits of this approach include the ability to ensure a consistent message and to review the message critically before it is presented. Drawbacks may include the price of the tapes and equipment, inaccessibility of equipment, and lack of teacher-learner interaction. Videotape instruction may be more effective if used in combination with other methods.[16]

Computer instruction is also becoming available for patient education. Benefits of this approach include interactive program capabilities and increased opportunities for "off-site" education. Drawbacks may include patient apprehension about computer equipment and its price.

Implementation

Good communication skills, teaching abilities, and organizational skills are key to the effective implementation of a teaching plan. The following recommendations are helpful for providing effective instruction:

- Establish rapport; reduce anxiety and fear.
- Incorporate a variety of teaching strategies (e.g., discussion, demonstration, written materials, audiovisual materials, return demonstration, peer instruction, restating) to respond to different learning styles and to take advantage of the synergy of complementary techniques.
- Speak the learner's language, avoid jargon, and clarify all terms.
- Divide the information into small steps.
- Be specific.
- Keep the information short, simple, and concrete.
- Address the most important information first.
- Stress the importance of instructions and expected benefits; explain the detrimental effects of inadequate treatment, but avoid fear tactics.
- Ask questions and encourage feedback to ensure comprehension of the information.
- Repeat the information as often as needed.
- Use verbal praise to reward learning.
- Take advantage of "teachable" moments when the learner is most likely to accept new information (e.g., when symptoms are present).
- Allow for the practice of a new skill or the use of new information without delay.
- Express enthusiasm and concern through voice and body language.
- Allow the patient to share knowledge about the subject.
- Be flexible; adjust learning goals as necessary.
- Summarize teaching frequently.

Evaluation

Evaluation of the effectiveness of the teaching plan and the accomplishment of patient (learner) objectives should occur throughout implementation and at the completion of the teaching sessions. The original teaching plan may be revised several times as a result of ongoing evaluation results. Evaluation can be analyzed in four major areas.

Reaction. Reaction involves measuring the responses of the learner to the content and the instructor through written forms or verbal expression. An example of a written response is having the learner complete a written evaluation form that asks questions about whether the teaching addressed all the learner objectives, and whether the instructor and instructional techniques were effective. An example of verbal expression may include discussion with the learner following the teaching session about the learner's reaction to the instruction.

Learning. Learning includes measuring the acquisition of knowledge through written and verbal testing.

Behavior. Behavior encompasses measuring the change in skills that occurs because of learning activities, as seen by return demonstration.

Results. Results involve measuring the life style changes resulting from the learning activities.[17]

DOCUMENTATION

As with all other nursing care provided to a patient, the action and results of patient education must be documented. Documentation is important for many reasons, including to provide a complete picture of the patient's condition and progress, communicate progress in patient education to other

CAREMARK
Affiliate Baxter Healthcare Corporation

Therapy		
☐ TPN	☐ CHE	☐ OTHER
☐ ENT	☐ WHC	(specify)
☐ ANT	☐ INP	
☐ PNM	☐ FLR	_____

THERAPY EDUCATION EVALUATION

☐ Initial   ☐ Follow-Up

Patient Name

Account Number

TOPIC Complete each category with appropriate dates and instructor initials.	N / A	ASSESSMENT / DISCUSSION / DEMONSTRATION	RETURN DEMONSTRATION WITH ASSISTANCE	RETURN DEMONSTRATION WITHOUT ASSISTANCE	ADDITIONAL COMMENTS
INTRO					
Purpose / Principle of Therapy					
Therapy Requirements					
Caremark Overview					
Rights / Responsibilities					
Plan of Care					
SAFETY / INFECTION CONTROL					
Handwashing					
Work Area					
Maintaining Asepsis					
Blood / Body Fluid Precautions					
Environmental Safeguards					
Waste Disposal					
SUPPLY MGMT					
Equipment / Supplies					
Inventory Control					
SOLUTION / MEDS / FORMULA					
Storage					
Inspection					
Additives					
Preparation					
Dosage / Concentration					
ADMINISTRATION PROCEDURES					
Administration Set					
Gravity / Bolus					
Pump: (specify)					
Operation					
Maintenance					
Alarm System					
Catheter / Tube Placement					
Connection Procedure					
Disconnection Procedure					
Rate of Administration					
Fat Administration					
CATH TUBE CARE					
Heparinization / Irrigation					
Site Care / Dressing Change					
SELF MONITORING					
Weight					
Temperature					
Intake / Output					
Urine Testing					
Documentation Requirements					
Other (specify)					
PSYCHO SOCIAL					
Integration of Therapy Into Lifestyle					
Community Resources					

COMPLICATIONS / EMERGENCY INTERVENTIONS

Including:

____ 24 Hour Emergency Number	____ Catheter Blockage	____ Electrolyte Imbalance	____ Infiltration
	____ Catheter Damage	____ Emergency Overstock	____ Nausea / Vomiting
____ Administration Set Malfunction	____ Catheter Disconnection	____ Emergency Resources	____ Oiling Out Phenomenon
____ Air Embolism	____ Catheter Displacement	____ Extravasation	____ Phlebitis
____ Air In Line	____ Dehydration	____ Fluid Imbalance	____ Phototherapy / eye patches
____ Allergic Reaction	____ Diarrhea / Constipation	____ Hypo / Hyperglycemia	____ Pump Malfunction
____ Aspiration	____ Distention	____ Incident / Grievance Handling	____ Signs and Symptoms PTL
____ Blood Back-up	____ Drug Specific Complication	____ Infection	

SPECIAL INSTRUCTIONS / COMMENTS

☐ Reviewed with Pharmacist   Date   ☐ NA
☐ Reviewed with other home support services   Date   ☐ NA

SIGNATURES

Instructor / Title   Date(s)

I / we _____ , (patient and / or caregiver) have received educational materials, and agree to undergo instruction in order to feel competent to safely and effectively perform the functions associated with the prescribed therapy. I / we understand that I / we will routinely perform these functions in a facility other than a hospital or medical institution.

Patient / Caregiver   Date

DISTRIBUTION: WHITE-Medical Record CANARY-Nurse PINK-Physician GOLDENROD-Patient

CS. 157 6/23/89 ©Copyright 1991, Caremark, Inc. All rights reserved.

MEDICAL RECORD

FIGURE 25–2. Example of patient education documentation checklist. (Courtesy of Caremark, Inc., Northbrook, IL.)

members of the health care team, and provide necessary information for reimbursement.

Complete documentation should include the assessment of patient knowledge deficit and readiness to learn, learning objectives, implementation of teaching plan, skills demonstrated, patient response to teaching, and an evaluation of the overall process.

Documentation can be accomplished in narrative form or on a checklist. Figure 25–2 shows the checklist format for documenting patient education. These provide easy reference for health care team members and patients to monitor progress.

THE TEAM APPROACH

Patient education is a collaborative effort of the health care team members, patient, family, and caregivers. Patient education begins with admission or diagnosis and continues throughout the patient's hospital stay and following discharge in the home or alternate care setting. Each member of the team has expertise and knowledge that can strengthen and enhance the total education plan. The intravenous nurse needs to be constantly aware of immediate and long-term patient learning needs, and should meet them through education or assist in planning patient instruction with other health care team members.

OTHER NURSING CONSIDERATIONS

Nursing Diagnoses

Nursing diagnoses are used to communicate patient assessments. Those related to patient education include the following:

- Alteration in health maintenance
- Impaired home maintenance management
- Knowledge deficit (specify)
- Learning need (specify)
- Noncompliance (specify)
- Compliance (specify)

Patient Outcomes

A compelling benefit of patient education is improved patient outcomes. Patient outcomes are both the goals for which the teaching plan is designed and the indicators of its success. Measurable patient outcomes related to patient education are as follows:

Improved adherence to a therapeutic regimen
Increased patient satisfaction
Enhanced patient self-determination with increased ability to handle symptoms
Enhanced patient recovery after surgery
Patient verbalization of understanding instructions and information given
Correct patient demonstration of learned procedures

Patient education is an important part of patient care provided by the intravenous nurse. Patient education must be a priority that takes precedence over non-nursing activities and is planned for in the patient plan of care. To be effective, patient instruction must be developed at the appropriate learning level, taking into consideration the age and cognitive abilities of the patient. The process of teaching patients must include a complete assessment of the learner and teacher, a comprehensive teaching plan based on learner objectives, effective implementation of the plan, and thorough evaluation of the teaching effectiveness and accomplishment of learner objectives. Complete documentation of patient education is necessary for communication of progress and results. Positive patient outcomes are the result of well-planned and implemented patient education.

References

1. Joint Commission on Accreditation of Healthcare Organizations. Accreditation Manual for Home Care. Oakbrook Terrace, IL: Joint Commission on Accreditation of Healthcare Organizations, 1991.
2. Joint Commission on Accreditation of Healthcare Organizations. Accreditation Manual for Hospitals. Oakbrook Terrace, IL: Joint Commission on Accreditation of Healthcare Organizations, 1992.
3. Intravenous Nurses Society. Intravenous Nursing Standards of Practice. Belmont, MA: Intravenous Nurses Society, 1990.
4. Smith CE. Overview of patient education: Opportunities and challenges for the twenty-first century. Nurs Clin North Am 1989; 24:583–587.
5. Oberst MT. Perspectives on research in patient teaching. Nurs Clin North Am 1989; 24:621–627.
6. Redman, BK. The Process of Patient Education, 7th ed. St. Louis: C.V. Mosby, 1993.
7. American Hospital Association. A Patient's Bill of Rights. Chicago, IL: American Hospital Association, 1980.
8. Knapp TA, Huff RL. Emerging trends in the physician's duty to disclose: An update of Cantebury v Spence. J Leg Med 1975; 3:41–45.
9. Fernsler JI, Cannon CA. The whys of patient education. Semin Oncol Nurs 1991; 7:79–86.
10. Whaley LF, Wong DL. Nursing Care of Infants and Children, 4th ed. St. Louis: C.V. Mosby, 1991.
11. Doak CC, Doak LG, Root JH. Teaching Patients with Low Literacy Skills. Philadelphia: J. B. Lippincott, 1985.
12. Jackson JE, Johnson EA. Patient Education in Home Care: A Practical Guide to Effective Teaching and Documentation. Rockville, MD: Aspen, 1988.
13. Humphrey CJ, Milone-Nuzzo P. Home Care Nursing: An Orientation to Practice. Norwalk, CT: Appleton & Lange, 1991.
14. Patterson O, ed. Special Tools for Communication. Chicago: Industrial Audio-Visual Association, 1962.
15. Bethea CD, Stallings SF, Wolman PG, Ingram RC. Comparison of conventional and videotaped diabetic exchange lists instruction. J Am Diet Assoc 1989; 89:405–406.
16. Curtis M. Videotapes: Are they helpful in a practice setting? J Am Acad Nurse Pract 1990; 2:172–173.
17. Haggard A. Handbook of Patient Education. Rockville, MD: Aspen, 1989.

Bibliography

Anderson C. Patient Teaching and Communicating in an Information Age. Albany, NY: Delmar, 1990.
Arndt MJ, Underwood B. Learning style theory and patient education. J Contin Ed Nurs 1990; 21:28–31.
Arnoldussen B, Coppin K, Schott L. Patient education as a quality indicator in critical care: Ischemic heart disease—recognition and response. AACN Clin Issues Crit Care Nurs 1991; 2:56–62.
Azarnoff P. Teaching materials for pediatric health professionals. J Pediatr Health Care 1990; 4:282–289.
Barnes LP. Commitment to patient education. Am J Matern Child Nurs 1991; 16:17.

Barrett C, Doyle M, Driscoll S, et al. Nurses' perceptions of their health educator role. J Nurs Staff Dev 1990; 6:283–286.

Belton AB. Reading levels of patients in a general hospital. Beta Release 1991; 15:21–24.

Berry RK. Home Intravenous Antibiotic Therapy: A Self-Study Module for Nurses. Lincolnshire, IL: Caremark, 1991.

Berry RK. Effective patient education: Communicating with children and families. Nurs Spectrum 1993; 23:12–14.

Berry RK. Effective patient education: Teaching adults. Nurs Spectrum 1993; 22:12–14.

Berry RK, Jorgensen S. Growing with home parenteral nutrition: Adjusting to family life and child development. Pediatr Nurs 1988; 14:43–45.

Blumberg BD, Gentry ED. Selecting a systematic approach for educating hospitalized cancer patients. Semin Oncol Nurs 1991; 7:112–117.

Boswell EJ, Pichert JW, Lorenz RL, Schlundt DG. Training health care professionals to enhance their patient teaching skills. J Nurs Staff Dev 1990; 6:233–239.

Bubela N, Galloway S, McCay E, et al. The patient learning needs scale: Reliability and validity. J Adv Nurs 1990; 15:1181–1187.

Caremark. Patient Education Manuals. Northbrook, IL: Caremark, 1994.

Dixon E, Park R. Do patients understand written health information? Nurs Outlook 1990; 38:278–281.

Frank-Stromborg M, Cohen R. Evaluating written patient education materials. Semin Oncol Nurs 1991; 7:125–134.

Greenberg LA. Teaching children who are learning disabled about illness and hospitalization. Am J Matern Child Nurs 1991; 16:260–263.

Harrison LL. Strategies to facilitate inpatient education. Am J Matern Child Nurs 1990; 15:255

Hiromoto BM, Dungan J. Contract learning for self-care activities: A protocol study among chemotherapy outpatients. Cancer Nurs 1991; 14:148–154.

Iyer PW, Camp NH. Nursing Documentation: A Nursing Process Approach. St. Louis: Mosby Year Book, 1991.

Knowles MS. The Modern Practice of Adult Education: From Pedagogy to Androgogy, 2nd ed. New York, Cambridge: Adult Education Company, 1980.

Kolb DA. Experiential Learning: Experience as the Source of Learning and Development. Englewood Cliffs, NJ: Prentice-Hall, 1984.

Kruger S. A review of patient education in nursing. J Nurs Staff Dev 1990; 6:71–74, 78.

Lipetz MJ, Bussigel MN, Bannerman J, Risley B. What is wrong with patient education programs? Nurs Outlook 1990; 38:184–189.

Lorig K. Patient Education: A Practical Approach. St. Louis: C.V. Mosby, 1992.

Luker KA, Caress A. The development and evaluation of computer-assisted learning for patients on continuous ambulatory peritoneal dialysis. Comput Nurs 1991; 9:15–21.

Masten Y, Conover DP. Automated continuing education and patient education. Comput Nurs 1990; 8:144–150.

Moora ME. Future trends in patient education. Semin Oncol Nurs 1991; 7:143–145.

Padberg RM, Padberg LF. Strengthening the effectiveness of patient education: Applying principles of adult education. Oncol Nurs Forum 1990; 17:65–69.

Padilla GV, Bulcavage LM. Theories used in patient/health education. Semin Oncol Nurs 1991; 7:87–96.

Rankin SH, Stallings KD. Patient Education: Issues, Principles, Practices, 2nd ed. Philadelphia: J. B. Lippincott, 1990.

Schofer KK, Ward CJ. The computerization of the patient education process. Comput Nurs 1990; 8:115–122.

Stevenson E, Crosson K. Patient education: History, development, and current directions of the American Cancer Society and the National Cancer Institute. Semin Oncol Nurs 1991; 7:135–142.

Theis SL. Using previous knowledge to teach elderly clients. J Gerontol Nurs 1991; 17:34–38.

Trent S, Free F, Weibel D. Home Total Parenteral Nutrition . . . A Self-Study Module for Nurses. Lincolnshire, IL: Caremark, 1991.

Tucker SM, Canobbio MM, Paquette EV, Wells MF. Patient Care Standards: Nursing Process, Diagnosis and Outcome. St. Louis: C. V. Mosby, 1992.

Villejo L, Meyers C. Brain function, learning styles, and cancer patient education. Semin Oncol Nurs 1991; 7:97–104.

Volker DL. Needs assessment and resource identification. Oncol Nurs Forum 1991; 18:119–123.

Wilson BW. Matching instructional methods to renal patients' learning abilities: The effect on knowledge and compliance with fluid restriction. J Renal Nutr 1991; 1:173–181.

Session 1: Introduction to Home TPN

Objective	Content	Teaching Method	Time Frame
On completion of teaching session, patient will be able to:			
Discuss goal and purpose of TPN therapy	I. TPN therapy A. Goals B. Purpose	Discussion: relate to usual eating habits	5 minutes
Discuss basic components of TPN solution	II. Components of TPN A. Protein B. Carbohydrates C. Vitamins D. Trace elements	Discussion: relate to oral nutrition	10 minutes
Explain roles and responsibilities of home TPN support team	III. The home care team A. Hospital B. Home care agency C. Nurse D. Physician E. Dietician F. Delivery person G. Home patient representative H. Pharmacist	Videotape from agency Discussion: relate to those people that patient has already met	15 minutes
List emergency phone numbers	IV. Emergency phone numbers	Develop a list together with Mr. and Mrs. Y	10 minutes
Session 1 evaluation		Ask questions regarding content of session	10 minutes

Session 2: Safety and Infection Control

Objective	Content	Teaching Method	Time Frame
	Review session 1		
On completion of teaching session, patient will be able to:			
Differentiate between "clean" and "sterile"	I. Definitions A. Clean B. Sterile	Discussion: apply to veterinary medicine Demonstration	5 minutes
Wash hands using proper technique	II. Hand washing A. Application to home TPN infusion B. Importance of handwashing C. Proper procedure D. How to accomplish this at home	Discussion Demonstration Videotape Printed materials with many pictures Return demonstration	15 minutes
Identify suitable home work and storage areas	III. Home work area A. Storage area B. Work space	Discussion regarding available work and storage space in home	10 minutes
Identify an appropriate means of medical waste disposal at home	IV. Equipment disposal A. Needles B. Syringes C. Other	Discussion Demonstration Return demonstration	10 minutes
Session 2 evaluation		Return demonstration of hand washing and equipment disposal Ask questions regarding clean versus sterile	10 minutes

Session 3: Solutions and Medications

Objective	Content	Teaching Method	Time Frame
	Review sessions 1 and 2		
On completion of teaching session, patient will be able to: Apply previously learned information and skills regarding solutions and medication	I. Review of solution and medication knowledge	Patient demonstration of previously learned skills Patient discussion of solution and medication knowledge	15 minutes
Handle solutions and medications correctly	II. Solutions and medications A. Storage and preparation B. Warming C. Prescription verification D. Expiration verification E. Visual inspection F. Additives G. Use of syringes, vials, and ampules H. Injecting additives into the solution container	Discussion Demonstration Return demonstration	25 minutes
Session 3 evaluation		Discussion and demonstration of all procedures	10 minutes

Session 4: Administration Techniques

Objective	Content	Teaching Method	Time Frame
	Review sessions 1, 2, and 3		
On completion of teaching session, patient will be able to: Prime tubing and filter	I. Priming A. Tubing B. Filter	Demonstration Discussion Return demonstration	15 minutes
Operate infusion pump	II. Infusion pump A. Operation B. Alarms C. Troubleshooting	Discussion Videotape from pump company Demonstration Return demonstration	35 minutes
Session 4 evaluation		Set up and operate pump	10 minutes

Session 5: Administration Techniques (continued)

Objective	Content	Teaching Method	Time Frame
	Review sessions 1 through 4		
On completion of teaching session, patient will be able to: Describe tapering	I. Tapering A. Rate B. Schedule	Discussion Demonstration Return demonstration	10 minutes
Administer fat emulsions	II. Fat administration A. Purpose B. Procedure	Discussion Demonstration Return demonstration	10 minutes
Connect TPN infusion	III. Connection procedure	Discussion Demonstration Return demonstration	10 minutes
Disconnect TPN infusion	IV. Disconnection procedure	Discussion Demonstration Return demonstration	10 minutes
Session 5 evaluation		Perform procedures without prompting	10 minutes

Session 6: Catheter Care

Objective	Content	Teaching Method	Time Frame
	Review sessions 1 through 5		
On completion of teaching session, patient will be able to:			

Perform catheter dressing change	I. Dressing change
	  A. Purpose
	  B. Supplies
	  C. Procedure
		Discussion
		Demonstration
		Return demonstration
			20 minutes

Heparinize central catheter	II. Heparinization
	  A. Purpose
	  B. Supplies
	  C. Procedure
		Discussion
		Demonstration
		Return demonstration
			20 minutes

Session 6 evaluation		Perform procedures without prompting	10 minutes

Session 7: Home Monitoring, Complications, and Emergency Interventions

Objective	Content	Teaching Method	Time Frame
	Review sessions 1 through 6		
On completion of teaching session, patient will be able to:			

Monitor TPN therapy at home	I. Home monitoring
	  A. Weights
	  B. Urine
	  C. Input and output
	  D. Documentation
		Discussion
		Demonstration
		Return demonstration of procedures and documentation
			20 minutes

Identify possible complications and interventions	II. Complications
	  A. Description
	  B. Interventions
		Discussion
		Review of written instructions
			20 minutes

Session 7 evaluation		Give correct answers to case study scenarios	10 minutes
	Sessions 1 through 7		
Total teaching evaluation		Written evaluation form Patient explains each aspect of care while demonstrating Question patient regarding emergency procedures—use case studies related to farm environment	25 minutes

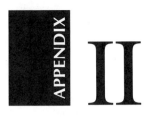

II SOURCES OF FREE PATIENT EDUCATION INFORMATION

Alzheimer's Disease and Related Disorders Association
919 North Michigan Avenue, Suite 1000
Chicago, IL 60611
800-272-3900

American Allergy Association
P.O. Box 640
Menlo Park, CA 94026
415-322-1663

American Diabetes Association
National Center
1660 Duke Street
Alexandria, VA 22314
703-549-1500

American Heart Association
7320 Greenville Avenue
Dallas, TX 75231
214-373-6300
(or local office)

American Liver Foundation
1425 Pompton Avenue
Cedar Grove, NJ 07009
800-223-0179
201-256-2550

American Lung Association
1740 Broadway
New York, NY 10019
212-315-8700
(or local office)

Association for the Care of Children's Health
7910 Woodmont Avenue, Suite 300
Bethesda, MD 20814
301-654-6549

Arthritis Foundation
1314 Spring Street, NW
Atlanta, GA 30309
404-872-7100

Crohn's and Colitis Foundation of America, Inc.
444 Park Avenue, South
New York, NY 10016
800-932-2423
212-685-3440

Cystic Fibrosis Foundation
6931 Arlington Road, #200
Bethesda, MD 20814
800-344-4823
301-951-4422

Leukemia Society of America
733 Third Avenue
New York, NY 10017
212-573-8484

National Association for Sickle Cell Disease
3345 Wilshire Boulevard, Suite 1106
Los Angeles, CA 90010
800-421-8453
213-736-5455

National Association of Anorexia Nervosa and Associated Disorders
(ANAD)
Box 7
Highland Park, IL 60035
708-831-3438

National Cancer Institute
Cancer Information Service
Building 31, Room 10A16
9000 Rockville Pike
Bethesda, MD 20892
800-4-CANCER

National Hemophilia Foundation
Hemophilia and AIDS/HIV Network for the Dissemination of Information
(HANDI)
110 Green Street, Suite 303
New York, NY 10012
800-42-HANDI
212-219-8180

National Kidney Foundation, Inc.
30 East 33rd Street
New York, NY 10016
800-622-9010
212-889-2210

North American Transplant Coordinators Organization
Executive Office
P.O. Box 15384
Lenexa, KS 66285-5384
913-492-3600

United Network for Organ Sharing
1100 Boulders Parkway, Suite 500
Richmond, VA 23225
804-330-8500

Documentation

Diane L. Baker, CRNI

OVERVIEW

Documentation of the nursing process has always been viewed as a necessary but time-consuming chore. In the past 20 years, nursing documentation has become more important and more reflective of the requirements of state and federal regulatory agencies, changes in nursing practice, determination of reimbursement fees, and legal ramifications.

Until around 3000 BC, when a system of writing was developed in Egypt, no formal records were kept by attendants to the sick. With the advent of Christianity, "patient care" records of nursing became organized and continuous. No one person contributed more to nursing than Florence Nightingale (1820 to 1910).[1] In her time, documentation was used primarily to communicate the implementation of physician's orders. Nurses notes were not viewed as an important part of the patient's medical record and were often discarded when the patient was discharged from the hospital. In her early writings, Nightingale advocated the recording of the patient's diet and environment as essential to the patient's chart, in an effort to collect and store data that could be used in the care of the patient.

In the 1930s, a written plan of care was developed. In 1951, nursing standards became formalized, and the Joint Commission on Accreditation of Hospitals was formed. In the mid 1960s, documentation in the nurses' notes evolved as an essential method of evaluating nursing care that met the requirements of regulatory agencies, provided testimony in litigations, and delineated professional responsibility. When diagnostic related groups were implemented in the early 1980s, the chart served as a mechanism for determining reimbursement guidelines. In the 1990s, the emphasis is on quality improvement, with a focus on evaluating organizational and clinical performance outcomes. Documentation is one way to evaluate outcomes.[2]

PRINCIPLES AND LEGAL ISSUES

The health care record is a factual, accurate, written account of the patient's history, present status, and progress toward goals. It should also contain physician's orders, prescription information, a care plan, financial information, a medication profile, and pertinent observations of the patient's physical and psychosocial condition. The medical record is a legal document and, as such, should contain objective statements that clearly promote and ensure that the nursing process is implemented by all clinicians. Only factual data are to be recorded; subjective conclusions by the care giver must be avoided. Descriptions of individuals as "strange," "uncooperative," and "weird" are not acceptable data. Such phrases as "IV running well" are not measurable and should be supported by facts, such as "5% dextrose in water infusing at 125/ml/hour."

Initial and ongoing assessments and nursing interventions must be documented in the record, as should communication of essential findings to the physician and others involved in the patient's care. Patient and care giver education must be accurately recorded in the chart in the case of a patient receiving home infusion therapy. Written instructions should be given to reinforce teaching, and the patient should acknowledge the receipt of this information by signing the form and keeping a copy.

Entries in the medical record should be made in a timely manner. Attempting to record an event a week after the fact usually results in faulty memory recall. If an entry is made in error, a line should be drawn across it and "mistaken entry" written on it in a way that does not obscure the original note. Any information that becomes illegible raises suspicion that a mistake was covered up. Correction fluid and erasures should never be used in a chart, and only permanent ink is allowed, preferably blue or black. Many charts are photocopied or faxed for various reasons, and some lighter-colored inks may not reproduce properly on a faxed or copied document.

Only those abbreviations that have been authorized for use by the facility or health care corporation should be used in the chart. Unusual abbreviations or acronyms can be misunderstood and may cause harm to the patient. This is particularly true if the abbreviation involves the administration of a drug. The abbreviation q.o.d. (every other day) can be misread as q.i.d. (four times a day) if the handwriting is not legible or if the abbreviation used is not accurate.

Documentation provides pertinent, accurate information to other clinicians involved in the patient's care. If others do not understand the language, then the medical record fails to convey information. In addition to performing this important function, charting allows essential data to be retrieved for legal purposes, reimbursement, and research. Proper documentation is a strong support for the quality of the care that is rendered. During litigation based on medical malpractice, the medical record becomes tangible evidence that is admissible in court. Caution should be taken that correct grammar and spelling are employed. Above all, entries must be signed by the clinician making the note.

PURPOSE AND SCOPE

In addition to being an American Nurses Association standard of nursing practice, documentation is also required by many state codes that were developed and approved in the 1980s. Several states have regulated the documentation of invasive procedures, such as intravenous (IV) therapy. The most important reason for these regulations is to protect the health care consumer by delineating professional responsibility and accountability. In 1985, the American Nurses Association stated: ''The nurse is responsible for data collection and assessment of the health status of the client; determination of the nursing care plan directed toward designated goals; evaluation of the effectiveness of nursing care in achieving the goals of care; and subsequent reassessment and revision of the nursing care plan.''[2]

Monitoring documentation is required to prove the delivery of quality care. Ongoing record reviews enable an auditor to track patient outcomes, monitor the quality of the nursing care being provided, measure the nurse's awareness of documentation policies, and identify and prevent problems before they occur. Of course, relying solely on documentation to prove quality of care has limitations. Incomplete or absent charting does not always mean that the care was not rendered. There may be several reasons why pertinent documentation was omitted: time constraints, inaccessibility of the records, lack of awareness, or poorly designed clinical forms. Record audits may simply point out the poor quality of the charting, not necessarily the poor quality of care. For all of these reasons, it is imperative that medical record forms be designed to promote accurate, complete, and timely entries.

Reimbursement by payers depends on documentation. Medicare is a federal insurance program for a large number of disabled or elderly health care consumers in the United States. Coverage determination is based on the review of properly completed forms. Managed care is the newest system of reinbursement provided by insurance companies who award benefits only when they receive complete and accurate documentation. IV therapy documentation can be simple and accurate, with dedicated forms that relate to the procedures being performed. In the hospital, this form might be an IV therapy flow sheet, on which all procedures, potential and actual problems, and nursing interventions can be included.[3]

Reimbursement from a Medicare provider is based on a diagnostic related group fixed price tag. For example, a patient admitted to the hospital is given a code based on the International Classification of Diseases developed by the US Department of Health and Human Services. If a patient is admitted with a diagnosis of acute appendicitis and undergoes a surgical procedure, such as an appendectomy, the code would appear thus:

540.9   Acute appendicitis
47.0   Appendectomy

If the fixed reimbursement rate for acute appendicitis is $1800 and the fixed rate for the surgical procedure is $4720, the hospital would be paid $6520 for the patient's care, regardless of how long a stay would be required. If the patient develops a severe phlebitis and requires an additional day in the hospital, an extra code would be added to the medical record: 996.5 phlebitis. This code might have a reimbursement value of $310. The only doccumentation of this adverse event might be in the IV therapy record. If the record of this event is not clear and accurate, the hospital might lose reimbursement dollars.

USING THE NURSING DIAGNOSIS IN DOCUMENTATION

At the 1990 conference of the North American Nursing Diagnosis Association, a definition of the term *nursing diagnosis* was accepted. It reads: ''A nursing diagnosis is a clinical judgment about individual, family, or community responses to actual or potential health problems/life processes. Nursing diagnoses provide the basis for selection of nursing interventions to achieve outcomes for which the nurse is accountable.''[2] The term nursing diagnosis has been in use for many years, but confusion has existed about its true meaning. Nursing diagnosis is an integral part of the nursing process and is a natural outcome of a systematic assessment of the patient's needs. Complete and accurate data are needed to formulate a concise nursing diagnosis. Data are gathered from the patient's history, physical examination, laboratory results, and members of the patient's family or significant others. Once the problems have been identified (nursing diagnoses), goals are established, and a plan is developed for nursing intervention. All of this information must be recorded in the medical record in a clear, organized manner.

PROBLEM-ORIENTED MEDICAL RECORD

The problem-oriented record consists of the same data that are present in the nursing process; the assessment, plan, implementation, and evaluation. The uniqueness of this type of documentation is that each problem is listed and numbered according to priority, with the date of onset and the date of resolution noted. The problems list is usually kept at the front of the chart and serves as an index. Information is then systematically entered on the multidisciplinary progress notes. The format is organized so that only the information that relates to a particular problem is noted. Thus, routine charting (IV patent, patient ambulating in hall) is eliminated. The following is an example of a problems list in this type of charting:

4/27/94	#1	postoperative pain
	#2	potential for pneumonia
	#3	high risk for chemical phlebitis

In this and the following scenarios, let us assume that a 62-year-old male has been admitted through the emergency department for a ruptured appendix and subsequent appendectomy. His postoperative orders include the administration of 1 L of 5% dextrose in Ringer's lactate solution every 8 hours and nafcillin, 3 g IV every 6 hours. He arrives in his room from the recovery room awake but drowsy. In his left hand, he has a 16-gauge IV cannula. The site is slightly edematous, with erythema extending from the puncture and along the vein for approximately 5 cm. He is moaning softly and complains of postoperative abdominal pain and a burning pain in the dorsal surface of his left hand.

Once the problems list has been developed, the multidisciplinary progress notes will address the problem with its corresponding number:

4/27	1600	#3	S:	My left hand burns. What's wrong with it?
			O:	Redness and swelling observed at the IV site on the left hand.
			A:	Inflammation of the vein caused by chemical and mechanical irritation.
			P:	Restart IV with smaller-bore cannula in a large vein.

This format (SOAP) was first introduced and recommended in the 1960s by a physician, Dr. Lawrence Weed. The acronym stands for subjective data (what the patient tells you), objective data (what you observe and inspect), assessment (what you think is happening based on the data), and plan (what you are going to do). Over the years, this format has been extended to include the nursing intervention and evaluation:

4/27	1630	I:	IV discontinued intact and restarted in the left forearm (LFA) with a 22-gauge × 1-inch cannula on first attempt. Warm moist compress placed on dorsum of left hand.
	1840	E:	No complaints of discomfort related to the infusion.

An advantage to SOAP (IE) charting is its predetermined format, which lends consistency to the documentation of patient care. A disadvantage is that SOAP (IE) charting is often redundant. The problems list and care plan are duplicated, and both identify the same problems and nursing diagnoses. The plan and interventions are also noted on both the care plan and the progress notes. Occasionally, different problems may have the same or similar interventions, resulting in repetitive documentation.

PIE CHARTING

Problems, interventions, and evaluation (PIE) charting, developed in 1984, is similar to SOAP documentation but arose from the nursing process. The PIE charting system consists of a daily flow sheet and progress notes. The 24-hour flow sheet lists specific needs, such as routine elements of care (activity, hygiene), as well as categories (behavior, skin, elimination). The flow sheet also provides space to record other information, such as dressings, IVs, and procedures. Any deviation from normal is identified by an asterisk and is described in the progress notes. After the initial assessment is completed, the nurse documents on the progress notes the specific problems that arise on his or her shift. Once stated, the problems are numbered and subsequently referred to only

by number in future entries. Each problem is evaluated once a shift and at the end of the day. The identified problems are carried from day to day until they are resolved (Table 26–1). The progress note addressing this problem might look like this:

4/27	1640	P#3	Redness and swelling of IV site, left hand, consistent with phlebitis. Patient complains of burning pain.
		IP#3	IV discontinued intact; restarted in LFA with 22-gauge × 1-inch cannula on first attempt. Warm moist compress to dorsum of left hand.
	1800	EP#3	Patient states IV infusing comfortably, left hand feels better.

As indicated, problem #3 is phlebitis of the left hand, which would have to be assessed and charted daily until resolved. One disadvantage of this type of charting is that it eliminates the planning step of the nursing process.

FOCUS CHARTING

Focus charting was developed in 1981 by a committee of nurses who were dissatisfied with the SOAP format. In this type of documentation, patient concerns are identified and organized to include data, action, and response in a narrative note. Thus, the identified concern is not a problem but a focus. It allows for a broader scope of assessment during an admission or a reassessment during the hospitalization. This format is usually in a column and separates the focus from the progress note. The acronyms used in this method describe similar steps to those used in SOAP:

Data:	Information and observation that identifies the focus
Action:	Nursing intervention
Response:	Patient's response to the intervention

4/27	1630	pain	D:	Complains of burning pain at IV site on left hand. Area red and swollen.

Table 26–1

Sample PIE Documentation

Shift	Time	Cannula/Site	Tubing Change	Appearance	IV Fluid/ Rate
7–3					
3–11	1600	16-gauge left hand	√	red/swollen	1 L D₅LR q8h
11–7					

D_5LR = 5% dextrose in Ringer's lactate solution.

A: Cannula discontinued intact. Restarted in LFA with 22-gauge × 1-inch cannula. Warm moist compress to dorsum of left hand.

1800   R: Patient states IV infusing comfortably.

If not monitored regularly, the focus chart can become a narrative note with no evidence of the patient's response to the intervention.

NARRATIVE CHARTING

Narrative charting is the type most commonly used and most familiar to nurses. It can be combined with flow sheets and is in a story format that documents patient care events that occur during each shift:

4/27   1630   Patient returned from operating room with a 16-gauge cannula in the left hand. 1 L of 5% dextrose in Ringer's lactate solution infusing well on pump at 125 ml/hour. Patient is moaning and complains of burning pain at the IV site. The area is slightly edematous, and erythema extends from the puncture along the vein for approximately 5 cm. IV discontinued intact and restarted in the LFA with a 22-gauge × 1-inch cannula on first attempt. Patient seems to be resting comfortably now.

This type of note is often lengthy, repetitive, time consuming, and unstructured. It includes normal assessment findings, and patient problems are often difficult to extrapolate from it. It is also task oriented and does not necessarily reflect the nursing process. Information from it is usually difficult to retrieve for quality improvement and auditing.

CHARTING BY EXCEPTION

In 1983, nurses at St. Luke's Hospital in Milwaukee, Wisconsin developed charting by exception.[2] Their motivation was to reduce documentation time, but specifically to make trends in the patient's status more obvious. Several key elements that constitute this type of charting: flow sheets, references to standards of practice and institutional protocols, nursing database, nursing care plans based on the nursing diagnosis, and SOAP progress notes. St. Luke's Hospital nurses use several types of flow sheets in their charting by exception, the most unique of which is the nursing/physician order flow sheet. Guidelines for the appropriate use of the flow sheet are printed on the back of the form. Unfortunately, the charting by exception system developed at St. Luke's

Hospital is cumbersome for the documentation of only one aspect of care, such as IV therapy. A modification of charting by exception may be used.

In 1987, the IV team at Highline Community Hospital in Seattle, Washington developed a form specific to IV therapy that combines a flow sheet with a nursing care plan (Fig. 26–1).[3] The reverse side of the flow sheet contains the parenteral fluid record (Fig. 26–2). This form can be left at the patient's bedside or on a clipboard at the nurses' station. When it is completed, the form is inserted into the patient's medical record and becomes a permanent part of the chart.

Because the patient's overall nursing care plan usually only cursorily mentions IV therapy, goals are not established in enough detail to assess and list the actual or potential problems that might occur to prevent the patient from achieving his or her goals. The flow sheet is checked once every 24 hours and whenever an IV-related procedure is performed, such as changing the administration set, restarting the IV, or establishing a second site for the administration of incompatible drugs. The checklist is simple and self-explanatory and encompasses standards of practice and institutional protocols. The IV nursing care plan is implemented by a member of the IV team but is readily available as a guideline for the staff nurses to review for the development of complications during routine care.

Regardless of the format developed for the documentation of IV therapy, basic requirements to the plan of care exist, including goals, actual and potential problems, nursing interventions, and outcomes. The care plan that includes these components can be modified for the hospital, home, or alternate site setting.

INTRAVENOUS NURSING CARE PLAN

The nursing care plan is a framework that enables nurses to objectively measure the nursing process. The nursing process is a deliberative problem-solving approach that requires technical, cognitive, and interpersonal skills and is aimed at meeting the specific needs of the patient. There are five components to the nursing process: assessment, diagnosis, plan, implementation, and evaluation. These elements remain constant, regardless of the type of nursing or the setting. The first step, assessment, is a systematic activity that gathers information on every aspect of the patient's status for the purpose of defining his or her needs. The next step, the nursing diagnosis, involves the analysis of the data that were collected during the assessment stage. This information allows the IV nurse to identify weaknesses, strengths, and problems that require intervention and resolution. Planning, the third step, is a means by which the needs are prioritized according to significance. The goals are formulated, and nursing interventions are described to resolve the problems and achieve the goals.

The next logical move, then, is to implement the plan. Without the implementation and completion of the interventions listed in the plan, the nursing process will fail. The IV nursing plan of care is a guide that clearly defines the activities that are required to achieve the desired outcomes of therapy. In the home setting, this plan can be used by the patient and family, as well as by the nurses. The activities that are defined in the plan of care must be documented on

YEAR: 19 DATE:							
TIME:							
NEW START							
O.R./E.R. START							
RESTART							
I.V. ACCESS FOR:							
FLUIDS							
MEDS VIA HEP LOCK							
BLOOD/COMPONENTS							
ACCESS ONLY							
CONVERT I.V. TO HEP LOCK							
FLUSHED W/SALINE & HEPARIN							
REASON FOR D.C.:							
ROUTINE SITE ROTATION							
PHLEBITIS: GRADE							
INFILTRATED							
OCCLUDED							
LEAKING							
POSITIONAL							
MEDIC START							
DR. ORDERS							
CATHETER D.C.'d INTACT?							
HOT PACKS APPLIED							
DEVICE/BRAND:							
GAUGE							
LENGTH							
# ATTEMPTS							
LIDOCAINE 1% S.C.							
SKIN PREP:							
ALCOHOL/BETADINE							
INSERTION SITE:							
DRESSING TYPE							
CHANGES:							
DRESSING							
TUBING							
FILTER							
SITE INSPECTION							
? PROBLEMS OBSERVED:							
COMMENTS:							
Pump Set-up							
Lab Draw							
INFUSION CONTROL DEVICE:							
PT. ED. VERBAL/BOOKLET							
NURSE INITIALS							

INTRAVENOUS NURSING CARE PLAN
(circle all that apply)

Date Care Plan Initiated:

SHORT TERM GOAL
(initial 72 hrs.): Establish I.V. access for: fluids, drugs, chemotherapy, blood/components, hyperalimentation, access only H.L.

LONG TERM GOAL (beyond 72 hrs.): Maintain safe access until physician discontinues.

POTENTIAL PROBLEMS: Phlebitis, occlusion, infiltration, limited access, confusion, electrolyte imbalance, circulatory overload, transfusion reaction, drug extrav. with tissue damage, sepsis, air embolism.

PLAN: AVI pump for accuracy, daily site check, tubing/filter chge. q 24-72 hrs., long-term cannula, 2nd line for incomp. drugs, restart PRN

ACTION: PCA set-up & instruc. with return demo., PIC line per physician order, intracath, landmark, S.C. line per physician, Infus-A-Port

OUTCOME: Completion of therapy; pt. discharged; cannula in place for: home, ECF.

COMMENTS:_____

PHYSICIAN CONTACTED_____ DATE:_____

INTRAVENOUS NURSE:_____

Figure 26–1. Form for intravenous therapy that combines a flow sheet and a nursing care plan.

DATE	BOTTLE NO RATE FLOW / INITIALS	TYPE OF FLUID	AMOUNT IN BOTTLE	ADDITIVES	TIME START	END	INFUSED VOLUME

PATIENT STAMP

IDENTIFY INITIALS WITH SIGNATURE

HIGHLINE COMMUNITY HOSPITAL
PARENTERAL FLUID RECORD

92

Figure 26–2. Reverse side of flow sheet shown in Figure 26–1 containing the parenteral fluid record.

the appropriate forms (hospital care plan, flow sheets, or visit reports) to enable objective evaluation of the efficacy of the plan. The evaluation is the final phase in the nursing process. At the evaluation, goals need to be reviewed and revised if they are not achievable.

If goals must be changed, then another strategy must be defined and implemented to meet the new goals. Criteria used in the evaluation of the plan include measurable, realistic goals related to the nursing diagnoses and interventions, including patient education. The IV nursing care plan developed and used at the Highline Community Hospital contains six components: short-term goals, long-term goals, potential problems, plan, action, and outcome. Each of these areas is addressed in the care plan based on the individual's diagnosis, prognosis, and type and duration of therapy.

Short-term goals usually consist of immediate actions taken as a direct result of the physician's orders. It is desirable to achieve this goal within 24 to 72 hours of the patient's admission to the hospital or to the home infusion service.

Long-term goals are tied closely to the desired outcomes, one of which is to ultimately maintain safe venous access until drugs can be administered orally, the course of antibiotics is complete, or the patient expires. Again, based on the prognosis, this goal is very individualized.

Potential problems are all possible local and systemic complications related to the therapy. They are listed to enable the care givers to use them as a tool for daily assessment of the patient's progress toward the goals.

The plan must outline measures to be taken to prevent potential complications that have been identified.

Action is a description of the actual steps taken as defined in the plan. Here, the word "implementation" or "intervention" can be substituted.

Outcome is the realization of the goals. In some cases, the outcome could be the peaceful death of a patient who requires patient-controlled anagelsia for a terminal illness. In most cases, the outcome would be successful completion of the therapy without complications. In the home or alternate site setting, IV therapy is not separated from the rest of the nursing documentation for a simple reason: the nurse who teaches or administers the therapy is also responsible for the complete assessment of the patient and the environment because usually no other nurses are involved in the patient's care. When a patient is admitted to a home infusion service, the primary nurse initiates the documentation process and must perform a complete assessment and review of systems. This assessment includes functional and psychosocial considerations, environmental safety, history and medication profile, list of problems or needs in addition to those related to the therapy, description of the therapy ordered, and goals. Teaching and compliance with the therapy are important issues in the home setting, and thorough documentation of these matters is required.

With the advent of health care reform, positive outcomes and continuous quality improvement tracking are of the utmost importance. Patients are often discharged from the hospital with venous access devices already in place either in the form of an implanted port, a tunneled central catheter, or a peripherally inserted central catheter. Initially, clear documentation of the IV access device should include the type of access, including the brand name of the device, if possible; location; gauge and length; insertion date; condition at discharge; and environment where the line was placed (e.g.,

hospital, clinic). Site care and condition should be assessed and accurately described at each subsequent home visit, and any procedures should be clearly documented. All of the sections that apply to the hospital IV nursing care plan may be used to develop a similar plan for home infusion therapy. However, the goals may differ slightly. The short-term goal may be to teach the patient or care giver to become independent in the administration of the therapy. A long-term goal may be to ensure compliance and to resolve the infection.

COMPUTERIZED DOCUMENTATION SYSTEMS

This chapter would not be complete without mentioning the latest trend in nursing documentation. Hospital information systems are becoming commonplace as computer systems are becoming more affordable and user friendly. Once the initial nursing documentation program is set up, data are easily entered and retrieved for outcome monitoring, ongoing quality improvement, utilization review, and reimbursement. The hospital may have its own mainframe or may be linked to a larger system in another state. Data can be entered into a system that uses a wand, a touch screen, a keyboard, a hand-held terminal, or a bar code reader. Based on the type of terminal available, the nurse may enter data in several ways: by filling in the blanks, by entering words or numbers to make complete sentences, by using free-form text, or by selecting choices that appear on the screen. A definite advantage of the computerized system is that the program contains prompts that prevent the entry of partial or incomplete information. Computerized clinical records are also more legible and concise than handwritten pages. Some of the disadvantages include computer "downtime," "crashing," slow response during peak hours of use, and cost. The key to the successful outcome of any documentation formula lies in the thorough education of the staff that will use it.

References

1. Donahue MP. Nursing: The Finest Art. St. Louis: C.V. Mosby, 1985.
2. Iyer P, Camp N. Nursing documentation, a nursing process approach. St. Louis: C.V. Mosby-Yearbook, 1991.
3. Baker D. Measuring outcome criteria, the intravenous nursing care plan. JIN 1990; 13(4):253–258.

Selected Reading

Bullard J, Ketchum K. Bar code systems justify staffing for I.V. Teams. JIN 1991; 14(5):345–349.
Coulter K. Intravenous therapy for the elder patient: Implications for the intravenous nurse. JIN (suppl) 1992; 15:518–523.
Hadaway L. Nursing diagnosis applied to I.V. nursing practice. JIN 1988; 11(2):109–111.
Joint Commission on Accreditation of Health Care Organizations, Chicago, IL, 1994.
Intravenous Nurses Society. Intravenous Nursing Standards of Practice. Belmont, MA: Intravenous Nurses Society, 1990.
Ketchum K. I.V. therapy and a bar code system. Infusion Management Update February 1992; 2(1):9–10.
Otto SE, LaRocca JC. Nursing diagnosis: Challenge for intravenous nursing practice. JIN 1988; 11(4):245–248.
Winskunas CA. A creative approach to comprehensive I.V. therapy documentation. JIN 1990; 13(2):115–118.

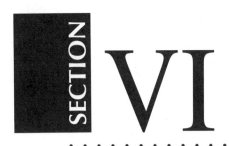

SPECIAL CONSIDERATIONS

CHAPTER 27 Intravenous Therapy in Children

Corinne Wheeler, CRNI, CPNP
Anne Marie Frey, BSN, CRNI

Starting and maintaining intravenous therapies in children poses unique challenges to the clinicians responsible for their care. Children are not only very different from adults, but they also display variations among their different age groups. These differences include physical, physiologic, developmental, cognitive, and emotional variables. When any type of infusion therapy is used in a child, a great responsibility is placed on the nurse. Accordingly, the nurse performing IV techniques in children should be skillful and knowledgeable in the basic IV therapy applications and in the child's development. Most of the basic principles of safe administration of IV solutions and medications are the same, regardless of the patient's age. However, special considerations are necessary to safeguard the child undergoing these procedures; these measures include the need to calculate small doses and low infusion rates, to choose appropriate venipuncture sites and equipment, and to develop creative measures to distract curious little minds and hands.

This chapter focuses on the children's needs as they relate to infusion therapy and on the unique aspects involved in the care of both the child and his or her family.

ANATOMIC AND PHYSIOLOGIC DIFFERENCES IN CHILDREN

Children present a wide variety of physical characteristics that are different from those in adults. In addition, premature infants and newborns vary greatly from older children in both their anatomic and their physiologic parameters. These characteristics affect their ability to cope with environmental stresses as well as to manage the metabolism, absorption, distribution, and excretion of medications and solutions. Although body systems in infants and children are different from those in adults, for the purpose of this text, only those related to infusion therapy are addressed in detail.

The newborn's adjustment to extrauterine life is a complex physiologic process. The first 24 hours of life are the most critical as the newborn makes the respiratory and circulatory transition to extrauterine life. During this period, there is a much higher incidence of death than in the remainder of the neonatal period. All of the body systems undergo change after birth, and most of them remain immature for a period of time. During infancy (birth to 12 months of age), physical and developmental changes occur more rapidly than during any other period. The infant's head and body grow very rapidly during this period, and major body systems undergo a progressive maturation process. In healthy infants, the birth weight is usually doubled at 6 months and tripled at 1 year. At this same time, certain critical developmental tasks that affect nursing care are mastered. However, each child has his or her own pace of development; no two children of the same age are at the same exact stage of development and maturation.

Changes in biologic development in the toddler period (12 to 36 months) are less dramatic than those in infancy. Body systems continue to mature, resulting in many children reaching full maturation by the end of the toddler period. Growth slows down during this time. Birth weight is quadrupled by 30 months, and the height at age 3 years is generally about half the adult height. Head circumference growth slows down, and chest circumference exceeds the measurement size of both the head and the abdomen. The toddler is able to participate in an increased number of activities as a result of gross and fine motor skill advancement. In toddlers, IV connections must be taped and secured and equipment kept outside of the child's reach.

Early childhood (36 months to 6 years), also referred to as the preschool period, is a time of growth stabilization. The average annual weight gain is about 5 lb (2.3 kg); the increase in height ranges from 2.5 to 3 inches (6.4–7.6 cm). Most of the height growth occurs in the legs, leading to a more slender physical appearance. The preschooler's more mature body system enables him or her to tolerate moderate physiologic stress. Skills mastered during the toddler period are refined during this time and include a rapidly developing ability to understand and use language. Successful achievement of expected levels of growth and development must be attained for the child to refine these skills and prepare him or her for the next stage of childhood, school age.

The school-age period (6 to 12 years of age) is a time of gradual growth and development, except for the end of this period, sometimes referred to as prepubescence. The school-age child will grow an average of 2 inches (5 cm) and gain 4.5 to 6.5 lb (2–3 kg) annually. Until prepubescence, little difference exists in size between males and females; toward the end of this stage, a growth spurt occurs. Girls first surpass the boys in both height and weight. Body proportions approach adult parameters by the end of the school-age period.

Adolescence is the period of transition from childhood to young adulthood. This period is divided into three substages: early adolescence (11 to 13 years), middle adolescence (13 to 15 years), and late adolescence (15 years and older). The changes occurring during adolescence are primarily puberty, growth, and personality. The central nervous system is inundated with hormonal activity, and dramatic and obvious growth changes are noted in both boys and girls. Both sexes develop secondary sexual characteristics and grow larger. Less obvious is the maturation of the reproductive system. This stage is often turbulent for adolescents because they are on a constant emotional roller coaster, attempting to master the developmental tasks for adulthood.

Biologic System Development in Children

Thermoregulation

The newborn's large surface area, thin layer of subcutaneous fat, and unique method for producing heat predispose it to excessive heat loss. The nurse responsible for any aspect of the newborn's care must take measures to protect him or her from hypothermia. Unlike the adult, the chilled neonate does not shiver but uses the mechanism of nonshivering thermogenesis to increase heat production. In response to hypothermia, norepinephrine is secreted by the sympathetic nerve endings. This action stimulates the breakdown of brown fat to generate heat, allowing distribution of the heated blood through the body.

Increased metabolism as a response to hypothermia results in higher oxygen and caloric requirements. A healthy infant can usually tolerate increased oxygen consumption; however, a sick infant is predisposed to cold stress and hypoglycemia. Cold stress begins as the infant requires an increase in oxygen and caloric consumption. The activation of norepinephrine stimulates the metabolism, and anaerobic glycolysis results. The lactic acid produced by this process, combined with the acid end products of brown fat metabolism, can lead to acidosis.[1]

This process of thermoregulation continues throughout the infant's first several months of life. During infancy, the child's ability to shiver increases. The older infant usually has acquired the benefit of insulation by the gradual growth of adipose tissue. By early childhood, the skin is thicker, and the body has a higher percentage of fat and a decreased surface area to volume ratio. These factors enable the preschooler to cope with environmental cold stresses much better than can the young infant.

The nurse performing such procedures as venipuncture on an infant must maintain a neutral thermal environment for that infant to prevent the possibility of cold stress. A neutral thermal environment is one that permits the infant to maintain a normal core temperature with minimum oxygen consumption and calorie expenditure. The neutral thermal environment for smaller infants is 35.4 plus or minus 0.5 C (95.7 plus or minus 1 F) and for larger infants is 32.5 plus or minus 1.4 C (90.5 plus or minus 2.5 F).[2]

Measures that nurses can take to assist the infant to maintain warmth include using radiant warming panels, incubators, cotton blankets, and head coverings (e.g., a piece of stockinette knotted at one end); keeping only the extremity of the IV insertion site exposed; and warming items that will have contact with the infant. Blankets can be warmed in warming units or in clean, unoccupied incubators. Gooseneck lamps effectively warm the treatment room table before the venipuncture procedure begins.

Vessel Size

The size of venous and arterial vessels in the infant and child are obviously smaller than those in the adult. Although the vessels are anatomically positioned in the same locations throughout life, their sometimes threadlike characteristics and tendency to hide make them difficult to locate for access in the young patient. Applying heat to the extremity before performing venipuncture facilitates venous identification and catheter insertion.

Renal Function

The newborn without congenital abnormalities has an anatomically complete renal system. However, all young kidneys have a functional deficiency in their ability to concentrate urine. Glomerular filtration in the infant younger than 6 weeks of age functions less precisely than that in the mature child. Mature kidney function is complete by approximately 2½ to 3 years of age. The young infant's renal system has difficulty coping with changes in fluid and electrolyte status; dehydration, conditions of hyperosmolality, and, sometimes, overhydration are problems for the infant. Not only are infants more prone to develop these conditions, but the effects also progress more rapidly. Infants have a greater urine volume per kilogram of body weight and a smaller bladder volume capacity than older children. Expected urine output with adequate intake should be 0.5 to 1.0 ml/kg/hour for the newborn and 1.0 to 2.0 ml/kg/hour for the infant.[1]

Hepatic Function

Decreased hepatic function due to liver immaturity in the newborn affects intravenous medication and/or solution administration. After the first few weeks of life, the liver has the capability to secrete bile and conjugate bilirubin. Throughout the first year of life, however, the liver remains immature in its ability to function. The ability to metabolize drugs is dramatically less than that of the adult, as is the formation of the plasma proteins and ketones, the storage of glycogen and vitamins, and the capacity to break down amino acids. Digestive and metabolic processes are usually complete by the beginning of toddlerhood.[1]

Endocrine Function

Like the renal system, the endocrine system in the newborn is fully intact anatomically; however, it functions at an immature level. The entire endocrine system interrelates and affects body homeostasis. Decreased functioning of this system affects the ability of the infant to cope with stress. For example, endocrine-secreted hormones that affect fluid and electrolyte equilibrium and metabolism include adrenocorticotropic hormone, antidiuretic hormone, and vasopressin. The immature endocrine system, in addition to some of the other immature body systems, predisposes the infant to such conditions as dehydration and unstable blood glucose levels.

Body Composition

Subcutaneous Fat

The percentage of body fat gradually increases over the first 6 months of life. As shown in Table 27–1, the highest percentages of body fat are seen in the toddler and prepubescent years. Additional adipose tissue may add to difficulty in vein location for IV access. In addition, the percentage of

Table 27–1	
Percentage of Body Fat by Age Group	
Age	**Percentage of Body Fat**
Newborn	12
Toddler	23
Preschooler	12
Prepubescent	20
Adult	15

body fat can affect therapeutic requirements of lipid-soluble IV medications such as diazepam (Valium), which is utilized as a sedative or anticonvulsant in children.

Circulating Blood Volume

In children, the circulating blood volume is much greater per unit of body weight than in the adult, but the absolute blood volume is small. Every child's total circulating blood volume should be calculated at admission to a pediatric intensive care unit (Table 27–2). In a small infant, hypovolemia can occur from only a small amount of blood loss. The following is an example comparing an absolute volume loss between a 7-kg infant and a 70-kg adult:

25 ml blood loss from 70 kg adult =
< 0.6% of total circulating blood volume (4150 ml)

25 ml blood loss from 7 kg infant =
5% of total circulating blood volume (500 ml)

When blood samples are obtained for laboratory examination, the smallest amount of blood required for accurate results should be removed. Blood replacement should be considered when blood loss is greater than 5 to 7% of the total circulating volume.[3] Blood sample amounts should be recorded in the output section of the intake and output record.

Fluid and Electrolyte Metabolism

The amount of fluid in body mass is greater in the newborn than at any other time and decreases with age (Table 27–3). The newborn has the largest proportion of free water in the extracellular spaces. This results in higher levels of total body sodium and chloride and lower levels of potassium, magnesium, and phosphate than in the adult. At a rate of exchange seven times greater than that of the adult, the infant exchanges approximately half of its total extracellular fluid daily. The basal metabolism rate is also twice as great in relation to body weight in the infant than it is in the adult.

Table 27–2	
Formula for Calculating Circulating Blood Volume in Children	
Age	**ml/kg of Body Weight**
Neonate	85–90
Infant	75–80
Child	70–75
Adolescent	65–70

From Hazinski MF. Nursing Care of the Critically Ill Child. St. Louis: CV Mosby, 1984.

Table 27-3
Body Water in Proportion to Age

Age	Percentage of Body Water		
	TBW	ECF	ICF
Premature infant (1.2 kg)	81	59	22
Term infant (3.6 kg)	69	42	27
1 year (10 kg)	60	32	28
Adult male (70 kg)	54	23	31
Adult female (60 kg)	49	23	26

TBW = total body water; ECF = extracellular fluid; ICF = intracellular fluid.
Data from Mahan LK and Arlin MT. Krause's Food, Nutrition, and Diet Therapy, 8th ed. Philadelphia, PA: W.B. Saunders Company, 1992:143.

Insensible water losses are greater in infants because of their larger body surface ratio per body weight. These factors, in addition to the inability of the kidneys to concentrate urine in infants, can cause dehydration, acidosis, and overhydration.[4]

The daily fluid requirement (per kilogram of body weight) for an infant is three times greater than that of an adult and increases under stress. With each centigrade degree of temperature elevation, an additional 50 to 75 ml of fluid replacement is required. The normal daily caloric requirements are also greater than those of the adult because of the child's increased basal metabolism rate and rapid growth rate. Children who are ill, especially those with fever or who have had major surgery, require more calories than those required for regular maintenance (Table 27–4).

PEDIATRIC DEVELOPMENTAL AND ASSESSMENT CONSIDERATIONS

Successful pediatric IV therapy relies on more than technical skill and knowledge about the physiologic differences between children and adults. An understanding of the psychological aspects of the child's growth and development and the application of appropriate interventions is essential when interacting with children. Table 27–5 outlines the various developmental stages of childhood and suggests nursing actions for each stage.

A complete health care assessment of a child has three main components: (1) health history, (2) physical assessment, and (3) review of diagnostic data. The urgency of the child's condition affects the order and the initial detail of these components. Occasionally, it may be necessary to obtain venous access and initiate IV therapy without a completed health care assessment. Routinely, however, the health care assessment is usually well under way before venipuncture, with the IV nurse contributing additional data.

History

Valuable information is collected not only during the initial assessment but also throughout the course of infusion therapy, whether it be in the hospital or in the home. In the younger child, questions are directed to the primary caregiver and include: (1) What are your concerns? (2) How is your child different from his or her normal or prior state? (3) What measures have been taken to alleviate the child's problem? (4) How effective were the measures? When developmentally appropriate and possible, given the child's condition, questions should be asked directly to older children and adolescents. This practice provides them with an opportunity to actively participate in the process and to respond according to their own perceptions.

Knowledge of the child's age, pre-illness weight, fluid and dietary habits, and elimination patterns is useful for determining the child's current hydration status. Asking the parents if the child is thirsty or nauseated may also provide valuable information. Thirst in a child can be indicative of a fluid volume deficit. However, nausea may blunt the desire to drink, even if the child is thirsty. The child's preferences for food and drink and any particular cultural and ethnic customs should also be acknowledged.

Physical Assessment

Before and during the course of infusion therapy, the clinical assessment of the child should include weight; height; vital signs; condition of skin, mucous membranes, and fontanelles; urine volume; and neurologic status. Some elements of the clinical assessment may be performed simultaneously with the nursing history interview. When possible, the young child should be allowed to sit in the parent's lap or the parent should be allowed to be in close proximity to the child. This helps the child to feel more secure and enhances the child's ability to cooperate.

Height and Weight

Height and weight measures are essential for accurate calculations to be made in fluid and medication administration. The comparison of prior weight with current weight is an accurate indicator of fluid volume deficit or fluid volume excess. Children under 2 years of age are more susceptible to weight changes resulting from fluid balance rather than from a change in body mass. In this age group, the proportion of body fluid to total body weight is greater, and most of this fluid is in the extracellular space (see Table 27–3).

Changes in weight must be monitored closely. Approximately 1 g of body weight is equal to 1 ml of body fluid. Thus, weight loss or gain of 1 kg (2.2 lb) within 24 hours represents a liter of fluid loss or gain. Weight changes in a 24-hour period of plus or minus 50 g in an infant, 200 g in a child, or 500 g in an adolescent may be significant, and the physician should be notified. Infants should be weighed without clothing and consistently on the same scale. With small

Table 27-4
Daily Caloric Requirements by Age

Age	Daily Caloric Requirement
High-risk neonate	120–150 cal/kg
Normal neonate	100–120 cal/kg
1–2 years	90–100 cal/kg
3–6 years	80–90 cal/kg
7–9 years	70–90 cal/kg
10–12 years	50–60 cal/kg

From Hazinski MF. Nursing Care of the Critically Ill Child. St. Louis: CV Mosby, 1984.

Developmental Stages of Childhood

Age Group	Developmental Characteristics	Child's Response to Illness or Procedures	Preparation of Child	Family Involvement	Nursing Implications
Infant (*birth to 1 year*)	Basic Trust vs. Mistrust Totally dependent on others for all needs. Trust develops as needs are consistently met. Mistrust develops as needs are not consistently met. Totally self centered at birth. During infancy, begins to separate self from others. Responses Random communication skills (3 mos). Simple gesturing (12 mos). Exhibits early memory. Fears Separation Strangers Rapid Motor Changes Head control from poor to stable. Moves hand to mouth (B–3 mos). Crawling (6–9 mos). Standing with support (12 mos).	Has the ability to resist with entire body. Recognizes primary caretaker and responds with fear of change. "Mirrors" emotional state of mother. Unpredictable response to repeated procedures. Uses cry to communicate all discomfort (not just pain)	Avoid feeding immediately prior to procedure (risk of vomiting and aspiration). Minimize separation from parents.	Encourage parental tactile and soothing verbal stimuli immediately after procedure and throughout duration of therapy. May be present during procedure but should not assist with restraining of child. Demonstrate safe handling of infant. Encourage questions. Education directed to family.	Physical comfort is most effective. Keep infant warm. Utilize a pacifier. Talk in soft voice and call by name; cuddle infant. Avoid extremity of infant's preference (finger sucking). Distract with bright toys, and prepare equipment out of older infant's view. *Safety* Utilize assistants other than family to restrain infant. Monitor color and respirations during procedure. Protect site with half-cup or stockinette. Utilize elbow restraints over wrist restraints. Do not restrain all four extremities. Secure IV equipment out of infant's reach. Avoid IV accessories with detachable parts.
Toddler (*1–3 years*)	Autonomy vs. Shame and Doubt *Preoperational thoughts:* Little understanding of past or present. Ritualistic. Explores self and world around him or her. Transitional objects provide comfort (blanket, toy). Differentiates self from objects. Can infer a cause while experiencing only the effect. Oppositional "No" stage. Early aggression and manipulative behavior. Has many fantasies. Enjoys new motor skills. Walking (12–15 mos) to running (24 mos) Indicates needs by pointing. Responds to sense of time.	Although frequently reminded "not to touch," is unable to comply. Gains comfort from parent's voice even if the parent is not in view. Misplaced objects of comfort lead to great emotional upset. Tolerates frustration poorly. Initial response to reason may be positive; however, without consistent effect. May regress to clinging, infant-like behavior. Attempts to "bargain" to avoid procedures.	Prepare immediately prior to procedure. Use concrete and immediate rewards. Use simple and honest explanations; tell child of impending "prick." Use calm, positive, firm approach. Do not give choices if a child does not have any.	Same as for infant. Encourage to decorate crib with pictures of family and pets. Utilize cassette tapes of family voices/songs/stories.	Restraining requires more than one person. Reassure during procedure with verbal and tactile stimulation. Provide toys to hit or throw. *Safety* Same as for infant. *Note:* Secure anchoring of IV site is essential for this age group. Use restraints minimally, since they may provoke increased fear and protest. Tape all IV connections and secure IV equipment out of reach, to avoid choking hazard. Assess IV site a minimum of every 2 hours.

Table continued on following page

Table 27-5

Developmental Stages of Childhood *Continued*

Age Group	Developmental Characteristics	Child's Response to Illness or Procedures	Preparation of Child	Family Involvement	Nursing Implications
Preschool (4–6 years)	Initiative vs. Guilt Exhibits general interest and fears mutilation. Makes decisions, seeks companionship. Able to follow directions. *Preoperational thoughts:* "Magical thinking." Egocentric. Animalistic. Short attention span. *Fears* Bodily injury. Loss of control. The unknown, the dark, and being alone.	Illness or pain often perceived as punishment. Needs support to cope with intrusiveness of IV procedure. Curious about IV but able to keep from touching with frequent reminders. May appear compliant but may be withdrawn and resistant.	Give control when possible; child should be active in decisions. Explain procedure in simple terms. Explain relationship between cause, illness, and treatment (IV is not a punishment). Prepare just prior to procedure. Use equipment to teach (with dolls and stuffed animals). Encourage assistance by child (open Band-aids, cleanse area). Explain that holding still is a big help and that it is "O.K. to cry." Never bribe or threaten ("If you don't drink, you'll get an IV.") Praise cooperation. Maintain privacy.	Parents should provide comfort and support but should not help restrain. Child may be more cooperative if parent is *not* present.	*Safety* Same as for toddlers. Needs minimal restraints; needs maximum mobility to master surroundings. Address fears and misconceptions even if not expressed. Allow child to identify with you. Understand resistance as fear and reassure. Do not participate in discipline of child.
School Age (6–12 years)	Sense of Industry Enjoys learning. Struggles between mastery and failure. Wants to participate. Needs to know how things work. Concrete Operational Thinking Understands rules and directions. Ability to understand relationship between illness and treatment. Increased awareness of danger. Improved concept of time. Increased self control. Peer group increasingly important. *Fears* Body mutilation. Loss of control. Inability to live up to expectations of others. Death.	Important for child to feel a sense of control. May interpret illness as a punishment. Does not accept illness because of fear of death. Develops "magical" sense of denial (healthy for age).	Prepare several hours in advance. Use diagrams, models. Explain each step. Offer choices as much as possible. Allow child to help. Reassure that crying is "OK." Reassure that you will help him or her to hold still. Games can be effective to gain cooperation. Give immediate tactile and verbal praise for cooperation. Provide distraction during procedure.	Parents present at child's choice. Prepare family and child together. Encourage family to arrange for peer visitation. Stress to parents child's need for independence with self care. Parent can be "silent partner" in helping child understand.	Provide privacy. Allow child to assist with procedure. Offer encouragement and praise for cooperation. Allow child to assist with recording intake/output. *Safety* Impulsivity and playfulness may lead to accident—remind child frequently of safe mobility with IV equipment connections. Provide distractions. Keep security objects close by. Allow as much mobility as possible.

Age	Developmental Characteristics	Response to Illness/Hospitalization	Preparation	Nursing Interventions	
Adolescence (13–19 years)	Sense of Identity Vacillates between dependence and independence. Questions authority figures. Strong need for privacy. Formal Operational Thought Able to understand abstract ideas. Able to consider alternatives. Little understanding of how body works. Peer acceptance important. Fears Loss of control. Altered body image. Separation from peers.	Hyper-responsive to pain; minor illness magnified. Regresses to lower developmental stage of behavior. Resistant to parent and authority figures. May be noncompliant with medication and treatment plan. Increased need for peer contact. Illness is threat to body integrity. Disease = ugliness.	Offer choices. Preparation several hours to days in advance is vital. Explain using adult terms. Show equipment, and explain function and allow time for questions.	Direct explanations to adolescent while parent is present. Reassure family of need for adolescent to participate and make decisions. Explain therapy as to an adult patient. Encourage family to bring friends.	Approach with sensitivity; adolescents react to "how" it is said rather than "what" is said. Provide privacy. Tolerate need to have "own stuff." Encourage to record own intake and output. Engage to help set up equipment. Set consistent behavioral limits, but allow some leeway in choices (e.g., if you want to take a shower now, I can start your IV later). Allow to wear own clothes. Safety May need supervision to ensure safety of IV site if "clowning around." Teach adolescent to report observations about IV. Monitor equipment; may tamper with pump rates.

infants, the IV equipment should be weighed before venipuncture, and that amount should be subtracted from the total weight obtained. Calculations for fluid replacement are based on the percentage of weight lost; the amount of fluid restriction is based on the amount of weight gained.[3, 5]

Vital Signs (see Table 27–6)

Temperature. Body temperature may initially be elevated during dehydration but becomes subnormal as the dehydration progresses. With each degree of rise or fall in body temperature, the basal metabolic rate increases. This increase in basal metabolic rate results in additional fluid and caloric maintenance requirements of 10 to 12% over maintenance requirements (see Table 27–4). Upon admission to the hospital or home health care agency, a baseline body temperature should be assessed. In many health care settings, the traditional method of using the rectal route has often been replaced by safer methods of body temperature recording. Rectal temperature assessment has the potential risk of perforating the wall of the rectum. This method is definitely contraindicated in conditions such as thrombocytopenia, neutropenia, and imperforate anus or postrectal surgery.[6] Oral temperature measurement should be assessed on children over 2 years of age who are cognitively able. More recently, devices that measure tympanic temperature in the ear may be used; these devices are very quick and comfortable but are accurate only if the probe fits well in the ear canal (usually in children older than 1 year of age). Axillary temperature measurements are frequently obtained in children up to 4 to 6 years of age or in any child who is uncooperative, unconscious, seizure prone, or has had recent oral surgery. The normal axillary temperature range is 36.5 to 37.0 C (97.9 to 98 F).

Pulse. The apical pulse is the best site for auscultation of the heart rate in an infant and child. Normal apical ranges for an infant are 120 to 140 beats per minute. As the child grows older, the heart rate decreases to adult values of 60 to 80 beats per minute. An apical rate in a resting infant of 80 to 100 beats per minute is considered to be bradycardia, and an apical rate of greater than 160 to 180 beats per minute is considered tachycardia. Changes in rate and rhythm may indicate changes in circulating blood volume or electrolyte imbalances. In the early stages of volume depletion, the pulse is usually tachycardiac and becomes more rapid, weak, and thready as the condition worsens. The pulse bounds during fluid overload.

Evaluations of the presence and the quality of peripheral pulses as well as the adequacy of end-organ perfusion are key elements in the clinical assessment of shock in children. The carotid, axillary, brachial, radial, femoral, dorsalis pedis, and posterior tibial pulses are all easily palpable in the healthy child. A discrepancy between the central (apical) and peripheral pulses may result from vasoconstriction associated with hypovolemia or may be an early sign of diminished stroke volume. The pulse volume is directly related to blood pressure. As shock progresses, the pulse pressure (systolic − diastolic = pulse pressure) narrows, resulting in a weak and thready pulse that may eventually become impossible to palpate. The rate of tachycardia also increases as the condition worsens. In septic shock or fluid overload, the pulse pressure widens and is represented by a bounding pulse.[7]

Respirations. The normal range of respiration in the infant is 30 to 60 breaths per minute, and the respiratory rate falls slowly during the toddler stage to near adult levels. An infant with a respiratory rate above 60 respirations/minute is generally considered to be tachypneic. Apnea is defined as a 15- to 20-second or longer period without respiration. The infant's respiratory rate may be increased in either fluid depletion or fluid overload. Alterations in respiratory rate may represent inadequate oxygenation or an attempt to compensate for metabolic acid-base imbalances (i.e., respiratory rate is increased in acidosis and is decreased in alkalosis). The child who is hyperventilating either from anxiety or from a disease process is likely to develop respiratory alkalosis.

The breath sounds as well as the rate should be noted when respirations are assessed. Moist breath sounds (rales) may be an indication of fluid overload.

Blood Pressure. Changes in blood pressure (BP) may be indicative of a change in circulating blood volume. In fluid volume deficit, the BP is usually decreased. When a fluid volume overload exists, the BP is generally elevated. In infants and children, however, the BP should *not* initially be relied on as an accurate measurement of shock. Normal BP may be maintained as the circulatory system compensates with vasoconstriction, tachycardia, and increased cardiac contractility. The other assessment signs discussed, including skin color, temperature, fluid volume, quality of peripheral pulses, mental status, heart rate, and urinary output, are the best status indicators. Hypotension occurs late and often suddenly, indicating a sign of cardiovascular decompensation. Once even a slight drop in BP occurs, it must be treated seriously because cardiopulmonary arrest often soon follows.[7]

To accommodate the various sizes of children, BP cuff sizes range from newborn to adult. To obtain an accurate reading, the appropriate sized cuff should be used. The width of the BP cuff should be sufficient to cover 75% of the upper arm between the top of the shoulder and the olecranon. There should be enough room in the antecubital fossa to accommodate the bell of the stethoscope. The length of the cuff must completely surround the circumference of the limb with or without overlapping. Sites other than the brachial artery that can be used to obtain a BP measurement include the radial, popliteal, dorsalis, pedis, and posterior tibial arteries.[5]

If an electronic BP monitor is used, the manufacturer's instructions and guidelines for correct cuff size should be followed. Even with an oscillometric device, movement interferes with the accuracy of measurement. The child should be quiet and the extremity stabilized during the procedure.

A listing of normal pediatric vital signs is provided in Table 27–6.

Skin

Skin color, turgor (elasticity), temperature, moisture, and texture all relate to the child's state of hydration and nutrition. With fluid volume deficit, the skin tends to be cool and dry and exhibits poor color return when pressure is gently applied to skin. Cyanosis and mottling usually occur in more advanced stages of fluid deficit. If fever is also present, the skin may be warm and moist. Assessment of skin turgor is generally a good indicator of fluid volume status. Skin turgor

Table 27–6

Pediatric Vital Signs (Normal Values)

Age	Heart Rate/Minute	Respiratory Rate/Minute	Blood Pressure Systolic	Blood Pressure Diastolic	Temperature Celsius	Temperature Fahrenheit
Infants	120–160	30–60	74–100	50–70		
Toddlers	90–140	24–40	80–112	50–80		
Preschoolers	80–110	22–34	82–110	50–78		
School-aged Children	75–100	18–30	84–120	54–80		
Adolescents	60–90	12–16	94–140	62–88		
Any Age						
Oral					36.4–37.4	97.6–99.3
Rectal					36.2–37.8	97–100
Axillary					35.9–36.6	96.6–98

From Testerman EJ. Current trends in pediatric total parenteral nutrition. J Intravenous Nurs 1989; 12(3):152–162.

is assessed by gently grasping the skin on the abdomen or inner thigh between the thumb and index finger and then quickly releasing. Good hydration is exhibited by an immediate return of the skin to its normal position. Fluid deficit may be present when the skin remains suspended for a brief period of time (called "tenting") after being released.

Usually, the skin begins to demonstrate some sign of tenting with mild (<5%) fluid deficit. However, tenting is not consistently a reliable sign of hydration status. Variables such as hypertonic dehydration may be evidenced by doughy or rubbery skin, and conditions such as obesity, abdominal distention, and malnutrition may also affect the elasticity of the skin.[8]

Edema is a sign of fluid volume overload or fluid shift from the intravascular space to the interstitial space. In infants, edema is most noticeable in the periorbital and scrotal areas, especially after the infant has been lying flat for a period of time. Occasionally, the eyes are so puffy that vision is impaired or eyelids are even swollen shut. As the child grows up, the locations of visible edema shift to the abdominal areas and extremities. The presence and severity of edema can be assessed by indenting this skin with a finger and then releasing. The severity is indicated by the indentation (pitting) left by the finger.

End-organ perfusion is assessed via the skin, brain, and kidneys. Decreased perfusion in the skin is an early sign of shock. In healthy white children, the hands and feet are pink, warm, and dry. As cardiac output decreases, the most distal extremities become cool. In African-American children and children of other cultures, a grayish pallor may be indicative of poor perfusion and decreased temperature. As the condition progresses, the coolness advances toward the trunk. After the skin is blanched, a slow capillary refill (>2 seconds) indicates low cardiac output. Poor perfusion is also indicated by mottling, pallor, and peripheral cyanosis, except in newborns, who normally have acrocyanosis. Severe vasoconstriction is represented by pallor in older children and grayish color in newborns.[7]

Mucous Membranes

Moistness of the mucous membranes provides information regarding the hydration status of a child. Dryness of the mucous membranes occurs early in dehydration. The area of the mouth where the gums and cheek meet is often the best place to assess moistness because it remains moist, even during mouth breathing. Longitudinal fissures on the tongue are an indication of dehydration, as is lack of tears in an infant older than 3 months of age. The lack of tears and the presence of dark circles around sunken eyes are signs of dehydration that occur later in the progression of the condition.[5, 8]

Fontanelles

The anterior fontanelle remains open until the child is approximately 2 years of age. This characteristic provides an additional tool with which the hydration status of infants can be assessed. When an infant is in a normal sitting position, the anterior fontanelle is either completely flat or slightly sunken. In states of fluid deficit, the fontanelle is depressed. A bulging fontanelle indicates increased pressure caused by either cerebral edema or fluid volume excess.

Urine

An accurate record of urinary output is an important element in the management of fluid balance. Urine output that is greater than or less than the intake suggests a fluid excess or deficit. The time, amount, and color of urine as well as its specific gravity should be documented in the medical record. The frequency of monitoring of urine output (ranging from every hour to every 8 hours) is determined by the seriousness of the child's condition. In fluid homeostasis, 1 to 2 ml of urine output per kilogram of body weight per hour is expected.

A specific gravity value between 1.002 and 1.030 is usually an indication of fluid balance. Fluid restriction or deficit is reflected by a high specific gravity, whereas a low measurement reflects fluid retention or overload. In young infants, however, the immature renal system is less able to concentrate urine, causing the results of the measurement to be less accurate. This fact should be considered when specific gravity results are assessed; a normal measurement of specific gravity in an infant with fluid volume deficit may be misleading.[5]

Children who are toilet trained present little difficulty in the monitoring of their urine output. Often, parents and older children can assist in the recording of the time and the amount. Children who are not toilet trained present the nurse with a greater challenge. Pediatric urine collection containers are available; however, they are not easily applied and can be irritating to the skin. When hourly output records are necessary in critical care units, the child usually has a ureteral or urethral catheter in place. In pediatric units, the usual practice is to weigh the diapers. The weight of the dry diaper is subtracted from that of the wet diaper, allowing the nurse to determine urinary output. The weight in grams equals the volume voided in ml. A simple way to keep track of pre-soiled diaper weights is to write the weight on the clean diaper before placing it on the child. With this method, should another caregiver change the diaper, the comparison weight is readily available.

Urine can be obtained from a wet diaper by several methods. It can be aspirated directly from a wet diaper by using a syringe without a needle. However, ultraabsorbent disposable diapers, which contain a gel, can alter the results of some laboratory tests. If cloth diapers or ultra-absorbent disposable diapers are used, cotton balls or small gauze pads can be placed into the diaper. The urine can then be extracted by either aspirating the material with a needleless syringe or expressing urine with a gloved hand from the gauze or cotton ball into a container.

Neurologic Status

In young children, neurologic status is more difficult to assess than in adults. Developmentally, young children are unable to respond verbally to questions regarding orientation to surroundings. Changes in behavior or mood, such as hyperirritability when touched or refusal to drink fluids, may indicate a change in the child's neurologic status. A child older than 2 months of age should be able to normally focus on his or her parent's face and be attracted by bright visual objects. Failure to recognize parents may be an early sign of hypoperfusion to the brain. The family is usually the first to detect this but may only be able to interpret this change as "something wrong." A usual sign of neurologic involvement in the infant is a high-pitched cry. Changes in the level of consciousness may be an indication of fluid volume or electrolyte imbalance. Infants are more sensitive to excess sodium concentrations in the blood (hypernatremia) and abruptly demonstrate signs of lethargy, somnolence, and hypersensitivity to noise and touch. Twitching, tremors, or convulsions may be noted in more advanced cases. Cerebral edema caused by fluid retention can be displayed by vomiting, restlessness, irritability, and even convulsions, as well as complaints of headache in older children.[5, 8]

Physician's Assessment and Orders

The nurse responsible for administering IV infusions to an infant or child must communicate bedside assessments to the physician and/or primary healthcare provider (e.g., nurse practitioner). The young patient has a narrower fluid balance range in which to tolerate any infusion errors stemming from miscommunications or a change in patient status. Therefore, open, ongoing communication between the nurse and primary healthcare providers is necessary to convey observations that may change the treatment plan.

Before an infusion is initiated or continued in an infant or child, the nurse should review the orders. These orders should be written legibly and should include the following:

Date order is written
Time order is written
Duration and frequency of infusion
Type of solution (in standard notation)
Rate of infusion in milliliters per hour
Amount of each additive per volume of solution
Physician/nurse practitioner signature
Cosignature of nurse reviewing order

FLUID VOLUME DEFICIT

Depletion of fluid in the extracellular and intracellular compartments can result from any abnormal fluid loss or reduction in fluid intake. The commonest cause of fluid loss in children is gastroenteritis. Children with diarrhea accompanied by nausea or vomiting are at a greater risk for developing dehydration. In these children, oral fluid intake is reduced and cannot balance the amount of fluid lost through the stools. A deficit of fluid volume results, and physiologic changes occur that progress as the condition worsens (Table 27–7).

Hypovolemic shock is a common problem in children who are in need of emergency care. Trauma and burns are obvious causes, but hypovolemic shock can also occur with gastroenteritis and diabetic ketoacidosis. Sepsis in a child can develop into septic shock, which is not classified as hypovolemic but equally requires fluid resuscitation. The initial therapies for hypovolemic and septic shock are similar, and both require immediate vascular access. In traumatic shock, large volumes of blood and fluid are required; therefore, the largest practical gauge and shortest IV needle should be inserted. The establishment of at least two IV lines is also recommended.[7]

The clinical assessment and the laboratory data determine the urgency and the type of therapy required. The degree of fluid loss is categorized according to the percentage of total body weight lost: mild (<5%), moderate (5 to 10%), and severe (>10%).

The infusion of IV fluids into infants and children with fluid volume deficit requires an understanding of the various types of deficit as well as the specific therapies required. Fluid volume deficit (dehydration) is categorized as isotonic, hypotonic, or hypertonic, depending on the changes in the child's serum sodium.

Isotonic

Isotonic fluid volume deficit is the commonest form of dehydration. In this form, the loss of solute and the loss of water are proportional. Dehydration is also considered isotonic when the losses are not proportional but the kidneys are able to compensate. Because the net fluid loss is isotonic, no redistribution between the intracellular fluid and the extracellular fluid occurs. The total loss is from the extracellular compartment, resulting in a reduction in plasma volume and circulating blood volume.

Correction of fluid and electrolyte imbalances is easily achieved in patients with this type of dehydration. Depending on the degree of severity of the imbalance, an initial bolus of 0.9% sodium chloride or Ringer's lactate solution may be

Table 27-7

Clinical Assessment and Infusion Treatment for Types of Fluid Volume Deficit (Dehydration)

Description	Isotonic	Hypotonic	Hypertonic
Type of Loss			
ICF and ECF fluid shift	Solute and water loss proportional	Greater solute loss than water	Greater water loss than solute
Plasma volume	None	From ECF to ICF	From ICF to ECF
Serum sodium level (mEq/L)	Decreased 125–150	Decreased <125	Maintained >150
Cause	GI fluid loss Urine loss Decreased oral intake	GI fluid loss with hypotonic oral intake (glucose in water, ginger ale)	GI fluid loss with hypertonic oral intake (boiled skim milk) Diabetes insipidus Fever Hyperventilation
Clinical Signs			
Skin	Poor turgor, cold, dry, dusky	Very poor turgor, cold, clammy, dusky	Fair turgor; cold, thick, and "doughy" skin
Eyes	Sunken	Sunken	Sunken
Mucous membranes	Dry	Slightly dry	Parched
Fontanelles	Depressed	Depressed	Depressed
Pulse	Rapid	Rapid	Moderately rapid
Blood pressure	Low	Very low	Moderately low
Neurologic status	Irritable or lethargic	Lethargic, coma, seizure	Hyperirritable, high-pitched cry, seizure
Fluid Replacement			
Resuscitation	Bolus of 0.9% sodium chloride or Ringer's lactate (20 ml/kg over 20 minutes)	Bolus of 0.9% sodium chloride or Ringer's lactate (20 ml/kg over 20 minutes)	None
Replacement	5% dextrose in water and 0.45% sodium chloride	5% dextrose in water and 0.9% sodium chloride If severely symptomatic, 3% sodium chloride (4 ml/kg over 10 minutes) with close monitoring	5% dextrose in water and 0.225–0.45% sodium chloride If hypertensive, 0.9% sodium chloride or Ringer's lactate solution (20 ml/kg) over 1 hour
Infusion	Half of deficit replaced in first 8 hours, remaining over next 16 hours	Half of deficit replaced in first 8 hours, remaining over next 16 hours	Slow and gradual over 48 hours
Sodium (mEq)	2–3 mEq/kg/24 hours	2–3 mEq/kg/24 hours plus replacement. Sodium should only be increased ≤ 2 mEq/L/hour up to a serum level of 120 mEq/L	Sodium should not be reduced >2 mEq/L/hr
Potassium	2–3 mEq/kg/24 hours	2–3 mEq/kg/24 hours	2–3 mEq/kg/24 hours

ECF = extracellular fluid; GI = gastrointestinal; ICF = intracellular fluid.

administered at 20 ml/kg of body weight. An infusion of maintenance fluids follows the bolus.

Hypotonic

Patients with hypotonic dehydration have a net loss that is hypertonic, that is, the loss of sodium is greater than the loss of water. This situation causes the extracellular fluid to shift into the intracellular space, where the fluid is less hypotonic. This phenomenon occurs most frequently when a hypotonic solution (glucose in water, ginger ale) is given orally to the child in an attempt to replace fluid lost through vomiting or diarrhea. The sugar is taken up by the cell and leaves the free water in the extracellular space. The child exhibits more severe signs and symptoms of deficit in hypotonic dehydration than in the other forms of dehydration.

Treatment for this type of dehydration is similar to that for isotonic dehydration, except that extra sodium is added. With the addition of this sodium, the dehydration changes from hypotonic to isotonic. Maintenance fluids and replacement fluids for ongoing losses are administered in a similar fashion to therapy for isotonic dehydration. In severe cases of hypotonic dehydration, the child is treated with 3% sodium chlo-

ride solution, which is administered until the plasma level reaches 120 mEq/L. Hyponatremia should be corrected slowly, raising the serum sodium level no greater than 2 mEq/L/hour.[4]

Hypertonic

Hypertonic fluid volume deficit has a proportionately greater loss of water than sodium; the net loss of fluid is hypotonic. Because of the hypertonicity of the extracellular fluid, the fluid in the intracellular space shifts out of the cell into the extracellular space. Circulating blood volume remains relatively stable. Oral fluids with a high concentration of sodium (i.e., boiled skim milk) fed to an infant with diarrhea, diabetes insipidus, fever, and hyperventilation can all cause hypertonic dehydration.

Classic signs present in a child with hypertonic dehydration include doughy skin, irritability, high-pitched cry, and seizures. Subarachnoid and subdural hemorrhage may occur in more severe cases. Hyperglycemia and hypocalcemia are often associated with this type of dehydration.

Rehydration is performed slowly—rapid rehydration can lead to serious neurologic complications, including seizures.

If the child is hypertensive, an infusion of 0.9% sodium chloride or Ringer's lactate solution is infused over 1 hour (20 ml/kg of body weight). If the child is not hypertensive, a hypotonic solution (0.225 to 0.45% sodium chloride in 5% dextrose) with added potassium is infused. The calculated fluid deficit is infused over 48 hours.[4, 8]

FLUID THERAPY

Maintenance Fluid Requirements

Maintenance fluid requirements for a 24-hour period are based on the child's weight in kilograms. The regimen for normal maintenance fluids is based on water and electrolyte output via insensible fluid losses, gastrointestinal fluids, and urine. Because the metabolic rate in infants and children is higher than that in adults, the fluid losses are greater than in adults, and maintenance requirements are increased. The amount of fluid lost before treatment is determined by comparison of pre-illness and current weight and by clinical signs of deficit. Maintenance fluid requirements for children are usually calculated by the following formula:

Newborn (0 to 72 hours)	60 to 100 ml/kg/24 hours
0 to 10 kg	100 ml/kg/24 hours
11 to 20 kg	1000 ml for first 10 kg + 50 ml/kg/24 hours for each kilogram over 10 kg
21 to 30 kg	1500 ml for first 20 kg + 20 ml/kg/24 hours for each kilogram over 20 kg

Example
Fluid maintenance for a 14-kg infant would be 1200 ml/24 hours:

Formula

$$\frac{1000 \text{ ml (for first 10 kg)} + 200 \text{ ml (50 ml} \times 4)}{1200 \text{ ml/24 hours}}$$

Once the 24-hour maintenance fluid requirement has been calculated, the need for additional fluids must be evaluated. Conditions in which fluid requirements are increased include fluid loss before treatment (e.g., gastroenteritis), increased metabolism (e.g., fever, hyperthyroidism), concurrent losses (e.g., wound drainage, nasogastric suction), or the need to dilute urine (e.g., before chemotherapy).[5, 8]

Replacement (Deficit) Therapy

Replacement therapy is divided into phases. The first phase is the initial or rapid delivery of fluid therapy; the second phase, the repletion or maintenance therapy; and the third, the early recovery.

Phase I: Initial Management

In children with fluid volume deficit, replacement of vascular volume is essential. These children require immediate infusion of fluids, especially when evidence exists of poor tissue perfusion or changes in vital signs and neurologic status. The presence of these symptoms or those associated with moderate-to-severe dehydration indicate the need for rapid fluid management.

A crystalloid solution (Ringer's lactate solution or 0.9% sodium chloride), 20 ml/kg, is infused as rapidly as possible over 20 minutes. If the child has a documented normal blood glucose level or is known to have diabetes, the dextrose solution should be omitted to avoid hyperglycemia, which may induce an osmotic diuresis. Otherwise, Ringer's lactate solution is preferred because it avoids hyperchloremic acidosis, which may result from the infusion of large volumes of sodium chloride. The child's condition is then reassessed. If the response to the therapy is poor, an additional bolus of the initial solution is given. The child continues to be evaluated for the need of additional boluses, invasive monitoring, or the implementation of repletion (maintenance) therapy.[4, 8]

The type of initial volume expansion for a child in hypovolemic shock is controversial. Crystalloid solutions are readily available, less expensive, and free from reactions and complications that can occur with blood and colloid products. Crystalloids expand the interstitial water space and replace sodium effectively; however, they are not efficient at expanding the circulating blood volume. Blood and colloids, such as 5% albumin, fresh frozen plasma, and dextran, are much more effective at expanding the circulating blood volume than crystalloids. The major disadvantage to these products is the cost and the risk of potential transfusion reaction or complication. Therefore, an initial bolus of 20 ml/kg is given, usually with a crystalloid solution. If further boluses are required, either a crystalloid or colloid solution may be given. Based on reassessment of the child's condition, repeated boluses are administered as needed. According to the *Textbook of Pediatric Advanced Life Support*,[7] a child with hypovolemic shock often requires at least 40 to 60 ml/kg in the first hour of resuscitation, and occasionally, up to 100 to 1000 ml/kg may be needed in the first few hours. In children with septic shock, at least 60 to 80 ml/kg is often required in the first hour. Frequent reassessment of the child's condition and infusion of sufficient amounts of fluid are the key to successful fluid therapy for hypovolemic shock.

Phase II: Repletion and Maintenance Therapy

During this phase (2 to 24 hours after onset of the deficit), replacement is combined with maintenance requirements. Acid-base and electrolyte disturbances are partially corrected. The following simple formula incorporates both replacement and maintenance requirements for mild, moderate, and severe volume deficit.

Amount of Deficit	Formula for Calculation of Amount of Fluid
Mild (5%)	Maintenance + (maintenance × 0.5)
Moderate (10%)	Maintenance + (maintenance × 1.0)
Severe (15%)	Maintenance + (maintenance × 1.5)

Example

A 10-kg infant has a maintenance fluid requirement of 1000 ml/24 hours. The replacement amount for 24 hours would be

Mild (5%)	Maintenance + (1000 ml × 0.5) 1000 + (1000 × 0.5) = 1500 ml/24 hours
Moderate (10%)	Maintenance + (1000 ml × 1.0) 1000 + (1000 × 1.0) = 2000 ml/24 hours
Severe (15%)	Maintenance + (1000 ml × 1.5) 1000 + (1000 × 1.5) = 2500 ml/24 hours

Note: The amount of fluid infused during the initial phase of replacement should be subtracted, and any ongoing losses sustained should be added to these amounts.

Phase III: Early Recovery

Early recovery, which can last from 24 to 96 hours, is aimed at correcting the remaining deficits occurring in hypertonic dehydration. These electrolyte deficits need to be corrected slowly so as not to impair neurologic status. Usually, by this time, the child is well enough to ingest some fluids orally.

OTHER INTRAVENOUS THERAPIES

In addition to administration of fluids, IV devices in children are also used for such therapies as medication administration, parenteral nutrition, and transfusion of blood products. An overview of these therapies as they relate to children is provided in this section; please refer to other chapters in this manual for additional information on transfusion therapy and parenteral nutrition (see Chapters 10 and 12).

Medication Administration

The most frequently used methods of calculation for pediatric medication administration are those based on body weight and body surface area (by use of a nomogram). Dosing of pediatric medications is usually recommended in terms of body weight, such as doses in milligrams per kilogram. This method is most frequently used to calculate drug dosages for infants and children. (See Chapter 19 for more details on IV dose calculations.)

Techniques

All methods of IV medication administration, such as IV bolus and intermittent and continuous infusion, are used in the pediatric patient. In children, however, the dose and volume can be different from those used in adults, depending on the age and the size of the child. In neonates and infants, medications are commonly calculated to the tenths of a milligram or milliliter. Continuous infusions are used primarily for replacement of fluid volume and nutrition, for administration of drugs that require maintenance of a steady blood level, or for administration of potent drugs that must be highly titrated to individual needs.

Intermittent infusions can be administered by several different methods. The in-line calibrated chamber is commonly used in general pediatric settings. The medication is injected into the in-line calibrated chamber and infused at a prescribed rate. At the completion of the infusion, the usual practice is to flush the chamber with 10 to 20 ml (depending on tubing volume) of the IV solution or a solution of 5% dextrose in water or 0.9% sodium chloride. The advantage of this method is simplicity; however, several disadvantages to this technique exist. This method is not practical for small infants whose infusion rates are slow. The drug must also be compatible with the primary solution, or a second tubing setup is required. Finally, flushing the chamber with a certain volume of solution is often not enough to clear the chamber from medication remnants, or it provides too much volume for the patient to tolerate.

The method of retrograde infusion is practiced both in the general pediatric area and in the neonatal intensive care units. A specific retrograde administration set is required for this purpose. The tubing volume varies but generally holds less than 1 ml. A three-way stopcock or access port is at each end of the tubing. The retrograde tubing is attached and primed along with the primary administration set. (Retrograde primary administration sets are also available.) The tubing functions as an extension set when it is not used to administer medication. To administer medications via the system, a medication-filled syringe is attached to the port most proximal to the patient, and an empty syringe is connected to the port most distal from the patient. The clamp between the port and the child is closed, and the medication is injected distally up the tubing (away from the child). The fluid in the retrograde tubing is displaced upward in the tubing into the empty syringe. Both syringes are removed, the lower clamp is opened, and the medication is then infused into the patient at the prescribed rate. The medication volume is then automatically incorporated into the regulated amount of fluid to be infused. This method is often used in infants or children who cannot tolerate a rapid infusion rate or additional fluid volume; in this method, the medication infuses at the same rate set for the IV infusion.

An increasingly popular and accurate method of IV medication administration in children is the syringe pump. The syringe pump can be connected via an extension set directly onto a heparin lock or in a "piggyback" fashion into the primary line. A syringe of diluted medication, prefilled by the pharmacy or by the nurse caring for the patient, is attached to microbore tubing, and the medication can then be infused at a prescribed rate. Syringe pumps have been discussed previously.

Parenteral Nutrition

IV nutrition is administered when patients cannot or will not use their gastrointestinal tract, or when they require supplemental calories for growth or healing. The goal of pediatric parenteral nutrition (PPN) is to meet anabolic needs as well as to provide for normal growth and development. Because the metabolic rate of children is greater than that of adults, children require greater fluid and caloric intake per kilogram (see Table 27–4). Some indications for PPN in children are congenital or acquired anomalies of the digestive tract, such as inflammatory bowel disease, Hirschsprung's disease, short-bowel syndrome, and pancreatitis, as well as possible disease states that may increase the risk of starvation, such as cancer, cystic fibrosis, and acquired immune deficiency syndrome. To identify potential candidates for PPN therapy, the following guidelines are used in conjunction with the physical examination and the nutritional evaluation:

- >5% weight loss
- Height/weight ratio below fifth percentile on growth chart
- Serum albumin level <3 g/dL
- Total lymphocyte count <1000/mm^3 (except in patients receiving chemotherapy)[9]

The parenteral nutrition solution is made up of several components, depending on the status of the child; these solutions can be individualized to fit specific pediatric calorie and nutrient needs. Table 27–8 lists the specific components of PPN.[10]

The amounts of electrolytes, minerals, and trace elements, as well as medications, are individualized for the growth and nutritional needs of each child. For children on long-term PPN, continued growth can change the nutritional requirements, so careful monitoring is essential. A difficult problem occurring in children is balance of fluid needs with calorie needs. A large volume would be necessary to infuse enough calories to meet the total needs of a child via the peripheral vein. Therefore, PPN is often concentrated in a smaller volume and is administered via a central vein. A concentration of greater than 10% dextrose must be delivered via a central venous catheter to avoid vein injury or extravasation, should infiltration occur. Fat emulsions or lipids provide a high-calorie content per volume, making them an ideal calorie source for the limited volume intake that can be tolerated by children.[9] Fat emulsions also buffer the irritating effects that glucose tends to exert on the vein. Lipids should be infused cautiously, however, in patients with infections, compromised renal function, or hyperbilirubinemia. In premature infants younger than 30 weeks of age with hyperbilirubinemia, lipid hydrolysis releases free fatty acids that can displace bilirubin from albumin and can increase the chance of kernicterus, or bilirubin encephalopathy. A smaller dose (1 g/kg/day) and a long infusion time (≥15 hours) tend to decrease this risk in premature infants.[9]

PPN can be administered in the hospital or the home; home PPN is usually administered via the central route and is cycled over 12 to 18 hours, usually at night, so that the child may function normally during the day. Home PPN is usually initiated in the hospital. When the child is stable and the education process for infusion of home PPN has been mastered by the caregiver or caregivers, with appropriate participation of the child (depending on his or her level of development), home PPN may be instituted.

Continuous monitoring is required to ensure safe, efficacious infusion of PPN that meets the changing needs of the child. This includes monitoring of the infusion itself and assessment of laboratory and nutritional parameters on a scheduled basis.

PPN has its share of complications, which, as demonstrated in Table 27–9, can be divided into metabolic and catheter related. A multidisciplinary team approach can result in successful clinical application and monitoring of PPN,

with a minimal number of complications. From the first documented success of infant PN in 1944,[11] on through the well-known efforts of Willmore and Dudrick in 1968,[12] the technique for infusion of nutrition via the venous system has been refined over the past 3 decades, greatly improving the quality of life and survival for children who undergo this therapy.

Transfusion Therapy

The basic principles of blood component therapy that apply to adults also apply to children (see Chapter 10). Children are unique with regard to maturation of their hematopoietic system and special requirements related to their smaller vein size and volume of blood products to be infused. During the last few weeks of intrauterine life, maternal gamma immunoglobulin (IgG) crosses the placenta into the fetus; therefore, the mother's serum is used for compatibility testing during the first few days of life. The fetus does not produce its own antibodies until it is exposed to foreign substances after birth. After about 1 week of life, or if the newborn underwent transfusion at younger than 1 week of age, serum from the baby is used for compatibility testing.[13] Other differences between children and adults include differences in blood volume (see Table 27–2), red cell life, and hemoglobin. The red blood cell of the premature newborn has a life span of 35 to 50 days, and the red cell of a term baby survives 60 to 70 days, compared with the red blood cell in an adult, which lives 100 to 120 days.[14] At birth, infants have a high percentage of hemoglobin F, or fetal hemoglobin, which has such a high affinity for oxygen that release of oxygen into the system is hampered. The level of hemoglobin F declines rapidly after birth, and by 6 months of age, hemoglobin F is replaced almost entirely with hemoglobin A, or adult hemoglobin, which lets go of oxygen more rapidly. In premature infants, persistence of hemoglobin F can result in hypoxia and respiratory distress. Interestingly, because hemoglobin A is a beta-chain molecule, beta-chain defects, such as sickle cell anemia and the beta thalassemias, were until recently not detected until 3 to 6 months of age; now, with genetic testing, earlier diagnosis of these disorders is possible.[13]

Specific indications for transfusion therapy are similar to those of adults and are outlined in Chapter 10. General indications for pediatric transfusion therapy include acute hemorrhage, anemia, abnormal component function (either congenital or acquired), and the presence of toxic substances, such as caused by a decrease in bilirubin levels by exchange transfusion. The most commonly used products for transfusion in children are packed red blood cells and platelets. Acute hemorrhage can be defined as reduction of blood volume by 30 to 40%, or a 20% blood volume loss with chance for recurrence. A 30% blood loss may be linked with systolic blood pressures as follows:[15]

- <65 mm Hg in children < 4 years of age (normal = 75 to 110)
- <75 mm Hg in children 5 to 8 years old (normal = 85 to 120)
- <85 mm Hg in children 9 to 12 years old (normal = 95 to 135)
- <99 mm Hg in adolescents (normal = 100 to 150)

Table 27-8.

Components of Pediatric Total Parenteral Nutrition

Component	Use	Deficiency	Recommended Daily Dose	Complications
Water	Vehicle for delivery of nutrients. Helps meet daily requirements.	Fluid deficit—decreased skin turgor, decreased weight, decreased tears, decreased CVP, lower temperature, increased heart rate, increased respirations.	< 10 kg, 100–150 ml/kg > 10 kg, 1500–2000 ml/m²	Fluid excess, dilutional hyponatremia.
Calories	Meet energy needs to promote growth and development (anabolism).	Catabolism—negative nitrogen balance, negative growth and development.	< 10 kg, 100–120 cal/kg > 10 kg, 2000 cal/m²	
Glucose (1 g = 3.4 kcal)—most important macronutrient	Maintain positive nitrogen balance (anabolism). Preferred energy source for CNS and RBC.	Protein catabolism, negative nitrogen balance.	< 10 kg, 20–30 g/kg > 10 kg, 25–30 g/kg	Phlebitis, diuresis, hyperglycemia, hypoglycemia, hyperosmotic, hyperglycemic nonketotic acidosis.
Protein (1 gm = 4.0 kcal) Essential: lysine, leucine, isoleucine, methionine, phenylalanine, threonine, tryptophan, valine arginine, histidine Nonessential: proline, alanine, serine, tyrosine, glycine, cystine	Growth and tissue synthesis. Provides energy if shortage of glucose and fat occurs. Buffer in the extracellular and intracellular fluids.	Kwashiorkor: edema, anemia, fatty degeneration of liver, scaling dermatitis, infection confirmed by serum transferrin. Marasmus: adipose and skeletal muscle atrophy, weight loss, depressed skin test reactivity to antigens, lethargy, dehydration. Mixed disorder: kwashiorkor and marasmus.	< 10 kg, 2–3 g/kg > 10 kg, 1–2 g/kg	Azotemia, hyperammonemia, abnormal plasma aminograms, hepatotoxicity.
Fats (1 gm = 9 cal) Components: soybean or safflower oil Fatty acids: linoleic, palmitic, oleic, steric acid, egg yolk, phospholipids, glycerol	Energy—prevent fatty acid deficiency and provide concentrated caloric source.	Mild diarrhea, dry and thickened desquamated skin, hair loss, brittle osteoporotic bones, thrombocytopenia.	0.5–4.0g/kg	Altered pulmonary function, deposition of pigmented material in macrophages, kernicterus, coronary artery disease, spurious hyperbilirubinemia, spurious hyponatremia. Adverse reactions: fever, chills, shivering, pain in chest or back, warmth, vomiting.
Insulin	Regulates serum glucose level.	Hyperglycemia.		Hypoglycemia, hypokalemia.
Potassium	Tissue synthesis. Transports glucose and amino acids across cell membranes. Regular heart rhythm. Nerve impulses.	Fatigue, drowsiness, decreased muscle tone, GI obstruction, flatulence, paresthesias.	2–4 mEq/kg	Hyperkalemia, tissue sloughing and necrosis if infiltration present, hypokalemia, cardiac arrhythmias.
Chloride	Acid-base balance.	Excessive sweating, diarrhea, clouded sensorium, hypotonicity of muscles, tetany, decreased respirations.	< 10 kg, 3 mEq/kg > 10 kg, 2–4 mEq/kg	Hyperchloremia, hypochloremia, metabolic acidosis or alkalosis.
Sodium	Fluid balance. Acid-base balance. Nerve impulses.	Abdominal cramps, diarrhea, increased heart rate, apprehension, decreased blood pressure, cold clammy skin.	3–5 mEq/kg	Hypernatremia, febrile response, hyponatremia, phlebitis.
Calcium	Clotting mechanism. Muscle contractions. Neuromuscular activity.	Numbness, paresthesias, tetany.	20–40 mg/kg	May cause tissue sloughing if infiltration occurs, hypercalcemic syndrome.
Magnesium	Metabolism of carbohydrates and protein, enzyme activity, nerve conduction.	Convulsions, tremors, increased blood pressure, increased heart rate, muscle cramps.	0.25–0.5 mEq/kg	Magnesium intoxication, impaired kidney function, flushing, sweating, hypotension, respiratory paralysis, hypothermia, hypocalcemia.
Folic acid	Cellular growth and development.	Megaloblastic anemia.	< 10 kg, 0.2 mg > 10 kg, 0.2 mg	Allergic reaction.

Table continued on following page

Table 27–8.

Components of Pediatric Total Parenteral Nutrition *Continued*

Component	Use	Deficiency	Recommended Daily Dose	Complications
Phosphates	Decrease paresthesias. Regulate calcium metabolism.	Muscle weakness, malaise, paresthesias, CNS irritability, confusion, seizures, obtundation, coma.	2–3 mEq/kg	Reciprocal hypocalcemic tetany, hyperkalemia with potassium compound, phosphate intoxication.
Acetate	Prevents acidosis.	Acidosis	1–6 mEq	Alkalosis.
Vitamin A	Prevents retardation of growth/visual adaptation.	Night blindness, xerophthalmia, pyoderma, mucosal carotenization, drying of skin, lowered resistance to infection.	1400 IU	Acute and chronic toxicity, anaphylaxis. Overdose: nausea, vomiting, anorexia, drying skin and lips, malaise, irritability, headache, loss of hair.
Vitamin B_1 (thiamine)	Absorption of protein and carbohydrates.	Peripheral neuropathy, deep tendon reflex increase or absence, muscle tenderness, muscle atrophy, fatigue, decreased attention span, beriberi.	0.3 mg	Warmth, pruritus, nausea, urticaria, weakness, sweating. Hypersensitivity reaction.
Vitamin B_2 (riboflavin)	Absorption of protein and carbohydrates.	Cheilosis: lip inflammation, oral fissures, seborrheic dermatitis, corneal vascularization. Ocular disturbances: itching, burning, corneal inflammation, dryness, dim vision, conjunctival redness, photophobia.	< 10 kg, 0.4 mg > 10 kg, 1.1 mg	
Vitamin B_3 (niacin)	Absorption of protein and carbohydrates.	Weakness, lassitude, anorexia, oral inflammation, indigestion, responsive dermatitis, irritability.	< 10 kg, 5 mg > 10 kg, 12 mg	Toxic reactions: decreased glucose tolerance, skin rash, elevated uric acid levels, postural hypotension, flushing.
Vitamin B_5 (pantothenic acid)	Absorption of protein and carbohydrates.	Possible symptoms: malaise, headache, nausea, vomiting, fatigue.	< 10 kg, 5 mg > 10 kg, 10 mg	
Vitamin B_6 (pyridoxine)	Absorption of protein and carbohydrates.	CNS disorders, sideroblastic anemia, greater tendency to develop deficiency with vitamin B_6 antagonists isoniazid, penicillamine, semicarbazide, cyclosporine.	> 10 kg, 0.3 mg > 10 kg, 0.3 mg	Paresthesia, somnolence, low serum folic acid levels.
Vitamin B_7 (biotin)	Absorption of protein and carbohydrates.	Fine-scale skin desquamation, anemia, anorexia, nausea, lassitude, muscle pain.	< 10 kg, 0.3 mg > 10 kg, 0.3 mg	
Vitamin B_{12} (cyanocobalamin)	Absorption of protein and carbohydrates.	Pernicious anemia, glossitis, neurologic symptoms, constipation.	< 10 kg, 0.3 μg > 10 kg, 1.5 μg	
Vitamin C	Wound healing.	Scurvy, hemorrhagic petechiae, gingivitis, slow wound healing.	< 10 kg, 35 mg > 10 kg, 40 mg	Large doses: diarrhea, renal stones.
Vitamin D	Promotes absorption of calcium and phosphorus	Osteomalacia, low serum calcium level, low serum phosphate level, elevated alkaline phosphatase level, tetany due to hypocalcemia, rickets.	< 10 kg, 400 IU > 400 kg, 35 IU	Weakness, headache, dry mouth, somnolence, nausea, vomiting, constipation, muscle pain, bone pain, metallic taste. Hypercalcemia, hypercalciuria, hyperphosphatemia.
Vitamin E	Protects red blood cells from hemolysis. Enhances vitamin A. Suppression of platelet aggregation.	Anemia, excessive creatinuria, skeletal muscle lesions, increased platelet aggregation.	< 10 kg, 4 IU > 10 kg, 9 IU	
Vitamin K	Promotes synthesis of active prothrombin.	Prolonged prothrombin, bleeding, hematuria.	< 10 kg, 1.5 mg > 10 kg, 2.5 mg	Anaphylaxis, pain and swelling at IV site, flushing, kernicterus.

Table 27-8.

Components of Pediatric Total Parenteral Nutrition *Continued*

Component	Use	Deficiency	Recommended Daily Dose	Complications
Chromium (trace mineral)	Glucose utilization and metabolism and pheripheral nerve function.	Insulin-resistant diabetes, neurologic changes (neuropathy).	0.14–0.2, µg/kg	Hypersensitivity, overdosage.
Copper (trace mineral)	Formation of transferrin, and RBC and white blood formation.	Anemia, leukopenia, neutropenia.	< 10 kg, 20 µg > 10 kg, 300 mg	Hypersensitivity, overdosage.
Manganese (trace mineral)	Activator for enzymes.	Weight loss, transient dermatitis, occasional nausea and vomiting, changes in hair color.	2–10 µg/kg	Hypersensitivity, overdosage.
Molybdenum (controversial, trace mineral)	Unknown (part of enzymes).	In humans: impaired amino acid utilization. In animals: growth retardation, dental caries.		Hypersensitivity, overdosage.
Selenium (trace mineral)	Protects cells from oxidative damage.	Muscle dysfunction (including cardiac muscle changes), muscle pain.		Hypersensitivity, overdosage.
Zinc (trace mineral)	Facilitates wound healing. Skin hydration, senses of taste and smell.	Scaling pustular rash, periorbital and nasolabial dermatitis, alopecia, change in taste or smell acuity, diarrhea, depression.	< 10 kg, 300 µg/kg > 10 kg, 5 mg	Hypersensitivity, overdosage.

From Testerman EJ. Current trends in pediatric total parenteral nutrition. J Intravenous Nurs 1989; 12(3):152–162.
CNS = central nervous system; CVP = central venous pressure; GI = gastrointestinal; IV = intravenous; RBC = red blood cell.

Hemoglobin and hematocrit values are considered less reliable indicators of blood loss. Activity level and cardiopulmonary status should be assessed before transfusion therapy is initiated in a child, because an unstressed child can tolerate hemoglobin levels of 3 to 6 g/dL without signs of heart failure or tissue hypoxia. Children usually undergo transfusion if hemoglobin levels fall below 6 g/dL.

Thrombocytopenia can result from maternally induced causes (e.g., aspirin ingestion during pregnancy), from acquired disorders (e.g., idiopathic thrombocytopenic purpura), from chemotherapy, or from congenital dysfunction of platelets. Platelet transfusions are indicated when bleeding time is longer than 15 minutes and/or the platelet count is less than 20,000/µl with active bleeding, less than 5000/µl with or without active bleeding, or less than 50,000/µl before surgery.[13]

Rarely is one whole unit used for a pediatric transfusion. Blood products are usually administered in increments of milliliters per kilogram that are based on body weight and estimated blood loss. Packed red blood cell dosage is 10 to

---

Table 27-9

Complications of Pediatric Total Parenteral Nutrition

Metabolic	Catheter Related	
	Central	*Peripheral*
Electrolyte imbalance	Bacterial or fungal sepsis	Sloughing of skin
Acid-base imbalance	Plugging or dislodgment	Phlebitis
Glycosuria	Local skin infections	Local infection
Hepatic disorders	Thrombosis of major vessel or embolism (vena cava syndrome)	
Cholestasis	Improper placement	
Postinfusion hypoglycemia	Hemorrhage	
Essential fatty acid deficiency	Extravasation of fluid	
Hyperlipidemia	Pneumothorax	
Hyperammonemia	Hemothorax	
Bone changes (demineralization)	Perforation and/or infusion leaks (pericardial, pleural, mediastinal)	
Trace element deficiency	Hydrothorax	
Azotemia	Arterial puncture	
Vitamin disorders	Brachial plexus injury	
Abnormal plasma aminograms	Catheter embolism	
Decreased pulmonary diffusion	Air embolism	
Eosinophilia	False aneurysm	
Bleeding	Cardiac arrhythmia	
Adverse reactions to components		
Anemia		

From Testerman EJ. Current trends in pediatric total parenteral nutrition. J Intravenous Nurs 1989; 12(3):152–162.

15 ml/kg; platelet dosage is 1 U (50 to 70 ml) per 7 to 10 kg of body weight.[16] Transfusion equipment is similar to that for an adult; differences for children include use of smaller gauge needles for transfusion (27-, 25-, or 23-gauge winged-steel needles or 22- or 24-gauge catheters). Studies show that 27-gauge needles can be used to give packed red cells at a rate of up to 50 ml/hour without significant hemolysis.[17] Packed red blood cells are not usually diluted with saline; rather, a saline flush is given through the IV line to avoid mixture of red cells with incompatible fluids that may cause hemolysis. In-line blood filters are used, which may be specially designed low-volume filters for children. In some cases, small aliquot bags or syringes of blood are transfused; these products are usually prefiltered by blood bank personnel during transfer to the smaller container. For accuracy, blood products are usually infused via an electronic infusion pump approved for use with blood and blood products. The rate of infusion for packed red cells is initially 5 to 10% of the total transfusion volume, given over 15 minutes.[13] If no adverse reaction is noted, the rate is then increased to 2 to 5 ml/kg/hour or as tolerated. Platelets are given by IV bolus or IV infusion over 30 minutes to 4 hours.[16] During transfusion, vital signs and monitoring parameters are similar to those recommended for adults. In addition, small infants should be monitored for cold stress and hypoglycemia, as well as for hypocalcemia. These reactions can occur because of the temperature of the blood product or the presence of a preservative in the blood, which can affect calcium and glucose levels. Another consideration in young infants is provision of blood that does not contain cytomegalovirus. Although adults may also contract cytomegalovirus, infants who contract it suffer much greater consequences that can lead to death.[18]

Immunosuppressed pediatric patients, such as premature infants and children with malignancies, end-stage renal disease, or acquired immune deficiency syndrome, are at risk of developing graft-versus-host disease if they receive transfusions of blood products that contain lymphocytes. Graft-versus-host disease can be avoided by giving these children transfusions with blood products that are rendered leukocyte poor, either by irradiating the product or by filtering or washing the cells before transfusion. Other transfusion reactions and complications are described in the chapter on transfusion therapy (see Chapter 10). Documentation of transfusion in children is similar to that used with the adult patient.

Exchange Transfusion

A type of therapeutic transfusion modality used almost exclusively in neonates and infants is exchange transfusion. The commonest indication for exchange transfusion is hemolytic disease of the newborn, which is caused by ABO or Rh incompatibility. Hemolytic disease of the newborn caused by ABO incompatibility occurs when a mother with blood group O carries a fetus with blood group A or B, resulting in anti-A or anti-B maternal antibodies crossing the placenta and causing hemolysis of fetal red cells and mild-to-moderate anemia. This phenomenon can occur in the first child; it is not usually severe enough for exchange transfusion but instead can be treated with phototherapy or a single transfusion of red cells. In hemolytic disease of the newborn caused by Rh incompatibility, an Rh-negative mother carries an Rh-

positive fetus. (The father must be Rh positive for this to occur.) At delivery, Rh-positive cells enter the mother's blood stream, and Rh antibodies form in the mother. With subsequent Rh-positive pregnancies, these anti-Rh antibodies can cause hemolysis of fetal red cells that is severe enough to require exchange transfusion. This disorder rarely occurs anymore because it is preventable by the administration of anti-D immunoglobulin within 72 hours of delivery, abortion, or miscarriage. A baby born with hemolytic disease of the newborn caused by Rh incompatibility has moderate-to-severe anemia and can rapidly develop high serum bilirubin (unconjugated or indirect) levels, which may cause kernicterus or deposits of bilirubin in the brain tissue.

The goals of exchange transfusion are to correct anemia, lower bilirubin levels in the serum, and remove sensitized erythrocytes. Exchange transfusion is considered when bilirubin levels increase more than 1 mg/dL/hour, or when they reach 15 to 16 mg/dL in the premature neonate or 20 mg/dL in the full-term infant. During exchange transfusion, part or all of the infant's blood volume is removed and replaced with plasma and red blood cells from one or several compatible donors. A two-volume exchange is usually performed, which replaces about 85% of the infant's blood volume and reduces the bilirubin level by about 50%. Albumin may be administered before the exchange to help bind bilirubin and increase the amount removed. One or two access sites, such as peripheral, central, or umbilical vessels, are used. Two sites are ideal, to allow simultaneous withdrawal and infusion of blood. Respiratory and cardiac status are closely monitored during the exchange, as is the potential for hypocalcemia and hypoglycemia. Complications of exchange transfusion include metabolic disorders, cardiopulmonary compromise, and catheter-related complications.

When transfusing a child, the child's and family's view of the transfusion, prior experience, and cultural and religious practices must be examined. Preparation should be age-appropriate, as outlined earlier in this chapter. With proper preparation and close monitoring and follow-up, IV nurses can ensure safe, efficacious transfusion therapy delivery to the pediatric patient.

PERIPHERAL ACCESS

Site Selection

Whether the prescribed therapy is infused via the central or peripheral route, the main goal of therapy is to provide the treatment with the maximum amount of safety and efficiency, while meeting the child's emotional needs and promoting his or her developmental tasks. The characteristics of the prescribed therapy and the patient's physical and developmental aspects are important when the intravascular site is chosen in a child.

Characteristics of the therapy itself to be considered include type and duration of therapy, rate of infusion, and expected site rotations. Physical considerations of the child include age, size, condition of the veins, reason for the therapy, general patient condition, and mobility of the child. Just as important, but often neglected, are the developmental considerations: level of activity (e.g., turns, crawls, walks); gross and fine motor skills (e.g., sucks fingers, plays with own hands, holds bottle, draws, and colors); sense of body image; fear of mutilation; and cognitive ability (i.e., understands and can follow directions).

The sites for peripheral IV site selection, as discussed pertaining to adults in Chapter 20, apply just as well to the pediatric patient. Although the anatomic location of the vessels are relatively the same in both children and adults, the child's smaller body and vessel size make it more difficult to successfully achieve access. The younger child, however, has the advantage of additional optional site locations, including the scalp and the foot. Along with the individual preference of the clinician, each site has its own characteristics and its own advantages and disadvantages. Table 27–10 lists peripheral IV site locations and associated advantages and disadvantages.

Peripheral Routes

Scalp

The use of the scalp vein for IV access in infants is controversial. The veins are readily visible and easily accessed, but the cannula can be more difficult to secure. Scalp vein infusions tend to infiltrate more easily, and if not detected immediately, can cause the infant's head to appear distorted. This phenomenon results from the lack of surrounding tissue (which would help absorb some of the fluid) on the scalp. This appearance is temporary, of course, but can be quite alarming to the family. The choice of the scalp for an IV line is often most traumatic for the parents. Removing the infant's hair is necessary for venipuncture. This practice not only interferes with parents' perception of their beautiful baby but can also interfere with their cultural beliefs and

practices. It is important to fully explain the procedure to the parents before proceeding with scalp vein access and to give the removed hair to them as a keepsake. Expectation of what the infant will look like once the scalp vein catheter is in place is important to include in the family teaching. To some parents, the visual impact of seeing a needle stuck into their baby's head is more traumatic than the reason for the treatment itself. Their lack of understanding can lead to additional anxiety and fear. Parents who do not fully understand the procedure commonly believe that the IV line is directly infusing into the child's brain.

Many pediatric and neonatal facilities choose the scalp vein as the preferred IV site (Fig. 27–1). The scalp IV site can be stabilized while the extremities remain free from restraints. The infant can play with his or her hands or suck his or her fingers without interruption. On a very tiny infant, the clinician monitors not only the IV line but also numerous other elements, such as oxygen saturation, cardiorespiratory status, and body temperature. Extreme care and very frequent site assessments must be made if irritating solutions, with the potential for causing extravasation injury, are infused via a scalp IV line. An injury in this area may cause lifetime disfigurement. In severely ill infants, placing the IV line in the scalp allows for maximum use of body space.

The superficial temporal, frontal, occipital, and preauricular veins of the scalp are most commonly used for IV access. Arteries are located near the veins and are sometimes hidden within the suture lines, which makes their pulsations difficult to feel. Scalp veins do not contain valves, a characteristic that reduces the risk of trauma to the vessel at insertion. Valves can obstruct the advancement of the IV catheter during insertion on a patient at any age.

The veins of an infant are fragile, especially the ones located in the scalp. Instead of a tourniquet, a rubber band

Table 27–10

Intravenous Sites in Children

Site	Patient Age	Veins Used	Advantages	Disadvantages
Scalp	Infant, toddler	Superficial temporal, frontal, occipital, postauricular, supraorbital, posterior facial	Easily visualized, readily dilates, no valves, hands kept free, head easily stabilized, allows accessibility to extremities	Hair must be shaved, arteries hidden, infiltrates easily, caudal disfigurement with infiltration, difficult to secure device, greater family anxiety
Foot	Infant, toddler	Saphenous, median, marginal, dorsal arch	Readily dilates, hands kept free, less rolling, more visible in chubby infants, easy to splint	Decreases mobility with walking, limited to smaller-gauge sizes, more difficult to advance cannula, near arteries, increased risk of phlebitis in older patients
Fingers	Toddler through adolescent	Digital	Useful if unable to access other sites, easily stabilized on tongue blade in older child	Infiltrates easily, limited to smaller gauge sizes, dependent edema masks infiltration, difficult to stabilize in small infant
Hand	All ages	Metacarpal, dorsal venous arch, tributaries of cephalic and basilic	Easily accessible, readily visible, large enough for larger size catheter, distal location, bones act as natural splints	Increased nerve endings means increased pain, difficult to anchor catheter on infant, interferes with child's activity
Forearm	All ages	Cephalic, basilic, median antebrachial	Same as for hand, keeps hands free	Difficult to visualize in chubby toddlers
Antecubital	All ages	Cephalic, basilic, median	Large veins visible and palpable, preferred site in infants	Elbow joint must be maintained in extended position, limits activity, limits sites for phlebotomy, limits sites for possible peripherally inserted central catheter placement

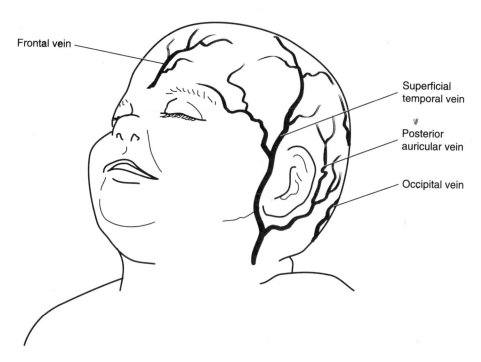

Figure 27–1. Scalp veins of an infant. These can be used as IV infusion sites.

with a piece of tape attached should be used as a tourniquet or pressure should be applied with the finger to distend the vein. During insertion, the needle or catheter should be aimed downward, toward the heart, so that the flow of the infusion can follow the same direction as the venous blood returning to the heart.

Scalp veins can be used in children as old as approximately 18 months, when hair follicles mature and the epidermis toughens.

Foot

This site is commonly used in children as old as 2 years. However, it is generally avoided in the child who has mastered walking. Several veins are highly visible and easily accessible. The most frequently accessed veins are the saphenous and median marginal veins and those of the dorsal arch. The curve of the foot, especially around the ankle, may make venous entry and catheter advancement difficult. The foot should be secured on a padded board, with its normal joint position maintained. Infants have great strength in their legs and kick their feet vigorously. The use of a sandbag to secure the extremity in place may assist in preserving the foot IV site.

Upper Extremity

As with adults, upper extremity sites are readily chosen for venous access in children. Similarly, the most distal part of the extremity is chosen first for access. The cephalic, median basilic, and median antecubital veins in the forearm are sometimes difficult to locate in children, especially chubby babies and toddlers. The veins of the hand, including the dorsal venous arch and tributaries of the cephalic and basilic veins, are generally easier to locate. The dorsal metacarpal veins are smaller but sometimes may be the only vessels visible in the hand.

Peripheral Access Devices

The guidelines for choosing the appropriate-gauge cannula are the same for children as for adults. Peripheral cannulas used in children range from 26 gauge to 21 gauge. Peripheral access devices are available from the manufacturers in various types and styles. Although personal preference for a certain type of device is a consideration, other factors, such as safety, patient comfort, type and length of therapy, and site of insertion are all important.

Winged-Steel Needle Set. This set is known also as a scalp vein needle or "butterfly" needle and is usually available in odd-number sizes from 27 to 19 gauge. Because these devices can easily become dislodged, causing injury to the child, they are best used for obtaining blood samples or for performing a one-time infusion of short duration. This set, once the only device available specifically for pediatric use, has been replaced by more contemporary types of peripheral venous access cannulas.

Over-the-Needle Catheter. These devices consist of a catheter over an internal stylet. They are commonly used in children for peripheral short-term or intermediate-term therapy. The gauge used depends on the child's age and vein size; most sites described previously accommodate this type of catheter, including scalp veins. Gauge sizes range from 26 to 14; the sizes most commonly used for neonates are 26 and 24 gauge, and for children, 24 and 22 gauge. Straight or winged-style catheters are inserted using the same technique; however, the winged-style may provide additional stabilization when the catheter is secured in place after insertion. Over-the-needle catheters are also available with built-in extension sets.

Peripheral cannulas are available in many materials, including polytetrathorethylene, polyurethane, and a polymer that softens and expands once it is in the vessel. The flexibility of over-the-needle catheters may add to the life span of the IV site. Peripheral IV sites should be rotated according to the *Intravenous Nursing Standards of Practice.*

Midline Over-the-Needle Catheter. This type of catheter is made of polyurethane or elastomeric hydrogel and is intended for use in patients who require therapy of intermediate duration, 2 to 6 weeks. It is inserted into a peripheral vein in the antecubital area and is advanced over a stylet into the upper arm veins. A commercially available variety of this cannula, made of elastomeric hydrogel, softens and expands once it is in the vein. Catheter care and site rotations for midline catheters are not specifically addressed in the current *Intravenous Nursing Standards of Practice.*[21] Manufacturers recommend infusing only isotonic and slightly hypertonic solutions and medications via midline catheters because the tip is still located in a peripheral vein. Because the midline catheter is still peripheral, site rotations related to peripheral cannulas still apply. More studies in children are indicated for this device.

Venipuncture

The actual method of venipuncture is the same for children as it is for adults. However, certain techniques facilitate successful venipuncture in a small infant or child. Peripheral IV access in children can be made easier by the following measures:

- Once the catheter is advanced into the vein and the stylet is removed, attach a small connector tubing and syringe that is prefilled with normal saline and flush a small amount into the vein. Correct position can be confirmed by nonresistant flushing and lack of evidence of swelling around the site at the tip of the cannula. The reason for this procedure is twofold. It confirms correct catheter placement, especially if a blood return was not present (in small infants, a blood return may not occur because of the size of the vessel and the gauge of the catheter), and it will keep the catheter from clotting before infusion is started.
- Collect laboratory specimens at the time of IV insertion, if possible, to prevent undue trauma and additional venipuncture.
- Surgical lubricating jelly works well as adhesive, helping to secure tape around a scalp IV. Apply a small amount under the tape. When you are ready to remove the tape, apply warm water and the tape will lift off easily.
- A flashlight or transilluminator device placed beneath the extremity helps to illuminate tissue surrounding the vein; the veins are then outlined for better visualization.
- Insert the cannula with bevel down. In very small veins, this can help in preventing puncture of the back wall of the vessel.
- Hold skin taut to cause less pain in the child and a smoother IV insertion.
- Spasms occur frequently in small veins; should "flashback" (blood return) cease, wait a second or two, then place a warm compress over the vein. Once the spasm stops, the cannula can be advanced.
- "Float" the IV cannula through the valves by flushing the catheter with normal saline solution as the cannula is advanced.
- Always have extra help.

- Padded tongue blades make excellent arm boards for little hands.
- Use rubberbands or ⅜-inch Penrose drains as tourniquets.
- If you are using the antecubital area, rotate the forearm while palpating. The tendon will roll, helping you distinguish the vein from the tendon.
- Wrap extremities in comfortably warm compresses before performing the venipuncture to assist in vein dilatation. (Commercially available warm packs or a warm, wet disposable diaper applied for 10 minutes works well.)
- Use stickers or drawings on the IV site as a reward.
- A stretch netting or a cut-off top of a sweat sock works well to protect the IV site or peripherally inserted central catheter site, especially for home IV patients.

Unlike adults, children fail to understand the need for venipuncture, may have a greater fear of pain, and generally do not hold still during the procedure. *Do not attempt to start an IV line on an infant or a young child without extra help or a passive restraint device.* Preferably, someone other than a family member is needed to assist with holding and positioning the child, as well as taping once venous access has been achieved. A papoose board or a tightly wrapped blanket around an infant (mummy wrap) serves well as a restraint during the procedure. Some clinicians secure the extremity to a padded board before performing the venipuncture. This technique aids with extremity stabilization during the procedure. Difficulties encountered during establishment of venous access in the infant or child include unsuccessful access at the first selected site, resulting in the need for the board to be removed and reapplied at the next attempted site; and active resistance from the child during the insertion, resulting in dislodging of the just-inserted catheter (often the tape is not strong enough to hold). With regard to local anesthesia before venipuncture, several options are available. Some institutions espouse the use of intradermal saline or lidocaine before venipuncture is performed in a child. The disadvantage to this practice is that an extra needle stick is involved. A eutectic mixture of anesthetic agents in cream form is now available for topical use 1 to 4 hours before the venipuncture is performed. Usually, the cream is applied to multiple sites in case the first attempt is unsuccessful. The length of time the cream must remain on the skin precludes its use in emergency situations.

The child's room is his or her "safe space." All attempts to start an IV line should occur in the treatment room or in an area separate from the child's room when possible. The need to explain the procedure and completely prepare the child and family was discussed earlier in this chapter.

Because venous access in children, especially in young infants, is limited, every effort should be made to decrease the number of venipunctures necessary. A highly recommended measure to reduce the number of additional punctures is to collect the necessary blood sample for laboratory tests at the time of venipuncture for the IV line. Once the blood sample has been collected, the catheter is flushed with 0.9% sodium chloride and connected to the prescribed therapy.

The challenge of pediatric IV therapy is not over once successful venipuncture has been established. Keeping the IV catheter securely in place in an infant or child can be more difficult than the initial insertion itself. Sterile transparent dressings or gauze protection are required to effectively maintain an IV catheter in place (Fig. 27–2); placing tape directly over the insertion site should be avoided. Clear plastic site protectors are available, but protectors can also be made simply by cutting a medicine cup or paper cup and lining the edges with tape. These protectors are secured over the site and help to prevent accidental dislodgement. Roller bandages should not be used to cover or secure the cannula site; the cannula site should remain readily visible for inspection. Although some IV complications, such as dislodgement and infiltration, are expected to occur in infants and children, careful securing of the IV device and frequent observation of the site can minimize these complications.

Dressing changes and site rotation follow the same standards as in the adult.[21] Limited venous access in the infant may result in the deferment of routine (every 48 to 72 hours) site changes. In *no* case should an IV line be left in place longer than 1 week. The condition of the site and the reason for not rotating the catheter must be documented in the child's medical record.

Restraints should be avoided if possible, but they are sometimes required to keep the IV catheter secure. Elbow restraints are preferred to arm restraints. The restraints can be muslin squares, with pockets to contain tongue blades, or tubular containers that have been padded and decorated creatively. Restraints are rarely needed on all extremities. Commercial restraints with Velcro closures are available, but a folded towel taped around an extremity works well also. Should clove-hitch restraints be used, caution must be taken to attach the restraint correctly and not impair the circulation to the extremity. In all cases, especially when restraints are used, site assessment should be completed and documented at least once every 2 hours.[21]

Heparin Locks Versus Saline Locks

In many adults, normal saline has replaced heparin solution for the maintenance of intermittent vascular devices. A recent study in children showed no significant difference in length of patency or reports of pain between saline and heparin solutions used for peripheral IV devices. However, these results cannot be applied to all subgroups (e.g., neonates) or all gauges of catheter.[22] In infants and children, caution must be exercised if normal saline is considered. Because of the tiny veins and small-gauge cannulas used in this population, clotting of the catheter can occur frequently. Often, in small infants, the catheter becomes clotted before it is completely advanced or connected to the IV tubing at insertion.

Effective heparin:saline ratios for maintaining the patency of peripheral IV lines range between 1 U of heparin per 1 ml of normal saline to 10 U of heparin per 1 ml of normal saline. Heparin solution that does not contain benzyl alcohol should be used in neonates weighing less than 1200 grams.

Complications

Complications related to IV therapy are discussed in detail in Chapter 24. Some complications occur more frequently or are more serious in the pediatric population. Because of children's small vessels and the smaller-gauge IV cannulas and the slow rates of infusion used in children, clotting of the catheter can occur more frequently than in adults. Because of the smaller vessels and the higher levels of activity in young children, infiltration can be a problem. In addition, as discussed earlier, fluid volume overload can be a serious complication in an infant and small child.

CENTRAL ACCESS

Central Venous Catheters

A central venous catheter (CVC) is a device whose tip is located in a central vein, defined by the *Intravenous Nursing Standards of Practice* as the subclavian, superior vena cava, and in children, the inferior vena cava.[21] Many catheter types and protocols for their care exist. Catheter type should be

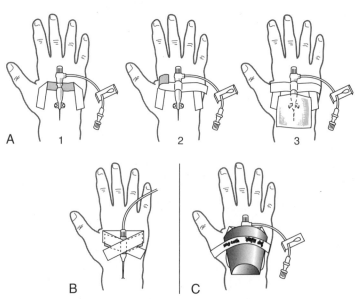

Figure 27–2. Taping techniques for keeping IV devices in place. *A*, Catheter. *B*, Butterfly needle.

based on the age and size of the child, his or her cognitive ability, the length of the therapy, the vein access, and body image considerations. Central catheters are usually considered when therapy is deemed necessary for longer than 2 to 3 weeks or when administration of hypertonic or irritating infusions is required.

Many controversies exist regarding flush protocols and dressing changes in central catheter care. Procedures described in the following section are based on manufacturers' recommendations and the current literature. Protocols should be based on this information as well as on catheter type and volume, fluid balance, and patient condition in both adults and children. More research is needed to substantiate uniform procedures that work for most patients.

Percutaneous Central Venous Catheters

Percutaneously placed central venous catheters are single or multiple lumen and are generally made of polyurethane. These catheters are placed directly into the superior vena cava by way of the right or left subclavian or the internal or external jugular veins. The femoral vein, with the catheter tip in the vena cava, is also a site utilized in pediatric patients. However, in the child who is still in diapers, use of the femoral area may result in an increased risk of infection. For percutaneously placed central venous catheters, jugular veins are the site of choice for neonates and infants, whereas subclavian entry is used in children.

Catheter volume:	Approximately 0.3 ml/lumen

Flushing Schedule

Intermittent (before and after medication administration):	3 ml of 0.9% sodium chloride followed by 1 ml of heparin solution (10 to 100 U/ml)
After blood infusion or withdrawal:	5 to 10 ml of 0.9% sodium chloride followed by 1 to 3 ml of heparin solution (10 to 100 U/ml)
Maintenance:	1 to 3 ml of heparin solution (10 to 100 U/ml) every 8 to 24 hours
Advantages:	Intended for short-term treatment, inpatient or outpatient insertion, usually secured with sutures, can be used for either intermittent or continuous infusion, access without needle stick to child.
Disadvantages:	Limited placement time, requires aseptic dressing change, daily heparinization is required, disturbance in body image, cost of maintenance and supplies.

Peripherally Inserted Central Catheters

The peripherally inserted central catheter is a thin, single- or double-lumen catheter inserted via a breakaway or peel-away introducer. Sizes used in children include 2, 3, and 4 French. These catheters are inserted peripherally into one of several sites, including the basilic, cephalic, and median cubital veins of the antecubital fossa. In newborns and small infants, other choices include the large saphenous vein, the superficial temporal vein, the external jugular vein, the popliteal vein, and the axillary vein.[19]

Catheter volume:	0.04 to 0.15 ml (depending on manufacturer)

Flushing Schedule

Intermittent (before and after medication administration):	2.5 ml of 0.9% sodium chloride, followed by 1 to 2 ml of heparin solution (10 to 100 U/ml)
After blood infusion or withdrawal:	5 to 10 ml of 0.9% sodium chloride, followed by 1 to 2 ml of heparin solution (10 to 100 U/ml)
Maintenance:	1 to 2 ml of heparin solution (10 to 100 U/ml) once or twice daily
Advantages:	Inserted at medical facility or in the home, longevity of catheters (weeks to months), accessed without needle stick to patient
Disadvantages:	Cost of maintenance supplies, disturbance in body image, child and family must learn catheter care, x-ray needed to confirm tip placement

Tunneled Catheters

Surgically placed tunneled catheters are single- or multiple-lumen catheters made of silicone elastic with one or two Dacron polyester cuffs. An example of this type of catheter is the Broviac catheter. These catheters are surgically tunneled under the skin of the chest into the superior vena cava. An alternate site is the inferior vena cava, with the catheter tunneled to the abdomen, thigh, or back.

Catheter volume:	1 ml or less (pediatric size)

Flushing Schedule

Intermittent (before and after medication administration):	3 ml of 0.9% sodium chloride, may be followed by 2 to 5 ml of heparin solution (10 to 100 U/ml)
After blood infusion or withdrawal:	5 to 10 ml of 0.9% sodium chloride, followed by 2 to 5 ml of heparin solution (10 to 100 U/ml)

Maintenance: 2 to 5 ml of heparin solution daily to weekly

Advantages: Reduced risk of bacterial migration after tissue adheres to Dacron cuff or cuffs, inpatient/outpatient placement, longevity of placement (months to years), clean dressing technique used, repair of catheter possible, easily accessed by patient, access without needle stick to patient, child may swim in chlorinated pool after several weeks, depending on immune system status, site healing, and physician order

Disadvantages: Daily-to-weekly flushing required, disturbance in body image, child and family must learn catheter care, catheter is at risk for accidental removal or breakage if child is very active

CLOSED TIP, PRESSURE VALVE

Another type of surgically placed tunneled catheter is a single-lumen or multilumen silicone catheter with a closed tip and a two-way sensitive pressure valve at the proximal end. The backflow of blood into the catheter is prevented when the valve is closed. The valve opens for infusion into the venous system or for blood aspiration that is dependent on the application of positive or negative pressure. An example of this type of catheter is the Groshong catheter.

Catheter volume: Approximately 1 ml or less

Flushing Schedule

Intermittent (before and after medication administration):   5 ml of 0.9% sodium chloride

After blood infusion or withdrawal: 5 to 10 ml of 0.9% sodium chloride

Maintenance: 5 ml of 0.9% sodium chloride every 7 days

Advantages: Same as for cuffed tunneled catheter, daily heparinization not required, reduced risk of air embolism, reduced risk of clot formation, no clamping needed, easily repaired

Disadvantages: Disturbance in body image, surgical procedure required, child and family must learn catheter care, potential for accidental removal

Implantable Port

An implantable port is also surgically placed and tunneled. It has a totally implanted metal or plastic dome that contains a self-sealing injection port. An implanted port may be sutured to the chest wall under the skin, and the catheter tip may be located in the superior or inferior vena cava. Alternately, another type of port can be implanted and positioned near the antecubital fossa in the arm. With the "arm" port, the catheter is threaded via the basilic or cephalic vein to the superior vena cava.

Reservoir volume: 0.33 to 1 ml

Flushing Schedule

Intermittent (before and after medication administration):   5 ml of 0.9% sodium chloride, followed by heparin solution (10 to 100 U/ml)

After blood infusion or withdrawal: 5 to 20 ml of 0.9% sodium chloride followed by 5 ml of heparin solution (10 to 100 U/ml)

Maintenance: 5 ml of heparin solution (10 to 100 U/ml) every 30 days or after each use

Advantages: Little site care and minimal flushing required, body image intact, longevity of placement (2 to 3 years), child may swim and bathe when needle is not in port, no catheter care required, low cost of maintenance supplies

Disadvantages: Skin pierced for access, pain associated with needle insertion unless topical anesthetic used, cost of surgical insertion and removal, possible displacement of port resulting from child's activity, vigorous contact sports (football, hockey) may not be allowed

OTHER INTRAVENOUS ROUTES

Umbilical Vein Versus Artery

The umbilical cord of the neonate provides an alternative route for vascular access. Because of the potential risks of complications associated with umbilical catheterization, it is reserved for emergency access in the delivery room and for hemodynamic monitoring in the neonatal intensive care unit. Three vessels are present in the umbilical cord: one vein (thin walled with a large-diameter lumen) and two arteries (thick walled with a small-diameter lumen). The goals of arterial catheterization versus venous catheterization differ, as do the techniques of insertion.

Because of its larger lumen, catheterization of the umbilical vein is easier than that of other veins. Although the vessel may be accessed during the infant's first 4 days of life, an umbilical venous catheter is usually inserted in the delivery room in an infant whose condition is compromised. The purpose of venous catheterization is primarily for emergency administration of medication and fluid, but central venous pressure measurement, venous blood sampling, and exchange transfusion are also accomplished through this line. The umbilical venous catheter is removed as soon as an alternative access route has been established, usually within 48 to 72 hours.

The main goals of arterial umbilical catheterization are (1) monitoring arterial pressure, (2) obtaining blood samples for arterial pH and blood gases, (3) performing aortography, and (4) performing exchange transfusions. Although parenteral infusion of medications and fluid can be performed via the arterial catheter, it is not the primary reason for this catheter's placement. Placement of an arterial catheter requires more time than venous cannulation and may not be the most appropriate choice for achieving access in an emergency.

With either umbilical access, aseptic technique is followed, with the operator, usually a neonatologist, scrubbed, gowned, masked, and gloved. Once the patient and equipment are prepared, the appropriate vessel is visualized, and a 3.5 or 5.0 French flexible, rigid-walled, radiopaque, umbilical catheter is advanced into the vessel. For venous catheterization, the umbilical catheter is introduced upward toward the liver for 5 to 8 cm or until a blood return is noted. The line is flushed with 1 ml of a heparinized solution and is secured in place by suture or tape. Tip placement is confirmed by x-ray before the catheter is used. In certain neonatal and delivery rooms, specially trained nurses are instructed in the technique of venous umbilical catheterization.

Before a catheter is inserted into one of the umbilical arteries, the proper catheter length must first be determined either by using a nomogram to estimate proper length or by multiplying twice the distance from the umbilicus to the midpoint of the inguinal ligament. The umbilical catheter is advanced 1 to 2 cm at a time until the required length of the catheter has been inserted. After arterial blood aspiration, the line is slowly flushed with 0.5 ml of a heparinized solution. The catheter is temporarily secured, pending verification of tip placement by radiologic examination. Appropriate catheter tip placement should be between L3 and L4. Once correct placement has been verified by x-ray, the therapy may proceed.[20] The umbilical artery catheter may be sutured in place, or secured with tape, or both.

Complications of umbilical catheterization include vascular compromise, hemorrhage, air embolism, infection, thrombosis, and vascular perforation. The risk of infection is greater with the venous catheter and becomes a significant hazard when the catheter is left in place more than 24 hours. The nursing assessment for potential complications of the newborn with an umbilical catheter should include the following:

- Frequently inspect lower extremities and buttocks for blanching or sudden cyanosis caused by spasm or embolism. Circulatory compromise may be observed initially in the toes; it then advances upward toward the buttock. The catheter should be evaluated and possibly repositioned or removed if lower extremity circulation is compromised. Occasionally, warming of the opposite extremity may result in improvement in circulation of the compromised limb.
- Monitor umbilical site frequently and ensure that the connections between attachments are secure.
- Monitor arterial waveforms. "Dampening," or alteration of waveforms from normal, requires re-evaluation of tip placement and line set-up.
- Closely monitor respiratory status and peripheral pulses and check for edema, which may indicate emboli formation.
- Monitor the umbilicus daily for signs of infection during the treatment and for 12 hours after catheter removal; provide routine cord care daily.

Intraosseous Routes

The intraosseous (into the bone) route is an important adjunct to emergency measures used in infant and child resuscitation. This technique, which is used by trained professionals (physicians, nurses, and emergency personnel), does not replace conventional methods of venous access. Instead, the intraosseous route provides immediate vascular access in emergency situations when access by the IV route is unattainable (i.e., after 5 minutes of attempts) and fluid or medication administration is essential to sustain life. The needle is inserted into the bone marrow (medullary) cavity of a long bone (Fig. 27–3). The solution injected into the bone marrow cavity is rapidly drained into the central venous channel and exits the bone into the systemic circulation via the nutrient and emissary veins.

The optimal sites for intraosseous needle placement in infants and children are the distal tibia, the proximal tibia, and the distal femur. The distal tibia is used with most reliability because of the flat area proximal to the malleolus and the thin covering of bony cortex. The proximal tibia, one to two fingerbreadths below the tibial tuberosity on the anteromedial surface, also works very well. As the child grows older, however, the cortex covering becomes tougher and can make penetration into the bone marrow more difficult. The distal femur is a larger bone to access, but it is usually padded more heavily with muscle and fat. The sternum is *never* used in children.

Lower extremities that have had recent fractures or trauma are to be avoided. Contraindications for needle placement also include skin areas with infected burns or cellulitis and bone disorders, such as osteoporosis or osteogenesis imperfecta.

In emergency situations, an intraosseous needle is not required; intraosseous infusions have been successful with the use of 16-gauge or 19-gauge straight needles. Certain needle features, however, are preferable and contribute to the success of insertion. These features include (1) a short shaft, (2) a stylet, (3) a sturdy needle, and (4) a handle. All of these

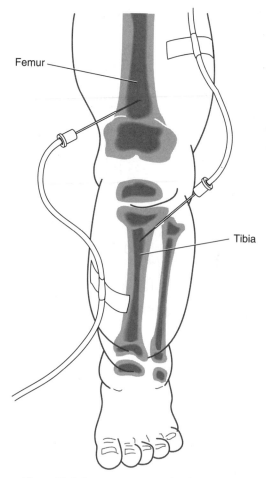

Femur

Tibia

Figure 27-3. Intraosseous access sites for IV infusion.

Osteomyelitis and sepsis, the complications that cause the greatest concern, are rare. When osteomyelitis does occur, the needle has been left in longer than 24 hours or the child had a previous case of bacteremia. Embolization of fat or bony fragments is a potential complication, but to date has not been reported.

The nursing responsibility regarding insertion of the needle varies from institution to institution. The primary role of the nurse is patient assessment, medication and fluid administration, and equipment monitoring.

ADMINISTRATION EQUIPMENT

Containers

Infants and children can have boundless energy and curiosity, which can result in the pulling and tugging of IV lines and IV poles. A plastic rather than a glass solution container should be used whenever possible to avoid breakage in case the container falls off its pole. To avoid the risk of fluid volume overload, the volume of the solution container should be based on the age and size of the child and should not contain greater than 500 ml of fluid.[21] In premature infants and neonates, smaller solution containers should be considered.

Administration Sets

The IV set-up for infants and children is different from that of adults in that flow rate requirements are minimal, necessitating proper choice of tubing. Precise infusion rates are required to avoid the possibility of medication overdose or fluid volume overload.

Microdrip tubing (60 gtt/minute) and microbore tubing are specific administration sets used for infants and children. IV tubing with an in-line calibrated volume control chamber (50-ml, 100-ml, and 150-ml sizes are available) should be used on all children whose prescribed fluid rate is less than 100 ml/hour.

Debate exists over whether this chambered IV set is required when an electronic infusion device is used. Manufacturers of electronic infusion devices may claim that their product is guarded against free-flow fluid. However, use of an in-line chamber constitutes an additional safety measure for monitoring and volume control and additionally provides a mechanism for medication dilution and administration.

Because acutely ill patients often need multiple therapies, extension sets with a three-way stopcock are frequently used in the critical care unit. However, on the general pediatric unit, such stopcocks can present concerns about infection and safety. In place of stopcocks, some institutions use multiple-arm connectors with two or more arms, each with its own clamp. These connectors provide a closed system for administration of multiple infusates via one IV site. In this case, consultation with pharmacy experts regarding compatibility issues is advisable.

Electronic Monitoring Devices

As discussed throughout this chapter, the nurse caring for the child undergoing infusion therapy has a grave responsi-

features are found on the commercially available intraosseous devices and on certain bone marrow aspiration needles.

The method of inserting the needle into the medullary cavity of a long bone and injecting a solution is both rapid and simple. The leg is restrained, cleansed with an antiseptic, and, in the awake child, 1% lidocaine is injected down to the periosteum. The needle is angled away from the joint space to avoid the growth plate, and it is introduced into the bone marrow with a downward screwing or boring motion, using firm pressure. Indications of proper placement include the feeling of a soft "pop" and a lack of resistance, the aspiration of bone marrow into a syringe, the needle standing upright without support, and a nonresistant flushing through the needle. Any standard syringe or IV administration set may be attached and medications or fluids infused by gravity or pressure. The rate of flow is regulated not necessarily by the gauge size of the needle but by the density and size of the bone marrow cavity. Medications as well as crystalloids and colloids can be administered via this route.

The intraosseous route is intended for short-term use only. Once resuscitation efforts have stabilized the patient, an alternative route of venous access must be used. Because of the risk of infection, the intraosseous needle should not be left in place for longer than 24 hours. The commonest difficulties encountered with the intraosseous technique are improper placement of the needle and needle obstruction from marrow.

bility to ensure that the prescribed treatment is delivered safely and effectively. Most complications occurring in infants and children are attributed to dosing or fluid administration errors. The nurse must possess the knowledge necessary not only to verify, calculate, and administer the therapy but also to accurately regulate the rate. The principles of safety and efficiency also apply to the home setting, where many children now receive their therapy intravenously. Today, infusion device technology is both sophisticated and simple. Ultratechnical devices found in critical care units can administer several infusions simultaneously or systematically, whereas small, portable, nonelectric infusion devices meet the needs of children at home. Infusion devices with an accuracy rate of 95% or greater are recommended for children.

Electronic infusion devices that assist with the regulation of fluid delivery are often used in infants and children. The volumetric controller operates under the same principles as gravity flow. These devices can regulate rate of flow and sound an alarm when the flow is interrupted. Volumetric controllers may manage fluid delivery in children; they control the flow rate and discontinue infusion when resistance is met. Volumetric controllers can be effective infusion devices for general pediatric use in older infants and in children who require infusion rates of 10 ml/hour or greater. This is a safety feature that is somewhat inconvenient because of the many occlusion alarms that occur from patient movement and activity. Unlike pumps, the controller stops infusing when resistance is met from an infiltration. The accuracy of the flow rate is reduced as the rate of the infusion is decreased. In addition, drop size varies from solution to solution, and therefore, volumetric accuracy may be compromised. This is an important consideration for neonatal and pediatric medication and fluid delivery. Dosage and flow rates in neonates and critical care patients are often in tenths of a milliliter per hour; therefore, accuracy is paramount. For this reason, and because of the need for additional pressure to override the higher intravascular pressure of small vessels and the resistance encountered with small-gauge catheters and microbore tubing, controllers may not be the best infusion device to use in children.

Infusion pumps are necessary in infants and children who require arterial lines, neonatal infusion, and infusion rates of less than 10 ml/hour or when large-volume infusions need to be administered over a short period of time. Pumps are available commercially in various styles and delivery options. Pumps are different from controllers in that they exert varying degrees of pressure when they meet resistance during infusion. Careful evaluation of pressure and alarm features is important when a device is chosen. Some pumps allow such high pressures that infiltration occurs without alarm. Considerations for the evaluation of pumps for pediatric use should include capability of the pump to infuse tenths of a milliliter, variable pressure limits, low alarm limits, ability to be programmed by milliliters per hour, and capability to be tamper proof.

Another type of volumetric pump used frequently in children is the syringe pump. This highly portable pump incorporates a syringe as the volume chamber to deliver the infusate. Most frequently, this type of pump is indicated in children for infusion of intermittent doses of medications, such as antibiotics. A syringe pump that has rate and volume

capabilities and can accommodate multiple-sized syringes (from 1 ml to 30 ml or larger) is most applicable for use in children.

Mechanical controllers, such as dial mechanisms on tubing, may assist with the regulation of flow rate; however, in the infant and child in whom flow rates are often only several

---

Table 27–11

Nursing Diagnoses and Desired Patient Outcomes in Children Receiving Intravenous Therapy

Nursing Diagnosis	Patient Outcome
Potential fluid volume deficit because of vomiting, diarrhea, burns, hemorrhage, wound drainage, or diabetic ketoacidosis.	The child's hydration status will demonstrate improvement by improved skin turgor, moist mucous membranes, stable weight, 1 mL/kg/hour of urine output, serum electrolyte values within normal limits. Oral fluids will be tolerated. Urine specific gravity will be between 1.000 and 1.010.
Potential fluid volume excess because of fluid overload, cardiac or renal disease, inappropriate secretion, or fluid shift.	The child's weight will return to pre-illness status, edema will decrease, vital signs will return to normal, and no audible rales will be present.
Potential alteration in sensory perception because of electrolyte imbalance, cerebral edema, or fever.	The child will respond appropriately for age (e.g, smile at parents, suck from bottle).
Potential impaired skin integrity because of diarrhea, edema, or dry skin.	The child's skin will be free of signs of breakdown, excoriation in diaper area will decrease, and skin turgor will return to normal.
Potential diversional activity deficit because of environmental lack of activity; frequent, lengthy treatments; or long-term hospitalization.	The child will participate in chosen activities and will express interest in surroundings and activity.
Potential fear because of separation from parent, unfamiliar environment, treatment, IV equipment, or normal developmental phobias.	The child will demonstrate reduced fear behaviors, e.g., crying, wide-eyed gaze, tension, or hiding.
Potential knowledge deficit because of lack of exposure, information misinterpretation, cognitive limitation.	The child and family will verbalize understanding of what was taught and will demonstrate ability to perform new skills.
Potential impaired physical mobility because of restraints and IV support boards and decreased endurance and strength.	The child will achieve maximum mobility within age and medical restrictions, no skin breakdown, no contractures, and maximum joint range of motion.
Potential altered nutrition resulting in less than body requirements because of nausea, vomiting, diarrhea, and inability to absorb nutrients.	The child will tolerate feedings via oral route, feeding tube, or IV line without side effects, gain ___ g/day, will experience an increased energy level, and will participate in diet decisions, if age appropriate.
Potential self-concept disturbance/ alteration in body image because of venous access device, illness, and effects of treatment (e.g., alopecia).	The child will participate in decision-making process about self-care, will take initiative to do tasks, will make eye contact, will interact freely with peers.
Potential altered patterns of urinary elimination because of fluid shift, diarrhea, inadequate intake, and chronic illness.	The child will have adequate output that is in balance with intake and will have urine specific gravity between 1.000 and 1.010.

Data from references 1, 3, and 5.

milliliters per hour, the accuracy of these devices cannot be guaranteed. In addition, these mechanisms often are accurate only when used in conjunction with larger-gauge IV devices. Complete manufacturer's information should be examined before these devices are used.

In the home, children are more mobile and active. The best infusion device is one that is portable, requires little or no programming, and is easy for the child and family to operate. Such systems include syringe pumps and positive-pressure devices. One such device is an elastomeric infusion device that incorporates a fillable latex balloon inside a plastic housing. This system eliminates gravity flow concerns and delivers antibiotic and chemotherapy infusions at a constant rate. Each system has a different delivery rate, based on the volume infused. Associated advantages to the child and family are that these devices come prefilled by the pharmacy, the set-up time is minimal, and the devices are small and lightweight, a characteristic that promotes ambulation. For school-aged children or adolescents, such devices can be hidden in their clothes or be carried in a user-friendly pouch.

For other infusion needs, ambulatory pumps are commercially available. Individual patient needs and family and clinician's preference determine which devices are best suited to the patient.

Examples of appropriate nursing diagnoses and desired patient outcome statements specific to the pediatric patient receiving IV therapy are detailed in Table 27–11. When documenting pediatric IV therapy, the care giver needs to include clinical information, such as size of catheter and patient response as well as desired outcome of therapy.

HOME INFUSION THERAPY

Home infusion therapy for the child is viewed as a positive alternative to hospitalization, but it certainly has its challenges for both the child and family, as well as for the professional team responsible for the family's care. After discharge criteria have been met, families and the child (if appropriate) begin education preparation for maintaining the prescribed IV treatment with their child at home. More so at home than in the acute care setting, the psychosocial and developmental needs of the child and family are an issue. The child may be returning to school and will need assistance on how to deal with the curiosity and remarks from peers. Return to a sport or other activity may be important to the child, and he or she will need help to do so. If siblings are in the home, they may feel neglected by their parents' attention to the child receiving therapy. Parents should be encouraged to spend private time with each of their children and to arrange for quiet, private time together. At home, parents do not have the security of the hospital unit nurses to rely on.

Alternate caregivers should be identified early in the process so that the parents can have respite periods.

The *Intravenous Nursing Standards of Practice* direct the practice of IV nursing in all settings in which IV therapy is delivered. Therefore, IV therapy services delivered in all environments are evaluated according to the same standards of practice. Individual policies and procedures in the home should be developed according to these standards.[21]

References

1. Whaley LF, Wong DL. Nursing Care of Infants and Children, 4th ed. St. Louis: Mosby-Year Book, 1991.
2. Merenstein GB, Gardner SL. Handbook of Neonatal Intensive Care, 2nd ed. St. Louis: Mosby-Year Book, 1989.
3. Hazinski MF. Nursing Care of the Critically Ill Child. St. Louis: CV Mosby, 1984.
4. Ichikawa I. Pediatric Textbook of Fluid and Electrolytes. Baltimore: Williams & Wilkins, 1990.
5. Mott SR, James SR, Sperac AM. Nursing Care of Children and Families, 2nd ed. Redwood City: Addison-Wesley, 1990.
6. Barrus D. A comparison of rectal and axillary temperatures by electronic thermometer measurements in preschool children. Pediatr Nurs 1983; 9: 424–425.
7. Chameides L. Textbook of Pediatric Advanced Life Support. Dallas: American Heart Association, 1988.
8. Barkin RM. Treatment of the dehydrated child. Pediatr Ann 1990; 19(10):597–603.
9. Hass-Beckert B. Removing the mysteries of parenteral nutrition. Pediatr Nurs 1987; 13(1):37–41.
10. Testerman EJ. Current trends in pediatric total parenteral nutrition. J Intravenous Nurs 1989; 12(3):152–162.
11. Helfrick FW, Abelson NM. Intravenous feeding of a complete diet in a child. J Pediatr 1944; 25:400.
12. Willmore DW, Dudrick SJ. Growth and development of an infant receiving all nutrients exclusively by vein. JAMA 1968; 203:860.
13. Rutman RC, Miller WV. Transfusion Therapy, Principles and Procedures, 2nd ed. Rockville, MD: Aspen Systems Corporation, 1985:179–183, 195–200.
14. Kelting S, Johnson C. Erythropoiesis and neonatal blood transfusions. Am J Matern Child Nurs 1987; 12:172–177.
15. Nathan D, Oski F, eds. Hematology of Infancy and Childhood. Philadelphia: W. B. Saunders, 1981:1491–1500.
16. Transfusion Therapy Guidelines for Nurses. National Blood Resource Education Program, Public Health Service, National Institutes of Health, US Department of Health and Human Services, 1990.
17. Herrera AJ, Corless J. Blood transfusions: Effect of speed of transfusion and of needled gauge on hemolysis. J Pediatr 1981; 99:757–758.
18. Yeager AS, Grumet FC, Hafleigh EB, et al. Prevention of transfusion acquired cytomegalovirus infections in newborn infants. J Pediatr 1981; 98:281–287.
19. Oellrich RG, et al. The percutaneous central venous catheter for small and ill infants. Am J Matern Child Nurs 1991; 16(2):92–96.
20. Sheldon RE, Dominiak PS. The Expanding Role of the Nurse in Neonatal Intensive Care. New York: Grune and Stratton, 1980.
21. Intravenous Nurse Society. Intravenous Nursing Standards of Practice. J Intravenous Nurs (suppl) 1990, S47.
22. McMullen A, Dutko-Fioravanti I, Pollack V, et al. Heparinized saline or normal saline as a flush solution in intermittent intravenous lines in infants and children. Am J Matern Child Nurs 1993; 18:78–85.

CHAPTER 28

Intravenous Therapy in the Older Adult

Beth Fabian, CRNI

● ●

● ●

As a result of the advances in medicine and the emphasis on good health and nutrition, the average life span is steadily increasing.[1] By the year 2000, over two thirds of the American population will be 65 years of age or older.[2] As the population ages, the medical community must attend to the special needs of the older adult. The term "older adult" describes a broad category that includes the 50-year old as well as the 80-year old because many physiologic changes associated with the older adult begin in the sixth decade of life. However, as with any age-related category, variations exist in individual physiologic responses that occur at any given age and in specific factors that influence these responses. These are important considerations to keep in mind when intravenous (IV) therapy principles related to this age category are examined.[3]

The older adult patient often requires administration of complicated IV therapies to treat multiple conditions that may occur simultaneously. In addition, when illness strikes, the older adult may be sicker for a longer time than a younger patient, requiring extensive technological, physiologic, and medical assistance.[2, 3] Therefore, considerations surrounding the initiation, delivery, and maintenance of IV therapies for the older adult are complex. As a result, an extensive clinical expertise and knowledge base are necessary for the IV nurse to competently evaluate and provide IV access for the older adult. The role of the IV nurse in the care of the older adult is anticipated to expand in the hospital, home, and alternative settings to meet the challenges of providing IV therapies to this population.

PHYSIOLOGIC CHANGES

The physiologic changes of aging are systemic and progressive, yet highly variable in each individual. Changes that occur in the skin, blood vessels, fluid balance, sensory systems, immune system, and mental status all affect the older

adult's response to IV therapy, and the IV nurse must be aware of these effects.

Skin

The skin is the first body system affected by venipuncture. The changes in the texture, depth, and integrity of the skin result from the natural process of aging as well as from the onset of certain disease states.[4] Changes that occur in the skin affect all layers of the skin, including the epidermis, the dermis, and the superficial fascia.[5]

The *epidermis* serves as a protective covering for the dermis. The characteristics of the epidermis may vary, depending on body location. For instance, the epidermis can be many layers thick over the palms and feet, and very thin over the inner arms. The epidermis is organized into 25 to 30 layers of dermal cells. The top one to five layers, called the *stratum corneum,* consists of overlapping cornified cells. The skin's normal resident bacteria flora exists beneath these overlapping epidermal cells.[4] Normal bacterial cell count can be 10,000 organisms/cm³.[6, 7] The outermost stratum corneum layer is composed of dead cells, which shed with contact friction. This layer will completely turn over every 1 to 4 days. The entire 25 to 30 layers of epidermal cells grow out from the basal layer up to the stratum corneum every 2 to 6 weeks.[7–9] A 30-year-old adult may lose and replace up to 45 cells per day. An older adult has a much slower turnover rate. After the age of 60 years, epidermal cell replacement may occur at a rate of only two per month.[2, 8] This slower rate can result in a marked thinning of the epidermis and an increase in the fragility of the skin.[9, 10] The thin epidermis results in a loss of skin moisture and resiliency. This dry, transparent, paper-thin tissue can tear and blister easily, it heals more slowly, it has decreased tolerance for ultraviolet light, and it has an increased tendency toward neoplasia.[2, 3, 7] The thinning cells have a slower rate of repair, resulting in delayed healing.[3, 9]

Beneath the epidermis lies the very vascular and sensitive layer of the *dermis.* The dermis consists of layers of connective tissue composed of collagenous fiber and elastic fiber. These fibers support the anatomic structures of blood vessels, nerves, glands, and hair follicles.[8] In the older adult, there is a decrease in the papillae, which hold the collagenous fibers to the epidermis.[7] This decrease results in a loss of stability in the epidermis and dermis. A decrease in the flexibility of the elastic fiber also occurs, resulting in a "loose" skin effect and wrinkles.[7, 9, 11] The aging process also results in a marked decrease in vascularity of the dermis. The skin becomes pale, and nerve endings lose their sensitivity.[7, 8] Because of this change, the older adult is at increased risk for hypothermia or hyperthermia as well as thermal skin injury.[3, 12, 13]

The subcutaneous connective tissue, or *superficial fascia,* lies below the dermis and acts as supportive tissue that contains many large superficial veins.[12] This layer is also affected by the aging process. The amount of subcutaneous fat decreases, especially in the extremities, and the production of sebum and sweat decreases.[7, 9]

Blood Vessels

The loss in dermal density that occurs with aging also affects the integrity of the blood vessels. The blood vessel changes can be as varied as the chronic diseases that affect the older adult population. In the older adult, arteriosclerosis and atherosclerosis occur, resulting in accumulations of lipid-containing materials as well as the thickening, hardening, and loss of elasticity of the walls of blood vessels. These changes may occur in the intima or the medial layers of the vessels and affect the vessels' ability to distend and contract.[9, 14, 15] Thickening of the intimal lining of the blood vessels results in a decrease in vessel lumen size, an increase in peripheral vascular resistance, a decrease in venous return and capillary refill, and ineffective venous valve actions.[4, 7, 8] Also, as the vein narrows and hardens, blood flow decreases and the circulatory system compensates by shunting more blood into smaller vein branches. These small, thin-walled, fragile surface capillaries are seen in the extremities and across the upper chest of the older adult.

Fluid Balance

Fluid homeostasis in the older adult is of significant concern. Fluid intake may not meet the body's demands, resulting in decreased saliva secretions, decreased absorption of calcium and vitamin B_{12}, decreased secretion of intrinsic factor, decreased peristalsis, increased constipation and diverticulosis. Additional factors affecting fluid homeostasis are decreased fiber intake and decreased exercise.[7, 8]

The changes that occur in the homeostatic organs that regulate fluid balance are also an important consideration in the evaluation of the fluid status of the older adult. For instance, the genitourinary system in the older adult shows a decrease in the number of nephrons, a marked decrease in blood flow, and a decreased ability to respond to stress that results from increased body needs in dehydration or fluid overload.[2, 8, 12] Renal changes result in the kidneys' reduced ability to concentrate and dilute urine in response to water or salt excess and to metabolize and excrete drugs.[8, 12, 15] Combine these factors with reduced cardiac efficiency, decreased vessel blood flow resulting from narrowing of the lumen, and uneven blood flow to the organs, and the older adult is precariously balanced between dehydration and fluid overload.[2, 3, 7, 8] The liver is also affected by a decrease in circulatory blood flow.[3] Medications that are metabolized in the liver and excreted by the kidneys may remain in the liver or kidneys for prolonged time periods resulting in potentially toxic drug levels.

The nurse must take all of these factors into account when preparing to initiate IV therapies in the older adult. For instance, IV rehydration must be performed with caution in the older adult because of the inability of this population to excrete fluids as rapidly as do younger patients. In addition, careful administration of salt-containing fluid is required for the volume-depleted older adult. If an excess of sodium is ingested, resulting in fluid overload, the kidney is less able

to compensate because of age-related changes.[16] Parenteral hydration should be considered only a temporary measure because of the associated risks of fluid imbalance in the older adult. When the underlying cause of fluid volume deficit is inadequate intake, then a program for ensuring adequate intake must be implemented.

Senses

Sensory deficits or disorders can also affect how the patient reacts and responds to the IV nurse and the delivery of IV therapies. In particular, the nurse must consider changes in vision, hearing, and tactile sensation when communicating with the older adult. Sensory deficits can dramatically affect older patients' understanding of procedures, their independence, and their ability to cooperate with prescribed therapies.[3] Therefore, these changes must be kept in mind so that a personal connection is established with the patient and successful IV therapies are administered.

The decreased visual and hearing acuity that occurs with aging affects the way nurses approach and instruct the older adult. Fifty percent of the legally blind population is over 65 years of age; therefore, vision may be impaired in many older adults.[7] Thus, the older adult must be aware of another person's presence either verbally or by touch. The nurse should look at the patient and speak slowly and clearly while facing the person directly.[14] Hearing is also often a problem in the older adult.[13] The nurse should be aware if the patient has a hearing aid or if visual story boards are needed to describe procedures. A clear, calm voice and a gentle touch carry a message of safety and reassurance.[14]

Tactile sensation is decreased and the skin is more susceptible to injury with aging. Infiltration may go unnoticed because of the skin's decreased integrity and loose skin folds.[8] A large amount of fluid may infuse subcutaneously before the patient experiences pain. Phlebitis may develop without pain but with significant vein inflammation resulting from the decreased sensitivity of the skin's nerve endings.[11, 15] Close monitoring of IV infusions, especially with potentially irritating medications, must be performed often because severe tissue necrosis, infection, or compartment syndrome can be the catastrophic result.[6, 11]

Immune System

As people age, their normal immune system changes by becoming hyporesponsive to foreign antigens and hyperresponsive to self.[7] These changes can result in decreased resistance to infection, increased incidence of cancers, and increased autoimmunity. Regarding IV therapy practice, the nurse must consider that the older adult may be more susceptible to infection and may not show the same signs and symptoms of infection that they did when they were younger.[14] Because of this change, the use of proper aseptic technique and appropriate use of antimicrobial agents with all IV therapy–related procedures are essential.

Psychological Changes

Psychological factors in the older adult can affect how the patient responds to IV therapy. The confused or demented patient may have problems determining recent versus remote memory.[2] For instance, the patient may understand the procedure while the IV catheter is inserted but an hour later may pull it out.[9] Difficulties with short-term memory may also dramatically affect the older adult who is receiving instruction for home infusion therapies. Depression may affect the older adult's attitude toward the IV line and decisions regarding the alternatives in the care and treatment of the illness. Causes for such behavior can be mental deterioration, administration of medications, thyroid disorders, Alzheimer's disease, stroke, or electrolyte imbalances.[3]

CONSIDERATIONS IN INTRAVENOUS THERAPY

Equipment selection for IV access in the older adult can be a key factor to successful delivery of IV therapies in these patients. Both the type of IV access device and related infusion delivery equipment should be carefully considered.

Vascular Access Device Selection

When a patient's vascular access device needs are evaluated, a judicious analysis of many factors is necessary, particularly the type and the duration of IV therapy. For instance, are hydration solutions, chemotherapy, antibiotics, total parenteral nutrition, or supplemental infusions, such as potassium piggyback solutions to be administered? The nurse must recognize agents that are potentially irritating and may require greater dilution or infusion into a larger vessel to promote hemodilution in the older adult.[11, 15] For example, continuous-infusion vesicant chemotherapy must be administered via a central access catheter to avoid the potential complication of peripheral extravasation. In addition, preparations containing greater than 10% concentrations of glucose, such as total parenteral nutrition solutions, must be administered through central venous access devices to avoid peripheral vein damage.[10] The duration of the therapy is also a factor in determining if a patient's needs are best met by a central or peripheral IV line. If therapy is required for several weeks, central venous access may be the most cost effective method of delivery, and it conserves the patient's peripheral access. Another indication for a central catheter is if the patient has no peripheral access available. The selection of the type of central catheter should be based on the evaluation of potential access sites and the anticipated duration of therapy.

In catheter selection, the skin and vein changes that occur with the older adult should be considered so as to enhance the successful placement and initiation of IV therapies. In particular, consideration should be given to catheter design and gauge size. The type of material the catheter is made of can make it more biocompatible as an indwelling IV device. This feature can determine where the catheter may be inserted and how long it may stay in place without the development of secondary complications. Catheters can be made of silicone, various polyurethane formulations, polytetrafluoroethylene (Teflon), or elastomeric hydrogel. Softer, more flexible materials and those that soften in the vein after insertion may allow increased dwell time and resist or reduce the

development of complications.[17, 18] Additionally, the needle–bevel tip design of a peripheral catheter should be considered when selecting an infusion access device to provide the least traumatic insertion.[19] When the gauge for insertion is selected, the smallest possible gauge size appropriate for the therapy to be delivered, and a vein that will provide adequate hemodilution around the catheter should be selected.[5, 9, 11] The use of 22- and 24-gauge catheters are appropriate for delivery of many IV therapies. These sizes are recommended whenever possible for the older adult to reduce insertion-related trauma and to provide greater hemodilution, thereby reducing vein intimal irritation resulting from catheter insertion trauma or from medications.

When a central venous access device has been determined to be necessary, the need for a long-term versus a short-term device should be evaluated, as should the older adult's ability to care for the device.[20] Percutaneously placed central venous catheters that are designed for short-term use may be appropriate for several weeks of therapy. The selection of a peripherally inserted central catheter may provide an excellent alternative for intermediate access and it may decrease the complications associated with subclavian and jugular insertions. Tunneled catheters may be appropriate when long-term, frequent access is required; however, associated catheter care needs should be carefully considered. The patient and or caregiver may have difficulty maintaining and coping with dressing and flushing procedures. In this instance, an implantable vascular access port may be a better alternative because of the limited catheter care requirements of this device.

Administration Equipment Selection

Because of the dangers associated with overadministration or underadministration of IV therapies, the type of infusion equipment selected should provide safe, consistent delivery of required medication or fluids. To prevent fluid overload, the use of microdrip administration sets, if appropriate for the delivery rate required, should be considered. When rapid flow rates or more exact delivery is required, the use of volume-controlled administration sets and electronic monitoring devices may be needed.

Advanced technology in IV therapy uses stationary and ambulatory electronic monitoring devices, such as controllers and pumps, of all types and sizes for the delivery of IV therapies. Because of the fragile nature of the veins of the older adult, the nurse must recognize the potential complications associated with pressures generated from mechanical infusion devices. Additionally, because of the dangers associated with overadministration or underadministration of prescribed therapies, monitoring devices must have safety features to protect the patient and still ensure delivery of the required medication or fluids.

An internal diagnostic system should evaluate the pump's basic programming to maintain a standard volume and rate of delivery. Variations from the required standard should trigger alarms and stop the infusion until the problem can be corrected. Pump infusion pressures should be carefully monitored to ensure the appropriate delivery of fluids and medications. A major area of confusion concerns the pressures that infusion pumps can generate. Pump line pressure can be calibrated in millimeters of mercury or pounds per square inch (psi). Normal peripheral venous pressure is between 10 and 30 mm Hg. Arterial pressure is much higher, at 100 to 140 mm Hg or higher, whereas central venous pressure is 6 to 9 mm Hg or less.[21]

Pump technical information may refer to pressure limits in terms of pounds per square inch. A pump with a fixed pressure alarm of 4 psi will sound an alarm when the peripheral venous pressure reaches 200 mm Hg (1 psi = 50 mm Hg). This setting can result in a significant infiltration before any pump alarm sounds. The IV nurse must recognize that an infiltrated site exerts a mean pressure gradient at 100 mm Hg or 2 psi. Dramatic infiltrations can occur when pumps simply continue to pump or when gravity infusion is used, because the loose peripheral skin of the older adult does not offer any peripheral tissue resistance to stop a subcutaneous infusion.[21]

An electronic flow control device is reliable only if it is used correctly. The device must not be so cumbersome that it inhibits the patient's movement. The older adult needs to maintain mobility to keep a sense of independence. If applicable to the type of pump and infusion, the pump should have a lock-out feature by key or code to prevent tampering with the programming once it has been set. This feature can be of significant importance with medications whose dosing can be critical.

Cost can influence the use of electronic monitoring devices. However, when these devices are used to provide more accurate delivery of needed therapies, the costs can be justified. Additionally, the use of smaller-sized or ambulatory pumps can increase patient mobility and independence, thereby potentially decreasing the length of hospital stay and the associated costs.[21] Hospitalization costs can be further reduced by the use of ambulatory and specialized programmable infusion devices for delivery of medications at home. The ultimate benefit is seen when patients are permitted to receive medication and fluid delivery while recovering within their own home environment. Both ambulatory and stationary devices can deliver drugs in various programmable models, are secured by built-in lock-out features, and do not inhibit the patient's mobility. Home infusion devices should be user friendly to make them readily acceptable by the nurse and the patient. The older adult may feel quite overwhelmed by the prospect of home infusion therapy, and one of the most intimidating components may be the high-technology electronic monitoring device.

Vein Selection

Appropriate vein selection for IV access in the older adult can provide the IV nurse with a great clinical challenge. The IV nurse must possess clinical and anatomic knowledge specific to the older adult and must have the physical dexterity and the high level of expertise needed to place an IV device into an appropriate vein.

Primary principles of IV site selection in the younger adult are applicable to the older adult. For instance, initial venipunctures should be in the most distal portion of the extremity, allowing for subsequent venipunctures to move progressively upward.[5, 6, 9] This method provides new IV access away from the previous site or area of complication. However, certain factors for site selection are specific to the older

adult. For instance, the veins of the hands may not be the best choice for the initial distal site because of the loss of subcutaneous fat and the thinning of the skin. An IV device inserted into such a site could quickly lead to mechanical inflammation of the vein and infiltration.[11, 12]

Vein selection begins by evaluation of the patient's peripheral access for potential sites that can accommodate the duration of the IV therapy. The entire surfaces of both arms should be inspected for potential sites. Whenever possible, sites should be selected that will not hamper the performance of activities of daily living. Physiologic changes in the skin and veins should also be considered when a site is selected. For instance, stabilization of an IV catheter may be affected by decreased skin turgor. Therefore, areas where sufficient tissue and skeletal support exists should be selected, if possible. The condition of the vein should be evaluated by careful palpation. The nurse should be aware of the more fragile nature of the vein and should begin at distal sites to preserve future access sites. The nurse should avoid previously used, bruised areas and articulating surfaces if possible. In choosing a site, the nurse should consider the need for a current as well as a future IV site; vein conservation is a serious concern for the IV nurse.[14, 19]

To enhance vein location, adequate lighting should be used. Bright, direct overhead examination lights may have a "washout" effect on the vein. Instead, the use of side lighting can add contour and "shadowing," which highlights the skin color and texture and allows visualization of the vein shadow below the skin.[9, 10]

The use of a tourniquet may be helpful in distending and locating an appropriate vein. However, important considerations surrounding the use of tourniquets on the older adult should be kept in mind. The tourniquet should be applied in a flat and snug fashion, but not too tightly. Venous distention may take a few moments longer in the older adult because of the slower venous return in this population. Excessive distention of the vein must be avoided because it might cause vein damage when the vein is punctured. This damage can result from blood back-pressure, which causes vein wall tearing at the needle insertion site.[5, 9] This phenomenon can create an immediate hematoma at the insertion site, and if the skin is loose, the blood will spread across the subcutaneous tissue layer.[14, 23] Additionally, the tourniquet itself may create bruising. Because of these factors, it may be preferable to eliminate the use of a tourniquet in the older adult, especially if the vein to be used is visible and already somewhat distended without the use of a tourniquet.[24]

During venous distention, the veins should be palpated to determine the condition of the vein. Adequate time should be taken to carefully evaluate all potential IV sites. Palpation is the key to determining which veins have soft, bouncy vein walls. These resilient veins feel very different from those that are sclerosed and hard. Veins that feel ribbed or rippled may distend readily when a tourniquet is applied. However, these corded veins are enlarged as a result of thickening of the vein wall, which may be so thick that the lumen may be extremely narrow or occluded.[6, 8, 23, 24] These sites are almost impossible to access, causing pain for the patient and frustration to the IV nurse.

The thickening that occurs in the vein wall also affects the function of the valves, which become stiff and less effective. In many elderly patients, these valves can be seen and palpated because of vessel sclerosis. The valves appear as small bumps along the vein path. The IV nurse must be aware of the potential problems associated with attempting vein access close to or through a valve area. For instance, venous circulation may be sluggish, resulting in slow venous return and distention, venous stasis, and dependent edema. These factors may inhibit the nurse's ability to thread a catheter into the vein. Inflexible valves can make catheter threading difficult or impossible. In these situations, it may be necessary to reduce catheter size by several gauges to thread a catheter through an inflexible valve. Sclerosed valves impede venous circulation and may result in slow or sluggish flashback, causing the IV nurse to advance the catheter too far, which can result in intima damage or vessel rupture.[9, 13]

Small, surface peripheral veins appear as thin, tortuous veins with many bifurcations. Only a few short, straight branches may sustain an IV catheter. Appropriate catheter gauge and length selection are critical to a successful IV access placement in these veins.

Venipuncture Issues

Skin Preparation

The first step in venipuncture is careful preparation of the proposed venipuncture site. The technique used to apply the cleansing agent can be as important as the antimicrobial effect of the agent. Application of cleansing agents should begin at the site and continue outward in a circular motion. Adequate friction is necessary to cleanse the skin, but older skin is more delicate, and too vigorous an action may damage surface skin tissue.

Appropriate cleansing agents for skin preparation include 70% isopropyl alcohol, iodophors, 1 to 2% tincture of iodine, and chlorhexidine.[11] Although practices vary, generally, preparatory cleansing with 70% isopropyl alcohol, followed by an iodophor that is allowed to dry for 30 to 60 seconds, is best for germicidal effect. For patients who are allergic to iodine, the site can be cleansed with alcohol pads until the pads no longer show soil after cleansing. Because older skin has lost some of its natural moisture as a result of aging, excessive use of alcohol may add to skin dryness and cracking.

Excessive amounts of hair over the IV site can be removed by clipping. Care must be taken to avoid nicking the skin. Shaving is not recommended to clean hair from potential IV sites because it causes microabrasions.[11] In the older adult, shaving could easily cause multiple cuts and nicks because of the fragile thinner skin layers; these cuts could provide an open pathway for bacteria to invade the tissue in and around the IV site.

Technique

A key factor for successful venipuncture for the older adult is absolute stabilization of the vein. In the older adult, the vessels may lack stability as a result of loss of tissue mass, and veins may tend to roll.[13, 14] Attempting to access such veins can result in the needle tip's nicking the vein or pushing the vein continually away. Skin tension is established by first determining the direction or axis of the vessel. Initial traction is accomplished by placing the thumb directly along the vein axis approximately 2 to 3 inches below the intended venipuncture site. The palm and fingers of the traction hand serve to hold and stabilize the extremity. The index finger of the traction hand can be used to further stretch the skin above the intended venipuncture site. Once traction has been initiated, it should be maintained throughout the venipuncture and catheter threading procedure.[22]

The directional line of the vein should be visualized. (Each vessel follows its own route). Through palpation, the IV nurse locates the vein and its route. When skin tension is established, palpating the vessel may be difficult or impossible. If the vein is a small, thin surface vessel, the venous distention may not be sufficient for extensive palpation. In these cases, the nurse should attempt to imagine the vein's track along the skin surface. This perceived path assists in aligning the catheter for insertion along the vein route after skin traction has been established.

The use of normal saline or lidocaine subcutaneously at the insertion site for anesthetizing the area is not recommended by the *Intravenous Nursing Standards of Practice*.[10] It is most commonly used in anesthesiology before large-bore 12-gauge, or 14-gauge catheters are inserted.[23, 24] In the elderly population, any additional needle puncture in the area for IV access may make successful venous access more difficult or impossible as a result of subcutaneous tissue swelling, vessel injury, or hemorrhage.[12, 23, 24]

An IV catheter with a sharp, atraumatic bevel tip should be selected. The contour cuts on the bevel tip are designed for sharpness and ease of skin penetration. With the vessel held securely and the vein track visualized, the catheter should be aligned parallel to the vein track. The catheter should be brought close to the skin directly above the potential insertion site. The angle of insertion should be lowered to 20° to 30° to reduce vein trauma on insertion.[5, 6, 9, 23, 24]

The insertion technique can be either a direct or an indirect technique. When a direct technique is used, once skin traction is established, the vein is directly accessed at a 20° to 30° angle in a single motion, thereby penetrating the skin and the vein simultaneously.[5, 6, 9, 11, 12] This method can be routinely used for patients with good vein access or those whose veins are easily stabilized.[19] For patients with small, delicate veins or whose vessels are difficult to secure, an indirect, or a two-step insertion technique, may be necessary.[5, 6, 9, 10, 11] With this technique, the skin is penetrated close to the vein, by the use of the same firm motion as that used for a direct-access method.[23, 24] If a stabbing or thrusting motion is used with the catheter, there is a danger of going too deep or accidentally damaging the vein. Once the surface of the skin has been penetrated, the insertion angle of the catheter should be lowered to 10° to 15°, the vein to be accessed should be restabilized, and the IV catheter bevel tip should be realigned to penetrate the vein wall. With a steady motion, the bevel tip should be advanced gently through the vein wall and into the lumen. The nurse should then check for backflow of blood into the flashback chamber of the catheter. As soon as the bevel and part of the catheter tip has advanced into the vein, the nurse should push the catheter forward off the stylet into the vein while stabilizing the stylet. During catheter-stylet separation, the nurse should observe the flashback chamber to ensure a continuing backflow of blood.[6, 12, 23, 24] The stylet should not be pulled out of the catheter; rather,

Special Techniques for Venipuncture

1. In patients with extremely delicate veins or those taking large doses of anticoagulants, the use of a tourniquet should be avoided.[19] The constriction of blood flow may overextend fragile veins, causing vein damage. When the catheter penetrates the vein wall, the back pressure may cause excessive tearing of the vein at the insertion site. In the patient who is taking anticoagulants, the tourniquet may cause vessel hemorrhages, resulting in subcutaneous bleeding.[9] An alternative method to slow venous return may be to use the hands of another nurse around the arm 6–8 inches above the potential venipuncture site. This pressure should be gentle, to provide minimal venous distention. The pressure should not cause discomfort and there should not be any residual bruising.

2. When a tourniquet is used and the vessel becomes excessively engorged, the tourniquet should be released and reapplied lightly. When vessel access is achieved, the tourniquet should be quickly released to reduce backflow pressure.[5]

3. For veins that are very hard with no elasticity, it may be necessary to use a technique of multiple tourniquets to gradually force the blood to distend smaller, previously undistended veins.

   - The first tourniquet should be placed on the mid–upper arm and the arm stroked downward toward the hand. After 1–2 minutes, a second tourniquet should be placed just below the antecubital fossa or at the middle of the forearm. The nurse should continue to stroke or gently tap the lower forearm in those anatomic areas.

   - In most patients, small veins will begin to be visible as a result of this forced blood distention. If no access can be found in 1–2 minutes, a third tourniquet should be placed just above the wrist. The first tourniquet at the mid–upper arm can be released. The inner wrist, thumb, knuckles, and fingers can be evaluated for suitable vein distention. No tourniquet should be left in place for longer than 5–6 minutes.

4. In patients with excessive peripheral edema, peripheral intravenous (IV) access may not be the best choice because of the increased danger of unrecognized infiltration and potential compartment syndrome. For some patients, the risk of complications during central line placement is too great, and peripheral IV access must be attempted.

   - Using anatomic landmarks, potential IV access sites should be located. The fingers or palm of the hand should be placed over the IV site, and firm, steady pressure should be applied for 10–20 seconds.

   - The hand should be removed and the displacement of the subcutaneous edema to either side of the pressure area should be noted. The flattened, edema-free area will permit easier vein visualization. This displacement will last for only a few moments, until the edema shifts back.

   - A tourniquet may not be necessary, because the tissue oncotic pressure resulting from the edema will appear to make the vessel bulge when the edema is displaced. If a two-step indirect approach is used, an immediate flashback of tissue fluid into the flash chamber will occur. The tissue fluid acts as a preflush when vessel penetration is achieved, causing the blood flashback to be rapidly diffused into the flash chamber.

5. A light finger should be used to tap in order to enhance vein dilation. The vein should not be slapped, because this action may cause vessel rupture.[9, 10]

6. Transillumination of the skin can be helpful in locating deep veins. Tangential side lighting can highlight skin contours and shadow the vein. Direct overhead examination spotlights may wash out visualization of veins in the extremity.[9, 10]

7. The catheter should be inserted with a steady motion. It may take a considerable amount of pressure to go through tough skin or a thick, scarred vein wall. Jabbing, stabbing, or quick thrusting should be avoided because such actions will increase the potential for going through delicate veins.[9, 23]

8. For patients with very small, spidery veins, the catheter should be preflushed before access is attempted. In veins with low blood pressure or slow capillary return, preflushing enhances the flashback, a characteristic that can be critical. It is important to know the instant the bevel enters the vein to avoid advancing the catheter through the vein wall or causing back wall trauma. The preflushed catheter rapidly diffuses the blood return at the instant of vein penetration from the bevel tip to the flash chamber.[12, 19, 24]

9. A two-step, indirect approach should be used for delicate veins that are difficult to stabilize.[5, 9, 23, 24]

10. After the bevel enters the vein and blood flashback occurs, the angle of insertion should be lowered and the catheter-stylet advanced together into the vein. This measure ensures that part of the catheter as well as the bevel has entered the vein lumen.[23] Once the catheter tip and bevel are in the vein, the catheter only should be advanced forward off the stylet into the vein ¼ to ½ inch. Blood should continue to backflow into the flash chamber.[12, 24]

11. A one-handed technique is recommended to advance the catheter off the stylet so that the opposite hand can maintain proper skin tension, thereby holding the vein in place.[6, 12] A two-handed technique can be used, but a greater chance of intimal damage and possible vessel rupture exists when a semirigid catheter is threaded into a nonstabilized vein.[23]

12. After the catheter is advanced off the stylet into the vein ¼ to ½ inch, a separation exists between the hub of the catheter and the hub of the stylet. The bevel tip is sufficiently retracted inside the catheter when a visible flashback of blood is seen within the unthreaded portion of the catheter. The hub of the catheter should be grasped and the catheter-stylet slowly advanced as a unit into the vein. The opposite hand maintains skin traction to keep the vein in alignment for threading.[5, 9] The tourniquet can be released immediately after catheter-stylet separation or after the catheter is threaded well into the vessel. Digital pressure is placed on the vessel at the tip of the threaded catheter to stop blood flow. Then, the stylet is removed.[19]

13. For narrow or tortuous veins, ''floating'' the catheter while threading it may be necessary. With these types of veins, the catheter may only partially advance.[23, 24] To float, the tourniquet, if used, should be released and the stylet removed from the catheter hub. A fully primed IV system or syringe filled with normal saline should be connected to the catheter. The catheter should be temporarily stabilized to prevent dislodgement while the vessel is dilated with fluid. The flow clamp should be slowly opened and a slow drip begun. The IV flow rate should be cautiously increased. As the rate is increased, the catheter should be gently advanced, if possible. If the flow has successfully dilated the vein, the catheter should be able to thread along with the fluid flow. Note: some catheters are designed to allow for preattachment to administration sets or syringes before insertion.

the catheter should always be pushed forward off the stylet into the vein. This method ensures that the bevel and part of the catheter are well into the vein before the stylet is removed.

If the veins are extremely fragile, it may be necessary to release the tourniquet as soon as a blood return occurs and catheter separation is achieved. This may avoid vein wall damage from high-pressure backflow of blood from the point where the catheter entered the vein.[5, 9]

A "hooded" technique can be effectively used to advance the catheter into the vein. In this technique, the catheter is advanced forward over the bevel tip into the vein. This measure retracts the stylet tip inside the catheter. Then, the nurse threads the catheter into the vein by grasping the hub of the catheter and advancing the catheter-stylet as one unit up the vein, with the blunt catheter tip leading the way up the vessel. This process reduces the possibility of an accidental penetration of the vein wall during the threading. Vein stabilization and skin tension must be maintained from the time of insertion throughout the threading of the catheter. Only after the catheter has been advanced as far as possible can the tension from stabilization be eased slowly.[5] The hooding technique can be essential to successful threading of the catheter without damage or rupture to the fragile vessels of the elder patient. If the skin tension is released before the catheter is threaded, the rebound of the skin and vein being released may cause the catheter to rupture the vein.[22, 23]

IV access in the older adult may test all of the skill and knowledge of the IV nurse. However, the use of special techniques may enhance the success of venipuncture in these patients.

Device Maintenance

Adequate stabilization of vascular access devices within the vein is essential to reduce the degree of mechanical irritation that results from the catheter's shifting inside the vein. The key to maintaining an IV site in an older adult is to anticipate all potential problems and to apply preventive measures before the problems occur. Many IV protective devices are available that can also be used to secure the catheter. The cost of these devices varies, and the degree of site protection must be carefully weighed on a cost-versus-need basis. Adaptations of products readily available can also be economically used to provide safe protection for the IV site.

Site care begins with careful stabilization and application of a dressing. The decrease in subcutaneous fat and tissue in the elderly results in the catheter being less stable and needing a secure dressing. To anchor the catheter, a ½-inch by 3-inch piece of tape with adhesive side up should be placed under the hub of the catheter. The edge of the tape should not be in contact with the IV site. The catheter rests on the adhesive strip, which helps anchor the catheter and protects the skin from the rigid plastic hub. The length of tape extending to each side of the catheter hub is then folded upward at a 90° angle to the catheter.[6, 12, 19, 22] This modified chevron taping technique can securely anchor the catheter with a minimum of tape. The use of soft-winged catheters also enhances the nurse's ability to stabilize and secure the catheter. IV devices that provide stiff wings or flanges must be used with caution on the delicate skin of the elderly. Hard, stiff edges can cause skin irritation, soreness, or even skin ulceration.[14] To prevent irritation when this type of device is used, any portion of the device that may cause irritation should be padded with a small gauze pad or sponge.

Securing the catheter to prevent accidental dislodgment is necessary; however, the amount of tape applied to the skin should be minimized in patients with delicate skin. Consideration should also be given to the type of tapes used on delicate skin. Some types of tapes may easily tear the fragile, thin skin of the older adult. Therefore, the patient should be carefully assessed for any reaction to the tape product used when the skin is thin and fragile. The patient should also be questioned about previous experiences with tape products before the tape is applied. Adaptations to the taping technique or product used should be implemented as necessary. To assist in decreasing irritation or damage to the skin of the older adult, the use of additional protection as provided in a skin polymer solution can be considered. This added skin barrier protects the skin from the effects of adhesives and from the drying nature of cleansing agents that occurs with repeated tape removal and dressing changes.[13, 14] While stabilizing the catheter, the nurse should apply the polymer solution in a circular motion around the site, starting ½ to ¾ inch out from the insertion point. The nurse should then allow the solution to air dry before applying the dressing. A gauze or transparent semipermeable membrane can be placed over the site to complete the dressing.[9, 11, 23]

The IV nurse must anticipate potential hazards that could affect the continued successful delivery of the necessary IV therapies. The older adult is not always as aware of his or her surroundings as other patients and is slower to adapt to environmental changes. These factors may result in accidents that might disturb or interrupt the patency of the IV catheter.[10, 13, 14] For example, the older adult may not remember that the IV device is in place or may not adequately visualize the set-up and may become tangled in the tubing, resulting in an accidental disconnection. Excessive lengths of IV tubing can become a physical hazard to the elderly patient who is trying to ambulate or to perform his or her own activities of daily living. The IV tubing should be long enough to give adequate range of motion but not to dangle on the floor or get caught under the IV pole or IV pump wheels. A segment of the IV tubing should be looped to the patient's arm so that inadvertent tugging pulls on the loop and not directly on the IV catheter site. Another important consideration is the type of administration sets connected to the IV catheter. A Luer-Lok connector provides a more secure connection and prevents more accidental disconnections than would a male-female interlock, which can easily pull apart.

Occasionally, the IV site may need to be covered to prevent the patient from inadvertently removing it. An alternative method used to stabilize the catheter is to stretch properly sized surgical burn mesh gauze over the IV site. This measure provides coverage and stability for the site and protects the catheter from snagging on bed clothes, pumps, or other encumbrances. The surgical burn mesh allows for unimpeded peripheral circulation for the IV site while stabilizing the IV catheter and dressing.[14] Appropriately sized, tube-shaped elastic gauze netting can be used to assist in stabilizing the device and minimizing the need for tape. However, roller-type gauze or any type of covering that is not easily removed and decreases the ability to observe the site should not be used. The *Intravenous Nursing Standards of Practice* do not recommend the use of any form of roller gauze bandage to secure IV dressing.[10]

Another approach to covering the IV site is to place the patient in a long-sleeved gown or pajamas. If the IV is covered from the patients' view, the patient may not disturb it and may forget that the IV is in place. A piece of tape can be wrapped around the sleeve at the cuff so that the sleeve cannot be pushed up the arm.[13, 14]

Armboards should be used with care to stabilize IV devices over areas of flexion. These boards must be padded with soft gauze or a washcloth and must support the hand or arm in a functional position. The fingers should be allowed some motion to encourage circulation and to decrease the potential for the development of dependent edema.[5, 10, 11] The tapes used to secure the board should be prebacked with gauze or tape so the adhesive does not contact the patient's skin, thereby permitting good control of the extremity without circulatory impediment. The IV site and the vein path above the site should still be visible for frequent evaluation. When any extremity is immobilized, increased peripheral edema may occur as a result of slowed venous return in the restricted extremity. This problem can be critical in the older adult with peripheral vascular changes, or limited mobility, or both. Any decrease in activity to an extremity increases venous stasis and the resultant dependent edema. Therefore, these IV sites must be monitored often and the observations documented at regular intervals.

Occasionally, some means of restraint must be used to prevent the patient from dislodging the IV device. A physician's order is required for use of the restraint. Restraint policies vary between institutions, but frequent monitoring and documentation are always required. Soft wrist restraints can be placed below the IV site but should never be placed directly over the IV site. If the IV site is in the wrist, hand, or fingers, the restraint should be placed around an armboard, and then the extremity should be secured on the armboard. The IV is secured by the board while the board takes the pulling stress of the restraint. Mittens can also be applied, if necessary.[6, 9, 11, 14] Dependent edema can develop below the restraint, where circulation can be impaired.

Site Monitoring

The IV site should be observed at regular intervals to ensure patency as set by hospital or extended care facility policy.[11] In many hospitals, nursing practice policy usually recommends observing the area every 1 to 2 hours and documenting to verify site patency, condition, and flow rate. Notation of IV site observations only once per shift is not sufficient to validate 8 hours of patent IV flow, because complications such as phlebitis and infiltration, could go unnoticed for several hours. With the older adult in particular, a small infiltrate could easily become a severe IV complication, such as compartment syndrome or extravasation.[10]

IV site rotation is recommended every 48 hours, according to the *Standards of Practice for Intravenous Nursing.*[11] Variations from this standard may be acceptable if they are justified through documented and statistically substantiated clinical practice. The incidence of complications or phlebitis should be less than 5%, using a 48-hour site change for the standard of care.[11] If a routine site change is not performed because of limited access or patient condition, a full description of the site evaluation, dressing change, and reasons for the inability to rotate the IV site should be well documented on the patient's record.

Legal Considerations

The initiation of IV therapy without consent is construed as assault and battery.[6, 11] The older adult does not give up the right to refuse treatment. Health care professionals must recognize that the elderly citizen needs to feel a sense of independence and control over his or her environment. In the acute care setting, so much of a patient's care and environment is out of his or her control. This circumstance must be met with reasoning and discussion, not force.[18]

The patient who is confused does not necessarily relinquish his or her rights to refuse treatment. The determination of what is best for the care and safety of the patient must be weighed against a careful evaluation of the patient's mental and emotional ability to make rational decisions.[6] The patient's life and safety are always the first priority to the health care provider. If a patient cannot make these judgments, the patient, the family, or the hospital representative can ask the court to appoint a patient advocate to oversee the best interests of the patient. The determination of who can speak for the patient must be made early in the course of care so that proper therapy can be continued with the appropriate consent.

As the population grows older, the use of advance directives in health care will increase. Patients now have living wills or special directives specifying the extent of life-saving medical technology to be used. These documents represent the desires of an individual and are legally binding. Each jurisdiction has its own interpretation of the legality of such directives. The health care provider who acts to extend or preserve life is not viewed as a criminal. In most states, families must go to court to ask permission to adhere to a patient's advance directive. This practice can only grow more complicated as advance directives become more common.[2]

PATIENT EDUCATION

The patient education process begins with the physician's order for IV therapy. It is important for the patient's self-esteem that all procedures be explained fully before they are performed. Such communication gives the patient a sense of participating in the process.[6, 13, 14]

The nurse should speak slowly, clearly, and directly to the older adult with sensory deficits. Additionally, the patient should be addressed by name, and anyone who is involved in performing the procedure should be introduced by name and identification.[13, 14] Steps in any procedure, such as IV catheter insertion, should be described as they are performed. The patient will be more cooperative if he or she can anticipate the elements of his or her care, and if trust is established.

Important ongoing IV therapy–related considerations should be clearly and simply explained to the patient. For instance, while cleansing and dressing the site, the nurse should provide the patient with instructions on basic care to protect the IV site from infection or dislodgment. In this way, the patient can become a partner in the maintenance of the IV site. If any pump or monitoring device is used, the nurse should explain potential alarms and how to avoid possible problems. The nurse should not use terminology that is unfamiliar but instead should use clear, concise phrases to leave no doubt as to the meaning.[6, 13]

HOME CARE

The IV nurse must balance many elements when planning the delivery of IV therapies in the home setting. The process begins with a physician's order for home IV therapy. The IV nurse's role includes evaluation of the type of therapy, the duration of therapy, and the associated IV access and infusion delivery equipment. These factors are all crucial to the determination of the appropriateness of home IV therapy. Careful evaluation of the home physical environment, the family members in the home, the designated home health provider and other care providers, and the cost and insurance coverage must be performed. If these physical needs cannot be met, then the environment for the patient and family may be too stressful for learning and retention.[6, 10]

Specific challenges exist in the education of the older adult in the administration of home infusion therapy. As people age, they less readily adapt to environmental changes,[7] especially those that they cannot easily control or affect their independence. The IV nurse must therefore have a high degree of motivation and patience when instructing the older adult. Teaching the older adult complex drug admixtures, tubing connections, IV maintenance, IV pump programming, and accessing and deaccessing various IV devices is a step-by-step, individualized process. A progressively organized training program should include a written teaching manual or a program module as well as direct demonstrations of specific procedures with return demonstration evaluated by the potential home care provider.[6, 12]

The amount of medical knowledge and nursing care thrust on a patient or family in a short time can be overwhelming. The IV nurse must evaluate the older adult for the ability to perform the skill in question. With the older patient or designated primary care provider, time must be spent evaluating the emotional stability, the intellectual capacity, and the physical ability to perform the required skills. For instance, is the patient emotionally able to cope with being cared for at home by a family member or a home health worker? The family members or significant others must be able to provide support for the patient as well as themselves. In addition, can the learner understand the necessary health care concepts? A gap in comprehension may result from language or cultural differences. The nurse should consider whether interpreters could be used to enhance learning. The use of pictorial step-by-step manuals can dramatically facilitate learning for those with a reading, language, or hearing deficit. Sign language interpreters and lip reading can help the hearing impaired. In addition, videotapes of procedures can permit the patient and family to refresh skills at home.

The number of IV nurses designated as patient educators should be limited to maintain continuity of the skills being taught. In patient education, the content must be taught in exactly the same way to each caregiver. Tasks can become easily confusing to the lay caregiver if different methods are used for procedures. Precise training examples should be used and repeated exactly the same way each time. This consistency and repetition will reduce the potential for errors or patient complications in the home.[6]

The patient and family should have an understanding of what complications or problems could occur and the appropriate interventions for these problems. This information should be included in the patient teaching module and should be reviewed several times before discharge or independent administration. The information should include care of the peripheral IV site or alternative access device (e.g., peripherally inserted central catheters, implanted ports, and tunneled catheters), various pumps (intermittent, continuous, patient controlled analgesia, ambulatory, stationary), medications and their side effects, total parenteral nutrition (cyclic or continuous), proper tubings and connections, medication incompatibilities, emergency procedures, emergency access to health care personnel, record keeping, storage of medical supplies, and proper disposal of medical wastes.

The impact of sensory changes that occur with aging, particularly changes in visual acuity, hearing, and manual dexterity, should also be considered. The importance of visual acuity is seen in the administration of small medication dosages for IV admixtures, the adjustment of pump rates, and the accessing of IV devices and tubing connections. The primary care provider must be able to see and read the directions for medication administration and for the care and maintenance of IV access devices. Changes in hearing may affect the patient's ability to hear and respond to pump alarms in a timely manner. Manual dexterity is another important requirement for many home infusion procedures. The older adult may have significant problems handling the necessary equipment for care because of illness-related changes resulting from arthritis, cardiovascular accidents, partial or full paralysis, amputation, or other physical impairments. For instance, the older adult may have difficulty attaching administration sets and handling the small caps attached to these sets. The older adult should be carefully observed working with the various devices, and alternatives should be used as are deemed appropriate. Needleless systems may be used with the older adult to eliminate the risk of needle sticks.

The IV nurse providing care in the home is a partner in the development of a safe IV home delivery system. The concerns of the home care provider include a clean, dry space for supplies; a clean work preparation area; special refrigeration needs; pets; parasites and infestations in the home; necessary electrical outlets; batteries and sufficient supplies; a telephone; and names of people to call in an emergency. The hospital and home care provider must evaluate all the home factors to determine if the home environment can provide a safe place for the administration of IV therapy.

The desired outcome for any course of IV therapy is to provide successful administration of a prescribed therapy for the duration required with no complications. The achievement of this goal is enhanced when care is provided by a highly skilled IV nurse. When the special needs of the older adult are addressed, the result will be atraumatic peripheral IV access; decreased complications through diligent IV site monitoring, care and maintenance; appropriate use of the newest techniques and care; quality patient education; and coordinated hospital or extended care facility to home transfers and delivery of home IV therapies. Only through awareness of the special concerns can the IV nurse attempt to provide and care for vascular access for the older adult requiring IV therapy.

References

1. Taylor S. Lost in the system. JIN 1992; 15:52–56.
2. Matteson RN. Gerontological Nursing Concepts and Practice. Philadelphia: W.B. Saunders, 1991:2–179.
3. Burke MM. Gerontologic Nursing. St. Louis: Mosby Yearbook, 1992:2–279.
4. Tortora G. Principles of Anatomy and Physiology, 5th ed. New York: Harper & Row, 1987:265–298.
5. Hadaway L. IV tips. Geriatr Nurs 1991; March/April:78–81.
6. Weinstein S. Plumer's Principles and Practices of Intravenous Therapy, 5th ed. Philadelphia: J.B. Lippincott, 1993:49–82.
7. Whitehouse MJ. The physiology of aging. JIN 1992; 15:S7–S13.
8. Price SA. Pathophysiology, 4th ed. St. Louis: Mosby Yearbook, 1992:64–70.
9. Enich M. Performing venipuncture in elderly patients. Nursing 91 1991; 21:32C–H.
10. Gardner C. I.V. specialization: Current issues. JIN 1989; 12(1):14–36.
11. Intravenous nursing standards of practice. JIN (Suppl) 1990; 13:S1–S98.
12. LaRocca J. Pocket Guide to Intravenous Therapy, 2nd ed. St. Louis: C.V. Mosby, 1993:14–36.
13. Andresen P. A fresh look at assessing the elderly. RN 1989; June:28–39.
14. Coulter K. Intravenous therapy for the elder patient: Implications for the intravenous nurse. JIN 1992; 15:S18–23.
15. Roth D. Intravenous Fluid Therapy Course for the Licensed Practical Nurse. Columbia, MO: University of Missouri Instructional Materials, 1988:383–389.
16. Metheny NM. Fluid and Electrolyte Balance, 2nd ed. Philadelphia: J.B. Lippincott, 1992:351–361.
17. Gaukroger PB, Roberts JG, Manners TA. Infusion thrombophlebitis: A prospective comparison of 645 Vialon and Teflon cannulae in anaesthetic and postoperative use. Anaesth Intensive Care 1988; 16(3):265–271.
18. Rasor JS. Review of catheter related infection rates: Comparison of conventional materials with Aquavene. JVAN 1991; 1:8–18.
19. Weinstein S. Memory Bank for I.V.'s. Baltimore: Williams & Wilkins, 1988:36–55.
20. Baranowski L. Central venous access devices: Current technologies, uses, and management strategies. JIN 1993; 16(3):167–194.
21. Thompson S. Instrument Assisted I.V. Site Management. IVAC, 1987:3–10.
22. Millam DA. Are nurses prepared to perform I.V. therapy? Nursing 88 1988; 18:43.
23. Millam DA. Starting I.V.'s. Nursing 92 1992; 22:33–46.
24. Channel S. Manual for I.V. Therapy Procedures, 3rd ed. Oradell, NJ: Medical Economics Co., 1993:19–22; 45–84.

Linda A. Grace, RN, BS, CRNI
Becky J. Tomaselli, CRNI, CNSN

This chapter gives a broad overview of home infusion therapy. It reviews basic concepts relative to the field and describes its evolution and history, including the original model for provision of home nutritional support and antibiotic therapy. It also describes the expansion of the original model by both the nursing and the pharmacy disciplines. This chapter gives a full description of the home care process and the roles and responsibilities of the service providers in-

volved. Because our health care environment demands justification for health care services, medical, professional, and financial benefits as well as reimbursement benefits are discussed. As this market segment grows at a projected rate of 25.9% annually, availability of qualified and experienced professionals has become a high-priority issue for this specialized high-technology field.[1] Along with discussion of personnel needs, a basic review of the most common infusion therapies provided in the home care environment as well as resources needed to provide these therapies are covered. This area includes the first home infusion therapies, total parenteral nutrition (TPN), antibiotic therapy, hydration, and pain management, as well as the newer therapies, complex chemotherapy, dobutamine therapy, transfusion therapy, α_1-proteinase inhibitor (Prolastin) and tocolytic therapy, and the newest of all, the biologic response modifiers. Finally, special considerations are suggested, as are future directions for the field of home infusion therapy and its place in our health care system.

EVOLUTION OF HOME INFUSION THERAPY

TEFRA/Diagnostic Related Groups

The concept of home visitation by medical personnel, including physicians and public health nurses, dates back many years, although home infusion therapy is a relatively new field as we know it today. Literature cites early cases in the late 1970s, in which the only reason for hospitalization was the extended need for intravenous nutritional support.[2] Only through the development of such technology as long-term indwelling catheters and ambulatory infusion pumps are we able to provide such services in the home setting today.

The credit for the impetus behind the provision of infusion services in the home goes to our government and its implementation of TEFRA, the Tax Equity and Fiscal Responsibility Act of 1982. This act shifted Medicare reimbursement from a retrospective case-per-day payment system to a prospective payment system based on a total fee that was fixed in advance.[3] In 1983, hospitals were provided with a list of 467 diagnostic related groups, which contained a fixed fee for each specific diagnosis. In other words, diagnostic related groups prospectively outline the exact amount that would be paid for a patient with a diagnosis such as small bowel obstruction. If the hospital could provide the service for less than the DRG allowable, the hospital would then make a profit. However, if care for a particular patient cost more than the amount allowable, then the facility suffered a loss.

In 1984, health care costs rose 4.5%. This percentage of growth was a decrease from that occurring in 1983, when costs rose 10%. The United States saw the first decline in the cost of health care in 20 years, leading one to the conclusion that a prospective payment system works.[3] For the first time, the health care system rewarded providers for efficiency and productivity and was penalizing for inefficiency. The emphasis of the health care system had changed from providing maximum quality whatever the cost to providing care in an atmosphere of efficiency, productivity, and cost-consciousness. In the earlier example of the patient with the small bowel obstruction, the hospital would now be encouraged to discharge the patient as soon as feasible. Moreover, if the only reason the patient was retained in the hospital was to receive TPN, financial reward existed for discharging the patient with a plan for home nutritional support. As the cost of health care has continued to rise over the years, the hospital-driven health care model of the 1980s is an option that is less sought after. Alternative sites, such as the patient's home, are now considered to be the treatment settings of choice.

Development of the Industry

The first two intravenous therapies to be self-administered in the home were TPN and antibiotics.[4, 5]

Home Parenteral Nutrition

In the 1960s, Professor Meng described the first results of experimental use of parenteral alimentation in dogs using a fat emulsion of 10%.[6] In 1968, Dudrick experimented with parenteral nutrition using beagle puppies. In Dudrick's study, growth curves of two male puppies from the same litter were compared after one was fed orally and one parenterally.[6] Results showed similar growth curves in both animals. The same results were later found in both the pediatric and adult patient population who, for whatever reason, could not use the gastrointestinal tract in the nutritional process. Along with advances in medicine, technologic advances of equipment, such as long-term catheters, pumps, and bags, have enabled patients to lead relatively normal lives by infusing essential nutrients parenterally. This advance, coupled with the need to control health care costs, led to the obvious alternative of providing infusion therapy in the home care setting.

Home Antibiotic Therapy

The first report of the successful use of parenteral antibiotics was published in 1974 by Harrison, who treated a cystic fibrosis patient for acute pulmonary infection.[5] In 1979, the Cleveland Clinic developed a program to train patients in the self-administration of antibiotics. Poretz reported on 150 patients in the Cleveland Clinic Home Antibiotic Program. Results showed mild and infrequent adverse reactions and more than a 90% treatment success rate.[2, 7] Based on these and other data, home parenteral antibiotic therapy was not only feasible but desirable. Frequently, patients were well enough to be either at home or at work while receiving their therapy and were bored and frustrated by prolonged hospitalization. The impetus for the development of home programs came in response to diagnostic related groups as well as the encouragement of federal and state governments and private insurers, who were seeking to reduce the cost of health care. Studies proved that providing antibiotic therapy in the home costs approximately 33% of the cost to administer the same drug in the hospital.[8]

Reimbursement

Private Insurance

Reimbursement for home infusion therapies has become more complex over the years because more and more therapies can be given safely and effectively in the home care setting. Each patient should be evaluated individually for coverage, and the coverage should be verified with the payer, including specific information on the therapy and services covered by the insurer. The diagnosis, therapy, drug, and full prescription, as well as covered services such as nursing and pharmacy, and others including laboratory, therapeutic monitoring, and diagnostics should be verified before providing a service.

Reimbursement for home care is based on a fee-for-services or per-unit basis. In the past, payment was made after the services were provided. More and more frequently, services are negotiated by indemnity insurers before the start of therapy. Insurers who are not using prospective methodology are reviewing cases for medical necessity and paying what is usual, reasonable, and customary once they have received invoices.[9, 10] Capitated agreements are going to be a methodology of payment in the future.

Medicare

Medicare pays for certain therapies based on very specific medical necessity. Short-term skilled nursing services are generally covered under part A, if the home care company is a certified home health agency. Covered under part B are infusion services, supplies, and some drugs. Payment for infusion medications has not been consistent to date and generally has been denied for antibiotics. It is based on a predetermined rate or a prevailing charge. A prevailing charge is calculated at a rate of 75% of charges for similar services provided in the same service area for the previous year. Part B also covers parenteral and enteral nutrition. Under the prosthetic device benefit, Medicare pays the prevailing rate for solutions and supplies, again, based on medical necessity. Specific details regarding medical necessity and Medicare benefit guidelines can be obtained through a Medicare intermediary.[9, 10]

Medicaid

Medicaid benefits vary from state to state. If Medicaid covers infusion therapies, reimbursement policies are restrictive. Reimbursement rates are low, and eligibility criteria are strict. Medicaid reimbursement is generally an unreliable source for financing home infusion services. Specific information about coverage can be obtained from the individual state programs.

OVERVIEW OF HOME INFUSION THERAPY

Pharmacy Home Infusion Therapy Model

The first to establish a multidisciplinary approach for providing home care was Montefiore Hospital in New York in 1947. The concept of the visiting nurse was married with the physician's house call. Physical, occupational, and speech therapists were added to the team to provide total care to the patient in the home. Unfortunately, a physician shortage resulting from World War II made house calling a less efficient way of seeing patients, and this practice ended, along with the multidisciplinary home care concept.

The pharmacy home infusion therapy model, which was conceptualized in the late 1970s by entrepreneurial health care providers with a vision for providing high-technology infusion services, employed a similar multidisciplinary team approach using pharmacy, nursing, and ancillary services.[11] Early descriptions of the home infusion therapy model included two simply defined processes—the admission process (Fig. 29–1) and the patient care process.[12] The admission process was the process by which the patient was admitted to the home infusion program. In the patient care process, the patient underwent the therapy and was discharged from the home infusion program at its completion. During the initial years of home infusion therapy, the number of diagnoses of these patients for which it was used was limited. Most of the patients were being treated with TPN for short bowel syndrome, Crohn's disease, or ulcerative colitis; with antibiotics for subacute bacterial endocarditis; with pain management for terminal cancer with intractable pain.[13–15]

Acceptance of home infusion therapy, largely as a result of community education and advances in pharmaceuticals, equipment technology, and medical treatment for chronic disease states, gave way to the development and complexity of the home infusion process we know today. The home infusion therapy "patient care management system" (PCMS) is an adaptation of the model described earlier (Fig. 29–2). Although the concept remains unchanged, additions have been made to the model to accommodate broader scopes of services necessary to provide care to the more acutely or chronically ill patient. It also accommodates reimbursement and regulatory demands as the industry continues to develop.

The PCMS is designed to provide a cohesive multidisciplinary team approach to patient care that respects the rights of patients, meets their needs, and effectively and efficiently manages quality and cost of care.

The objectives of the PCMS are to

- Facilitate a smooth transition from the hospital to the home.
- Anticipate problems, thereby allowing for early intervention on the part of the care providers and preventing or minimizing need for rehospitalization.
- Encourage patient comfort by allowing patients to receive care in a familiar environment and to live according to the life style to which they are accustomed.
- Maximize independence and self-sufficiency by educating patients or caregivers on the administration and under-

standing of the therapy with minimal assistance from the clinicians.
- Ideally, facilitate the return to optimum health and independence.

Realizing that return to optimum health and independence may not always be possible, PCMS aims to provide the same high-quality medical services that are found in acute care facilities to prevent illness; promote, maintain, and restore health; or minimize the effects of illness, disability, and mortality.[11, 17] The system, which is described in detail later under "Home Infusion Patient Care Process," integrates clinical pharmacy and nursing services through four processes: the admission process, the planning process, the patient care process (including implementation, monitoring, and evaluation), and the termination of care.

The Role and Responsibilities of the Home Infusion Clinician

INTRAVENOUS NURSE

The intravenous (IV) nurse's role and responsibilities include initial patient assessment, review of systems, development of nursing diagnosis, review of current and past medical history, psychosocial assessment, evaluation of available support systems, and assessment of functional limitations, environment, and cognitive and technical skills. Recommendations are formulated based on nursing impressions. Ongoing responsibilities include patient training, visitation for therapeutic monitoring and evaluation, assessment of compliance with medication regimen, performance of technical procedures of infusion therapy, psychosocial support, and 24-hour emergency availability.

PHARMACIST

In some geographic locations, the pharmacist as well as the IV nurse visit the patient when necessary for evaluation and assessment. Whether the pharmacist provides home care depends on the philosophy of the organization and the demands of the marketplace. The role and responsibilities of the pharmacist include reviewing medical records for current and past medical, nutritional, and medication history; reviewing laboratory data; obtaining physician orders; and conducting interviews with patients. The pharmacist's role also includes preparing, dispensing, and delivering medications, solutions, supplies and equipment; planning patient care; monitoring therapeutic response; performing ongoing analysis of laboratory data; and being available 24 hours a day for emergencies. A therapeutic evaluation is made based on patient assessment (when possible); on the physical examination and history; and on consultative information conveyed by nursing staff as well as from conversation with patients, family members, caregivers, and other members of the health care team.

Through a collaborative and consultative effort, the nursing and pharmacy staff formulate clinical impressions that are communicated to the physician. This process ensures that the best possible decisions are made for patient care and services and the highest quality of care is provided.

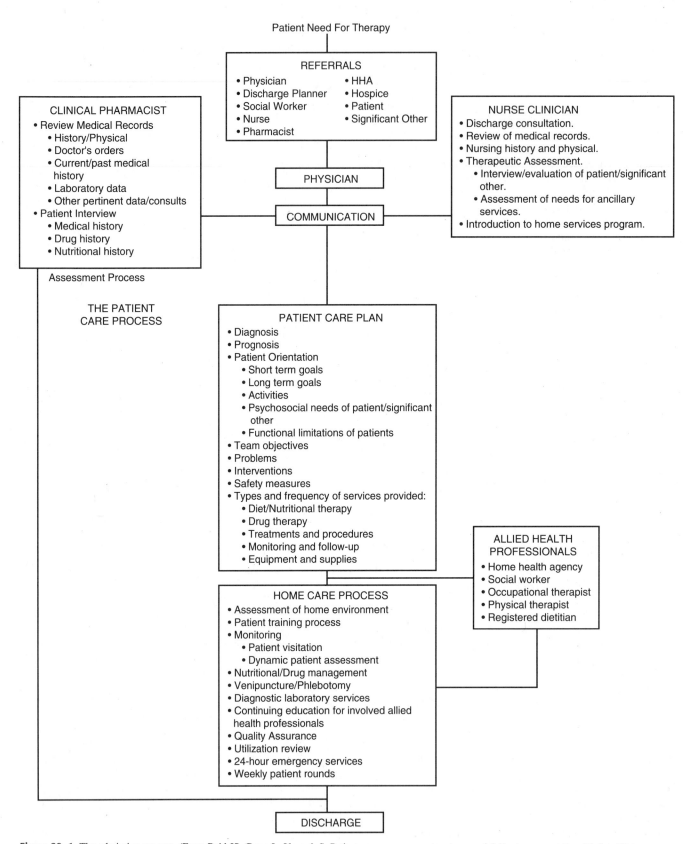

Figure 29–1. The admission process. (From Reid JS, Grace L, Venook S. Patient care management system model. Poster presentation. National Intravenous Therapy Association, Nashville, TN, May 1987.

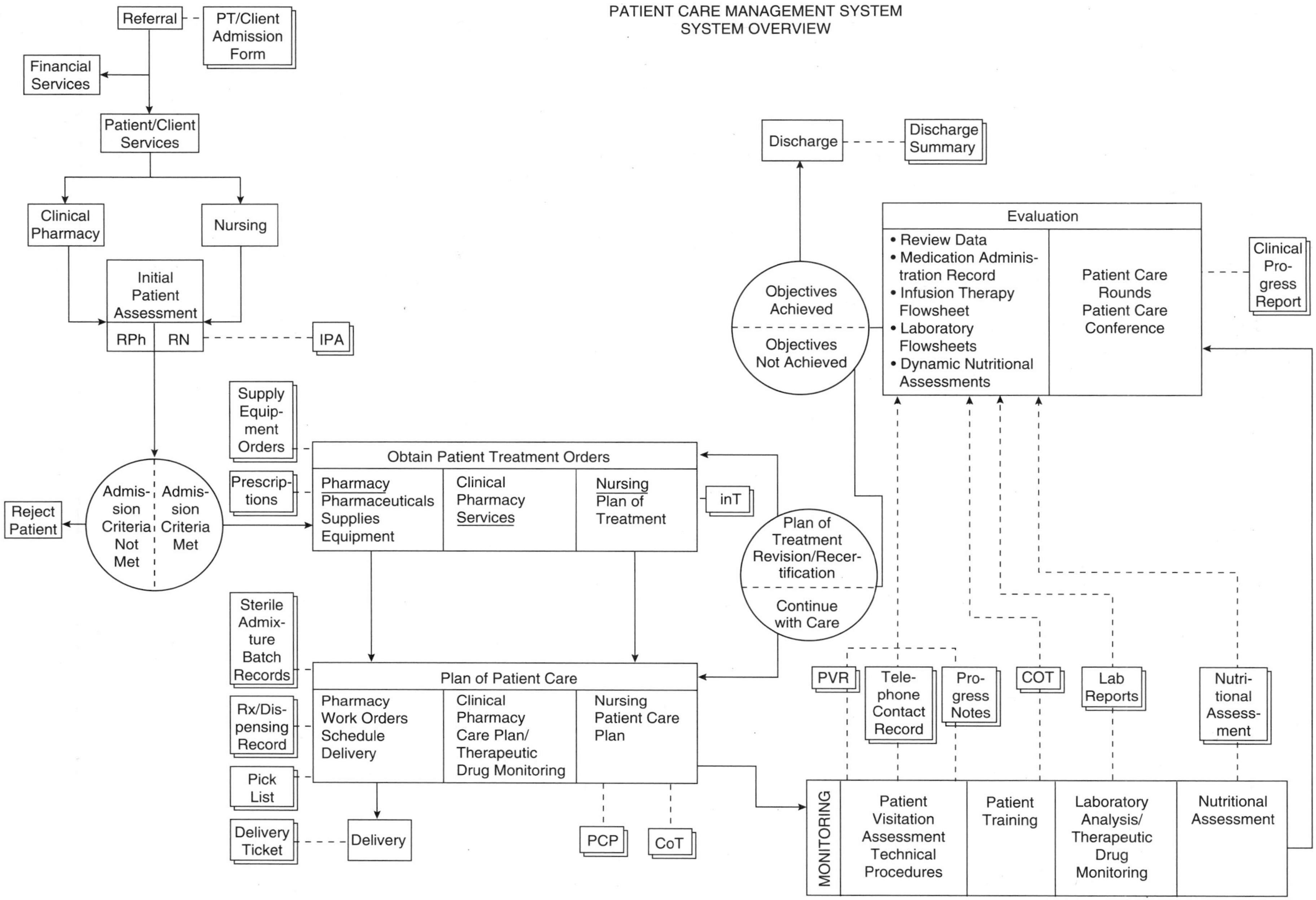

PATIENT CARE MANAGEMENT SYSTEM
SYSTEM OVERVIEW

Figure 29–2. Home infusion therapy patient care management system (PCMS).

OTHER MEMBERS

A very important member of the health care team is the patient financial services representative, who is responsible for the financial aspects of services, such as verifying insurance coverage, negotiating with case managers, and discussing their financial obligations with patients. Another member is the pharmacy technician, whose job responsibilities depend on the benefits provided in a particular state. Some state pharmacy laws allow trained technicians to perform drug preparation duties, whereas others do not. Individual state pharmacy law can be reviewed by obtaining state pharmacy laws, rules, and regulations from the local state boards of pharmacy. A very visible and important member of the team is the delivery technician or driver. This member interacts with the patient on a frequent basis to deliver medications, supplies, and equipment.

Overall, the goal of this model is to promote collaboration as a multidisciplinary team. Consultation eliminates duplication of services and lends itself to efficiency and cost effectiveness while still allowing for a more complete approach to patient assessment than that provided by other methods. Through an integrated assessment, a more accurate evaluation of the patient's overall status can be determined, and better recommendations for patient care can be made. This process, in turn, improves the quality of care and services received by the patient.

Nursing Agency Home Infusion Therapy Model

The nursing agency home infusion therapy model has only recently evolved. With the diminishing profit margins of nursing services, largely as a result of the high cost of professional services, agency administrators saw home infusion therapy as an avenue of survival.[18] This market would generate not only revenue but also the need for services in the way of visits to be provided by their agencies' nurses and therapists. This model typically subcontracts for pharmacy services with a pharmacy providing product only, or with a home infusion pharmacy providing a full complement of services, as described earlier. More recently, nursing agencies have begun to employ the concept of an on-site pharmacy as described in the original Pharmacy Home Infusion Therapy Model. In addition, more pharmacies are seeking nursing agency licensure and certification, leading to the possibility that the two models are merging to become yet a new and third model for home infusion therapy.

Involvement of Ancillary Services

Ancillary services are considered to be those services not provided directly by the home infusion therapy agency; the services most often include durable medical equipment (with the exception of infusion pumps), respiratory therapy, and in some cases medical social work and physical therapy. These services are commonly provided, either by referral or subcontract, through the home care pharmacy or nursing agency that provides the infusion therapy. A list of direct and ancillary services can be found in Table 29–1. As the models

merge, any combination of these services can be offered directly or indirectly. The multidisciplinary team concept for the management of health care (Figure 29–3), in which the patient is central and all team members interact collaboratively, best accommodates the goal of quality patient care and services.

BENEFITS OF HOME INFUSION THERAPY

Many benefits of home infusion therapy exist for patients, their family and caregivers, the home care clinicians, and the health care system.

Patient

Patients experience psychosocial, emotional, financial, and health benefits. They are able to return to their own environment, which in itself is a major benefit because the risk for acquiring nosocomial infections decreases. Patients are also more comfortable in the privacy and familiarity of their own home than the hospital. Another benefit for patients is the ability to maintain a higher degree of control over their therapy and their lives with home care. Often, patients are able to return to work or other activities and still maintain their therapy regimen. Patients also experience financial benefits: home treatment is 25 to 75% less expensive than hospital therapy.[8] This fact is extremely important in light of insurance costs and capitation, as well as the increasing life expectancy of patients with chronic or acute diseases.

Family Members and Caregivers

Home infusion therapy reduces the stress experienced by family members and caregivers when their loved ones are

Table 29-1
Direct and Ancillary Services

Direct Services
Consultation for predischarge evaluation
Discharge planning and case management
Complete patient training (hospital/home program)
Patient visitation in the home, clinic, SNF
Dynamic patient assessment and monitoring, including the following:
    Nutritional and physical assessment
    Therapeutic monitoring
Psychosocial support
Parenteral, intramuscular, epidural, and subcutaneous medication administration
Technical procedures by infusion specialists
Infusion control device implantation, monitoring, and removal
Ancillary Services
Diagnostic and laboratory services
Social services
Diet counseling services
Physical therapy
Home health services, including the following:
    Skilled nursing care
    Home health aides
    Durable medical equipment

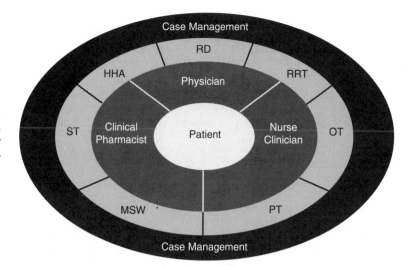

Figure 29–3. Home infusion therapy multidisciplinary team. (From Reid JS, Grace LA, Tomaselli B. Patient Care Management System. Lecture Presentation: National Association for Home Care, San Francisco, CA. Curaflex Health Services, 1991, Ontario, CA.

hospitalized. Often the family member, whether a parent, spouse, or friend, is the primary caregiver. Home care involves and requires family participation. The home infusion program allows them to be active in the care of the patient to whatever degree they feel most comfortable and appropriate. Assistance with care may be obtained based on the acuteness of the illness and the financial resources of the patient. These options may include companions; skilled nursing care, either intermittent or continuous; and home health aides. The availability of assistance with care reduces time lost from work for the family members and caregivers.

In addition to the reduced cost of infusion therapy provided in the home, other financial benefits may be experienced by the family. As the patient is treated in the home setting and the clinicians come to the home, the family members are no longer burdened with making special arrangements to transport their loved one for treatments and evaluations. Home infusion allows the family to spend time in their own home and eliminates the need to make special arrangements for child care and other responsibilities often made difficult during periods of hospitalization. The home environment and activities return to as near normal a state as possible.

Home Infusion Clinician

The IV nurse and pharmacist benefit from the home care environment because it allows more autonomous clinical practice and involvement in emerging home infusion therapies. Work schedules are often flexible and based on patient needs, visits, and therapies. Clinicians are allowed to expand their traditional roles and become more self-fulfilled. Nurses and pharmacists function as a team to provide highly technical, high-quality patient care in the home.

Health Care System

The health care system benefits from home infusion therapy because it provides a cost-effective alternative for medical treatment. Payers are constantly searching for ways to

reduce cost, and hospitals are attuned to diagnostic related groups and early discharge. Home infusion therapy has allowed an increasing number of patients to be treated without ever being admitted to the hospital, once again avoiding unnecessary costs and unnecessary psychological stress related to hospitalization.

QUALIFICATIONS OF HOME INFUSION THERAPY CLINICIANS

Home infusion therapy is a highly specialized technical field; therefore, more specific qualifications exist for the nursing and pharmacy clinicians who are members of the home infusion team.

Educational Requirements

Educational requirements for IV nurses include graduation from an accredited school of nursing and professional licensure from the state in which they will be practicing. Most IV nurses are registered nurses because limitations still exist on the role of the licensed practical nurse/licensed vocational nurse in infusion therapy. Many state boards of nursing are closely reviewing the expanded role of licensed practical nurses/licensed vocational nurses, with the possibility of including more infusion therapy–related procedures in their scope of practice. In general, no established requirements exist regarding the degree or certification held by the home IV nurse. The Intravenous Nurses Society (INS) recommends a Bachelor of Science degree in nursing as the entry level degree. At present, however, criteria are set by individual organizations or agencies based on job description and responsibilities.

Educational requirements for home infusion pharmacists include a Bachelor of Science degree in pharmacy from an accredited school of pharmacy and professional licensure from the state in which they will be practicing. Many clinical home infusion pharmacists have obtained higher or additional degrees, such as a Doctor of Pharmacy or Master of Science in pharmacy. Many pharmacy doctoral programs offer the pharmacist the opportunity to participate in specialized residencies that include nutritional support or home infusion therapy. Once again, the educational requirements are established by the individual organization or agency based on job description and responsibilities.

Experience

One of the key areas of qualification for both nursing and pharmacy personnel is previous experience in infusion therapy. The entry level home IV nurse should have experience in administering infusional therapies and in inserting and managing venous access devices, as well as knowledge of the various infusion devices used to deliver the therapies. This experience may come from previous nursing positions on hospital infusion teams, in the critical care areas (intensive care, cardiac care, neonatal intensive care), or in specialty areas (oncology, pediatrics, hemodialysis, or outpatient infusion clinics). This background in general infusion therapy provides the IV nurse with a solid foundation on which to build home infusion experience. When practicing in home care, IV nurses must realize that although the standards of care are the same, they will be practicing in an environment that is more autonomous and less structured than the hospital or clinic. Independent decision making and effective communication skills are always required. Some nurses find it difficult to make the transition to home practice and are not successful as home IV nurses.

There are two levels of managers in home infusion therapy, the director and the supervisor. Whether an infusion center has need for one or both depends on the size of the center and the number of staff needing supervision. In addition to the qualifications discussed earlier, the home IV nurse manager should possess management skills obtained through previous experience as a charge nurse, head nurse, supervisor, or possibly the director of a specific department in nursing, as well as home care experience. Organizational skills, time management, communication, and personnel management are extremely important skills that ensure the cohesiveness and effectiveness of the nursing component of the team. Home infusion pharmacy managers should also possess management skills. They must be able to identify and prioritize operational and clinical issues to ensure successful operation in the home infusion pharmacy. Home care experience is also required.

Previous home infusion management experience is required for these managers to hold a director position. Many organizations require at least 6 months to 1 year of home infusion management experience for the director of nursing or pharmacy. Experience in the delivery of complex therapies is desirable, as is advanced clinical experience in specialty areas, such as chemotherapy, care for patients with acquired immune deficiency syndrome, and nutritional support.

Personal Attributes

Personal attributes and behavioral characteristics affect one's ability to become a successful home IV nurse or pharmacist. The home IV nurse should be independent, self-motivated, and flexible. Good decision-making abilities are important because clinical judgments must often be made independently. Impeccable communication skills are a must. The physician and other members of the home health care team rely on the home IV nurse and pharmacist for sound, thorough clinical assessment and communication of their findings. Prompt attention to detail is important. Home IV clinicians must be compassionate and empathetic. The ability to be a patient advocate is especially important in the home care setting, where the patient has more control over his or her therapy. The rules are no longer set by the clinician, but by the patient. The home IV clinician must always keep in mind that active patient participation and decision making is key to comprehensive home care.

The home IV clinician has a strong, well-rounded knowledge of general practice as well as his or her specialty area. Providing expertise with a generalist's perspective allows for a holistic approach to home infusion therapy. The home IV nurse must possess excellent physical assessment skills. Highly developed teaching skills are required, particularly the ability to present information clearly and confirm that it is understood. This educational process often extends to the medical community to provide information relative to available infusion therapies in the home.

Certification

An advanced credential for home infusion clinicians is the certified specialist, whose certification requirements vary depending on the professional organization, infusion provider, hospital, or agencies. Some require national certification by a professional organization, whereas others require their own internal certification.

What are the advantages of national certification? National certification promotes professional recognition and identification of clinicians. Because home IV nurses function autonomously, certification validates advanced knowledge, skills, and competency that patients, as educated health care consumers, regard as a patient right rather than a privilege. National certification can provide better employment opportunities, personal development, and career advancement. It allows organizations hiring and employing nurses as well as individuals and organizations referring for services to compare qualifications. Therefore, the home IV nurse is not the only beneficiary of certification. The health care consumer, the employer, and indirectly, the manufacturers of infusion products benefit from the credentialling process.[19]

Several professional organizations offer national certification related to home infusion therapy. The Intravenous Nurses Certification Corporation (INCC) provides certification. By documenting work experience and passing a comprehensive examination, the credentials CRNI (Certified Registered Nurse, Intravenous) are awarded. The certification period is 3 years, at which time you may recertify by retesting or obtaining recertification units at designated INS educational programs.

The American Society for Parenteral and Enteral Nutrition provides certification for nurses, dieticians, and most recently, pharmacists who desire to specialize in nutritional support. Certification is obtained by passing a comprehensive examination. The certification period for nurses and dieticians is 5 years, and for pharmacists, 7 years. Recertification for all disciplines is obtained by retesting. The Oncology

Nursing Society also offers a credentialling exam for Oncology Certified Nurses. This certification is obtained by passing a comprehensive examination. The certification period is 4 years, at which time recertification is obtained by retesting.

Many home infusion companies and home health care agencies maintain their own internal certification programs to validate and document basic competency in the highly technical services they offer. One of the internal certifications most frequently required is IV certification. The INS recommends provision of theoretical aspects in the following areas: fluid and electrolyte balance, infection control, oncology, pediatrics, pharmacology, quality assurance/risk management, technology and clinical application, parenteral nutrition, and transfusion therapy.[20] The home IV nurse's knowledge of the theory is assessed by a comprehensive examination. Along with the didactic portion of the program, a practicum should be completed to demonstrate technical proficiency. Other internal certifications that may be offered to clinicians by home infusion organizations are transfusion therapy, chemotherapy, placement of peripherally inserted central catheters (PICCs), sterile admixture, and pharmacokinetics. Theory and practical experience are recommended by the above-named professional organizations to be a part of these internal programs.

Some home infusion companies and agencies provide advanced internal certifications that focus on advanced theory in certain specialty areas, such as complex home chemotherapy regimens, nutritional and metabolic support, and immunomodulating agents. The home infusion company or agency decreases risk management concerns and provides assurance to the patient that he or she will receive qualified, competent care.

HOME INFUSION PATIENT CARE PROCESS

Although the medical community is equipped to provide home infusion therapy to almost any patient, not every patient is a home care candidate. The criteria that a patient must meet to be accepted into the home infusion program include clinical, financial, and technical issues, which are described further in the section titled "Parameters for Patient Selection."

Therapies Seen in the Home Setting

Historically, the commonest therapies provided in the home care setting have been TPN, total enteral nutrition, antibiotics, chemotherapy, hydration, pain management, aerosolized pentamidine, and catheter care. Recently, however, advances in medicine and technology have opened the door for the provision of several new home therapies, including biologic agents and blood modifiers, human growth hormone, immunoglobulin, blood products and blood factors, α_1-proteinase inhibitor, deferoxamine mesylate (Desferal), cardiologic agents, and continuous and complex chemotherapies. With the rapid progression of research in the 1990s, one can predict that this list will only continue to grow. A list of common home infusion diagnoses and suggested therapies is provided in Table 29–2.

Patient Admission Process

The patient admission process begins with the referral. Many potential referral sources exist, including physicians, case managers, discharge planners, medical social workers, nurses, pharmacists, patients, and caregivers. Although anyone can refer a patient, an order from the physician for pharmaceutical agents must always be obtained and verified by the pharmacy providing the therapy.

Parameters for Patient Selection

Each patient undergoes an admission criteria evaluation process to determine his or her appropriateness for the program. This process includes evaluation of clinical, technical, and financial criteria. On meeting the criteria, the patient is then admitted for services.

Clinical Criteria

The patient must be considered to be medically stable for home infusion therapy as determined by his or her physician[7, 21]; however, because care at home has become so advanced, the criteria for medical stability have become very vague. *Medically stable* is usually defined as a status that does not require continuous intensive medical monitoring and intervention. Because we are now able to provide services and care to the more acutely ill patient in the home, each patient's needs are evaluated individually along with the ability of the organization to provide services that meet those needs in the home care environment. The benefits of provision of services in this setting are evaluated as well.

Even though geographic location is somewhat of a technical issue, it becomes a clinical issue when the accessibility of emergency medical services is evaluated. Moreover, proximity to the health care team is important, if not essential, for providing ongoing assessment to evaluate therapeutic progress and for performing intervention to prevent complications and emergencies. If clinical criteria are not met, ancillary services may be arranged. The patient is then reevaluated for meeting the criteria of the home infusion program. The patient acceptance/rejection model describes this process (Fig. 29–4).

Technical Criteria

A vital component of successful home infusion therapy is the patient's desire and willingness to receive therapy at home. This element goes hand in hand with the patient's ability to learn to administer the therapy or to mobilize the support system to aid in the process if the patient is not able to administer the therapy. The home environment must also be appropriate and must have a telephone, electricity, hot and cold running water, refrigeration, and a clean area for preparation of medications and solutions.

Table 29–2

Potential Home Infusion Diagnoses and Suggested Therapies

Diagnosis/ICD9 Description Code	ICD9 Code	Suggested Therapy	Diagnosis/ICD9 Description Code	ICD9 Code	Suggested Therapy
Abscess, general	682.9	Antibiotic	Histoplasmosis	115.9	Anti-infective
Abscess, brain	324.0	Antibiotic	Hodgkin's disease	201.9	Chemotherapy
Abscess, pelvic	614.4	Antibiotic	Human immunodeficiency virus	044.9	Anti-infective/TEN/TPN
Achalasia, digestive organs congenital	751.8	TPN	Hyperalimentation	783.6	TPN
Achalasia, esophagus	530.0	TPN	Hyperemesis gravidarum	643.0	TPN/Hydration
Acquired immune deficiency syndrome	279.3/D43	Anti-infective/TPN	Hypogammaglobulinemia	279.0	Gamma globulin
Actinomycosis	039.9	Anti-infective	Ileus	560.1	TPN
Adhesions, intestinal with obstruction	560.81	TPN	Infarct, bowel	557.0	TPN
Amyotonia	728.2	Antibiotic/TPN	Infection	136.9	Antibiotic
Anemia	285.9	Blood	Infection, atypical mycobacteria	031.9	Antibiotic
Aphagia	783.0	TEN	Infection, bacterial	041.9	Antibiotic
Arthritis, bacterial	040.89	Antibiotic	Infection, brain	323.9	Antibiotic
Arthritis, infective	711.9	Antibiotic	Infection, cytomegalovirus	771.1	Anti-infective
Asthma	493.9	Aminophylline	Infection, skin	686.9	Antibiotic
Atresia, alimentary organ or tract	751.8	TPN	Ischemic, bowel	557.1	TPN
Bacteremia	790.7	Antibiotic	Ixodiasis	134.8	Antibiotic
Bacteremia caused by organism	038.8	Antibiotic	Kaposi's sarcoma	173.9	Chemotherapy
Blastomycosis	116.0	Anti-infective	Labor, premature	644.2	Tocolytics
Blood transfusion	V58.2	Blood	Leukemia	208.9	Chemotherapy
Bronchiectasis	494.0	Antibiotic	Leukemia, acute myelogenous	205.9	Chemotherapy
Bronchitis	491.0	Antibiotic	Lymph node removal	088.8	Chemotherapy
Cachexia caused by cancer	199.1	TEN/TPN	Lymphoma	202.8	Chemotherapy
Cachexia caused by malnutrition	261.0	TEN/TPN	Malabsorption	579.9	TEN/TPN
Candidiasis	112.9	Anti-infective	Malnutrition	263.9	TEN/TPN
Carcinoma	194.3	Chemotherapy	Melanoma	172.9	Chemotherapy
Celiac disease	579.0	TEN/TPN	Meningitis	322.9	Antibiotic
Cellulitis	682.9	Antibiotic	Metaplasia, agnogenic myeloid	289.8	Antibiotic/TEN
Chemotherapy	V58.1	Chemotherapy	Mycobacterium avium–intracellulare	031.0	Antibiotic
Coccidioidomycosis	114.9	Anti-infective	Mycosis	117.9	Anti-infective
Colitis	558.9	TEN/TPN	Myeloma	203.0	Chemotherapy
Colitis, ulcerative	556.0	TEN/TPN	Myocarditis	429.0	Antibiotic
Congestive heart failure	428.9	Dobutamine	Neoplasm	199.1	Chemotherapy
Cooley's disease	282.4	Deferoxamine mesylate	Neoplasm, alimentary tract	159.9/197.8	Chemotherapy
Crohn's disease	555.9	TEN/TPN	Neoplasm, bone	170.9/198.5	Chemotherapy
Crush injury with infection	929.9	Antibiotic	Neoplasm, breast	174.9/198.81	Chemotherapy
Cryptococcoses	117.5	Antibiotic	Neoplasm, digestive organs	159.9/197.8	Chemotherapy
Cytomegalovirus	363.2	Antibiotic	Neoplasm, esophagus	150.9/197.8	Chemotherapy
Deficiency, α_1-antitrypsin	277.6	Prolastin	Neoplasm, intestine	159.0/197.8	Chemotherapy
Deficiency, antihemophilic factor	286.0	Blood product	Neoplasm, large intestine	153.9/197.5	Chemotherapy
Deficiency, growth hormone	253.3	Growth hormone	Neoplasm, larynx	161.9	Chemotherapy
Deficiency, immunoglobulin	279.0	Gamma globulin	Neoplasm, lung	162.9/197.0	Chemotherapy
Decubitus ulcer	707.0	Antibiotic	Neoplasm, metastatic	275.4	Chemotherapy
Degenerative heart disease	429.1	Dobutamine	Neoplasm, neck	195.0/198.89	Chemotherapy
Dehydration	276.5	Hydration	Neoplasm, prostate	185.0	Chemotherapy
Diabetes	250.0	Antibiotic	Obstruction, intestine	560.9	TPN
Diabetes with gangrene	250.7	Antibiotic	Osteomyelitis	730.2	Antibiotic
Diabetic ulcer	250.8	Antibiotic	Otitis, external malignant	380.14	Antibiotic
Diarrhea, chronic	558.9	TEN/TPN	Pain, bone	733.9	Pain
Diarrhea, infectious	009.2	TEN/TPN	Parkinson's disease	332.0	TEN/PEN
Disease, pelvic inflammatory chronic	614.4	Antibiotic	Pneumonia	486.0	Antibiotic
Embolism, pulmonary	415.1	Antithrombolytic	Pneumonia, Pneumocystis carinii	136.3	Anti-infective
Encephalitis, viral	049.9	Anti-infective	Prematurity	765.1	PEN
Encephalitis, viral, arthropod borne	064.0	Anti-infective	Prostatitis	601.9	Antibiotic
Endocarditis, infectious	421.0	Antibiotic	Pseudomonas	250.8/682.6	Antibiotic
Enteritis, viral	008.6	Anti-infective	Pseudo-obstruction, intestinal	564.8	TPN
Enteritis, bacterial	008.5	Antibiotic	Pulmonary disease, chronic obstructive	416.9	α_1-Proteinase inhibitor
Fibrosis, cystic	277.0	Antibiotic/TEN/TPN	Purpura, idiopathic thrombocytopenic	287.3	Biologics
Fistula, abdomen	569.8	TEN/TPN	Pyelonephritis	590.8	Antibiotic
Fracture, open	829.1	Antibiotic	Septicemia	038.9	Antibiotic
Fungal disease	117.9	Anti-infective	Short-bowel syndrome	579.2	TPN
Gangrene	785.4	Antibiotic	Sinusitis, chronic	473.9	Antibiotic
Gonococcal joint infection	098.5	Antibiotic	Stomatitis	528.0	PEN
Gonococcal pelvis infection chronic	098.39	Antibiotic	Thalassemia	282.4	Deferoxamine mesylate
Hemophilia	286.0	Blood products	Thrombophlebitis	451.9	Anticoagulants
Herpes simplex, complicated	054.8	Anti-infective	Wound, complicated	879.8	Antibiotic

ICD = International Classification of Diseases; PEN = partial enteral nutrition; TEN = total enteral nutrition; TPN = total parenteral nutrition.

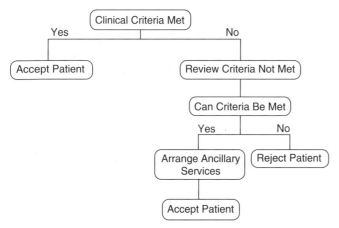

Figure 29–4. Patient acceptance/rejection model.

Financial Criteria and Considerations

Once the referral is made, the patient financial services representative evaluates the reimbursement potential for the therapy prescribed, verifies insurance coverage, and arranges payment plans with the patient or guarantor of payment. If the therapy is not covered by insurance, the patient could pay for the therapy, receive the therapy in the hospital or physician's office, or obtain funding through charitable organizations. Patient financial service representatives are trained in assisting the patient in exploring reimbursement possibilities as well as negotiating with insurance companies. Because insurance policies differ, this service assists the patient by interpreting and clarifying policy limits and negotiating rates and services covered under the policy as well as those not covered.

Initial Patient Assessment

The initial patient assessment (IPA) is the baseline evaluation of the patient against which all subsequent and future evaluations are compared. The assessment includes a medical, drug, and nutritional history; analysis of laboratory data and trends; a therapeutic assessment; a complete physical examination; a psychosocial and cognitive assessment; and evaluation of the admission criteria mentioned earlier. Ideally, this assessment is initiated before the start of care during a conference at which all members of the health care team, including the patient and family, discuss and develop the plan for care and services at home. The IPA is most commonly concluded at the first home visit, when the home environment and technical skills are observed.

The traditionally short interval from the referral to the initial infusion visit is an issue that frequently prevents the luxury of a preadmission conference. More frequently than not, preadmission coordination of care and services occurs via telephone between the members of the health care team. The patient is not fully accepted into the program until all admission criteria have been evaluated and met, the IPA is complete, and the home environment is considered to be safe and appropriate for home infusion therapy. The nurse and/or pharmacist visits the patient and family members or caregivers to develop this plan in the hospital, the home, or both, to complete the IPA.

Patient Care Planning and Initiation of Therapy

Obtaining Orders

Although a referral can come from any discipline, most states require that physician's orders for prescriptions be verified by a pharmacist. An order can be taken from a physician's designated representative, and in most states, a verbal order taken by the pharmacist does not need a physician's signature. On the other hand, verbal orders taken by nurses must be signed in accordance with state nursing law and practice acts. If the organization is a state-licensed or Medicare-certified agency, state and Health Care Finance Administration licensure rules must be followed and a physician plan of treatment, addendum and updates (Health Care Finance Administration forms 485, 486, and 487) must be completed as required.

Developing the Plan of Care

Patient care planning begins at the time the referral is communicated and the physician's order obtained. It is ongoing throughout the course of therapy, and in some cases, occurs even while the patient is not undergoing therapy. The most integral piece of the patient care process, the care plan, is multidisciplinary and provides a road map for technical procedures and schedules, therapeutic monitoring, evaluation, treatment, and patient teaching. It specifies parameters and goals for each individual patient, as well as scheduling and delivery system needs, and is updated as needed. Therapy scheduling should be planned with the patient, and it should be as convenient as possible for both the patient and the caregivers while still meeting the goals of therapy. If feasible, procedures should occur during waking hours and should interrupt the patient's rest period as little as possible. Long, cyclic infusions should be administered during sleeping hours, and short, intermittent infusions should be scheduled during waking hours. Delivery systems and equipment should be user friendly, safe, and trouble free. Lightweight ambulatory equipment should be used if the patient is mobile or needs round-the-clock infusion.

Initiating the Plan: Interdisciplinary Communications and Coordination of Care

Interdisciplinary communication and coordination are two important components to the success of the home infusion program, second only to the patient component. Only through collaborative efforts, diligent management of the case coordinator, and interdisciplinary case conferences does quality communication occur. Such communication enables a clear definition of the roles and responsibilities of each provider, ensuring the provision of quality patient care and services. Such technology as telephone conferencing, communication via facsimile machines, and computers with modems have all enhanced our communication abilities and should be advocated for use in the home infusion therapy program.

Performing the Initial Patient Visit

As mentioned earlier, during the initial patient visit, the IPA is usually completed. The patient receives an intensive orientation to the service and a lesson on the procedures to be performed. The patient's psychological status should be considered at this time; the patient likely has other issues on his or her mind besides the technical aspects of the home infusion visit, including issues related to a newly diagnosed illness or a reoccurrence of an illness, and family, work, or other responsibilities. Although it is difficult to determine how much each patient can handle, only approximately 30% of what you tell a patient will be retained.[22] For this reason, a teaching plan should be developed after the IPA is performed and before the second visit. Important instructions should be addressed, repeated, and reviewed, along with simply written step-by-step instructions. Simply written references and telephone contacts should be left with the patient in case he or she has questions or needs assistance. Overwhelming a patient can be counterproductive; less important issues and details should be addressed on subsequent visits.

Orientating Patient to Service

General issues to be discussed during orientation include components of the service, roles of clinicians, ordering and delivery of equipment and supplies, and important telephone numbers and contacts. Addressed at this time are the more formal issues, such as service consents, assignment of benefits, receipt of goods, rights and responsibilities, and access to services in case of a medical emergency or a natural disaster.

As of December 1, 1991, it is mandatory that advanced directives be addressed with each patient. This mandate came about as a result of the Patient Self-Determination Act passed by the United States Congress as a part of the Omnibus Reconciliation Act of 1990. It requires that home health care providers inform their patients of their rights to make decisions about their health care and to execute advanced directives. Advanced directives are documented instructions made by the patient that relate their wishes for the provision of health care when they become incapacitated. It defines their choices and designates an individual who will make decisions on their behalf at a point of which they are no longer able to make their own decisions. These documents include a durable power of attorney for health care and a declaration pursuant to the Natural Death Act. Written handbooks about the information discussed should be left with patients for their reference.

Teaching the Patient

Teaching the home infusion therapy program involves lessons related to technical procedures as well as monitoring of therapy. Technical procedures that the patient is expected to learn and perform depend on several factors, including the patient's cognitive ability, his or her willingness to learn, the technique being taught, the philosophy of the organization, the number of available visits, the remoteness of the patient, and the standard of practice. Patients or their caregivers are commonly expected to administer solutions and medications, change dressings and infusion tubing, and give injections. They would not routinely be expected to start IV lines or draw blood. The training process should be progressive according to the prescribed therapy. Although no set standards exist for the number of visits required to teach a patient to

administer therapy, some broad guidelines are provided in Table 29–3.

The length of teaching is customized and adjusted based on the patient's abilities and progress and should be documented on the care plan. Not all clinicians are equally experienced in communication and teaching techniques of home infusion therapy. Some therapies are more complicated than others, such as those using programmable infusion devices, and take more time to teach and to learn. Therefore, the teaching period should be as long or as short as both patient and clinician feel is appropriate. When both feel comfortable, they sign a statement documenting competency. This document is usually in the form of a patient teaching checklist.

Monitoring and Evaluating Patient Care

Monitoring is specific to the type of therapy, the patient's condition, and the goals of treatment. The patient or caregiver is generally expected to monitor and report any changes in condition or status. Therapy-specific areas addressed in the patient teaching sessions are also monitored and include vital signs, intake and output, weight, urine or blood glucose level, treatments, and medication or solution administration. A list of potential problems and complications is usually provided in the patient teaching material (Table 29–4).

The strategy for clinical therapeutic monitoring and evaluation of patients may vary depending on which model of home infusion therapy is being employed. Ultimately, however, the outcome should be the same. In the case of the pharmacy home infusion therapy model, the nurse, or the pharmacist, or both, visit and communicate with the patient and caregivers to assess the patient's physical condition and the therapeutic progress. They also evaluate the appropriateness of the prescribed therapy. The pharmacist analyzes laboratory data and reviews observations and physical findings. The pharmacy also completes an assessment of appropriateness of the formulation or prescribed medication. Comparison of data collected allows for assessment of outcome or progression toward expected goals. At the same time, the nurse analyzes physical assessment findings, symptomatology, laboratory data, and therapeutic response. The two then collaborate to make clinical recommendations for adjusting the plan. In the nursing agency home infusion therapy model, the process is the same; however, collaboration usually occurs via telecommunications or during scheduled interdisci-

---

Table 29–3

Progressive Training for the Home Infusion Therapy Patient*

Visit No.	Teaching Action
1	The clinician gives demonstration of preparation and administration of therapy.
2	The patient prepares the equipment and gives demonstration with clinician's assistance and intervention.
3	The patient prepares the equipment independently. The clinician reviews the preparation and observes the demonstration with minimal intervention.
4	The patient prepares the equipment and gives demonstration using good technique without clinician intervention. The clinician observes.

*Each step in the process may be repeated as many times as necessary.

Table 29-4

Potential Problems and Complications Encountered in Home Infusion Therapy

Problem	Potential Complications
Mechanical	
• Blood back-up in tubing	• Pump alarming
• Inability to flush catheter	• Nonrunning IV line
• Fluid leakage	• Pain or swelling at site
• Redness or warmth at site	
Systemic	
• Shortness of breath	• Coughing
• Respiratory distress	• Chest pain
• Rash	• Itching
• Fever	• Chills
• Muscle aches	• Weakness
• Exit site drainage	• Lethargy
Metabolic	
• Dizziness or fainting	• Heart pounding
• Increased thirst	• Sugar in urine
• Increased urination	• Cold sweats
• Abdominal or leg cramp	• Flushing
• Double vision	• Headache
• Confusion	• Nervousness
• Numbness	• Twitching
• Tingling in extremities	

plinary meetings. In either case, the physician is contacted to communicate findings, to obtain new orders, or to change orders.

Ongoing Dynamic Assessment

Physical Systems

Clinical monitoring should be ongoing and dynamic. A commonly used tool for facilitating assessment is a physical systems review, during which the clinician reviews each system for subjective and objective signs and symptoms and changes in condition. The current status is then measured against the baseline IPA evaluation.

Nutrition

No one good measurement exists for nutritional assessment in the home patient. Methodology for assessing nutritional status is highly controversial even among clinicians. Nutritional status is usually measured using a combination of measurements or assessments,[15, 23, 24] such as laboratory analysis of visceral proteins, including total protein and albumin levels, as well as evaluation of somatic proteins, measured by anthropometric measurements and ideal body weight, usual body weight, and percentage of weight gain or loss over a period of time. Other measures, such as transferrin levels and creatinine height index, are not usually performed in the home. Physical evaluation is also an important component of nutritional status. A course on general nutrition equips a clinician with the basic knowledge for determining signs and symptoms of nutritional deficiencies. For proficiency in the area of nutritional support, a residency or training period with a nutritional support team is recommended. Overall, the most reliable and commonly used ongoing meas-

urement of nutritional status in the home patient is weight gain or loss.

Outcome

A fairly new concept to home infusion therapy is outcome monitoring. The Joint Commission on Accreditation of Healthcare Organizations (JCAHO) made voluntary accreditation available to this industry only in the past three years. A requirement for accreditation is ability to monitor outcome.[25] A home infusion therapy company must monitor two indicators for each service provided: nursing, pharmacy, equipment, and one patient satisfaction indicator. Outcome for each subcontracted service, such as rehabilitation therapist, social worker, and dietician, must also be evaluated. These can be indicators that are cross-disciplinary. A common outcome indicator seen in home infusion is "The patient has achieved the goals of therapy as stated on the plan of care." As the patient's condition or status changes, so must the plan. The plan is altered so that either the original goals of therapy are more realistic or the overall goals of therapy are redefined based on changes in patient status.

For organizations not seeking accreditation, outcome monitoring is not yet mandatory. Although JCAHO accreditation is a voluntary process, some third-party payers have recently made accreditation a requirement for reimbursement. As hospitals and physicians progress toward an outcome-based reimbursement system rather than a diagnostic related group system, home care should also expect to follow suit.[26, 27] The JCAHO is currently beta testing several outcome indicators. Home infusion companies should begin to prepare themselves for monitoring the outcome of the care and services they provide to their patients.

Reporting and Communications

Communication is the key to the success of the home infusion therapy program. Because the health care team and record may be located in several places (e.g., the physician's office, the home infusion pharmacy, the nursing agency, the durable medical equipment/respiratory therapy supplier), alternate methods of communication should be used. Interdisciplinary team meetings, although ideal, cannot be conveniently held often enough to achieve the necessary results. Advanced telecommunications have contributed to enhanced communications in the home infusion industry. Progress reports, physician's orders, and laboratory results are commonly faxed between doctor's offices, infusion companies, nursing agencies, and laboratories. The telephone is used as the main mode of communication for patient status, new or changed orders, scheduling and coordination of home visits, and various other activities.

Weekly patient care rounds should be held to discuss new patients and changes in plan for patients already on service. Concise patient updates can be presented by each patient's primary clinician. Therapy, acuteness of illness, and status should all be determinants of how often a patient is discussed. For instance, a patient undergoing monthly intravenous gamma globulin therapy should be discussed the week before and after the monthly visit and additionally when changes in status or condition warrant. This method keeps weekly rounds manageable even if patient census is large.

More informal communication, within as well as outside of the hospital, needs to occur between all members of the health care team. The better the communication, the greater the continuity of care and service the patient receives. The central documents for communication between all of the different parties are the clinical progress notes. In these notes, weekly patient care rounds, communication with the physician, nursing agencies, patient, patient caregivers, and interoffice communication should be documented. The clinical progress notes may also contain laboratory analysis, clinical assessments, and documentation of progress toward outcomes. Communication boards or computerized programs tracking schedules for deliveries, patient visits, and routing may be used; however, nothing replaces verbal communication between the pharmacist, nurse, delivery technician, and reimbursement coordinator.

Patient Discharge and Termination of Care

Discharge planning should begin the day the patient begins therapy; this process takes time and should not be postponed until the last day of therapy. Discharge planning begins when the duration of therapy is determined and discussed with the patient. It continues as the nurse discusses discontinuation of therapy, postdischarge plans, and follow-up care or services. At a point close to discharge, usually the second or third visit from the discharge date, plans are finalized and the patient is provided with a written plan. Services are coordinated according to the physician's orders for postdischarge services as necessary. A written report evaluating the course of therapy and summarizing the discharge instructions is then sent to the physician and other appropriate members of the health care team.

Postdischarge follow-up depends on the diagnosis and the therapy the patient is receiving. For instance, a patient with acquired immune deficiency syndrome who has received a course of antibiotics may be closely monitored after therapy for reoccurrence of infection. After infusion, a chemotherapy patient may be monitored during the nadir of the white blood cell count for signs and symptoms of neutropenia-induced sepsis. Conversely, a patient who has had a course of antibiotics for subacute bacterial endocarditis may never be seen again by the home infusion clinician once therapy is discontinued. More and more, however, the more acute patient in the home who needs postdischarge follow-up is seen to identify the potential for complications and prevent reoccurence.

THERAPIES APPROPRIATE FOR HOME CARE

Antibiotics and Anti-Infective Agents

The administration of antibiotics and anti-infective agents in the home care setting originated in response to the demand for reduction of treatment costs to patients, third-party payers, and hospitals. Many patients have been trained to successfully administer their infusion antibiotics at home since the late 1970s.[7]

The most common diagnoses treated in the home care

setting are disease states in which chronic or deep-seated infections are not effectively eradicated by the use of oral antibiotics.

Common Diagnoses for Which Home Intravenous Antibiotic and Anti-Infective Agents Are Used

- Abscesses
- Acute leukemia
- Bacterial endocarditis
- Candidiasis
- Cellulitis
- Chronic urinary tract infections
- Coccidioidomycosis
- Cryptococcal meningitis
- Cryptosporidiosis
- Cystic fibrosis
- Cytomegalovirus retinitis
- Hairy leukoplakia
- Histoplasmosis
- Lyme disease
- Mycobacterium avium–intracellulare
- Osteomyelitis
- Pelvic inflammatory disease
- Pneumocystis carinii pneumonia
- Sepsis
- Toxoplasmosis
- Wound infections

Most Commonly Prescribed Antibiotic and Anti-Infective Agents

The selection of the antibiotic or anti-infective agent is of critical importance. Criteria reviewed by the physician and home infusion pharmacist when the medication is selected include efficacy of the medication against the offending pathogen or pathogens, tolerance of the patient to the medication, frequency of administration, stability of drugs and solutions, severity of toxicities, patient allergy history, presence of organ failure, duration of therapy, monitoring requirements, potential drug interactions, and availability of venous access.[7] Many antibiotic and anti-infective agents have been administered successfully in the home. The most frequently administered IV medications are the cephalosporins.

Scheduling, dose frequency, and ease of administration are much more important considerations for home antibiotic therapy than for IV therapy administered in the hospital. Several of the newer cephalosporins have extended half-lives that allow once- or twice-daily dosing, making it convenient for the patient and causing minimal interruption of daily activities. Antibiotics that have an increased ability to cause phlebitis should be considered carefully for home peripheral administration because of the increased frequency of rotating peripheral IV access. Several options exist in this situation, including inserting a central venous access device, diluting the medication, and slowing the infusion rate or changing to another, less caustic, medication that is equally effective against the causative pathogen.

Common Antibiotics and Anti-Infective Agents Used in Home Care

- Acyclovir (Zovirax)
- Amikacin (Amikin)
- Amphotericin B (Fungizone)
- Azlocillin (Azlin)
- Aztreonam (Azactam)
- Carbenicillin (Geopen, Geocillin)
- Cefazolin (Ancef, Kefzol)
- Cefoperazone (Cefobid)
- Cefotaxime (Claforan)
- Cefotetan (Cefotan)
- Cefoxitin (Mefoxin)
- Ceftazidime (Fortaz, Tazicef)
- Ceftizoxime (Cefizox)
- Ceftriaxone (Rocephin)
- Ciprofloxacin (Cipro)
- Clindamycin (Cleocin)
- Cotrimoxazole (Bactrim)
- Erythromycin lactobionate (Erythrocin)
- Foscarnet (Foscavir)
- Ganciclovir (Cytovene)
- Gentamicin (Garamycin)
- Imipenem/Cilastatin (Primaxin)
- Metronidazole (Flagyl)
- Mezlocillin (Mezlin)
- Nafcillin (Unipen)
- Netilmicin (Netromycin)
- Oxacillin (Bactocil)
- Penicillin G
- Piperacillin (Pipracil)
- Ticarcillin (Ticar)
- Ticarcillin/Clavulanate (Timentin)
- Tobramycin (Nebcin)
- Vancomycin (Vancocin)

Common Concerns and Issues

A common concern of home infusion antibiotic patients and home infusion providers is reimbursement. Medicare payment has generally been denied for antibiotic therapy, although legislation is in process to change this. Many third-party payers allow for reimbursement of home infusion antibiotics after close review of the statement of medical necessity, the charges for the antibiotics and supplies, and the type of coverage that the patient has. Because home antibiotic and anti-infective agents are prescribed based on culture and sensitivity tests and diagnosis, respectively, a statement of medical necessity is completed to document the need and the appropriateness of the medication and the causative organism. Because of the ever-changing environment and the complexity of reimbursement issues, the home infusion provider must have an experienced billing and reimbursement staff person work with the patient, third-party payer, and home infusion team to obtain the best reimbursement possible.

A major concern for the patient and the health care team is achievement of therapeutic goals. For this reason, time should be taken to teach the patient the importance of maintaining therapeutic blood levels of the prescribed medication. This goal can be accomplished only by diligent compliance with administration of dosages as scheduled. The home care

team can assist the patient with scheduling to minimize interruptions of daily activities and rest periods. For multiple daily infusions, an infusion pump may be suggested, if appropriate for the drug. Hypersensitivity and allergic reactions are always of major concern, and these are discussed in detail under ''First-Dose Guidelines.''

Some other concerns of home infusion antibiotic patients include their ability to self-administer medications and problem solving, the frequency of rotating peripheral venous access sites, the frequency of administration, and the support available from the home infusion provider. Patients should receive thorough training by the home nursing and pharmacy clinicians regarding their diagnosis, the medication prescribed, the goals of therapy, aseptic technique, the care and maintenance of their specific access device, the set-up of supplies and equipment, and the initiation and termination of infusion. Information regarding possible side effects and complications, the process of delivery of supplies and medication, and the frequency of nursing visits should also be reviewed. This information is provided verbally and in writing.

First-Dose Guidelines

Many patients are able to avoid hospitalization because of the advent of home infusion antibiotic therapy. This practice raises the controversial issue of first-dose administration in the home. In the past, the first dose of antibiotic or anti-infective agent could be given only in a controlled clinical environment, such as the hospital, physician's office, clinic, outpatient infusion suite, or emergency room. A controlled clinical environment is still the location of choice for first-dose administration; however, today, first dosing is administered more frequently safely and effectively in the home setting. This change largely results from advances in technology and pharmaceuticals as well as specialization of home IV nurses and pharmacists. The availability of first-dose administration in the home does not negate the necessity to perform it in a controlled environment for highly sensitive or allergic patients. All patients who are to receive antibiotic or anti-infective agents need to have a thorough allergy history evaluation. The home infusion pharmacist reviews this information and performs a risk analysis. If the patient is determined to have low or minimal risk and no history of allergic response or cross allergies, the pharmacist may recommend the first dose to be administered in the home under the continuous supervision of the IV nurse. However, a reaction can occur even though risk is low. For this reason, an anaphylactic order and protocol should always be obtained and available. A few antibiotics, such as penicillin and cotrimoxazole (Bactrim), are extremely likely to cause allergic reactions, and clinicians should carefully evaluate their use when considering giving a first dose in the home. Patients with allergies to penicillin may also have an allergic response to cephalosporins.

Allergic and anaphylactic reactions can occur not only on the first dose, but at any time during antibiotic therapy. The home IV nurse must be able to identify and differentiate allergic responses from anaphylactic reactions. IV nurses must train their patients to recognize and report signs and symptoms of allergic reactions and access emergency medical services in the event of anaphylaxis. The provision of anaphylaxis kits for every home antibiotic patient is controversial. Anaphylaxis kits should be provided and readily accessible for all first-dose administrations. The kit should include epinephrine, diphenhydramine (Benadryl), hydrocortisone (Solu-Cortef), acetaminophen, 0.9% sodium chloride solution, an IV administration set, and the required needles, syringes, and swabs. There are several commercially prepared kits available. The home infusion pharmacist must review with the physician the anaphylactic kit and protocols and must obtain orders to dispense the kit and its contents. The home IV nurse must have knowledge of each medication in the anaphylactic kit and the protocols for intervention, as well as ongoing education on this issue. It is extremely important that the home infusion provider develops and implements policies and procedures for first-dose administration.

Delivery Systems

Home infusion antibiotics can be administered via peripheral heparin lock, central venous catheter, PICC, tunneled central venous catheter, or implantable port. The route of administration is determined by the patient, physician, and home infusion clinician based on diagnosis, duration of therapy, frequency of administration, venous access available, and medication prescribed. Generally, home antibiotics are given by gravity infusion that uses minibags. Ambulatory infusion devices may be used for medications that need to be accurately controlled, such as amphotericin B, when patient compliance is a concern or if the frequency of the dose would lend itself to the use of such a device. In some situations, the infusion device is connected only intermittently. The access device is flushed after administration. In other situations, the infusion device may be connected continuously, with intermittent infusion of the medication at preprogrammed intervals. During the ''off'' cycle, the infusion device maintains positive pressure and administers a minute amount of medication to keep the infusion access device patent. Some pumps are also capable of delivering multiple antibiotics at independently timed schedules. The cost versus benefit must be evaluated to identify the most appropriate and cost-effective method of administration.

Clinical Monitoring

Clinical monitoring of patients receiving antibiotics is based on the same standards, regardless of the treatment environment, i.e., home, hospital. Geographic logistics need to be considered. Routine home visits by the home IV nurse are completed based on access device and acuteness of the patient's illness. During this visit, the home IV nurse performs technical procedures related to the infusion access device and equipment, reinforcement of training, compliance monitoring by inventory count, blood drawing, and clinical assessment. Clinical assessment focuses on the antibiotic prescribed in relation to the development of adverse reactions and complications, symptoms related to the patient's disease process, and progress toward the goals of therapy. Laboratory monitoring may include complete blood counts with differential, renal profile, electrolyte, liver enzyme, and antibiotic drug levels.

Some adverse reactions and complications include direct tissue toxicities, such as irritation to the veins (phlebitis) or intramuscular injection sites (pain, swelling, or hematomas). The gastrointestinal tract can also be irritated, causing nausea, vomiting, or diarrhea. Organs of metabolism or elimination can be directly affected (e.g., liver, kidney), which can result in reversible or permanent damage. Superinfections, such as yeast infections, can also occur from nonsensitive organisms allowed to grow unchecked. Hypersensitivity reactions of either the immediate or delayed type may also occur and must be closely monitored. Patients should be cautioned against ingestion of alcohol or medication containing alcohol when taking some cephalosporins, such as cefamandole, cefoperazone, moxalactam, and cefotetan, because they may experience a disulfiram-like reaction. This reaction is an alcohol intolerance response and is exhibited by flushing, headache, nausea, vomiting, and tachycardia.

Total Parenteral Nutrition

TPN, also known as hyperalimentation and as home parenteral nutrition when given in the home setting, was one of the first infusion therapies to be administered outside of the acute care setting. Initial indications for TPN were conditions in which nutritional deficiencies occurred as a result of the patient's inability to properly use the digestive system, resulting in prolonged administration of TPN. These patients either shortly recovered after initiating TPN, or their only medical needs were for TPN administration. Hospitalization purely for the administration of TPN became an issue both financially and psychologically for the patient.[8, 18] An alternative for the patient was to receive TPN in his or her home, and thus home parenteral nutrition was born.

Indications

Indications for TPN have expanded over the last 10 years. Initially, TPN, a total nutritional source providing all of the body's daily nutritional requirements, was prescribed in cases in which the patient could not eat because of a functional impairment, such as short-bowel syndrome or small-bowel obstruction, or in cases in which the patient was restricted from eating when bowel rest was indicated, such as in the treatment of ulcerative colitis or Crohn's disease. As medical and technologic advances progressed and research found other indications for TPN, terms of reimbursement became more strictly defined by medical necessity. TPN was now being prescribed based on functional impairment and symptomatology rather than purely on diagnosis.[9, 10] For example, not all patients who have a short bowel need TPN. However, a percentage of bowel resection patients have short-bowel syndrome and failure to thrive secondary to malabsorption, necessitating TPN administration.

Common diagnoses, therefore, include short-bowel syndrome, massive bowel resection, mesenteric infarction, radiation enteritis, inflammatory bowel disease, intestinal obstruction, and motility disorders, such as intractable nausea and vomiting or diarrhea. In addition, the patient must be unable to absorb sufficient nutrients to maintain height and weight.

Routes of Therapy

Central venous access is generally the most common route used for administration of home parenteral nutrition. TPN can be given both centrally and peripherally. The peripheral route may be used provided that the final dextrose concentration is not greater than 10%.[20] However, peripheral administration in the home setting is not generally recommended. With the advent of the PICC and the advances in permanent long-term access devices, use of peripheral access for TPN is rarely indicated in the home setting. There is no longer a need to subject the patient to increased risks of infiltration and phlebitis and repeated infusion restarts.

Types of Parenteral Nutrition

In addition to TPN, other parenteral nutrient admixtures prescribed for home infusion include partial parenteral nutrition and total nutrient admixture, also known as three-in-one or all-in-one. Partial parenteral nutrition provides a portion of the body's requirements and is prescribed as a supplement to oral or enteral nutrition. Although most commonly administered intermittently, three times a week or every other day, partial parenteral nutrition may be prescribed daily based on the patient's fluid needs. Total nutrient admixture is the same as TPN; however the term indicates that patients are receiving part of their caloric source in the way of a fat emulsion and that a single administration container system is being used. This system is recommended in the home care setting because it is easier to teach and to learn. The risks of contamination are reduced because there is only one line to manipulate.[6, 28]

Intradialytic parenteral nutrition, parenteral nutrition administered during hemodialysis (provided by the home infusion company), has been limited to date largely because of reimbursement issues. Intradialytic parenteral nutrition is administered over a 3- to 4-hour period, three to four times per week in conjunction with dialysis treatments. Other specialized formulas for hepatic or renal failure are less frequently seen in the home setting.

Common Issues and Concerns

TPN in the home setting is one of the more complex therapies for several reasons, including TPN vascular access availability, duration and frequency of administration, mobility of the patient, complexity of the delivery system, and clinical and patient monitoring issues. As with any home infusion therapy, psychosocial support and compliance are always important issues, especially in therapies of extended duration. Permanent vascular access devices, such as tunneled catheters and ports, are generally recommended for long-term TPN administration.[29] Intermediate vascular access devices, such as PICCs, can be used as well.[30]

Home parenteral nutrition is generally cycled or given over a 12- to 16-hour period, and most of the administrations occur during the sleeping hours. Ideally, the less time it takes for the patients to receive their TPN safely, the less interruptive it will be and the easier it will be to integrate into the patient's life. Depending on the patients' diagnosis or disease process, their level of activity ranges from being completely bedridden to participating in normal daily activities, including work or school. Recent advances in ambulatory pump technology have minimized the concern about the use of such equipment while having an active lifestyle. A small pump can now be programmed to turn on, taper up, taper down,

and turn off TPN and can be slipped into a backpack that even a small child can carry.[31]

Clinical monitoring is one of the major concerns depending on the status and stability of the patient. The more acutely ill the patient is, the closer the monitoring needs to be. Both the nurse and the pharmacist need to pay particular attention to laboratory values, physical status findings, fluid requirements, and signs and symptoms of infection. The patient as well as the physician depends on these clinicians to communicate information related to observation between the patient's doctor visits. Thorough training courses in advanced nutrition, physical and nutritional assessment, laboratory analysis, therapeutic monitoring, and nutritional support are recommended for home care clinicians caring for TPN patients.

Patient self-monitoring is as important as clinical monitoring. The patient must be taught to monitor vital signs, fluid status, urine glucose level, and weight, and the patient must be given parameters for reporting outer limits.

Psychosocial support is another concern. As with any long-term therapy, family, friends, and caregivers provide an important means for assisting and supporting the patient through difficult times. Not all patients need assistance with the administration of their therapy, but most need some psychosocial support because nourishment by the IV route is not the norm. Patients who are more acutely ill or are diagnosed with a terminal illness may eventually need a full-time caregiver. It is generally recommended that along with the patient, a primary caregiver as well as an alternative caregiver learn and become involved in the home infusion program.

Because home infusion patients are not in a controlled setting, compliance to scheduling and daily administration is a concern. An excess number of bags in the refrigerator is usually the telltale sign of noncompliance. However, gross noncompliance may also be noted by fluctuations in laboratory values, both upward and downward, and loss of or failure to gain weight. Continual reinforcement and support as well as involving the patient and caregiver in the treatment plan reduces the chance of noncompliance.

Initiating TPN in the Home Setting

Initiating TPN in the home setting requires the availability of skilled clinicians, especially a pharmacist with experience and education in the field of nutritional support and a higher level of service. The patient is initially evaluated for nutritional and physical status as well as all other components of the IPA. Baseline laboratory values are obtained and evaluated, and recommendations for TPN formulations are made. A modified formulation may be initiated, depending on the results of the evaluation of the patient. The modified formulation is then adjusted upward to the final formulation as the patient's clinical condition permits. One or two bags are compounded at a time to limit waste. Obtaining laboratory values before the next bag is used allows one to make adjustments in the formulation until a stabilization point is reached. If uncomplicated, this process generally takes about one week. If complicated, stabilization can take several weeks. TPN is usually compounded for 7 days, at which time the laboratory values are obtained and evaluated. Depending on the patient's stability, laboratory values may be obtained and TPN compounded twice a week, or in the case of the stable, long-term TPN patient, once a month.

Delivery Systems

TPN is always administered by an infusion device in the home. The complexity of the therapy as well as the ambulation status of the patient determines which pump is chosen. Generally, for the administration of TPN, a programmable, variable-rate, volumetric pump that is safe, accurate, user friendly, and easy to troubleshoot is the device of choice.

Clinical Monitoring

Clinical monitoring of home TPN patients should be no different from monitoring hospitalized TPN patients. However, although the areas monitored are the same, the logistics are quite different. Patients are taught to monitor vital signs, fluid intake and output, weight gain or loss, and blood and/or urine glucose levels. They are also taught to report outer limits to the home infusion clinicians. These outer limits commonly include temperature increases, weight gain of more than a half pound per day, spilling of glucose in the urine or abnormal fingerstick glucose level, and any changes in overall status. The home infusion clinician tracks and analyzes this information along with physical findings and laboratory analyses to evaluate progress, prevent potential complications, and make recommendations for achieving the goals of therapy. Areas that are generally monitored, tracked, and analyzed include vital signs, urine glucose level, weight, fluid status, complete blood count, and full chemistry panel (Table 29–5).

Chemotherapy

Chemotherapy has been prescribed for the treatment of cancer since the 1960s. Over the past 10 to 15 years, single chemotherapeutic agents have been administered by infusion in the home setting.[18] Those most commonly administered include fluorouracil and floxuridine. In the past few years, complex chemotherapy or multiple-agent chemotherapy reg-

Table 29–5

Laboratory Monitoring for the Home TPN Patient

Complete Blood Count		Chemistry
White blood cells	Sodium	Uric acid
Red blood cells	Potassium	Cholesterol
Hemoglobin	Chloride	Triglycerides
Hematocrit	Carbon dioxide	Bilirubin
Segmented neutrophils	Glucose	Alkaline phosphatase
Lymphocytes	Blood urea nitrogen	Lactic dehydrogenase
Band neutrophils	Serum creatinine	Aspartate aminotransferase
Eosinophils	Calcium	Alanine aminotransferase
Platelets	Phosphorus	Magnesium
	Total protein	Ionized calcium
	Albumin	

Table 29–6

Common Indications for Chemotherapeutic Drugs Prescribed in the Home Complex Chemotherapy Program

Bone cancer	Metastatic cancer
Breast cancer	Multiple myeloma
Chronic lymphocytic leukemia	Head and neck cancer
Hodgkin's disease	Non-Hodgkin's lymphoma
Intestinal cancer	Ovarian cancer
Leukemias	Prostate cancer
Lung cancer	Stomach cancer

imens have been administered in the home under the care of trained oncology infusion specialists. It is no longer necessary to admit these patients to the acute care setting for therapy, provided that the support of clinical oncology specialists is available.

Indications

Chemotherapy is prescribed in the home for patients with cancer. Agents and their route of administration are prescribed based on the type, location, and stage of cancer as well as the age, medical history, and physical status of the patient.[32] Prior treatment effectiveness and other diagnostic tests are also taken into account. In the past, the diagnoses most commonly seen in the home were those for which continuous fluorouracil and floxuridine were prescribed. With advances in medical and clinical applications, as well as in technology, many patients with cancer are seen in home chemotherapy programs (Table 29–6).

Routes of Therapy

Chemotherapy can be given to the home infusion patient safely and cost effectively through many routes. This particular therapy, unlike some other therapies, demands close monitoring not only while the patient is undergoing therapy but even closer while the patient is not undergoing therapy. Chemotherapy infusions are most commonly given intravenously; however, they can be given by the intra-arterial, intrathecal, intraperitoneal, or subcutaneous route. These infusions may be given by bolus, continuous infusion, or periodic continuous infusion (5-day infusions). All chemotherapeutic drugs can be administered in the home care setting with the appropriate level of specialized clinical oncology support. A list of common chemotherapeutic drugs and combination regimens can be found in Table 29–7.

Common Issues and Concerns

Patients are generally concerned with their quality of life while undergoing therapy as well as after therapy. Issues related to side effects, such as nausea, vomiting, and hair loss, are the most common initial concerns. These concerns largely result from anticipation of the unknown and the media attention that these side effects receive. Other concerns that arise later include susceptibility to infection as the patient reaches the nadir (the point at which the white blood cell count is at its lowest), nutritional status, and ability to carry on routine activities of life without interruption.

T a b l e   2 9 – 7

Commonly Used Chemotherapeutic Drugs and Combination Regimens

Common Therapeutic Drugs Used in the Home CURAFLEX Complex Chemotherapy (CCC) Programs

Bleomycin	Carboplatin	Cisplatin	Cyclophosphamide	Cytarabine
Doxorubicin	Etoposide	Fluorouracil	Ifosfamide	Leuprolide depot
Levamisole	Methotrexate	Mitomycin C	Mitoxantrone	Tamoxifen
Vinblastine	Vincristine			

Combination Chemotherapy Regimens Prescribed in the Home CURAFLEX Complex Chemotherapy (CCC) Program

Acronym	Drugs	Cancer
PEF	Bleomycin, etoposide, cisplatin	Genitourinary
CAF (FAC)	Cyclophosphamide, doxorubicin, fluorouracil	Breast, metastatic disease
CAP	Cisplatin, doxorubicin, cyclophosphamide	Lung, non–small cell
CF	Cisplatin, fluorouracil	Head and neck
CFL	Cisplatin, fluorouracil, leucovorin	Head and neck
CHOP	Cyclophosphamide, doxorubicin, vincristine, prednisone	Non-Hodgkin's lymphoma
CV	Cisplatin, etoposide	Lung, non–small cell
CVI (VIC)	Carboplatin, etoposide, ifosfamide, mesna	Lung, non–small cell
EVA	Etoposide, vinblastine, doxorubicin	Hodgkin's lymphoma
FAC	Fluorouracil, doxorubicin, cyclophosphamide	Breast, metastatic disease
FAM	Fluorouracil, doxorubicin, mitomycin C	Colon, lung, non–small cell
FCE	Fluorouracil, cisplatin, etoposide	Gastric
F-CL	Fluorouracil, calcium leucovorin	Colon
FLE	Levamisole, fluorouracil	Colon
FMV	Fluorouracil, methyl-CCNU, vincristine	Colon
IMF	Ifosfamide, mesna, methotrexate, fluorouracil	Breast
mPFL	Methotrexate, cisplatin, fluorouracil, leucovorin	Genitourinary
MVAC	Methotrexate, vinblastine, doxorubicin, cisplatin	Genitourinary
PFL	Cisplatin, fluorouracil, leucovorin	Gastric, head and neck, lung, non–small cell
VAC	Vincristine, doxorubicin, cyclophosphamide	Lung, small cell
VIP	Vinblastine, etoposide, ifosfamide, cisplatin, mesna	Genitourinary
Wayne State	Cisplatin, 5-fluorouracil	Head and neck

From CURAFLEX Infusion Services Home Infusion Therapy Resource Guide 1991.

While patients are not undergoing chemotherapy, a clinical concern is monitoring the nadir period. Approximately 14 to 21 days after therapy begins, depending on the drugs being administered, the patient reaches the nadir. From the point of nadir until the white count rises again is a very critical period; during this time, the patient is most susceptible to infections. Neutropenic precautions, including scrupulous hand washing and hygiene, sterile accessing of device and infusion therapy technique, as well as crowd, injury, and dietary precautions, must be adhered to.[33] Several new biologic drugs, such as the colony-stimulating factors and monoclonal antibodies, have recently been introduced to treat and prevent complications related to chemotherapy administra-

tion.[34, 35] These agents, along with medical research findings that suggest new clinical applications and the reduction in risk of catheter-related infection resulting from advances in catheter technology, make home chemotherapy less intimidating and more acceptable.

Permanent vascular access is usually a subject encountered early on for the home chemotherapy patient. The choice of access device is usually based on the frequency and duration of therapy, the medications prescribed, and the patient's preference. Peripheral access for the administration of vesicant agents in the home is discouraged. Psychosocial and physical support is important with the patient on chemotherapy. A new or reoccurring disease process places a major stress on the patient and family members. Toxicities and side effects also pose a potential for debilitation and a need for both physical and psychological support. For this reason, a strong support system as well as an alternate caregiver is recommended.

Agents Commonly Used in the Home Curaflex Chemotherapy Programs

Bleomycin	Leuprolide depot
Carboplatin	Levamisole
Cisplatin	Methotrexate
Cyclophosphamide	Mitomycin C
Cytarabine	Mitoxantrone
Doxorubicin	Tamoxifen
Etoposide	Vinblastine
Fluorouracil	Vincristine
Ifosfamide	

Delivery Systems

Advances in technology that allow multiple drug regimens to be delivered on multiple schedules via ambulatory devices have made chemotherapy administration in the home more easily achievable and acceptable to the patient.[32] Whereas some patients receive their chemotherapy by rapid infusion (bolus), a one-time rapid injection, others receive administration by continuous infusion that can last several days to several months. To date, the optimal schedule for most antineoplastic agents has not been established. New studies of many drugs are revealing a marked schedule dependency, with a prolonged infusion yielding a greater tumor cell kill response than a short or bolus infusion.[36] This finding will increase the need for provision of this service in the home setting.

Clinical Monitoring

Chemotherapy demands close monitoring while the patient is undergoing therapy as well as between courses of therapy. Vital to the prevention of complications is ongoing monitoring of laboratory values, physical status, fluid status, and drug-related side effects and toxicities. Education and certification in chemotherapy administration and monitoring are strongly recommended. Specific knowledge about the drugs prescribed assists clinicians in better monitoring their home chemotherapy patients. Although side effects are to be expected with this therapy, complications related to these side effects can be prevented. Therefore, protocols and reporting parameters should be established for physical and therapeutic assessment as well as for side effects and toxicities management. Protocols for use in home chemotherapy include hydration, therapeutic monitoring, antiemetic, laboratory, and patient monitoring. Extravasation, or escape of chemotherapeutic agents into the tissue, is not expected. However, protocols should be readily available to treat extravasation promptly if it occurs.

Complex Chemotherapy

A recent advance is the provision of the complex chemotherapy regimens in the home. This therapy includes hydration before and after therapy, antiemetic regimens, multiple chemotherapeutic agents, adjuvants, and, if needed, biologic agents. Laboratory results and physical findings are monitored closely during and between therapy by pharmacists and nurses specializing in oncology infusional therapy. Adjustments in therapy regimens and medications are made when complications and toxicities occur. Crisis can be avoided and preventive measures implemented only through diligent monitoring by clinicians specially trained in the field of oncologic infusional therapy. Provision of home complex chemotherapy should not be an undertaking for the novice home care clinician. An oncology residency or advanced oncology and chemotherapy certification, or both, are strongly recommended.

With the publication of new medical advances in continuous and complex chemotherapy regimens and the introduction of new drugs, chemotherapy is increasingly being administered in the home care setting. As patients become more acutely aware of the availability of home chemotherapy, coupled with the success of new regimens, patients will seek not only quality of life but also an uninterrupted lifestyle. Predictably, referral sources will also realize the cost benefit of administration of these complex therapies in the home versus the hospital, and the demand for cost containment will steer referrals into the home care program.

Pain Management

Management of pain has always been an important focus in the hospital setting and has now become just as important in home care. Some of the rationales for its use in home care include the existence of unrelieved pain in the progression of chronic terminal diseases, the advances in technology, and the increasing knowledge of health care professionals regarding the causes and successful treatment of pain.[37] It is now accepted that pain can cause physical harm to the patient and that patients need to have more involvement in the control of their pain.

Indications

Some of the most common diagnoses for home pain management include intractable pain in patients with cancer or acquired immune deficiency syndrome and those with postoperative pain, and chronic pain from causalgia, neuralgia, or reflex sympathetic dystrophy. The traditional management of debilitating pain associated with terminal disease progression consists of administration of oral medications, usually narcotic analgesics. When oral pain management results in poor pain control, other routes should be explored. Narcotic analgesics can be safely administered in the home by subcutaneous, intravenous, epidural, or intrathecal routes. These infusions may be intermittent, continuous, or continuous with patient-controlled bolus capabilities.[38, 39] Better pain control and decreased central nervous system effects are experienced with a continuous infusion of a low-dose medication. Patients are able to manage their "breakthrough" pain by self-administering preset bolus doses.

Most Commonly Prescribed Pain Medications

The most common medications administered in the home for pain management are morphine sulfate, meperidine (Demerol), and hydromorphone (Dilaudid). The home infusion pharmacist collaborates with the physician to obtain the appropriate dose based on the route of administration. Thorough pain assessment by the home IV nurse should include location and distribution, timing and pattern, onset and duration, and quality and severity of the pain experienced (rated by the patient using an established scale). The home IV nurse uses these data to assist the home infusion pharmacist and physician to titrate the dose to maintain adequate pain control. It is extremely important that the home infusion pharmacist, home IV nurse, physician, and patient work closely together to obtain optimal pain management when medications or routes are changed. The home infusion pharmacist makes recommendations on equianalgesic doses to help stay within the relatively same analgesic range. This analysis prevents inadvertent underdosing or overdosing, causing the recurrence of pain or resulting in excessive sedation.

Common Issues and Concerns

A successful home pain management program requires a motivated patient or caregiver, a conducive home environment, adequate support, and an appropriately prescribed medication, dose, and route of administration. Careful consideration should be given to the admission of patients with known intravenous drug abuse or those in a situation in which the home environment poses a potential for drug abuse. Alternative arrangements need to be explored in these cases. Nursing management of the patient in pain is virtually the same regardless of the health care setting. Education plays an extremely important role in caring for the home pain management patient. The patient and caregiver should be given instructions on the specific medication being administered, the route of administration, and the side effects. Explanations of pain control, the pain rating system, and home self-monitoring should be given. The teaching may include giving bolus dosing, determining precipitating events to pain, and handling specific side effects.

Many home pain management patients and caregivers have concerns regarding the administration of narcotics. One of the most common concerns is addiction. At this point in their disease progression, many patients have been on narcotics orally for some time. Conversion to the parenteral route of administration does not lead to addiction, as some patients fear. Patients and caregivers should be reassured that addiction is of minimal concern and that bolus dosing should be administered as needed. Physical dependence and tolerance are expected and are easily managed by adjusting the dose upward according to need, or conversely, slowly decreasing the dose over time before discontinuing the narcotic.

Patients are also very concerned about maintaining their mental capabilities. Through education, patients will learn that by using the parenteral route, with the medication infusing continuously, a much lower dose is required, therefore decreasing sedation. They are instructed to notify the home IV nurse if sedation does occur or if their pain is not being controlled. Such signs may be an indication to adjust the dose or to switch to another route. The route of administration is another patient concern. Patients are instructed on the various parenteral administration routes. The patient and the physician decide on the route of administration that will be most effective for the degree of pain experienced and the disease state of the patient. The home IV nurse provides instructions for the care and maintenance of the selected route.

Patients are instructed on the clinical adverse effects of narcotics. Because constipation, nausea, and vomiting are relatively consistent side effects and are anticipated, they are treated concurrently with such drugs as stool softeners, laxatives, and antiemetics. Respiratory depression is not of great concern, because when doses are titrated for pain relief, respiratory depressant effects of narcotics lie above the sedation threshold, which lies above the pain relief threshold.[40] Patients also develop a tolerance to the sedative and respiratory depressant effects. Patients and caregivers are instructed that if the respiration rate decreases to half of what has been normal for that patient, the rate of infusion needs to be decreased and the home IV nurse notified.

Delivery Systems

Many technologic advances in infusion devices have occurred, making administration of narcotics in the home relatively safe. These devices are designed for ease in ambulation. They have a built-in safety mechanism (lock-out function) to prevent the rate of infusion and the programmed dose from being changed by unauthorized persons. They have the capability of infusing intermittently or continuously and allowing the patient to administer bolus doses during the continuous infusion. The remainder of the delivery system simply consists of the appropriate administration tubing for the infusion device, supplies, and a dressing change kit that is appropriate to the route of administration.

Clinical Monitoring

Clinical monitoring performed by the home infusion pharmacist and the IV nurse includes physical assessment, pain assessment, compliance check, equipment check, and psychosocial support.

Cardiac Therapies

Chronic congestive heart failure and its progressive degenerative course affects millions of people. Because of its prevalence, interest has increased in identifying alternative methods of treatment that are relatively safe and cost effective.

Indications and Medications Prescribed

The use of parenteral inotropic agents in the home setting for the management of terminal congestive heart failure was reported as early as 1984. The literature on this topic contains documentation of successful home IV infusions of dobutamine, dopamine, and amrinone for the management of decompensated, terminal congestive heart failure in patients in whom conventional therapy was unsuccessful or for those who were awaiting heart transplantation.[41-44]

Common Issues and Concerns

The success of a home IV inotropic program depends on several factors. The first is patient stability before discharge. The patient must have responded in the acute care setting to the IV inotrope and the dosage regimen to be administered at home. Another area of significant importance is the psychosocial evaluation, including assessment of patient acceptance, involvement, and compliance; identification of a patient caregiver to assist in the therapy; and knowledge of the limitations of the therapy. The patient, family, and caregiver must understand that this therapy is not a cure, but rather an attempt for improved quality of life compared with that which may be experienced in the cardiac care unit. Reimbursement for the therapy in the home care setting should be verified before acceptance into the program.

Patient and caregiver training, as with any home infusion therapy, includes provision of information regarding the disease state, the prescribed medication, and the goals of therapy. Education of the medication regimen includes expected therapeutic effects of the drug, side effects, and home self-monitoring. This information enables the patient to understand the rationale for increased urine output and the need for monitoring. Patient-specific information is provided regarding aseptic techniques and care and maintenance of their infusion access device. The patient and caregiver need to master set-up and initiation of therapy using an ambulatory infusion device. Troubleshooting for malfunctions in the pump is also covered during training. Written patient training information is provided, and competency is documented on a patient training checklist.

Some of the common concerns of the home infusion inotrope patient are adverse reactions, such as increased heart rate and blood pressure and ventricular ectopic activity; support from family and the home health care team; and home self-monitoring. Early identification of concerns and development of a plan will assist in allaying these concerns. Routine nursing visits for physical and vital sign assessment, blood drawing, technical procedures, and reinforcement of teaching also decrease concerns.

Delivery Systems

Central venous access is preferred because of the need for continuous administration of the medication. It is also more practical and cost effective for this long-term home infusion therapy. The pharmacist needs to dilute the drug to a concentration that is likely to be more concentrated than that used in the hospital. This strength facilitates the use of ambulatory infusion devices and the need to restrict the fluid in these patients because of their congestive heart failure.

Clinical Monitoring

The provision of infusion inotropes at home mandates monitoring by the patient or caregiver and the home infusion clinician. Baseline vital signs are obtained and are used for comparison to all future vital signs, especially heart rate and systolic blood pressure. Once stable, vital signs are monitored three times a day or as per physician order. Patients record their intake and urine output as well as their daily weight. The venous access site is monitored for signs of infection as well as signs and symptoms suggestive of catheter occlusion or subclavian vein thrombosis. The clinician closely assesses for peripheral edema (location and severity) and determines respiratory status, heart sounds, daily weights, vital signs, and intake and output. Laboratory monitoring is dictated by the physician and the disease state and may include complete blood counts and electrolyte and chemistry profiles. Complications documented in the literature for home infusion inotropic therapy are primarily infectious and are related to the infusion access device. Cases of drug tolerance have also been reported.

Biologic Therapies

Relatively new to home infusion are the biologic therapies. Advances in recombinant DNA technology have made therapies such as the hematopoietic growth factors (granulocyte colony stimulating factor and granulocyte macrophage colony stimulating factor), erythropoietin, and interferon available for home use. This group of therapies, commonly called biologic, target specific areas of the immune or hematopoietic systems that have been adversely affected by disease or a drug used in the treatment of a disease.[35] The biologics stimulate the proliferation or differentiation of specific cells in the hematopoietic system. Figure 29–5 describes the biologics and diagnoses common to home infusion therapy.

Transfusion Therapy

Home transfusion is a safe and effective treatment modality for providing blood and blood products to individuals whose disease state is such that the patient requires frequent transfusion but hospitalization is not otherwise indicated. Blood transfusions can be performed at home provided that specific criteria are met.

As early as 1982 and 1983, home health care agencies were receiving inquiries regarding the availability of providing transfusions in the home care setting.[45] The American Association of Blood Banks formally recognized the use of home transfusion in 1988 when their Transfusion Practice Committee published a brochure entitled ''Out-of-Hospital Transfusion.'' This brochure provided recommendations for the development of protocols and documentation of a home transfusion service.[46] Since that time, an increasing number of home infusion companies and agencies offer home transfusion therapy as a complement to their other high-technology infusion services.[47]

Blood Components Prescribed

The commonest blood or blood products transfused in the home care setting include packed red cells, washed packed red cells, frozen deglycerolized red cells, platelets, plasma, and cryoprecipitate or plasma derivatives. Other components need to be evaluated on an individual basis to determine their safety for administration in the home.

Indications

During the referral process and pretransfusion home visit, the home infusion clinician assesses the patient's candidacy for the home transfusion program. Specific admission criteria must be met before the patient is accepted into the program. The appropriateness of the diagnosis for transfusion must be assessed. The patient's cardiopulmonary status and medical condition must be stable. The patient should be alert, cooperative, and able to respond appropriately to body reactions and relate this information to the home transfusion nurse. There should be a conducive home environment in which a capable adult is present during the transfusion and telephone access is available. Usually, the patient has physical limitations that make travel outside the home difficult. Lastly, there should be ready access to emergency medical services and the primary physician during transfusion.

Diagnoses Appropriate for Admission to Home Transfusion Program

- Chronic gastrointestinal bleeding
- Anemia resulting from
  Bone marrow failure
  Malignancy
  Chronic renal failure
  Sickle cell
  Thalassemia
  Acquired immune deficiency syndrome
  Chronic congestive heart failure
- Thrombocytopenia
- Bleeding related to congenital or acquired deficiencies in coagulation factors

Figure 29-5. Biologics and diagnoses common to home infusion therapy.

GM-CSF

DRUG
Sargramostim
(Granulocyte Macrophage Colony Stimulating Factor-GM-CSF)
Leukine (Immunex)
Prokine (Hoechst-Roussel)

DOSAGE
250 mcg/m² over 2 hours for 21 days or until ANC reaches 20,000/mm³ or platelet count exceeds 500,000/mm³

COMMENTS: Caution in CHF or fluid retention, pre-existing cardiac, renal or hepatic disease. Therapy should begin two to four hours following autologous bone marrow infusion and not less than twenty-four hours following cytotoxic chemotherapy or twelve hours following radiation therapy.

ACTIONS
A glycoprotein that stimulates the proliferation and differentiation of white blood cells in the granulocyte-macrophage pathways.

MONITORING
• CBC with differential twice weekly
• Physical assessment
• Patient interview

INDICATIONS/USE
1. Acceleration of myeloid recovery in patients with non-Hodgkin's lymphoma (NHL), acute lymphoblastic leukemia (ALL) and Hodgkin's disease undergoing autologous bone marrow transplantation. 2. Bone marrow transplantation failure or engraftment delay. *Unlabeled uses:* a. Increase WBC counts in AIDS patients receiving AZT and patients with myelodysplastic syndrome. b. Correct neutropenia in aplastic anemia. c. Decrease nadir of leukopenia secondary to myelosuppressive chemotherapy.

ADVERSE REACTIONS
Fever, headache, bone pain, chills, diarrhea, rack, malaise and asthenia

G-CSF

DRUG
Filgrastim (Granulocyte Colony Stimulating Factor-G-CSF)
Neupogen (Amgen)

DOSAGE
5 mcg/kg/day SQ or IV × 2 weeks or until ANC reaches 10,000/mm³

COMMENTS: Filgrastim should not be administered within 24 hours prior to or following the administration of cytotoxic chemotherapy.

ACTIONS
A glycoprotein that stimulates the production of neutrophils

MONITORING
• CBC with differential twice weekly during therapy
• Physical assessment
• Patient interview

INDICATIONS/USE
Neutropenia in patients with non-myeloid malignancies receiving myelosuppressive anticancer agents.

ADVERSE REACTIONS
Bone pain—24%; Less frequently: Exacerbation of some pre-existing skin disorders (psoriasis, alopecia), hematuria, proteinuria, thrombocytopenia and osteoporosis; spontaneously reversible elevation in uric acid, lactic dehydrogenase and alkaline phosphatase have also occurred.

EPO

DRUG
Epoetin alfa
(Erythropoietin; Epo)
Epogen (Amgen)
Procrit (Ortho Biotech)

DOSAGE
Starting dose: 50 to 100 U/kg 3 times weekly, IV: dialysis patients, IV or SC: non-dialysis CRF patients.
Reduce dose when: (1) Target range is reached or (2) Hematocrit increase > 4 points in any two week period.
Increase dose if: Hematocrit does not increase by five to six points after eight weeks of therapy and hematocrit is below target range.
Maintenance dose: Individualize. General dosage change: 25 U/kg/(3 times weekly).
Target hematocrit range: 30% to 33% (maximum, 36%)

COMMENTS: 1. Requires refrigeration at all times. 2. Patient may require iron supplementation.

ACTIONS
A glycoprotein that stimulates red blood cell production

MONITORING
• Baseline CBC and H/H and twice weekly
• Physical assessment
• Patient interview
• Monitoring BP closely on CRF patients

INDICATIONS/USE
1. Anemia secondary to chronic renal failure.
2. Anemia secondary to AZT therapy in HIV infected patients.
3. Unlabeled uses: a. Anemia in cancer patients receiving chemotherapy. b. Procurement of blood in presurgical patients.

ADVERSE REACTIONS
CRF patients: Hypertension 24%, headache 16%, arthralgias 11%, nausea 11%, edema, fatigue and diarrhea 95%, vomiting 8%, seizure 1.1%.
AZT treated HIV patients: Pyrexia 38%, fatigue 25%, headache 19%, cough 18%, diarrhea 16%, rash 16%, respiratory congestion 15%, nausea 15%, SOB 14%

INTERFERON

DRUG
Interferon Alfa 2a & 2b
Intron-A (Schering)
Roferon-A (Roche)

DOSAGE
Roferon-A—Hairy cell leukemia—Induction dose: 3 M.I.U. for 16–24 wks SC or IM.
Maintenance dose: 3 M.I.U. 3 times per week
AIDS related Kaposi's sarcoma—Induction dose: 36 M.I.U. daily for 10–12 wks, SC or IM.
Maintenance dose: 36 M.I.U. 3 times a week
Intron-A—Hairy cell leukemia—2 M.I.U. per M² 3 times a week, SC or IM (maintain dose unless disease progresses rapidly or severe intolerance)
Condylomata acuminata—1 M.I.U. per lesion 3 times a week intralesionally for 3 weeks.
AIDS related Kaposi's sarcoma—30 M.I.U. per M² 3 times a week, SC or IM (maintain dose unless disease progresses or severe intolerance develops)
Chronic hepatitis non A, non B/C—3 M.I.U. 3 times a week SC or IM for 6 months

COMMENTS: 1. Category C for pregnancy (potential risk to fetus). 2. Safety in children < 18 not established. 3. Interferon may have additive myelosuppressive activity with other antineoplastic drugs or radiation therapy. 4. Caution with aminophyllin. May decrease metabolism and increase aminophyllin levels.

ACTIONS
A sterile protein that has immunomodulatory and tumor antiproliferative activity.

MONITORING
• Baseline CBC with differential and throughout therapy.
• Baseline liver function tests and renal function test, and throughout therapy.
• Physical assessment with close attention to: a. Cardiac status. b. Fever, sore throat, c. Signs of infection, d. Signs of bleeding, e. Neurologic status.

INDICATIONS/USE
Intron-A, Roferon A — Hairy cell leukemia in patients > 18 yrs old.
AIDS-related Kaposi's sarcoma in patients > 18 yrs old.
Intron-A — Chronic hepatitis, non A, non B/C.
Intron-A — Condylomata acuminata.
Non-approved use: Treatment of various tumors.

ADVERSE REACTIONS
1. Flu-like syndrome.
2. Fatigue, dizziness, depression, sleep disturbances, paresthesia, nervousness, confusion, anxiety/agitation.
3. Nausea, vomiting, diarrhea, anorexia.
4. Rash, pruritus, alopecia, dermatitis, chest pain, arrhythmias.
5. Taste alteration, vision disorders.
6. Hypotension, edema, hypertension, chest pain, arrhythmia.
7. Anemia, leukopenia, thrombocytopenia.

527

Arrangements with Blood Bank

Each home infusion company and agency involved in providing transfusion therapy must identify a local blood bank from which to obtain their blood products. In some areas, state regulations require the home infusion company or agency to be a licensed blood bank for limited transfusion services. The blood bank should be provided with a copy of the company or agency transfusion program protocols, policies, and procedures for their review and recommendations. Clarification should be obtained regarding the blood bank's requirements for patient identification and use of identification bracelets, transportation, and storage of blood products, as well as any specific equipment and supplies, such as microaggregate or leukocyte-depleting filters. The company or agency must ensure that their home IV nurses are qualified in transfusion therapy.

Common Issues and Concerns

Home blood transfusion carries with it the same liability risk as hospital transfusion. During the pretransfusion visit, the informed consent and any other company-specific forms should be signed and the patients educated on the purpose of the transfusion, their rights and responsibilities, and possible adverse reactions. A complete medical history is obtained, and a thorough physical examination, including evaluation of vascular access is performed. An identification bracelet with the patient's full name and identification number is attached to the patient's wrist. The home IV nurse also obtains blood samples for baseline chemistry (if ordered), complete blood count, and type and crossmatch assessments. All blood tubes must be labeled with the same full name and identification number that is found on the patient's bracelet and returned to the blood bank for testing.

The blood product must be transported in a container that has an appropriate coolant for the component. The temperature should be recorded at the time of delivery or per blood bank or agency policy. Transportation of the blood products from the blood bank to the patient's home can be conducted by the nurse performing the transfusion or the blood bank. Regardless, the blood product must be checked against the requisition by the blood center personnel and the home IV nurse. When the blood product is to be administered, the home IV nurse verifies with the caregiver the information on the blood product against the patient's identification bracelet. All verifications should be documented on the transfusion visit form.

Clinical Monitoring

Once peripheral venous access has been established, or verified in the case of an existing access device, and baseline vital signs are obtained, the transfusion is initiated. Accurate records of vital signs and general patient condition should be maintained (Fig. 29–6). The home IV nurse remains with the patient during the entire transfusion and for at least 30 to 60 minutes after completion of the infusion. Vital signs should be taken before the transfusion, with close monitoring every 15 to 30 minutes (depending on agency or organization pol-

icy) throughout the duration of the transfusion, and for 30 to 60 minutes after the completion of the transfusion. Each unit of packed red cells is usually transfused over 1 to 2 hours, with a maximum time of 4 hours. If the transfusion must be performed slowly, then the units should be split to decrease the risk of bacterial proliferation, which occurs at room temperature. Usually, no more than 2 units of packed red cells or 10 units of platelets are transfused in a day. However, under certain circumstances, and under a physician's direction, more than 2 units have been administered.

Thirty to 60 minutes after the completion of the transfusion, the peripheral IV access device is removed, or the central line is flushed. The blood container, administration set, and any other blood-contaminated supplies must be properly disposed of as per Occupational Safety and Health Administration, city, and state waste management regulations. Post-transfusion follow-up should be conducted either via telephone contact or via a home visit. The physician may order follow-up laboratory studies. The patient and caregiver should receive further instructions on observation for transfusion reaction. Written information should be left with the patient.

Any transfusion carries with it the potential for adverse reactions that result from the uniqueness of each patient and each unit of blood. Patients are monitored frequently during the transfusion for symptoms of transfusion reaction. The medications and supplies for the home transfusion reaction kit are the same as those for hospital transfusion. It usually includes diphenhydramine, hydrocortisone, acetaminophen (Tylenol), and epinephrine. The supplies include normal saline, an IV administration set, syringes with needles, blood-drawing supplies, urine specimen containers, and alcohol wipes. Orders for the transfusion reaction procedure should be obtained from the physician before the transfusion is performed.

Symptoms of Transfusion Reaction

- Chills
- Chest tightness
- Headache
- Myalgia
- Pruritus
- Nausea
- Pain at infusion site, chest, or flank
- Fever
- Hemoglobinuria
- Restlessness
- Dyspnea
- Cough
- Vomiting
- Pink sputum
- Hypotension
- Tachycardia
- Bradycardia

A transfusion reaction kit and protocol should be available in the home during the transfusion. In the event of an urticarial reaction not accompanied by other adverse effects, an antihistamine is usually ordered by the physician and administered. If the urticaria resolves, the physician may order the transfusion to be resumed slowly. Other nonhemolytic reactions may subside with prescribed therapy without requiring hospitalization.

TRANSFUSION PATIENT VISIT/SHIFT RECORD

PATIENT NAME		PATIENT ID NO.	DATE		EMPLOYEE NUMBER	☐ ☐ ☐ ☐ ☐

CLINICIAN NAME	CLINICIAN SIG.	VISIT TIME IN HOURS (Round to nearest ¼ hr.)	TIME ARRIVED	TIME LEFT	TO

CAREGIVER NAME	CAREGIVER SIGNATURE X	TRAVEL TIME IN HOURS (Round to nearest ¼ hr.)	TO	FROM	TO

SERVICE TIME: ☐ WD ☐ WED ☐ WE ☐ WEE ☐ WN ☐ WEN

SERVICE TYPE: ☐ INF NSG ☐ INF

LOCATION: ☐ HOME ☐ HOSP ☐ MD OFFICE/CLINIC

☐ ECF/SNF ☐ OTHER _____

IPA DONE: ☐ YES ☐ NO

MILEAGE   TO _____   FROM _____   TO

CHARTING   MINUTES   SIG. PT.

☐ BILLABLE ☐ NON BILLABLE   PAYOR SOURCE

DESCRIPTION

GENERAL: BASELINE H & H _____ V/S _____ PATIENT BLOOD TYPE _____

VENOUS ACCESS/CONDITION OF SITE _____

PHYSICAL ASSESSMENT _____

RX: NUMBER OF UNITS ON HAND _____

UNIT NO. ONE: TYPE _____ RH _____ BLOOD BANK NUMBER _____

UNIT NO. TWO: TYPE _____ RH _____ BLOOD BANK NUMBER _____

TRANSPORT: METHOD: _____ TIME _____ TEMPERATURE _____

TRANSFUSION

IV SOLUTION _____

BLOOD (No. of units, time started, time ended, rate, amount infused for each unit)

MEDICATIONS GIVEN _____

ANAPHYLAXIS KIT ORDERED? ☐ YES ☐ NO   PRESENT IN HOME? ☐ YES ☐ NO

V/S p̄ first 15 minutes, X2, then every 30 minutes, then 30 minutes after each unit.

	TIME	TEMPERATURE	PULSE	RESPIRATION	BLOOD PRESSURE		TIME	TEMPERATURE	PULSE	RESPIRATION	BLOOD PRESSURE
1						8					
2						9					
3						10					
4						11					
5						12					
6						13					
7						14					

TRANSFUSION REACTIONS

TRANSFUSION REACTION: ☐ YES ☐ NO   REACTION DESCRIPTION _____

ACTION TAKEN: _____

LABS DONE: _____

FOLLOW UP: _____

RESPONSE TO TRANSFUSION

FOLLOW UP LABS: _____

PATIENT EDUCATION

Figure 29–6. Record of vital signs and patient's general condition.

Transfusion Reaction Procedure

1. If reaction is suspected or observed, stop transfusion.
2. Change intravenous tubing and maintain patient's intravenous line with 0.9% sodium chloride solution.
3. Take vital signs and continue to monitor the patient until stable.
4. Administer medications as prescribed.
5. Verify blood product identification and requisition with patient's identification bracelet.
6. Notify physician, as soon as patient's condition permits, for further instructions. Notify blood bank. Access local emergency services if a medical emergency arises.
7. Obtain necessary laboratory specimens:
   Freshly collected urine
   Blood samples—red top tube without separator gel and purple top tube
8. Monitor the patient until the reaction subsides or the patient is transferred to an emergency facility.
9. Document incident on transfusion flow sheet and transfusion reaction report.

Reimbursement

Reimbursement for home transfusions varies from carrier to carrier. Medicare part A or part B does not currently reimburse for the blood products themselves. To verify coverage, each insurance carrier is contacted before service is initiated to describe the therapy, the required nursing visit, the associated equipment, and the supplies. Many insurance carriers will reimburse for this therapy if it is "in lieu of hospitalization." A thorough investigation of resources is made, and all concerns (i.e., appropriate diagnosis, ability to transport) should be addressed. Only then can options be presented to the patient and the payers.

MISCELLANEOUS THERAPIES

Deferoxamine Mesylate Therapy

Deferoxamine mesylate is an iron-binding agent that combines with the iron in the body to produce a red-colored chelate called ferrioxamine, which is then excreted in the urine and feces. Deferoxamine is prescribed for the reversal of iron overload. A common diagnosis for which the agent is prescribed in the home is thalassemia, which is also known as erythroblastic anemia, Mediterranean anemia, or Cooley's anemia. This disorder includes a group of hereditary hemolytic anemias in which the red blood cells are very thin and fragile. These anemias are thought to be caused by a deficit in hemoglobin synthesis, and they occur more frequently in people from the Mediterranean, South Asian, and North and Central African areas. The anemic symptoms of thalassemia usually present before the child reaches the age of 18 months. Frequent periodic transfusions (every 3 to 4 weeks) of red blood cells, depending on hemoglobin levels, are required to correct the anemia. Iron overload occurs as a result of the blood transfusions and unless reversed can cause damage to such vital organs as the heart and liver and can even be fatal.[48–50]

Deferoxamine is prescribed based on the laboratory values of serum ferritin. It is most commonly administered via the subcutaneous routes and less commonly via the intravenous route by an ambulatory infusion pump over an 8- to 12-hour period. This therapy is lifelong, and patients are generally trained to mix and administer the drugs themselves. Side effects, although rare, may include disturbances of vision and hearing, vertigo, and respiratory difficulties. Average life expectancy for the thalassemia patient is largely dependent on early detection of the disease, diligent monitoring, treatment on an ongoing basis, and patient compliance with therapy. Home care has allowed these and other long-term therapy regimens to be administered with minimal disturbances of daily activities.[50]

α_1-Proteinase Inhibitor

α_1-Proteinase inhibitor is an enzyme indicated in the treatment of severe α_1-antitrypsin (AAT) deficiency with clinically demonstrable panacinar emphysema. AAT deficiency is an autosomal hereditary disorder characterized by low serum and lung levels of AAT. AAT is a protease inhibitor responsible for inhibiting neutrophil elastase. Emphysema is believed to result from an imbalance between the neutrophil elastase in the lung, which is capable of destroying elastin and other connective tissue components, and the antielastases that function to protect the lung from the elastase. Therefore, persons with AAT deficiency are at high risk for developing severe panacinar emphysema between the ages of 30 to 50 years. They are also at an increased risk for developing liver disease; however, this problem is usually seen in children. The first clinical symptom in adults is dyspnea on exertion and lower lung involvement.[51]

Treatment of this disorder is aimed at replacement therapy with α_1-proteinase inhibitor. Long-term replacement therapy should be considered only in patients who exhibit early evidence of the disease. It is not indicated in those with emphysema that is associated with cigarette smoking who lack the positive phenotype. α_1-Proteinase inhibitor is prepared from large pools of fresh human plasma, usually from paid donors. It is heat treated to reduce the potential for transmission of infectious agents, such as the human immunodeficiency and hepatitis viruses. No cases of human immunodeficiency virus transmission have been reported thus far. It is recommended by physicians, however, that before patients undergo α_1-proteinase inhibitor therapy, they be immunized for hepatitis using hepatitis B vaccination as per the manufacturer's recommendations.

α_1-Proteinase inhibitor is administered intravenously via peripheral heparin lock, tunneled catheter, PICC, or implanted port. The recommended dosage is 60 mg/kg once weekly to increase and maintain AAT levels. This dose can be administered at a rate of 0.08 ml/kg/min or greater.[51, 52] The average infusion time is 30 minutes. An infusion device may be used if ordered. The drug concentrate must be refrigerated; the bottles should be brought to room temperature and then reconstituted with the sterile water for injection that is provided. It may be diluted in 0.9% sodium chloride if necessary. The drug should not be refrigerated after reconstitution and should be used within 3 hours. Any unused solution should be discarded appropriately.

α_1-Proteinase inhibitor therapy is lifelong and may cause patient concerns. Lung function will not improve, but it is hoped that the progression of the disease can be halted with replacement therapy. Patients must learn to deal with the chronicity of their disease, and compliance often becomes an issue. Routinely skipped doses can lead to worsening of the disorder. The home IV nurse should educate the patient on the IV access devices available for their therapy. Some may decide to use a peripheral heparin lock or a long-term access device, such as a PICC or a tunneled catheter. Care and maintenance of their IV access device is a very important part of patient education. Because of the limited drug stability time, patients are educated on aseptic reconstitution procedures and IV administration. Some patients express concern over the possibility of acquiring hepatitis or human immunodeficiency virus as a result of the method of preparing α_1-proteinase inhibitor. Educating the patient on the availability of the hepatitis B vaccine assists in decreasing the fear and the risk of acquiring hepatitis B.

Periodic pulmonary function tests may be needed to determine the progression of the disease and the patient's response to therapy. Effectiveness of therapy is demonstrated by slowing of the destructive process on lung tissue, as measured by increased serum α-proteinase inhibitor levels. Minimum serum concentration is 80 mg/100 ml.

Tocolytic Therapy

Premature births are considered to be a major cause of morbidity and mortality. In the United States, 10% of births are delivered before term ($<$ 37 weeks of gestation); 25 to 50% of these births result from preterm labor. Over the past 15 years, several drugs have been prescribed for the prevention of preterm labor, including magnesium sulfate, terbutaline, and ritodrine. Recent studies using continuous subcutaneous infusion of terbutaline have proved it to be both efficient and cost effective. Study results show lowered rates of side effects, improved prolongation of pregnancy, decreased recurrence of preterm labor, and reduced intensive care nursery admissions as compared with the results of other drugs and routes of administration. These effects are attributed to lower dosing levels, improved absorption into the subcutaneous tissue, and automatic and continuous delivery of the prescribed therapy.[53]

Home terbutaline therapy is given via a portable infusion pump, which is programmed to administer a continuous basal rate (0.05 mg/hour), scheduled bolus doses (0.25 mg) 4 to 6 times per day for peak periods of contractions, and unscheduled bolus doses (0.25 mg) should the patient experience two contractions in 10 minutes or four contractions in 60 minutes. The subcutaneous site is rotated every 3 to 4 days. The total daily terbutaline dose rarely exceeds 3 mg. The patient is instructed on caring for and maintaining the infusion site, reloading and reprogramming the pump, and self-monitoring, including counting fetal heart rate and uterine self-palpation for detecting contractions. The patient remains on bed rest for the duration of therapy. The home care nurse visits the patient weekly and as necessary to perform a physical assessment, including blood pressure, vital signs, weight gain, evaluation of clinical cervical dilatation, and uterine contractions. The goals of tocolytic therapy are to stop labor, suppress contractions, and prolong gestation to at least 36 weeks. Terbutaline therapy is generally discontinued at the end of week 37.

Hydration

Hydration therapy has been successfully prescribed within the past decade for use in the home. Various conditions result in dehydration and fluid and electrolyte imbalance. Home hydration therapy has eliminated the need for hospitalizing patients with these conditions as long as they are medically stable and meet patient acceptance criteria. Hydration solutions are ordered by the physician based on the patient's diagnosis. Electrolytes may be added to correct electrolyte imbalance as indicated by laboratory data. The route of administration that is most effective for meeting the patient's needs is determined by the physician, the patient, and the home infusion clinicians.

Commonest Diagnoses for Home Hydration Therapy

- Dehydration
- Fluid and electrolyte imbalance resulting from
    Cardiopulmonary disorders
    Fistulas
    Gastrointestinal dysfunction
    Hyperemesis gravidarum
    Intractable diarrhea
    Chemotherapy (before and after therapy)
    Radiation enteritis
    Short-bowel syndrome

Short-term therapy, lasting from 1 to 7 days, is administered via a peripheral heparin lock unless a long-term access device is available, such as in the chemotherapy patient. The delivery system is quite simple, consisting of the hydration solution and the IV administration set. The physician may order an electronic infusion device to regulate the rate of infusion. In most situations, an in-line flow regulator is all that is required. Hydration therapy patients are educated in the necessity for therapy, aseptic technique, set-up and administration of their solution, and possible complications.

Clinical monitoring of the patient consists of conducting a physical assessment, paying close attention to weight and hydration status, and reviewing laboratory results. Laboratory tests should be performed on a routine basis; however, the frequency depends on the diagnosis. The commonest concern of the hydration patient is recovery from the causative factor. Based on the degree of the patient's physical debility, other caregivers may be required to administer the therapy. Patients must be assessed for compliance as well because many patients discontinue their therapy before the prescribed duration because they are feeling better. Education and reinforcement will help eliminate this tendency.

Special Pharmaceutical Issues

Pharmaceutical issues can be broken down in two types. The first, patient care management, has been an added value until the past few years, when some state pharmacy laws and the Joint Commission on Accreditation of Healthcare Organizations have made it a requirement of retail and home infusion pharmacies. The clinical role of the pharmacist in patient care management has recently expanded and is discussed in more detail under "Future Directions." The second issue relates to pharmacy operations management and has recently become increasingly important. As profit margins are squeezed, pharmacists need to become experts in small business administration. Areas needing particular attention are procurement of pharmaceuticals and supplies, asset and inventory management, and cost of goods and services as compared with revenue generated. In other words, without sacrificing quality, the pharmacist must buy the best products at the lowest cost, produce and distribute them in the most cost-effective manner at the highest level of productivity, while getting the highest return on the dollar invested in the shortest period of time. Nurses also need to be astute in business and administrative issues and in cost containment of services and supplies through prudent product selection.

What does all of this mean to the home infusion industry? Not only will pharmacists have to be superior clinicians but they will also have to master interactions and negotiations with insurers, case managers, and referral sources, while at the same time addressing the issues of small business management. Some state pharmacy laws already allow the use of pharmacy technicians and others are following suit. Soon, the impetus will be to use technicians in an effort to reduce cost of service. This trend will force us to educate pharmacists on personnel management. With the inevitability of cost containment, the home infusion industry will no longer be able to afford the luxury of an all-pharmacist staff in the foreseeable future.

SPECIAL CONSIDERATIONS

Documentation

Documentation is the primary communication tool among members of the home care team. Documentation has always been an accepted duty of the nurse in any health care setting. The home infusion pharmacist is responsible for documentation as well. This may be an expanded area of responsibility for many pharmacists entering the clinical realm of home infusion therapy. Continuous communication with all members of the team facilitates thorough documentation.

Nursing and pharmacy documentation includes initial and ongoing patient assessment and development of a patient care plan. Pharmacy documentation focuses on medication evaluation, therapeutic outcome monitoring, laboratory analyses, and recommendations to the physician. Nursing documentation focuses on physical and therapeutic assessment, especially as it relates to the disease process and the prescribed therapy, patient training, medication administration, skilled nursing services and technical procedures, and psychosocial evaluation and support. Both disciplines document communication with each other, members of the health care team, and the patient and caregiver. Routine patient care rounds and patient case conferences require documentation in the patient's medical records as well.

Documentation is a key component for securing reim-

bursement. In addition to serving in the reimbursement process, documentation has legal ramifications. The phrase "If it is not documented, it was not done," carries special emphasis for the home infusion team.

Standards of Care

Standards of care have been in existence for approximately 10 years. National standards have been developed to address infusion therapy in general as well as subcategories, such as parenteral nutrition and chemotherapy administration.[20, 54, 55] Although the settings for patient care may vary during a disease process, standards of care do not. Integration of nationally recognized standards in the development of policies and procedures helps facilitate the maintenance of appropriate, safe, high-quality care in the home as well as any health care setting.

Reimbursement

Patient acceptance criteria includes review of reimbursement for services. Many insurance policies cover home care; however, some policies limit services, such as nursing visits or equipment and supplies. Patients with Medicare coverage need a thorough review of diagnosis and therapy to determine reimbursement. The managed care environment continues to grow rapidly, exerting its impact on reimbursement. Some payment systems are based on subjective review, which solidifies the need for meticulous and thorough documentation. Even with thorough documentation, this subjectivity still leaves many uncertainties. During the insurance verification process, the carrier should be questioned regarding the required documentation, such as statement of medical necessity, physician orders or prescriptions, and clinical notes. This communication will assist in decreasing the denial rate and expedite the reimbursement process.

Patients are provided with information regarding their portion of financial responsibility, which can often be a burden to the patient and family. The home infusion team works with the patient to develop financial arrangements and to research alternate sources of financial assistance.

Quality Assurance Issues

The primary mission of home infusion providers is the provision of high-quality home care. Each home infusion provider needs to be able to demonstrate that it has a systematic approach to the identification of problems and methods for resolution. Quality assurance should focus on patient outcome criteria and reflect activities that occur frequently, affect large numbers of patients, and are at high risk for creating either patient or clinician problems. There may come a time when selection of providers and payment for services will be made on the basis of patient outcomes as opposed to cost effectiveness alone. Some examples of outcome criteria are unscheduled inpatient admission, infection rates of central lines, patient monitoring, and appropriate intervention in patients receiving parenteral nutrition.

All home infusion providers should be challenged to move

beyond quality assurance and embody quality improvement. Quality improvement is the process by which problems and opportunities for improvement are identified, root causes are determined, and improvement and prevention systems and corrective actions are implemented on a continuous basis to ensure that quality care and services are provided to patients.

Translators

Many patients speak English as a second language or do not speak English at all. It is the home infusion providers' responsibility to ensure the patients receive and understand their therapy. This goal can be accomplished through the use of bilingual clinicians, family members, or friends as interpreters. A professional translator may also be used. A thorough assessment of the cultural populations in the providers' geographic service area will assist in identifying translation needs and will also provide the information necessary to obtain appropriate translator consultants.

Accreditation

The JCAHO and the National League for Nursing have defined and issued home care standards. They both offer a voluntary accreditation. One of the benefits of accreditation includes national recognition of compliance to standards. Recently, the Health Care Finance Administration has awarded deemed status to both organizations. With slight alteration in the accreditation process, the accrediting body may survey organizations for Medicare certification. Some payers have begun to award preferred provider status to organizations that are accredited, therefore it would behoove home infusion organizations to become accredited.

Legal Issues

The 20th century has been described as an era of professional autonomy. Along with autonomy have come regulations and legislation to assist in defining the boundaries of practice. In spite of those activities, many gray areas still remain. Organizations and staff must be cognizant of the potential liabilities in the home as responsibilities and therapies increase in number and acuteness. Only clinicians trained and skilled in these new complex therapies should be undertaking treatment of these patients. Home infusion providers are responsible for documenting basic competency and advanced training of their clinicians.

Accurate assessment, ongoing communication, and meticulous documentation, coupled with strong problem-solving abilities, are minimum requirements for the home infusion clinician. Although the home lacks the resources needed to manage medical emergencies, the home infusion clinician must use prudent clinical judgment in the management of such situations. Anticipating potential problems and taking proactive measures to prevent crises are qualities of a good home infusion clinician. Patient and family education also assist in the process of early problem detection and intervention.

All home infusion providers should have a system for risk management and incident, infection control, and adverse drug reaction reporting. These reporting mechanisms will indicate problem areas and allow for early intervention and establishment of a prevention system. This diligence, in turn, will reduce liability exposure.

Professional Competition Versus Sharing

With a change in practice settings from the hospital, where clinicians were to some extent insulated from competitive pressures, to the home, where competition is a daily reality, traditional, professional interaction has been challenged. Clinicians from different acute care institutions have historically exchanged supplies, pharmaceuticals, and information in a manner that benefited the institutions in the area, and in fact, tended to improve the overall quality of care in the community. In the home care setting, where smaller organizations are in direct competition, the exchange of supplies, pharmaceuticals, and information may not be as readily available.

As the home infusion industry has grown and matured in recent years, the level of cooperation and exchange of information has steadily increased. This trend can be observed in professional organizations, such as the INS and the American Society of Hospital Pharmacists, whose meetings, journals, posters, and presentations provide forums for exchange of information, education, research, and networking. As clinicians find comfort in a new professional environment, sharing of information and knowledge will continue, and the overall quality of care will improve.

FUTURE DIRECTIONS

Home infusion is just now coming into its own at a time when our current health care model is faltering. As the condition of the home care patient becomes more acute, the clinical pharmacist and IV nurse will have to sharpen their skills. Therapeutic monitoring and patient care management by the nurse as well as the pharmacist are being demanded and even required by law in some cases. One can only assume that as the industry grows, so will opportunities for the home infusion clinician. Although it is difficult to predict what our health care model will look like in the future, one thing is certain: because we can no longer afford to exhaust our health care budget on the high cost of hospital care, a cost savings of 25 to 75% will make home infusion therapy a viable alternative for the future.

References

1. Biomedical Business International (BBI). Home and Alternate Site Infusion Therapy Markets in the U.S. Report #2822, March 1992.
2. Poretz DM. High tech comes home. Am J Med 1991; 91:453–454.
3. Darrow C. Hospitals seeking ways to cut costs. La Crosse City Business 1985; 3(19).
4. Paris E. Home remedies. Forbes, January 1989:58,62.
5. Rehm SJ. Home intravenous antibiotic therapy. Cleve Clin J Med 1985; 52:333–338.
6. Joyeux H. Background and development of the AIO concept. Nutrition 1989; 5(5).
7. Poretz DM. Home management of intravenous antibiotic therapy. Bull N Y Acad Med 1988; 64(6):570–576.

8. Stiver HG, Trosky SK, Cote DD, et al. Outpatient (home) intravenous antibiotic administration. Can Med Assoc J 1982; 127:207–211.

9. Health Care Finance Administration. Medicare Program Payment for Home Intravenous Drug Therapy Services, 42CRF Part 414 (BPD-618-P) RIN 0938-AE00, 1989.

10. Giglione L. Home IV therapy—Who pays? JIN 1988; 11(5):294–296.

11. Reid JS. Clinical Management Resources Guide. Community Alimentation Services. Department of Clinical Services, Chattsworth, CA, 1983.

12. Reid JS, Grace L, Venook S. Patient care management system model. Poster Presentation, National Intravenous Therapy Association's Annual Meeting, Phoenix, 1985.

13. Brown RB, Sands M. Outpatient intravenous antibiotic therapy. Am Fam Physician 1989; 40:157–162.

14. Herfindal ET, Bernstein LR, Kuzida K, Wong A. Survey of home nutritional support patients. JPEN J Parenter Enteral Nutr 1989; 13(3):255–261.

15. Ross Laboratories. Applying New Technology to Nutritional Assessment: Report on the Ninth Ross Roundtable on Medical Issues. Columbus, Ohio, 1989, pp 1–41.

16. Reid JS, Grace LA, Tomaselli B. Patient Care Management System, NACH, 1988.

17. Grace LA. Panel Presentation, National Association for Home Care, Annual Meeting. San Francisco, 1988.

18. LaBell L, O'Neil K, Bing CM. Overview of home healthcare programs. J Pharm Pract 1990; 3(1):4–10.

19. Crudi C. Credentialing for I.V. nurses. NITA 1984; 7:233–239.

20. Intravenous Nurses Society. Standards of practice. J Intravenous Nurs (suppl) 1990; 13:S1–S60.

21. New PB, Swanson GF, Bulich RG, Taplin GC. Ambulatory antibiotic infusion devices: Extending the spectrum of outpatient therapies. Am J Med 1991; 91:455–461.

22. Cross RP. Adults as Learners. San Francisco: Jossey-Bass Publishers. 1983:152–156, 186–215.

23. Grant JP. Handbook of Total Parenteral Nutrition. Philadelphia: W.B. Saunders, 1992.

24. Losoya F, Carder A. Total Parenteral Nutrition Guidelines For Administration. Memorial Medical Center, Long Beach, CA, June 1986.

25. Joint Commission on Accreditation of Healthcare Organizations. Home Health Standards. Oakbrook Terrace, IL: Joint Commission on Accreditation of Healthcare Organizations, 1992.

26. Report On Medical Guidelines and Outcomes Research. 1991 Handbook on Medical Guidelines and Outcomes Research. Health and Sciences Communications, Washington, DC, 1991.

27. US Department of Health and Human Services. Report To Congress: The Feasibility of Linking Research-Related Data Bases To Federal and Non-Federal Medical Administrative Data Bases. Agency for Health Care Policy Research, Rockville, MD, 1991.

28. Meguid MM. Clinical Applications and Cost Effectiveness of AIO Nutrition. Nutrition 1989; 5(5).

29. Pomp A, Caldwell M, Albina JE. Subcutaneous infusion ports for administration of parenteral nutrition at home. Surg Gynecol Obstet 1989; 169:329–333.

30. Brown JM. Peripherally inserted central catheters—Use in home care. JIN 1989; 12(3):144–150.

31. Hirsch J. Portable IV Frees Patients. The Orange County Register, Business Section, November 1991.

32. Dollinger M, Rosenbaum EH, Cable G. Everyone's Guide to Cancer Chemotherapy. Kansas City, MO: Universal Press Syndicate Company, 1992.

33. Schwartz C, Roy A. Neutropenia Precautions. Department of Health and Human Services, National Cancer Institute, Bethesda, MD, 1991.

34. Montague MJ. Biotechnology and the future of medicine. Pharm Prac News, January 1992, pp 3–4.

35. Ruef C, Coleman D. Granulocyte-macrophage colony stimulating factor: Pleiotropic cytokine with potential clinical usefulness. Rev Infect Dis 1990; 12(1):41–62.

36. Lokich JJ, ed. Cancer Chemotherapy by Infusion. Chicago, IL: Precept Press, 1990.

37. St. Marie B. Narcotic infusions—A changing scene. JIN 1991; 14(5):334–344.

38. Wilkie DJ. Cancer pain management: State-of-the-art nursing care. Nurs Clin North Am 1990; 25(2):331–343.

39. American Pain Society. Principles of analgesic use in the treatment of acute pain and chronic pain. Clin Pharm 1990; 9:601–611.

40. Tartaglia MJ. The management of chronic cancer pain. JIN 1988; 11(2):79–87.

41. Applefeld MM, Newman KA, Grove WR, et al. Intermittent, continuous outpatient dobutamine infusion in the management of congestive heart failure. Am J Cardiol 1983; 51:455–458.

42. Baptista RJ, Mitrano FP, Perri-LaFrancesca J. Home intermittent amrinone infusions in terminal congestive heart failure. Ann Pharmacother 1989; 23:59–62.

43. Applefeld MM, Newman KA, Sutton FJ, et al. Outpatient dobutamine and dopamine infusions in the management of chronic heart failure: Clinical experience in 21 patients. Am Heart J 1987; 114:589–595.

44. Collins JA, Skidmore MA, Melvin DB, et al. Home intravenous dobutamine therapy in patients awaiting heart transplantation. J Heart Lung Transplant 1990; 9:205–208.

45. Monks ML. Home transfusion therapy. JIN 1988; 11(6):389–396.

46. American Association of Blood Banks. Out-of-Hospital Transfusion. Arlington, VA: American Association of Blood Banks, 1988.

47. Crocker KS, Coker MH. Initiation of a home hemotherapy program using a primary nursing model. JIN 1990; 13(1):13–19.

48. Katzung BG. Basic and Clinical Pharmacology. Los Altos, CA: Lange Medical Publications, 1984.

49. Curaflex Health Services. Home Infusion Therapy Resource Guide. Ontario, CA: Braunwald E, Isselbacher KJ, Petersdorf RG, et al, eds. Curaflex Health Services, 1991.

50. Harrison's Principles of Internal Medicine, 2nd ed. New York: McGraw-Hill Book Company, 1987:1525–1527.

51. Cutter Biological. Production Information: Prolastin. West Haven, CT: Cutter Biological, 1988.

52. Deglin JH, Vallerand AH, Russin MM. Davis Drug Guide for Nurses, 2nd ed. Philadelphia: F.A. Davis, 1991:25–26.

53. Lam F, Gill PJ. Terbutaline Pump Therapy Guide. San Francisco, CA: Lam-Gill Children's Hospital of San Francisco, 1987.

54. American Society of Parenteral and Enteral Therapy. Standards for home nutrition support. Nutr Clin Pract 1992; 7:65–69.

55. American Nurses Association; Oncology Nurses Society. Standards of Practice. Kansas City, MO: American Nurses Association, 1987.

CHAPTER 30

Intravenous Therapy in Alternative Settings

Debbie Benvenuto, CRNI
Donna Baldwin, MSN, CRNI
David Schuetz, PharmD

- -

■■■■■ Intravenous Therapy in Emergency Settings
Intravenous Therapy in Ambulatory Settings
Intravenous Therapy in Nursing Homes
Conclusion

- -

Over the past decade, it has been demonstrated that the delivery of intravenous (IV) therapies in alternate settings can be safely and effectively accomplished while overall health care expenditures are reduced. This trend has resulted in a paradigm shift of the delivery of IV therapies from the traditional acute care hospital to various alternative settings. Some of the areas in which IV therapy is now successfully delivered include outpatient infusion centers, physician office–based programs, home care programs, extended care facilities, nursing homes, and psychiatric facilities. IV therapy may also be delivered in emergent situations before hospitalization, to provide prehospitalization care. The IV therapies delivered in these alternative settings often occur on a continuum. IV therapy may be initiated in any one of these areas and then continued or completed in another.

The shift in the delivery of IV therapies to alternative settings has been accelerated by numerous factors, including (1) fixed or declining reimbursement for inpatient care (e.g., diagnostic related group, per diem, capitation, and managed care), (2) need to reduce financial loss by decreasing length of stay, (3) re-emphasis of preventive care, (4) patient desire to avoid hospitalization if possible, (5) potential revenue generation from outpatient clinic or home health care, (6) availability of highly sophisticated vascular access and electronic ambulatory infusion devices, (7) evolution of scientific data supporting prolonged parenteral drug stability, (8) newer antimicrobial agents with extended biologic half-lives, and (9) studies demonstrating the safe delivery of multiple IV regimens in alternative settings. All of these factors support the potential for a comfortable transition of a medically stable patient from the hospital into the alternative setting for the completion of therapy.

Regardless of the setting, both federal and state regulatory agencies mandate that individuals who deliver such specialized care be properly oriented, competent, and proficient in the skills of initiating, administering, and terminating IV therapy. In addition, patient safety is the primary consideration of clinicians administering IV therapy in all practice settings. The *Intravenous Nursing Standards of Practice* forms the foundation of the standard by which the delivery of care may be measured.

Practitioners who may be involved in the delivery of IV therapies in alternative settings include emergency medical technicians and paramedical personnel, licensed practical and licensed vocational nurses, registered nurses, and physicians.

The authors would like to acknowledge the contributions of Maxine Acevedo, CRNI, in the preparation of this manuscript.

Organizations that regulate IV therapy include the Departments of Public Health, the Departments of Health and Hospitals, the Registries for Licensure, and specialty practice and professional regulatory organizations on both the federal and state levels.

This chapter provides an overview of the delivery of IV therapy in alternative settings, as opposed to the established or traditional acute care setting. In addition, current practice issues affecting the specialty in these settings are explored. Home infusion therapy is discussed in detail in Chapter 29 and therefore is not specifically addressed herein.

INTRAVENOUS THERAPY IN EMERGENCY SETTINGS

The delivery of IV therapies in emergency settings may involve IV access and administration of medications and solutions at the scene, en route to the hospital, or at the emergency room. IV therapies may be initiated for support for critical situations, or for less critical situations in which IV administration of the medication is desired, such as in antibiotic administration for infectious diseases. Increasingly, patients are seeking medical care in emergency departments and urgent care centers, often requiring the administration of IV medications.

Current practice in prehospital stabilization and resuscitation of traumatized patients contains a fair amount of controversy.[1, 2] Many reports question the usefulness of IV therapy initiated in the field versus in the transport vehicle en route to the acute care facility or in the emergency department of the hospital. Several authors advocate minimal-to-no paramedical prehospital involvement, whereas others maintain that on-site airway control and fluid replacement can be life-saving.[2] These sources seem to corroborate data obtained in rural areas, where transport times may be prolonged, and avoidance of delay in transport is paramount. Speed combined with efficiency is essential in this setting.

At the site of an accident, one must remember prioritization of the victim's treatment, if necessary. Because it is imperative that no time be lost in the transport of the victim, the IV line may be placed en route, except in cases such as entrapment. Even if sufficient volume cannot be delivered during transport, the presence of a functioning IV line as the patient arrives in the emergency department is a major advantage.[1] Some investigators believe that no trauma surgeon would object to an IV line being started if it did not delay transport.[2]

Standard procedure at the accident scene includes scene evaluation, assessment of emergency mechanism or precipitating illness, rapid physical examination, and paramedic intervention. The decision to insert an IV line is based on the paramedic's assessment of the patient's physiologic status, the injury mechanism or underlying medical disease, and the distance to the hospital.[1]

Standardization of policy and procedures must be well defined for those participating in prehospitalization emergency care. In many instances, individuals may be certified and licensed to initiate routine advanced life support procedures, including endotracheal intubation, IV access, fluid administration, and defibrillation. Protocols should address the various vascular access devices available. In some regions, emergency medical technicians are allowed to access central line catheters already in place. Careful consideration and education are imperative to ensure that these clinicians are able to identify existing devices and access them appropriately.

Emergency personnel assigned to an air transport unit are usually allowed to use the external jugular and femoral veins for access, if necessary. Intraosseous infusion can also be initiated by both emergency medical technicians and registered nurses in emergency settings. This route is indicated in extreme situations in which attempts at peripheral access are unsuccessful.

At the successful admission of such a critically ill patient, the IV nurse should ensure that all IV devices placed in the field (i.e., before admission to the hospital) are removed and new devices inserted, according to hospital policy and procedures, within 24 hours of admission. Further venous assessments should be performed for determination of expected duration of therapies. If long-term treatments and infusions are to be expected, the team approach, including a physician, a pharmacist, and other ancillary members, should be used to coordinate all the patient's IV therapy. This therapy may include the use of such devices as centrally placed multilumen catheters or long-term indwelling devices.

Safety to both the patient and the person delivering the care is a major consideration. Usually, no clinical information is available about these patients; therefore, as in standard practice, universal precautions are uniformly employed without exception. Protective clothing and face gear should be worn, in case large volumes of body fluids are lost or aerosolization of these fluids occurs. These products must be made available at the scene of a trauma and in the emergency department.

To prevent accidental exposure or injury to the care giver, violent or belligerent patients should not be approached with any sharp device or tool. Containers must also be made available for rapid but efficient disposal of sharp and contaminated devices (e.g., stylets, scissors, needles) as well as the disposal of contaminated dressing materials and clothing. Provisions must be made available to decontaminate these specialists in the event of their inadvertent contamination.

Means of recording and documenting all events at the scene of the rescue, en route to the medical facility, and on arrival at the emergency department further enhance the subsequent medical care the patient will receive.

In addition to emergent care, the treatment of appropriate conditions, such as common infectious diseases, has been accomplished on an outpatient basis through the emergency room.[3] Such care can be particularly successful for IV administration of medications that require only once-daily dosing. The daily doses can be administered in the emergency department, and when a satisfactory clinical response is obtained, oral medications can be prescribed to complete the course of therapy, as appropriate.

INTRAVENOUS THERAPY IN AMBULATORY SETTINGS

The delivery of IV therapies in ambulatory settings, often accomplished in conjunction with home care, has had a major impact on reducing the length of stay for patients requiring IV medications. The ambulatory setting may include physician office–based programs and hospital-based or freestanding outpatient infusion centers. The evolution of physician office–based programs followed by the hospital-based approach has been prompted by pressures from the health care industry.

The transition of IV therapy into the ambulatory setting was accomplished originally through physician office–based programs. These programs initially thrived on physician's visits after the patient was discharged from the hospital, coupled with continued antibiotic administration. Within a short time, other therapeutic modalities followed including chemotherapy, pain management, and parenteral nutrition. Frequent office visits facilitated the need for ongoing clinical assessment and laboratory monitoring, thereby fulfilling the requirement that the physician bear the primary responsibility for the continuity of patient care while securing payment for the physician's services.

Several different models for delivery of outpatient IV therapies have evolved in addition to the physician office–based programs. These infusion centers can be freestanding entities that incorporate physician's offices; laboratory and treatment facilities; and nursing, pharmacy, and financial services. The advantages of this type of infusion center include easier access for patients as compared with that of the hospital, centralized services for one-stop shopping, and the on-site physician's control over the program.[4]

Hospital-based infusion centers are another alternative. The hospital-based program works well to provide a continuum of care from the hospital to the outpatient arena. Regardless of the outpatient setting, 24-hour staff coverage is necessary to respond to off-hour patient needs. With hospital-based programs, many of these off-hour needs can be supported by an in-house 24-hour IV team that can provide services for ambulatory outpatients.

Specialized infusion therapies in the clinic or home environments may include catheter care; blood component administration; antimicrobial, antifungal, or parenteral nutrition therapies; IV or subcutaneous pain management infusions; continuous or intermittent chemotherapy; intramuscular and subcutaneous injections of varied nature; or IV gamma globulin administration. As previously mentioned, the rapidly growing availability of sophisticated vascular access devices has supported both short-term and long-term infusions in these alternative settings.

At each visit to an infusion center, the patient's access devices are assessed, dressings are changed, and medication- and equipment-related supplies are given to the patient. Current literature reveals a low incidence of phlebitis in the alternative care milieu. The reduced occurrence appears to be directly attributable to (1) thorough patient education by the IV nurse and (2) reduced device manipulation during the alternative site infusions.[5–7]

Significant cost can be saved when IV therapy is delivered in infusion centers rather than in other types of outpatient or home infusion programs or in hospitals.[4] Infusion centers allow for excellent coordination of resources and efficient delivery of services. For example, in infusion centers, depending on the type of therapy being delivered, several patients can be monitored at the same time, which cannot occur in the home setting.

Several important factors should be contemplated before successful alternative site infusion programs are established, including:

1. A knowledgeable certified IV nurse who is well versed in all aspects of patient assessment, parenteral therapies, vascular access devices, and ambulatory infusion pumps
2. A knowledgeable and supportive clinical pharmacist who is well versed in the pharmacologic aspects of parenteral therapies, the appropriateness of their use, their compounding, and the selection of germane monitoring parameters to reduce toxicity and promote positive therapeutic outcomes
3. The provision of available nursing care coverage, 24 hours a day, seven days a week
4. The availability of support services, including clinical laboratory, radiology, vascular surgery, and business services departments
5. The provision of a high-quality continuum of care from the inpatient to the outpatient environment, as prescribed by the *Intravenous Nursing Standards of Practice*
6. The ready access to the prescribing physician for the development of an interdisciplinary plan of care and appropriate plans for future communication and orders, as required by changing, or lack of, patient outcomes during the course of therapy
7. The research and development of legally approved instruments to document such patient interactions as consents to therapy, consents for placement of specific vascular access devices, statements of patient rights and responsibilities, information on advance directives, patient education regarding prescribed therapies, physician's orders, and after-hours emergency contact guidelines for patients.

The patient referral process is as complex and varied as the specialized infusion therapies. Each program should have specific guidelines and back-up policy and procedures for referred patients who reside outside the agency service area or who do not meet an individual agency's admission criteria. The Joint Commission on Accreditation of Healthcare Organizations recommends specific considerations for the review of a referral for acceptance:[8]

1. Receive and screen preliminary referral.
2. Determine if the requested service can be provided.
3. Perform individualized, comprehensive patient assessment.
4. Determine specific patient needs and educational requirements and assess the psychosocial status of the home environment, including available transportation and residence within the geographic service area.
5. Conduct insurance verification for authorization of prescribed care and then discuss and document the potential financial impact of the therapy on the patient.
6. Assess the appropriateness of therapy and develop an interdisciplinary plan of care with the prescribing physician.
7. Determine if therapy can be provided.

8. If service can be provided, interdisciplinary team develops and agrees on therapeutic goals and service plan of care.
9. Determine appropriate delivery system and supplies required.
10. Initiate patient and primary care provider education and assess learning capability of patient.
11. Continue comprehensive instruction as appropriate.
12. Assess patient's or primary care provider's final return demonstration of technique to self-administer prescribed therapy.
13. Document patient's readiness to self-administer therapy in a safe, timely, and effective manner. Release patient to the selected alternative setting.
14. Monitor and evaluate the patient's response to therapy based on established plan of care.
15. Perform scheduled tests to assess the patient's clinical status.
16. Intervene as appropriate.
17. On completion of the prescribed therapy, assess whether the patient's therapeutic goals have been fulfilled, and if so, discharge the patient from the service.
18. If the patient's therapeutic goals have not been fulfilled, ask the prescribing physician if the plan of care requires revision and if the therapy should be continued. Determine if the current agency can provide the service.
19. Obtain new physician orders or transfer patient to new agency that is capable of providing the prescribed service.
20. If the current agency can provide amended service, develop new plan of care and proceed with steps 8 through 17.

The responsibilities of the clinical pharmacist are extensive. The pharmacist should be acting in concert with the IV nurse to act as a liaison in interpreting and implementing alternative infusion site services for patients; physicians; hospital staff, where appropriate; allied health professionals; and third-party payers. In addition, the pharmacist should participate in the initial and ongoing clinical evaluation, including:

1. Collecting, analyzing, interpreting, and evaluating appropriate clinical data and patient history necessary to identify nutritional, fluid, and drug therapy requirements.
2. Setting therapeutic objectives and monitoring and evaluating therapeutic response.
3. Developing practical alternative infusion site therapy protocols.
4. Evaluating the significance of signs or symptoms related to the disease process and making recommendations for therapy modification.
5. Monitoring for potential adverse reactions and complications associated with infusion therapies, contributing to their prevention or resolution, and reporting such occurrences through established continuous quality improvement pathways.
6. Participating in the interdisciplinary health care team preparation and implementation of the patient's plan of care, and as appropriate to the patient's health care setting:

   • Participating in the discharge planning process, patient and family education, review and assessment of the patient's complete medication profile, follow-up visits, and on-call rotation pertaining to the alternative infusion site.

- Coordinating the preparation and delivery of pharmaceuticals.

7. Maintaining records and preparing reports on the alternative infusion site program.
8. Establishing and managing the continuous quality improvement aspects of the alternative infusion site program as they relate to pharmaceutical care.

Experience suggests that most patients adjust to their new responsibilities in an admirable manner. They also appear to enjoy the psychosocial interchange associated with periodic visits to the physician's office or infusion center for follow-up monitoring and evaluation of their therapy. A small percentage of patients prefer daily visits to the office or clinic for both professional administration of therapy and applicable monitoring. In either instance, the office or clinic visit allows the patient to interact with the members of the support team, as the medical and psychosocial situation demands.

Studies suggest that patients readily adapt to the alternative site programs.[9, 10] They respond to the positive benefits of the programs, which include a reduced length of hospital stay and associated costs, and they benefit from having a near-normal lifestyle, whether at home, in the workplace, or in the academic setting. In a broader sense, alternative infusion site care promotes patient healing and cost containment, while fostering a high degree of quality care. However, inherent risks to patients do exist. Some other considerations for a complete plan of patient care ought to include addressing patient rights and responsibilities, safety management, infection control, continuous quality improvement, equipment management, patient response to damaged vascular access devices, illicit use of vascular access device by patient, limited patient transportation that restricts emergent access to medical attention, and an infusion and visit schedule that interrupts the patient's lifestyle. However, attention to complete initial patient and family assessment followed by appropriate education often resolves potential deterrents to patient transition to the alternative care setting.

Reimbursement issues for alternative site infusion abound. Medicare coverage for home infusion therapy was disallowed with the defeat of the 1988 Medicare Catastrophic Coverage Act. Medicaid remuneration varies from state to state, depending on established formularies and the degree of restriction of the treatment authorization request process. Potential payment for outpatient infusion services varies widely with each third-party payer and managed care agency; this variability requires individual patient insurance verification of benefits for all prescribed therapies. Many states are now implementing legislation that restricts physician referrals to agencies in which they retain financial interest.[11]

INTRAVENOUS THERAPY IN NURSING HOMES

The population of Americans older than 65 years has more than tripled since the beginning of this century, and it is projected to represent approximately 20% of the population by the year 2000.[12] The aging of the population has been accompanied by an increased utilization of health care services. Although the elderly represented only 12% of the population in 1985, they accounted for 39% of the acute hospital census and 31% of the overall health care expenditures.[13] The total health care expenditures for the elderly, including nursing home costs, are expected to reach $40 billion by the year 2000.[14]

Approximately 5% of Americans older than 65 years currently reside in nursing homes, and 20% of those 65 years or older can expect to reside in a nursing home at some point in their lives.[15] The major focus of nursing homes has been custodial care, but reimbursement changes have resulted in increased provision of skilled services in the nursing home.[16] Medicare's implementation of the prospective payment system to hospitals in 1983 shortened hospital stays for the elderly, and earlier discharge of these patients necessitated the provision of complex, high-technology treatment modalities in alternate settings.[17] As a result, nursing homes began to offer skilled services that were previously limited to the acute care setting.

Skilled care is defined by Medicare as "care that can be performed only by or under the supervision of licensed nurses or professional therapists pursuant to a doctor's order." In the nursing home, skilled care qualifications for Medicare reimbursement require that the physician certify the need for daily provision of care, the care must relate to a condition for which the patient was hospitalized for a minimum of 3 days, and nursing home placement must occur within 30 days of discharge from the hospital.[18] Although Medicare reimbursement for these services is limited, more nursing homes are offering such services.

A primary example of a nursing activity that qualifies as skilled care is IV therapy. Studies regarding the increased acuity of nursing home residents have demonstrated the need for such services.[19, 20] However, the increased need for provision of IV therapy is not always met. Researchers in California have documented that almost half of the hospitalizations of nursing home residents could have been avoided and that 70% of these residents could have been treated in a nursing home if the nursing staff had been trained to administer IV therapy.[21]

Because IV therapy qualifies as skilled care, it is provided in a type of nursing home known as a skilled nursing facility (SNF). Nursing care is the major service provided in the SNF, but federal regulations require that the facility employ only one registered nurse, in addition to the director of nursing, regardless of the size of the facility. Researchers have cited this lack of professional staff as a factor in the failure of SNFs to meet their residents' need for IV therapy.[21]

Another factor that has contributed to the inconsistencies in the provision of IV therapy is the variety of settings in which skilled care may be delivered. The commonest type of nursing home offers skilled services that do not require 24-hour licensed nursing coverage. This type of facility may admit patients requiring IV therapy, but the complexity of the procedures and the sporadic need for such services may hamper the proficiency of the nursing staff. A second setting for skilled services are "swing" beds in small, rural hospitals. Because of the limited availability of SNFs in rural areas, several beds may be classified as either hospital or SNF beds, depending on the patients' needs. The same nursing staff are responsible for the IV nursing care, regardless of the bed classification. The third type of skilled nursing setting is the hospital-based SNF. IV therapy is a common admission criterion when the SNF is established within a major medical center and, when the institution has an IV team, the SNF patients receive the same quality of IV nursing care as the hospital patients.[22]

Although IV therapy is a skilled nursing service, little emphasis has been placed on the evaluation of the quality of such care in SNFs. The Health Care Financing Administration, which certifies nursing homes, considers IV therapy a complex treatment modality but stipulates only that residents require "proper care for parenteral fluids."[23, 24] Little explanation is offered as to what constitutes proper care. In fact, when the Health Care Financing Administration released its 93-volume report on the quality of nursing home care in 1990, IV therapy was grouped in a single category with injections, fluids supplied by tube, ostomies, tracheostomy and respiratory care, and tube feedings. The report was labeled as unreliable by the American Health Care Association, but, significantly, almost 15% of the nursing homes surveyed failed to meet federal requirements for this broad category.[25]

A definite and increasing need exists for IV therapy in the SNF setting. To meet this need and provide high-quality IV nursing care, several strategies need to be initiated. First, nursing home providers must understand that the *Intravenous Nursing Standards of Practice* are applicable to all health care settings, including nursing homes. The standards must serve as the foundation for policy and procedures for IV nursing and the criteria by which the quality of IV nursing care is evaluated. Second, the Health Care Financing Administration must place greater emphasis on IV therapy as a complex treatment modality. Listing possible problems is insufficient; instead, opportunities for improvement must be specifically identified and plans for correction initiated. Third, the Joint Commission on Accreditation of Healthcare Organizations, which surveys long-term care facilities, must develop standards specific to the provision of IV nursing care. Voluntary accreditation through the Joint Commission would then require that nursing home providers assess and improve the quality of IV nursing care for their residents. Last, IV nurses must contribute to the quality of IV care in nursing homes by developing educational programs and providing resources for the nursing home staff.

CONCLUSION

In summary, the delivery of IV therapies in alternative settings has been characterized by extraordinary growth. Patients will continue to seek treatments in alternative settings as medical technology and health care maintenance issues evolve. The demand for alternative site infusion therapies will continue to grow as hospitals maintain an emphasis on cost control to remain viable. To provide a true continuum of care, a seamless transition of services must be provided.

As a result of the transition of care to the alternative setting, health care professionals in many settings are now incorporating IV skills into their practice. In addition, because of the inevitable changes that will occur in health care delivery, more participants in the practice will emerge. The roles of the licensed practical/vocational nurse, registered care technicians, and other ancillary health care providers will expand as a result of these future health care reforms. The continued goal will be to ensure the provision of ambulatory IV therapy services by competent care providers.

The role of the IV nurse specialist has never been more apparent. The complexity of alternative site infusion necessitates that the IV nurse becomes the pivotal clinical element to coordinate and provide patient care, as mandated by state statute, thus ensuring the highest quality of care within the alternative setting. The *Standards of Practice* established by the Intravenous Nurses Society has laid a solid foundation for the nursing professional practicing within the specialty of IV therapy. Ongoing risk management and quality improvement initiatives will remain essential to the evaluation of competency.

References

1. O'Gorman M, Traubulsky P, Pilcher DB. Zero-time prehospital I.V. J Trauma 1989; 29:84–86.
2. Pons PT, Moore EE, Cusick JM, et al. Prehospital venous access in an urban paramedic system—A prospective on-scene analysis. J Trauma 1988; 28:1460–1463.
3. Lindbeck G. Outpatient parenteral antibiotic therapy: Part II. Amenable infections and models for delivery. The emergency department and urgent care center. Hosp Pract (Off Ed; suppl 2) 1993; 28:44–47.
4. Poretz D. Outpatient parenteral antibiotic therapy: Part II. Amenable infections and models for delivery. Infusion center, office and home. Hosp Pract (Off Ed; suppl 2) 1993; 28:40–43.
5. Brown J. Innovative antibiotic therapy at home. JIN 1988; 11:397–401.
6. Corky D, Schad RF, Fudge JP. Intravenous antibiotic therapy: Hospital to home. Nurs Manage 1986; 17:52–61.
7. Intravenous Nurses Society. Revised intravenous nursing standards of practice. JIN (Suppl) 1990.
8. Joint Commission on Accreditation of Healthcare Organizations. Joint Commission Perspectives. March/April 1991:7.
9. Poretz D. The infusion center: A model for outpatient parenteral antibiotic therapy. Rev Infect Dis (suppl 2) 1991; 13:S142–146.
10. Tice A. An office model of outpatient parenteral antibiotic therapy. Rev Infect Dis (suppl 2) 1991; 13:S184–188.
11. Grimaldi PL. Medicare covers home I.V. drug therapy. Nurs Manage 1989; 20:14–17.
12. Ad Hoc Committee on Special Care for the Elderly. Report of the Ad Hoc Committee on Special Care for the elderly. Chicago: American Hospital Association, 1989.
13. American Association of Retired Persons. A Profile of Older Americans. Washington, DC: American Association of Retired Persons, 1986:1–5.
14. Abrams WB, Berklow R, eds. The Merck Manual of Geriatrics. Rahway, NJ: Merck & Co., 1990:1116.
15. Dychtwald K. Age Wave. New York: St. Martin's Press, 1989:6–8.
16. Shaughnessy PW, Kramer AM. The increased needs of patients in nursing homes and patients receiving home health care. N Engl J Med 1990; 322:21–27.
17. Lytes YM. Impact of Medicare diagnosis-related groups (DRGs) on nursing homes in the Portland, Oregon, metropolitan area. J Am Geriat Soc 1989; 34:573–576.
18. Vogel RL, Palmer HC, eds. Long-Term Care: Perspective from Research and Demonstrations. Rockville, MD: Aspen Systems Corp., 1989:133–166.
19. Stull MK, Veron JEA. Nursing care needs are changing in facilities with rising patient acuity. J Gerontol Nurs 1986; 12:15–18.
20. Chambers JD. Predicting licensed nurse turnover in skilled long-term care. Nurs Health Care 1991; 11:474–477.
21. Kayser-Jones JS, Wilener CL, Barbaccia JC. Factors contributing to the hospitalization of nursing home residents. Gerontologist 1989; 29:502–510.
22. Baldwin DR. Provision of intravenous therapy in a skilled nursing facility. JIN 1991; 14(6):366–370.
23. Department of Health and Human Services. Health Care Financing Administration. US Federal Register. Vol. 54, No. 21. Washington, DC: US Government Printing Office, February 2, 1989.

24. Department of Health and Human Services. Health Care Financing Administration. Interpretive guidelines for skilled nursing facilities and intermediate care facilities. Washington, DC: US Government Printing Office, 1989.

25. Department of Health and Human Services. Health Care Financing Administration. Nursing home guide. Washington, DC: US Government Printing Office, 1990.

Selected Reading

Balinsky W, Nesbitt S. Cost-effectiveness of outpatient parenteral antibiotics: A review of the literature. Am J Med 1989; 87:301–305.

Brown R. Selection and training of patients for outpatient intravenous therapy. Rev Infect Dis (suppl 2) 1991; 13:S147–151.

Green S. Practical guidelines for developing an office-based program for outpatient intravenous therapy. Rev Infect Dis (suppl 12) 1991; 13:S189–192.

Grizzard M, Harris G, Karns H. Use of outpatient parenteral antibiotic therapy in a health maintenance organization. Rev Infect Dis (suppl 12) 1991; 13:S174–179.

Handy C. Vascular access devices—Hospital to home care. JIN (suppl 1) 1988; 12:S10–18.

MAST and IV infusion: Do they help in prehospital trauma management? Ann Emerg Med 1987; 16:565–567.

CHAPTER 31 ## Ethics

Lorys Oddi, Ed D, RN

The increasing complexity of biomedical decisions has created many ethical issues in health care. The unique role played by nurses in the health care system intimately involves nurses in these ethical issues. Long recognized as patient advocates, nurses sometimes feel uncomfortable with decisions made about patient care or with how the care is carried out. They may feel powerless, however, to articulate their concerns or may be uncertain of how, or if, they have a right to raise their concerns.

This chapter provides an overview of the unique role of nurses in recognizing and addressing questionable ethical practices, the multiple forces that affect nurses' ethical decision making, a sample framework that is useful for resolving ethical dilemmas, and some actions that can be taken by intravenous (IV) nurses to constructively address the ethical aspects of nursing practice.

UNIQUE ROLE OF NURSES IN ETHICAL ASPECTS OF PRACTICE

Ethics consists of moral judgments about the rightness or wrongness of actions in a specific situation. The nursing

The author acknowledges the contributions of Lynda Trauner, practitioner of intravenous nursing, for examples in practice, and of her aunt, Mary E. Schell, a registered nurse for more than 60 years, for historical insights related to practice and education.

literature abounds with reports of situations encountered in nursing practice that raise questions about the "right" course of action that a nurse should take. In addition, ample evidence in the literature indicates that nurses may be unable to recognize ethical conflicts; even if conflicts are recognized, nurses may lack the knowledge and skill to approach such conflicts in a constructive way.

The involvement of nurses in ethical decisions has changed dramatically since Florence Nightingale introduced modern nursing in the latter part of the nineteenth century. The "Nightingale Pledge," which can be regarded as an embryonic form of the American Nurses' Association Code of Ethics, reflected society's view of nurses and the subordinate role they were expected to play in health care delivery. Prominent ideas expressed in the pledge were the need for nurses to be obedient and to aide the physician in his work. Today's nursing ethics has moved beyond concerns about etiquette to emphasis on nurses' responsibility to society and to patients or clients, professional colleagues, employers, self, and family.

From its inception, nursing has continued to examine and articulate the importance of ethics to nursing practice. Furthermore, the development of professional ethics has evolved to meet the changing needs of health care.

Some individuals question whether or not such a thing as nursing ethics really exists; they suggest that the moral issues confronting nurses are identical to those of physicians and other health care workers. Nurses, however, because of their intimate and ongoing contact with patients, their position in the health care hierarchy, and their opportunity to perceive the health care situation of patients and families, are placed in unique ethical positions. Nurses must appreciate the ethical aspects of such practices as organ donation and transplantation, artificial prolongation of life, genetic engineering, and other biomedical advances. In addition, nurses are confronted by many critical issues for which they have professional autonomy to choose a course of action. For example, the nurse must decide how, when, or if they should enhance the autonomy of a patient; whether to intervene if a professional colleague (nurse, physician, or other health care worker) is violating the rights of other individuals or is endangering patients or clients; or how they can balance legitimate self-interest against the demands of the institution, patients, or physicians.

The nature of IV nursing and the different organizational structure under which IV nurses practice may further complicate their participation in ethical decision making. For this reason, IV therapy nurses must develop knowledge and skill to analyze the ethical aspects of care if they are to effectively fulfill their professional responsibilities.

INFLUENCES ON NURSES' PARTICIPATION IN ETHICAL DECISIONS

The activities and responsibilities of nurses in ethical dilemmas have their roots in the traditional patterns of nursing education and service. Although many changes have occurred since modern nursing began, the vestiges of outdated values and practices are still capable of affecting nursing behaviors. Some insight into these influencing factors may help nurses analyze their own behavior when they encounter ethical dilemmas and may provide a means of clarifying their ethical responsibilities in specific situations.

Patterns of Education and Service

Modern nursing was born in a military hospital, a fact that has traditionally exerted a strong influence on the practice of nursing. The military model of a hierarchy of command, with nursing at the bottom, has tended to dominate nursing. Nurses were, in effect, required to be "good soldiers" who obeyed orders without question and were prepared to make heroic personal sacrifices, if needed or ordered to do so.

This early association with the military exerted a pervasive influence on patterns of education and service, traces of which are found in nursing education and practice today. The early training of nurses took place in hospital schools of nursing, which awarded a diploma on completion of an apprenticeship. Students, who may have come from lower socioeconomic strata of society, were provided with training, room and board, and various necessities, such as uniforms and books, at little or no cost. Through their nurses' training, they were afforded an opportunity to earn a living and to advance their socioeconomic status after graduation. In exchange, the hospital had access to a source of relatively inexpensive labor that was totally subject to its control.

The reliance on student labor made it unnecessary for hospitals to hire graduate nurses to provide patient care. Instead, graduate nurses were independent practitioners of "private duty nursing" and obtained employment through registries and referral by individual physicians. Once employed by a patient, the nurse may have been put in a position of carrying out domestic tasks, such as baby sitting and laundering the family's clothes, in addition to nursing duties. Thus, from their entry into training, nurses were subject to rigid control from the hospital school, on which they were dependent for education and sustenance, and from patients, who had considerable power to control the nurse through job opportunities. The need to submit to others' demands became a pervasive force in nursing.

Physicians also exerted a great deal of influence over nurses. Most physicians were men, who were viewed by society as having a dominant role over women. Physicians also were better educated and exercised strong authority in the hospital. Student nurses were expected to be deferential to physicians at all times, even to the point of standing whenever physicians came into a room. Such codes of behavior were rigidly enforced by the teachers and supervisors responsible for the training school. Moreover, after graduation, nurses were frequently dependent on physicians for their very livelihood: nurses perceived as being rebellious or disrespectful would not be recommended for private duty cases or could be removed arbitrarily from a case; future employment could thus be jeopardized. Nurses learned early to conform to the system and to placate physicians to survive.

The professional values stressed during the early development of nursing included loyalty to the physician and the hospital where one received training, and self-sacrifice. The most important value, however, was unquestioning obedience to authority. The echoes of these early patterns of education and service still linger to a variable degree in nurses' education and employment environments today. Such influences exert an inhibiting effect on nurses' ability to participate meaningfully in ethical decisions in health care. Nurses who adopt bureaucratic values of the work place may view involvement in ethical aspects of care as antithetical to their role. They may have exaggerated views of physicians' authority in nonmedical decisions and may hesitate to question interventions about which they feel uncomfortable. They may fear that "making waves" will jeopardize their future.

Multiple Expectations in Contemporary Nursing

Another potential influence on nurses' participation in ethical decisions lies in the fundamental expectations that nurses encounter in their personal and professional lives. These expectations create moral roles and duties that may exert opposing demands and may create ethical conflicts for the nurse. In addition to the expectations of the physician and the employing institution, the profession, the greater society, and the families of nurses have different claims on nurses' time and energy—to say nothing of nurses' duty to themselves.

Over the years, the nursing profession has been increasingly articulate in professing the need for nurses to have autonomy in their professional practice. Improved education and broadening of the nurse's responsibilities have certainly contributed to increasing this autonomy. Professional organizations also stress that nurses' primary responsibility is to their clients or patients. Nurses are exhorted to be patient advocates. This professed autonomy model, which states that patients come first, may cause conflict if nurses practice in a situation in which they are expected to conform to institutional routines and practices, regardless of their views of appropriate courses of action for patient care.

Whether the nurse is employed in a hospital, the community, a clinic, or a home, the employing institution exerts a significant effect on professional practice. While overtly promoting the ideal of patients' needs as their primary concern, institutions may actually expect nurses to be primarily concerned with the agency's welfare. In today's climate of cost containment, nurses may feel pressure to ''cut corners'' in delivering care, to accept understaffing that they feel may jeopardize patient care, and to sacrifice their personal welfare and that of their families to work double shifts or forego earned days off when low staffing exists. An employer does have certain legal and ethical rights that should be respected by the nurses they employ. However, when the demands of the institution appear to be excessive or in conflict with what the nurse feels are legitimate rights of patients or family, the nurse is placed in the uncomfortable position of having to choose whose rights are met. The institution expects the nurse to be trustworthy and loyal and to work within its system. At times, these expectations conflict with the needs of patients, which puts nurses in the middle of two opposing demands.

Although their attitude toward nurses as collaborators in care has undergone remarkable improvement since the inception of modern nursing, physicians still may be more comfortable when nurses carry out their orders without question and refrain from questioning decisions they consider to be strictly their domain. Nurses who raise questions about ethical aspects of patient care with a physician may risk personal reprimand, verbal abuse, or disciplinary action within the institution or by the licensing board. Although physicians legitimately need nurses to carry out some medical aspects of patient care, they are not entitled to interfere with aspects of nursing practice that lie outside of their medical expertise, or to expect nurses to abandon their responsibilities to the patient or to the institution because of a physician's demands.

Society's expectations of nurses can be somewhat ambiguous. Whereas general expressions of support for a more independent role for nurses in health care and of trust and respect for nurses' expertise are documented in the literature, nurses are still frequently expected to function as ''the lady with the lamp,'' to practice with limited financial reward, and to assume a subservient role to physicians in areas that society views as ''medical.'' In the current economic environment, nurses may feel pressured to incorporate unlicensed personnel into the health care scene because of public concerns about the cost of health care. If the use of such personnel is viewed by the nurse as hazardous for patients, nurses are again in a dilemma. To the extent that nurses feel they cannot fulfill the expectations of society, they may also experience confusion and conflict about such activities as providing artificial feeding, resuscitating terminal patients, and engaging in other life-prolonging efforts when such efforts appear futile.

The traditional view that nurses must sacrifice personal and family interests and concerns to meet the demands of patients and the employing institution may occasionally place nurses in ethical dilemmas. A nurse could feel obliged to work extra shifts and holidays to such an extent that primary commitments to family members (e.g., spouse, children, or aged parents) would suffer. In these situations, the nurse's physical and psychological health and well-being could also be impaired. Nurses may also feel they are forced to give up other values and responsibilities to maintain the appearance of being a ''good nurse.'' The era of nurses' not being permitted to marry or not enjoying the benefits of a well-rounded life is gone. Although they are obliged to fulfill their professional responsibilities to their employer by reporting punctually for their shift and by carrying out assigned tasks,

nurses should realize that there are limits to how far they should go to compensate for their employer's deficiencies in planning and staffing. Rather than feeling guilty, angry, and devalued, nurses should refuse to engage in ''codependent behavior'' and should take constructive action to improve the working environment. Such action will ultimately benefit not only the nurse but also professional colleagues and patients.

In summary, the traditional patterns of education and service and the conflicting expectations of the multiple roles of the nurse as professional, employee, family member, and individual place nurses in ethical dilemmas. Nurses may feel they are obliged to be ''all things to all people'' and are adversely affected when they are unable to please everyone in a given situation. Feeling caught between opposing duties is stressful and demoralizing for the nurse, who may retreat into inaction in an effort to escape psychological conflict.

CAN NURSES FUNCTION AUTONOMOUSLY?

The multiple professional demands on nurses lead to conflict. Because of legitimate rights of all parties involved in a situation, nurses cannot act with complete autonomy in every situation (which is true for any individual). Furthermore, if nurses fail to comply with demands or cannot meet the expectations of others, they may suffer consequences in their personal and professional lives.

Failure to act in accordance with one's beliefs violates one's conscience and places one in moral jeopardy. Unfortunately, the correct course of action is not always obvious. In addition, numerous other factors come into play, such as the seriousness of the violation of another's rights and well-being; the harshness of the consequences for all concerned; and the scope of authority, control, and responsibility of the nurse. For example, if a nurse risks negative repercussions from the institution or the physician because he or she fulfills perceived obligations to the patient, the nurse may be tempted to avoid the risk and act in self-interest and for self-protection. Failure to act in accordance with one's conscience can cause acute discomfort and, as discussed later, can be very detrimental if it develops into an ongoing pattern of behavior. Conflicting demands and potentially serious consequences mitigate nurses' moral responsibility for actions taken or avoided in a situation, however.

Conversely, nurses should not be required to be heroic in their disagreements with an institution. Nurses need to develop a realistic view of others' duties in ethical dilemmas and to recognize the limits of their own responsibility. The consequences to all parties involved should be considered before any action is taken by the nurse, and the nurse must make every effort to make sound ethical decisions before choosing a course of action. Incurring a reprimand or the displeasure of a colleague is a small price to pay for taking appropriate action. However, harsh personal sacrifices, such as losing one's job or facing legal or professional disciplinary action, should not ordinarily be required to maintain one's moral integrity, unless the ethical violation involved is sufficiently grave to warrant such sacrifice. In other words, an important question to ask in nurses' ethical decision making may be ''How far must I go to resolve this situation?'' In some situations, the demands of other parties may be so unreasonable, and the consequences of failure to comply with those demands so drastic, that nurses may have to make a conscious choice about whether or not to continue to work in a given situation.

Fortunately, heroic sacrifice is not routinely required. Even if nurses cannot always successfully and openly confront issues, engaging in ethical analysis can clarify the issue and can open the door for realistic efforts at resolution. In any situation, nurses can and must critically examine questionable health care decisions, analyze the constraints and contingencies involved, and ask for reasons or justification for actions taken. The nurse is not justified in standing by passively when ethical dilemmas arise.

If, therefore, nurses are responsible for recognizing and dealing appropriately with ethical conflicts, they must sensitize themselves to the ethical climate in which they work, recognize when ethical violations occur, and be prepared to take an active, constructive role in ethical decision making. Nurses who have knowledge and skills in ethical analysis can make a critical difference to health care. They are role models for colleagues, they enhance the sensitivity of professional colleagues to the rights of others, and they contribute significantly to changing the status quo in the ethical aspects of care.

EFFECTS OF VIOLATIONS OF ETHICS ON NURSES

Evidence exists in the literature that ongoing violation of nurses' values and beliefs has severe and far-reaching effects. Nurses who feel forced to act in opposition to their conscience develop a sense of moral outrage. Internally, they are subject to feelings of rejection, disillusionment, hostility, and despair; their sense of frustration and powerlessness may be overwhelming. These negative feelings may pervade every aspect of life and interfere with the nurse's well-being.

Such intense emotions are capable of affecting the professional life of the nurse as well. To cope with the pain and guilt that accompany moral outrage, nurses may abdicate their professional ideals and ethical responsibilities and become totally compliant with the existing system, with detrimental consequences for the patient. The nurse's self-esteem and self-confidence suffer as a result. Some withdraw and regard patient care as "just a job"; they avoid any commitment and make no effort to go beyond the minimal requirements of the job. Others may make no conscious decision to withdraw. Instead, they drift into a series of small decisions to tolerate decisions with which they disagree. Before they realize it, such nurses have developed a pervasive pattern of apathy and insensitivity to the ethical aspects of their practice. They can grow to tolerate almost any violation, regardless of its severity, and regardless of the consequences. Finally, some nurses either quit the job or leave the profession entirely. Although finding a new job may be a necessary choice in some situations, a repeated inability to resolve conflicts that leads to quitting a job is not a viable solution. Whatever the cause, repeated violations of one's integrity are harmful to oneself and, ultimately, to patient care. The whole reason for the existence of nursing is to contribute to the health of patients. Ultimately, all activities undertaken by the nurse must be measured against this standard.

PROCESS OF ETHICAL DECISION MAKING

Much of the process of ethical decision making is already familiar to nurses. The nurse need not be intimidated by this process but rather should transfer already acquired skills to the ethical decision-making process and build on them.

Like the nursing process, ethical decision making requires a systematic approach of collecting facts from many sources, analyzing the facts, and arriving at a conclusion. What may not be recognized by nurses is that values, which are inherent in ethical decision making, are also involved in the nursing process. Nurses ask themselves, "What *should* I assess?" "How *should* I do this procedure?" "*Should* I consult the physician about this lab test?" "Should" questions are value questions. Within the nursing process, the nurse uses values that have been acquired through education and experience in nursing; these values are involved, perhaps unconsciously, in the day-to-day decisions the nurse makes about nursing practice.

The values involved in the ethical decision-making process may not be obvious to the nurse. Many of these values have their origins in the nurse's religious, cultural, and ethnic childhood experiences. They are an integral part of the nurse's personality, and they play a major role in the nurse's intuitive response to ethical dilemmas encountered in practice; furthermore, each nurse has a different value system. Many of the beliefs, assumptions, and attitudes that contribute to the value system may need to be examined systematically before they are put into action in ethical decision making.

The process skills that nurses bring to ethical decision making are not sufficient to enable nurses to make sound ethical decisions. Ethics is not intuition, personal preference, or what is popular in the culture at a particular time. Theories of the ethics of human actions have been studied for more than 2000 years in Western civilization. Individuals involved in the ethics of health care need to develop a basic understanding of this body of knowledge if they want to make sound, moral decisions. Following is a brief overview of fundamental concepts in ethics. Readers are encouraged to use this overview to orient themselves to the field of ethics so that they can deepen their knowledge by further study.

Fundamental Questions

Veatch and Fry[2] present a detailed discussion of the four fundamental questions that lie at the heart of any ethical decision. These questions address the nature of "right" actions, the kinds of actions that are right, the use of ethical principles, and decisions about actions to take.

What Is Right?

The nature of right actions focuses on what determines the "rightness" of an action. Veatch and Fry conclude that the answer lies in the reasons for acting, according to universal values that consider others' welfare on an equal basis with one's own welfare.

Western culture is based on certain universal values, such as the value of human life and the harmful effects of lying or stealing. All humans are regarded as having worth and dignity, regardless of attributes such as race, religion, ethnicity, and wealth. Although humans may have the ability to commit an act (e.g., murder another person), concern with universal values says that they should not put this capacity into action.

KINDS OF RIGHT ACTIONS

Much is written in ethics literature about the kinds of actions that are right. The two broad approaches among philosophers are that either the consequences of actions determine whether an act is right or wrong (*consequentialism*) or the nature of the action itself determines if an act is right or wrong (*deontologism*). The first approach tends to emphasize goals, or ''the end justifies the means.'' The second approach focuses more on doing one's duty and respecting the rights of individuals, while emphasizing the nature of the act that is taken. In reality, aspects of both views may be needed in any ethical dilemma. Neither approach satisfactorily resolves all ethical conflicts, and both approaches can also be absurd if carried to extremes. Nurses who develop only a superficial understanding of these two approaches and try to apply them without sufficient analysis may become confused and frustrated. For this reason, the reader is encouraged to consult a basic ethics text, such as the ones listed at the end of this chapter,[3–5] to develop more insight into fundamental ethical theories.

USE OF ETHICAL PRINCIPLES

Ethical principles should be used by nurses as a general guide to making decisions in a specific situation. As mentioned previously, no theory satisfactorily applies to all ethical conflicts. In other words, no ''cookbook'' exists to tell us step by step what to do and when to do it. This ambiguity is what makes the process of ethical decision making so frustrating for health care professionals. Each situation we encounter is unique, because each patient and relevant circumstances are unique. A set of rules cannot be rigidly and automatically applied, or unethical decisions may result. The inability to apply rules rigidly leads some nurses to draw the erroneous conclusion that all ethical decisions are arbitrary and subject to personal whim. Nothing could be further from the truth: exercise of arbitrary and capricious decisions in the ethical aspects of care can create much harm and injustice. A consistent, thoughtful approach is mandatory for those responsible for the care of patients and clients.

What Action Should Be Taken?

The final question that underlies all ethical decision-making processes is ''How can we decide what action should be taken in a specific case?'' To answer this question, one must systematically collect all the relevant facts and apply the ethical principles that one believes are appropriate to the situation. In short, one must systematically address the conflict.

Steps in the Process

Numerous models and approaches to ethical decision making are available in the nursing literature. These models and approaches vary in their complexity, practicality, and ease of application. For nurses engaged in active clinical practice, the steps suggested by Benjamin and Curtis,[4] outlined in this section, are the most practical for the nonspecialist in ethics because they form a common-sense approach that uses the analytical skills already possessed by nurses.

Step 1. Determine If an Ethical Issue Exists

Not every decision in health care involves ethics; those that do may not require in-depth analysis to determine a course of action. Most nursing actions can be implemented without fear of ethical violations. Nurses should sort out such actions and devote time to serious ethical concerns.

An initial question for the nurse to ask is ''Is this strictly a matter of technical expertise?'' Some matters do not fall within the realm of ethics because they relate solely to technical expertise. Diagnosis and prognosis are matters of technical expertise that require medical decisions, and physicians are educated to make such decisions. Such straightforward technical questions in themselves do not present ethical problems. Ethical problems may arise, however, when communication of technical information is indicated. Nurses need to recognize that ethical issues arise, for example, if physicians use medical jargon that patients cannot understand, if they fail to provide enough information so that patients can make appropriate decisions, or if they covertly or overtly discourage patients from asking questions about their diagnosis or treatment. Patients have the right to be informed so that they can make necessary decisions about their care. Any nurse has the expertise to recognize and address the ethical issues in this situation.

In health care, many patients and health care workers label all or most matters as ''medical.'' Patients and health care workers may regard physicians, because of their medical expertise, as the best or the only individuals who should make all decisions. In reality, if the issue is nonmedical, there is a need to decide who has the right to make the decision. Without sound ethical analysis, personal values of health care personnel who make the decisions about patient care may be imposed wrongfully on others, especially the patient.

A second question for the nurse to ask is ''Is a conflict of values operating in this situation?'' As detailed in the preceding discussion of factors influencing nurses' participation in ethical decision making, physicians, patients, administrators, and colleagues bring different values to any situation. If a situation exists in which fundamental values are in conflict, ethical analysis must be undertaken to resolve conflicts so that important rights of those in the situation are not violated. One example concerns the withdrawal of fluids from a dying patient. Although a nurse may value the patient's right to ''die with dignity,'' the physician may value a perceived duty to preserve life at all costs; discussing these different positions may facilitate a resolution of the issue in a way that respects the values of all concerned.

The key to identifying whether or not an ethical issue exists in a specific case, then, lies in the identification and elimination of questions that require only medical expertise to answer them. Next, nonmedical issues should be examined to identify conflicts in human values; when a conflict in values exists, ethical analysis must be performed to ensure that the most ethical approach to resolving the conflict is determined.

Step 2. Engage in Ethical Analysis

To analyze an ethical conflict is to reflect critically on the facts and principles of the situation. Such reflection must be interactive rather than linear. That is, the nurse must evaluate the facts, consider different scenarios about the outcomes of different courses of action, and sort major issues from minor ones. The process requires that the nurse be able to use imagination, see the situation as others may see it, analyze how different facts change the situation, avoid making hasty judgments until all available aspects of the situation have been taken into account, and try to obtain a comprehensive perspective of the situation. Throughout the analysis, the nurse should be open to opposing views. (In fact, opposition should be welcomed because it broadens one's view and forces one to examine other perspectives more thoroughly.) A nurse may be angry that a physician provides what the nurse considers futile treatment for a terminal patient; however, talking to the physician may reveal that the patient requested such treatment in the hope of living to see a new grandchild. The nurse should be flexible enough to change position on an issue if convincing new evidence is presented that renders the position erroneous.

Collect and Examine Relevant Facts. Sometimes a conflict exists because individuals have different facts or do not have all the facts that bear on an issue. When the relevant facts are available, the conflict may disappear. Facts are not sufficient to resolve ethical problems, but they can alter significantly the ethical claims (rights and duties) of the individuals in the situation. Arriving at a decision without examining all the facts that are available is foolish and may result in significant violation of patients' rights. For example, a nurse may fail to determine in advance whether or not a patient desires to be resuscitated should a cardiac arrest occur. Without knowing the patient's wishes, any course of action (to provide or withhold resuscitation) could violate the patient's wishes.

Clarify Terms. The use of cliches and emotionally charged language, such as "right to die," "unfair," and "doctors cure, nurses care," can inhibit or prevent sound ethical analysis of a situation. Nurses may use terms imprecisely or assume that they understand what someone else means by a word or phrase, when, in reality, assumptions about what is meant may differ from individual to individual. So-called conflicts may evaporate when individuals in opposition discover that they both mean the same thing. For example, both physicians and nurses may believe that they know what a "good quality of life" means, but discussion to clarify this term may reveal very different perceptions. Clarifying meaning helps resolve ethical conflict.

Determine the Pros and Cons of Positions. Developing and justifying various positions on an ethical issue requires the ability to think logically or to engage in philosophical analysis. Courses in logic or critical thinking may be required to improve one's ability in this respect. Nonetheless, logical thinking is necessary if nurses are not to rely solely on intuition to decide on a course of action, which would create

the probability of treating others unethically. Such questions as "Are there good grounds to support this action?" "Are my assumptions valid and true?" "Is there a logical connection between these facts and my conclusions?" help to sharpen thinking and clarify issues throughout the analysis.

Use a Systematic Framework. A framework is necessary to provide a common basis for discussion of everyone's rights and duties in any health care dilemma and of the goals to be achieved by any course of action. A framework is developed from the two major approaches to ethics described earlier: consequentialism and deontologism. Nurses should study the basic tenets of these approaches and clarify their own beliefs and guiding principles. Defending a position based on principle rather than on intuition and impulse gives credibility to that position. Others involved in the discussion can then learn how the nurse views the situation and can examine the logic of the nurse's position. In turn, they can then clarify their own positions to the nurse. Nurses, for example, may emphasize patients' rights to make autonomous decisions about receiving costly treatments although the patients are receiving public aid. Management, however, may emphasize the "big picture" of allocation of scarce resources as well as the goal of having a financially viable institution.

Acting on principle is necessary if nurses are to exhibit integrity, which requires that one's actions be consistent with one's beliefs. People who lack integrity, who vacillate from one value system to another, quickly become known as unreliable, capricious, or untrustworthy among professional colleagues. They are dangerous because their intuitive actions can violate the rights of those with whom they come in contact.

Re-examine Your Position as Needed. Individuals must always remember that they may have inadequate or incorrect information about a situation. They may have engaged in faulty reasoning or may lack insight or experience necessary to make the decision. Furthermore, health care situations are dynamic, and new developments may change the ethical aspects of any situation we encounter. These limitations mean that nurses must remain flexible and open to consider new information. Nurses must, furthermore, respect others as moral agents who also have legitimate values and concerns. Respect for others is absolutely critical. If nurses enter ethical conflicts with a rigid and judgmental attitude, satisfactory resolution of conflicts will be delayed, inhibited, or prevented. In addition, interpersonal conflicts will develop if others feel devalued by the nurse's negative attitudes.

APPLICATIONS TO INTRAVENOUS NURSING PRACTICE

An examination of the nursing literature reveals that many rules, principles, and philosophies are available to help nurses in their ethical decision-making endeavors. Sometimes, this variety of information can be more of a hindrance than a help because the resulting detail and complexity can overwhelm the reader and lead to a sense of paralysis and despair. Each nurse should study and adopt a coherent approach that makes sense to him or her. It is useful, however, to have a starting point.

The principles comprising the framework presented in this chapter are not discussed comprehensively in the following paragraphs. Rather, essential elements of each principle, an overview of its importance, and examples of types of situations where the IV nurse may encounter conflicts relating to the principle are presented.

A Framework for Health Care Decisions

Two recognized experts in the ethics of health care, Beauchamp and Childress[3] have evolved a "composite theory of ethical principles" that they believe is useful in most health care settings. The composite theory consists of four ethical principles: autonomy, nonmaleficence, beneficence, and justice, which the authors encounter most frequently in their research in health care situations.

The composite theory is a useful starting point for nurses in their study of ethical decision making because these four principles are easily understood, and their underlying concepts are familiar and generally accepted in Western cultures. The principles also are broad in their application, in that they apply to patients and clients as well as health care workers. A very practical feature of the composite theory is its flexibility; the relative priority given to each principle is determined by the context of the particular situation in which it is applied. Such flexibility is essential if the complex ethical dilemmas encountered in clinical practice are to be approached in a practical manner. Finally, using a framework consisting of only four principles reduces the number of variables juggled by the nurse in what may be an already extremely complex dilemma, thus making the analysis more manageable. In addition, the principles are interrelated and frequently overlap.

Autonomy

The principle of *autonomy* is familiar to most nurses because it is the basis for the legal doctrine of informed consent. The American culture values independence and the right of individuals to be autonomous, that is, to be free from control by others and free from personal limitations that interfere with their ability to make meaningful choices in their lives.

Freedom from control by others means that one should not be coerced, forced, deceived, or manipulated into doing what another desires. Freedom from personal limitations means that one must have the mental capacity to consider the risks and benefits of any action, to anticipate the potential consequences of actions, and to choose in one's perceived best interests. Lack of adequate information, psychological stress, and inadequate time to explore alternative courses of action are examples of personal limitations that interfere with autonomy.

The right of autonomy implies that others have a duty to respect and not interfere with the ability of an individual to exercise that right. Although health care professionals formerly de-emphasized the autonomous rights of patients because health care professionals believed that *they* should always act to promote patients' physical well-being, current trends in the legal and ethical aspects of health care are to give priority to patient autonomy. However, no one's autonomy is necessarily absolute. The rights of others and the inherent limitations in any situation make it necessary to balance individual autonomy against others' rights and duties.

As mentioned previously, nurses have the right of autonomy in their practice, and others should respect that right. Nurses exercise this autonomy in relation to ethical conflicts in health care by analyzing the facts in a situation, resisting others' attempts to force them to comply with unacceptable procedures, and obtaining information necessary for them to make an informed decision. Remember, the nurse can always raise questions about any practice that causes discomfort or concern.

IV nurses may encounter potential violations of patients' rights of autonomy with every patient contact. Some obvious areas that may be questionable include the initiation, continuation, or discontinuance of total parenteral nutrition or experimental drugs; unusual dosages or combinations of drugs; artificial hydration; and similar procedures. To make autonomous decisions about undergoing any of these procedures, patients must be informed about the risks associated with them, the available alternative treatments, the benefits anticipated from the treatment, and the consequences of accepting or rejecting the treatment. Patients must be given adequate information with which to make their decisions; in addition, they must have adequate time to consider their choices without being pressured to comply by the staff, even if the staff believes that a certain treatment is the only choice a patient has. Remember, only the patient can choose what is best for him or her. The health care worker can only create the appropriate climate within which the decision can be made.

If patients lack decision-making capability (e.g., because of changes in level of consciousness, emotional distress, effects of age, inability to understand and judge alternatives), an attempt should be made to ascertain what the patient would choose, if he or she were able. Advance directives, documentation of patient wishes before mental impairment, and information provided by significant others offer means of promoting respect for patients' autonomy. Furthermore, these resources are available to IV nurses, regardless of the site of practice.

Health care workers must recognize that patients do not lose their rights of autonomy merely because their capacity to make decisions is impaired; therefore, every effort must be made to find out the preferences of the patient to the greatest extent possible. In cases in which the patient's wishes cannot be determined, the health care workers must rely on other ethical principles to guide care.

IV nurses have brief encounters with patients over varying lengths of time. In some respects, the nature of this contact is a disadvantage because the IV nurse may lack vital insight and opportunity to determine whether or not autonomy has been respected. Alternatively, these brief encounters over a period of time enable the IV nurse to view the situation from a fresh perspective, free from activities on the unit that may have a desensitizing effect on the unit staff. In the community or home situation, the IV nurse may be the only health professional available to note changes in patients' conditions or attitudes. The IV nurse in any setting may be viewed by the physician as a collaborator whose expert opinion is valued because of his or her extensive knowledge and experience.

Thus, IV nurses are frequently in a position to enhance the

autonomy of patients they care for. The nature of their contact with patients and their unique perspective requires that they be sensitive to situations in which patients' rights of autonomy are in jeopardy. Sometimes, the conversation of a patient will suggest to the IV nurse that the patient does not fully understand the implications of a particular procedure. Or, a patient's chance remark (e.g., ''I don't want to go through all of this'') triggers a question about the patient's desire to continue or begin a course of therapy. A patient who lacks mental capacity (e.g., obviously doesn't understand what is being explained) may appear to be suffering without hope of benefiting from a procedure. In all such instances, the IV nurse should explore the situation more fully, with the patient, if possible. Raising questions on the basis of personal observations and collecting relevant data can help clarify the existence of an ethical problem and provide additional facts with which the situation can be analyzed. Ethical analysis can then be used to resolve conflicts associated with the violation of a patient's autonomy.

Nonmaleficence

Nonmaleficence refers to the right of individuals to be free from the infliction of actual harm or the risk of harm by another person. Harm refers to both physical or emotional damage. Often, health professionals may focus on avoiding actual harm, while forgetting that it is a violation of the right of nonmaleficence to act in a way that causes a *risk* to others. The requirement of avoiding harm to patients has been a very strong mandate in health care for centuries. The mandate to avoid harm or the risk of harm is obviously not absolute in health care, because numerous procedures can be ''harmful,'' at least in the short term, but have an ultimately beneficial effect on the patient.

IV nurses can avoid physical harm to their patients by exercising care in the performance of procedures, by ensuring that proper dosages of IV medications and nutrients are administered, by keeping current with developments in their field, and by remaining alert to signs of untoward effects of treatments and intervening early to prevent further damage. Educating the patient, caregivers, and other staff to the specific care required for treatments provided by the IV nurse is another way of preventing harm. Physical harm may also be prevented when the IV nurse raises questions about poor care that he or she observes and takes action to promote safe care for patients. One group of IV nurses in a community setting was instrumental in changing policy regarding home administration of a chemotherapeutic agent that had a greater than 50% risk of systemic anaphylaxis. Their concerns about patient safety and their own ability to handle such a complication were expressed to their management and the ordering physician, leading to a resolution that was satisfactory for all.

Psychological harm is a broad area of concern that may be less obvious than the threat of physical harm. Patients may be harmed psychologically by being cared for by nurses who convey a lack of concern and compassion for them. Indifference to patients as individuals can result in the patients' experiencing loneliness, despair, grief, anger, and many other negative emotions, all of which are harmful or risk harm. The fidelity, veracity, and commitment of the nurse contribute to the avoidance of psychological harm for patients. If

nurses break faith with patients or deceive patients by lying to or misleading them, patients lose trust in their care givers—a disastrous situation when the patient is in most need of support.

Nurses should also appreciate the need for confidentiality in their relations with patients. Although nurses are strictly mandated to protect patients from unwarranted disclosure of intimate facts that are revealed in the patient-nurse relationship, idle talk or interest in sensational aspects of patients' lives may lead nurses to talk to other individuals who have neither the need nor the right to know such details. The nurse should also not assume that the patient wants family members or significant others to know what has been told to the nurse. Much harm can result if a nurse inadvertently reveals sensitive information, such as a seropositive human immunodeficiency virus status, without the expressed consent of the patient. The nurse should, if disclosure is regarded as essential to the patient's care, obtain the permission of the patient to reveal the information to the appropriate individuals on the health team or should encourage the patient himself or herself to make the disclosure. When disclosure of confidential information is mandated, such as the legal requirement to report suspected child abuse, the patient needs to know that the nurse will report information to the appropriate individuals.

Beneficence

The principle of *beneficence* goes beyond the mere avoidance of harm to taking positive action to help another person or to contribute to the well-being of that person. The principle of beneficence has long been the guiding force in health care. In fact, the past emphasis placed on beneficence over autonomy led to paternalism in health care: physicians and nurses felt justified in doing things to and for patients, even if patients objected, because it was ''for the patient's own good.'' The fallacy of paternalistic thinking is that no one knows for sure what action is best for another individual; only that individual can weigh the positive and negative aspects of any recommended course of action to determine the best choice, which is one reason why autonomy has become an important consideration in health care.

Nonetheless, beneficence overlaps considerably with autonomy. Providing sufficient information about the risks and benefits of a proposed course of treatment, as well as the consequences of choosing alternatives, is an essential element of respecting a patient's autonomy. It also promotes the well-being of the patient by seeing that all available information is brought to bear on the decision.

IV nurses can provide for the well-being of their patients by carrying out the patient's care in a safe, caring manner. Questioning management's decision to use less expensive peripheral lines with public aid patients needing prolonged therapy, in an effort to control costs incurred by using more expensive central lines, is a beneficent action. Listening to patients' concerns and providing follow-up for anticipated problems also promotes beneficence. Intervening to ensure that the patient receiving nursing at home or in the hospital obtains the services of physicians, chaplains, or other resource personnel is also a means of actively promoting the welfare of patients.

Justice

Justice is the fourth, and last, principle comprising the composite theory of Beauchamp and Childress.[3] The principle of justice, as used here, involves fairness in dealing with others, or giving them that to which they are entitled or deserve. Treating all patients with respect is one manifestation of acting justly. IV nurses may encounter patients from diverse racial, ethnic, religious, and socioeconomic backgrounds—all of whom should be approached with a professional standard of care and concern. IV nurses may not personally approve of the lifestyles of some patients, and they may react with fear and repugnance when various situations (e.g., gay lifestyles, acquired immune deficiency syndrome, or criminal records) are encountered. Nonetheless, they must go beyond their personal preferences and deliver the same standard of care to all patients. Employers may endeavor to have the IV nurse provide a lesser standard of care to patients who lack financial resources, in which case the nurse must take steps to ensure that the patient is not treated unfairly.

If IV nurses are aware of dishonesty in billing patients or governmental agencies for services, they may be required to take action to have such practices investigated. Ultimately, such practices may result in a loss of essential services to all because of the legal and professional sanctions that may result.

Actions To Promote Ethical Practice

IV nurses can take many actions to improve their ability to practice ethically and to ensure ethical care of their patients. First and foremost, IV nurses should actively improve their knowledge of, and sensitivity to, the ethical aspects of patient care. Attendance at workshops and conferences dealing with ethics is a valuable means of learning more about ethics. Continued independent learning is essential, for example, through reading texts such as those listed at the end of this chapter, to learn about the theoretic basis for ethics. Professional nursing journals are increasing their publication of articles that deal with specific ethical conflicts through the presentation of case studies. Application of approaches for resolving ethical conflicts, such as that presented by Benjamin and Curtis[4] and summarized in this chapter, are useful; reviewing situations in which they have been involved by using such approaches will increase nurses' proficiency in analyzing ethical conflicts. Actions needed to promote ethical practice range from increasing one's ability to answer ethical violations to informing relevant staff or organizations when ethical violations are identified.

Assessment

IV nurses need to develop insight and sensitivity to questionable practices that they encounter. Such insight requires a willingness to investigate further when one feels a sense of discomfort or questions some aspect of care. The nurse must embark on a systematic process of ethical analysis to determine if an ethical conflict truly exists and to define the nature of the conflict.

Reliance on a sense of discomfort is, however, only one aspect of assessment. Serious violations of ethics may go unrecognized by the nurse whose value system does not include the area of the violation. Thus, the nurse is obliged to go beyond an intuitive sense that ethical concerns exist to a conscious effort to learn more about ethical implications of nursing practice. Such efforts include a thorough review of the literature dealing with nursing ethics, attendance at meetings, discussions with colleagues, follow-up investigations of ambiguous areas, and consultation of journal articles.

Role Modeling of Ethical Practice

IV nurses must show respect and faith in all members of the team as ethical practitioners who share concern for ethical care of patients. In addition, the IV nurse must raise questions where doubt or insufficient information exists. Silence may result in the violation of another's rights. On the other hand, the nurse must appreciate the complexity of any health care situation and must not leap to conclusions without being certain that unethical practice is being used. The IV nurse's efforts to explore further any situation in which a patient's rights may be threatened or violated are an invaluable asset for ensuring ethical practice. Simple actions, such as asking questions to see if patients understand and accept their therapy, reminding physicians and other personnel to explain options fully to patients and families, and asking whether advance directives are available and encouraging their use, are all means of anticipating and preventing ethical dilemmas later in the course of an illness.

IV nurses should be especially alert to patients' comments that indicate their states of mind in relation to such measures as prolonging life by use of technology; such comments are invaluable should a patient lapse into coma and be unable to make necessary choices at a later time. Verbatim documentation of such comments in the chart is essential in case evidence of the patient's state of mind is required at a future date.

Problem Solving

Ample evidence in the literature indicates that nurses are often reluctant to intervene when confronted with violations of ethics in health care. When IV nurses encounter practices that seem suspect, they should raise constructive questions about such practices. Further investigation may reveal that, indeed, an ethical problem needs to be resolved; conversely, the nurse may find that other colleagues have different ethical principles, that additional factors unrecognized by the nurse are influencing the situation, or that appropriate steps to resolve the issue have already been implemented. An open, problem-solving approach and avoidance of hasty judgments are necessary to promote the resolution of ethical dilemmas, as is persistence in confronting such dilemmas.

A useful approach that will increase sensitivity to ethical aspects of care is to copy chapters and articles dealing with ethics for distribution and discussion among peers on the IV team. Group discussion can help sensitize everyone to the range of ethical issues involved in an area of practice. Open discussion may encourage a cohesive approach to resolving problem issues and is a means of developing consensus among the staff.

Resources available in the agency should be used to help define and address ethical concerns. Hospitals and nursing homes may have access to ethicists, legal counsel, or pastoral staff who can help clarify and facilitate resolution of ethical dilemmas. Nurses practicing in the community, who may not have ready access to such personnel, nonetheless can consult religious leaders in the community or the staff of the local hospital to obtain referral for such problems.

Volunteering to serve on the agency's ethics committee is an excellent way to gain knowledge and experience in the ethical aspects of care. Networking, which can widen the nurse's awareness or knowledge of persons who are available as resources, is an added bonus to such service. The creation of unit-based ethics committees, either for the IV team itself or for members of the unit staff with the IV nurse in attendance, may also be helpful. Such local ethics committees may improve problem solving, communication, and support for all individuals involved in patient care.

A critical mechanism for helping the individual nurse address ethical concerns in a systematic and constructive way is a personal diary. Any perceived problems or concerns should be fully and objectively described by the nurse. The situation, the dates, the times, and the people involved should be included. Diary entries can provide evidence of the prevalence and seriousness of problems. The continuing occurrence of some types of problems will become obvious through content analysis of the entries and can serve as an impetus for corrective action. When the IV nurse has prepared such an analysis, the next step is to ask a representative of the ethics committee or pastoral team or a risk manager to meet with the appropriate administrator to discuss the issue and to devise an approach for its resolution. Another important contribution of a diary is that it provides a reliable record of events that have transpired; thus, it has a protective function for the nurse. The diary is a valuable legal record should litigation ensue from a breach of ethics in care.

SUMMARY

The willingness and ability of IV nurses to participate in ethical decision making in clinical practice is influenced by numerous historical and organizational factors. Both the types of ethical dilemma nurses encounter and their ability to intervene as autonomous practitioners are affected by the values and the power of colleagues in the work situation. Nurses must be alert to the influence of these factors on their willingness and responsibility to intervene. At all times, the nurse's primary obligation is to act to safeguard the patient's welfare, although other aspects of the situation must be investigated and balanced so that an ethically acceptable resolution is reached.

Although a concern for ethics is evident throughout the history of nursing, nurses may lack the knowledge and skills in ethical decision making that provide them with confidence or credibility to be full participants in this process. Nonetheless, nurses can and must always raise questions about the ethics of clinical practice. They should embark on a conscious effort to improve their knowledge of ethical theory and their ability to engage in ethical analysis. This chapter provides an overview of introductory material and suggestions for further study to improve the knowledge base of IV nurses in this area.

The pivotal position of IV nurses provides them with opportunity to recognize ethical problems in care that may not be evident to others on the health care team. Especially in the community, the IV nurse may be the only professional contact who has insights relating to ethical concerns. Hence, IV nurses must assess care situations for the potential for developing ethical problems, act as a role model for ethical care, and adopt a problem-solving approach in situations that give rise to ethical concerns. IV nurses, like other nurses, have a critical role to play in ensuring ethical practice in today's health care environment.

References

1. American Nurses' Association. The Code for Nurses with Interpretive Statements. Kansas City, MO: American Nurses' Association, 1985.
2. Veatch RM, Fry ST. Case Studies in Nursing Ethics. Philadelphia: J. B. Lippincott, 1987.
3. Beauchamp TL, Childress JF. Principles of Biomedical Ethics, 3rd ed. New York: Oxford University Press, 1989.
4. Benjamin M, Curtis J. Ethics in Nursing, 3rd ed. New York: Oxford University Press, 1992.
5. Edge RS, Groves JR. The Ethics of Health Care. Albany, NY: Delmar Publishers, 1994.

Carol Bolinger, MSN, CRNI, OCN
Donna R. Baldwin, MSN, CRNI

A profession is identified by the unique body of knowledge from which its members practice. Continual development of this knowledge base is fundamental to the profession. When the knowledge evolves from systematic inquiry based on the scientific approach, it is known as research. Research, therefore, enhances a profession by broadening the scientific body of knowledge essential to its practice.[1]

For nurses, research is vital to extend the base of nursing knowledge. Nursing intervention has traditionally been task oriented, that is, nurses perform nursing activities. Nursing research provides an investigatory pathway to improve patient care through identification of the unique properties of nursing. As a result, research may substantiate traditional nursing interventions or may reveal the need to alter them.

The specialty practice of intravenous (IV) nursing requires research for the validation and improvement of IV nursing care, treatment modalities, and advancement of the professional practice.[2] Through research, nurses may validate current and future practices to facilitate optimal patient care outcomes. To promote IV nursing research, however, the nurse must understand basic research concepts and relate them to practice. The intent of this chapter is to broaden nurses' knowledge of research by applying research principles to IV nursing.

RESEARCH TERMINOLOGY

Scientific research has its own language and terminology. An understanding of this terminology is necessary to participate in the research process and to comprehend the findings of others.

Concepts, Constructs, and Theories

Scientific research is usually concerned with abstract rather than tangible phenomenon. *Concepts* are abstractions that help identify emotions or sensations characterized by a particular constellation of behaviors.[3] Examples of concepts are ''pain'' and ''distress.'' In the research process, concepts are indirectly, rather than directly, measured.

Constructs are singular ideas that encompass many related ideas. However, constructs differ from concepts in that they are deliberately constructed by the researcher for a specific scientific purpose.[4] Conceptual frameworks in nursing contain constructs that describe an abstract structure of the human response. For example, Dorothea Orem developed the construct of ''self-care'' to describe one's ability to care for oneself.

Polit and Hungler defined *theory* as ''an abstract generalization that presents a systematic explanation about the interrelationship among phenomena.''[1] A theory integrates findings to explain, predict, and control phenomena. In this way, the findings become meaningful and generalizable. For example, Selye's theory of stress presents a systematic explanation of adaptation to stress.

Variables

A *variable* is something that assumes different values.[1] *Quantitative variables* can be measured in specific units of measure. Catheter gauge, cannula length, and number of attempts to cannulate a vein are examples of quantitative variables. In contrast, *qualitative variables* differ in quality or degree. They are not measured in numeric form but are described in terms of increased or decreased intensity.[5] An example of a qualitative variable is pain.

The purpose of most research is to establish a cause-and-effect relationship by distinguishing between the independent and dependent variables. The *independent variable* is the variable that is manipulated; it is the presumed cause. The *dependent variable* is the quality or unit of measure the investigator is studying to determine the presumed effect.[5] For example, the researcher investigates the effect of saline flushes (independent variable) on the maintenance of patency of an IV catheter (dependent variable). Additional examples of independent and dependent variables from published literature are listed in Table 32–1.

The term *criterion variable* is sometimes substituted for dependent variable when criteria must be established to assess the success of an intervention.[1] For example, a phlebitis scale (criterion variable) measures the effects of a new IV catheter material (independent variable).

In research, all possible influences on the dependent variable must be controlled so that the true relationship between the independent and dependent variables is understood. Competing influences that interfere with identification of the underlying cause are known as *extraneous variables*, and failure to control these variables affects the validity of the research conclusions.[1] For example, an investigation of the dwell time (dependent variable) for five brands of peripheral IV catheters (independent variable) would be influenced by extraneous variables, such as catheter gauge and length, insertion procedure, site maintenance, and patient characteristics. Such extraneous variables may be controlled by standardizing catheter size, nursing procedures, and the type of patients included in the study.

Table 32–1

Examples of Independent and Dependent Variables

Research Question	Independent Variable	Dependent Variable
What is the effect of extravasation of 5% dextrose in water?[9]	Intentional infiltration of 5% dextrose in water	Pain at insertion site
What is the effectiveness of 70% isopropyl alcohol as a disinfectant agent for IV latex injection ports?[8]	Injection ports cleansed with 70% isopropyl alcohol	Microbial growth on injection ports
What are the potential risks of prolonged PICC insertion?[19]	Length of time PICCs remained in place	Catheter-related colonization
What are the benefits of multiline IV infusion systems?[12]	Use of multiline infusion device	Equipment costs
What are the success rates for repositioning the tip location for PICCs?[26]	Repositioning tip location for PICCs	SVC tip location confirmed by x-ray
What is the impact of an IV team on the management of CVCs?[27]	CVCs maintained by members of IV team	CVC-related complications
Is 10 U/ml heparin flush adequate to maintain PICC patency?	Heparin (10 U/ml) flushes	Catheter patency

CVC = Central venous catheter; IV = intravenous; PICC = peripherally inserted central catheter; SVC = superior vena cava.

Quantification of Variables

Numbers may be used to represent measurements of the variable. The assignment of numbers to attributes of the objects follows a well-defined set of rules known as the *scale of measurement.* Four major scales used in research are nominal, ordinal, interval, and ratio. In a *nominal scale*, numbers are used to sort characteristics into categories. Demographic characteristics are frequently classified in this manner. For example, a male may be classified as a 1 and a female as a 2. When degrees of an attribute can be identified, an *ordinal scale* is used to order the objects on a continuum. This scale may be used to classify catheter dwell times as (1) less than 12 hours, (2) 12 to 23 hours, (3) 24 to 47 hours, (4) 48 to 72 hours, and (5) greater than 72 hours. *Interval scales* are used when both the different levels of an attribute and the equal distances between them can be identified. An example of an interval scale is the Fahrenheit scale for measuring temperature. The last scale of measurement, the *ratio scale*, has the characteristics of an interval scale, but it also has a meaningful zero.[5] A pain evaluation scale in which 0 represents the absence of pain and the numbers 1 to 10 depict increased pain intensity is an example of a ratio measurement.

Research Process

By means of the scientific approach, research moves in logical progression from posing a question to obtaining an answer. The question is reduced to its observable components so that possible answers may be tested and conclusions drawn. The research process consists of multiple steps that may be grouped into five sequential stages: conceptualization, planning, data collection, data analysis, and dissemination.[1] For clarification, the study presented in the box illustrates each phase of the research process.

Double-Blind, Randomized, Two-Way Crossover Trial in Healthy Male Volunteers to Compare the Efficacy of 0.9% Sodium Chloride Versus Heparin Sodium Solution (10 U/ml) in Maintaining Intermittent Dwelling Catheter Devices for the Purpose of Repetitive Blood Sampling

This study compared the overall efficacy of 2 ml of 0.9% normal saline flush solution with 10 U of heparin sodium in the maintenance of patency of an intermittent catheter device (INT) used for repetitive blood collection. The INT was a peripheral intravenous catheter to which an injection cap with latex injection port had been attached by a Luer lock.

Ninety volunteers were used to detect differences in the flush solutions used with INTs. The volunteers had INTs placed in their arms for blood collection as part of their participation in the study. Volunteers were randomly assigned to receive either normal saline or heparin flush solution in period I and then receive the other flush solution in period II, 14 days later. Over two separate 24-hour periods, the INTs were flushed with either 2 ml of normal saline or 2 ml of heparin sodium (10 U) every 2 hours. By the end of the second 24-hour period, each volunteer had received both types of flush solution. Both the investigators and the subjects were blinded to the type of flush solution used during the study. The pharmacist was responsible for mixing the flush solutions and maintaining the double-blind dosing procedure.

Evaluation of the INT was conducted at times corresponding to the flushing schedule, and catheters were routinely checked for clot formation on removal. All data were recorded on standardized flow sheets. Analysis of the data using the chi-square test determined differences between normal saline and 10 U of heparin flush relative to catheter patency.

From Frisco R, Bolinger C. Unpublished data, 1991.

Phase I: Conceptualization

The research study begins when the researcher develops the question within a conceptual framework. Specific steps in this phase include identifying and describing the problem, reviewing the literature, developing the conceptual framework, and formulating the hypothesis.

Identifying the Problem

Selecting a problem for study requires identification of a question from an area of interest. Nursing situations that cause the staff to question their actions are a good basis for the formulation of research questions. When a nurse analyzes patient care quality or questions the standard, delivery, or outcome of care, the nurse is formulating a research question.

The most difficult step in research is the development of a feasible research question. For years, IV nurses have been asked how much air is fatal if it is infused intravenously. Techniques are scrupulously followed to prevent any air from entering the IV line, but anecdotal accounts exist of air being infused without adverse patient outcomes. Investigation of this issue, however, would not be feasible because of the unethical demands it would place on study participants. Other considerations relevant to the feasibility of a research problem are timing, availability of subjects, cooperation of others, availability of facilities and equipment, finances, and experience of the researcher.[3] Based on the properties listed in the box, the following example illustrates a researchable problem.

Properties of a Researchable Problem

- The outcome of the research will contribute to nursing practice and patient care in a meaningful way.
- The problem studied occurs frequently in a definable population.
- The methods currently used to address the problem are inadequate.
- The problem involves variables capable of being precisely defined and measured.
- The investigation of the problem is feasible.
- The research question is of interest to the researcher.

Describing the Problem

The research question is typically written as a problem statement which summarizes the problem and identifies the key study variables. The problem may be written as either a declarative or an interrogatory statement.

Researchable Problem
The efficacy of normal saline in maintaining intermittent catheter devices used for blood sampling.

Declarative Statement
The purpose of this research is to determine the efficacy of normal saline versus heparin sodium in maintaining intermittent dwelling catheter devices for the purpose of blood sampling.

Interrogative Statement
What is the efficacy of normal saline as compared with heparin flush in maintaining intermittent dwelling catheter devices for the purpose of blood sampling?

Reviewing the Literature

Once the problem is formulated, the researcher needs to become familiar with previous investigations on the same or related topics. A review of the literature assists the researcher in developing a more specific question or in dealing with data more effectively. Often, the review reveals that the question has been adequately answered in the past, and further research may replicate and validate previous work on the subject. Replication studies are critically needed in nursing research because they add support to research findings.

Researchers may complete a literature review using sources listed in the *Index Medicus* and *Cumulative Index of Nursing and Allied Health Literature* (CINAHL), as well as

social and psychological indices. Computerized access to these indices is available, such as the Medical Literature and Retrieval System (METLARS) and MEDLINE, which drastically reduces the time invested in the literature search.

Once a cumulative list of articles of interest is developed, the laborious tasks of accumulating and reviewing these references ensue. The method of organization of the reference articles is unique to each researcher. Many find it helpful to record on index cards certain key points, such as the statement of the problem, the hypothesis, the methodology, the findings, and a full citation. It is also helpful to record any deficiencies noted by the reader or the author. These cards are then filed by topic and used as a reference for preparing the written literature review.

A written literature review is required for both the research proposal and the future publication of the study results. It summarizes consistencies and inconsistencies in previous research findings. Presentation of inconsistencies does not weaken the researcher's support of the hypothesis; instead, it strengthens and defends the hypothesis by demonstrating that all previous work has been considered in the formation of the current research methodology.

Literature Review Excerpt

The most common solution used for maintenance of intermittent infusion devices (INTs) has been heparin sodium. However, there is disagreement regarding the optimal concentration of heparin to be used. Recent studies have not successfully illustrated that heparin solution is necessary, and the use of only normal saline has been proposed (Stang et al., 1987; Taylor et al., 1989). Deeb and DiMattia (1976) reported inconsistency in hospital protocols for flushing of INTs varying from the use of normal saline to the use of 1000 U. S. P. units of heparin sodium for the maintenance of INTs.

Developing the Conceptual Framework

The next step involves placement of the problem within a theoretical or conceptual framework. Nursing scholars, such as Orem, Roy, and Neuman, have developed theoretical frameworks for nursing practice that describe the relationships between nursing, health, patients, and the environment. Theories allow nurses to make presumptions about the interaction of these elements so that the outcome of nursing interventions can be predicted.

Conceptual frameworks are less fully developed than are theories, but they also guide research. For example, Biggert and colleagues described the framework for pediatric home care in their article "Home Infusion Services Delivery Systems Model: A Conceptual Framework for Family-Centered Care in Pediatric Home Care Delivery."[6] This model can serve as a basis for research on the interrelationship of resources for families who care for their sick children at home.

Formulating the Hypothesis

Initially, a researcher may have an intuitive feeling regarding the outcome, but the hypothesis is not finalized. The hypothesis is derived after the problem is identified and the related literature is reviewed, and it predicts what the researcher expects to find.[1] Characteristics of a hypothesis, as defined in the box, are illustrated in the following example.

Hypothesis

A flush solution of 0.9% sodium chloride injection is as effective as a flush solution of 10 U/ml of heparin sodium for preventing loss of catheter patency over 24 hours.

A null hypothesis, as its name implies, is not what the hypothesis states. Dempsey has described a null hypothesis as "a statement of no difference or no relationship between the variables."[7] It states the lack of a relationship between the dependent and independent variables and is used as a tool to explain the statistical significance of study results. The null hypothesis for the preceding example is as follows:

Null Hypothesis

There will be no difference in the catheter patency when two different treatment flush solutions are used.

Characteristics of a Hypothesis
- The hypothesis is in the form of a statement rather than a question.
- The hypothesis states the relationship between the independent and dependent variables.
- The hypothesis is testable.

Requirements for Experimental Studies
- The study must be prospective so that data are collected under experimental conditions as they occur.
- The researcher must be able to both control and manipulate the variables. *Control* implies that extraneous variables are eliminated or controlled so that they do not affect the dependent variable.
- The population must be randomized.

Phase II: Planning

The second phase in the research process involves planning the methodology to be used in the study. Methodology is simply the path the researcher plans to follow to get from the question to the answer. Formulation of the methodology depends on key factors related to the research problem. What type of study design best suits the question? What types of comparisons are being made? How often are the subjects available to the researcher? What type of conclusion is the researcher attempting to support? Answers to these questions determine the study design, the sampling methods, and the measures for research variables.

Study Design

The term *study design* describes the framework the researcher plans to use to answer the research question. Many types of study designs exist, but some are more appropriate for certain types of questions and deal more effectively with

certain types of data. The two main approaches in research are experimental and nonexperimental, and each has specific advantages and disadvantages.

An *experimental study design* is considered by many to be classic research because it meets stringent requirements. The variables are under the control of the researcher and may be manipulated, one at a time, to enable evaluation of causal relationships.[1] Extraneous variables are present, but they are not studied. Examples of experimental research published in the *Journal of Intravenous Nursing* are "Effectiveness of Disinfectant Techniques on Intravenous Tubing Latex Injection Ports" and "Differences Among Intravenous Extravasation Using Four Common Solutions."[8, 9]

When the researcher is able to control the extraneous variables, the relationship between the independent and dependent variables is more pronounced. Identifying or controlling all the extraneous variables is often impossible, and such control may not always be necessary. Only those variables that occur simultaneously with the independent and dependent variables require controls. The inability to regulate significant extraneous variables, however, introduces a contaminating effect on the data and produces misleading results. Examples of extraneous variables and controls in the saline-versus-heparin study are listed below.

Extraneous Variables	Controls
Catheter gauge	All catheters will be 20 gauge
Catheter brand	All catheters will have the same manufacturer
Catheter length	All catheters will be 1¼ inch
Experience of registered nurse	All registered nurses will have minimum of 3 years IV experience
Insertion site	All sites will be cephalic on the flat portion of the forearm
Blood-drawing techniques	All blood-drawing techniques will be standardized
Number of blood drawings	12 blood drawings will occur over each 24-hour period

Investigation of relationships requires comparison. In an experimental study, a *control group* is compared with an experimental group. The control group of subjects participates in a study but never has the independent variable manipulated. In contrast, the independent variable is manipulated in the experimental group. Individuals are assigned to the two groups randomly so each person has an equal chance of being in either group. Once the study is completed the results of the two groups are compared.

Blinding is a control method used to correct for investigator or participant bias. When both the investigator and the participants are unaware of the independent variable manipulation, the study is labeled double-blind. If only the subject or investigator is blinded, the study is considered single-blind.[10] In the saline-versus-heparin trial, the investigators were blinded to the type of flush solution to prevent them from acting on preconceived ideas about the efficacy of the flush solutions. Because the participants were also unaware of flush solution used, this study is double-blind.

In nursing research, ensuring that the sample is randomized is often difficult. Because subjects may not be assigned to experimental or control groups on a random basis, each member of the sample may not have an equal chance of receiving the experimental treatment. When this occurs, the study is considered *quasiexperimental*. The research involves manipulation of the variables but lacks randomization. To compensate for the lack of random sampling, quasiexperimental designs introduce controls over the extraneous variables. An example is Loughran and colleagues' comparative study of the use of guidewires versus nonuse of guidewires for insertion of peripherally inserted central venous catheters. The researchers introduced controls by selecting study sites that had initiated their peripherally inserted central catheter programs at the same time. In this way, the site not using guidewires was comparable with the site in which guidewires were used.[11]

Although the experimental and quasiexperimental designs are highly effective for testing hypotheses concerning causal relationships between variables, some situations may prohibit the use of experimentation. In such situations, the *nonexperimental study design* is more appropriate. Because the variables are not controlled by the researcher, causality cannot be established; however, associative relationships may be revealed.

The two broad classifications of nonexperimental research are descriptive and ex post facto. *Descriptive studies* do not focus on relationships between variables, but rather, they observe and describe phenomena. Bostrom and Batina's comparison of single-line and multiline IV infusion systems is an example of a descriptive study. In this study, the researchers observed the impact of each type of system on nursing time, equipment costs, and personnel safety.[12]

Ex post facto studies examine relationships after the natural course of events, but they differ from experimentation because of the lack of researcher intervention in the former studies. A type of ex post facto design frequently used in IV nursing research is the retrospective study. For example, Anderson and Holland[13] used a retrospective study to evaluate the effectiveness of maintaining patency of peripherally inserted central catheters with 10 U/ml versus 100 U/ml of heparin.

Sampling Plan

A *population* is the entire group of objects or people that are to be studied. Examples include all registered nurses working on hospital-based IV teams, all patients receiving total parenteral nutrition at home, or all patients receiving peripheral IV therapy. Because a population is generally too large for investigation of each subject, the study is limited to a subset of the population, known as a *sample*. *Sampling* refers to the method by which this sample is drawn from the population, and it determines the extent to which the sample represents the entire population.[1]

Two classifications of sampling techniques are probability and nonprobability sampling. *Probability sampling* involves random selection of subjects from the population so that each individual in the population has an equal chance of being selected. This is different than randomization, which is the random assignment of subjects to control and experimental groups. *Nonprobability sampling* relies on nonrandom selection procedures.[1] The probability approach is preferred, but most samples in nursing research are based on nonprobability techniques.

Three methods of nonprobability sampling exist. The first is *convenience sampling*, which relies on the subjects that are most available to study. The nurse who conducts an observational study of all peripherally inserted central catheters inserted in a metropolitan hospital during a 1-month period is relying on a convenience sample, as was the study that used volunteers in the saline-versus-heparin trial. With the second method, *quota sampling*, the researcher specifies characteristics of the sample to increase its representation of the population. The sample is subdivided into groups based on attributes such as age, sex, and diagnosis, and a specified number of subjects are selected from each group. For example, Moldowan divided the sample into men and women to study the outcomes of patients receiving intermittent bupivacaine by ambulatory infusion pump after undergoing thoracotomy.[14] The third method, *purposive sampling*, relies on the researcher's knowledge of the population to hand pick the sample. An example of purposive sampling is the Delphi technique, which is a tool for short-term forecasting. In this technique, a panel of experts is asked a series of questions in an effort to combine the expertise of the entire group.

To maintain homogeneity of the sample, the researcher may use inclusion and exclusion criteria, which limit the sample by including and excluding subjects who meet or do not meet the qualities defined by the researcher. A small sample is believed to be adequate if it is relatively homogeneous. For most nursing studies, however, a fair degree of heterogeneity is preferred. In the saline-versus-heparin study, the inclusion and exclusion criteria were as follows:

Criteria for Selection
- Male between the ages of 18 and 40 years
- Nonsmoker for at least 1 year and no evidence of pulmonary disease
- Within 20% of ideal body weight
- Judged to be in good health based on physical examinations and routine laboratory data

Criteria for Exclusion
- Under the age of 18 or over the age of 40 years
- History of asthma or other pulmonary disease, gastrointestinal abnormalities, or cardiovascular, hepatic, neurologic, endocrine, hematologic, or renal disease
- Has donated a unit of blood within past month
- Smoker or heavy consumer of coffee
- Clinically significant findings on prestudy physical examination or laboratory data

Once the sampling method is determined, the next issue is the sample size. Most researchers recommend that the sample be as large as possible because if the sample size is not large enough, the results may not reflect the characteristics of the population. In the saline-versus-heparin study, the sample size of 90 subjects was determined by means of a sophisticated statistical determination known as power analysis.

Measurement of the Research Variables

Research requires the measurement of critical attributes of the object being studied. Because these characteristics need to be qualified, operational definitions of each attribute are developed. An *operational definition* is a description of the variable in terms of the procedures by which it will be measured.[1] Examples of the operational definitions in the saline-versus-heparin study are as follows:

Catheter Patency
Patency is defined as the investigators' ability to obtain 9 ml of blood by aspirating with a 10-ml syringe through a latex injection cap.

Phlebitis
Criteria for evaluation of phlebitis are based on the Intravenous Nurses Society *Standards of Practice*. For the purpose of this study, a score of 1+ or greater is defined as phlebitis.

Measurement of the variable based on the operational definition may be accomplished by several methods. The three types most used by nurse researchers are self-report, observation, and physiologic measures. *Self-reported data* are collected by directly questioning the subjects using an oral interview or a written questionnaire. Interviews and open-ended questions are unstructured means of data collection, whereas closed-ended and fixed-alternative questions limit the number of responses from which the respondents may choose. *Observational data* are obtained by direct examination and interpretation of the phenomena being studied. LaFortune used observational data to confirm tip position in her study on peripherally inserted catheters. In her study, radiographic examinations were observed, such as temperature, blood pressure determinations, and blood tests, and interpreted to determine catheter tip position.[15] *Physiologic measurements* are frequently used in clinical studies because of their objectivity and validity.

In the saline-versus-heparin study, observational methods were used. Catheter sites were observed for symptoms of phlebitis; catheter patency was measured by observation of no clot formation after catheter removal.

Regardless of the measurement method used, the instrument used to collect data must possess certain attributes to obtain quality measures. *Reliability* is the ability of a tool to provide an accurate measurement each time it is used. The higher the reliability of a tool, the greater the accuracy of the data it obtains.[3] For example, a numeric phlebitis rating scale is frequently used to assess phlebitis. Because such scales are based on the assumption that the signs and symptoms observed at each stage always succeed those observed in preceding stages, researchers have questioned the reliability of a phlebitis scale as a measurement tool.[16] In fact, Maki and Ringer have suggested a more reliable alternative that defines phlebitis as the presence of two or more signs and symptoms from a standardized list.[17]

Validity refers to the ability of a tool to measure what it is intended to measure. Validity depends on reliability to the extent that an unreliable tool cannot produce valid results.[1] *Content validity* is the degree to which the tool adequately represents the content, and it is based on the investigator's judgment. For example, Kaufman established content valid-

ity of an interview questionnaire regarding IV therapy education in associate degree nursing programs by having nursing faculty review the measurement tool.[18] In contrast, *construct validity* refers to the ability of the instrument to measure the abstract construct of interest. The more abstract the concept, the greater the difficulty in establishing construct validity.[1]

Validity is associated with the measurement tool, but it also reflects the adequacy of the research design. The validity of many published studies is questioned not because of the tools used for measurement but because of interpretation of the findings. In this situation, the research study must be evaluated in terms of the internal and external validity. *Internal validity* means that the study measures what it is intended to measure. If a study has internal validity, the findings are the result of the independent variable and do not reflect the effects of extraneous variables. For example, internal validity for a study of a new dressing material would require that extraneous variables, such as age, diagnosis, and dressing technique, be controlled so that the effects of the dressing may be determined. *External validity* is the extent to which the research findings may be generalized to the population. A study has external validity if the sample is representative of a broader population.[5] In the saline-versus-heparin study, internal validity was ensured by control of the extraneous variables. However, because the sample was limited to healthy male volunteers, the external validity of the study may be questioned.

Protection of Human Rights

An important consideration in the planning process is protection of the human rights of potential subjects. Because researchers may not be objective in their evaluation of the safety of the subjects they enroll in study protocols, institutional review boards (IRBs) may be used to objectively review the intended research before initiation. All research conducted by hospitals and universities that accept federal funding must satisfy guidelines set by their IRB to obtain funding. The IRB functions as an unbiased referee to assess the risk to participants and the benefit to scientific knowledge of research conducted in their domain. Legal and ethical implications of the proposed research are evaluated, and, based on IRB recommendations, researchers may be required to modify portions of a project.

In situations in which an IRB is not available to the researcher, such as a non–federally funded institution or an independent nurse researcher, the researcher may seek peer review from a professional organization or a research committee. The Intravenous Nurses Society has an ethics committee geared to assist nurse researchers who are interested in the review of projects relative to IV nursing.

Nursing research that involves the cooperation of human subjects requires the consent of the subjects. Just as a hospitalized patient signs an informed consent before a procedure is performed, research subjects must also sign an informed consent to be observed, questioned or exposed to experimental situations. Informed consent is obtained in the subject's native language and in language easily understood by nonmedical participants. All medical and legal terminology is reduced to simple terms, and subjects are fully informed about the nature of the research and its potential risks and benefits.[1] Basic components of an informed consent statement are listed in Table 32–2.

Because consent is voluntary, subjects have the right to withdraw from the study even after investigation has begun. In such instances, information obtained from the subject may signal the need for minor protocol variations. If the variations can be made without affecting the outcome of the study, the subject may remain enrolled. However, if the subject declines to give reasons for withdrawal, it is considered ethically improper to attempt to coerce the subject to remain in the study. Subjects must be allowed to withdraw without change in the quality of their care or fear of retaliation.

Phase III: Data Collection

Collection of data is based on the planned methodologies and procedures of the study. It may include obtaining the necessary consents, training those involved in data collection, scheduling subjects for measurements, and coding the results. In the saline-versus-heparin study, data collection procedures were as follows:

Before Study
One to 2 weeks before the study, potential subjects were evaluated to determine that they met entry requirements. Volunteers were informed of the nature of the study and its requirements and restrictions, and informed consents were obtained.

Study Day
The volunteers reported to the clinic at 6:00 AM on the study day, and a 20-gauge, 1¼ inch polytetrafluoroethylene (Teflon) catheter was inserted into a cephalic vein in the forearm. Immediately after the catheter was inserted, an injection cap with latex port and Luer lock connection was connected to the catheter hub. This plastic catheter and cap, referred to as the INT, was inserted by one of six IV nurses employed by the clinic. The first 2 ml of allocated treatment solution was instilled into the INT at this time.

Treatment
Blood samples were obtained, and subsequent flushes with treatment solution were performed at 2-hour intervals. Treatments were administered by piercing the hub of the INT with a needle attached to a 10-ml syringe that contained the treatment solution and by pushing the solution into the INT and vein. Assessment for phlebitis according to the operational definition also occurred at these intervals.

Measurement
Catheter patency was defined as the ability to withdraw 9 ml of blood through the INT using the standard blood sampling procedure. The catheters remained in place for 24 hours, unless removal was required because of evidence of phlebitis or lack of patency for blood collection. At removal, each catheter was checked for clot formation, by instillation of 0.5 ml of normal saline through the catheter onto a gauze pad. The research data were recorded on standardized flow sheets.

Methodology
The study was conducted in two periods with volunteers randomly assigned to receive either normal saline or heparin flush solution in period I and the other flush solution in period II. Period I consisted of the first study day; the second period occurred 14 days later.

Phase IV: Data Analysis

Data are collected to enable the investigator or investigators to draw conclusions about the population. To accomplish this, the data must be organized, summarized, and analyzed so that patterns and relationships may be detected. The analysis consists of statistical techniques that process both qualitative and quantitative data. *Qualitative analysis* refers to the organization and interpretation of nonnumeric observations to determine themes or patterns. In contrast, *quantitative analysis* involves the manipulation of numeric data through statistical procedures.[1] These methods range from the simple to the complex and may be classified as descriptive or inferential statistics.

Descriptive Statistics

Descriptive statistics are used to organize, summarize, and describe collections of data in tabular, graphic, or numeric form.[5] One of the easiest such methods is frequency distribution, which organizes data according to the number of occurrences of a phenomenon. Values are ordered from lowest to highest, and the frequency of each value is determined. Bar graphs and histograms are graphic representations of frequency distribution.

Measures of central tendency are also used to describe the data. The three measures commonly used are mode, median, and mean. The *mode* is the value that occurs most frequently in the distribution; the *median* is the middle score of a group that is arranged from lowest to highest scores; and the *mean* is the average distribution.[5] For example, Pauley and coworkers used measures of central tendency to describe catheter-related colonization. In their study, the most common reason

Table 32–2

Components of Informed Consent

Component	Explanation
Subject status	Subjects are informed that information they provide is solely for the purpose of research.
Study purpose	The purpose of the research is stated in lay terms.
Potential risks	Any foreseeable risks associated with participation in the study are listed.
Potential benefits	Specific benefits from participation in the study are described.
Confidentiality	Subjects are assured that their privacy and anonymity will be protected.
Voluntary consent	Subjects are informed that participation in the study is voluntary and that consent may be withdrawn without fear of retaliation.
Procedures	All procedures that will be used to collect research information are described.
Contact information	Information is provided regarding whom to contact for questions.

for catheter removal (mode) was discontinuation of therapy (in 83 of 100 catheters), but the average catheter dwell time (mean) was 15.4 days.[19]

Measures of central tendency report the average, but they do not describe the variability or dispersion of the values. The distribution, therefore, also needs to be described in measures of variability, such as the range and the standard deviation. The *range* is the distance between the highest and the lowest values. For example, in the study by Pauley and associates, the range for catheter dwell time was 2 to 43 days. The *standard deviation*, the most commonly used measure of variability, is an index of the spread of scores around the mean of a distribution (Fig. 32–1). It indicates how much the scores deviate from the mean. The further the value is from the mean, the more varied are the data. A small standard deviation implies tightly clustered data, whereas widely dispersed data are represented by a large standard deviation.[5]

Brown and colleagues[20] reported measures of variability in their study comparing patient-controlled analgesia versus traditional intramuscular analgesia. In the study, the duration of the patient-controlled analgesia therapy ranged from 8 to 210 hours, the average length of therapy was 41.44 hours, and the standard deviation equaled 3.659. These results indicate that there was a wide range in the length of therapy and a significant variation in the scores in relation to the average length of therapy.

The significance of the standard deviation can be illus-

trated by the results from the saline-versus-heparin trial. In phase I of the study, the mean (average) dwell time was 14 hours for catheters flushed with saline. When each dwell time for this group is plotted on a graph, the values form a "normal curve."

When a curve is normal, 68% of the population fall within one standard deviation (34% above the mean and 34% below the mean), 95% fall within two standard deviations, and 99.7% within three standard deviations. The standard deviation in the heparin-versus-saline study was 2.2, implying that 68% of catheters were patent for 11.8 to 16.2 hours, 95% were patent from 9.6 to 18.4 hours, and 99.7 were patent from 7.4 to 20.6 hours.

Descriptive statistics are also used to describe the correlation between two variables. The statistic that describes the relationship and strength of association between the variables is the *correlation coefficient*. Many correlation coefficients exist, but the most widely used measure is the Pearson r, or the Pearson product-moment correlation coefficient. For example, a researcher studying the correlation of IV nursing experience and venipuncture proficiency would most likely use the Pearson r.

Inferential Statistics

Inferential statistics refers to procedures by which the researcher may draw inferences about the population based on data collected from the sample. Values are not simply de-

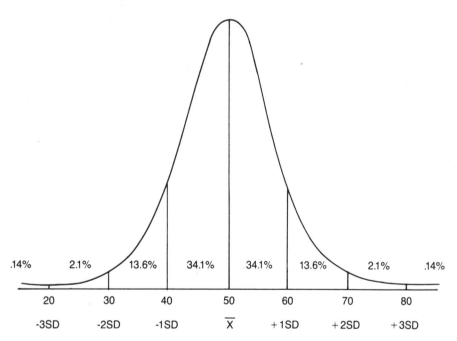

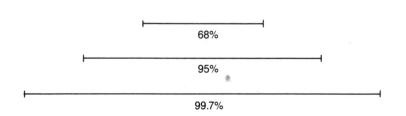

Figure 32–1. Standard deviations in a normal distribution. (From Polit DS, Hungler BP. Nursing Research: Principles and Methods, 4th ed. Philadelphia: J. B. Lippincott, 1991, 20.)

Table 32-3

Decisions Regarding the Null Hypothesis

Decision	Null Hypothesis (H_0) True	Null Hypothesis (H_0) False
Fail to reject H_0	Correct decision	Type II error
Reject H_0	Type I error	Correct decision

scribed but rather are used to make conclusions regarding the population. In this type of statistics, the validity of the inferences rests on the representation of the population in sample.

Hypothesis testing is a statistical approach by which the researcher objectively analyzes the results of the study. The null hypothesis, not the research hypothesis, is used to measure the significance of the findings. Rejection of the null hypothesis lends support to the research hypothesis; the findings are not significant if the researcher fails to reject the null hypothesis. However, errors may occur. Failure to reject the null hypothesis when it should be rejected is a *type II error*. In contrast, a *type I error* refers to rejection of the null hypothesis when it should not be rejected (Table 32–3).

Type I errors may be controlled by establishing levels of significance. The *level of significance* describes the risk of committing a type I error and is commonly referred to as the p value. The p value ranges from zero to one and describes the probability that the findings are the result of chance.[5] The smaller the number for the level of significance (p value), the less the chance of a type I error occurring. The two most common levels of significance are 0.05 ($p < 0.05$) and 0.01 ($p < 0.01$). For a significance level of 0.05, the researcher is at risk of rejecting a null hypothesis that is true five of 100 times. When the 0.01 level of significance is used, the probability of a type I error decreases to one of 100. However, as the probability of a type I error decreases, the probability of a type II error increases.[5]

Research results are reported as either statistically significant or statistically nonsignificant. If the results are statistically significant, they are unlikely to be the result of chance. Nonsignificant findings imply that the results may be attributable to chance fluctuations. However, the p value measures only biases and not necessarily the proposed research hypothesis.

Knowledge of the level of significance (p value) and the sample size (N) are important in the evaluation of the findings. A direct correlation exists between the magnitude of the p value and the size of the sample.[16] In the study on catheter performance relative to pain perception performed by Ahrens and associates,[21] both values may be evaluated. Seven catheter brands were studied, and sample sizes ranged from 59 to 62 for each brand. Only one brand of catheters approached the significant level for inducing less pain on first insertion ($p = 0.068$, $p < 0.5$ statistically significant). Although the samples were comparable in size for the purpose of the study, the small sample size prohibits generalization of findings to the entire population.

Statistical Tests

The procedures used in inferential statistics may be classified as parametric and nonparametric. *Parametric statistics* test the significance of the differences between group means. They involve estimation of at least one variable, measurement of interval or ratio data, and assumptions about the variable under consideration. The two commonest parametric tests are the t test and the analysis of variance (ANOVA).[5]

The *t test* is used in two-group situations, such as studies involving control groups, pretest/posttests, or paired samples. The means of each sample are compared to determine if a statistically significant difference exists between them. If a significant difference exists, it is assumed to result from the influence of the independent variable. For example, Loughran and co-workers used the t test to compare patient outcomes when peripherally inserted central catheters were inserted with and without guidewires. The variable of duration of catheter placement was found to be statistically different ($t = -2.7628$, $p < 0.01$) between the use and the nonuse of guidewires.[11]

When the study involves three or more groups, as well as more than one independent variable, *ANOVA* is used. ANOVA contrasts variation *between* treatment groups with variation *within* the treatment groups to determine the F ratio. If the differences between the groups are large relative to fluctuations within the group, it is possible to establish the probability that group differences are related to, or result from, the treatment.[1] For example, ANOVA would be the appropriate statistical technique to determine if three different catheter materials contributed to phlebitis.

Nonparametric tests are used for nominal or ordinal data or when the normality of distribution cannot be assumed. The commonest nonparametric technique is the *chi square test*, which tests the presence of an association between two variables on the same subject. The chi-square statistic is computed to determine whether the observed frequencies in the categories differ significantly from the expected categories. If the chi-square value is substantially larger than what would be expected by chance, the value is determined to be statistically significant.[5] Chi-square contingency analysis was used by Mukau and associates[22] in their study of risk factors for central venous catheter–related vascular erosions. Large-diameter catheters were found by the researchers to significantly increase the risk of vessel erosion. Chi-square statistics were also used in the saline-versus-heparin trial to determine if differences existed between flush treatments with normal saline and with 10 U of heparin in terms of catheter patency and phlebitis ($p \leq 0.05$).

Although the chi-square test is appropriate for samples of more than 30, *Fisher's exact test* may be used for smaller samples. Data are collapsed into cells to test the significance of differences in the size of the groups.[5] Bozzetti and colleagues[23] used the Fisher exact test to analyze groups of patients in their study of central catheter sepsis. The relationship between the results of hub cultures and clinical demonstrations of sepsis was found to be statistically significant.

Because the phenomena of interest to nurses are generally complex, advanced statistical procedures, known as *multivariate tests*, may be used. There is increasing use of such tests because of the need for such analysis and the availability of computers to calculate the statistics. Two examples of multivariate statistical procedures are factor analysis and multiple regression.

When a large set of variables is being analyzed, *factor analysis* reduces them into a smaller, more manageable set of dimensions known as factors.[5] This multivariate procedure involves a higher degree of subjectivity, but it is, nonetheless, a widely used statistical technique. Yucha and associates[9] used factor analysis in their investigation of extravasation using common IV solutions. Differences in extravasation of the solutions were determined over time and were significant for factors such as pain, area of induration, and infiltrate volume.

Multiple regression analysis is used to study the relationship between a dependent variable and two or more independent variables. This method allows the researcher to make predictions about phenomena. From a set of independent variables, the researcher tests hypotheses about the relationship between the dependent and independent variables.[5] Lucas and co-workers[24] used multiple regression in their study of nosocomial infections in patients with central venous catheters. Among the study variables, the length of hospitalization and the number of intermittent infusions were found to be the best predictors of central venous catheter infections.

Another procedure that may be used in research is *meta-analysis*. The literature review typically is a preliminary step in the research project. However, meta-analysis applies statistical methods to the findings from research reports. The results of each study represent a single piece of data, so that multiple studies may be analyzed and the findings regarding the effectiveness of the interventions integrated.[1] Such an approach may assist in demonstrating the effectiveness of IV teams on quality (i.e., phlebitis, infection, infiltration rates) of patient care outcomes.

For statistical methods to render the quantitative data meaningful, the results must be understood. In this chapter, computation of the actual statistics was not discussed. Because explanation of the various techniques is far beyond the scope of this text, emphasis has been placed on the appropriateness of statistics in different research situations and their significance in regard to the findings. Table 32–4 is a summary of research problems and the appropriate statistical tests for each. Often, one statistical method is insufficient based on the study design, and the answer to the research problem may require several statistical tests. For example, Senefeld and Patterson used the t test, the ANOVA, the chi-square test, and the Fisher's exact test in their comparative study of manual-versus-computerized drug delivery systems.[25]

Interpretation

Analysis of the data provides the "results" of the study. However, this information must be interpreted to determine the implications of the findings within a broader context. Failure to reject the null hypothesis means that the findings support the research hypothesis. In the saline-versus-heparin example, the null hypothesis (no differences in catheter patency relative to flush solutions) was not rejected; therefore, the findings lend support to the research hypothesis (normal saline is as effective as heparin flush in preventing loss of catheter patency). If the null hypothesis is rejected, the research hypothesis is not supported. In this situation, methodologic weaknesses must be considered.

Statistical significance should not be confused with clinical significance. If the study is statistically significant, the results have occurred more frequently than if they had occurred by chance. In contrast, clinical significance would cause a change in nursing practice based on the findings. All too often, the statistical data reported have little effect on clinical practice and nursing interventions.

Phase V: Dissemination

Publication in journals is the most effective route of dissemination for research findings. Journals reach a target group of professionals interested in the research topic and findings. For example, research studies relative to IV therapy would be expected to be published in the *Journal of Intravenous Nursing*. Often, it appears that a researcher has published the same article in several journals. Close inspection, however, reveals that minor alterations in the text have been made in a manner that does not infringe on the original copyright.

Professional meetings and conferences are another avenue for dissemination of information. Such meetings allow the researcher to target professionals who will be affected by the findings. The presentations may be formal lectures, abstracts, or poster presentations; the type of presentation selected depends on the material being presented and the preference of the researcher.

OVERCOMING BARRIERS TO RESEARCH

A comparatively small number of nurses perform research, frequently because of lack of experience, insufficient resources, inadequate funding, and time constraints. All of these reasons are obstacles that can be overcome.

Research has become a component of nursing curricula, and nurses are learning how to apply research principles to their practice. Once the nurse identifies a problem for investigation, statisticians are available to assist with planning the research design and methodologies, as well as analyzing the results. Simply because the nurse is the principal investigator

---

Table 32-4

Research Problems and Appropriate Statistical Tests

Research Problem	Statistical Method
Cleansing the site with chlorhexidine will have an effect on decreasing the incidence of CVC site infections.	T test
Catheter dwell time differs in pediatric, adult, and elderly populations for two specific types of polymers.	ANOVA
Urban nurses are more satisfied with IV therapy responsibilities.	Factor analysis
Compliance regarding routine site rotations is higher in hospitals with IV teams than those without IV teams.	Chi-square test
A relationship exists between the use of an IV team and patient care outcomes, e.g. • Phlebitis rate • Catheter dwell time • Infiltration rate • Patient satisfaction	Pearson's r test

ANOVA = Analysis of variance; CVC = central venous catheter; IV = intravenous.

does not mean that all components of the research process must be performed by the nurse. Experts are available to assist the nurse in ensuring the study validity so the results may be applied to practice.

In 1993, nursing gained a powerful ally when the National Institute of Nursing Research (NINR) was established at the National Institutes of Health in Bethesda, Maryland. The goal of the NINR is to promote excellence in nursing science by offering opportunities for continuing research training, career development, and research awards. The NINR meets these goals by offering assistance to nurses who conduct research. Fellowships offered by the NINR, as well as scholarships and grant funding, also encourage nurse researchers to expand their horizons.

The greatest obstacle to nursing research is, therefore, the lack of time and motivation to conduct it. For many nurses, encounters with research have been unrewarding and uncompensated in terms of resources and time. Nonetheless, the need for research far exceeds the dedication and commitment required. Only by participating in research can nurses achieve their objective of high-quality patient outcomes. The beneficiaries of our efforts are the patients and, ultimately, the nursing profession.

References

1. Polit DF, Hungler BP. Nursing Research: Principles and Methods, 4th ed. Philadelphia: J. B. Lippincott, 1991.
2. Intravenous Nurses Society. Intravenous Nursing Standards of Practice. Belmont, MA: Intravenous Nurses Society, 1990.
3. Woods NF, Catanzaro M. Nursing Research: Theory and Practice. St. Louis: CV Mosby, 1988.
4. Wilson HS. Research in Nursing, 2nd ed. Menlo Park, CA: Addison-Wesley, 1989.
5. Shavelson RJ. Statistical Reasoning in the Behavioral Sciences, 2nd ed. Boston: Allen & Bacon, 1988.
6. Biggert R, Watkins J, Cook S. Home infusion service delivery systems model: A conceptual framework for family-centered care in pediatric home care delivery. JIN 1992; 15(4):210–218.
7. Dempsey P, Dempsey A. Nursing Research with Basic Statistical Applications, 3rd ed. Boston: Jones & Bartlett, 1992.
8. Ruschman KL, Fulton JS. Effectiveness of disinfectant techniques on intravenous tubing latex injection ports. JIN 1993; 16(5):304–308.
9. Yucha CB, Hastings-Tolsma M, Szeverenyi NM. Differences among intravenous extravasations using four common solutions. JIN 1993; 16(5):277–281.
10. Jacobsen B, Meininger J. Seeing the importance of blindness. Nurs Res 1990; 2(1):54–57.
11. Loughran SC, Edwards S, McClure S. Peripherally inserted central catheters: Guidewire versus nonguidewire use. JIN 1992; 15(3):152–159.
12. Bostrom J, Batina M. A comparison of costs, labor time, and needle use associated with single- and multi-line intravenous infusion systems. JIN 1993; 16(3):140–147.
13. Anderson KM, Holland JS. Maintaining the patency of peripherally inserted central catheters with 10 units/cc heparin. JIN 1992; 15(2):84–88.
14. Moldowan C. Improved outcome for post-thoracotomy patients using intermittent bupivacaine with epinephrine by CADD-Plus ambulatory infusion pump. JIN 1992; 15(6):333–337.
15. LaFortune S. The use of confirming x-rays to verify tip position for peripherally inserted catheters. JIN 1993; 16(4):246–250.
16. Stoddard GJ, Ring WH. How to evaluate study methodology in published clinical research. JIN 1993; 16(2):110–117.
17. Maki DG, Ringer M. Evaluation of dressing regimens for prevention of infection with peripheral intravenous catheters. JAMA 1987; 258:2396–2403.
18. Kaufman MV. Intravenous therapy education in associate degree programs. JIN 1992; 15(4):238–242.
19. Pauley SY, Vallande NC, Riley EN, et al. Catheter-related colonization associated with percutaneous inserted central catheters. JIN 1993; 16(1):50–54.
20. Brown ST, Bowman JM, Eason FR. A comparison of patient-controlled analgesia versus traditional intramuscular analgesia in postoperative pain management. JIN 1993; 16(6):333–338.
21. Ahrens T, Wiersema L, Weilitz PB. Differences in pain perception associated with intravenous catheter insertion. JIN 1991; 14(2):85–89.
22. Mukau L, Talamini MA, Sitzmann JV. Risk factors for central venous catheter-related vascular erosions. JPEN J Parenter Enteral Nutr 1991; 15(5):513–516.
23. Bozzetti F, Bonfganti G, Regalia E, et al. A new approach to the diagnosis of central venous catheter sepsis. JPEN J Parenter Enteral Nutr 1991; 15(4):412–416.
24. Lucas JW, Berger AM, Fitzgerald A, et al. Nosocomial infections in patients with central catheters. JIN 1992; 15(1):44–48.
25. Senefeld P, Patterson A. A comparative study: Manual versus computerized automated drug delivery systems. JIN 1991; 14(5):291–295.
26. James L, Bledsoe L, Hadaway LC. A retrospective look at tip location and complications of peripherally inserted central venous catheter lines. JIN 1993; 16(2):104–109.
27. Gianino MS, Brunt M, Eisenberg PG. The impact of a nutritional support team on the cost and management of multilumen central venous catheters. JIN 1992; 15(6):327–332.

CHAPTER 33

Future of Intravenous Therapy

Leslie Baranowski, CRNI
Judy Terry, BSN, CRNI

- -

- -

As demonstrated throughout this textbook, intravenous (IV) therapy and the specialty of IV nursing have grown at a tremendous rate as a result of rapid advances in medicine and technology. IV therapy has established itself as an integral and essential component of the medical treatment of a large percentage of patients in all practice settings. Approximately 90% of hospitalized patients now receive IV therapy, and it is probably not far fetched to speculate that close to 100% of hospitalized patients will receive IV therapy in the near future. Outside of the traditional acute care setting, we have also witnessed an explosion in the delivery of IV therapies in the alternative or home care settings. With the extraordinary growth in IV therapy, it is reasonable to assume that the IV nursing specialty will thrive in the future. However, to survive in today's health care environment, which is challenged by cost-containment pressures, all health care delivery settings and specialties have had to closely evaluate avenues to contain cost and restructure services.

There is little doubt that both the structure and the process for delivery of patient care will continue to change in the future.[1] The health care environment will continue to be affected by increased complexity in patient care and higher-risk patients and by the emphasis on health care reform and cost control. The patient population is getting older, which also presents special challenges. In addition, as more patients immigrate to America, it is necessary to deal with an increased number of foreign-speaking consumers and address issues of cultural diversity. The number of people who are homeless or do not have medical insurance will also affect the financial picture of health care. Diseases such as acquired immune deficiency syndrome or infections related to bacteria-resistant medications will present many clinical and legal problems.

We are currently facing the challenges of managed care and capitation. One can only speculate on where health care reform will lead us from here. All health care environments are clearly challenged by the reality of lower profit expectations and the possible elimination of charge-based reimbursement. In particular, the hospital environment has been dramatically affected. The fiscal foundation on which hospitals were built has been turned upside-down and has forced hospitals to closely scrutinize methods to more efficiently deliver patient care and to redesign itself.[2] To remain viable, hospitals are faced with increased pressures to discharge patients

as soon as their condition warrants and to decrease inpatient costs. As a result, we have witnessed significant downsizing, restructuring of internal operations, and emergence of new patient care delivery models. The alternative site and home infusion arena has not been immune to these changing forces and has had to significantly restructure as well. In all health care delivery settings, further trends toward restructuring and consolidation of the health care industry can be anticipated, including integrated service networks, mergers, and acquisitions.

The health care environment in the 1990s has presented the specialty of IV nursing with unprecedented challenges that at times seem insurmountable. However, at the same time, it is providing us with opportunities never before available. The future of IV nursing revolves around the IV nursing specialties' response to these opportunities. The successful IV therapy services program embraces and incorporates these opportunities rather than drowns in the challenges. Anyone associated with IV nursing would have difficulty not being affected by the dramatic change in our roles in the past 5 years. We have to learn to embrace this change, to find the positive aspects of the change, to truly understand what is driving these changes, to strategically incorporate these changes into our practice, and to allow it to drive us in a positive direction. Unfortunately, this is easier said than done. There are demands for us to change and find new and more efficient ways to perform our services regardless of how successful our previous paradigms were. Changes are unsettling but are essential for the profession to evolve. In all practice environments, the IV therapy service program must be innovative, must be adaptable, must maximize capabilities, and must analyze complimentary practice roles and multidisciplinary care.

EXAMINING THE PRESENT TO BUILD FOR THE FUTURE

It is essential to carefully examine what is driving current changes in our profession to strategize for the future. In the hospital setting, the major change affecting the IV therapy team concept has been work redesign models, which hospitals are implementing in response to increased cost-containment pressures. No universal model is currently incorporated by health care institutions for redesign; however, they are all aimed at improving continuity and reducing fragmentation through patient-centered care delivery.[1, 2] With these new patient-care delivery models, a trend toward greater instances of cross-training and the use of nonlicensed personnel has occurred, with a focus on centering of patient care services around the patient on the nursing unit. As a result, the use or need for ancillary services, such as IV teams, is now strongly scrutinized and questioned. However, although these care delivery models maximize the capabilities of every level of employee in an institution, ancillary services need not be made extinct. Many professional ancillary services, including IV teams, can be successfully integrated into these patient care models if they can demonstrate the benefits of their service in supporting the registered nurse as well as nonlicensed technical personnel care team members. To demonstrate this support, however, the IV department must carefully evaluate the benefits and how they fit into the new structure. This analysis requires careful evaluation of current services and exploration of opportunities for new and more efficient ways to perform our services, regardless of how successful our previous patterns of success were. All patient care departments must analyze their work and suggest changes that would improve patient care as well as reallocate workload. Processes need to be carefully assessed, problems diagnosed, and action plans formulated to strategically direct an IV therapy service program.

Patient Care Outcomes

The members of the IV team need to re-evaluate their current responsibilities to see if the tasks they perform are still pertinent and relevant. The survival of ancillary professional departments depends on the profession's focusing on patient care outcomes rather than on the completion of specific tasks. Tasks performed by technical versus professional staff that make no contribution to desired patient care outcomes need to be carefully evaluated. In addition, an ongoing annual review of all department tasks and activities forces professionals to identify irrelevant tasks, prioritize key activities, and evaluate the appropriate skill mix required to attain the desired outcomes. The roles of the licensed practical/vocational nurse, and nonlicensed technicians should be carefully assessed to take greater advantage of the registered nurse's professional knowledge, skills, and guidance.

Throughout restructuring, the benefits associated with the specialty that have already been well established must not be forgotten but rather must be clearly demonstrated in the process. Considering that the scrutiny in the 1990s revolves around whether specialization impedes the organization from delivering quality care, the IV nurse specialist can demonstrate the quality care benefits associated with his or her practice. Also, even with new care delivery models, IV teams can reduce hospital costs through decreased use of labor and materials. Labor represents the largest component of the cost associated with IV services. The key to the success of an IV team is its ability to improve labor efficiency through the use of IV team specialists. Further, IV teams reportedly use materials more efficiently. Material savings can be achieved when supplies are handled by professionals with familiarity with each product and its function, thereby maximizing use of appropriate equipment and minimizing waste. Length of stay has become a critical measure of hospital success; each additional day in the hospital adds significantly to the costs. IV teams have contributed to decreased length of stay by ensuring delivery of ordered therapies, better use of supplies, and decreased IV-related complications.[3] Now more than ever, the IV team should be actively consulting with the patient-centered care teams regarding recommendations for IV therapy–related plans of care. Consultation would include assessment for, and coordination of, outpatient services if appropriate.

Full Continuum of Services

With the evolution of alternative and home infusion programs, IV therapy has developed into a multifaceted specialty in multiple practice settings. The development of IV delivery in alternative settings has been characterized by extraordinary growth, not only in the numbers of patients treated but also in the number of different therapies provided. The demand for alternative sites will continue to grow as hospitals are increasingly pressured to discharge patients as soon as warranted by clinical conditions. Payment methodologies are projected to change to a capitated system in which financial risk for patient care is shifted from the payers to the providers. Health care systems that are capable of providing the full continuum of services will benefit under this system. Therefore, the focus is now on establishing processes so that the patient passes seamlessly from the inpatient setting to outpatient services. Hospital networks and integrated health care systems are already in an advantageous position in the new health care environment. These networks will be able to provide continuous care delivery as patients are shifted between multiple care settings based on patient needs and cost differentials. Hospitals are increasingly recognizing the importance of outpatient and home infusion and are expanding into this area of business.[4] This trend provides hospitals and IV therapy service programs with an incredible opportunity. The members of the hospital-based IV team need to shift their thinking from the acute care model because these clinicians will be involved in the care of patients who transition to other settings for IV care even when the clinicians work exclusively in the acute care setting. The hospital-based IV nurse plays an integral role in the planning of patients' care to promote transition to the other practice settings. In addition, opportunities exist for the IV therapy program to provide all aspects of care in both the inpatient and the outpatient settings. One example of these expanding opportunities is the delivery, care, and training of most patients who require outpatient or home IV therapies in an ambulatory clinic setting versus the traditional home infusion model. If non–bed-bound patients come to an infusion center for IV-related teaching or care, staffing efficiency is maximized. The full-service IV team concept can make this an even more efficient system. The IV therapy program that can support delivery of IV therapy in all settings fits well with the future of health care and maximizes its benefit to the organization. A full-service program is also a benefit in that it closely follows the patient-centered care philosophy of decreasing the obstacles to patient care and decreasing the number of people involved with the patient. Specific benefits also include

- Decrease in length of stay through more efficient, timelier transfer from inpatient to outpatient settings.
- Consistency in personnel, procedures, and equipment used throughout all care delivery settings.
- Increased patient satisfaction, seeing the same faces, understanding the system.
- Efficient use of highly skilled staff. Adjustments in staffing from the inpatient or outpatient environments as the need dictates.
- Justification of a 24-hour IV therapy service to answer the calls of the ambulatory outpatient.

- On-call back-up would then be necessary only if the patient is homebound.

Great growth will continue to occur in outpatient and home care settings as cost-effective alternatives to hospitalization. Providers now have incentive to control overall health care costs as well as access to, and utilization of, alternative infusion services, which is an important component to helping manage these costs. Other areas that home infusion providers need to address are the more sophisticated information needs that will now be required, including quality monitoring, outcomes studies, and patient satisfaction surveys, as well as better cost control and reporting. As health care comes more and more under the managed care umbrella, decisions on reimbursement and provider selection will be increasingly based on quality and cost. Providers will be required to supply these data.

TECHNOLOGY

If the advances over the past 40 years in technology related to IV therapy are any indication of the advances that will occur over the next 40 years, one cannot even begin to imagine what the future may hold. Continued advances and new technologies can be anticipated to affect the IV nursing practice.

Flexibility

The key to survival in the future is flexibility. Successful programs have now incorporated therapies other than the delivery of fluids and medications by the IV route. For example, IV nurses are commonly involved with subcutaneous, intraspinal, and intraosseous therapies. IV nurses need to be open to the possibility that other innovative therapies or delivery routes may affect their practice in the future.

Increased complexity of practice often parallels advanced technology. The IV therapy staff, therefore, will need to be prepared to safely deliver new therapies and to understand their application to each patient, as well as to educate staff, patients, families, and alternative site personnel. The practice of IV therapy will need to be defined through policies and procedures, and competency will need to be monitored by newly developed assessment protocols.

Flexibility in relation to technology necessitates that the IV nurse stay in tune with all aspects of patient care. The IV nurse manager should have an awareness and thorough understanding of patient needs, expertise of the IV therapy staff, and the mission of the health care facility. IV nursing leaders should incorporate this information and determine if there are additional services that could be better provided by the IV staff.

Involvement in Product Development

Advances in technology include the equipment and supplies used to provide therapy. IV nurses should continue to play a significant role in product development and should continually be aware of practice issues and should work with the health care industry to meet practice needs. Because of diminishing staffs, multiple care settings, and sicker patients, the industry will be challenged to develop more sophisticated equipment that is user friendly and provides necessary safety features. Regarding the introduction of new technology, it is more important than ever for IV nurses to use a multidisciplinary approach. As new products are being considered, personnel safety should also be considered and patient care should not be compromised.

As the level of technology increases, so do the costs. With the decrease in health care funds, will the IV nurse be caught in the dilemma of rationing care? The IV nurse will be challenged to help develop more creative strategies to provide a more complex level of care for the acutely ill patient.

Changes in technology, whether services or products, are inevitable for successful IV therapy programs. Therefore, it is necessary for IV personnel to understand the importance of change and the effects of change that will be experienced by staff and patients. Changes necessary for success will occur as IV nurses continue to analyze opportunities and incorporate these into IV therapy practice.

QUALITY IMPROVEMENT

Quality of patient care and positive patient outcomes will remain paramount in the future of IV therapy. As cost factors continue to drive changes in health care delivery, all personnel must consider how far to push these changes before quality is adversely affected. Therefore, it is more important than ever to develop and maintain quality monitoring programs.

IV nurses need to be responsible for the quality of IV therapy–related services. In assuming this responsibility, the nurse must remember that patient care crosses all disciplines. Therefore, the nurse should incorporate the expertise of individuals from other areas and disciplines, including pharmacy, nursing, laboratory, oncology, and outpatient units. This corroboration can be accomplished through multidisciplinary committees and by continuous monitoring.

Multidisciplinary committees may take several forms. An IV therapy committee may be used that is composed of members from many departments. Another alternative would be the participation of IV nurses on institutional committees that might affect IV-related services. Many health care facilities use the continuing quality improvement concept, also known as the total quality management concept, to measure and achieve customer satisfaction. Therefore, IV nurses must become familiar with this concept, participate on quality teams, and be proactive in initiating teams to look at IV therapy issues.

In addition to attending committees, the nurse must review and update the IV therapy program to monitor and evaluate continuing quality improvement. This annual process encourages institutions to keep the system current because it includes reviewing the scope and important aspects of care.

Focusing on patient outcomes will continue to help determine the viability of IV nursing. Positive outcomes are important because customers continue to shop for quality care at the best price. IV nurses need to be aware that these customers may be patients, physicians, fellow health care workers, hospitals, alternate care facilities, and payers. These customers need to be familiar with the quality of care that is delivered by IV nursing programs.

As health care costs are decreased, there will be even further increases of complicated IV therapy treatments and procedures that move patients to outpatient and home infusion services. Routine monitoring of IV care will be vital as this transition continues. IV nurses need to remain flexible and need to carefully look at where their expertise will have an impact on patient care no matter what setting is involved.

Further emphasis on prevention is anticipated. Therefore, the need for community services provided by qualified health care practitioners will increase. These settings may include performing central line dressings on outpatient dialysis patients, providing IV services for extended care facilities, or teaching basic venipuncture skills to industrial nurses. IV nurse specialists also need to search for opportunities to use their expertise in the area of prevention.

IV nurses need to market their services to clinics and dialysis units, where the volume of professional staff may be limited. Providing a program for central line dressing procedures may be effective in the clinical and financial arenas. Developing educational programs to help alternate care facilities maintain quality IV services may also be cost effective and may help meet staff education requirements.

COMPETENCY AND EDUCATION

Nurses in today's health care environment must understand change to be able to function effectively. Thus, the process of change should be included in the IV nurse's continuing education program. Nurses involved in increasingly complex roles will also need to be educated and competent to assess, deliver therapy, monitor care, and evaluate patients. The challenge will be to ensure that staff feel competent in light of the rapid, multiple changes that will occur.

Nursing education must keep pace with the changes in health care. Significant changes will occur in curricula and continuing education programs. Nurses will need to be prepared to provide high-technology care within hospitals, as well as in alternative care settings.

Health care agencies will need to determine how to ensure that their staff is competent. New nurse orientation programs will need to be streamlined while remaining all-inclusive (i.e., policies, procedures, equipment, anatomy, physiology, etc.). Innovative ways to update staff in regard to procedural changes, including self-study packets, computer programs, or audiovisual techniques, will also be needed.

With the rapid technologic advances, it is also going to be a challenge to provide IV equipment related in-services in an efficient, effective manner. This task will need to be addressed by the health care industry and by health care organizations.

As patients migrate from the hospital setting, IV nurses will need to have a better understanding of the principles of education. They will need to ensure that patients, families, or significant others are competent to provide care and will need to educate them on the necessity of compliance if patients are to remain outside the hospital setting. Patients need to be educated about when and what questions to ask regarding their therapy. IV nurses need to be prepared to be challenged by a more knowledgeable consumer. Patients are reading more and are taking a more active role in their own care. Therefore, tomorrow's consumers will more likely challenge their caregivers. Today's consumer is also very aware of the large medical malpractice verdicts. The increased patient knowledge and expectations of quality increase the need for the specialist in IV therapy.

As the rigid departmental boundaries become more fluid, the IV nurse's role will take on more importance. It will be necessary for IV nurses to continue to focus on maintaining standards of quality IV care while yielding to a much-needed multidisciplinary approach to meeting the total needs of the patient.

The necessity of containing cost continues, and the possibility of restructuring responsibilities of health care personnel remains. IV nurses should be alert to the potential for acquiring new tasks. Therefore, IV therapy managers must establish programs to ensure that the staff is competent to deliver services that will yield positive outcomes.

Competency-based orientation and training programs must be developed on the local level. However, "Given the diverse educational preparation, experience, and training of nurses, it simply is no longer realistic to hold the view that 'a nurse is a nurse is a nurse.'"[5]

"There are a number of forces and influence, both external and internal, driving the development of formal nurse credentialing and privileging programs."[5] These include the Joint Commission on Accreditation of Health Care Organizations, the Departments of Health, State Nurse Practice Acts, the legal system, and the nursing profession.

The disparity in education preparation is probably one of the best-known and most problematic internal forces. Licensure to practice nursing may be acquired through associate degree programs, hospital-based programs, or baccalaureate programs. With the increasing complexity of health care, the assurance of quality practice based solely on entry level licensure is becoming more difficult. Therefore, national certification programs have been developed in an attempt to address the competency issue. Specialty organizations have been in the forefront of trying to protect the patient through ensuring competency via certification programs.

This approach has certainly been true in the profession of IV nursing. IV nurses are following their patients into many alternate care sites. Often, the setting in alternative care facilities is less structured and less supportive when patient care problems present. Therefore, validating competency through national certification will continue to be valuable and possibly essential to help ensure that patient care will be provided by competent practitioners.

CONCLUSION

The IV nursing specialty has established itself as an integral component of the multidisciplinary approach needed to provide the quality care that our patients deserve. From the critically ill neonate to the cancer patient receiving supportive therapy at home, the IV nurse's role in supporting multiple, extensive IV therapies has been well established. The challenge for the specialty of IV nursing in the coming years is to respond to the changes affecting health care and to design the new look of IV nursing. As demonstrated throughout this chapter, the future of IV nursing appears to depend on the profession's response to the rapidly evolving changes. The IV nurse of the future needs to think strategically and to establish goals that closely reflect the institution's mission. The successful IV therapy programs of the future will adapt to changing paradigms and will keep in step even when the pace of change accelerates. However, as we become overwhelmed with the changes and challenges ahead of us, we need to keep in perspective the accomplishments of our profession and the true focus of our role—the patients who need us.

References

1. Henderson J, Williams J. The people side of patient care redesign. Health Care Forum 1991; July/August:44–49.
2. Strasen L. Redesigning hospitals around patients and technology. Nurs Econ 1991; 9(4):233–238.
3. Burik D, Cramton CW, Holtz J. A workbook approach to justifying I.V. therapy teams under prospective payment. NITA 1984; 7:411–418.
4. Gannon K. Reach-out programs: Hospitals expand into home care. Hosp Pharm Rep 1994; 8(6):1–12.
5. Archibald PJ, Bainbridge DD. Capacity and competence: Nurse credentialing and privileging. Nurs Manage 1994; 25:49–56.

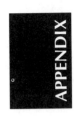

ANNOTATED BIBLIOGRAPHY

American Association of Blood Banks. Technical Manual, 10th ed. Arlington, VA: 1990. This manual describes all types of blood and blood components, indications, and procedures for transfusion therapy. Types of and signs and symptoms of transfusion reactions, as well as treatment parameters for transfusion reactions, are discussed. There is also information on immunology, blood types and blood typing, blood banking procedures, and quality assurance parameters for transfusion services.

American Society of Hospital Pharmacists. American Hospital Formulary Service Drug Information. Bethesda, MD: 1993. The formulary is an in-depth discussion of all pharmacologic preparations available in the United States. It is published yearly, with quarterly updates available. Administration guidelines and descriptions of all parenteral solutions available are included.

Baird SB, McCorkle R, Grant M. Cancer Nursing: A Comprehensive Textbook. Philadelphia: W.B. Saunders, 1991. Written by leading experts in the field, this text is the definitive reference for oncology nursing. It integrates social, psychologic, and basic science considerations in a multidisciplinary approach. Family communication and education, as well as professional collaboration, are addressed.

Bennett JV, Brachman PS. Hospital Infections, 3rd ed. Boston: Little, Brown and Co., 1992. All aspects of infection, its causes and preventative measures, are discussed in depth. The text contains a section specific to intravenous therapy and delineates intrinsic and extrinsic causes of contamination, associated organisms, and recommendations for the prevention of IV-related infection.

Black JM, Matassarin-Jacobs E. Luckmann and Sorensen's Medical-Surgical Nursing: A Psychophysiologic Approach, 4th ed. Philadelphia: W.B. Saunders, 1993. This is a complete medical-surgical text that discusses nursing process and practice as well as holistic approaches in health care and nursing practice. Health promotion, health assessment, and physical examination are presented, as well as the nursing care of patients with various disease states and conditions. The information is organized by body system. A unique feature of the text is the presentation of information within the chapters that provides ''bridges'' to care of the patient in the home and critical care settings. Ethical issues are also presented throughout the text, as is the application of nursing research to patient care. The topics of fluid and electrolyte balance, acid-base imbalance, and pain assessment and intervention are discussed in separate chapters.

Burke B. Oncology Nursing Homecare Handbook. Boston: Jones and Bartlett, 1992. This handbook covers various aspects of the home care of the person with cancer. Also discussed are clinical trials in home care, bone marrow transplantation from the home care perspective, anti-infective therapy, nutritional management, vascular access devices, and antineoplastic agents frequently used in the home. The handbook is supplemented with tables, charts, and assessment tools.

Burns N, Grove SK. The Practice of Nursing Research: Conduct, Critique and Utilization, 2nd ed. Philadelphia: W.B. Saunders, 1993. This is a comprehensive textbook on research methods for nursing. It includes quantitative research, qualitative research, and triangulation. The text provides a background for critiquing quantitative and qualitative studies, developing a research proposal, and conducting the actual research.

Corbett JV. Laboratory Tests and Diagnostic Procedures with Nursing Diagnoses, 3rd ed. Norwalk, CT: Appleton and Lange, 1992. The text discusses laboratory tests and nursing functions in laboratory testing. The purpose and clinical indications for each test are given, as are potential nursing diagnoses consistent with a given laboratory result. ''Normal'' laboratory reference values are given in the body of the text and in the tables.

Covino BG, Scott DB. Handbook of Epidural Anesthesia and Analgesia. Orlando, FL, Grune and Stratton, 1985. This handbook discusses the principles of epidural anesthesia and analgesia. Topics covered include spinal anatomy and physiology, techniques of catheter insertion, pharmacologic considerations of spinal drug administration, clinical considerations, and a discussion of complications. This text is currently out of print, but is a useful resource if it can be obtained.

Crudi C, Larkin M. Core Curriculum for Intravenous Nursing. Philadelphia, J.B. Lippincott, 1984. This text defines the nine content areas specific to the specialty practice of intravenous nursing and outlines the content within each core topic.

Dienemann J. Nursing Administration: Strategic Perspectives and Application. Norwalk, CT: Appleton and Lange, 1990. This text discusses the ethical framework that underlies health care delivery, legal aspects of nursing administration, decision making systems, and organizations as open systems. Also discussed are such issues as professional development, program evaluation, and performance appraisal.

Fischer JE. Total Parenteral Nutrition, 2nd ed. Boston, Little, Brown and Co., 1991. A thorough discussion of the rationale for the provision of parenteral nutrition is presented, along with the types and uses of various components and formulations. Care of the patient receiving total parenteral nutrition and associated equipment are described.

Gahart, BL. Intravenous Medications, 9th ed. St. Louis: C.V. Mosby, 1993. This book discusses only those drugs that are administered by the intravenous route. Dosages, actions, indications, contraindications, side effects, administration techniques, and nursing implications are presented in a concise format.

Grant JP. Handbook of Total Parenteral Nutrition, 2nd ed. Philadelphia: W.B. Saunders, 1992. All aspects of total parenteral nutrition are covered, including nutritional assessment, patient selection for total parenteral nutrition, vascular access (techniques and complications), catheter care, metabolism, parenteral nutrition solutions, and preparation of those solutions. Additionally, septic and metabolic complications and their recognition and treatment are discussed, along with a chapter on home total parenteral nutrition.

Handbook of Pediatric Drug Therapy. Springhouse, PA: Springhouse, 1990. Drugs are presented specifically as they apply to the pediatric patient. Dosages, actions, side effects, administration techniques, and nursing implications are discussed.

Horne MM, Heitz UE, Swearingen PL. Fluid, Electrolyte, and Acid-Base Balance: A Case Study Approach. St. Louis, Mosby Year Book, 1991.   Fluid, electrolyte, and acid-base balance are reviewed in depth from a nursing perspective. A case review format is used to assist in synthesizing the material. A companion pocket guide is also available from the same publisher.

Intravenous Nurses Society. Intravenous Nursing Standards of Practice. Belmont, MA: Intravenous Nurses Society, 1990. The Intravenous Nursing Standards of Practice delineate those nursing actions and interventions that direct the nurse in delivering safe, effective patient care to those requiring parenteral therapies.

Jarvis C. Physical Examination and Health Assessment. Philadelphia: W.B. Saunders, 1992.   The author describes the art and science of physical assessment. The process of obtaining a health history is presented, along with developmental considerations across the life span. Mental assessment and nutritional assessment parameters are provided. The physical assessment techniques begin with an overview of the general assessment followed by a body systems approach to physical assessment. Tables of select abnormal findings are presented with each body system.

Katz J, Green E. Managing Quality: A Guide to Monitoring and Evaluating Nursing Services. St. Louis, Mosby Year Book, 1992.   The authors use an approach called ''The Blueprint'' to create a framework for quality management. The process is described and operationalized within this blueprint context.

Kirk R, Kranz D. Home Care Management: Quality-Based Costing, Pricing, and Productivity. Rockville, MD: Aspen, 1988.   This text explores the development of standards and delivery of quality care and then demonstrates how to cost out various services to meet the desired standards and quality. Topics such as pricing home care services by service line labor contribution, pricing of home care services, and implementing new costing, pricing, and productivity plans are delineated.

Koch MW, Fairly TM. Integrated Quality Management. St. Louis, C.V. Mosby, 1993.   The authors approach quality management as an integration of quality assessment and improvement, risk and safety management, utilization management, and infection control to measure and achieve quality management synergy. The individual components of the model within a nursing context are presented and explained.

Kokko JP, Tannen RL. Fluids and Electrolytes, 2nd ed. Philadelphia: W.B. Saunders, 1990.   This comprehensive clinical reference encompasses the differential diagnosis and management of fluid, electrolyte, and acid-base disorders, and fluid and electrolyte abnormalities of disease. The book also includes discussions on drug-induced electrolyte disorders and the use of diuretics, fluid and electrolyte problems in surgery, trauma, and burns, and acid-base, fluid, and electrolyte aspects of parenteral nutrition.

Maffei LM, Thurer RL. Autologous Blood Transfusion: Current Issues. Arlington, VA: American Association of Blood Banks, 1988.   This book contains the proceedings of a conference that addressed the issues, concerns, and increased knowledge of autologous transfusions. Information is given about who should be an autologous donor, when to transfuse donors, whether autologous blood should be tested for infectious disease markers, and the labelling, shipping, and accountability of autologous units.

Martin KS, Scheet NJ. The OMAHA SYSTEM: Applications for Community Health Nursing. Philadelphia: W.B. Saunders, 1992.   The OMAHA SYSTEM resulted from 15 years of research, development, and refinement by the VNA. It is a classification system that is designed to manage and improve patient care in the community setting. It covers a problem classification scheme, an intervention scheme, and a problem rating scale for outcomes. The text describes the systems application approach in the public health, home, school health, and alternative site settings, as well as its use in nursing education and quality assurance programs. Sample forms and data collection records are included.

Martin KS, Scheet NJ. The OMAHA SYSTEM: A Pocket Guide for Community Health Nursing. Philadelphia: W.B. Saunders, 1992.   This work is a quick reference guide that accompanies the above-noted text.

McCorkle R, Grant M. Pocket Companion for Cancer Nursing. Philadelphia: W.B. Saunders, 1994.   This handy, pocket-sized companion to Baird et al.: Cancer Nursing (see earlier) is an excellent clinical tool for the nurse at the bedside. It condenses all the essential content found in the textbook and is organized by cancer site and common clinical problems, making it easy to reference.

Meisenheimer CG. Improving Quality: A Guide to Effective Programs. Rockville, MD: Aspen, 1992.   Meisenheimer describes the move from quality assurance into the realm of quality improvement and total quality management. The text delineates the quality process, methodology selection, reporting mechanisms, and evaluation techniques. Topics are included that assist in the integration of quality with other disciplines, such as risk management and utilization review, home health care, long-term care, and managed care.

Meisenheimer CG. Quality Assurance for Home Health Care. Rockville, MD: Aspen, 1989.   This text covers the principles of quality assurance and applies them to the home health care setting. Included are many sample forms useful in a home care quality assurance program. There is a section dedicated to high-tech home care, inclusive of IV therapy.

Metheny NM. Fluid and Electrolyte Balance: Nursing Considerations, 2nd ed. Philadelphia: J.B. Lippincott Co., 1992.   All aspects of fluid and electrolyte balance and the role of individual electrolyte replacement therapy are reviewed. The text discusses disease processes and conditions that affect fluid and electrolyte balance, as well as appropriate nursing interventions.

Phillips L. Manual of I.V. Therapeutics. Philadelphia: F.A. Davis, 1993.   The author presents information that incorporates pretest, post-test, worksheet, quality assessment, and activity journal formats. The manual discusses fluid and electrolyte balance, parenteral fluids, and equipment and techniques for peripheral IV therapy. Also included is information on complications of therapy, transfusion therapy, central venous access, nutritional support, and administration of intravenous medications.

Rombeau JL, Caldwell MD. Clinical Nutrition: Parenteral Nutrition, 2nd ed. Philadelphia: W.B. Saunders, 1993.   This clinical reference covers the complete range of topics concerning parenteral nutrition, from nutrients and their metabolism to interventions for specific disorders. Included are discussions of catheter access, nutrition support teams, computers, cost effectiveness of TPN, home parenteral nutrition, and individual chapters addressing stages of the life span.

Silver H, Kemp C. Handbook of Pediatrics, 16th ed. Norwalk, CT: Appleton and Lange, 1991.   This handbook discusses general pediatric care from the medical perspective. It includes information pertinent to the fluid and electrolyte status of the pediatric patient and treatment for related disease states and conditions. Growth and development information is addressed, as is nutritional information useful to the nurse delivering IV therapy to the pediatric patient.

Smith E. Kinsey M. Fluids and Electrolytes: A Conceptual Approach, 2nd ed. New York: Churchill Livingstone, 1991. The subject of fluids and electrolytes is presented in a story board format. The pictorial approach and accompanying text can enhance understanding of a complex subject matter.

Snyder EL, Menitove JE, eds. Home Transfusion Therapy. Arlington, VA: American Association of Blood Banks, 1986. This text describes the process for carrying out transfusion therapy in the home. Criteria for patient acceptance, medical and legal aspects, and insurance industry perspectives are included. Nursing protocols are delineated for all aspects of transfusion therapy, including the management of transfusion reactions in the home and patient identification criteria.

Tenenbaum L. Cancer Chemotherapy: A Reference Guide, 2nd ed. Philadelphia: W.B. Saunders, 1994. This guide to chemotherapy and biotherapy reports on more than 80 agents now in use, and provides essential information on their preparation, administration, disposal, and toxicities. The tables in the book provide comparisons of various agents. New chapters on biologic response modifiers, chemoprevention, and PICC lines make this book a valuable reference for the intravenous nurse.

Troyer GT, Salman LS. Handbook of Health Care Risk Management. Rockville, MD: Aspen, 1986. This text discusses the discipline of health care risk management in the hospital environment. One chapter is devoted to nursing and risk management, covering topics such as nursing liability, documentation, standards of practice, and the nurse as defendant.

Weinstein S. Plumer's Principles and Practice of Intravenous Therapy, 5th ed. Philadelphia: J.B. Lippincott, 1993. This text presents many aspects of parenteral therapy administration, describing techniques and equipment used in the delivery of various therapies. Practice issues such as risk management, quality improvement, and legal implications are discussed. Fluid and electrolytes, parenteral fluids, transfusion therapy, parenteral nutrition, antineoplastic therapy, and pain management are also covered. There is also information regarding home infusion therapy, care of the pediatric infusion patient, and the role of the IV nurse and IV teams.

Wilson BA, Shannon MT. A Unified Approach to Dosage Calculations, 2nd ed. Norwalk, CT: Appleton and Lange, 1991. The text begins with a review of basic arithmetic skills and working with decimals, fractions, and percentages. Using an approach called dimensional analysis, the authors demonstrate dosage calculations for both nonparenteral and parenteral medication administration and intravenous solutions. Two sections describe calculations specific to the pediatric patient.

Workman ML, Ellerhorst-Ryan J, Hargrave-Koertge V. Nursing Care of the Immunocompromised Patient. Philadelphia: W.B. Saunders, 1993. This text discusses basic concepts of immunology, conditions that cause immunosuppression; syndromes of immunodeficiency, including acquired immunodeficiency syndrome; immunodeficiency secondary to medical treatment (cancer treatment, solid organ, and bone marrow transplantation); and immunodeficiency associated with aging. A nursing care plan for the immunocompromised patient is also presented.

INDEX

Note: Page numbers in *italics* refer to illustrations; page numbers followed by t refer to tables.

O

P

ISBN 0-7216-4267-5

90038